Arrhythmias

Arrhythmias

SECOND EDITION

John A. Kastor, M.D.
Professor of Medicine
University of Maryland School of Medicine
Baltimore, Maryland

W.B. Saunders Company
A Division of Harcourt Brace & Company
Philadelphia London Montreal Toronto Sydney Tokyo

W.B. SAUNDERS COMPANY
A Division of Harcourt Brace & Company

The Curtis Center
Independence Square West
Philadelphia, Pennsylvania 19106

Library of Congress Cataloging-in-Publication Data

Arrhythmias / John A. Kastor.—2nd ed.

p.   cm.

Includes index.

ISBN 0–7216–7647–2

1. Arrhythmia.   I. Kastor, John A.

[DNLM: 1. Arrhythmia.   WG 330 A7743 2000]
RC685.A65T37   2000

616.1′28—dc21

DNLM/DLC   99–19076

Arrhythmias   ISBN 0–7216–7647–2

Printed in the United States of America.

Last digit is the print number: 9   8   7   6   5   4   3   2   1

To Elizabeth, Anne, & Peter

Welcome to the second edition of *Arrhythmias,* a text designed for physicians, nurses, and other health care workers with interest in the subject and the opportunity to care for patients with cardiac arrhythmias.

Based on the assumption that arrhythmias are more than electrocardiograms and electrophysiological studies, I have discussed at some length the clinical effects of these disturbances. This is not an easy task because subjects such as history and physical examination are not particularly fashionable topics in this era of the clinical electrophysiological study. Some of the best descriptions in our specialty appear in the writings of leaders from a previous generation. I have reprinted what they wrote in several cases.

I should add that *Arrhythmias* has not been specifically written for clinical or basic electrophysiologists, although I hope that many of them will find parts of it useful. I have discussed clinical electrophysiology but not in sufficient detail to ensure that candidate electricians will pass their subspecialty examinations. Nevertheless, all pertinent references on clinical electrophysiology are included, in some cases listed in paragraphs called "advances"; interested readers can find the sources there to answer their questions. I have not discussed basic electrophysiology because I am not qualified to do so.

As you can see from the table of contents, the book is organized by arrhythmias and does not include chapters on electrophysiological mechanisms, drugs, or devices. These subjects are covered in each chapter as applicable to the particular arrhythmias under discussion. Most of the information on pacemakers is found in Chapter 15, "Atrioventricular Block," and Chapter 16, "Sick Sinus Syndrome," and on implantable cardioverter-defibrillators in Chapter 14, "Ventricular Fibrillation." Ablation turns up in several chapters as the application of this technique grows. The discussions on these technical subjects are not extensively detailed, so operators will need to look elsewhere to learn how to install pacers and defibrillators and ablate arrhythmias. Perhaps I will tackle them in the third edition.

As for the references, reviewing and listing all relevant publications for the 30 years preceding the summer of 1998 is one of my purposes in writing this book, and I hope that the bibliographies will prove useful to workers who need this information. Accomplishing this has been made immeasurably easier for the author and his secretary in this edition by the use of Medline and Reference Manager, one of the computerized reference management systems. I had to draw the line somewhere, and, therefore, include, for the most part, only clinical studies, no references in languages other than English—except for a few of the greatest historical interest—and few abstracts or letters to the editor.

Here are a few technical points about the references:
- Whenever possible, each fact is supported by at least one reference. Research reports are referenced with statements, reviews and editorials with topics.
- On several occasions, I refer to the third edition (1968) of Paul Wood's superb *Diseases of the Heart and Circulation.* Wood fans, and there are many, will know that this edition, which was revised and enlarged by Dr. Wood's friends and colleagues, appeared after his untimely death of ischemic heart disease in 1962 "at the height of his powers."[a]
- To keep the references in the footnotes in sequence, the bibliographic system I used requires that the references also be identified in the body of the text, even though their presence there may seem otherwise obscure.

Arrhythmias does contain footnotes, an uncommon practice in most medical texts. Here you will find the data supporting the facts so that you may concentrate, if you wish, on the text and bypass the numbers in the footnotes. I hope, however, that you will not completely ignore the footnotes. They contain historical notes, differences of opinion, deductions that have not been proved, intriguing irrelevancies, and a few now outdated conclusions reached by our distinguished predecessors to remind us of the rapidity with which favorite discoveries and theories become amusing when no longer authoritative.

[a]Anonymous. Paul Wood's *Diseases of the Heart and Circulation,* 3rd ed. Philadelphia; JB Lippincott, 1968, p. xxxv.

Readers familiar with the first edition, published in 1994, will recognize that this time I have written all the chapters except for Bruce Fye's superb history of arrhythmias. This means that eight of the thirteen chapters on arrhythmias are completely new, two are mostly new, and three have been revised as extensively as increasing knowledge during the past five years dictates.

Caught up in historical enthusiasm by Dr. Fye's chapter, I have reprinted and updated a biographical sketch, first published in 1989, about Michel Mirowski, the developer of the implantable cardioverter-defibrillator, and I have added notices, written when they died, about Kenneth Rosen and Alfred Pick, two outstanding contributors to arrhythmology and clinical electrophysiology. Thanks to the translating skill of Dr. Jan-Michael Klapproth, my colleague at the University of Maryland, readers will find an obituary on the life of Woldemar Mobitz, who first defined the two types of atrioventricular block.

I thank the authors of the chapters in the first edition for the use of several of their illustrations—each one is identified—and for the help that their writing gave me in constructing the new chapters. E. William Hancock, Robert A. O'Rourke, and James A. Shaver sent me new illustrations and references, and I am grateful to them. Hugh Calkins, Michael R. Gold, and Arthur J. Moss reviewed several of the chapters and saved me from making some monumental gaffes; the mistakes that remain can only be blamed on me.

Eugene Rhim and Ravi M. Lala, members of the class of 2000 at the University of Maryland School of Medicine, were superb research assistants. Phyllis Farrell, executive secretary to the Department of Medicine, kept the whole project together, as she did for the first edition; she worked at length with the bibliographic system and proofread all the copy. I cannot thank her enough for her help and support. Molly Lutz and Rosalind Robinson also contributed greatly.

I thank Professor Philip A. Poole-Wilson for making it possible for me to research and write some of the text as a visiting principal fellow at the National Heart and Lung Institute in London during the fall of 1995. Dr. Donald E. Wilson, Dean of the University of Maryland School of Medicine, arranged that I have more time to write beginning in the spring of 1997, thereby allowing me to finish the book sooner than expected.

At W.B. Saunders, Richard Zorab, Senior Medical Editor, and his colleague, Jennifer Shreiner, provided much needed support and advice. I thank Holly Lukens who carefully edited the copy.

Contents

A History of Cardiac Arrhythmias

W. Bruce Fye[a]

During the past few decades, advances in basic and clinical electrophysiology and pharmacology, the development of noninvasive and invasive electrophysiological diagnostic procedures, the introduction of surgical and catheter ablation techniques for the treatment of arrhythmias, and the invention of electronic therapeutic devices have revolutionized the diagnosis and management of cardiac arrhythmias. So much is new that it is easy to forget that these advances emerged gradually from a long tradition of research and clinical observation. This chapter provides a historical framework in which to view recent developments in the field of cardiac arrhythmias. Concepts that have emerged and techniques that have been developed since about 1960 are not discussed in this historical chapter; they are included in the other chapters of this book.

Much of our current understanding of cardiac arrhythmias can be traced to experiments performed and clinical observations made between 1850 and 1950.[1] Midway through that period, owing mainly to the introduction of electrocardiography, disorders of cardiac impulse formation and conduction took on new relevance for clinicians. Three quotations from the turn of the century reflect the dynamic state of arrhythmia research in that era and its implications for medical practice. Writing in 1899, Scottish physiologist Arthur Cushny observed: "The physiology of the mammalian heart has advanced with such rapid strides of late years, that clinical observers have apparently had difficulty in keeping pace with it, and but little attempt has been made to adapt the theories of the experimen-

tal investigators to the observations made on the diseased heart."[2]

The clinical relevance of scientific discoveries regarding the heartbeat was becoming apparent, however. In 1904, Dutch physician and clinical investigator Karel Wenckebach claimed: "The facts which we have obtained from physiology towards an explanation of the irregularities of the heart will form the groundwork on which the future study of these irregularities must be based, and will be bound to lead to a better classification and a logical nomenclature for the various clinical forms of arrhythmia."[3]

In 1909, just following the introduction of the electrocardiograph, American physician and researcher Samuel Meltzer declared: "Keen investigators and leading clinicians throughout the world are now paying a great deal of attention to the study of cardiac arrhythmias, and the literature on the subject has already assumed large proportions."[4] The literature on cardiac arrhythmias has grown steadily since Meltzer made these claims. In this brief historical survey, I have had to select only a small sample of the many discoveries and observations that have led to our current understanding of the pathophysiology and treatment of arrhythmias.

Speaking of significant discoveries, Thomas Lewis, a British cardiologist and pioneer of electrocardiography, said in 1921 that ". . . a successful issue does not depend upon the work of this or that group of researchers, it is a natural outcome of progressive work stretching over many years and undertaken by many workers in the same field."[5] Julius Comroe and Robert Dripps made the same point in 1978. In their comprehensive study of 10 major clinical advances in cardiovascular medicine, they concluded that "in every in-

[a]Clinical Professor of Medicine, Adjunct Professor of the History of Medicine, University of Wisconsin, Madison; Medical Director of Non-Invasive Cardiology, Cardiology Department, Marshfield Clinic.

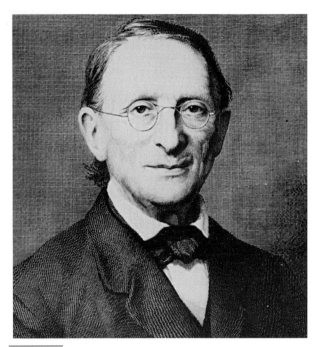

FIGURE 1.1 Carl Ludwig (1816–1895), a German scientist who made numerous important contributions to cardiovascular physiology. In 1847, he invented the kymograph, an instrument that made it possible to record hemodynamic events over time. (From the National Library of Medicine, with permission.)

stance . . . previous work by scores or hundreds of competent scientists was essential to provide the basic knowledge necessary for the widely known clinical advance, usually attributed to one man."[6]

I was aware of this concept as I selected themes, specific discoveries, and individual scientists and physicians for inclusion in this historical chapter. I had to be highly selective, and many arbitrary decisions were required. Usually, the physicians and scientists whose contributions are mentioned spent several years—occasionally decades—pursuing the research or making clinical observations that ultimately resulted in a significant advance in our understanding of cardiac arrhythmias. The names of their predecessors and co-workers are generally not noted, nor are the contributions of others whose efforts led, in some small way, to a more complete understanding of disorders of the heartbeat. Some readers may be surprised to find that the observations of a few early researchers whose conclusions eventually proved wrong are mentioned in this chapter. It is important to recognize that some discoveries, although originally misinterpreted, were of great significance in the subsequent elaboration of theories that are now accepted as correct.

PULSE LITERATURE

Although cardiac arrhythmias were poorly understood until the twentieth century, physicians have palpated the pulse since antiquity.[7, 8] Galen (AD 132–201) emphasized the importance of feeling the pulse and taught that an intermittent pulse carried a poor prog-

nosis and could be a harbinger of sudden death. The teachings of this ancient physician dominated Western medical thought until the seventeenth century. Most of the pulse literature that appeared up to the nineteenth century is irrelevant in terms of our modern conception of cardiac arrhythmias, however.

Following the 1628 publication of William Harvey's account of his discovery of the circulation, occasional observations reflected growing insight into the relationship between the character of the pulse and a patient's symptoms. For example, in his 1674 work, *Pharmaceutice Rationalis,* British physician Thomas Willis noted an intermittent pulse in a patient who complained of palpitations. He attributed this physical finding to a failure of the heart to contract.[9] Italian physician Giovanni Lancisi, in his 1707 study of sudden death, argued that an intermittent pulse without shortness of breath or other symptoms did not imply the dire prognosis that had been accepted since the time of Galen.

Although pulse counting can be traced to the fifth-century Alexandrian physician Herophilus, who used a water clock for this purpose, until the eighteenth century it was rare for physicians to count the pulse. In 1707, British physician John Floyer invented a watch that ran for 60 seconds, an invention that made accurate evaluation of the heart rate possible. Floyer's work attracted little attention, and few used his invention,

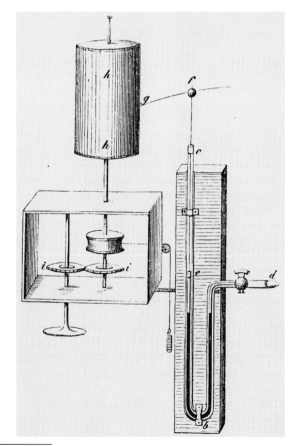

FIGURE 1.2 Carl Ludwig's kymograph. (From Ludwig C. Lehrbuch der Physiologie des Menschen. 2nd ed., vol. 2. Leipzig: CF Wintersche, 1861, p. 122.)

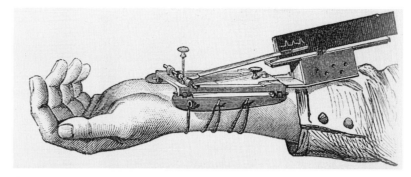

FIGURE 1.3 Marey's sphygmograph. (From Marey EJ. La circulation du sang. Paris: G Masson, 1881.)

however.[10] In their valuable summary of the ancient pulse literature, Schechter, Lillehei, and Soffer published excerpts from several pre-1900 works in which abnormalities of the rate and character of the pulse were reported.[8] The significance (or irrelevance) of these early clinical observations became more obvious with the introduction of sophisticated experimental approaches and graphic techniques during the second half of the nineteenth century.

SPHYGMOGRAPH AND ELECTROCARDIOGRAPH

The development of instruments of precision and graphic techniques to record cardiac events greatly stimulated cardiovascular research during the nineteenth century.[11] In 1835, French physician Julius Hérisson invented the sphygmometer, an instrument that transmitted the movement of the peripheral pulse wave to a column of mercury. Carl Ludwig (Fig. 1.1), a pioneering German physiologist, invented the kymograph in 1847.[12] This instrument included a pen attached to a float on top of a mercury column (Fig. 1.2). When the pen was placed on smoked paper that moved on a revolving drum, Ludwig could record hemodynamic events over time. Seven years later, German physiologist Karl Vierordt published a description of his sphygmograph, which consisted of a spring-mounted lever attached to a revolving drum that made it possible to record arterial pulsations. Vierordt's in-

strument was cumbersome, and the first practical sphygmograph (Fig. 1.3) was invented by the French physiologist Étienne Marey in 1860 (Fig. 1.4).

Before the invention of the sphygmograph, there was no reliable way to record the pulse. Subjective descriptions of the pulse were becoming ever more suspect. In 1772, British physician William Heberden (Fig. 1.5), best known for his description of angina pectoris, denounced the dozens of pulse types that had been differentiated over the centuries. He believed that they "exist chiefly in the imagination" of the authors who described them.[13] The sphygmograph made it possible to record pulse tracings that could be studied, stored, repeated, and compared. Scottish physician James Mackenzie pioneered the use of these newer graphic recording techniques in his studies of the cardiovascular system. In 1892, Mackenzie invented a polygraph that enabled him to record simultaneously the arterial and venous pulses as well as the apical impulse. From these combined tracings, Mackenzie made several important observations on the electrical activity of the human heart and the mechanical functions of the cardiac chambers and valves.

For nearly half a century, investigators had recognized that the heart had intrinsic electrical activity. Continental physiologists Rudolph von Kölliker and Eduard Mueller first showed, in 1856, that an electric current was associated with the contraction of the heart when they recorded a cardiac action potential. In 1887, British physiologist Augustus D. Waller (Fig.

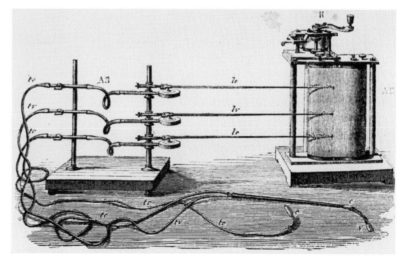

FIGURE 1.4 Marey's three-channel cardiograph. (From Marey EJ. Physiologie médicale de la circulation du sang. Paris: Adrien Delahave, 1863, p. 54.)

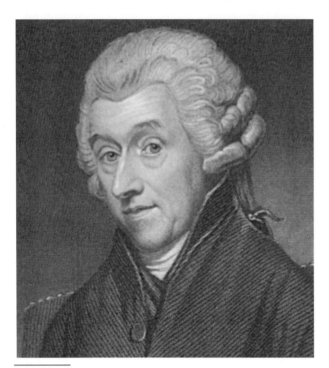

FIGURE 1.5 William Heberden (1710–1801), a British physician who first described angina pectoris. Heberden published a paper in 1772 that questioned the value of the traditional classification of pulse types. (From Pettigrew TJ. Medical Portrait Gallery, vol. 3. Fisher, London, 1839.)

1.6) recorded the first human electrocardiogram—he later coined the term.[14] Waller connected electrodes strapped to a man's chest to a capillary electrometer, an instrument invented 15 years earlier by French physicist Gabriel Lippmann. By photographing the moving column of mercury, Waller recorded the electrical activity of the human heart for the first time (Fig. 1.7).[15]

Although the capillary electrometer was used to study cardiac electrophysiology, it was of limited value because of its poor frequency response. Dutch physiologist Willem Einthoven (Fig. 1.8) tried to refine this instrument, but he eventually turned to another approach that appeared more promising. He adapted a recent invention, the Ader string galvanometer, to record the electrical activity of the heart. Einthoven's string galvanometer, first described fully in 1902, allowed scientists and clinicians to record the electrical impulses of the human heart directly. This invention was a crucial step in the development of clinical electrocardiography.[16–18] Those few medical scientists and clinicians interested in disorders of the heartbeat quickly recognized the significance of Einthoven's invention.

In 1908, the first Einthoven string galvanometer was installed in Great Britain, in Edward Schäfer's physiological laboratory at the University of Edinburgh. The following year, modified versions of the instrument were installed in Thomas Lewis's laboratory at University College Hospital in London and in Alfred Cohn's cellar workroom at Mt. Sinai Hospital in New York. Lewis systematically studied many patients using the

electrocardiograph, and in 1911 he published a classic work on the mechanism of the heartbeat in which he described the electrocardiographic patterns of many arrhythmias.[19] Einthoven characterized Lewis as "the first man in England who applied electrocardiography to clinical investigations."[20, 21] Workers in Great Britain, Europe, and the United States used the electrocardiograph to investigate arrhythmias in experimental animals and in human patients. With this instrument, disorders of cardiac impulse formation and conduction that had long defied explanation could be studied and characterized with great precision.

ORIGIN OF THE HEARTBEAT

The incessant rhythmic action of the heart is a remarkable phenomenon of nature.[22] Three centuries ago, scientists began to debate whether the heartbeat was the result of a property of the heart muscle itself (the myogenic theory) or whether it depended on the influence of nerves that supplied the organ (the neurogenic theory). Although it was not universally accepted until the twentieth century, the myogenic theory of the heartbeat can be traced to Galen. Experiments on the nervous control of muscular function undertaken by seventeenth-century anatomists and physiologists led to the elaboration of the neurogenic theory of the heartbeat. English physician Thomas Willis argued that a "nervous liquor" originating in the cerebellum was carried to the heart through nerves

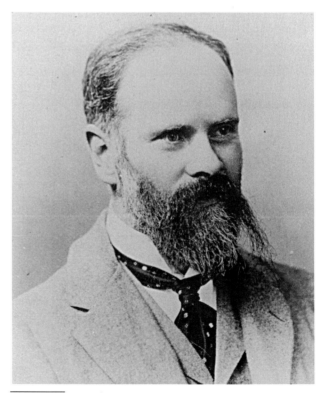

FIGURE 1.6 Augustus D. Waller (1856–1922), a British physiologist who first recorded an action potential from the heart. He also recorded the first human electrocardiogram in 1887. (From the National Library of Medicine, with permission.)

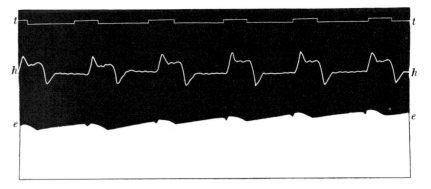

FIGURE 1.7 First published recording of the human electrocardiogram (using a capillary electrometer). (Reproduced from Waller AD. A demonstration on man of electromotive changes accompanying the heart's beat. J Physiol 1887; 8:229–234.)

and, once it reached the organ, stimulated it to contract.

Swiss physiologist Albrecht von Haller presented experimental evidence in the eighteenth century that led many to reject the neurogenic theory of the heartbeat in favor of the myogenic hypothesis. During the first half of the nineteenth century, several workers in Europe studied the problem. Simple observation and experiments based on destruction of the connections between the heart and nervous system were replaced gradually by more elegant histological and physiological studies. Although some of their conclusions and hypotheses are now known to have been wrong, the observations of these nineteenth-century investigators are worth recounting because of the role their discoveries played in others' elaborations of theories that are now universally accepted.

As understanding of the sympathetic nervous system grew, a new theory of the heartbeat was proposed that attributed the rhythmic action of the organ to the ganglia that had been discovered in its substance. French physiologist François Magendie, a master of vivisection, found that the heart continued to beat rhythmically even after he had carefully dissected away all the sympathetic nervous connections to the organ. Using improved microscopes, other workers reported previously unrecognized specialized tissues in the heart. In 1839, German histologist Robert Remak, a pupil of Johannes Müller, reported his discovery of ganglia in the heart. In a series of studies published over the next decade, Remak showed that ganglia were most prevalent in the region of the sinus venosus and argued that they could explain the automatic action of the heart. This hypothesis seemed reasonable, because French pathologist Xavier Bichat had shown several decades earlier that ganglia were capable of independent discharge.[23]

In 1848, another of Müller's pupils, Friedrich Bidder, identified similar specialized cells at the atrioventricular junction. He also demonstrated that these cells received fibers from the vagus nerve. The same year, Carl Ludwig identified ganglia in the interatrial septum. These observations lent credence to the neurogenic theory of the heartbeat. It was proposed that the ganglia in the sinus venosus caused the heart to beat by sending out stimuli at regular intervals. An analogy was drawn to the accepted mechanism of the automatic nature of respiration, which was attributed to periodic stimuli arising in the nerve cells of the respiratory center of the brain. Based on these observations and his experiments, Johannes Müller proposed that the sympathetic nervous system was the source of a constant stimulus that acted on the heart to trigger a contraction. To explain how a constant nervous stimulus could result in periodic muscular contractions, Müller drew an analogy to recent discoveries in electricity. He claimed that a certain amount of nervous energy had to accumulate in the ganglia before a threshold was reached that would trigger a heartbeat.

One of the most important discoveries in cardiovascular physiology during the nineteenth century was the recognition by German physiologists Eduard and Ernst Weber (Fig. 1.9) of the effect of the vagus nerve

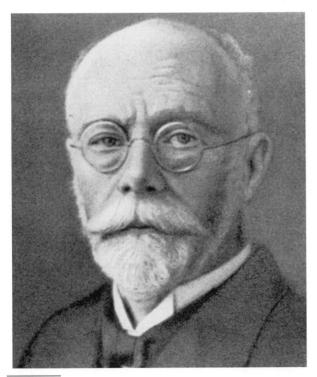

FIGURE 1.8 Willem Einthoven (1860–1927), a Dutch physiologist who invented a string galvanometer that he used to record the electrical activity of the heart, thereby inaugurating clinical electrocardiography. (From Fischer: Biographisches Lexikon der Hervorragenden Artze der Letzten Fünfzig Jahre. Berlin: Urban & Schwarzenberg, 1932, I:368).

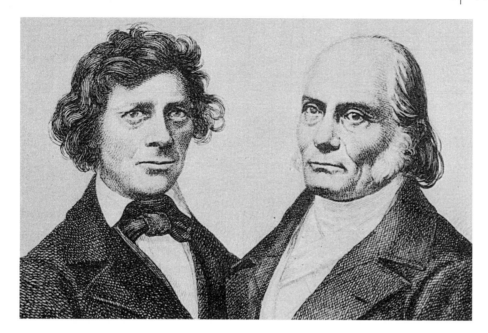

FIGURE 1.9 Eduard Weber (1806–1871) and Ernst Heinrich Weber (1795–1878), German physiologists who discovered the cardioinhibitory effects of the vagus nerve in 1845. (From Sterling W. Some Apostles of Physiology. London: Waterlow & Sons, 1902.)

on the heart.[23] They demonstrated, in 1845, that electrical stimulation of the vagus nerve led to slowing or even cessation of the heartbeat. From a series of experiments, the Webers concluded that the sympathetic nerves were the motor nerves of the heart and that they acted through the intercardiac ganglia they innervated. Recognition by the Webers of the cardioinhibitory influence of vagal stimulation encouraged other investigators to study the mechanism of the heartbeat. German physiologist Moritz Schiff (Fig. 1.10) demonstrated the phenomenon of the refractory

period of cardiac muscle in 1850. When his results were verified by European physiologists Hugo Kronecker and Étienne Marey, the concept of the refractory period gained widespread acceptance.

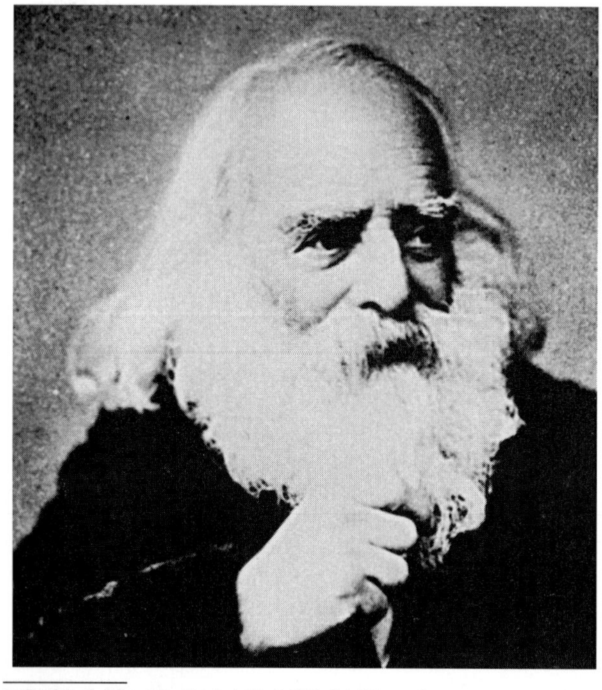

Clinical observations seemed to confirm the important role of the vagus nerve in the regulation of the heartbeat. Bradycardia as a result of carotid pressure was first reported by British physician Caleb Parry in 1799. Joseph Czermak published his observations on massage in the region of the carotid artery in 1866. Czermak performed the maneuver on himself and noted a dramatic decrease in his heart rate, which he attributed to direct stimulation of the vagus nerve.[24] The mechanism by which carotid massage caused bradycardia was not elucidated until the twentieth century, when Heinrich Hering reported his observations on the carotid sinus reflex.

In 1852, German physiologist Hermann Stannius showed that the heartbeat could be interrupted by placing a ligature between the sinus venosus and the body of the right atrium. By electrically stimulating the tissue near the atrioventricular junction, Stannius demonstrated that it was possible to restore the rhythmic action of the heart. He also showed that the atrium was much more susceptible to electrical stimulation than the ventricle.[25] These experiments, combined with the discovery of the cardiac ganglia, reinforced the belief that the ganglia in the region of the sinus venosus controlled the heartbeat. Still, many questions regarding the origin of the heartbeat remained.

The mechanism of the heartbeat became the prime research focus of Michael Foster (Fig. 1.11), Britain's leading physiologist during the second half of the nineteenth century.[26, 27] By 1869, Foster had concluded that the rhythmicity of the heart was due to some intrinsic property of cardiac muscle. He knew, however, that proof was necessary to convince the many scientists who still adhered to the neurogenic theory. For several decades, Foster and his associates tried to explain ap-

FIGURE 1.10 Moritz Schiff (1823–1896), a German physiologist whose observations led to the concept of absolute and relative refractory periods. (From the collection of W. Bruce Fye.)

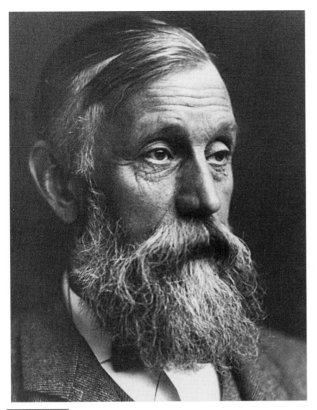

FIGURE 1.11 Michael Foster (1836–1907), a British physiologist whose research (conducted with several of his pupils) resulted in general acceptance of the myogenic theory of the heartbeat. (From the collection of W. Bruce Fye.)

liam Porter of the United States, now showed that many of Gaskell's observations could be reproduced in mammals. In a series of experiments that extended over 2 decades, German physiologist Theodor Engelmann (Fig. 1.13) provided compelling evidence in support of the myogenic theory of the heartbeat. By 1897, his work, with that of Gaskell and others, had led to almost universal acceptance of the myogenic hypothesis. Three years later, Gaskell provided the scientists and clinicians of the new century with a concise yet comprehensive summary of the theory.[30]

A major advance in understanding the origin of the heartbeat occurred in 1907, when British anatomist Arthur Keith and medical student Martin Flack identified in humans a differentiated system of muscular fibers in the region of the sinus venosus. These investigators concluded that it was within this specialized cardiac muscle "that the dominating rhythm of the heart normally begins."[31] Physiological events that had been elucidated through decades of research could now be viewed in a comprehensive morphological framework.

Once a specific site of origin for the heartbeat had been proposed based on histological studies, Thomas Lewis sought to confirm in mammals that the electrical impulse triggering atrial contraction originated there. In an innovative series of experiments, Lewis recorded epicardial electrograms from anesthetized dogs and subsequently studied the atrial tissue histologically. This electrophysiological-histological study led him to conclude that the "pacemaker" in the dog was located

parent inconsistencies in earlier observations and attempted to develop a comprehensive myogenic theory of the heartbeat.

Foster was convinced that the myogenic theory was correct. He claimed, in his widely used physiology text, first published in 1877: "The beat of the heart is an automatic action; the muscular contractions which constitute the beat are caused by impulses which arise spontaneously in the heart itself."[28] Foster's pupils Albert Dew-Smith, George Romanes, and Walter Gaskell (Fig. 1.12) extended his work on the heartbeat. Using newer physiological and histological techniques, and building on Francis Darwin's discovery of a muscular connection between the atrium and the ventricle in the snail heart, Gaskell provided conclusive proof of the myogenic theory. In an 1883 paper he explained: "The ventricle contracts in due sequence with the auricle because a wave of contraction passes along the auricular muscle and induces a ventricular contraction when it reaches the auriculo-ventricular groove."[29] Gaskell also proposed the concept of heart block to explain the phenomenon of some atrial contractions not being transmitted to the ventricle under certain experimental conditions.

To this point, the experiments to explain the origin of the heartbeat and the physiology of the conduction of the cardiac impulse had been performed in cold-blooded animals. Several researchers, including William Bayliss and Ernest Starling of England and Wil-

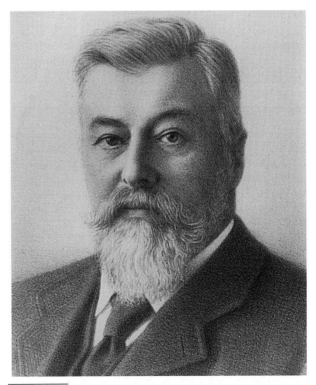

FIGURE 1.12 Walter Gaskell (1847–1914), a pupil of Michael Foster. This British physiologist provided experimental proof of the myogenic origin of the heartbeat. (From the collection of W. Bruce Fye.)

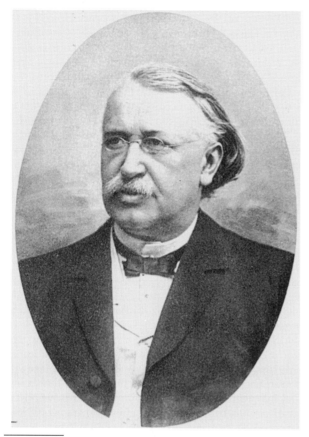

FIGURE 1.13 Theodor Engelmann (1843–1909), a Dutch physiologist. Using the extrastimulus technique in animals, Engelmann made classic observations on extrasystoles, a term he coined. (From the collection of W. Bruce Fye.)

at the site of the sinoatrial node recently described by Keith and Flack.[32] The myogenic theory of the heartbeat had been proved unequivocally.

CARDIAC CONDUCTION SYSTEM

While some researchers were trying to elucidate the origin of the heartbeat, others were making discoveries that would eventually provide an anatomical and physiological framework for understanding the conduction of the cardiac impulse. That the atria contracted before the ventricles had long been recognized. In his 1628 monograph, *De Motu Cordis*,[33] English physician William Harvey (Fig. 1.14) reported the results of experiments and observations that led him to propose his theory of the circulation: that the heart propelled blood in a circle through the blood vessels in the body. From many vivisections, Harvey concluded that the atria and the ventricles did not beat simultaneously: "the movement seems to start in the auricles and to spread to the ventricles."

Harvey also observed the phenomenon of heart block: "When the heart slows in approaching death . . . there is a pause between the two movements, and the heart seems to respond to the motion as if aroused, sometimes quickly, sometimes slowly. At length, nearly dead, it fails to respond to the motion,

and it stirs so obscurely that the only signs of motion are pulsations of the auricle. . . . The heart thus stops beating before the auricles." He also claimed: "While the heart gradually dies, it sometimes responds with a single weak and feeble beat to two or three pulsations of the auricles."[33]

During the nineteenth and early twentieth centuries, anatomical and physiological studies gradually led to an understanding of the relationship of atrial and ventricular contraction and the phenomenon of heart block. Often, anatomical observations preceded physiological discoveries, and workers tried to identify electrical or mechanical events that might be related to the structures they had found. The converse was sometimes true: A physiological phenomenon was recorded and an anatomical substrate for it was sought.

In 1839, Polish anatomist Johannes Purkinje reported the discovery of a network of fibers in the subendocardial region of the ventricle. Although it would be several decades before the physiological significance of this discovery was appreciated, Purkinje is remembered eponymically for his description of the distal part of the cardiac conduction system.[34] The first description of a muscle bundle connecting the atria and the ventricles was published in 1893 by German physician Wilhelm His, Jr.[35] Familiar with the research of Engelmann and Gaskell and their support of the myogenic theory, His had undertaken a series of physiological and histological studies of mammalian (including human) hearts. He identified "a muscle bundle which unites the auricular and ventricular septum . . . in a grown mouse, a newborn dog, two newborn and one adult (30-year-old) human."[36, 37]

Working independently, British physiologist Stanley Kent was studying the same problem. He reported, in

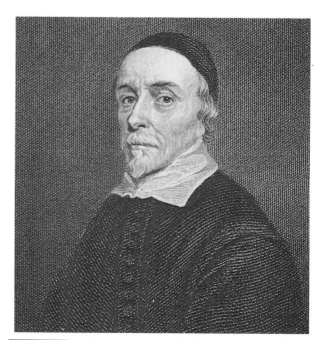

FIGURE 1.14 William Harvey (1578–1657). A description of heart block appeared in Harvey's 1628 book on the circulation. (From the collection of W. Bruce Fye.)

1893, the discovery of a muscular connection between the atria and the ventricles that he thought could conduct the cardiac impulse.[38] Because of the discoveries of His and Kent, it was no longer necessary to assume that the cardiac impulse passed from the atria to the ventricles over nervous connections. These discoveries led His to propose, in 1899, that heart block could be the result of damage to the atrioventricular muscle bundle he had described 6 years earlier.[8]

As the new century dawned, the pace of discovery quickened. Sunao Tawara, a recent Japanese medical graduate working in Ludwig Aschoff's pathological laboratory in Marburg, reported his detailed study of the cardiac conduction system in 1906.[39] Tawara identified a region of specialized muscular fibers that he termed the "Knoten des Verbindungsbündels." He claimed that the atrioventricular bundle of His had its origin in this specialized structure. Besides his description of the atrioventricular node, Tawara demonstrated that the bundle of His merged distally with the Purkinje network in the ventricular musculature.

James Mackenzie was following these developments closely. In 1905, he encouraged Arthur Keith (Fig. 1.15) to study the bundle of His. Initially, Keith could not identify any structure such as His described. He told Mackenzie in January 1906 that he had "given up the search for His's bundle—having come to the conclusion that there is not and never was any such thing."[40] Mackenzie responded by sending Keith a copy of a recent paper on the subject by Aschoff and Tawara. Now Keith found that he could identify the

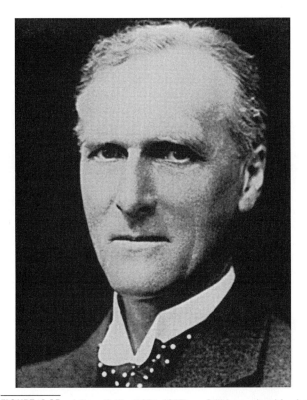

FIGURE 1.15 Arthur Keith (1866–1955), a British anatomist who first identified the sinus node in which the heartbeat originates. (From the National Library of Medicine, with permission.)

structures described by His and Tawara in every instance. He confessed to Mackenzie, "I must be a great duffer not to have seen it before—let alone question its existence."[40] Keith extended his study of the cardiac conducting system, and, as noted earlier, he and Martin Flack discovered the sinus node in 1907. The fundamental structures related to the origin and conduction of the cardiac impulse had been discovered. It now remained for physicians and scientists to explain the mechanisms of the many cardiac arrhythmias that occurred in humans.

BRADYCARDIA AND HEART BLOCK

As physicians became aware of these scientific discoveries, they sought to explain complaints and events that had long been recognized but were poorly understood. Variations in the heart rate had been noted since antiquity. Beginning in the early eighteenth century, physicians claimed that some symptoms and signs could be due to bradycardia. In 1719, European physician Marcus Gerbezius reported the case of a man with profound bradycardia and episodes of dizziness and minor epileptic attacks.[41, 42] Subsequently, other physicians described patients with a slow or intermittent pulse accompanied by symptoms that included dizziness, seizures, syncope, and sudden death. Early reports of such patients were published by Giovanni Morgagni (1761), Thomas Spens (1793), William Burnett (1827), Robert Adams (1827), Herbert Mayo (1838), John Gibson (1838), Thomas Holbertson (1841), and William Stokes (1846).[8, 43] French physician Henri Huchard first used the eponym Stokes-Adams disease for the condition of recurrent syncopal or epileptic attacks associated with bradycardia.[44]

In 1846, Irish physician William Stokes (Fig. 1.16) published his classic paper on the syndrome that bears his name. He described seven patients, three of whom he had seen, who had bradycardia and recurrent syncopal attacks. Several of these patients had evidence of aortic stenosis, but Stokes believed that this was not causally related to their symptoms. In one of his patients, whose heart rate was consistently 28 to 36 beats per minute, Stokes noted a striking abnormality of the jugular pulse. His description is consistent with complete heart block with occasional cannon waves.[45]

The first case of graphically documented heart block in a human was reported in 1875 by British physician Alfred Galabin.[46] Among the many apical pulse tracings he published in an extensive paper on "cardiographic tracings" was one recorded from a 34-year-old man with a 2-year history of lightheaded spells associated with bradycardia. Galabin's tracing is consistent with complete atrioventricular dissociation with a normal atrial rate and a ventricular rate of 25 to 30 beats per minute (Fig. 1.17). Galabin was uncertain of the mechanism and significance of this unusual finding, however. A decade later, French physiologist Auguste Chauveau published similar tracings from another patient who had recurrent syncopal attacks. He correctly concluded that the tracings reflected atrioventricular dissociation.[8]

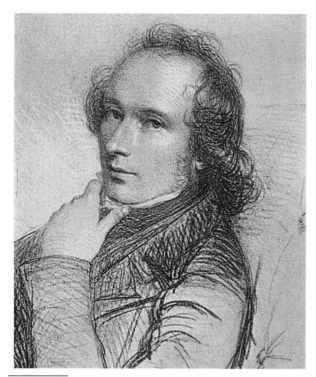

FIGURE 1.16 William Stokes (1804–1878), an Irish physician, was one of the earliest proponents of auscultation. He made classic observations on patients with syncopal attacks associated with bradycardia. (From Stokes W. William Stokes: His Life and Work. London: T Fisher Unwin, 1898.)

At this time, two recent medical graduates were performing experiments in Carl Ludwig's physiological laboratory in Leipzig that would provide insight into the phenomenon that Galabin and Chauveau had documented. Leonard Wooldridge of England and Robert Tigerstedt of Sweden showed that they could cause dissociation of the atria and ventricles in mammals by ligating or sectioning the atrial wall near the atrioventricular groove or the interatrial septum. Wilhelm His, Jr. (Fig. 1.18) repeated their experiments and reported, in 1894, that the same result could be obtained by damaging the atrioventricular muscle bundle he had recently described. These observations proved that there was functional continuity between the atria and the ventricles.[37]

Other workers refined His's approach and extended his experiments. Ewald Hering produced heart block experimentally in dogs by cutting the atrioventricular bundle and showed that sectioning the boundary between the atrium and the ventricle at sites other than the bundle did not lead to heart block. Unlike His, whose observations relied on visual inspection of the beating heart, Hering recorded the activity of the dissociated atria and ventricles.

By the end of the nineteenth century, several investigators had shown that the atrioventricular bundle was responsible for conduction of the cardiac impulse between the atria and ventricles and that its destruction would lead to heart block. Their observations provided an explanation for the clinical syndrome of Stokes-Adams attacks. In 1899, His published a polygraph tracing that revealed atrioventricular dissociation in a patient with recurrent syncope. Karel Wenckebach (Fig. 1.19) claimed that this case led to the recognition of heart block in humans. Shortly after His's article appeared, Wenckebach published a case report supported with polygraph tracings that he thought represented heart block.

Further insight into the pathophysiology of heart block was gained from histological studies and physiological experiments performed early in the twentieth century. In 1905, British physician John Hay, who had studied with Wenckebach, published an article on the pathology of bradycardia in which he demonstrated histological changes in the atrioventricular bundle in the heart of a patient who had documented heart block. At the same time, physiologist Joseph Erlanger of the United States devised a clamp that could be used to apply variable pressure to the bundle. Using this technique, Erlanger produced what we now term first-degree, second-degree, and third-degree heart block. He showed that the heart block that resulted from his interventions was accompanied by microscopic evidence of physical damage to the bundle.[47] In 1906, Einthoven published the first electrocardiographic tracing depicting experimental heart block in a dog.[48] As Einthoven's string galvanometer and refinements of it became available in Europe and the Americas, electrocardiographic tracings of many conduction disturbances were published. They included complete heart block with ventricular bigeminy (Lewis, 1909), the effect of exercise on complete heart block (Nicolai, 1909), complete heart block with atrial fibrillation (Cohn and Lewis, 1912), and atrioventricular dissociation with digitalis excess (Cohn and Fraser, 1913).[16]

Italian physiologist Luigi Luciani, working in Carl Ludwig's laboratory in 1872, observed the phenomenon of grouped beats in the frog heart. The phenomenon of the "regular falling out of a beat" resulting from a disturbance of atrioventricular conduction was first described in humans by Wenckebach in 1899. Although he termed the phenomenon "Luciani peri-

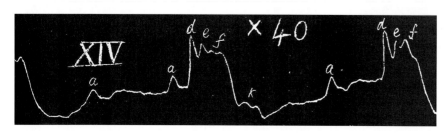

FIGURE 1.17 First published tracing (apex cardiogram) depicting complete heart block. (From Galabin AL. On the interpretation of cardiographic tracings. Guys Hosp Rep 1875; 20:260–314.)

Hollman and Burch and DePasquale summarized the early confusion that existed regarding the electrocardiographic patterns of left and right bundle branch block and the difficulty of distinguishing them from those that resulted from ventricular hypertrophy.[16, 50] The observations during the 1920s of George Fahr and Frank Wilson, pioneers of electrocardiography in the United States, eventually led to the correct association of the underlying defect in the conduction system with the corresponding typical electrocardiographic patterns of bundle branch block.[16, 50]

PREEXCITATION

Frank Wilson was aware of Rothberger's studies on bundle branch block when he published a case report, in 1915, that included the first electrocardiogram reflecting what is now recognized as preexcitation, a term coined in 1944 by R.F. Öhnell. Although Wilson commented on the short PR interval (0.10 sec) and the bundle branch block pattern, he did not appreciate the origin or significance of these electrocardiographic findings.[51] In 1930, Louis Wolff, John Parkinson, and Paul White (Fig. 1.20) described a clinical syndrome consisting of "the combination of bundle-branch block, abnormally short P-R intervals, and paroxysms of tachycardia" (Fig. 1.21). Of the 11 patients they reported, only 2 had evidence of heart disease apart from the abnormal electrocardiograms and epi-

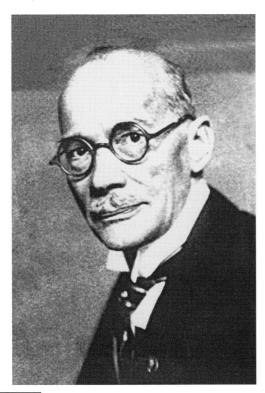

FIGURE 1.18 Wilhelm His, Jr. (1863–1934), the German physician and anatomist who first described the atrioventricular bundle in 1893. (From the National Library of Medicine, with permission.)

ods," today it is known as Wenckebach periodicity. Wenckebach's conclusions regarding the mechanism of these "groups of contractions" were drawn from careful study of radial pulse tracings. He hypothesized that such grouped beating occurred when "conduction is arrested in the auriculoventricular groove."[3] Other investigators extended Wenckebach's studies and confirmed his conclusions. In 1924, European physician and electrocardiographer Woldemar Mobitz described the form of atrioventricular block for which he is remembered eponymically.[49]

BUNDLE BRANCH BLOCK

Bundle branch block is a physiological phenomenon that is clinically silent (unless it is bilateral) but is readily detected by electrocardiography. This technique proved invaluable to investigators who tried, in the early twentieth century, to study the conduction of the cardiac impulse. Austrian Carl Rothberger, a pioneer of electrocardiography, and Hans Eppinger, Jr., used the technique to document the results of their experiments on the branches of the bundle of His. In 1910, they reported that sectioning of both bundle branches resulted in complete heart block. The same year, Rothberger and Heinrich Winterberg published the first electrocardiographic tracings of experimental bundle branch block.[50] These investigations supported Tawara's claim that the electrical impulse of the heart was conveyed to the ventricles through the His-Purkinje system.

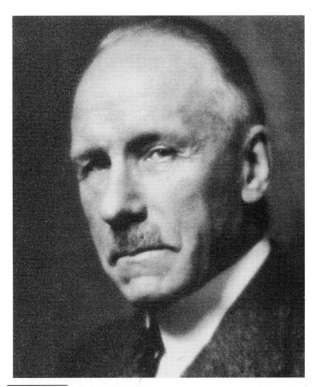

FIGURE 1.19 Karel Wenckebach (1864–1940), a Dutch physician who made many important contributions to our understanding of arrhythmias. Especially important were his observations on extrasystoles and heart block. (From Lindenboom GA. Karel Frederik Wenckebach (1864–1940): Een Korte Schets van Zigan Leven en Werken. Haarlem: DeErven F. Bohn, NV, 1965).

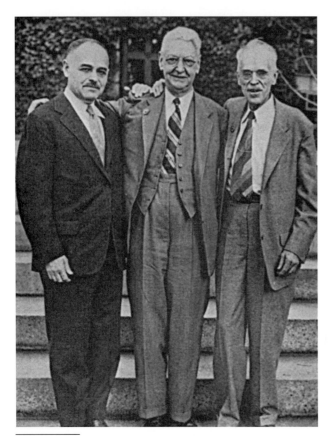

FIGURE 1.20 Louis Wolff (1898–1972), John Parkinson (1885–1976), and Paul Dudley White (1886–1973), the physicians who described, in 1930, the syndrome of paroxysmal tachycardia associated with a short PR interval and bundle branch pattern. (From the National Library of Medicine, with permission.)

sodes of tachycardia. The authors did not speculate on the mechanism of the tachycardia, but they attributed the abnormal electrocardiographic pattern to "vagal stimulation."[52]

Two years later, in 1932, German physicians M. Holzmann and David Scherf (a pupil of Rothberger) proposed the concept of preexcitation to explain the peculiar electrocardiographic features of the syndrome.[53] Working independently, Charles Wolferth and Francis Wood of Philadelphia hypothesized the following year that "an accessory pathway of auriculo-ventricular conduction" could permit retrograde conduction from the ventricle to the atrium, thereby setting up a reentry tachycardia. They thought that the bundle of Kent was the most likely anatomical substrate for this accessory pathway. Wolferth and Wood acknowledged, however,

that "other analogous auriculo-ventricular connections" could exist to explain the phenomenon.[54]

Cambridge physiologist George Mines had advanced a similar theory 2 decades earlier. In 1914, he postulated that some episodes of tachycardia induced in experimental animals "might best be explained as circulating excitations, the impulse passing from auricle to ventricle by one path and returning from ventricle to auricle by another path." Mines reported that "some instances of paroxysmal tachycardia observed in man . . . might conceivably be explained along somewhat similar lines." He thought that the muscular connections demonstrated by Stanley Kent provided the substrate for the mechanism he proposed.[55]

In 1942, J.C. Butterworth and C.A. Poindexter provided experimental proof of the theory of preexcitation. Additional observations in support of the hypothesis were reported by Frank Wilson's group 3 years later. As electrophysiological techniques became more sophisticated, additional discoveries caused investigators to reinterpret earlier observations and conclusions and to put forth new hypotheses regarding the relationship of accessory anatomical connections between the atria and ventricles and preexcitation. It had become clear that the anatomical structures identified by Kent and others were insufficient to explain these complex phenomena.[38]

EXTRASYSTOLES

As graphic methods were applied to the study of the pulse and the electrical impulses of the heart a century ago, it became apparent that several mechanisms could explain an irregular heartbeat or bradycardia. While scientists and clinicians were investigating the phenomenon of heart block, another explanation for these physical findings was proposed. Investigators argued that premature cardiac contractions could account for an irregular pulse, and, if they occurred in a bigeminal pattern, they could result in an apparent halving of the pulse rate.

In the late eighteenth century, Italian scientist Felice Fontana recognized the phenomenon that became known as the refractory period.[56] In 1850, German physiologist Moritz Schiff reported that during the latter portion of the refractory period a strong electrical stimulus could induce a contraction. This phenomenon eventually led to the concept of absolute and relative refractory periods, largely because of the work of physiologist Anton Carlson of the United States in the early twentieth century.[49]

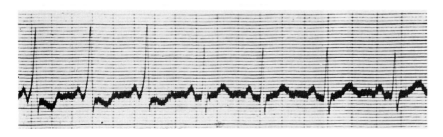

FIGURE 1.21 First published electrocardiograph of intermittent preexcitation, recorded in 1926. (From Wolff L, Parkinson J, White PD. Bundle-branch block with short P-R interval in healthy young people prone to paroxysmal tachycardia. Am Heart J 1930; 5:695–704.)

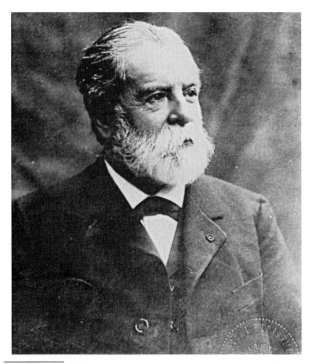

FIGURE 1.22 Étienne Marey (1830–1904), a French physiologist who invented, in 1860, the first practical sphygmometer. This instrument, which graphically recorded the pulse, was used by several investigators in their efforts to study cardiac arrhythmias during the nineteenth century. (From the National Library of Medicine, with permission.)

Schiff's studies of the refractory period were extended in the 1870s by French physiologist Étienne Marey (Fig. 1.22), who first used graphic techniques to record the phenomenon. Marey also described the compensatory pause, an observation that was critical for the development of the concept of the extrasystole. Marey's findings, which he summarized in an 1876 article, impressed Theodor Engelmann, whose studies and conclusions provided the critical link between the experimental observations made by Marey and others and the clinical phenomena of irregular and bigeminal pulses.[57]

Using an isolated frog heart preparation, the extra-stimulus technique, and sophisticated recording apparatus, Engelmann showed, in 1895, that an extrasystole (a term he coined) induced by electrically stimulating the ventricle did not reset the atrial rhythm. An electrically induced ventricular extrasystole was followed by a compensatory pause. When Engelmann produced an atrial extrasystole, he found that the interval to the next systole was shorter than would be expected if a full compensatory pause had occurred. He hypothesized, therefore, that an atrial extrasystole reset the atrial rhythm.[9]

Karel Wenckebach related these experimental observations to clinical medicine and proved that the so-called intermittent pulse was often due to extrasystoles. Wenckebach had worked in Engelmann's laboratory at the University of Utrecht and was familiar with his mentor's experiments on the isolated frog heart. Shortly after he entered practice in 1891, Wenckebach was struck by the irregularity of the heartbeat in an elderly woman whose heart he was auscultating. What set this case apart in his mind was the apparent periodicity of the irregularity of her heartbeat. Wenckebach was reminded of Engelmann's experiments in which an induced ventricular extrasystole was followed by a compensatory pause, and he wondered whether his patient's arrhythmia could represent frequent extrasystoles. When Wenckebach returned to Utrecht to resume his electrophysiological research, he attempted to prove that this was the case.[58]

In 1898, Wenckebach reported the results of experiments in which he proved that extrasystoles accounted for some cases of intermittent pulse. The following year, he published pulse tracings to support his claim that this arrhythmia occurred in humans. Arthur Cushny, a Scottish physiologist then working at the University of Michigan, was studying the same phenomenon and independently concluded that extrasystoles were a common cause of cardiac irregularity in humans.[2] James Mackenzie also held this belief. In an 1894 monograph on venous pulse tracings, he claimed that bigeminal rhythm was due to "the early occurrence of an imperfect systole following a normal systolic contraction of the left ventricle."[59] He based this conclusion on his observations and the earlier studies of Marey, Ludwig Traube, and Franz Riegel. Mackenzie followed the work of Wenckebach and Cushny with interest and lent support to their conclusions about extrasystoles when he published several pulse tracings that represented the phenomenon in humans.[60] The following year, Wenckebach published his monograph on cardiac arrhythmias in which he urged physicians "not to attach much significance to extrasystoles in themselves."[3]

Einthoven published the first electrocardiographic recordings of extrasystoles in 1906 (Figs. 1.23 and 1.24).[48] Five years later, Thomas Lewis summarized contemporary understanding of the phenomena of atrial, junctional, and ventricular extrasystoles.[19] Augustus Hoffmann, a German pioneer of electrocardiog-

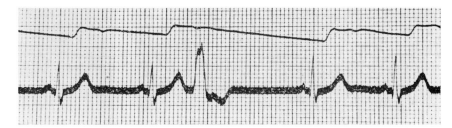

FIGURE 1.23 First published electrocardiograph of a premature ventricular contraction. (From Einthoven W. Le télécardiogramme. Arch Int Physiol 1906; 4:132.)

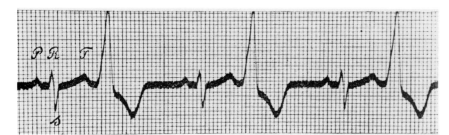

FIGURE 1.24 First published electrocardiograph of ventricular bigeminy. (From Einthoven W. Le télécardiogramme. Arch Int Physiol 1906; 4:132.)

raphy, reported his observations on the experimental induction of extrasystoles in humans in 1914. His subject had undergone rib resection, and the heart was covered only by soft tissues. When Hoffmann electrically stimulated the left ventricle, he found that the electrocardiographic pattern recorded was consistent with bundle branch block.[50]

ATRIAL FIBRILLATION

Extrasystoles were identified as a cause of cardiac irregularity in humans before it was appreciated that atrial fibrillation could also explain this physical finding. Atrial fibrillation was observed in experimental animals almost 300 years before investigators realized that this arrhythmia could be of clinical significance. It was not recognized as a distinct entity in humans until the early twentieth century. In 1628, William Harvey described peculiar movements of the right atrium, probably reflecting atrial fibrillation, in dying experimental animals.[61] Early clinical descriptions of patients with grossly irregular pulses (which we now recognize as consistent with atrial fibrillation) were published by French physician Jean-Baptiste Senac (1749) and Irish physician Robert Adams (1827). Adams also commented on the unusual pattern of jugular venous pulsation he observed in one case, a finding that would eventually be shown to reflect ventricular contractions without normal atrial activity.[62] In his classic 1854 monograph on heart disease, Irish physician William Stokes described the case of a woman with long-standing attacks of paroxysmal tachycardia "during which the action of the heart became greatly excited, extremely irregular, and attended by a loud bellows murmur."[63] Stokes and other nineteenth-century clinicians commented on the association between a grossly irregular pulse and mitral valve disease.

Atrial fibrillation was first graphically depicted in 1863 in Marey's book on the application of graphic techniques to the study of the circulation.[64] Nine years later, French physiologist Edme Vulpian noted rapid irregular motion of the atria in a dog and termed the condition "mouvement fibrillaire."[65] In 1899, Arthur Cushny (Fig. 1.25) noted the similarity of arterial pulse tracings from patients with "extreme irregularity of the heart known clinically as delirium cordis" and those from dogs recorded "when the auricle is undergoing fibrillary contractions." Although Cushny was reluctant to conclude that the arrhythmias were identical, he claimed "the resemblance is certainly striking."[2] Seven years later, Cushny was convinced that the arrhythmias were the same. Meanwhile, other clinical investigators tried to explain the cause and significance of this peculiar arrhythmia known by many names, including delirium cordis. It is not surprising that these investigators sought explanations for it that would conform to contemporary theories of cardiac electrophysiology.

In 1903, Heinrich Hering reported his studies of the condition he termed "pulsus irregularis perpetuus." Although Hering was the first to claim that this was a distinct arrhythmia in humans, he did not appreciate that the unusual findings were the result of atrial fibrillation. His explanation of the mechanism of the arrhythmia was based on the idea of the extrasystole. Hering thought that the rapid and irregularly irregular pulse resulted from "an extra stimulus or a stimulus arising prematurely at the place of normal formation." Although Hering argued that this was a distinct arrhythmia and that it was of cardiac origin and not due to the "indirect influence of the extra-cardial nerves," he did not attribute it to fibrillation of the atria.[42]

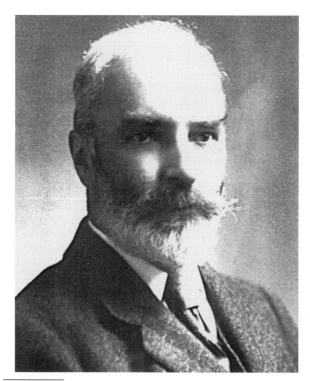

FIGURE 1.25 Arthur Cushny (1866–1926), a Scottish physiologist who was the first to claim that atrial fibrillation occurred in humans. (From the National Library of Medicine, with permission.)

Cushny and Charles Edmunds published an article on "auricular fibrillation" in 1906 in which they argued that this arrhythmia, long recognized in experimental animals, existed in humans. They described their experiments on dogs in which atrial fibrillation was observed occasionally when the heart was exposed. When they reviewed a series of arterial pulse tracings recorded from dogs with atrial fibrillation, Cushny and Edmunds noted a similarity between those recordings and pulse tracings from a 64-year-old woman with gross cardiac irregularity. They concluded that it was likely that the woman's rapid, irregular pulse was due to atrial fibrillation.[66]

Without appreciating its mechanism or its clinical significance, James Mackenzie (Fig. 1.26), in the early 1890s, had recorded in humans what became recognized as atrial fibrillation. Because he could not identify atrial activity in his pulse tracings, Mackenzie thought that the atria were paralyzed. Despite this erroneous conclusion, he made the important observation that gross irregularity of the pulse was frequently associated with a specific type of jugular pulse tracing that he termed the "ventricular form of venous pulse," because it was characterized by a prominent systolic wave. By 1907, Mackenzie had studied several hundred patients with this peculiar form of jugular pulse and had come to accept Cushny's hypothesis that the condition represented atrial fibrillation.[67]

Mackenzie credited Cushny with first suggesting that atrial fibrillation could be of clinical significance. He recalled that "on a visit Professor Cushny paid to me

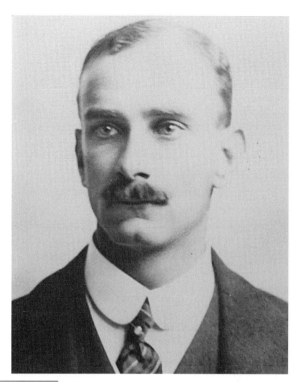

FIGURE 1.27 Thomas Lewis (1881–1945), a British physician who was among the first to use the electrocardiograph to study cardiac arrhythmias. Using this technique, he made many classic observations on disorders of impulse formation and conduction. (From the National Library of Medicine, with permission.)

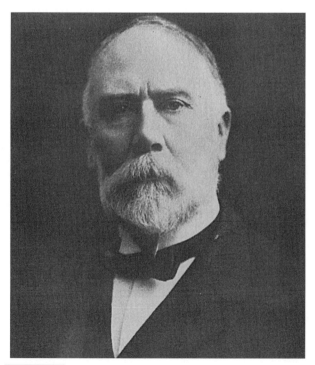

FIGURE 1.26 James Mackenzie (1853–1925), a Scottish physician who published many classic observations on cardiac arrhythmias based on his careful study of pulse tracings. (From Wilson RM. The Beloved Physician, Sir James Mackenzie. New York: Macmillan, 1926.)

in Burnley in 1906, he discussed with me the probability of auricular fibrillation being the cause of the irregular heart action in certain cases of 'nodal rhythm,' and he agreed that certain small waves which I recognized in the jugular pulse of one case were due to the fibrillation of the auricle." Mackenzie admitted that at first he failed to recognize the significance of the concept of atrial fibrillation. He credited Thomas Lewis (Fig. 1.27), who used the electrocardiogram to study the disorder, with finally convincing him of its clinical significance.[68]

Although the importance of Lewis's observations on atrial fibrillation is difficult to exaggerate, he was not the first to use electrocardiography to document the existence of this arrhythmia in humans. Even Einthoven, who published the first electrocardiogram depicting atrial fibrillation in 1906, did not correlate this tracing with any specific clinical condition (Fig. 1.28). Three years later, two continental pioneers of electrocardiography, Carl Rothberger and Heinrich Winterberg, used the new technique to prove that atrial fibrillation existed in humans. Based on electrocardiographic tracings, these investigators argued that the arrhythmia known as atrial fibrillation in experimental animals was the same as the rhythm disturbance in humans termed (among many other names) delirium cordis and arrhythmia perpetua. They showed that electrocardiograms from experimental animals and patients with what they believed to be the same arrhythmia—atrial fibrillation—shared three distinc-

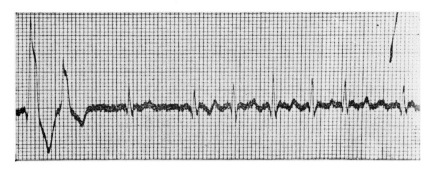

FIGURE 1.28 First published electrocardiograph of atrial fibrillation. (From Einthoven W. Le télécardiogramme. Arch Int Physiol 1906; 4:132.)

tive features: a totally irregular ventricular rate, an absence of P waves, and the presence of oscillations of the string galvanometer representing fibrillary waves.[69]

Working independently, Thomas Lewis reported, in 1909, his electrocardiographic studies of patients with grossly irregular rhythms. He concluded that atrial fibrillation was the usual cause of this arrhythmia and declared that it was "a common clinical condition."[70] This discovery demonstrated the utility of the new technique of electrocardiography. Lewis explained: "Although auricular fibrillation has been regarded by certain isolated observers as a possible phenomenon in clinical pathology, its association with anything beyond rare cases of paroxysmal tachycardia has not been seriously attempted until the last few months. The introduction of the string galvanometer as an aid to diagnosis has facilitated a much wider conclusion."[71]

Some investigators had attempted to elucidate the mechanism of this dramatic arrhythmia that they observed in experimental animals in the late nineteenth century. One theory advanced to explain fibrillation was that it resulted from a disturbance of a hypothetical "coordinating center" of the heart thought to be located in the proximal interventricular septum. This theory, supported by Swiss physiologist Hugo Kronecker and others, was proved false by Scottish physiologist John MacWilliam and American physiologist William Porter.

Another theory, advanced by Theodor Engelmann in 1895, attributed fibrillation to multiple ectopic foci beating independently at their maximum intrinsic rate. This theory influenced Hering in his attempt to explain the arrhythmia. In 1905, Rothberger and Winterberg reported on their study of atrial arrhythmias in which they were the first to apply electrodes directly to the surface of the fibrillating atria. They proposed the theory of "tachysystole," which held that fibrillation was due to the extremely rapid (3000–3500 times per minute) discharge of a single focus.[72]

Thomas Lewis, because of his experiments, rejected these theories. In a series of articles published in the early 1920s, he developed the circus hypothesis to account for atrial fibrillation and flutter. He explained: "Clinical fibrillation of the auricle is a condition in which a *single* excitation wave circulates continuously through the auricular muscle." Atrial fibrillation was "a state of advanced impure flutter, and both arrhythmias have as their underlying basis a single circulating wave; they differ from each other in that in flutter this wave follows a constant anatomical path, while in

fibrillation this varies in greater or lesser degree from cycle to cycle."[5]

Lewis's elaboration of the circus theory was stimulated by the work of other investigators. American zoologist Alfred Mayer, studying the umbrella of the jellyfish, first demonstrated the phenomenon of circus movement in 1908. He found that an extrastimulus applied to the muscular ring of the jellyfish would induce an excitation wave that continued to circulate for several minutes.[73] Cambridge physiologist George Mines extended Mayer's experiments and claimed, in 1913: "If a closed circuit of muscle is provided, of considerably greater length than the wave of excitation, it is possible to start a wave in this circuit which will continue to propagate itself round and round the circuit for an infinite number of times." Mines made the important observation, later to have therapeutic implications, that "the condition is readily upset by an extra systole."[74] Lewis also credited American physiologist Walter Garrey with observations that helped to establish the circus theory of fibrillation.[72, 75]

Some European workers, most notably Rothberger, were reluctant to accept the circus theory of atrial fibrillation. Based on experiments performed in the 1920s, German (later American) physician David Scherf argued for the heterotopic foci theory. This minority view received further support from American Myron Prinzmetal and his coworkers, who used the technique of high-speed cinematography to study atrial arrhythmias in the late 1940s.[76] As invasive electrophysiological techniques emerged, other mechanisms, including the theory of intra-atrial reentry and the multiple wavelet hypothesis, were proposed to explain atrial fibrillation.

ATRIAL FLUTTER

Atrial flutter was first reported in an experimental animal by Scottish physiologist John MacWilliam in 1887. He induced the arrhythmia by applying a faradic current to the atrium: "The application of the current sets the auricles into a rapid flutter. . . . The movements are regular; they seem to consist of a series of contractions originating in the stimulated area and thence spreading over the rest of the tissue. The movement does not show any distinct sign of inco-ordination; it looks like a rapid series of contraction waves passing over the auricular walls."[77]

The first pulse tracings documenting atrial flutter in a human were published in 1906 by Edinburgh physician William Ritchie. After administering atropine to a man with chronic heart block, Ritchie recorded a regular atrial rhythm at a rate of 275 and a regular ventricular rhythm at a rate of 37 beats per minute. He did not comment on the significance of the extreme atrial rate, however.[78] Einthoven published the first electrocardiographic tracing of atrial flutter in 1906 (Fig. 1.29).[48] Three years later, Ritchie, with his colleague William Jolly, recorded the same arrhythmia in this patient using an electrocardiograph.[79, 80] They recognized the similarity between their patient's arrhythmia and that described by MacWilliam in the experimental animal nearly 2 decades earlier. They adopted MacWilliam's term "flutter" to describe their subject's arrhythmia, because they believed that it should be distinguished from atrial fibrillation. At this time, London physicians Arthur Hertz and Gordon Goodhart reported another case of atrial flutter that led to Thomas Lewis's interest in the arrhythmia.

In 1912, Lewis described the characteristic clinical, polygraphic, and electrocardiographic features of 16 patients with atrial flutter, an arrhythmia he characterized as "curious and not uncommon." He found that 2:1 atrioventricular block was the most common degree of block in atrial flutter and reported that digitalis and vagal stimulation increased the block and that exercise decreased it. Lewis advocated digitalis for control of the ventricular response and noted that it was occasionally associated with conversion to sinus rhythm.[81]

PAROXYSMAL TACHYCARDIA

Investigators have long recognized that tachycardias are either regular or irregular, but only in the twentieth century was it discovered that regular tachycardias have multiple mechanisms. In a 1909 article on paroxysmal tachycardia, Thomas Lewis noted that the advent of electrocardiography made it possible to distinguish "at least two definite and distinct forms of the affection, and in the future they will require separate consideration."[82] Soon, the clinical and electrocardiographic features of supraventricular and ventricular tachycardia were differentiated by workers in several countries. Over the past several decades, it has become apparent that tachycardia has many distinct forms.[65]

London physician Richard Cotton first reported paroxysmal tachycardia in 1867. He described the case of a 42-year-old man who had the sudden onset of rapid heart action accompanied by faintness and dyspnea. Using a sphygmograph, Cotton's colleague John Bur-

don-Sanderson recorded a radial pulse tracing during an attack. This revealed a regular rhythm at a rate of 232 beats per minute. Cotton was impressed with the sphygmograph, because it enabled him to count the pulse accurately and to prove that it was regular. In his report, he emphasized that his patient's tachycardia always began and ended abruptly.[42, 83]

In an 1888 article, British neurologist John Bristowe reported nine patients with paroxysmal tachycardia. He was aware of Cotton's description of the condition as well as recent case reports by James Edmunds and Thomas Watson. Several of Bristowe's patients had evidence of congestive heart failure and most had died, often suddenly. A review of his cases suggests that they included examples of supraventricular tachycardia, ventricular tachycardia, and atrial fibrillation. Surprisingly, Bristowe concluded that the episodes of tachycardia had "no special connection with cardiac disease."[84]

French physician Léon Bouveret used the term "tachycardie paroxystique essentielle" in an 1889 article in which he reported three patients who suffered sudden attacks of rapid heart action lasting a few hours to several days. Bouveret emphasized several characteristics peculiar to paroxysmal tachycardia: the abrupt onset, the episodic nature, the regularity of the pulse during the attacks, and the absence of any evidence of cardiac dysfunction between the spells.[42]

In 1900, German physician Augustus Hoffmann published a comprehensive monograph that described 135 cases of paroxysmal tachycardia and listed 336 references. He believed, as did James Mackenzie, that paroxysmal tachycardia represented runs of extrasystoles rather than ordinary contractions.[85] Two years later, Hoffmann claimed that "attacks of paroxysmal tachycardia are really attacks consisting of long continued series of premature systoles."[60] Wenckebach was reluctant to speculate on a mechanism because, as late as 1903, he had not seen a "typical case" of paroxysmal tachycardia.[3]

In 1909, Thomas Lewis proposed a classification of arrhythmias in which he differentiated paroxysmal atrial tachycardia from paroxysmal ventricular tachycardia. Unlike Hoffmann, who attributed paroxysmal tachycardia to a disturbance of the nervous system, Lewis claimed that it, as well as most other arrhythmias, was "probably as a result of an irritable lesion" in the heart.[82] Based on a series of elegant experiments, George Mines proposed, in 1913, that "circulating excitation," later termed reentry, was "responsible for some cases of paroxysmal tachycardia as observed clinically."[74]

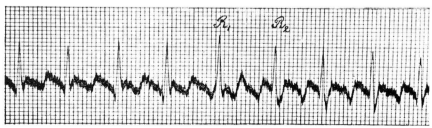

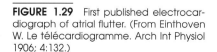

FIGURE 1.29 First published electrocardiograph of atrial flutter. (From Einthoven W. Le télécardiogramme. Arch Int Physiol 1906; 4:132.)

VENTRICULAR TACHYCARDIA

Undoubtedly, some cases of paroxysmal tachycardia reported during the late nineteenth century were ventricular in origin. As Thomas Lewis noted, the modern distinction between supraventricular and ventricular tachycardia had to await the arrival of electrocardiography. Some nineteenth-century investigators discovered that they could induce tachycardia in experimental animals by interrupting coronary blood flow.[49, 86] The significance of these observations gradually became apparent during the early twentieth century as insight into the pathophysiology and clinical implications of coronary thrombosis grew.[87]

Although the possibility of ventricular tachycardia had been suggested by James Mackenzie and Karel Wenckebach, proof of its existence in humans was first provided by Lewis in 1909. He reported the case of a seaman who suffered from chest discomfort and dyspnea on exertion. Using Augustus Waller's electrocardiographic apparatus at South Kensington, England, Lewis documented recurrent episodes of 3 to 11 "successive extrasystoles" that he thought were of ventricular origin (Fig. 1.30). Lewis claimed that his electrocardiographic documentation of the arrhythmia "placed occurrence and recognition in man beyond question."[88, 89]

The same year, Lewis published the results of a series of experiments in which he ligated the coronary arteries in animals in an attempt to induce arrhythmias that could shed light on the pathophysiology of "the two main types of paroxysmal tachycardia known to occur in the human subject." From these experiments, Lewis argued that the tachycardia induced by coronary ligation originated in the ventricular walls, arising independent of "all central nervous system control," and that the "ventricular rhythm is independent of impulses received from the auricle."[90] By 1911, Lewis had concluded that ventricular tachycardia had a bad prognosis and was often rapidly fatal.[19]

The following year, New York physician Stuart Hart published a case report of a man with symptomatic paroxysmal ventricular tachycardia documented by electrocardiography. Based on the patient's clinical picture and his electrocardiogram, Hart concluded that the arrhythmia was probably caused by "myocardial changes due to coronary disease possibly following a syphilitic infection and the prolonged use of alcohol." He was impressed by the similarity between the electrocardiographic tracings from his patient and those recorded by Lewis from dogs in which he had ligated the left anterior descending coronary artery.[91]

In 1921, American physicians Canby Robinson and George Herrmann reported four patients with electrocardiographic documentation of ventricular tachycardia. They were familiar with the recent animal studies of American physicians James Herrick and Fred Smith on the electrocardiographic manifestations of experimental coronary occlusion. One of the patients studied by Robinson and Herrmann died and was found to have a thrombus in the left anterior descending coronary artery that supplied a bulging area of myocardium that was discolored. Robinson and Herrmann proposed that coronary occlusion was responsible for some cases of ventricular tachycardia in humans. They also suspected that the ventricular tachycardia could "pass over into ventricular fibrillation, which usually means permanent cessation of the circulation and death," although they did not have proof of this transition.[92, 93]

The following year, in 1922, French physician Louis Gallavardin described repetitive monomorphic ventricular tachycardia. He distinguished this form of ventricular arrhythmia from the more rapid and chaotic type that he believed was associated with a worse prognosis, because it could herald ventricular fibrillation.[88] In 1930, Maurice Strauss summarized 63 published cases of ventricular tachycardia and added 2 of his own. This important review included a summary of the clinical, electrocardiographic, and pathological features of the arrhythmia. Most patients had angina or symptoms of congestive heart failure. From his review of the literature, Strauss concluded that the prognosis of ventricular tachycardia without evidence of organic heart disease was good.[94]

VENTRICULAR FIBRILLATION

In 1683, Dutch physician Johannis Pechlin described the terminal motions of the heart in a man dying of an open chest wound. In his classic 1749 monograph on heart disease, French physician Jean-Baptiste Senac claimed that Pechlin was describing fibrillation of the ventricles, a condition Senac had observed in the hearts of dying experimental animals.[61] In 1850, Carl Ludwig and his pupil Moritz Hoffa showed that it was possible to induce ventricular fibrillation in experimental animals by applying a strong constant or faradic current to the heart.[95, 96]

John MacWilliam, who had studied with Ludwig, claimed, in 1887, that ventricular fibrillation was "familiar to all who have worked much with the mammalian heart." He was aware of the work of French physician Germain Sée, who had reported that he could induce ventricular fibrillation in dogs by occluding their coronary arteries. Based on 2 years of mammalian experiments, MacWilliam concluded that ventricu-

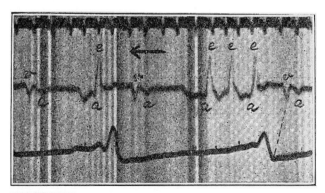

FIGURE 1.30 First published electrocardiograph of ventricular tachycardia. (From Lewis T. Single and successive extra-systoles. Lancet 1909; 1:382–385.)

lar fibrillation was "due to certain changes occurring within the ventricles themselves." He rejected the theories that the arrhythmia was due to "abnormal nerve impulses" or was caused by a disturbance of a hypothetical coordinating center in the interventricular septum, a concept championed by Hugo Kronecker.[77, 97]

In an 1889 article, MacWilliam argued that sudden death in humans was often the result of ventricular fibrillation.[98, 99] Moreover, he claimed: "In the great majority of cases where sudden death is caused by cardiac failure, there is, no doubt, an altered and impaired state of nutrition in the cardiac tissues, sometimes rendered palpable by degenerative changes recognisable with the microscope or pointed to by the presence of disease in the coronary arteries." Although ventricular fibrillation was usually fatal in experimental animals, MacWilliam found that he could occasionally restore normal rhythm by applying "rhythmic compression of the ventricles with the hand" and administering pilocarpine intravenously.[100]

In 1911, Augustus Hoffmann published an electrocardiogram that he believed represented ventricular fibrillation in a human. Review of the tracing suggests that the rhythm was polymorphic ventricular tachycardia, a view held by several of Hoffmann's contemporaries. Besides, the patient survived, further evidence that the rhythm, which terminated spontaneously in sinus rhythm, was not ventricular fibrillation.[101] The following year, Canby Robinson reported on the electrocardiograms recorded at the time of death of seven patients. Two of his subjects had tracings consistent with ventricular fibrillation.[102]

Thomas Lewis offered an explanation for the delay in documenting ventricular fibrillation in humans in 1915. "It is a remarkable fact," Lewis claimed, "that practically every form of irregularity, which has been produced experimentally in the mammalian heart, has now been recorded frequently in clinical cases. But there is one notable exception. . . . Why is fibrillation of the ventricles so uncommon an experience? For a good reason: fibrillation of the ventricles is incompatible with existence. . . . If it occurs in man, it is responsible for unexpected and sudden death."[103]

TREATMENT OF ARRHYTHMIAS

Except for digitalis, effective and practical therapeutic approaches to the management of cardiac arrhythmias did not become available until the twentieth century.[104] Chronic, symptomatic bradyarrhythmias could not be treated effectively until the advent of permanent pacemakers. Although MacWilliam anticipated the development of the pacemaker more than a century ago and New York physician Albert Hyman invented a machine that he termed an "artificial pacemaker" in 1927, technology that made permanent pacing practical in humans did not emerge until the 1950s.[105, 106]

In 1950, Canadian surgeons Wilfred Bigelow and John Callaghan described their investigation of electrical stimulation of the heartbeat. Boston physician Paul Zoll extended their studies and reported, 2 years later, the successful stimulation of the heart of a patient with ventricular asystole by a transthoracic pacemaker. Zoll claimed that "a simple, effective and apparently safe means is therefore available of arousing the heart from ventricular standstill and keeping it beating until internal pacemakers revive."[107] The subsequent development of the field of pacemakers is beyond the scope of this review, but this technology revolutionized the treatment of symptomatic bradyarrhythmias.

For many decades, extrasystoles have been viewed as generally benign. In 1916, American physician J.E. Greiwe advised an audience of American Medical Association members: "Base your prognosis not on the presence of premature ventricular systoles, but rather on the underlying cause."[108] Fifteen years later, Paul White explained that isolated extrasystoles were often triggered by tobacco, alcohol, and fatigue. He claimed that they usually required no treatment and urged physicians to reassure their patients that the palpitations caused by this arrhythmia were insignificant. If the extrasystoles were so symptomatic as to require treatment, White advocated digitalis, quinidine, or triple bromides.[109]

Digitalis has been used in the treatment of heart disease for more than 2 centuries. William Withering's 1785 book, *An Account of the Foxglove, and Some of Its Medical Uses,* was based on his experience with the drug in 160 patients.[110] In 1835, French physician Jean-Baptiste Bouillaud noted the beneficial effect of digitalis on the irregular pulse in a patient with mitral stenosis.[111] Long before investigators recognized that this form of cardiac arrhythmia was due to atrial fibrillation, digitalis became the mainstay of therapy for patients with the condition.

Quinidine also has a long history as a therapeutic agent. The cinchona bark (which contains quinine and its isomer quinidine) was first advocated for the treatment of palpitations by the French physician Jean-Baptiste Senac in 1749. The modern use of quinidine can be traced to Karel Wenckebach, who claimed, in 1914, that quinine was sometimes of value in patients with atrial fibrillation. In response to this observation, German clinical investigator Walter Frey undertook a systematic study of the value of various cinchona alkaloids as antiarrhythmic agents. In 1918, he reported that quinidine was the most effective antiarrhythmic derived from cinchona.[112, 113] The value of quinidine in the management of patients with atrial fibrillation was quickly acknowledged, and it was often used with digitalis in patients with this arrhythmia.[109]

Quinidine was first advocated for the treatment of ventricular tachycardia in 1922 by American physician Roy Scott.[114] He considered the arrhythmia to be a manifestation of reentry and found that quinidine often suppressed it. By the end of the decade, quinidine was the standard treatment for ventricular tachycardia. Paul White claimed, in 1931, that quinidine could "help to prevent fibrillation of the ventricles . . . in spite of the fact that overdosage can induce it." Speaking of sudden cardiac death, the Boston cardiologist noted: "There is here a mystery to solve and with its solution may come light, leading perhaps to the resuscitation of these victims."[109] Scientists and clinical investigators shared White's conviction that cardiac arrhythmias provided a fertile ground for research.

In 1936, American physician Frederick Mautz reported his empirical observation in animals that intravenous administration of the local anesthetic procaine hydrochloride increased the likelihood of successful countershock.[115] The clinical use of this drug was limited by its short half-life and side effects, however. Systematic study of other procaine compounds led, in 1951, to the introduction of procaine amide by Lester Mark and his colleagues. A year earlier, J.L. Southworth and his associates had reported the efficacy of intravenous lidocaine for the treatment of ventricular arrhythmias.[116]

While these pharmacological discoveries provided physicians with agents that were effective in treating ventricular tachycardia, work on cardiac resuscitation using electrical and mechanical approaches was coming to fruition. Elsewhere, I have reviewed the development of cardiac resuscitation.[98] The efforts of scientists and clinical investigators in Europe and the Americas during the first half of the twentieth century culminated in the first successful human heart defibrillation by Cleveland surgeon Claude Beck and his colleagues in 1947. This procedure was performed during a cardiac operation, and the current was applied directly to the heart.[117] Nevertheless, it stimulated great interest in defibrillation as a component of attempts at cardiac resuscitation.

In 1956, Paul Zoll and his colleagues reported that ventricular fibrillation could be terminated by a countershock delivered transthoracically. They described the successful termination of 11 episodes of ventricular fibrillation in 4 patients and concluded that "external countershock is an immediately effective, safe and clinically feasible procedure."[118] Soon, this technique was combined with external cardiac massage by William Kouwenhoven and his colleagues at the Johns Hopkins Hospital in Baltimore, and the modern era of cardiac resuscitation began.[119]

POSTSCRIPT

The period following World War II witnessed dramatic growth of biomedical enterprise in the United States.[120] Discoveries by American scientists and clinical investigators, together with important contributions by workers in many other countries, have led to an explosion of basic knowledge about cardiac arrhythmias. Some groups have focused on the mechanisms underlying arrhythmias; others have sought effective treatments for this important class of disorders. As newer diagnostic techniques emerged and efficacious therapies were introduced, a new discipline arose—clinical cardiac electrophysiology.

In recent decades, the diagnosis and management of cardiac arrhythmias have undergone remarkable changes as a result of many discoveries that have resulted from basic research.[121, 122] Clinical cardiac electrophysiology has grown dramatically as noninvasive and invasive diagnostic techniques such as Holter monitoring, His bundle electrocardiography, intracardiac mapping, programmed electrical stimulation, and signal-averaged electrocardiography were developed.[123, 124] Creative nonpharmacological approaches to the management of arrhythmias have also been introduced, including surgical and catheter ablation techniques and the automatic implantable defibrillator.[125–127] Pharmacological therapy of arrhythmias has also advanced dramatically in recent decades.[128]

These newer diagnostic and therapeutic modalities are beyond the scope of this historical review. They are discussed in other chapters that summarize the dynamic field of cardiac arrhythmias. As you read this book, I urge you to reflect on this provocative question: "Where does medical history end and a review of the literature begin?"

REFERENCES

1. Krikler DM. The development of the understanding of arrhythmias during the last 100 years. Med Hist 1985; 5:77–81.
2. Cushny AR. On the interpretation of pulse-tracings. J Exp Med 1899; 4:327–347.
3. Wenckebach KF. Arrhythmia of the Heart: A Physiological and Clinical Study. Edinburgh, William Green, 1904.
4. Meltzer SJ. The neurogenic and myogenic theories and the modern classification and interpretation of cardiac arrhythmias. Med Rec 1909; 75:873–883.
5. Lewis T. Observations upon flutter and fibrillation. IX. The nature of auricular fibrillation as it occurs in patients. Heart 1921; 8:193–227.
6. Comroe JH, Dripps RD. The top ten clinical advances in cardiovascular-pulmonary medicine and surgery 1945–1975. Washington, DC: US Government Printing Office, 1978.
7. Horine EF. An epitome of ancient pulse lore. Bull Hist Med 1941; 10:209–249.
8. Schechter DC, Lillehei CW, Soffer A. History of sphygmology and of heart block. Dis Chest 1969; 55:535–579.
9. Scherf D, Schott A. Historical remarks. In Scherf D, Schott A (eds). Extrasystoles and Allied Arrhythmias. London: William Heinemann, 1953, pp. 1–26.
10. Townsend GL. Sir John Floyer (1649–1734) and his study of pulse and respiration. J Hist Med Allied Sci 1967; 22:286–316.
11. Borell M. Extending the senses: the graphic method. Med Heritage 1986; March-April:114–121.
12. Fye WB. Carl Ludwig and the Leipzig Physiological Institute: a factory of new knowledge. Circulation 1986; 74:920–928.
13. Heberden W. Remarks on the pulse. Med Trans College Phys London 1772; 2:18–33.
14. Waller AD. A demonstration on man of electromotive changes accompanying the heart's beat. J Physiol 1887; 8:229–234.
15. Frank RG. The telltale heart: physiological instruments, graphic methods, and clinical hopes, 1854–1914. In Coleman W, Holmes FL (eds). The Investigative Enterprise: Experimental Physiology in Nineteenth-Century Medicine. Berkeley, CA: University of California Press, 1988, pp. 211–290.
16. Burch GE, DePasquale NP. A History of Electrocardiography. Chicago: Year Book Medical Publishers, 1964.
17. Katz LN, Hellerstein HK. Electrocardiography. In Fishman AP, Richards DW (eds). Circulation of the Blood: Men and Ideas. New York: Oxford University Press, 1964, pp. 165–351.
18. Burnett J. The origins of the electrocardiograph as a clinical instrument. Med Hist 1985; 5:53–76.
19. Lewis T. The Mechanism of the Heart Beat. London: Shaw & Sons, 1911.
20. Einthoven W. The different forms of the human electrocardiogram and their signification. Lancet 1912; 1:853–861.

21. Snellen HA. Two Pioneers of Electrocardiography: The Correspondence Between Einthoven and Lewis from 1908–1926. Rotterdam: Donker Academic Publications, 1983.
22. Fye WB. The origin of the heart beat: a tale of frogs, jellyfish and turtles. Circulation 1987; 76:493–500.
23. Hoff HE. The history of vagal inhibition. Bull Hist Med 1940; 8:461–496.
24. Pick J. From William Harvey to the "explorer," some comments on the carotid sinus and other vascular reflexes. Am Pract Dig Treat 1959; 10:451–464.
25. Fulton JF, Wilson LG. Selected Readings in the History of Physiology. Springfield, IL: Charles C Thomas, 1966.
26. French RD. Darwin and the physiologists, or the medusa and modern cardiology. J Hist Biol 1970; 3:253–274.
27. Geison G. Michael Foster and the Cambridge School of Physiology: The Scientific Enterprise in Late Victorian Society. Princeton, NJ: Princeton University Press, 1978.
28. Foster M. A Text Book of Physiology. London: Macmillan, 1877.
29. Gaskell WH. On the innervation of the heart. J Physiol 1883; 4:43–127.
30. Gaskell WH. The contraction of cardiac muscle. In Schafer EA (ed). Text-Book of Physiology. New York: Macmillan, 1900, pp. 169–227.
31. Keith A, Flack M. The form and nature of the muscular connections between the primary divisions of the vertebrate heart. J Anat Physiol 1907; 41:172–189.
32. Lewis T, Oppenheimer BS, Oppenheimer A. The site of origin of the mammalian heart-beat; the pacemaker in the dog. Heart 1910; 2:147–169.
33. Harvey W. Exercitatio Anatomica. De Motu Cordis et Sanguinis in Animalibus [reprint]. Springfield, IL: Charles C Thomas, 1928.
34. Wiktor Z. Purkyne's research on the structure of the heart. In Kruta V (ed). Jan Evangelista Purkyne, 1787–1869: Centenary Symposium. Brno, Czechoslovakia: University Jana Evangelistâ Purkyne, 1971, pp. 237–244.
35. James TN. The development of ideas concerning the conduction system of the heart. Ulster Med J 1982; 51:81–97.
36. His W. The activity of the embryonic human heart and its significance for the understanding of the heart movement in the adult [1893]. J Hist Med Allied Sci 1949; 4:289–318.
37. His W. The story of the atrioventricular bundle with remarks concerning embryonic heart activity [1933]. J Hist Med Allied Sci 1949; 4:319–333.
38. Anderson RH, Becker AE. Stanley Kent and accessory atrioventricular connections. J Thorac Cardiovasc Surg 1981; 81:649–658.
39. Tawara S. Das Reizleitungssystem des Saugetierherzens. Jena, Germany: Gustav Fischer, 1906.
40. Mair A. Sir James Mackenzie, M.D., 1853–1925, General Practitioner. Edinburgh: Churchill Livingstone, 1973.
41. Flaxman N. The history of heart-block. Bull Hist Med 1937; 5:115–130.
42. Major RH. Classic Description of Disease. Springfield, IL: Charles C Thomas, 1945.
43. Leibowitz JO, Ullmann DT. Early references to heart block. J Hist Med Allied Sci 1965; 20:43–51.
44. MacMurray FG. Stokes-Adams disease, a historical review. N Engl J Med 1957; 256:643–650.
45. Stokes W. Observations on some cases of permanently slow pulse. Dublin Q J Med Sci 1846; 2:73–85.
46. Galabin AL. On the interpretation of cardiogenic tracings, and the evidence which they afford as to the causation of the murmurs attendant upon mitral stenosis. Guys Hosp Rep 1875; 20:261–314.
47. Erlanger J. A physiologist reminisces. In Luck MJ (ed). The Excitement and Fascination of Science. Palo Alto, CA: Annual Reviews, 1965:93–106.
48. Einthoven W. Le télécardiogramme. Arch Int Physiol 1906; 4:132–164.
49. Shapiro E. The electrocardiogram and the arrhythmias: historical insights. In Mandel WJ (ed). Cardiac Arrhythmias: Their Mechanism, Diagnosis and Management. Philadelphia: JB Lippincott, 1980, pp. 1–11.
50. Hollman A. The history of bundle branch block. Med Hist 1985; 5:82–102.
51. Wilson FN. A case in which the vagus influenced the form of the ventricular complex of the electrocardiogram. Arch Intern Med 1915; 16:1008–1027.
52. Wolff L, Parkinson J, White PD. Bundle-branch block with short P-R interval in healthy young people prone to paroxysmal tachycardia. Am Heart J 1930; 5:685–704.
53. Burchell HB. Ventricular preexcitation: historical overview. In Benditt DG, Benson DW (eds). Cardiac Preexcitation Syndromes: Origins, Evaluation, and Treatment. Boston: Martinus Nijhoff Publishing, 1986, pp. 3–19.
54. Wolferth CC, Wood FC. The mechanism of production of short P-R intervals and prolonged QRS complexes in patients with presumably undamaged hearts: hypothesis of an accessory pathway of auriculo-ventricular conduction (bundle of Kent). Am Heart J 1933; 8:297–311.
55. Mines GR. On circulating excitations in heart muscles and their possible relation to tachycardia and fibrillation. Proc Trans R Soc Can 1914; 8:43–53.
56. Hoff HE. The history of the refractory period: a neglected contribution of Felice Fontana. Yale Biol Med 1942; 14:635–672.
57. Marey EJ. Des excitations électriques du coeur: Physiologie experimentale. Travaux du Laboratorie de M Marey 1876; Paris, Masson, 2:63–86.
58. Fye WB. Karel Frederik Wenckebach, 1864–1940. Clin Cardiol 1990; 13:146–148.
59. Mackenzie J. The venous and liver pulses, and the arrhythmic contraction of the cardiac cavities. J Pathol Bacteriol 1894; 2:84–154.
60. Mackenzie J. The Study of the Pulse, Arterial, Venous, and Hepatic and the Movements of the Heart. Edinburgh: Young J. Pentland, 1902.
61. McMichael J. History of atrial fibrillation 1628–1819: Harvey—de Senac—Laennec. Br Heart J 1982; 48:193–197.
62. Bloomfield AL. A bibliography of internal medicine: auricular fibrillation. Arch Intern Med 1958; 102:302–313.
63. Stokes W. Diseases of the Heart and Aorta. Dublin: Hodges and Smith, 1854.
64. Marey EJ. Physiologie médicale de la circulation du sang. Paris: Adrien Delahaye, 1863.
65. Reddy CP, Surawicz B. Terminology of tachycardias: historical background and evolution. Pacing Clin Electrophysiol 1983; 6:1123–1142.
66. Cushny AR, Edmunds CW. Paroxysmal irregularity of the heart and auricular fibrillation. In Bulloch W (ed). Studies in Pathology. Aberdeen, Scotland: University of Aberdeen, 1906, pp. 95–110.
67. Mackenzie J. The interpretation of the pulsations in the jugular veins. Am J Med Sci 1907; 134:12–34.
68. Mackenzie J. Diseases of the Heart. 3rd ed. London: Oxford University Press, 1913.
69. Rothberger CJ, Winterberg H. Vorhofflimmern und Arhythmia perpetua. Wien Klin Wochenschr 1909; 22:839–844.
70. Lewis T. Auricular fibrillation: a common clinical condition. BMJ 1909; 2:1528.
71. Lewis T. Auricular fibrillation and its relationship to clinical irregularity of the heart. Heart 1910; 1:306–372.
72. Garrey WE. Auricular fibrillation. Physiol Rev 1924; 4:215–250.
73. Mayer AG. Rhythmical pulsation in Scyphomedusae. Papers of the Tortugas Laboratory, Carnegie Institution 1908; 1:115.
74. Mines GR. On dynamic equilibrium in the heart. J Physiol 1913; 46:349–383.
75. Roth IR. The mechanism of auricular flutter and fibrillation, an historical survey. J Mt Sinai Hosp N Y 1942; 8:965–979.
76. Prinzmetal M, Corday E, Brill IC, Oblath RW, Kruger HE. The Auricular Arrhythmias. Springfield, IL: Charles C Thomas, 1952.
77. MacWilliam JA. Fibrillar contraction of the heart. J Physiol 1887; 8:296–310.
78. Ritchie WT. Complete heart-block, with dissociation of the action of the auricles and ventricles. Proc R Soc Edinburgh 1906; 25:1085–1091.

79. Jolly WA, Ritchie WT. Auricular flutter and fibrillation. Heart 1911; 2:177–221.

80. Ritchie WT. Auricular Flutter. New York: Paul B. Hoeber, 1914.

81. Lewis T. Observations upon a curious and not uncommon form of extreme acceleration of the auricle. "Auricular flutter." Heart 1912; 4:171–220.

82. Lewis T. Paroxysmal tachycardia. Heart 1909; 1:43–72.

83. Cotton RP. Notes and observations upon a case of unusually rapid action of the heart (232 per minute). BMJ 1867; 1:629–630.

84. Bristowe JS. On recurrent palpitation of extreme rapidity in persons otherwise apparently healthy. Brain 1887; 10:164–198.

85. Hoffmann A. Die Paroxysmal Tachycardie. Wiesbaden, Germany: JF Bergmann, 1900.

86. Fye WB. Acute coronary occlusion always results in death, or does it? Circulation 1985; 71:4–10.

87. Fye WB. The delayed diagnosis of acute myocardial infarction: it took half a century. Circulation 1985; 72:262–271.

88. McGovern B, Schoenfeld MH, Ruskin JN, Garan H, Yurchak PM. Ventricular tachycardia: historical perspective. Pacing Clin Electrophysiol 1986; 9:449–462.

89. Lewis T. Single and successive extra-systoles. Lancet 1909; 1:382–385.

90. Lewis T. The experimental production of paroxysmal tachycardia and the effects of ligation of the coronary arteries. Heart 1909; 1:98–137.

91. Hart TS. Paroxysmal tachycardia. Heart 1912; 4:128–136.

92. Robinson GC, Herrmann GR. Paroxysmal tachycardia of ventricular origin, and its relation to coronary occlusion. Heart 1921; 8:59–81.

93. Fye WB. Classic Papers on Coronary Thrombosis and Myocardial Infarction. Birmingham, AL: Classics of Cardiology Library, 1991.

94. Strauss MB. Paroxysmal ventricular tachycardia. Am J Med Sci 1930; 179:337–345.

95. Hoffa M, Ludwig C. Einige neue Versuche uber Herzbewegung. Z Rationelle Med 1850; 9:107–144.

96. Schechter DC. Early observations of ventricular fibrillation. In Schechter DC (ed). Exploring the Origins of Electrical Cardiac Stimulation. Minneapolis, MN: Medtronic, 1983:138–149.

97. Schechter DC. Theories on the pathophysiology of ventricular fibrillation. In Schechter DC (ed). Exploring the Origins of Electrical Cardiac Stimulation. Minneapolis, MN: Medtronic, 1983:150–158.

98. Fye WB. Ventricular fibrillation and defibrillation: historical perspectives. Circulation 1985; 71:858–865.

99. DeSilva RA. John MacWilliam, evolutionary biology and sudden cardiac death. J Am Coll Cardiol 1989; 14:1843–1849.

100. MacWilliam JA. Cardiac failure and sudden death. BMJ 1889; 1:6–8.

101. Hoffmann A. Fibrillation of the ventricles at the end of an attack of paroxysmal tachycardia in man. Heart 1912; 3:213–218.

102. Robinson GC. A study with the electrocardiograph of the mode of death of the human heart. J Exp Med 1912; 16:291–302.

103. Lewis T. Lectures on the Heart. New York: Paul B. Hoeber, 1915.

104. Fye WB. Cardiology in 1885. Circulation 1985; 72:21–26.

105. Zoll PM. Historical development of cardiac pacemakers. Prog Cardiovasc Dis 1972; 14:421–429.

106. Schechter DC (ed). Exploring the Origins of Electrical Cardiac Stimulation. Minneapolis, MN: Medtronic, 1983.

107. Zoll PM. Resuscitation of the heart in ventricular standstill by external electric stimulation. N Engl J Med 1952; 247:768–771.

108. Greiwe JE. Premature ventricular systoles, their clinical significance. JAMA 1916; 67:1072–1076.

109. White PD. Heart Disease. New York: Macmillan, 1931.

110. Aronson JK. An Account of the Foxglove and its Medical Uses, 1785–1985. London: Oxford University Press, 1985.

111. Meijler FL. An "account" of digitalis and atrial fibrillation. J Am Coll Cardiol 1985; 5:60A–68A.

112. Frey W. Ueber Vorhofflimmern beim Menschen und seine Beseitigung durch Chinidin. Berl Klin Wochenschr 1918; 55:450–452.

113. Wenckebach KF. Cinchona derivatives in the treatment of heart disorders. JAMA 1923; 81:472–474.

114. Scott RW. Observations on a case of ventricular tachycardia with retrograde conduction. Heart 1922; 9:297–309.

115. Mautz FR. Reduction of cardiac irritability by the epicardial and systemic administration of drugs as a protection in cardiac surgery. J Thorac Surg 1936; 5:612–628.

116. Szekeres L, Papp JG. The discovery of antiarrhythmics. In Parnham MJ, Bruinvels J (eds). Discoveries in Pharmacology: Hormones and Inflammation. New York: Elsevier Science Publishers, 1984, pp 185–215.

117. Geddes LA, Hamlin R. The first human heart defibrillation. Am J Cardiol 1983; 52:403–405.

118. Zoll PM, Linenthal AJ, Gibson W, Paul MH, Norman LR. Termination of ventricular fibrillation in man by externally applied electric countershock. N Engl J Med 1956; 254:727–732.

119. Safar P. History of cardiopulmonary-cerebral resuscitation. In Kaye W, Bircher NG (eds). Cardiopulmonary Resuscitation. New York: Churchill Livingstone, 1989, pp. 1–53.

120. Fye WB. The origin of the full-time faculty system: implications for clinical research. JAMA 1991; 265:1555–1562.

121. Denes P, Ezri MD. Clinical electrophysiology: a decade of progress. J Am Coll Cardiol 1983; 1:292–305.

122. Fisch C. Electrocardiography of arrhythmias: from deductive analysis to laboratory confirmation: twenty-five years of progress. J Am Coll Cardiol 1983; 1:306–316.

123. Scherlag BJ. The development of the His bundle recording technique. Pacing Clin Electrophysiol 1979; 2:230–233.

124. Corday E. Historical vignette celebrating the 30th anniversary of diagnostic ambulatory electrocardiographic monitoring and data reduction systems. J Am Coll Cardiol 1991; 17:286–292.

125. Sealy WC. The case of the fisherman with the fast pulse and the beginning of arrhythmia surgery. N C Med J 1983; 44:489–490.

126. Kastor JA. Michel Mirowski and the automatic implantable defibrillator. Am J Cardiol 1989; 63:977–982.

127. Kastor JA. Michel Mirowski and the automatic implantable defibrillator. Am J Cardiol 1989; 63:1121–1126.

128. Surawicz B. Pharmacologic treatment of cardiac arrhythmias: 25 years of progress. J Am Coll Cardiol 1983; 1:365–381.

Michel Mirowski and the Implantable Cardioverter-Defibrillator[a]

In one of the operating rooms at the Johns Hopkins Hospital in Baltimore, a large group of people crowded the floor and the overhead viewing booth on February 4, 1980 to watch the first installation of an automatic implantable defibrillator in a human patient.[3] The patient was a 57-year-old woman who had had a myocardial infarction and coronary artery bypass graft operation for angina. She had lost consciousness several times from ventricular tachycardia and fibrillation, and antiarrhythmic drugs had not controlled her symptoms. A fatal outcome from a future episode seemed inevitable. She had flown to Hopkins from California for the procedure with her cardiologist, Dr. Roger Winkle of Stanford University Medical School.

The operation was performed by Dr. Levi Watkins, a young Hopkins cardiothoracic surgeon. Assisting him was Dr. Philip R. Reed, a cardiac electrophysiologist and head of the arrhythmia service at Hopkins, and Dr. Morton Mower, a cardiologist from Sinai Hospital of Baltimore and one of the developers of the defibrillator. Close to the operating table, in unaccustomed surgical scrub suit and mask, was Dr. Michel Mirowski, at 55 years of age the man whose waking hours had been dominated by his efforts to build the electronic device now being applied for the first time to treat a patient.

Michel Mirowski (Fig. 2.1) believed that he began learning how to construct the automatic implantable defibrillator when he was 15 years old. At that time, there were no pacemakers, no external defibrillators, no clear understanding, in fact, of how to resuscitate a patient from cardiac arrest. Mirowski was certainly not considering then how to invent a defibrillator, but he was about to have experiences that would teach him how to accomplish what seemed impossible.

EARLY YEARS

Mieczyslaw (Michel) Mirowski was born Mordechai Friedman, the son of Israel Lieb Friedman and Genia Handelsman Friedman, on October 14, 1924 in Warsaw, Poland. His parents operated a delicatessen and "factory," as Mirowski remembered the establishment, where much of the kosher food they sold was manufactured. "My parents worked long hours," he recalled. "I don't think my father ever took a vacation. My mother and I would leave Warsaw for a week or so in the summer and stay in a *pension* outside the city."

Warsaw was then a city of a million people, one-third of whom, including the Mirowskis, were Jewish. Earlier generations of the family had been quite religious, but his parents' attitude was less orthodox, his father somewhat more traditional than his mother. Michel Mirowski, although deeply aware of his cultural heritage, was never religious.

Mirowski and many Warsaw Jews found the Polish culture attractive and tried to enter the more general Polish life. For this reason, Mirowski did not learn Yiddish as a boy, even though the family spoke Yiddish as well as Polish in the home. His father had been raised speaking only Yiddish, and Mirowski's paternal grandfather could probably speak no Polish at all. Later, to honor the traditions of his family, Mirowski learned to speak and write Yiddish well.

Mirowski's mother's sister had become a lawyer, a significant accomplishment for a woman and a Jew in the 1920s. The members of Mirowski's own generation and that of his father had slightly less difficulty becoming members of the professional class because all were boys. When Mirowski and his wife later had daughters, a "family tradition" was broken.

To Mirowski and his family and to many of Poland's 3 to 4 million Jews—the total population of Poland in

[a]Adapted from Kastor,[1, 2] with permission.

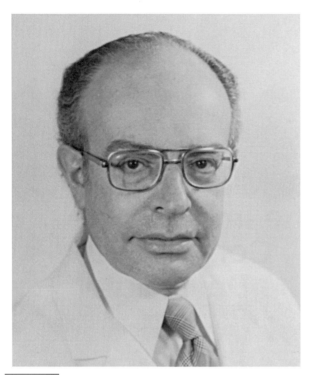

FIGURE 2.1 Michel Mirowski, M.D. (From Kastor JA. Michel Mirowski and the automatic implantable defibrillator. Am J Cardiol 1989; 63:977–982, with permission.)

the early 1930s was about 30,000,000—their country seemed conservative, almost fascist and definitely anti-Semitic. He remembered, "Even the police were sympathetic to right-wing trends. They stood aside when fascistic toughs beat and even killed Jews, and this was before the Nazis arrived."

The traditional restrictions still applied to the education of Jews. A *numerus clausus* limited the number of Jews who could study at the universities. Those Jews who were admitted had to sit in a special part of the classrooms. Rather than do so, they stood through the lectures.

Mirowski's formal education started at the age of 7, when he began attending a Jewish private school because of limited access to the public schools of Warsaw. The classes were taught in Polish. By the age of 11, he was in a private gymnasium, a school that prepared brighter students for the university. "We studied French, Latin and Hebrew. We read Sholom Aleichem in Polish, not in the Yiddish that Aleichem used," Mirowski remembered. "Though his work was obviously fine literature, I could not then relate myself to it, set, as the stories were, in the rural *shtetls*. In view of my career, it was probably significant that I was attracted to Paul de Kruif's *Microbe Hunters*. But the book which always seemed to have the greatest influence on me was *Martin Eden* by Jack London."[4]

In *Martin Eden*, written in 1909 when the author was 33 years old, London tells much about himself, a self-taught working man, deeply distressed by the effects of poverty and the life of the laborer. Eden, who supports himself, as London did, as a sailor and laborer, falls in love with Ruth, the college-educated daughter of an Oakland, California lawyer. She teaches him how to speak properly and what to learn to become a member of her class, to which he always feels an outsider. Martin has a talent for writing, and after years of repeated rejections, his work is finally published. When he becomes famous and acceptable to Ruth's parents, however, he rejects the life they offer, becomes increasingly depressed, goes back to sea, this time as a first-class passenger, slips out of his cabin porthole, and drowns himself.

It was Martin Eden, the outsider who succeeded, that appealed to Mirowski. He also saw himself able, by self-discipline and application of his own abilities, to overcome the most degrading difficulties. Eden's resolution of his conflicts, however, would not have been suitable for Mirowski.

By September 1938, Mirowski was almost 14 years old and was well aware of the great political events occurring in Europe. The Munich settlement was followed 1 year later by the von Ribbentrop–Molotov nonaggression pact that provided the political terms leading to the simultaneous German invasion of Poland from the West and the Russian assault from the East.

Mirowski's family survived the bombing of Warsaw, which opened the Second World War in September, 1939, but by 1945, only he was alive.

> Six of the 30 members of my high school class, all boys of course, survived the War and the Holocaust, which is rather surprising. Some even got out with their families. We stay in contact. Two are in New York City, 2 in Paris, 1 in Geneva, and I am here in Baltimore. How did we make it? More luck than intelligence, probably, but good sense didn't hurt. Each of us has had a rather successful career, so stress and adversity need not necessarily have a negative effect.

In November, 1939, Mirowski's mother, who was 34 years old, died of heart failure, probably from rheumatic heart disease. On December 1, all Jews were ordered to wear yellow stars on their clothes to identify themselves to the occupying Germans.

> When the war started, I had a liberal view of the world which was in conflict with the traditional Jewish reality in Poland. I thought I was, first of all, Polish—obviously a mistaken impression. I was committed, even then, to a life of study and education.
> Then the Nazis came. The schools were closed, and the persecution began. I remember German officers cutting off the *payess* [the long hair traditionally worn by Orthodox Jewish men] to humiliate them. I told my father that I wouldn't wear the yellow star and that it seemed foolish to stay in Warsaw. Worse things were obviously coming—although I can't say that I imagined what was really ahead. I had to continue my education since I knew I had some contribution to make, although I had no idea what it would be. Even then, I felt that I could overcome all difficulties. This was, and is, an irrational idea. In retrospect, it seems completely crazy that at the age of 15, I should leave my family, my town and my country.

At this point, his father gave him a new name in the hope that the change would help to protect him from the deadly anti-Semitism of the time. Mordechai Friedman, now Mieczyslaw Mirowski—later, his wife, Anna, would call him Michel, by which he became known—never saw his father or his younger brother Abraham again.

ESCAPE AND SURVIVAL

On December 5, 1939, Mirowski started east toward Russia. He traveled with a friend, heading toward Lvov, about 200 miles from Warsaw. Another friend of his had relatives there. They walked, rode in trucks and trains, and slept in railroad stations. They spent many days in trenches, traveling at night to avoid capture. In Lvov, Mirowski lived in a house set up for war victims. Lvov had been incorporated into the Soviet Union soon after the beginning of World War II. Although Ukrainian was still the official language and much Polish was spoken there, Mirowski began learning Russian.

Lvov had been part of Poland since 1340, and, by the end of the 14th century, had become the most important and populous Polish city. Later, it was ruled by Swedes, Austrians, Russians, and briefly after World War I by Ukrainian nationalists. Lvov was one of the first large cities to fall to the Germans after their attack to the east in June, 1941. The Russians recovered it in July, 1944, and transferred most of the resident Poles to western Poland. The Jews, who built their first synagogue in Lvov in 1582, had been annihilated. Early in the 20th century, the Jews had constituted almost one-third of the city's population.

While Mirowski was in Lvov, the Soviet government ruled that refugees from German-conquered territories had to live in cities and villages with populations of less than 100,000 that were at least 100 kilometers from the front. Refugees were expected to carry passports, but most did not want them because they feared that accepting passports would acknowledge possession of Russian citizenship. Those who were caught without passports were exiled to Siberia, many to labor camps. Mirowski recalled:

> In July 1940, I was arrested by an officer whom I presumed at the time to be a general from the NKVD, the secret police He seemed, to my eyes, so powerful that he *must* have been a general. I told him that I wasn't yet 16 years old and—such *chutzpah*—was too young to be issued a passport. It is true that I was 3 months short of my 16th birthday, but I had no idea whether such a rule existed. Anyway, he bought the story plus my claim that there were a few more of us kids, each less than 16. So none of us was sent away. I later realized that my chances of survival would have been greater in Siberia than if I were captured by Germany, Russia's great ally at the time.

That alliance lasted less than 2 years. On June 22, 1941, Germany attacked Russia, the day before the anniversary of Napoleon's invasion in 1812. Mirowski tried to enlist in the Russian army but was rejected for being too young, the same reason that the "general" had been led to believe he had no passport. Now he had to flee the advancing German army and continue

an odyssey that would cover more than 9,000 miles in 4½ years.

The next stop was Kiev, the great city of the Ukraine on the Dnieper River, where Mirowski remembered sleeping in a park. When he and his friends saw officials burning papers, they knew the German army was approaching—the Germans entered Kiev in September, 1941—and they continued east. "We tried to take trains. Of course, one never had a ticket and rode both inside and on the roofs of the cars. My daughter once asked me what we ate. I can't really remember. We just ate."

Mirowski settled briefly in Rostov on the Don River just northeast of the Sea of Azov. There he worked on a building crew in the countryside. The next stop was Krasnodar, 150 miles to the south, a quiet town, as he remembered it, with schools for electricians, plumbers, and tool makers. Krasnodar, under its former name of Ekaterinodar, had been the seat of the White Russian government during the Civil War. The Germans eventually captured it after much devastation. Mirowski remembered:

> In Krasnodar, I engaged in my first commercial venture, and in communist Russia at that, but this was war time. My friends and I manufactured cigarettes and made some additional money cleaning up at the schools after classes were done. But I heard on the radio that the Germans had taken Rostov and were heading toward Baku. It was time to move east again. One of my friends named Ernst stayed behind with his newly acquired Russian girlfriend who told him they would be safe there. I never saw him again.

East was to Baku—ahead of the Germans—a city important for its oil wells and refineries on the western shore of the Caspian Sea. It was in Baku that Mirowski remembered hearing the Polish national anthem played on the radio in honor of General Sikorski, who was raising a Polish army in exile.

Then by ship and train, Mirowski traveled through Tashkent to Andijan, an agricultural town in which factories had recently been built presumably beyond the Germans' reach. Mirowski was now more than 2,500 miles from Warsaw in a city that lies less than 200 miles from India and Afghanistan to the south and China to the east. In Andijan, Mirowski worked up to 11 hours per day in an airplane factory and thereby made, as he put it, "my first contribution to beating the Nazis, and I did it with pleasure. Even though I was gainfully employed and somewhat more comfortable physically, each day was a test in survival. A pickpocket once cut my pocket and took my papers, but not my wallet so I still have some pictures. An honest pickpocket!"

Malnutrition was commonplace throughout Russia at this time. Everything was rationed. Mirowski, along with many others, contracted tropical infections for which little treatment was available. Nevertheless, he went to the public library every day to read books and newspapers. By now, Polish nationals were fighting the Germans in Iran, Palestine, and Italy. Mirowski read that Stalin had created the first Polish Communist Army and that it was training at a camp near Moscow.

"I was freed from the factory and sent to Moscow to join the army. When I got there and was asked for my nationality, I said 'Jewish'—I should have said Polish—and I was sent back to Andijan."

Mirowski then took a different job working for a traveling group of singers, story tellers, and an orchestra. At first, the work was prosaic; he put up signs and posters. Within 2 weeks, however, he was made an administrator, and life became somewhat more pleasant. He now had time to study and became, in the terms of that time, relatively rich. He could travel and had more coupons for food. One bread coupon was worth 2 weeks' salary.

In 1944, Mirowski volunteered successfully for the army—this time as a Pole—and became a junior officer in the support forces. He had a heart murmur and therefore was not assigned to a fighting branch.

MEDICAL SCHOOL

By the fall of 1945, Mirowski was back in Poland and registered as a medical student at the University of Gdansk. The war was over, but signs of it were everywhere.

> There was no shortage of cadavers—or soap. I saw the camp near Gdansk where the Germans had converted human corpses into soap, and there was a lot of it still available. Warsaw had been completely destroyed, including its ghetto. None of my family was left; I couldn't even find our old home. Two of my friends had survived, hidden by Poles. Their purpose, however, wasn't heroic; they were handsomely paid for it. Their motivation was pure greed.
>
> I stayed in medical school there for a year but gradually came to believe I had to leave Poland. Many Poles still felt that Hitler hadn't finished the job. I had been a local fighter; now I became a Zionist. After all that had happened and that I had seen, the Jews had to have a country of their own to survive. As far as Poland was concerned, it had become a cemetery for me. I told myself that I would never return.

With a friend who now lives in Paris, Mirowski set off again, this time for Palestine. It was illegal then to emigrate there, but, he said somewhat defiantly: "That didn't deter me. For 6 years I had stretched the law. This was necessary simply to survive the war and seemed justified because so many laws were directed specifically against Jews."

Friends had arranged the transport of Jews through Austria, and Mirowski was preparing to leave for Salzburg when his asthma recurred. This had happened previously, the first time when he left his family in 1939 and fled to Russia, and later on two or three other occasions when he was about to cross national borders. He was sufficiently ill to miss the group's departure, but later, acting on his own, he entered Germany on the way to France. In Paris, Mirowski lived with a few surviving former classmates and their relatives. Although it was particularly difficult to travel from France to Palestine, he managed to obtain a visa.

In the spring of 1947, he arrived in Tel Aviv, where his paternal grandfather had settled many years previously. Mirowski stayed at the home of his cousins, who found him a job as a shoe salesman. He asserted: "I wanted to continue my education. I was committed to becoming a doctor, if for no other reason than to honor my father's last words to me, 'Be a physician, be a Jew.'"

No medical schools were operating in Israel in the early postwar years, so Mirowski decided to return to France and seek admission there. "Even on the boat going back to France, I didn't know where I would study. It couldn't be Paris; my friends were there. They weren't studying, and I needed to be where I would not be distracted." On the ship, Mirowski met a couple from Lyon. He liked what he heard about the city, traveled there and entered the medical school in the fall of 1947. His French was poor, and his English was almost nonexistent. He listened to the lectures and demonstrations in French and studied medical texts in English as he taught himself both languages.

The French medical schools were greatly overcrowded. Five hundred students started in his class. The amphitheater did not have enough seats, no one knew the professors, and the faculty knew none of the students. Medical school in France took 7 years and included some subjects taught in premedical courses at colleges in the United States. Contact with patients was limited, and most students graduated without the clinical clerkships and subinternships typical in the United States and Great Britain. Most graduates then proceeded to their permanent jobs. Only the best 10% of the graduates were appointed to the equivalent of house staff positions to prepare themselves for academic or specialty careers. Mirowski remembered:

> As a student, I had the unusual opportunity of getting to know one of the members of the faculty, not well of course. He was Professor Roger Froment, a leading cardiologist. In the French system you could start specializing even as a student. Of course, this might get you nowhere, and you'd wind up a general practitioner in the provinces. Anyway, I became a cardiologist, before I became an internist.

Froment's field greatly appealed to Mirowski, who was enchanted by cardiology, which seemed suitable to his way of thinking. The specialty had become extraordinarily exciting. Cardiac catheterization was being applied to the study of congenital and valvular heart disease. Every case seemed to reveal some new knowledge. Surgery of the heart was now possible. Repair of patent ductus arteriosus and coarctation of the aorta had been performed just before the war. Taussig and Blalock had developed extracardiac shunts for tetralogy of Fallot, and in 1947, successful operative relief of mitral stenosis was announced. Extracorporeal circulation was applied for the first time in the repair of an atrial septal defect in 1953, the year Mirowski graduated. He also found cardiology, at least in France, satisfying for very practical reasons. "I could learn cardiology independently. In surgery, for example, you had to be part of the system, or you could never operate. All my life I have never been part of the system."

Every medical student was required to write a thesis, which could range from very simple to exceedingly involved. Mirowski reviewed the patients from Froment's clinic who had undergone mitral commissurotomy. Eventually, his thesis reached 157 pages.[5]

On graduating, Mirowski had to decide where to take further training and where to practice. "I knew I wouldn't be staying in France. I would always be a second-class citizen there. Only in Israel or the United States could someone like me be a first-class citizen."

POSTGRADUATE TRAINING

So in January, 1954, Mirowski returned to Israel, to a country overpopulated with physicians, many of whom were refugees who had been professors and well-known consultants in Europe before the Nazis. Nevertheless, Mirowski found a job in the heart station at Tel Hashomer Hospital. He became first assistant to Dr. Harry Heller, the chief of medicine, whom Mirowski saw as "very firm, a typical German professor, but every day that we made rounds together was a holiday for me. Heller was smart but very Nietzschean and not personally helpful. I think he didn't care much about people. He'd fire someone by putting a letter on his desk. I saw him as a stereotype of the German culture of his time."

Nevertheless, Mirowski described Heller as "the best internist I ever met."

We used English titles left over from the British occupation—I was known as a registrar, for example. Although our books were in English, everyday conversation was usually in Hebrew. Actually one could find a person who spoke almost every European language. Yiddish, of course, competed with Hebrew especially among the patients. Hebrew and service in the army unified the country. Israel was more of a melting pot in the 50s than America had ever been.

Mirowski liked what he was doing, and he particularly liked being right about what he was doing. He still enjoys telling the story of a 30-year-old patient who was admitted with hemoptysis and had a systolic murmur and a large heart with right ventricular and left atrial hypertrophy evident on the electrocardiogram. A fellow registrar, later a well-known cardiologist in Israel, diagnosed Eisenmenger's syndrome; Mirowski suggested silent mitral stenosis. The catheterization showed pulmonary hypertension with a normal wedge pressure, apparently confirming the colleague's diagnosis, thus ruling out an operation and defining a limited prognosis. The competitor in Mirowski remembered, "It didn't fit. Why should the left atrium be large if he had Eisenmenger's?" Unfortunately for the patient, Mirowski was proved right, at the autopsy. "There must have been something technically wrong with the catheterization. A mitral commissurotomy might have saved his life."

In 1958, a physician from the Cardiological Institute in Mexico City visited Mirowski's hospital. As soon as he heard the visitor lecture, Mirowski knew he had to go to Mexico. The creator of the Institute was Dr. Ignatio Chavez, but the most famous member of the group was Dr. Demetrio Sodi-Pollares, who was known particularly for his research in electrocardiography.

Travel had become more complex because Mirowski had a family. In 1950, as a medical student, he had married the sister of the woman from Lyon whom he had met on the boat from Israel to France 3 years earlier. Their first daughter was born in 1959.

About his Mexican experience, Mirowski said:

The person I really wanted to work with was Sodi's associate, Enrique Cabrera, the only genius I've ever known. He played the piano like a virtuoso, knew archeology better than many professionals and made basic contributions to electrocardiography and vectorcardiography. Remember the business of systolic and diastolic overloading? We don't use the concepts much today, but at the time they made a lot of sense. Cabrera, whose father had been Foreign Minister of Mexico, was already a communist. I heard some of his lectures on Marxism-Leninism and had wild debates with him about the 1956 Sinai war. His politics didn't fit with Sodi's conservative Catholicism. In 1962, Cabrera went to Cuba; I think he may have lost his job. Soon afterwards he developed a brain tumour, went to Russia for an operation and died. He was still quite young.

Even though Mirowski had not learned Spanish previously, he picked up enough to write his first article 2 months after arriving in Mexico City.[6] The time he spent there was exceedingly satisfying, but by 1½ years, he sought different experiences.

I wanted to know how leading people did their work. To my surprise, I was offered a fellowship with Dr. Helen Taussig at Hopkins, and so we came to Baltimore for the first time. Dr. Taussig gave me 10 days to learn to speak English and then put me to work in her clinic. From 8 to 6 I worked for her; after 6, I did my research. My name was on 14 papers from the 2½ years with her. I felt then, and have always felt, an internal need to investigate and create. One should enter academics because of the drive to make contributions, not for advancement—although it's nice when it comes. Dr. Taussig was a great lady and made tremendous contributions, like the blue baby operation, but I think that Dr. Sodi challenged me more intellectually.

That period in Baltimore was difficult for the family. They were new to the United States, they did not have much money, and Mirowski worked very long hours. By then, he and his wife had 3 young children. So in 1963, Mirowski returned to Israel. He felt a duty to live there, that leaving Israel would constitute a desertion. At the time, he did not even consider remaining in the United States.

CARDIOLOGIST IN ISRAEL

For the next 5 years, Mirowski was the sole and, therefore, the chief cardiologist at Asaf Harofeh Hospital, 15 miles from Tel Aviv. Asaf Harofeh is a community hospital and provided Mirowski with his own carpeted, air-conditioned office, considerably more generous accommodations than his academic colleagues enjoyed at Israeli teaching hospitals. He did not have a secretary or a typewriter, and, moreover, he was not the hospital director's most popular doctor.

I was always asking him for things. He said that if they gave me a typewriter, every other chief would want one—a perfect bureaucratic response. Well if you can't get into the room through the door, you get in through the window. I convinced the librarian to lend me his typewriter and with 2 of my fingers turned out 18 papers. Once I asked for a leave to finish some research and was told to use vacation time. I am afraid my colleagues didn't have much use for me either, but that didn't matter. One can produce and create anywhere even in the intellectual desert to which I had returned.

In 1966, my old boss, Professor Harry Heller, started having bouts of ventricular tachycardia. He was repeatedly hospitalized and treated with quinidine and procainamide. My wife asked me why I was so concerned. 'Because he will die from it,' I told her. And he did, 2 weeks later while at dinner with his family.

From Heller, Mirowski had learned the virtues of logical thinking, and the first step was to read what was known about sudden death. He was unaware then of the magnitude of the problem and the ineffectiveness of contemporary therapy. Coronary care units were then being built in many hospitals. Conversion of ventricular tachycardia and ventricular fibrillation by countershock and prevention of cardiac arrest by suppression of ventricular ectopy were generally accepted forms of therapy. However, preventing sudden death after the patients left the hospital seemed hopeless. Cardiologists in the United States had been alerted to the importance of ventricular fibrillation in the post–coronary care period by investigators such as Dr. Bernard Lown, who had developed synchronized cardioversion and had popularized the prevention of ventricular tachycardia and fibrillation in the coronary care unit with the use of lidocaine. The oral antiarrhythmic drugs then available were relatively ineffective, however, and no medical, surgical, or electrical method of treatment had been shown to prevent cardiac arrest outside the hospital. A few patients could be saved by doctors and nurses in mobile coronary care units that operated in a few cities, but unless these workers reached the patient soon, treatment failed. Mirowski wondered:

How could we have prevented Heller's death at that time: keep him forever in the CCU, or follow him around with a defibrillator? Both solutions were obviously impossible. Implantable pacemakers were then becoming available. So, I reasoned, let's create a similar kind of implantable device to monitor for ventricular fibrillation and automatically shock the patient back to sinus rhythm. Should be simple enough.

I talked to some cardiologists who knew more about such devices. They all told me that debrillators couldn't be miniaturized. In those days, a defibrillator weighed 30 to 40 pounds; it was preposterous to reduce it to the size of a cigarette box. But I had been challenged by the problem, initially because of the death of a man I admired very much, but also because people told me it couldn't be done. Thank goodness I wasn't an engineer because then I would certainly have realized that the idea was crazy.

Mirowski found himself in an unlikely place to accomplish the impossible. Israeli medicine was run by the government and the trade union Histadrut, the 2 organizations that owned the hospitals and employed the doctors. Asaf Harofeh was a government-run community hospital. Research was conducted in the university teaching hospitals and seldom in community hospitals. "As I saw it, there were three prerequisites to developing the device: the concept, technology, and funding. I had the concept—strenuously questioned by leading cardiologists and engineers—but neither of the other two. I was outside the university system and had no access to engineering or financial support."

Mirowski concluded that only in the United States could he assemble what was needed to make the defibrillator, the building of which had clearly become an obsession and was to remain the principal goal for the rest of his professional life. He recalled:

In retrospect, moving back to America was one of the most reckless acts of my life. My compulsion now involved my family which had lived in Israel for the last 5 years, and we had become quite comfortable. I had job tenure, my own office and, what is available to relatively few Israeli doctors, a flourishing private practice. It isn't easy for physicians to do well financially in Israel, but we were OK. We had a house in Savyon, the Beverly Hills of Israel, 2 cars and a full-time maid. I was 44 years old. There are some people who are beginning to think of retirement then.

Mirowski was better known in the United States than in Israel. He usually published in American medical journals and presented papers at American cardiology meetings. He wrote to some friends in the United States and received several inquiries about staff positions. In the spring of 1968, he flew to San Francisco to attend the annual meeting of the American College of Cardiology and to participate by invitation in a seminar on arrhythmias, about which he had written several articles.

There Mirowski spoke with Dr. Bernard Tabatznik, the chief of cardiology at Sinai Hospital of Baltimore. Mirowski knew about Sinai. Two of his children had been born there when he was working at Hopkins. Sinai was a successful community hospital, actively supported by the philanthropic Jewish community of Baltimore. It had a close academic affiliation with the Johns Hopkins Medical School and had been located across the street from the Johns Hopkins Hospital for many years. Recently, Sinai had moved into new buildings, close to the suburban residential areas where most Baltimore Jews then lived.

The offer letter from Sinai, which traveled slowly by surface mail, arrived in Israel after the Mirowskis had reached Baltimore. He would become director of the Coronary Care Unit (Fig. 2.2), and, most significantly for him, half of his time would be dedicated to research. Sinai had a dog laboratory and a clinical engineering department in addition to a sympathetic director of medicine in Dr. Albert Mendeloff, who assured Mirowski of the time and support needed for his work. Mirowski, who greatly admired Mendeloff, said:

Al and I never had a contract. I still don't have one with the hospital. Our deal was simple; if things didn't work out, I'd leave.

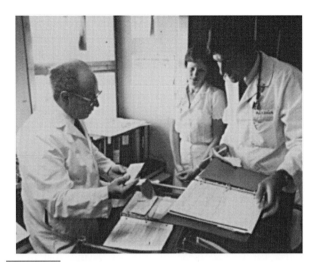

FIGURE 2.2 Dr. Michel Mirowski conducting rounds in the Coronary Care Unit at Sinai Hospital of Baltimore. (From Kastor JA. Michel Mirowski and the automatic implantable defibrillator. Am J Cardiol 1989; 63:977–982, with permission.)

We sold what we owned and after the taxes cleared $6,000 to start our new life. Don't let me overdramatize the move. My wife and eldest daughter had fond memories of the United States and were not unhappy to return. Of course in my unreasonably optimistic way, I knew that this was the right move. America was the only place to do what I wanted to do. Although I might meet hostility there also, and some people were bound to say that my idea was nonsense, you still had a chance to succeed. I couldn't have done it in Israel, France, Britain or Russia.

BACK IN BALTIMORE

On September 3, 1968, Michel Mirowski, his wife Anna, and their 3 children, Ginat, 9, Ariella, 7, and Doris, 6, returned to Baltimore. They rented a house in a northwest suburb of the city, and the children entered the local schools. Mirowski was 44 years old as he and his family began their second life in the United States. At last he had found security and professional opportunity after years of flight and turmoil.

By the time he moved to Baltimore, Mirowski had written or was the coauthor of 29 articles published in leading American, European, Israeli, and Mexican medical journals. Most of those in which he was the principal investigator reported clinical studies on electrocardiography and cardiac arrhythmias. Research was really what Mirowski admired. "The creators, of whatever stripe, are my heroes. Recognition by peers, compensation, praise are secondary."

From his earliest days, Mirowski wanted to be a scientist, not the practitioner his father had in mind for him. "There is nothing wrong with practice, or for that matter with being a musician or whatever, but they're not for me." In research, one has no guarantee that the project will succeed, so the investigator must keep up his or her spirits. Mirowski strongly believed this and recalled a favorite barnyard fable on this point he enjoyed telling his daughters. Two children are

together in a room. One is an optimist, the other a pessimist. One of them sniffs the air and says, "I smell horse manure." The optimistic child says, "I think there's a horse outside." Mirowski concluded: "I would always dream about the horse rather than smell the manure."

On first appearance, Sinai Hospital of Baltimore would not seem to be the ideal place for Mirowski to accomplish the impossible. It was, and is, a community hospital, not a primary teaching hospital, although Sinai has been affiliated with the Johns Hopkins Medical School for decades. "I was always slightly outside the mainstream of academic medicine," Mirowski recognizes. "There are those who are accepted, whose futures are planned, whose promise is appreciated. But that's not me. Nobody nursed me along."

Mirowski recalled Dr. Harry Heller, his favorite professor in Israel. It was Heller who, unknowingly, inspired Mirowski to his life's work. Heller had developed ventricular tachycardia and, as Mirowski predicted, had died suddenly soon afterward. It had been 2 years since Heller's death, and the automatic implantable defibrillator seemed as far from reality in 1968 as when Mirowski swore he would develop a device that could treat the arrhythmia that killed his former chief.

Although comfortably established at a fine hospital and enjoying the strong support of his chief, one vital part of his dream was still missing. For all Michel Mirowski's creativity and persistence, he was not a particularly avid experimenter. At this point, Mirowski spoke with Dr. Morton M. Mower, whom Mirowski had met before arriving at Sinai. Mower, a junior member of the hospital staff, ran the hospital's heart station and was starting a private cardiology practice. Morty Mower, a self-described tinkerer, had led a very different life from the man who was to become his collaborator. He had traveled outside the United States only once while an army medical officer in Germany and had lived in the vicinity of Baltimore for the rest of his 36 years. He had graduated only 7 years previously from the University of Maryland Medical School and then had trained in medicine and cardiology at the University of Maryland and Sinai Hospitals.

"'Could I build an automatic implantable defibrillator?' Michel asked me in July 1969," Mower remembered. "Mirowski wasn't the only one to have suggested such a device. I had actually thought about it myself—the idea had crossed my mind—but I had considered the whole thing impractical. Now here it was thrown back at me. I'd better not reject it out-of-hand twice." Mower asked for a day or so to think about the project. However, he had already decided to work with Mirowski and was elated by the extraordinary coincidence that two people with an identical enthusiasm should find themselves in the same institution.

DESIGNING THE DEFIBRILLATOR

It was almost a year after Mirowski moved to the United States before he discussed his concept of the automatic implantable defibrillator with Mower. During this time, Mirowski recalled:

> I had concluded that one could not miniaturize the conventional bulky defibrillator because of constraints in capacitor technology and the need to deliver some 400 joules to terminate ventricular fibrillation. Therefore, I formulated a working hypothesis that most of the energy used for external defibrillation is wastefully dissipated in the tissues surrounding the heart. One should be able to significantly reduce the energy needed for defibrillation by delivering the shock from within or close to the heart, and, consequently, reduce the size of the capacitor sufficiently to build a device suitable for implantation in man. I believe that this initially purely theoretical concept of internal defibrillation in closed chest subjects was the crucial breakthrough which allowed the development of the implantable defibrillator.

As they began their work together, Mirowski and Mower seemed to have a fundamental disagreement. Mirowski was convinced that cardioversion could be accomplished with intravascular electrode catheters that could be inserted without thoracotomy or general anesthesia. Mower was equally convinced that catheters would not work. "When Morty agreed to work with me on this project," Mirowski recalled, "his reaction to the concept of catheter defibrillation was very negative. It required more than gentle persuasion to convince him to go to the lab and test my hypothesis."

For their first experiment, Mower and William Staewen, the director of the Sinai bioengineering laboratory, inserted a plate from a broken defibrillator paddle subcutaneously into the chest wall of a dog. A catheter was used for the other electrode, but its resistance of about 50 ohms seemed prohibitively high. To decrease this electrical property, they soldered together the connections from several catheters and threaded this multicatheter rig into the dog's superior vena cava. They then fibrillated the dog's heart and successfully converted it with the first shock of 20 joules. This was early in August 1969 and less than 1 month since Mirowski and Mower had begun working together. It was an auspicious beginning, but their first patient would not be treated for 11 years.

After a moment of elation, the pair looked more dispassionately at the problems they faced. Mower recalled: "The components of a workable defibrillator are huge 'space-occupying lesions.'" Chief among the larger parts of standard defibrillators at the time were capacitors to store the charge and inductors to change certain characteristics of the current. "We wanted to get rid of the inductor if possible. This would require use of a pulse with a narrower duration and probably more power than was usually employed for standard cardioversion."

Electrical relays, standard equipment in contemporary cardioverters, could not be used because arcs of current produced during switching could interfere with the sensing circuits located adjacent to the power circuits in implanted units. Solid-state technology would be needed at a relatively early stage in its application to medical instrumentation. "We had to make the two circuits work as one, and this required some

pretty fancy electronics," Mower said. "I thought, mistakenly as it happens, that we would have trouble using the electrocardiogram to sense from. So in our early models we used pressure-filled catheters connected to extracardiac pressure transducers, just like in the cath lab, and triggered the shock from the absence of right ventricular pressure." The first breadboard they built for the circuits "worked like clock-work, just as it was supposed to" (Fig. 2.3).

Mirowski and Mower now thought they had something specific to report, and they published their first experiences in a general medical journal in 1970.[7] They were not entirely prepared for the difficulty they then encountered securing acceptance for their early work in the cardiology literature, however. The reviewers were critical of their manuscripts. "I had always looked on reviewers as helpful by giving instructive criticism to improve the manuscript," Mower said, but in the early 1970s, that is not how they appeared to Mirowski and Mower.

The team was particularly distressed by an editorial published in 1972 by Dr. Bernard Lown, director of the Coronary Care Unit at the Peter Bent Brigham Hospital in Boston and a faculty member at the Harvard School of Public Health.[8] Dr. Lown was, as Dr. Mirowski recalled, "the guru of sudden death at the time," and his pronouncements were extremely influential. After describing the difficult technical problems well known to Mirowski and Mower, Dr. Lown wrote:[8]

> The very rare patient who has frequent bouts of VF is best treated in a coronary care unit and is better served by an effective antiarrhythmic program or surgical correction of inadequate coronary flow or ventricular malfunction. In fact, the implanted defibrillator system represents an imperfect solution in search of a plausible and practical application.

Dr. Lown was not alone with his reservations. "Everybody thought it unfeasible," said Mirowski. "Someone actually called it a 'bomb inside the body.' I remember

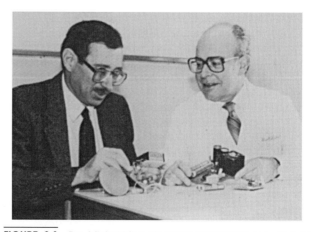

FIGURE 2.3 Drs. Michel Mirowski (*right*) and Morton Mower reminisce about the events of 1969 with the first working breadboard model of an automatic implantable defibrillator developed for use in dogs. This photograph was taken in 1985. (From Kastor JA. Michel Mirowski and the automatic implantable defibrillator. Am J Cardiol 1989; 63:1121–1126, with permission.)

a successful inventor in the pacemaker field who asked me, 'Do you know why a defibrillator is so large? It's because you must store energy in capacitors, and to store 400 joules, you'll need capacitors at least 4 inches in each dimension.'" Mirowski and Mower never resolved their colleague's objections. Because their device defibrillated inside the chest rather than externally through the chest wall, much less power was needed, and smaller capacitors could be used.

In retrospect, Mirowski and Mower see the rejection of their work during the early 1970s as useful. Many of the objections were helpful and drove the investigators to find solutions they would not perhaps otherwise have emphasized, but the general skepticism kept others out of the field. "There was virtually no competition," Mirowski recalled, but consequently, there were no others working in the area with whom Mirowski and Mower could discuss their problems.

FINANCING THE WORK

Furthermore, the unconventional nature of the device and the reservations of consultants kept Mirowski and Mower from obtaining money from the usual federal and foundation sources. Because funding was unavailable, Mirowski and Mower had to support their work from their own limited resources. Frequently, unconventional solutions were needed, such as obtaining experimental animals directly from the pound at $1.00 per dog. Mower observed that, as could be anticipated by those who know Mirowski, "Michel shows his badge of 'No Grants Asked for or Received' with some pride. At times of adversity, Michel's logical mind gives way. Many of his vital decisions have been illogical, even reckless. The word 'No' is not in his vocabulary." Mower remembered Mirowski's frequently saying: "It's not that it can't be done; you haven't found a way to do it. It's a question of mind, not facts."

Constructing further models of their defibrillator required Mirowski and Mower to seek additional collaboration. In the spring of 1970, about 1½ years after Mirowski had moved back to the United States, a senior officer from a leading pacemaker firm visited the laboratory for a demonstration. After a dog with an early model of the defibrillator had been resuscitated, the visitor asked what would happen if the device had not worked. "So we disconnected the defibrillator and refibrillated the animal," Mower recalled. "The dog died, of course. The executive was impressed."

Mirowski and Mower made an agreement to develop their device with the firm, which then proceeded to repeat the Baltimore experiments at the company's laboratories. "They wanted to use their own electrode catheters," says Mower. "They also didn't much like our pressure catheters which could be clogged by fibrous material."

"Actually," said Mirowski, "we, ourselves, did not like and did not intend to work with pressure catheters beyond the initial period."

Meanwhile, Mirowski and his group studied different defibrillating waveforms for safety and efficacy, but "the upshot was that none of the discharge patterns was particularly damaging," Mower recalled.

As the pacemaker company continued with its experiments, Mirowski and Mower came to believe that, as Mower put it, "They weren't moving fast enough." The company had conducted a marketing survey that convinced them that "few doctors had an interest in an implanted defibrillator or even in sudden death. Michel and I felt that a realization of the need by M.D.s had to be created. The company decided we weren't worth the effort, and we parted. Michel got his patent rights back."

The pair considered forming their own company, but in the meantime a mutual friend introduced Mirowski to Dr. Stephen Heilman at a conference in Singapore in 1972. Heilman, a physician turned engineer, had formed a small company called Medrad in Pittsburgh. Mower described it as "a garage-type enterprise, but even then the world's largest supplier of angiographic injectors." The firm had several innovative engineers who could help solve the technical problems that plagued the project at this time.

TECHNICAL PROBLEMS

By then, Mower had accepted the value of sensing arrhythmias electrically rather than hemodynamically. "Why had it taken so long to go the ECG route?" Mower speculated: "Probably because we knew too much about electrocardiography." Mirowski had specialized in the subject, and Mower directed his hospital's heart station. "We kept seeing the artifacts and horrendous problems of noise in the ECG" that are familiar to all clinical cardiologists.

Heilman's group translated some of Mirowski's concepts about identifying ventricular fibrillation into a mathematical formula called the probability density function (PDF), a reflection of the amount of time that an electrical signal avoids the baseline. "With PDF," Mower explained, "the ECG signal spends quite a bit of time near or on the baseline in sinus rhythm. During ventricular fibrillation, however, the signal is always away from the baseline." Circuits that sense such characteristics can reliably distinguish normal rhythm from fibrillation while ignoring nonphysiological artifacts. "In 2 years—the same time we had spent with the large pacemaker firm—this tiny angiographic injector company came up with a working implantable unit. They had to learn a whole new technology. Wonderful! They really busted leather," Mower recalled with enthusiasm.

Mirowski and Mower then had to decide whether to develop an all electrode catheter–based system, which Mirowski favored because it could be inserted without a thoracotomy, or to concentrate their efforts on the use of electrode patches to be sewn directly to the heart. Heilman advised that the pericardial patches be used because of seemingly insurmountable technical problems that prevented the equipment's consistently and reliably delivering a therapeutic defibrillation shock through intravascular electrodes alone. Transvenous catheters, however, would be used as one of the electrodes and to detect physiological signals for the sensing circuits.

ANIMAL STUDIES: THE FILM

By 1975, the team had built a model that was small enough to be completely implanted in dogs. They had also by then been able to publish a few descriptions of their work as investigators and clinicians became more aware of the importance of sudden cardiac death.[9–11] Mirowski and Mower remembered how the demonstration of an earlier unimplanted unit had impressed the pacemaker company executive. So they made a movie, a silent movie, which showed a dog equipped with both the defibrillator and a coil attached to the heart through which a fibrillating current could be transmitted from the surface of the skin. The humans seen in this production are Mower, hobbling across the screen with a cane because of knee injuries from skiing, William Staewen, the bioengineer, and Mirowski.

The dog, a healthy-appearing mongrel, stood still as the inducer was placed on the coil. The animal's heart fibrillated, cardiac output disappeared, and, in a few seconds, the dog lost consciousness. The defibrillator sensed the loss of normal cardiac electrical activity and charged the capacitors. The dog was next seen to shudder slightly as the device discharged and, in a few more seconds, was standing again (Fig. 2.4).

When they first showed the film, "A wag in one of our audiences asked if the dog had been trained to do what we filmed—in some Pavlovian way," Mower recalled. So they added the dog's electrocardiogram

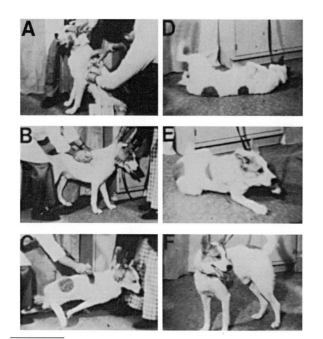

FIGURE 2.4 Demonstration of a dog (**A**) being fibrillated (**B**), losing consciousness in ventricular fibrillation (**C**), shocked by the automatic implantable defibrillator (**D**), and recovering (**E** and **F**). A continuously running electrocardiogram was superimposed on the film produced from these pictures. (From Kastor JA. Michel Mirowski and the automatic implantable defibrillator. Am J Cardiol 1989; 63:1121–1126, with permission.)

along the bottom of the film synchronized to the action. The arrhythmia and the conversion could be clearly correlated with the dog's collapse and recovery. This touch of Hollywood proved to be extraordinarily persuasive. Mirowski and Mower showed it on the increasing number of occasions when they were invited to speak about their work.

READY FOR HUMANS

Soon thereafter, the group converted the canine unit into a device suitable for human implantation. Its hermetic seal was improved, and toxicity tests were conducted. Defibrillators were installed on a long-term basis in 25 dogs, who survived an average of 3 years.[12] About every 3 months, the dogs were fibrillated, and the device was discharged. "In this period," Mower remembered, "we lost some dogs because of electrode troubles which prevented defibrillation. This led us to make design changes, but nothing conceptual."

To satisfy the United States Food and Drug Administration (FDA) that the defibrillator was safe and practical, another company, with which the developers had no relationship, conducted protracted trials. The unit's function exceeded the specifications required for pacemakers in avoiding interference from vibration and electromagnetic energy.

Mirowski and Mower were then ready to implant their first unit in a human patient. For this step, they went to the Johns Hopkins Hospital because Sinai Hospital had no cardiac surgical program. At Hopkins, Dr. Myron Weisfeldt, the chief of cardiology, and Dr. Philip Reed, the clinical electrophysiologist, helped to guide the device through the Hopkins institutional review board. After approval was obtained, the first patient was treated successfully in February, 1980.[3, 13]

During the next 5 years, the automatic implantable defibrillator (AID) was installed in 800 patients in several university hospitals. "For our first 50 patients," Mower said, "the mortality from arrhythmias was less than 10%. It would have been 40% to 50% in the patients we treated if they hadn't received the device. The FDA was very cooperative during the premarket clinical trial. We wanted to be more Catholic than the Pope and would do even more than the FDA wanted." The FDA encouraged Mirowski and Mower to seek full approval before the developers actually wanted to do so. "We would have preferred more premarket testing," recalled Mower. They were worried about the clinical results at hospitals where they could no longer exercise close control, and "It would be easier to keep track of 2,000 rather than 50,000 devices."

With release of the AID from clinical trials, demand for the units increased rapidly and quickly surpassed the manufacturing capacity of Medrad, the "garage-type enterprise" that had developed and produced the earlier units. In 1985, Medrad assigned all its rights and knowledge about the defibrillator to CPI, an established pacemaker company and a division of Eli Lilly since the 1970s.

With the AID becoming an accepted method of treatment, the roles of Mirowski and Mower changed from developers to refiners. The automatic implantable defibrillator became the automatic implantable cardioverter-defibrillator, which could detect ventricular tachycardia as well as ventricular fibrillation and could cardiovert as well as defibrillate. The weight of the devices decreased from 225 grams in 1980 to 90 grams in 1998, and the size over the same period diminished from 250 to 48 cubic centimeters. Models using electrode catheters rather than myocardial patches, and therefore implantable, like pacemakers, with local anesthesia and no thoracotomy, were developed and have now become standard. Mirowski has been proved correct here as well. "We're smart people, but we don't pretend to know everything," Mower acknowledged. (One can hear Mirowski making the same statement as well.) "There comes a certain point in time when no one can louse it up. So the 'child' left its parents. We knew it was in good hands, and we'd continue to have a role as consultants."

The prediction made by Mirowski and Mower that their "child" would shrink further as even smaller batteries, capacitors, and inductors were developed came to pass. Software replaced hardware, so that current devices perform more specialized functions such as detecting a wider range of arrhythmias and converting by pacing as well as by shock. Physicians can now program many features of the device's sensing and discharging functions transcutaneously.

By the beginning of 1998, 197,000 units had been implanted worldwide, 44,000 during 1997 alone. As Mirowski and Mower had predicted,[14] physicians are now beginning to implant cardioverter-defibrillators prophylactically in patients who have not as yet suffered ventricular tachycardia and fibrillation but who are at high risk of developing these arrhythmias.

ILLNESS

In the mid 1980s, Mirowski became ill. In retrospect, his family believes that the first symptoms appeared while the family was vacationing at a beach. Using her father as the subject, Ariella was demonstrating the chest examination to Doris. She touched him in the ribs, a tap that should not have hurt as much as it did. In typical fashion, Mirowski medicated himself for the pain, which gradually became severe. Finally, he agreed to be admitted to Johns Hopkins Hospital, and multiple myeloma was diagnosed. Treatment relieved his symptoms for several years. However, in 1989, plasma cell leukemia developed. Mirowski insisted on receiving the most intensive chemotherapy, fighting against the odds as usual. When the disease stopped responding, his oncologist raised the possibility of a bone-marrow transplant, then in experimental development for the treatment of myeloma. A near relative as donor would be needed; did he have a brother? This would have been Abraham, lost in the Holocaust. When Mirowski died on March 26, 1990, at the age of 65 years, he had more than 20 pathological fractures.

For years, but particularly during his final illness, Mirowski was tortured by regret that he had not adequately honored the name of his parents. (On becoming a United States citizen, he had officially adopted the name Michel Mirowski.) He ordered that his gravestone read: "Michel Mirowski son of Israel Lieb Friedman and Genia Handelsman."

FAMILY AND REPUTATION

In his sixties, by then a leading figure in international cardiology, Mirowski appeared as a man of his years, of medium height, slightly overweight, with thinning gray hair and the demeanor of a scholar. His speech was highly articulate, laced with classical and literary references. A listener was always surprised when Mirowski could not find the precisely correct English word to express what he wished to say. He would then recall the *mot juste* in some other language. Mirowski's English had a slight accent, clearly European, but difficult for the American ear to localize further. Always wanting to know what was happening everywhere, Mirowski compulsively read *The New York Times* every day and was clearly uneasy until his copy arrived.

Anna, his wife of 40 years, continues to maintain a European ambiance in their Baltimore home, where she still lives. She projects warmth and sensitivity with an elegance and formality of speech and manner from her European background. Food always mattered to Anna and Michel Mirowski, but probably for different reasons. Michel observed from less happy times that fat people survive. So one should eat a lot, and Mirowski, more than his wife, was likely to offer the second helping. Of the two, however, Anna Mirowski is the more practical and the more sentimental. When she talks about him, Mirowski is always "my Michel" or "my dear Michel." She claims that she started using this title to distinguish her Michel from another Michel, also a refugee in Lyons.

Each of Anna and Michel's daughters is now a physician. Mirowski insisted that he "bent over backwards" not to push his children into medical careers: "I tried to be supportive but neutral. The worst way to get them to do something is to tell them to do it." When his children complained about their work, Mirowski liked to respond: "The bumps in the road are not bumps, they are the road. You're not being punished; you do it because you want to." Anna, however, encouraged the children to be doctors almost from infancy. She wanted them to have professions, "not be just a housewife like me," and, she had observed that doctors usually prospered even in difficult times because of the value of their work. Their daughters have six children, whose names honor Michel and other members of the Mirowski family, as well as their husbands' families.

The last 5 years of his life brought Mirowski the recognition that was not his in earlier times. Professional societies and leaders of academic medical institutions honored him. He received invitations to write more articles and to give more lectures than he could accept. So he picked and chose, accommodating his friends and those who had supported him in darker times. Often with his wife or children, he traveled where he wished because he had become welcome everywhere.

When he spoke overseas, Mirowski usually lectured in English, but he often discussed his papers during the question-and-answer period in the language of the country he was visiting. He spoke French, Hebrew, Polish, Russian, Spanish, and Yiddish fluently, but he never learned Italian and would not learn German. Some things cannot be forgotten.

REFERENCES

1. Kastor JA. Michel Mirowski and the automatic implantable defibrillator. Am J Cardiol 1989; 63:977–982.
2. Kastor JA. Michel Mirowski and the automatic implantable defibrillator. Am J Cardiol 1989; 63:1121–1126.
3. Mirowski M, Reid PR, Mower MM, et al. Termination of malignant ventricular arrhythmias with an implanted automatic defibrillator in human beings. N Engl J Med 1980; 303:322–324.
4. London J. Martin Eden. New York: Macmillan, 1957.
5. Mirowski M. A propos de 29 observations de commissurotomie mitrale. M.D. thesis, Faculty of Medicine, University of Lyon, Lyon, France. Trevoux: J. Patissier, 1953, pp. 1–157.
6. Cabrera E, Piccolo E, Hernandez Y, Mirowski M. Correlación vectocardiografica y hemodinamica en la communicación interventricular. Arch Inst Cardiol Mex 1960; 30:387.
7. Mirowski M, Mower MM, Staewen WS, Tabatznik B, Mendeloff AI: Standby automatic defibrillator: an approach to prevention of sudden coronary death. Arch Intern Med 1970; 126:158–161.
8. Lown B, Axelrod P. Implanted standby defibrillators. Circulation 1972; 46:637–639.
9. Mirowski M, Mower MM, Gott VL, Brawley RK, Denniston R. Transvenous automatic defibrillator: preliminary clinical tests of its defibrillating subsystem. Trans Am Soc Artific Intern Organs 1972; 18:520–525.
10. Mirowski M, Mower MM, Gott VL, Brawley RK. Feasibility and effectiveness of low-energy catheter defibrillation in man. Circulation 1973; 47:79–85.
11. Mower MM, Mirowski M, Spear JF, Moore EN. Patterns of ventricular activity during catheter defibrillation. Circulation 1974; 49:858–861.
12. Mirowski M, Mower MM, Langer A, Heilman MS, Schreibman J. A chronically implanted system for automatic defibrillation in active conscious dogs: experimental model for treatment of sudden death from ventricular fibrillation. Circulation 1978; 58:367–371.
13. Watkins L, Jr, Mirowski M, Mower MM, et al. Automatic defibrillation in man: the initial surgical experience. J Thorac Cardiovasc Surg 1981; 82:492–500.
14. Mirowski M, Mower MM. The automatic implantable defibrillator: some historical notes. In Brugada P, Wellens HJJ (eds). Cardiac Arrhythmias: Where Do We Go From Here? Mt. Kisco, NY: Futura, 1987, pp. 655–662.

CHAPTER

3

Biographical Sketches

WOLDEMAR MOBITZ[a]

On November 4, 1951, after an arduous illness, Professor Dr. Woldemar Mobitz ended a life filled with quiet scholarship and remarkable scientific achievements. Born the son of a renowned surgeon in St. Petersburg in 1889, Mobitz and his family moved to Tubingen when he was 6 years of age. His father having died young, the youth was raised by his mother and a sympathetic uncle who provided for his education and upbringing.

Mobitz studied medicine in Freiburg and in Munich, apprenticed with Romberg, with whom he later became a resident, was promoted to a rank comparable to attending physician, and was granted tenure with the publication of "About the incomplete disruption of conduction between atrium and ventricle of the human heart." This early work exemplified the basis of Mobitz's scientific work and intellectual direction.

Lonely and introverted by nature, Mobitz had a mind equipped with a mathematical precision that lent itself to the study of conduction abnormalities. "It might seem strange to the clinician, that the aforementioned results are seemingly based on pure mathematical calculations," his thesis concludes almost apologetically. From his precise observations, we gained further understanding about the different types of conduction disturbances, especially interference dissociation, a concept that established Mobitz's reputation in cardiology. Later, he moved on to study mathematically derived features of the circulation such as stroke and

minute volume. This work, it appears, led to Eppinger's invitation to join the faculty at his Freiburg Clinic.

Mobitz also demonstrated an ability to analyze purely clinical problems closely. As early as 1924, he produced an exemplary description of primary pulmonary stenosis and developed advanced bedside technology with experiments on action potentials and alveolar air, among others.

That such a career, with its versatile, intelligent, and ingenious achievements, was not acknowledged with the ultimate honors, was, assuredly, not due to a lack of scientific or medical maturity that raised him far above more visible colleagues. The principal reasons were his debilitating illness, possibly acquired in the care of patients, and his delicate sense of justice, rooted in his entire way of thinking, which conflicted with his environment. Although he was considered several times for senior appointments—Bonn and Magdeburg, for example—these characteristics hindered his receiving such positions. A short assignment as head of the Medical Clinic in Magdeburg ended with the invasion of the Russians in 1945.

Members of the Freiburg faculty who had the privilege of discussing scientific, particularly cardiological, problems with Mobitz during his final years came to admire his outstanding scholarship, brilliant thinking, knowledge of many fields in addition to medicine, and extraordinary capabilities. On behalf of the entire Department of Internal Medicine, we emphasize, while mourning his unanticipated death, these unique characteristics and express our gratitude for the opportunity of knowing this important and significant contributor to medical knowledge.

ALFRED PICK[b]

Dr. Alfred Pick (Fig. 3.1), the distinguished electrocardiographer, died in Chicago of carcinoma of the pancreas on January 8, 1982 at the age of 74 years.[4] When

[a]In 1975, Dr. Gerhard C. Meier of Newport, R.I. sent me this obituary written by Dr. Heilmeyer, former director of the Department of Internal Medicine at the University of Freiburg in Breisgau. Jan-Michael Klapproth, M.D., of the University of Maryland School of Medicine translated the text from the German. I hope that my editing into colloquial English accurately reflects the intent of Dr. Heilmeyer. Dr. Klapproth remembers being told during his education in Germany that the "arduous illness" of Mobitz was tuberculosis.

Unlike Wenckebach, whose name is familiar to many physicians, English-speaking cardiologists and their students perhaps would never have heard about Mobitz, were it not for the popularization of his description of the 2 types of block[1,2] by Drs. Richard Langendorf and Alfred Pick of Chicago[3] (see later).

[b]Originally published in 1982[4] and reprinted with permission.

35

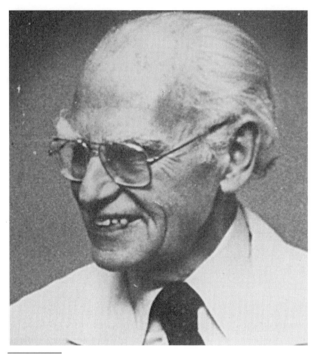

FIGURE 3.1 Alfred Pick, M.D. (From Kastor JA. Alfred Pick. Int J Cardiol 1982; 2:151–155.)

he died, Dr. Pick was professor of medicine at the Pritzker School of Medicine of the University of Chicago and senior consultant to the Michael Reese Hospital and Medical Center.

Dr. Pick was born in Prague in 1907 and was educated at the gymnasium and at the German University of Prague, where he received his M.D. degree in 1932. He was in charge of electrocardiography departments at the First University Medical Clinic of Prague from 1935 to 1937, at the Priessnitz Sanatorium in Graefenberg, Czechoslovakia from 1937 to 1939, and at the State Hospital of Prague from 1947 to 1949. In 1949, he came to the United States and began an association with the Michael Reese Hospital and Medical Center in Chicago, where he worked for the rest of his career. He served a second internship there from 1950 to 1951 and was then appointed director of the Heart Station. He was also associate director of the Cardiovascular Institute at the Michael Reese Hospital from 1958 to 1969 and was acting director from 1969 to 1971.

Dr. Pick was one of the world's leading scholars of cardiac arrhythmias, which he studied for more than 45 years. Virtually all topics in the field attracted his attention. He wrote definitive papers, continuously cited despite their having been written more than 15 years ago, on aberrant conduction, reciprocal beating, parasystole, preexcitation, digitalis intoxication, the supernormal phase of atrioventricular conduction, and the diagnosis of supraventricular versus ventricular tachycardias. He and his colleagues first defined and described nonparoxysmal atrioventricular nodal tachycardia, atrioventricular nodal tachycardia with block,

and the phenomenon of depression of cardiac pacemakers by premature impulses. Our understanding of atrioventricular dissociation was greatly clarified by Dr. Pick's studies. With Dr. Louis N. Katz, he wrote one of the most renowned books in cardiology, *Clinical Electrocardiography. Part I: The Arrhythmias* in 1956.[5] Dr. Pick's admirers awaited part II patiently, and in 1979, with his long-time collaborator Dr. Richard Langendorf, he published the text, *Interpretation of Complex Arrhythmias.*[6]

For several decades, Drs. Pick, Katz, and Langendorf conducted their famous postgraduate course in electrocardiography at the Michael Reese Hospital. The students included trainees and professors. The teaching technique that the directors developed was unique and highly effective. Students would be called, one by one, to the front of the room to analyze electrocardiograms. Slowly but surely, understanding replaced confusion, and by the end of the week, the class could be seen muttering in unison "concealed conduction" and other concepts they had learned. Through this course, many cardiologists who subsequently made contributions to the study of cardiac arrhythmias received their introduction to the field under the tutelage of Dr. Pick and his colleagues.

Dr. Pick was a member of many professional organizations in the United States and was a corresponding member of the Cardiological Society of Peru. He served on the editorial boards of the *American Heart Journal* and the *Journal of Electrocardiology* and was a member of the International Scientific Board of *Coeur et Médicine Interne (Paris).*

Dr. Richard Langendorf, Dr. Pick's long-time colleague at the Michael Reese Hospital, wrote:

Fred Pick was my friend and co-worker, going back to the time when we both graduated from the German University of Prague, Czechoslovakia in 1932. After our graduation we both were active in the Medical Department of the University Hospital of the German University in Prague. There we came under the strong and lasting influence of Dr. Max Winternitz, an excellent clinical cardiologist with special interest in electrocardiography and outstanding skill in the interpretation of arrhythmias.[7] We included Winternitz as co-author of our paper dealing with the "Rule of Bigeminy" published 3 years after his death.[8] He had used the term already while we were working with him in the nineteen thirties. We also dedicated our book to the memory of Max Winternitz and Louis Katz.[6]

The first paper I published with Fred was on "ECG Findings in Pulmonary Embolism"[9] followed by "The ECG of Acute Nephritis"[10, 11] and "The Use of Chest Leads in the Diagnosis of Myocardial Infarction."[11] All of our subsequent 48 joint publications dealt with arrhythmias.

Fred Pick and I were separated during the war years, when I was able to obtain a visa to the United States and was extremely fortunate to be accepted by Louis Katz to join his department at Michael Reese Hospital, while my friend Fred and his wife, Dr. Ruth Pick, suffered greatly as victims of the Nazi persecution.

After their return to Prague following the end of

World War II we resumed our contact, and I succeeded in my efforts to convince Louis Katz that Fred and Ruth would become valuable members of his department. Fred's impressive interpretation of an unusual and difficult arrhythmia observed at Michael Reese Hospital and sent to him by me convinced Louis that Fred was indeed an arrhythmia expert. It is of interest that Fred kept my wire of congratulations, with the ECG strip attached to it, framed on the wall of his office. After Fred arrived in this country in 1949, the ECG of the telegram became the subject of our first joint report.[12]

For Ruth Pick, who was to specialize in pathology, we also had some work waiting, namely the heart of a patient with W.P.W. syndrome to be examined for the presence of an accessory A-V pathway.[13]

Fred had a regular internship at Michael Reese Hospital and then became a full time member of the Cardiovascular Institute. He was Dr. Katz's co-author of the highly successful textbook on *The Arrhythmias*.[5] Fred and I maintained our friendship and close cooperation that culminated in our book on *The Interpretation of Complex Arrhythmias* in 1979.[6]

We enjoyed our advanced arrhythmia courses given at Michael Reese Hospital for 26 consecutive years until 1980, attended by a number of physicians who by now have become prominent cardiologists whose main interest is electrocardiography or electrophysiology. We also "exported" our one-week course to Holland (Prof. Durrer's Department at the Wilhelmina Hospital), to Sweden (Dr. Lars Mogensen), and to France (Prof. Grosgogeat at the Salpetriere). In addition Fred lectured in Japan and Australia.

Fred Pick will be remembered and greatly missed as a devoted friend, a loyal member of the Michael Reese Cardiovascular Institute, as a productive and scrupulously honest investigator and an outstanding teacher.

KENNETH M. ROSEN[c]

Dr. Kenneth M. Rosen (Fig. 3.2), the clinical electrophysiologist, died suddenly on March 6, 1982 in Vail, Colorado. He was 44 years old.[14] Dr. Rosen seemed well and had lectured and skied the day before he died. Examination later revealed that he had severe coronary artery disease. When he died, Dr. Rosen was professor of medicine and chief of cardiology at the Abraham Lincoln School of Medicine of the University of Illinois in Chicago.

In his short but extremely productive career, Dr. Rosen made many important contributions to the developing field of cardiac electrophysiology, in which he was an early worker. He first described dual atrioventricular nodal pathways in humans, pseudoatrioventricular block from concealed His bundle depolarizations, and the location of atrioventricular block in myocardial infarction. His studies increased our understanding of intraventricular block, sinus node disease, cardiac refractoriness, supraventricular tachycardia, and preexcitation. Dr. Rosen and his colleagues first reported the method of repeated electrophysiological testing to assess the effectiveness of antiarrhythmic

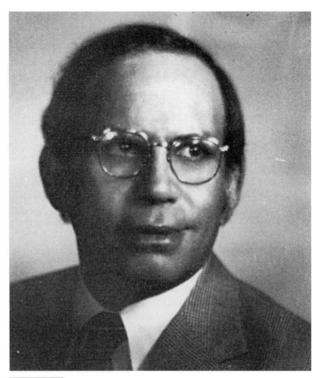

FIGURE 3.2 Kenneth M. Rosen, M.D. (From Kastor JA. Kenneth M. Rosen. Int J Cardiol 1982; 1:465–466.)

drugs, and he collaborated to particularly good effect with cardiac pathologists.

Dr. Kenneth Rosen was born in New York City in 1937, attended the local public schools, and graduated from the Bronx High School of Science. He received his B.A. degree from New York University and his M.D. degree from the Chicago Medical School. He then trained in internal medicine and cardiology at Cincinnati General Hospital and at Mt. Sinai Hospital in New York City, where he was chief resident physician. Dr. Rosen learned the techniques of intracardiac electrocardiography at the United States Public Health Service Hospital in Staten Island, New York, where a group of investigators under the leadership of Dr. Anthony N. Damato developed the contemporary approach to investigation of cardiac arrhythmias in the United States. In 1969, Dr. Rosen joined the faculty of the University of Illinois and 3 years later was appointed full professor. He was also professor of physiology in the School of Basic Sciences.

Dr. Rosen was associate editor of *Chest* and assistant editor of the *Archives of Internal Medicine* and served on the editorial boards of 8 journals. He belonged to many professional organizations, including the American Heart Association, American Federation for Clinical Research, American Society for Clinical Investigation, Association of University Cardiologists, American College of Cardiology, Central Society for Clinical Research, and Chicago Heart Association, and he served on important committees of several societies. In 1980,

---

[c]Originally published in 1982[14] and reprinted with permission.

he received the Distinguished Alumnus Award from his medical school.

Dr. Pablo Denes[d] wrote:

Kenneth M. Rosen's outstanding achievements in the field of human electrophysiology will always remain with us, through his many publications and through his teachings. He died at a very young age, at the height of his career. His life was like an explosion of energy, touching everyone around him. His enthusiasm was contagious, capturing all who worked with him. There are many facets to Kenneth Rosen's life. He was an outstanding researcher, teacher, clinician, a music lover, an avid reader.

For Kenneth Rosen, research was a giant puzzle which had to be solved. He loved to ask the questions, how and why. He also loved to teach. Through his lectures, he was able to transmit to the audience his great enthusiasm, clear thinking and straight logic. He was a nationally and internationally recognized speaker on cardiac arrhythmias. His efforts in teaching students, residents and fellows resulted in the recruitment of many of his collaborators: Ramesh Dhingra, Delon Wu, Fernando Amat-y-leon, Christopher Wyndham, Robert Bauernfeind, Steven Swiryn and Boris Strasberg.

His interest was not restricted to science. Oftentimes, I saw him at the symphony totally absorbed by the music he loved. He was a good piano player. He was an avid reader of biographies and history. Above all he was a generous human being and a friend. We have suffered a great loss. His legacy will survive in his children and in those of us who learned so much from him.

[d]Currently (1998) at the Michael Reese Hospital and Medical Center, Chicago.

REFERENCES

1. Mobitz W. Uber die unvollstandige Storung der Erregungsuberleitung zwischen Vorhof und Kammer des menschlichen Herzens. Z Ges Exp Med 1924; 41:180.
2. Mobitz W. Uber den partiellen Herzblock. Z Klin Med 1928; 107:450.
3. Langendorf R, Pick A. Atrioventricular block, type II (Mobitz): its nature and clinical significance. Circulation 1968; 38:819–821.
4. Kastor JA. Alfred Pick. Int J Cardiol 1982; 2:151–155.
5. Katz LN, Pick A. Clinical Electrocardiography. Part I: The Arrhythmias. Philadelphia: Lea & Febiger, 1956.
6. Pick A, Langendorf R. The Interpretation of Complex Arrhythmias. Philadelphia: Lea & Febiger, 1979.
7. Langendorf R. Necrologia: Dr. Max Winternitz (1900–1952). Cardiologia 1953; 22:62–63.
8. Langendorf R, Pick A, Winternitz M. Mechanisms of intermittent ventricular bigeminy. I. Appearance of ectopic beats dependent upon length of the ventricular cycle, the "rule of bigeminy." Circulation 1955; 11:422–430.
9. Langendorf R, Pick A. Ekg: Befunde bei Lungenembolie. Acta Med Scand 1936; 90:289–304.
10. Langendorf R, Pick A. Elektrokardiogramm bei akuter Nephritis. Med Klin 1937; 126–136.
11. Langendorf R, Pick A. Elektrokardiogramm bei akuter Nephritis. Acta Med Scand 1938; 94:1–58.
12. Pick A, Langendorf R. A case of reciprocal beating with evidence of repetitive and blocked reentry to the cardiac impulse. Am Heart J 1950; 40:13–29.
13. Langendorf R, Lev M, Pick R. Auricular fibrillation with anomalous A-V excitation (WPW syndrome) imitating ventricular paroxysmal tachycardia. Acta Cardiol 1952; 7:241–260.
14. Kastor JA. Kenneth M Rosen. Int J Cardiol 1982; 1:465–466.

CHAPTER

4

Atrial Fibrillation[1-29]

Although we have known for almost 100 years that atrial[a] fibrillation occurs in humans, the cardiac diseases with which it is associated have changed as the incidence of rheumatic fever in Western countries has waned. Monitoring units have revealed that atrial fibrillation occurs more often during acute myocardial infarction than was previously thought. We now recognize the frequent presence of atrial fibrillation in the "holiday heart." Cardiac surgery, first applied successfully to the treatment of rheumatic mitral stenosis in the 1940s, has relieved much of the distress and has prolonged the lives of patients with the valvular heart disease often associated with atrial fibrillation. However, cardiothoracic surgery itself can also produce the arrhythmia, at least temporarily. We continue to observe some patients with atrial fibrillation who, as yet, have no definable structural heart disease.

During the past 25 years, beta-adrenergic and calcium-channel–blocking drugs and powerful antiarrhythmic drugs such as amiodarone have greatly improved the medical treatment of atrial fibrillation. Two centuries after its introduction into clinical medicine, digitalis still has value for treating atrial fibrillation, but we have become more aware in recent decades of its limitations and of the cardiac manifestations of its toxicity. The more widespread use of anticoagulation and the better understanding of its value have reduced the incidence of disabling strokes in patients with atrial fibrillation.

Thirty years have passed since the introduction of synchronized electrical cardioversion, the most successful method for restoring sinus rhythm. Although enthusiasm for this method decreased when the high frequency of reversion became known, cardioversion remains the treatment of choice for reestablishing a normal rhythm. It is significantly safer and more effective than drugs such as quinidine, the use of which was first described soon after the arrhythmia was defined.

Implantable pacemakers, first available in the 1960s, provide sufficiently rapid heart rates when bradycardia complicates atrial fibrillation, and the more recently developed rate-adaptive units further increase cardiac function and patients' well-being.

Except for the subject of Wolff-Parkinson-White syndrome during atrial fibrillation, clinical electrophysiologists almost ignored the arrhythmia during the 1970s and 1980s as they concentrated on such arrhythmic afflictions as atrioventricular block, supraventricular tachycardia, ventricular tachycardia, and ventricular fibrillation. In the past 10 years, however, interest in studying atrial fibrillation has grown rapidly, as documented by the attention given to the subject at the annual scientific meetings of the American Heart Association (Table 4.1) and in the literature.[30-32]

SOME ADVANCES SINCE THE FIRST EDITION OF THIS BOOK

- Transesophageal echocardiography to determine whether patients need to be anticoagulated before elective cardioversion to sinus rhythm.
- Greater emphasis on sustaining sinus rhythm in patients with chronic atrial fibrillation.
- Development of intra-atrial cardioversion and early application of its use.

Table 4.1	ABSTRACTS ON ATRIAL FIBRILLATION PRESENTED AT THE ANNUAL SCIENTIFIC MEETINGS OF THE AMERICAN HEART ASSOCIATION		
Year and Reference	Abstracts on Atrial Fibrillation	All Abstracts	Percentage of All Abstracts on Atrial Fibrillation (%)
1984[30]	10	1,852	0.54
1990[31]	22	3,064	0.72
1997[32]	97	4,286	2.26

[a] Formerly called "auricular."

PREVALENCE[33, 34]

Although atrial fibrillation is the most common sustained disorder of the heartbeat[35, 36], the arrhythmia occurs infrequently in the general population.

- The occurrence of atrial fibrillation was barely perceptible,[37] only 0.004%,[38] in 122,043 healthy men aged 16 to 50 years in the United States Air Force and in 0.2%[39] of 757,693 flyers with valid Federal Aviation Administration medical certificates.
- The arrhythmia was detected in 0.3% to 0.4% of subjects in each of 3 series: in 5,138 men and women who constituted 85% of the adult population of Tecumseh, Michigan;[40] in 9,067 persons 32 to 64 years of age from Reykjavik, Iceland;[41] and in 18,403 British male civil servants aged 40 to 64 years.[42]
- In the Framingham study of 5,191 adult men and women, chronic atrial fibrillation developed in 2% during 22 years of follow-up.[43]

Atrial fibrillation occurs rarely in fetuses,[44–46] infants, and children.[47–54] Only 35 cases were collected from 1 children's hospital during 22 years.[55–58, b]

AGE[34]

"The most important single factor encouraging the onset of atrial fibrillation in those conditions that are prone to it is the advancing age of the patient."[59] This statement, from the third edition (1968) of Paul Wood's cardiology text, emphasizes the effects of age on the development of atrial fibrillation in the general population,[40, 42, 43, 60] in men,[61] and in patients with[62–67] or without[1, 68, 69] heart disease, with stroke,[70] and undergoing coronary artery surgery.[71, 72]

The range of prevalence of atrial fibrillation reported in elderly patients is wide:

- 2.3% of 1,770 people older than 60 years of age in Bussleton, Western Australia.[73]
- 2.4% of 87 patients aged 62 to 90 years in Edinburgh, Scotland.[74]
- 3.7% of 819 asymptomatic patients older than 65 years of age.[75]
- 4% of 500 patients in Indianapolis who were older than 70 years.[76]
- 5% of patients who were older than 72 to 75 years.[77, 78]
- 4.8% of women and 6.2% of men more than 64 years old who enrolled in a study of risk factors for coronary heart disease and stroke in the United States.[79]
- 10% of a group of healthy, elderly people in Sussex, England who were at least 75 years of age and who were leading active, independent lives.[80]
- 11% on entering the study and 17% by the age of 84 years in 101 healthy, elderly subjects living

independently in Jersey, Channel Islands, who were studied with 24-hour ambulatory electrocardiographic recordings.[81]
- 17% of 559 patients 85 years of age or older in Tampere, Finland; the study included 83% of the population of this age.[82]
- 16% of 31 men and 69 women each older than 90 years of age (mean age, 93.1 years) in a report from Buffalo, New York.[83]

Although rare, atrial fibrillation has been observed in fetuses and newborns.[84]

GENDER[34, 85, 86]

Men develop atrial fibrillation more often than women,[41, 43, 71, 87–88, c] as much as 1.5 times as often, according to the Framingham Heart Study.[89] Consequently, myocardial infarction is significantly associated with the development of atrial fibrillation in men, whereas valve disease is more frequently the etiological factor for the arrhythmia in women.[89]

GENETICS[90]

A few cases of atrial fibrillation have been found to occur with familial association in patients with no obvious organic heart disease.[84, 91–95, d] The genetic locus for familial atrial fibrillation inherited as an autosomal dominant trait has been mapped to chromosome 10q.[96]

CLINICAL SETTING[97]

Most clinicians refer to atrial fibrillation as paroxysmal or chronic, depending on whether the arrhythmia is short-lived or continuously present. Investigators have suggested that we classify the temporal aspect of the arrhythmia into three components:[29, 98, 99, e]

- *Paroxysmal:* recurrent episodes of the arrhythmia that spontaneously revert to sinus rhythm.
- *Persistent:* atrial fibrillation for more than 48 hours or until cardioversion is performed.
- *Permanent:* atrial fibrillation refractory to cardioversion, which will no longer be attempted.

Most patients with atrial fibrillation have structural heart disease[36] (Table 4.2). Those patients with no

---

[b] The atria of the human infant and young child may be too small to sustain fibrillation. Atrial mass determines which animals develop atrial fibrillation.[55, 58] The arrhythmia occurs in large breeds of dogs and horses but rarely in small dogs and never in cats.[55, 56, 58]

[c] "Perhaps because men are generally subject to greater strain than are women,"[87] observed Paul D. White, one of the founders of American cardiology, 50 years ago. (Despite his knowledge and many contributions, White was, quite obviously, a physician from a previous generation.)

[d] A striking report, published in 1957, describes the presence of the arrhythmia in 5 generations of a family. Twenty-one members who lived to the age of 40 developed paroxysmal and, occasionally, chronic atrial fibrillation.[93] In the first and second generations, all who lived into or beyond the sixth decade had atrial fibrillation.

[e] Although not all agree.[29]

Table 4.2	**PROMINENT CAUSES OF ATRIAL FIBRILLATION**

Mitral valve disease
  Stenosis
  Regurgitation and prolapse
Coronary heart disease
  Myocardial infarction
  Angina
  Prinzmetal's angina variant
  Chronic coronary disease
Hypertension
Wolff-Parkinson-White syndrome
Thyrotoxicosis
Congenital heart disease
  Atrial septal defect
Cardiomyopathy and myocarditis
  Alcoholic
  Amyloid
  Congestive
  Hypertrophic
  Peripartum
  Sarcoid
  Viral and idiopathic myocarditis
Rheumatic fever
Lung disease
Cardiac and thoracic surgery
Infective endocarditis
Pericarditis
Tumors
Alcohol
Lone or idiopathic fibrillation

organic abnormalities are said to have lone atrial fibrillation.[100, f]

Valvular Disease

Mitral stenosis.[101] Many older physicians remember when mitral stenosis was the most common cause of atrial fibrillation in Western countries. In the preoperative era, it was present in 20% of patients when they were first seen,[102] and it developed during the course of the illness in 40%[103] to 50%.[104] Increasing age, not the degree of stricture, is chiefly responsible for the fibrillation.[65, 103–106]

The mean age of onset in unoperated patients is about 37 years.[104] Women predominate.[102, 103] When effective mitral surgery became available, atrial fibrillation had developed in 42%[105] to 65%[107] of patients who presented for operation. Ambulatory monitoring reveals that transient and asymptomatic paroxysms of atrial fibrillation frequently develop in patients with mitral stenosis.[108]

Mitral regurgitation and mitral valve prolapse. The

likelihood that atrial fibrillation will complicate mitral regurgitation increases with age[64, 109, 110, g] and with severity of illness.[111] By the time patients with mitral regurgitation are evaluated in cardiology units, many already have atrial fibrillation.[112–117, h]

However, atrial fibrillation develops less often in association with mitral regurgitation than with mitral stenosis;[117] only 16% of those with isolated mitral regurgitation in one series had the arrhythmia. Moreover, patients who have mitral valve prolapse without significant regurgitation seldom have atrial fibrillation,[118, i] although the incidence of the arrhythmia grows when mitral regurgitation develops and worsens.[116]

In a review written in 1972 about patients with atrial fibrillation resulting from mitral regurgitation, the cardiac lesion was rheumatic heart disease in 57%, ruptured chordae tendineae in 23%, and coronary heart disease in 8%.[110, j] Seventy-five percent of those with rheumatic mitral regurgitation who required mitral valve surgery had atrial fibrillation. When operation was required for mitral regurgitation resulting from rupture of chordae tendineae, 27% had atrial fibrillation.[110]

In a more recently compiled series of patients requiring mitral valve replacement who were severely disabled by the effects of isolated regurgitation, atrial fibrillation occurred more often in patients with coronary heart disease than in those with mitral valve prolapse, infective endocarditis, or rheumatic heart disease.[115] Pure mitral regurgitation was formerly[119] thought to be caused by rheumatic heart disease.[115]

Mitral annular calcification. Atrial fibrillation is present in many patients with severe calcification of the annulus of the mitral valve.[120, 121] This disease occurs predominantly in the elderly.

Aortic stenosis. Atrial fibrillation occasionally complicates the course of pure aortic stenosis.[122–124, k]

Coronary Heart Disease and Myocardial Infarction

Atrial fibrillation is rare in uncomplicated coronary heart disease[41] and occurs infrequently during most of the illness.[41, l] Atrial fibrillation occurs more frequently

---

f Before reading about the current relationships between clinical heart disease and atrial fibrillation, the reader may be interested in the results of an analysis reported more than 70 years ago of 3,000 patients in New England who sought medical attention because of cardiac symptoms.[100] Atrial fibrillation occurred in 376 cases (12.5%), 309 of which were permanent and 67 paroxysmal. In 42%, rheumatic heart disease was the primary organic lesion; in 38%, findings of atherosclerosis and/or hypertension were present; hypertension alone accounted for only 4%. Hyperthyroidism appeared to cause atrial fibrillation in 4%. In 8%, no organic lesions could be found.

g Paul Wood observed: "The great majority of patients [with mitral regurgitation] over 50 years of age fibrillate."[1910]

h One hundred-one (30%) of 335 patients in 6 series.[112–117] The etiology and severity of illness among the patients varied, and the series included 2 relatively large groups of 194 who were referred for mitral valve replacement.[114, 115]

i Six of 114 patients, all of whom were male and 5 of whom were older than 50 years of age.

j Before hemodynamic and echocardiographic studies were performed on patients with mitral valve disease, many patients reported to have mitral regurgitation probably also had significant amounts of stenosis.[110, 111]

k Atrial fibrillation was present in 39 (10%) of 397 patients with aortic stenosis.[124]

l Atrial fibrillation was present in only 2.5% of 916 patients with clinical evidence of coronary disease[1911] and in 0.6% of 18,343 patients in the Coronary Artery Surgery Study (CASS),[67] and in only 11 of 1,671 patients in 2 large series.

when congestive heart failure is present and, paradoxically, when fewer than three major coronary arteries are occluded by 70% or more.[67]

Coronary heart disease. Coronary heart disease, often associated with hypertension, nonetheless occurs in patients with atrial fibrillation.[61, 125, 126] In one study, atherosclerotic cardiovascular disease was the most common form of heart disease present in patients coming to an emergency room with atrial fibrillation.[127] According to the Framingham study, coronary heart disease is a significant precursor of both chronic and paroxysmal atrial fibrillation in men, although it exhibits no relation to chronic atrial fibrillation among women.[128] However, hypertensive cardiovascular disease,[61] cardiac failure, and rheumatic heart disease are more strongly associated with atrial fibrillation than is coronary disease.[128] New coronary events occur sooner in elderly patients with heart disease and atrial fibrillation than in those in sinus rhythm.[129]

Myocardial infarction. Atrial fibrillation develops during the course of myocardial infarction in 11% of patients.[66, 130–144, m] This incidence, observed since the introduction of electrocardiographic monitoring, is slightly higher than the rate of 7% reported in the premonitoring era.[137, 145, n]

Compared with those without atrial fibrillation, patients with myocardial infarction who develop the arrhythmia tend to be older,[66, 138, 139, 142, 143, 146–148] to be in a worse Killip class,[146, 148] to have had more severe myocardial damage,[142, 146, 147, 149] and to have the following features:

- Increased heart rate.[148]
- ST segment elevations of at least 5.0 mm.[150]
- More right bundle branch block.[142]
- More ventricular tachycardia[142, 146, 151] and fibrillation.[142, 151]
- Higher peak levels of serum glutamic-oxaloacetic transaminase[141] and creatine kinase.[148]
- Higher pulmonary capillary wedge and right atrial pressures.[66, 149, 152]
- Three-vessel coronary disease and initial TIMI (Thrombolysis in Myocardial Infarction) flow grade lower than 3[148] or occlusion of the right or left circumflex coronary artery just proximal to the origin of the artery to the sinus node.[153]

Time of onset. The arrhythmia appears soon after symptoms of myocardial infarction develop.[66] It was present on admission in 11% of patients in one series.[138] Twenty percent of patients monitored within 1 hour after the first symptoms of myocardial infarction develop atrial fibrillation, an incidence significantly higher than in other patients whose monitoring begins

at different times after the beginning of symptoms.[154] Most episodes—87% in one report[137]—start within 48 hours after the illness begins. Atrial fibrillation that develops more than 12 hours after the infarction begins predicts worse coronary disease, more complications, and an unfavorable prognosis[147] (Table 4.3).

Atrial fibrillation during acute myocardial infarction is usually brief.[130, 132, 137, 139, 142, 152] Most patients who develop the arrhythmia and survive the infarction spontaneously return to sinus rhythm.

Pericarditis. According to some reports, pericarditis occurs more frequently in those patients with myocardial infarction who develop atrial fibrillation;[140, 141, 152] other reports do not support this finding.[66, 154]

Inferior infarctions. Patients with inferior myocardial infarctions who develop atrial fibrillation are more likely to have the following:

- Pericardial friction rubs.[152]
- Decreased cardiac output.[152]
- Elevated mean right atrial pressures.[152]
- Right ventricular dysfunction[155] or infarction.[152]

In one report, occlusion of the left circumflex coronary artery proximal to the origin of the left atrial circumflex branch was characteristic of patients with inferior infarction who developed atrial fibrillation.[156] In another report, no significant dominance of lesions in the proximal right coronary artery or left circumflex artery was found.[152]

Admissions with atrial fibrillation. About 11% of patients admitted to cardiac and medical intensive care units because of new-onset atrial fibrillation have acute myocardial infarction.[157] Patients with myocardial infarction are more likely to have left ventricular hypertrophy, electrocardiographic evidence of an old myocardial infarction, typical cardiac chest pain, and cardiac symptoms lasting less than 4 hours.

Hypertension

Hypertension is often found in patients with atrial fibrillation, as would be expected in view of the high

---

*m Six hundred sixty (11.1%) of 5,969 patients in 16 series.[66, 130–144] In another series, by far the largest reviewed, 16% of 4,108 patients had atrial fibrillation, but in some patients the arrhythmia may have been unrelated to the myocardial infarction.[1907]

*n For inexplicable reasons, the occurrence of atrial fibrillation during admission with myocardial infarction to a coronary care unit in Copenhagen (Denmark) County increased from 11% to 18% from 1979 to 1988.[145]

Table 4.3	**CHARACTERISTICS OF MYOCARDIAL INFARCTION AND TIME OF ONSET OF SUPRAVENTRICULAR TACHYARRHYTHMIAS, MOSTLY ATRIAL FIBRILLATION**[147]

Characteristics of Infarction	Within 12 Hours (%)	Between 12 Hours and 4 Days (%)
Three-vessel coronary disease	4	31
Inferior infarctions	61	—
Anterior infarctions	—	50
Killip class III–IV congestive heart failure	11	63
Died during first month	7.6	32
Died during 47 months	15	24

(Adapted from Serrano CV Jr, Ramires JA, Mansur AP, Pileggi F. Importance of the time of onset of supraventricular tachyarrhythmias on prognosis of patient with acute myocardial infarction. Clin Cardiol 1995; 18:84–90, with permission.)

prevalence of hypertension in the population.[43] The arrhythmia, however, is seldom present in patients who have hypertension without myocardial dysfunction.[43]

Wolff-Parkinson-White Syndrome and Supraventricular Tachycardia

Prevalence. Atrial fibrillation was observed in 11%[o] of patients with Wolff-Parkinson-White syndrome studied before electrophysiological evaluation[158–160] and in 35%[o] of patients studied after electrophysiological evaluation.[161–166, p] Atrial fibrillation was the first arrhythmia to be clinically documented,[167] in 9% of patients with the Wolff-Parkinson-White syndrome. One episode of atrial fibrillation in patients with Wolff-Parkinson-White syndrome predicts that other episodes will follow.[168] Patients with concealed accessory pathways, and thus without the preexcitation characteristic of Wolff-Parkinson-White syndrome, infrequently have clinical atrial fibrillation.[166, q] Atrial fibrillation rarely occurs in children with the Wolff-Parkinson-White syndrome,[169–175] although the arrhythmia was documented in a fetus in the thirty-second week of gestation.[44]

Associated cardiac diseases. About 25% of patients with atrial fibrillation associated with the Wolff-Parkinson-White syndrome have structural heart disease.[163–165, 176] The diagnoses in 114 patients were as follows:

- Valvular heart disease, 8.
- Cardiomyopathies, 8.
- Ebstein's anomaly of the tricuspid valve, 5.
- Coronary heart disease, 4.
- Hypertension, 2.

Most patients with atrial fibrillation and Wolff-Parkinson-White syndrome also have supraventricular tachycardias, and the development of atrial fibrillation is functionally related to the presence of supraventricular tachycardias. In those relatively few patients without supraventricular tachycardias, organic heart disease is common.[164]

Atrioventricular nodal reentrant supraventricular tachycardia. Atrial fibrillation occurs more frequently in patients with supraventricular tachycardia resulting from atrioventricular nodal reentry than in those without the tachycardia.[177]

Metabolic Disorders

Thyrotoxicosis.[178, 179] Although thyrotoxicosis is seldom the cause of atrial fibrillation,[180, r] between 16%[63,] 181, 182 and 25%[62, 183] of patients with thyrotoxicosis develop atrial fibrillation.[s] Toxic doses of thyroid hormone can produce atrial fibrillation in euthyroid subjects.[39, 184]

Atrial fibrillation occurs more frequently among men than among women with thyrotoxicosis and is more common in older thyrotoxic patients.[62, 63, 185–188, t] The higher incidence probably relates to the concurrent presence of coronary heart disease.[189] Atrial fibrillation rarely complicates hyperthyroidism in children.[190–193] Hyperthyroidism is relatively common in elderly women with atrial fibrillation.[194, u]

Hypothyroidism. Hypothyroidism and atrial fibrillation may coexist, and the thyroid malfunction may cause the arrhythmia.[195]

Hypoglycemia. This disorder has been incriminated in producing atrial fibrillation.[196]

Congenital Heart Disease[197]

Atrial fibrillation is relatively uncommon in children with congenital heart disease, but it develops in adults with such lesions as they grow older.

Atrial septal defect. Atrial fibrillation is present in 20% of adults with atrial septal defect.[198–208, v] The incidence of atrial fibrillation increases as patients age.[204, 209–212] For example, in a series of 66 patients with atrial septal defect 60 years of age or older, 52% had atrial fibrillation.[213]

Other congenital lesions. Atrial fibrillation occurs occasionally in congenital coronary arterial fistula,[214] Ebstein's anomaly of the tricuspid valve,[215–217] Eisenmenger syndrome,[218, 219] Lutenbacher syndrome,[220] and ventricular septal defect.[221]

Cardiomyopathy and Myocarditis

Atrial fibrillation is said to occur in 15%[222] to 25%[223] of adult patients with all types of cardiomyopathies.[w] The arrhythmia also develops in a few children with cardiomyopathy.[57]

Alcoholic cardiomyopathy. Atrial fibrillation has

---

[o] From 295 patients in 4 series. This incidence of atrial fibrillation in patients with Wolff-Parkinson-White syndrome referred to electrophysiological laboratories is almost certainly higher than occurs among all patients with the Wolff-Parkinson-White syndrome.[998]

[p] Louis Wolff and Paul D. White recorded paroxysmal atrial fibrillation in 23% (3 of 13) of their first cases in whom electrocardiographic records of tachyarrhythmias could be obtained.[161]

[q] One (3%) of 33 patients.[166]

[r] Overt hyperthyroidism was found in only 1% of patients with atrial fibrillation in the Canadian Registry of Atrial Fibrillation (CARAF), but laboratory abnormalities and a history of thyroid dysfunction occurred in 19%.[180]

[s] The smaller figure, 49 of 302 patients, was reported from 3 general hospitals,[63, 181, 182] whereas the larger number, 322 from 1,307, derived from 2 large series of patients referred for treatment with radioactive iodine.

[t] The arrhythmia was found in 31% of patients with hyperthyroidism older than 40 years of age and in none of those younger than 40.[188]

[u] Five (31%) of 16 women with atrial fibrillation in a nursing home had laboratory evidence or history of hyperthyroidism.[194]

[v] Two hundred twenty-seven (20%) with atrial fibrillation from 1,154 patients with atrial septal defect in 11 series.[198–208]

[w] These figures are presented unreferenced in a frequently cited review[222] and a leading cardiology text. Specific reports on the subject, except as noted in the text, are relatively imprecise, often grouping atrial fibrillation together with atrial flutter under the general title of "supraventricular tachycardias."

been recorded in 24% of patients with alcoholic car-diomyopathy.[224-227, x] The arrhythmia appears more commonly in older patients,[225] as well as when the heart dilates and hypertrophies.[228]

Amyloid cardiomyopathy. Paroxysmal and chronic atrial fibrillation occurs occasionally in cardiomyopathy resulting from amyloidosis.[229-231]

Dilated congestive cardiomyopathy. Atrial fibrillation has been observed in 24% of patients with this condition.[232, 233, y] According to an autopsy study, the arrhythmia appears only in those patients with electro-cardiographic signs of myocardial damage and left ventricular scars.[234]

Rapid, persistent atrial fibrillation, as well as other atrial tachyarrhythmias, can produce reversible, in some cases, recurrent[235] cardiomyopathy with cardio-megaly and congestive heart failure.[235-239] Recognizing that the tachyarrhythmia produces the cardiomyopathy is vital because treatment of the arrhythmia cures the myocardial disease.

Hypertrophic cardiomyopathy.[240] Chronic atrial fib-rillation, which is present in 10% of patients with hypertrophic cardiomyopathy, usually appears late in the course of the disease and is associated with severe clinical deterioration.[241, 242, z] Contrary to expectation, most patients with hypertrophic cardiomyopathy and chronic atrial fibrillation have relatively mild left ventricular hypertrophy and no obstruction to left ventricular outflow when compared with patients with hyper-trophic cardiomyopathy in sinus rhythm.[243]

Paroxysmal atrial fibrillation also occurs and has been recorded during 24-hour electrocardiographic monitoring in patients with obstructive and nonob-structive hypertrophic cardiomyopathy.[244-246] Of 100 such patients, 7 had a clinical history of intermittent atrial fibrillation, and in 2 others, the arrhythmia was first documented by monitoring.[244] Two patients with supraventricular tachycardias eventually developed chronic atrial fibrillation.[244]

Myocarditis. Atrial fibrillation occasionally occurs during active inflammation of the heart.[247] Atrial fibril-lation developed in a patient with psittacosis, which may have produced myocarditis.[248]

Peripartum cardiomyopathy. The cardiomyopathy that develops in the puerperium is seldom associated with atrial fibrillation.[249, 250]

Rheumatic fever. The age when children first have rheumatic fever does not correlate with the subsequent development of atrial fibrillation.[104, aa]

Sarcoid. Atrial fibrillation seldom complicates sar-coidosis even when the heart is affected.[251]

Lung Disease

Atrial fibrillation occurs relatively infrequently in pa-tients with pulmonary disease.[43, 125, 128, 252-254] The ar-rhythmia developed in 7% of patients admitted to hospitals because of respiratory failure,[255-257, bb] some of whom also had coronary and other forms of heart disease that could have caused the arrhythmia.[256] Of 40 patients admitted to a hospital with atrial fibrilla-tion, lung disease was found to be the principal con-tributing factor in 10% and was associated with other contributing factors in an additional 13%.[258]

Surgery[259, 260]

Coronary artery bypass graft operations.[261-263] Atrial fibrillation, the most frequently occurring sustained tachyarrhythmia after cardiac surgery,[264-267] appears in as many as one-third of patients after coronary surgery who were in sinus rhythm before the operation.[71, 265, 267-275] Patients who develop atrial fibrillation tend to be older than those who maintain sinus rhythm after surgery,[71, 273-280] and they have at least one of the follow-ing features before the operation:

- Atrial fibrillation.[275]
- Atrial premature beats[279] (and after the operation[280]).
- Cardiomegaly.[277]
- Congestive heart failure.[275]
- Demonstrable myocardial ischemia.[281]
- Hypertension.[274]
- Left atrial enlargement.[277]
- Previous myocardial infarctions.[282]
- Stenosis of the right coronary artery.[283]

Features of the operations in patients who develop atrial fibrillation postoperatively include the following:

- Heart rate of more than 100 beats per minute before bypass.[275]
- More bypass grafts and, consequently, longer periods of cardiopulmonary bypass.[276]
- Longer time for cross-clamping[275] and of myocardial ischemia.[271]
- Bicaval venous cannulation.[275]
- Venting of the pulmonary veins.[275]
- Use of crystalloid cardioplegia compared with blood cardioplegia.[284]
- Intraoperative intra-aortic balloon support.[274]
- Assisted ventilation for more than 24 hours.[274]

---

[x] From 151 cases in 4 series in which the incidence ranged from 10% to 50%.

[y] In 31 (24%) of 129 patients in 2 series. Atrial fibrillation was also present in 24% (7 of 29) of patients with idiopathic congestive cardiomyopathy.

[z] In 167 patients followed in the Cardiology Branch of the National Institutes of Health.

[aa] "Children who are afflicted with rheumatic fever in the first decade of life are just as likely to develop this arrhythmia as are patients first affected in later life provided they live long enough," according to Arthur C. DeGraff and C. Lingg in 1935.[104]

[bb] Sixteen of 234 patients in 3 series.

- Postoperative pacing.[275]
- Postoperative pneumonia.[274]
- Return to the intensive care unit.[274]
- Longer duration of atrial activity during cardioplegic arrest, possibly because of poor atrial protection during arrest.[285]
- Induction of atrial fibrillation after stimulation of the atria with alternating current.[286]

Anemia, type of venous drainage,[287] temperature,[288] or amount of potassium[287] in the cardioplegic solution, creatine kinase levels, and even perioperative myocardial infarction do not appear to influence the development of atrial fibrillation after surgery.[71, 273, 282, cc] Patients with atrial fibrillation after coronary surgery develop stroke more often than those who remain in sinus rhythm.[289] Compared with patients without atrial fibrillation, those who develop the arrhythmia after coronary surgery spend an average of 13 hours longer in the intensive care unit,[275] 2 days longer on the ward,[275] and 4.9 days longer in the hospital.[274]

Congenital heart disease.[290] Atrial fibrillation develops in some, particularly older, adults with atrial septal defect who were in sinus rhythm preoperatively,[201, 202, 208, 291–293] and it may persist, despite general clinical improvement, in those who had paroxysmal atrial fibrillation preoperatively.[294] Few patients with atrial septal defect and atrial fibrillation before operative repair revert to sinus rhythm after surgery.[207, 295] Atrial fibrillation seems to occur more frequently after operation in those patients whose atrial septal defect is associated with abnormal pulmonary venous return.[296] The arrhythmia also appears in a few children after surgical correction of congenital heart lesions, particularly transposition of the great vessels (Mustard procedure),[57, 296] the Fontan procedure,[297] and tetralogy of Fallot.[298]

Valvular surgery. Atrial fibrillation develops in 24% to 47% of patients with mitral stenosis after valvulotomy,[299, 300] and in 32% after valve replacement.[301] Patients who fibrillate after valvulotomy tend to be older, to have had prior episodes of atrial fibrillation, and to have some degree of mitral insufficiency.[299] The arrhythmia appears most frequently on the second day after operation.[302]

The most common arrhythmias after aortic valve replacement are atrial fibrillation and accelerated idioventricular rhythm, atrial fibrillation being the more frequent in patients older than 60 years of age.[303] Atrial premature beats herald the appearance of atrial fibrillation in these patients.[303]

Cardiac transplantation. Atrial fibrillation occasionally complicates the postoperative course of patients who receive cardiac transplantations.[304]

Cardioverter-defibrillator implantation. Implanting cardioverter-defibrillators by the epicardial technique,

which requires thoracotomy, produces atrial fibrillation; the incidence of the arrhythmia when the units are placed by the transvenous technique is very low.[305, dd]

Noncardiac surgery. Some patients also develop atrial fibrillation in association with noncardiac major surgery in the thoracic region[306–315] and elsewhere.[316]

Discharge in atrial fibrillation. Patients discharged in atrial fibrillation that has developed for the first time after cardiovascular surgery tend to be older and to have had valvular surgery, rather than coronary artery bypass graft surgery.[317]

Infective Endocarditis

Atrial fibrillation occurs infrequently,[318] but more than rarely, in patients with infective endocarditis.[319–322, ee]

Pericarditis

Atrial fibrillation develops frequently in constrictive pericarditis, in which it has been found in about 35% of patients[323–327, ff] and in up to 70% of those older than 40 years.[328] The arrhythmia rarely occurs in acute pericarditis.[329, 330, gg]

Tumors[331–336]

Atrial fibrillation is said to occur relatively frequently when primary and secondary tumors invade the heart and the pericardium.[337, hh] Patients with cardiac myxomas seldom develop atrial fibrillation despite the location of most of the tumors in the left atrium.[338–341, ii]

---

cc Some of the patients from whom these conclusions were derived received antianginal therapy, including beta-adrenergic blocking drugs, preoperatively but not during or after surgery.

dd New atrial fibrillation developed in 15% of 119 patients receiving their cardioverter-defibrillators by the epicardial technique but in only 1% of 110 patients when the transvenous method was used.[305]

ee In 14% of 427 cases reported when rheumatic valvulitis was the most common associated cardiac lesion.[318, 321] Wood correctly states: "There is no evidence that the two conditions are mutually antagonistic."[1912] As was suggested by Emanuel Libman more than 80 years ago:[319] "The observation that auricular fibrillation and active subacute infective endocarditis are mutually exclusive (save in an exceptional instance) is of diagnostic value."[320]

ff From 5 series reporting 235 patients.

gg Only 5 cases were observed in 100 consecutive patients with acute pericarditis, each of whom had some additional type of heart disease.[330] Not a single example of atrial fibrillation was detected in another series of 50 patients with acute pericarditis studied with Holter monitoring.[1913] Paul Wood suggests: "The difference between [constrictive pericarditis and acute pericarditis] is so remarkable that in differential diagnosis not only does atrial fibrillation suggest inactive disease of long duration but also normal rhythm actually favors activity."[325]

hh Although according to Davies and Pomerance (1972), "Atrial fibrillation is a well-known clinical complication of involvement of the heart by secondary carcinoma,"[337] there are few primary data on the incidence of the arrhythmia in patients with cancer. Standard texts and review articles discuss the coincidence without referencing to specific studies.[331–336]

ii Atrial fibrillation was present in only 9% of 141 patients with atrial myxoma from 4 series.[338–341]

Alcohol Ingestion

Ingestion of alcohol[342, *jj*] can induce arrhythmias in patients without overt manifestations of alcoholic cardiomyopathy.[343, 344] Atrial fibrillation is the most common of the sustained arrhythmias produced.[343, 345, *kk*]

Alcohol intoxication was the most frequent cause of new-onset atrial fibrillation in 40 patients admitted to a public hospital; alcohol played a substantial role in 35% and was the sole cause in 23%.[258] Alcohol causes atrial fibrillation more commonly in younger patients, whereas coronary heart disease and pulmonary disease contribute more frequently in patients older than 65 years of age.[258] Alcohol consumption is an independent risk factor for recurrences of the arrhythmia in men younger than 65 years old.[346]

Alcohol-induced atrial fibrillation occurs more frequently in males.[347] Men are less likely to complain of palpitations, possibly because of the intoxication itself, than are women with the arrhythmia.[347]

Atrial fibrillation can develop during alcohol withdrawal as well as during intoxication.[347] Patients in whom alcohol intoxication has been associated with paroxysmal atrial fibrillation seem more likely to develop findings of alcohol withdrawal than patients with a history of heavy alcohol intake without atrial fibrillation.[347]

The association of paroxysmal arrhythmias with weekends and holidays has led to use of the phrase "holiday heart" to characterize such cases.[345, 348] Arrhythmias, including atrial fibrillation, appear to occur in both regular, heavy drinkers and in usually sober individuals who celebrate too emphatically on special occasions.[349] Alcohol-induced atrial fibrillation, of course, is not limited to drinking on weekends or holidays.[39, 258, 347, 350, 351, *ll*] The experimental administration of alcohol has converted paroxysmal to sustained atrial fibrillation.[352]

Procedures

Cardioversion[353–355] and discharge of implantable cardioverter-defibrillators[356–361] to treat ventricular arrhythmias can occasionally induce atrial fibrillation. Ablating the atria to treat atrial flutter produces transient or sustained atrial fibrillation in some patients.[362, 363] Carotid sinus pressure can occasionally induce atrial fibrillation.[364–368]

Lone Atrial Fibrillation

Idiopathic or lone atrial fibrillation is a diagnosis of exclusion,[369] assigned to patients with the arrhythmia when no cause can be established.[370] The arrhythmia has also been called benign, functional, senile, and atrial fibrillation of unknown origin or without heart disease.[370]

Prevalence. No overt cardiovascular disease or precipitating illness was observed in 2.7% of 3,623 patients with atrial fibrillation at the Mayo Clinic in Rochester, Minnesota[371] and in 11% of 376 patients in the Framingham study.[69] In patients older than 64 years, most patients with atrial fibrillation have structural heart disease; consequently, lone atrial fibrillation is uncommon at this age.[79]

The most frequently missed diagnoses in patients given the presumptive diagnosis of lone atrial fibrillation are probably cardiomyopathy[328] and thyrotoxicosis.[187, 372] However, asymptomatic coronary artery disease can easily be overlooked. In a study conducted in 1961 of 12 patients thought to have lone atrial fibrillation by clinical criteria, 7 had moderate to severe coronary atherosclerosis at postmortem examination.[373] Today, with more sophisticated invasive and noninvasive diagnostic techniques, organic heart disease may be recognized in patients formerly thought to have lone atrial fibrillation.[374]

Patients with lone atrial fibrillation seldom also have supraventricular tachycardia resulting from reentry in the atrioventricular node or accessory pathways.[375] Most,[57] but not all,[376] children with atrial fibrillation have organic heart disease.

Gender. All series that included both men and women with lone atrial fibrillation report a predominance of men.[43, 69, 92, 127, 236, 371, 377, 378, *mm*]

Risk factors. The usual risk factors for the development of heart disease—systolic blood pressure, serum cholesterol, diabetes, body mass, ethanol consumption, coffee consumption, and use of cigarettes—were not different for patients with or without lone atrial fibrillation in the Framingham study.[69] In electrocardiograms taken before atrial fibrillation developed, abnormal ST and T waves occurred twice as often and intraventricular block occurred four times as often as in patients who developed atrial fibrillation.[69]

Autonomic influences.[379, 380] The autonomic nervous system can dramatically affect the arrhythmia in patients with lone atrial fibrillation.[381–382] Bradycardia from heightened vagal activity can favor the development of paroxysms of atrial fibrillation.[383–389] The patients, usually between the ages of 40 and 50 years and predominantly men (4:1), develop paroxysms that occur weekly, or more or less frequently, and last from a few minutes to several hours. Episodes usually occur when the patient is resting, either during sleep or after the evening meal. The shorter the paroxysms, the more frequent the attacks. The P waves are abnormal, a finding suggesting intra-atrial conduction defects, and the F waves often are coarse or have the form

---

jj Or even inhalation of frosty peppermint Binaca breath spray, 60% of which is 120-proof standard denatured alcohol.[342]

kk "This form is more apt to evolve in high-strung people."[343]

ll "After all, ethanol is the culprit instead of Saturdays, Sundays, or holidays," M. Kupari and P. Koskinen remind us.[351]

---

mm Seventy-nine percent of 310 patients in 7 series.[43, 69, 92, 236, 371, 377, 378]

of flutter-fibrillation. The arrhythmia seldom becomes chronic.

Paroxysms of atrial fibrillation have also been related to adrenergic stimulation, particularly in the morning or during exercise or emotional stress.[387, 390, 391, nn] Autonomic influences presumably participated in the production of atrial fibrillation in two patients with elevated intracranial pressure, one of whom had a subarachnoid hemorrhage;[392] the other had no cardiac lesions at autopsy.[393] Vagal tone decreases and sympathetic tone increases before paroxysmal atrial fibrillation begins in patients after coronary artery bypass graft surgery.[280]

Circadian Influences

Atrial tachyarrhythmias, most often atrial fibrillation according to one study, begin in the morning and evening and least frequently during the night.[394] Other investigators, who have found circadian cycles, report that atrial fibrillation begins slightly more often from 12 midnight[395] to 2 a.m.[396] or after lunch[395] than at other times of the day or night.[397, oo]

Beta-adrenergic blocking drugs reduce the morning frequency and increase the preference for paroxysms to start during the night.[394] In the absence of these drugs, adrenergic stimuli may predispose the patient to paroxysms in the morning, whereas vagal stimuli may predominate in patients taking these drugs.[394]

Miscellaneous Conditions and Situations

Atrial fibrillation has been observed in the following situations:

- In heredofamilial neuromyopathic disorders such as the muscular dystrophies.[398]
- With an intrapericardial lipoma compressing the left atrium.[399]
- From fat infiltration of the myocardium.[400]
- In cold weather, which increases the likelihood that patients will develop paroxysmal atrial fibrillation.[401, pp]
- From swallowing frozen yogurt.[402]

Emboli and Stroke[403–409]

Patients with atrial fibrillation are more likely to develop emboli and stroke[410, 411] than are patients in sinus rhythm.[64, 70, 233, 412–426, qq] Those with chronic fibrillation are more often affected than patients with paroxysms.[371, 427, 428]

Prevalence. About 22% of patients with atrial fibril-

lation sustain systemic emboli.[102, 106, 126, 183, 415, 427, 429–431, rr] When stroke occurs in patients with atrial fibrillation, embolism from the heart is the mechanism in about 75% of cases.[432] About 17% of patients with stroke[433, 434, ss] and 75% of patients with peripheral emboli[418, 435] have atrial fibrillation.

Embolism develops, in patients with chronic atrial fibrillation, at a rate of about 5% per patient-year.[411, 415, 436] Computed tomographic scans reveal that many patients with nonrheumatic atrial fibrillation sustain silent cerebral infarction.[437]

The risk of emboli in patients with atrial fibrillation is higher in those who have had a previous stroke[438, 439] or are female,[440] hypertensive,[439] or older.[413, 414, 425, 439, 441, 442, tt] Atrial fibrillation itself is the single most important characteristic associated with stroke in women older than 70 years,[424] it is more important than hypertension in producing cerebral infarction in the aged, and it may contribute to the development of dementia in older patients.[443]

Time of occurrence. Embolic complications cluster at the onset of paroxysmal atrial fibrillation[434] and after paroxysmal fibrillation converts to chronic fibrillation.[427] In patients with coronary heart disease, 40% of emboli occur when atrial fibrillation begins,[126] and in patients with rheumatic heart disease, one-third of emboli occur within 1 month and two-thirds occur within 12 months.[415] Emboli develop more frequently in patients who have recently sustained emboli than in those who have not.[435, 444, 445] Some patients with atrial fibrillation who present with strokes have had asymptomatic cerebral infarctions previously.[446] Although the incidence is low, emboli also occur when sinus rhythm is reestablished spontaneously, by drugs, or by electrical cardioversion.[447] Stroke that develops just *before* the onset of atrial fibrillation may cause the arrhythmia to appear.[448]

Etiology of heart disease. In patients with atrial fibrillation, emboli develop more often in the presence of structural heart disease,[440] such as the following:

- Mitral valve disease, 35%.[436]
- Ischemic and hypertensive disease, 18%.[436]
- Hyperthyroidism, 11%.[183, 436, 449–451, uu]

At autopsy, the frequency of emboli is higher in patients with atrial fibrillation and valvular disease than in those with other causes of heart disease.[429, 447, vv]

---

nn And after such extraordinary stresses as having been bitten by a black widow spider, which produced high levels of urinary catecholamines.[390]

oo Another study found no characteristic time of day when paroxysms start in most patients.[397]

pp Researchers from a hospital in Helsinki, Finland found that admission for new-onset atrial fibrillation was 2 to 3 times higher in winter than in summer among 100 consecutive patients.[401] They suggested that greater use of alcohol during cold weather may have contributed to the higher incidence.

qq This complication led one worker to observe: "Atrial fibrillation is indeed a neurological problem."[419]

rr From several series reporting a total of 3,106 patients. A wide range of incidence has been found because the different series include patients with paroxysmal or chronic fibrillation; from medical, neurological, pathological, and other inpatient and outpatient services; with fibrillation for different periods of time; and with different types of heart disease.

ss One hundred thirty-seven (17%) patients with atrial fibrillation among 817 with stroke in 2 large series.

tt The Framingham Study found that the risk of patients with atrial fibrillation having a stroke rises from 1.5% for those aged 50 to 59 years to 23.5% for those aged 80 to 89 years.[425]

uu Forty-one patients with emboli from 373 with thyrotoxicosis and atrial fibrillation.[183, 436, 449–451]

vv Forty-five percent in those with mitral valve disease and 35% in those with ischemic and hypertensive disease.[429]

The emboli arise from clots in the left atrium and its appendage,[337, 452] which, when larger, are more likely to produce thromboembolism.[64, 417, 439, 453, 454, ww]

Valvular disease. Compared with the risk of stroke with sinus rhythm, the risk of stroke when chronic atrial fibrillation complicates rheumatic heart disease is 17 times greater and 5 times greater in other types of heart disease.[455] Emboli develop more often when the mitral lesion is stenosis than regurgitation,[456] but the incidence does not relate to the severity of the obstruction.[414] Predominant mitral regurgitation, however, does cause emboli in patients with atrial fibrillation.[64, xx]

Isolated mitral regurgitation, however, may not increase,[427] and may even decrease,[457, 458] the production of emboli in patients with nonvalvular atrial fibrillation.[yy] Atrial fibrillation further increases the risk of stroke in patients with mitral annular calcification.[459]

The operative mortality of patients with atrial fibrillation after mitral commissurotomy is higher than when sinus rhythm is present, mostly because of systemic emboli.[106] Although emboli occur more frequently in older patients with mitral valve disease and atrial fibrillation, the incidence is not inconsequential in younger patients.[64, 413] Mitral annular calcification does not increase the risk of stroke in patients with atrial fibrillation.[460]

Myocardial infarction. Although atrial fibrillation increases the risk of stroke during myocardial infarction,[148] this complication infrequently occurs, whether or not anticoagulation has been given.[66, 130, 135, 137, 139–141, 143, zz]

Nonvalvular disease. Stroke, probably resulting from emboli, which also occurs with nonvalvular paroxysmal[427] and chronic atrial fibrillation,[427, 455, 461–463] develops in 35% of patients[424] at a rate of 2.98% per year.[464] The risk of a second stroke rises to as much as 20% per year in patients with atrial fibrillation who have had one cerebrovascular event.[465] The incidence of fatal cerebral infarction in the elderly is high.[466]

The risk of stroke when atrial fibrillation develops increases in patients with any of the following factors:[467, aaa]

- Acute[148] or previous myocardial infarction.[468]
- Congestive heart failure[469] within 3 months.
- Hypertension.[463, 469]
- Previous arterial thromboembolism.[462]

Patients without diabetes have a low risk of embolism, and those with no risk factors who are under the age of 60 have no thromboembolism.[467]

Some,[467, 470–472] but not all,[473] reports suggest that left atrial enlargement increases the risk of ischemic stroke in patients with nonvalvular heart disease and atrial fibrillation. Patients with left ventricular hypertrophy[460] and dysfunction[467] also have more strokes.

Cardiomyopathy. Atrial fibrillation increases the likelihood that patients with idiopathic dilated cardiomyopathy will develop systemic emboli.[233, 420] Systemic emboli occur at a rate of 2.4% per patient-year in those with hypertrophic cardiomyopathy and atrial fibrillation. Cardiomegaly, left atrial enlargement, and decreased cardiac index[420] also contribute to the development of atrial fibrillation in these patients.

Atrial septal defect. Atrial fibrillation, age, and pulmonary hypertension increase the number of emboli that may develop in patients after surgical repair of atrial septal defects.[206]

Lone atrial fibrillation. Emboli seldom develop in patients with lone atrial fibrillation,[92, 236, 350, 370, 474–477] particularly when these patients are younger than 60[371] or even 70[477] years of age. However, the Framingham Study revealed that patients with lone atrial fibrillation have more emboli than similar patients in sinus rhythm.[69]

Coronary surgery. Patients who develop atrial fibrillation after coronary artery bypass graft operations have more strokes than those patients who remain in sinus rhythm.[289]

Congestive heart failure. Despite the increased incidence of thromboembolic events when atrial fibrillation appears in many settings, a large study of patients with congestive heart failure found that morbidity from embolic events did not increase when atrial fibrillation developed.[478, bbb]

Thyrotoxicosis. Patients who develop atrial fibrillation during thyrotoxicosis are not immune to developing emboli.[450, ccc]

Resolution of intra-atrial thrombi. Transesophageal echocardiography of patients with nonrheumatic atrial fibrillation reveals that thrombi in the left atrium and its appendage resolve after 3 weeks of treatment with warfarin, thereby permitting cardioversion to be conducted without danger of emboli.[452] These observations suggest that the mechanism of such treatment is resolution of the current thrombus and prevention of new thrombus formation, not thrombus organization.[452]

---

ww Before echocardiography resolved the question, workers differed on whether the size of the left atrial appendage influenced the incidence of emboli.[64, 417, 453]

xx Twenty-two percent in one series.[64]

yy The presence of mitral regurgitation reduces the levels of blood factors favoring coagulation in patients with nonrheumatic atrial fibrillation.[458]

zz Furthermore, one can infer that the incidence of emboli is low from the many reports that do not specifically mention emboli in patients with acute myocardial infarction who develop atrial fibrillation.[66, 139–141, 143]

aaa Rates of thrombosis per year per factor (not including previous myocardial infarction): 2.5% per year, no factors; 7.2% per year, 1 factor; 17.6% per year, 2 or 3 factors.[467]

bbb The Veterans Affairs Vasodilator-Heart Failure Trial (V-HeFT).[478]

ccc Emboli complicated the course of 5 (24%) of 21 patients with thyrotoxicosis who developed atrial fibrillation.[450]

OTHER ARRHYTHMIAS IN PATIENTS WITH ATRIAL FIBRILLATION

Atrial Flutter[407]

One-fourth of patients with atrial fibrillation also have periods of atrial flutter.[479, ddd] The frequency of this association is particularly high after open-heart surgery and in patients taking antiarrhythmic drugs.[479]

Atrial Dissociation

Rarely, atrial fibrillation may coexist with sinus rhythm or arrhythmias such as atrial flutter or atrial tachycardia either in the contralateral atrium or even within the same chamber and may produce the condition known as atrial dissociation.[480–491, eee] Atrial dissociation usually occurs in very ill patients with severe heart disease.[492]

Atrial dissociation has been recognized from surface electrocardiograms and has been established with intracavitary recordings from the right atrium, left atrium, coronary sinus,[487, 493] and esophagus,[484, 493] from which signals in the adjacent left atrium can be recorded.

In some cases, coarse atrial fibrillation may be due to interatrial dissociation in which a regular arrhythmia with more uniform depolarizations appears in one chamber and a faster and more irregular arrhythmia appears in the other.[484] "Flutter-fibrillation," in which forms suggesting both arrhythmias appear in the same electrocardiographic recording, may develop from interatrial dissociation.[487] This requires the presence of a rapid regular tachycardia in one of the atria,[493] and it is not present when atrial fibrillation is the only rhythm in both atria.[493]

Sick Sinus Syndrome[494]

Atrial fibrillation is present in 8% of patients when the diagnosis of sick sinus syndrome is made.[495, fff] It developed during the course of sick sinus syndrome[496, 497] in 16% of patients followed for 38 months[495, ggg] and in 7% (or 1.4% per year) of patients who received atrial pacing for sick sinus syndrome.[498] Atrial fibrillation occurs more frequently in patients with sick sinus syndrome than in those with atrioventricular block.[499]

Supraventricular Tachycardia

Atrial fibrillation develops in about 12% of patients with paroxysmal supraventricular tachycardia over the course of 1 year.[500] Its occurrence is unrelated to their age,[501] the number of years of supraventricular tachycardia,[501] the heart rate during tachycardia,[500, 501] or coexistent heart disease.[501] Atrial fibrillation develops

whether the supraventricular tachycardia is sustained within the atrioventricular node or through accessory pathways.[500] Among patients with paroxysmal atrial fibrillation, the next tachycardia is regular and presumably supraventricular tachycardia in about 12% of recurrences, and among those with supraventricular tachycardia the next paroxysm of tachyarrhythmia is atrial fibrillation in about 6.5%.[397]

Spontaneous supraventricular tachycardia occurs in 38% of patients with Wolff-Parkinson-White syndrome and atrial fibrillation.[164] Supraventricular tachycardia, sustained through accessory pathways, often precedes the onset of atrial fibrillation and produces fibrillation in susceptible atria by rapid stimulation of those chambers.

His Bundle (Junctional) Escape Beats

His bundle escape beats usually have a normal QRS complex and terminate the longest RR intervals.[502] They arise when the bundle of His is called on to discharge the ventricles after a pause of varying length produced by atrioventricular nodal block.

His Bundle Rhythm

When His bundle escape beats dominate the rhythm of the heart, His bundle or junctional rhythm is said to be present. His bundle rhythms are regular, and their presence implies that a relatively high degree of atrioventricular nodal block has developed that prevents atrial impulses from reaching the bundle of His. The rhythm of the ventricles under these circumstances is unaffected by atrial electrical activity, and cardiologists say that atrioventricular dissociation is present.

His bundle rhythms can arise in the presence of both atrioventricular nodal block and acceleration of His bundle pacemakers. Digitalis, acute inferior myocardial infarction, cardiac surgery, or myocarditis most frequently produce these rhythms in the presence of atrial fibrillation.[503–505] His bundle escapes and rhythms in patients with atrial fibrillation may be associated with periodic apnea, as in Cheyne-Stokes respiration.[504, 505]

Atrioventricular Block

The ventricular rate in atrial fibrillation depends primarily on the quality of conduction through the atrioventricular node. Atrioventricular block, however, may coexist with atrial fibrillation,[506, 507] and it is detected by a slow ventricular response or a long PR interval after conversion to sinus rhythm.[35, 508–510] Slight first-degree atrioventricular block is frequently found at this time.[35]

Patients with paroxysmal atrial fibrillation during acute myocardial infarction may display long PR intervals before the arrhythmia develops and after return to sinus rhythm.[511] Atrioventricular block also occurs in many patients with lone atrial fibrillation;[236] the ventricular response in untreated patients may be rela-

---

ddd According to one study of 96 patients.[479]

eee Some electrocardiographers have suggested that the findings called atrial dissociation in some cases may have been due to potentials from the diaphragm or accessory muscles of respiration.[482, 485]

fff From a comprehensive review of 21 studies with 958 patients.

ggg From 1,171 patients compiled from 19 studies.

tively slow and does not increase much with exercise.[92, 370, hhh]

When intrinsic atrioventricular block develops in patients with atrial fibrillation and the ventricular rate decreases, one cannot grade the block as first or second degree if sinus rhythm has not been observed. Third-degree, or complete, atrioventricular block, however, can be recognized by a regular ventricular rate. The ventricles are then driven by intrinsic pacemakers in the specialized conducting tissues of the His bundle, bundle branches, or Purkinje network. The atria were fibrillating in one-fourth of patients with complete atrioventricular block in a series compiled before pacemakers were available.[512]

When the intrinsic pacemaker is located in the bundle of His, the form of the QRS complex is normal, so long as concurrent bundle branch block is absent. Wide QRS complexes suggest that the pacemaker arises within the ventricles. Ventricular pacemakers tend to discharge more slowly than do His bundle pacemakers.

Partial or complete heart block in patients with atrial fibrillation may be permanent or transient. Atrioventricular nodal inflammation from inferior myocardial infarction, myocarditis, or cardiac surgery, transient increases in vagal tone, and the effects of atrioventricular nodal depressing drugs such as digitalis and amiodarone can all produce temporary atrioventricular block in patients with atrial fibrillation, as well as those in sinus rhythm.

Ventricular Tachycardia and Fibrillation

Dangerous ventricular arrhythmias develop concurrently in patients with atrial fibrillation who have advanced structural heart disease. In patients with coronary heart disease, the atrial arrhythmia may incite the ventricular tachyarrhythmias when the rapid ventricular response produces ischemia.

Atrial fibrillation produces ventricular fibrillation in a few patients with Wolff-Parkinson-White syndrome because of rapid conduction in their accessory pathways.[158, 173, 513–520] Even patients without preexcitation may occasionally develop ventricular fibrillation from transmission of atrial fibrillation through rapidly conducting atrioventricular nodes[518, 520] or perinodal tissues, as in the Lown-Ganong-Levine syndrome.[521, 522, iii]

Paced Rhythms

Many patients whose ventricles are being permanently paced have atrial fibrillation, the presence of which is frequently overlooked.[523, jjj]

SYMPTOMS[524]

Rapid beating of the heart is the symptom that patients with atrial fibrillation observe most often when the arrhythmia first appears. They sense the tachycardia as palpitations in the chest, but they may, or may not, perceive that the rhythm of the beats is irregular[525] or that the intensity of the beats varies. In addition to palpitations, patients may sense characteristic symptoms of reduced cardiac output, congestive heart failure, or ischemia. Dyspnea, lightheadedness, weakness, sweating, pallor, chest pain, and, rarely, fainting[526, 527] can all appear.[528, kkk]

Syncope and Dizziness

Patients seldom faint from a paroxysm of atrial fibrillation, although atrial fibrillation may be present when people become dizzy or faint.[529] Syncope, however, occurs not infrequently in young subjects with Wolff-Parkinson-White syndrome and rapid ventricular rates during atrial fibrillation,[526, 530] and occasionally it results from neurocardiogenic influences.[527]

Perception of the Arrhythmia

Many patients observe when a paroxysm of atrial fibrillation replaces sinus rhythm,[42, 92, 395] but most perceive fewer episodes than actually occur.[531] Patients are less likely to detect the arrhythmia when the ventricular rate is relatively slow.[395] Slight decrease in cardiac output or irregularity of the pulse at a relatively slow rate can easily be overlooked, particularly by patients who tend to be unaware of changes in the function of their bodies, who are intoxicated,[347] or who have limited mental capability to perceive such changes. In such cases, the patients may be surprised when physicians tell them that they have an arrhythmia.

In general, the more severe and persistent the symptoms, the faster the heartbeat and the greater the structural cardiac disease.[532] Consequently, a young person with paroxysms of lone atrial fibrillation and an otherwise normal heart may have few symptoms other than palpitations.[350] Conversely, a patient with coronary, valvular, or myocardial disease may develop alarming symptoms of congestive heart failure, ischemia, and even myocardial infarction when paroxysmal atrial fibrillation appears at a relatively slow rate.

Paroxysmal Atrial Fibrillation

Paroxysms of atrial fibrillation, lasting from seconds to days, usually precede the establishment of chronic or permanent atrial fibrillation. Although paroxysms can last for more than 2 weeks,[533] in only about 20% do attacks last longer than 2 days.[534, 535, lll]

[hhh] "Thus, in our series [W. Evans and P. Swann in 1954] it was never as rapid as 100 per minute. In only two cases was it 90 or over during the first clinical examination. It was 70 or under in 11 and 60 or under in three. The slower rate was natural for each patient and not the result of digitalization."[370]

[iii] Short PR interval, normal QRS complex, atrial arrhythmia.[521]

[jjj] Fifty-three (48%) of 110 consecutive patients attending the pacemaker clinic at a university hospital had atrial fibrillation.[523]

[kkk] About two-thirds of 69 patients with atrial fibrillation or supraventricular tachycardia considered their symptoms to be at least moderately disruptive to their lives.[528]

[lll] "The immediate attack . . . will seldom persist more than two days. But if it lasts a week, permanent fibrillation becomes much more likely, and after two weeks almost certain. . . . Rheumatic heart disease makes permanent fibrillation more likely. The absence of any underlying heart disease makes it much less likely," observed John Parkinson and Maurice Campbell in 1941.[534]

Seventy percent of paroxysms of atrial fibrillation lasting less than 72 hours convert spontaneously to sinus rhythm.[536] Twenty-two percent of patients spontaneously return to sinus rhythm within 2 hours[537, mmm] and about half return to sinus rhythm within 24 hours.[535] Presentation with symptoms lasting less than 24 hours best predicts spontaneous conversion.[536]

The older the patient, the sooner paroxysmal atrial fibrillation first recurs.[397] Paroxysms sometimes develop during or after certain activities such as the following:

- Sleeping.[381, 383]
- Smoking.[39, 350]
- Swallowing.[39, 538]
- Excessive intake of food,[39, 535] coffee,[371] cola,[371] or alcohol.[39, 345, 347, 350, 371]
- Nausea and vomiting from gastroenteritis and other acute abdominal illness.[39, 350]
- Strenuous physical activity.[39, 350, 371, 535]
- Overwork or mental stress.[39, 350, 371]

Progression to chronic fibrillation. About one-fourth of patients with paroxysmal atrial fibrillation eventually develop permanent arrhythmia.[533, 535, nnn] Patients with lone atrial fibrillation, however, often have many paroxysms over years or decades and seldom develop the permanent form.[69, 126, 253, 328, 374, 477, 533, ooo]

Nonrheumatic paroxysmal atrial fibrillation will most likely become chronic within 1 year when four of the following are present:[539]

- Age 65 years or older.
- Cardiothoracic ratio 50% or greater.
- Congestive heart failure.
- Diabetes mellitus.
- Electrocardiographic F-wave amplitude 2.0 mm or greater.
- Echocardiographic left atrial dimension 38 mm or greater.
- Left ventricular ejection fraction less than 77%.

Classification.[540] To define the clinical features of paroxysmal atrial fibrillation better, hospitalized patients with this arrhythmia can be categorized into three classes:[541]

I. First attack
 A. With spontaneous termination
 B. Requiring pharmacological or electrical conversion because of associated symptoms
II. Recurrent attacks without treatment with antiarrhythmic agents to prevent recurrences

A. No symptoms during the attack
B. Less than one symptomatic attack every 3 months
C. One symptomatic attack every 3 months
III. Recurrent attacks despite treatment with antiarrhythmic agents to prevent recurrences
 A. No symptoms
 B. Less than one symptomatic attack per 3-month period
 C. More than one symptomatic attack per 3-month period

Delayed Spontaneous Conversion

A few patients who have had chronic atrial fibrillation for many years convert spontaneously to sinus rhythm.[542–554, ppp]

PHYSICAL EXAMINATION

The most obvious sign of atrial fibrillation is an irregular pulse[555] or heartbeat in which no repetitive pattern can be discerned.[48, qqq] The irregularity of the heartbeat, the changing periods of ventricular diastolic filling, and the post-extrasystolic potentiation[556] produce variations in the pulse and the heart sounds.

Arterial Pulse

During atrial fibrillation, ventricular filling varies, and the left and right ventricular contents of each beat are not transmitted to the pulmonary or systemic circulation with the same force.[557] Consequently, the blood pressure changes from beat to beat.[558] One may also hear more beats from the heart than one can detect as Korotkoff sounds when taking the blood pressure or when feeling at the wrist.[559–561] This difference, known as the pulse deficit, is characteristic of atrial fibrillation, although it occurs in other irregular supraventricular arrhythmias such as multifocal atrial tachycardia.

The pulse deficit is greater when the ventricular response is rapid and severe myocardial or valvular dysfunction is present. The contents of the left ventricle or the force that ejects the blood may be inadequate to open the aortic valve.[562] Then, of course, no pulse is felt. Moreover, for other weak beats, the operator may feel no pulse, even though interarterial and external recordings of flow reveal that some blood has been propelled beyond the aortic valve. Large pulse deficits occur infrequently in patients with lone atrial

---

mmm Seven of 32 patients given a placebo in a trial of the effects of 2 antiarrhythmic drugs.[537]

nnn This was Maurice Campbell's observation more than half a century ago.[535] In another series of patients studied almost 2 decades ago, 19 (25%) of 75 patients with paroxysmal atrial fibrillation who were followed for more than 12 months developed the permanent form.[533] Data from other reports on how often paroxysmal atrial fibrillation becomes permanent vary, however, because most series include patients with different types and severity of organic heart disease.

ooo Half of the 70 cases of lone atrial fibrillation in Paul Wood's series were paroxysmal.[328]

ppp Of 45 cases collected from the reviewers' personal experience and the literature in 1980, 39 had significant rheumatic mitral valve disease.[553]

qqq Sir Thomas Lewis wrote in 1934: "Characteristically, the pulse is turbulent, or grossly irregular; it consists of a medley of beats, varying in force and most unevenly spaced."[48] An old diagnostic aid of uncertain provenance uses the foot as if it were a metronome. While palpating the pulse, the operator starts tapping his or her foot to what appears to be the rhythm. Because the foot tends to beat regularly, comparison with the pulse can help one to differentiate sinus rhythm with premature beats and compensatory pauses from atrial fibrillation.

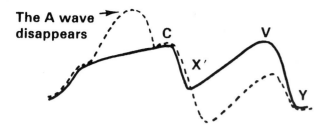

The A wave disappears

FIGURE 4.1   Atrial fibrillation causes the A wave in the venous pulse to disappear. The A wave in sinus rhythm requires right atrial contraction *(dotted line)* and is absent during atrial fibrillation *(solid line).* (Adapted from Constant J. Bedside Cardiology. 3rd ed. Boston: Little, Brown, 1985, p. 108, with permission.)[564]

fibrillation[92] because the ventricular rate even in untreated cases is relatively slow and the heart is structurally normal. Because of the pulse deficit, treatment to slow the heart rate must be guided by examination of the apical pulse or the QRS complexes of an electrocardiographic monitor and not by the impulses felt or recorded at a peripheral vessel. Ambulatory blood pressure monitoring devices provide data comparable to those obtained with the stethoscope and mercury manometer in patients with atrial fibrillation.[563]

Venous Pulse

The A wave, produced by right atrial contraction, disappears during atrial fibrillation[564] (Fig. 4.1). Consequently, one can overlook the presence of tricuspid stenosis because the characteristic large A waves from right atrial contraction against stenotic tricuspid valves are absent in patients with atrial fibrillation.[565]

Heart Sounds

The rhythm of the heart sounds is characteristically irregular in atrial fibrillation. The intensity of the first sound, in particular,[566] and of the second heart sound can vary greatly. The rate may be so rapid and ventricular filling so small that the atrioventricular valves are not driven shut quickly so as to produce an easily audible first sound, or the semilunar valves are not opened so that they may close and produce the second heart sound. A characteristic exception occurs in mitral stenosis, where the snapping first sound often,[567] but not always,[568] maintains the same intensity from beat to beat during atrial fibrillation. The first sound, however, may be louder in some patients when diastole is short.[568] When the regular rhythm of complete atrioventricular block coexists with atrial fibrillation, the intensity of the first sound is constant.

Third heart sounds may be present when the usual causes such as youth, congestive heart failure, or mitral regurgitation are present. Fourth heart sounds, of course, are not heard because of the absence of atrial contraction.[rrr] Additional diastolic sounds are occasion-

ally heard in patients with "coarse" atrial fibrillation. The cause of this finding has not been established.[569]

The interval between the aortic closure sound and the opening snap of the mitral valve in patients with mitral stenosis varies with the different cycle lengths of atrial fibrillation.[570] This finding can seldom be detected by auscultation, however. The pericardial knock that is characteristic of constrictive pericarditis can be confused with an opening snap of the mitral valve when atrial fibrillation is present.[571]

Murmurs

The systolic murmurs that originate from abnormal pulmonary and aortic valves and from their outflow tracks are characteristically louder after long diastolic periods and softer after shorter periods. The systolic murmurs of mitral or tricuspid regurgitation, however, change little with variations in the length of diastole.[572, 573] This difference provides a useful clue in distinguishing aortic stenosis from mitral regurgitation when the heartbeat is irregular.

The presystolic accentuation of the diastolic rumble of mitral stenosis may disappear when atrial fibrillation develops because of the loss of atrial contraction that produces this auscultatory finding. However, when the ventricular rate is rapid and a diastolic gradient from left atrium to left ventricle persists, the mid-diastolic murmur may occur sufficiently close to the first heart sound to simulate presystolic accentuation.[574–577] Even in the absence of mitral stenosis, a presystolic murmur may appear during atrial fibrillation because of early closure of the normal mitral valve[577] or the initial effects of ventricular contraction.[578]

ELECTROCARDIOGRAM DURING ATRIAL FIBRILLATION

Irregularity of the rhythm of the QRS complexes and the absence of uniform atrial activity are the electrocardiographic features most useful for making the diagnosis of atrial fibrillation.

Rate

The ventricular rate in patients with untreated atrial fibrillation, normal atrioventricular conduction, and no preexcitation ranges from 100 to 200 beats per minute.[579–582, sss] The average rate tends to decrease as patients age[583] (Fig. 4.2).

Ventricular rate. The ventricular rate, which is faster at the onset of paroxysmal atrial fibrillation than in sinus rhythm immediately before the paroxysm begins,[584, ttt] decreases spontaneously as time passes.[584] The

---

[rrr] Many a teacher has tried to confound many a medical student presenting a case of atrial fibrillation by asking, "And could you hear S₄?"

[sss] According to cardiology textbooks, 120 to 150[581] and 100 to 160[582] in chronic atrial fibrillation, and up to 180 to 200 in paroxysmal atrial fibrillation.[579] Intervals of at least 6 seconds should be analyzed to gauge the average heart rate accurately at rest and during exercise in patients with atrial fibrillation.[580]

[ttt] An average of 80 beats per minute in sinus rhythm and 124 beats per minute in atrial fibrillation in 18 subjects.[584]

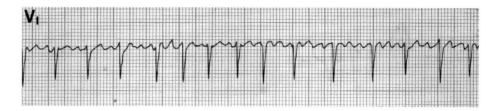

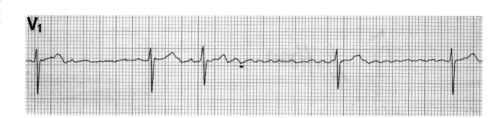

FIGURE 4.2 Different ventricular responses to atrial fibrillation. The rapid average ventricular rate is 150 beats per minute *(upper panel)*, and the rate in the slow example 45 beats per minute *(lower panel)*.

mean ventricular response in untreated patients is faster during paroxysmal than in chronic atrial fibrillation,[583] and it tends to be slower in patients with lone atrial fibrillation[92, 370] than in patients with structural heart disease. The ventricular rate in a patient with spontaneous subarachnoid hemorrhage and atrial fibrillation slowed to 40 beats per minute, probably from autonomic stimulation.[392]

Wolff-Parkinson-White syndrome. The ventricular response in patients with atrial fibrillation and Wolff-Parkinson-White syndrome is characteristically faster than in patients without accessory pathways. Rates of more than 200 beats per minute are frequently encountered, although the range of rates in untreated patients is wide.[164] Children with preexcitation may sustain ventricular rates of more than 300 beats per minute.[173]

P Waves and F Waves

Atrial fibrillation is characterized by the absence of P waves between T waves and QRS complexes. The fibrillating atria produce a continuous undulating baseline made up of what are often called F waves, the amplitude and form of which vary (Fig. 4.3). The peaks of these deflections appear at irregular intervals. F waves are often best seen in right precordial leads,[585] and they are seen least well in leads I, aVL, and the left chest leads.

The size of the F waves decreases as the duration of atrial fibrillation increases[510, 560, 586, *uuu*] and as patients with atrial fibrillation grow older.[587] Atrial volume is

---

uuu Or as D. S. Brachman put it in 1921: "The auricles will continue to fibrillate until they become completely exhausted. The auricle waves in the electrocardiogram then become very small and fine, and ultimately disappear almost entirely."[560]

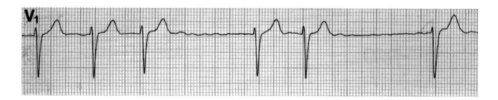

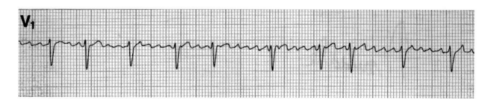

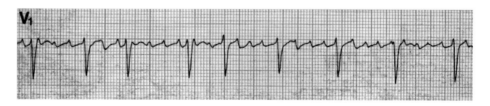

FIGURE 4.3 F waves during atrial fibrillation. "Fine" F waves *(upper panel)* may be barely visible. "Coarse" F waves *(middle panel)* have greater amplitude. In "flutter-fibrillation" *(bottom panel)*, the large F waves appear to be regular, but measurement will indicate their irregularity. The F waves of atrial fibrillation are best seen in lead V₁, whereas flutter waves tend to be largest in leads II, III, or aVF.

greater in chronic atrial fibrillation that has persisted more than 3 months than in transient atrial fibrillation lasting 1 month or less.[586] Youth and normal PR intervals in sinus rhythm are associated with large F waves.[510] In patients whose left atria are small but who have large F waves, the arrhythmia can be converted to sinus rhythm relatively easily.[510]

The form and size of the F waves in atrial fibrillation tend to remain constant, but in a few cases, the size grows or diminishes as the patient's disease progresses.[588] Digitalis may,[588] or may not,[589] decrease the size of F waves; possibly, it relieves congestive heart failure and consequently reduces cardiac size.[590]

Other factors postulated to affect the size of F waves are degeneration of atrial muscle,[586] increase in fibrosis with aging,[586] tissue edema,[586] lung volume,[586] posture,[586] respiration,[586] chest size,[586] intra-atrial conduction defects,[591] increased left atrial pressure,[592] left atrial hypertrophy,[593] right or biatrial enlargement,[590] and the ratio of atrial hypertrophy to dilatation.[594]

Controversial determinants of size of F waves. Larger or "coarse" F waves have been reported to be associated with rheumatic heart disease,[588, 589, 592-595] particularly when left atrial enlargement is present[594] or when mitral stenosis is severe.[588] In lone atrial fibrillation, even in patients without left atrial enlargement, large F waves have been said to predominate.[594]

Small or "fine" F waves have been reported to characterize many patients with coronary[588, 592, 594, 595] and hypertensive[594, 595] heart disease. In patients with atrial fibrillation caused by thyrotoxicosis, large[594] or small[588] F waves have been found.

Echocardiographic,[591] radiological,[593] and autopsy[586, 589] studies, however, do not support the suggestion that larger left atrial size or volume produces bigger F waves. Furthermore, echocardiographic data show no correlation between the size of the F waves and the cause of the heart disease,[591] and electrophysiological studies demonstrate that the size of the F waves reflects the complexity of endocardial atrial activation.[596]

Return of sinus rhythm. The amplitude of the P waves tends to be small in those few instances in which sinus rhythm spontaneously returns after years of chronic atrial fibrillation.[553]

PR Intervals

The electrocardiograms of patients in atrial fibrillation, of course, do not have PR intervals. However, when such patients are in sinus rhythm, the PR interval may bear an inverse relation to the ventricular rate when they return to atrial fibrillation because the longer the PR interval, the slower the atrioventricular nodal conduction. This characteristic has been observed in patients with abnormally short PR intervals but no preexcitation.[521, 597-602, vvv] Their ventricular rates in atrial fibrillation are faster than in patients with normal PR intervals.[601]

Patients with rheumatic carditis and persistently prolonged PR intervals more often develop atrial fibrillation than those whose PR intervals are normal.[603] Conversely, first-degree atrioventricular block with prolonged PR intervals is frequently present in those patients who spontaneously return to sinus rhythm after many years of chronic atrial fibrillation.[553]

QRS Complexes

Other than the fibrillatory or F waves, the most characteristic electrocardiographic feature of atrial fibrillation is the irregularity of the QRS complexes. The rhythm is frequently called "irregularly irregular" because no pattern for the rhythm, such as in bigeminy or other forms of group beating, can be discerned.

Aberrancy. The QRS complexes during atrial fibrillation usually have a normal duration. Although bundle branch blocks and intraventricular conduction disturbances may coexist, the irregular rhythm of atrial fibrillation can, in addition, produce intermittent bundle branch block resulting from beat-by-beat loss of conduction, usually in the right bundle branch (Figs. 4.4 and 4.5) and occasionally in the left bundle branch (Fig. 4.6). Such aberrancy occurs when a beat conducted through the atrioventricular node finds part of the intraventricular conduction system to be refractory.[559, www] The diagnostic dilemma that then arises is differentiating temporary right, or occasionally left, bundle branch block from ventricular premature beats or ventricular tachycardia.[604-607, xxx]

The problem is common. Abnormally formed QRS complexes can be found in almost 60% of electrocardiograms of atrial fibrillation.[608]

Form of lead V₁. Much can be learned by inspecting lead V_1[608-611] or modified chest lead MCL_1.[612]

- Aberrantly conducted beats with the form of right bundle branch block tend to be triphasic, whereas ventricular ectopic beats are usually monophasic or biphasic.
- The initial 0.02-second vector of an aberrant beat is

---

vvv Some patients with short PR intervals, normal QRS complexes, and tachyarrhythmias (Lown-Ganong-Levine syndrome)[521] have paroxysmal atrial fibrillation. Conduction through the atrioventricular node in these patients is characteristically rapid.[597-602]

www Sir Thomas Lewis proposed 85 years ago: "The phenomena . . . should be termed, 'aberration of the supraventricular impulses' or more simply 'aberration'; the anomalous beats may be conveniently spoken of as 'aberrant beats' or 'aberrant ventricular contractions.'"[559]

xxx The phrase "Ashman's phenomenon" is frequently assigned to this finding. The eponym derives from the name of Richard Ashman, Ph.D., at the time professor and chairman of the Department of Physiology at Louisiana State University in New Orleans, who described how aberrancy begins when a short RR (QRS-to-QRS) interval follows a long interval, a sequence that increases bundle branch refractoriness.[604, 605] He postulated that the aberrancy was perpetuated by what later came to be recognized as repetitive retrograde concealed conduction into the right bundle branch from the ventricle depolarized by the left bundle branch.[606] The value of the Ashman phenomenon is low in predicting whether an abnormally formed QRS complex is aberrantly conducted or originates in the ventricles.[607]

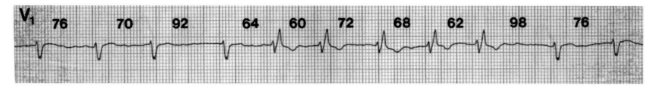

FIGURE 4.4 Tachycardia-dependent right bundle branch block during atrial fibrillation. When the RR intervals are equal to or less than 0.72 second, conduction in the right bundle branch fails. (Numbers indicate RR intervals in hundredths of a second.)

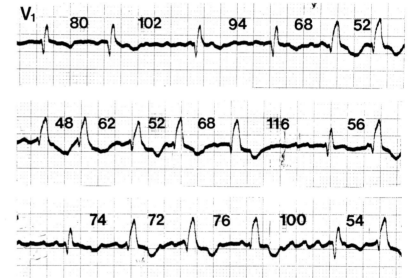

FIGURE 4.5 Conversion of incomplete to complete right bundle branch block during atrial fibrillation. Tachycardia further decreases conduction in the right bundle branch, already conducting abnormally. Complete right bundle branch block aberrancy develops when the preceding RR intervals are 0.76 second or shorter. (Numbers indicate RR intervals in hundredths of a second.)

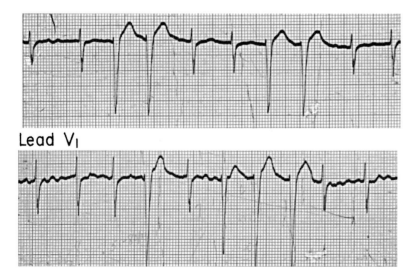

Lead V₁

FIGURE 4.6 Tachycardia-dependent left bundle branch block during atrial fibrillation. The abnormally wide QRS complexes are conducted aberrantly because of temporary block in the left bundle branch, which occurs less frequently than rate-related right bundle branch block. Notice the absence of a ``compensatory-like'' pause after the last of the abnormally conducted beats (*bottom panel*). Ventricular beats, unlike aberrantly conducted beats, produce such pauses by penetrating the atrioventricular junction in retrograde fashion. The presence or absence of such pauses can help in diagnosing the origin of abnormal beats during atrial fibrillation.

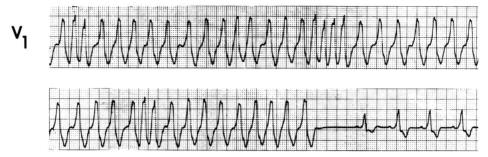

FIGURE 4.7 **Aberrant ventricular conduction during atrial fibrillation in a patient with Wolff-Parkinson-White syndrome.** Conduction from the fibrillating atria through an accessory pathway produces the rapid rate, irregular rhythm, and wide QRS complexes *(upper panel)*. The last four QRS complexes *(lower panel)* have short PR intervals, delta waves, and abnormal ST and T waves and, thereby, reveal the presence of ventricular preexcitation.

identical to that of the normally conducted beat in about half of cases. The first portion of the QRS complex of a ventricular beat seldom looks like a conducted beat. Thus, although a changed initial vector is of little or no use in distinguishing between ventricular ectopy and aberrancy, an identical initial vector strongly favors aberration.

• Aberrancy is more likely when one observes progressive increase in the abnormality of the QRS complexes as the rate increases.[613]

Compensatory pause.[614–616] Ventricular premature beats, even in the presence of atrial fibrillation, are followed by relatively long pauses because ectopic impulses in retrograde manner penetrate the atrioventricular node, thus making it temporarily refractory to the conduction of antegrade impulses.[606, 611, 613, 615, 617, 618, yyy] Aberrantly conducted beats are seldom[616] followed by compensatory pauses.

"Long-short" intervals. Refractoriness, like the QT interval, increases at slow rates and after long preceding RR intervals. Thus, in atrial fibrillation, aberrancy is favored when a short RR interval follows a long RR interval.[604, 608] However, this finding also applies to ventricular premature beats that more likely arise after long RR intervals.[619, 620, zzz] Anomalous beats that appear after short preceding RR intervals are almost always ectopic.[608, 611]

Bursts of beats. Repetitive bigeminy, often with fixed coupling of the anomalous beat to the normal beat, characterizes ventricular premature beats, whereas supraventricular beats in atrial fibrillation often feature repetitive aberrancy; of course, ventricular tachycardia may need to be considered in such cases. When ventricular tachycardia coexists with atrial fibrillation, the diagnosis may be made when fusion (Dressler) beats are seen.[621] However, the nature of a wide QRS complex may not always be recognizable from the surface electrocardiogram. In such cases, the diagnosis can be confirmed only with a clinical electrophysiological study.[622]

RR interval scattergram. Review of the data developed from this technique can help to differentiate aberrant ventricular conduction from ventricular beating in patients with atrial fibrillation.[623]

Carotid sinus pressure. In slowing the ventricular rate, carotid sinus pressure may, by facilitating conduction in the bundle branches, narrow the width of aberrantly conducted beats, thereby revealing the mechanism of such beats.[624]

Wolff-Parkinson-White syndrome. Rapid rhythms with wide QRS complexes that stimulate ventricular fibrillation appear in patients with atrial fibrillation and preexcitation (Fig. 4.7).[159, 161, 162, 522, 625–629, aaaa] The QRS complexes can be so bizarre and variable that ventricular flutter or fibrillation may be suspected,[630] an unlikely explanation in a patient who seems otherwise well except for rapid heart action.

The peculiar QRS morphologies are produced by abnormal ventricular activation when atrial impulses conduct through an accessory pathway. The abnormality of the QRS complexes is greater when more of the ventricular activation is produced by conduction through the accessory pathway than through the atrioventricular node–His bundle system. Normally con-

---

yyy The phrase "compensatory pause," also used in describing the rhythm of the pulse during physical examination, refers to the time that elapses from a ventricular premature beat to the next sinus-driven ventricular beat. It is obviously longer than the sinus interval. When used in reference to atrial fibrillation, the observation might best be described as a "post-extrasystolic" or "compensatory-like" pause, because the duration does not relate to sinus rhythm. In atrial fibrillation, pauses[615] after single[615] or multiple[616] ventricular ectopic beats are always longer than the *average* cycle length of the supraventricular beats. However, a patient may, and frequently does, demonstrate *individual* RR intervals during atrial fibrillation that are longer than a compensatory pause.[616] Even a paced signal that does not activate the ventricles may delay appearance of the next supraventricular beat by concealed retrograde discharge of the conducting system.[614]

zzz In introducing the concept, Richard Langendorf and colleagues wrote in 1955: "The term 'rule of bigeminy' is proposed as a short designation of this phenomenon";[619] see Figure 11.2 in Chapter 11.

aaaa The first patient described by Louis Wolff, John Parkinson, and Paul Dudley White[1319] had "Abnormal beats which occurred at a fast rate during paroxysmal atrial fibrillation . . . simulated paroxysmal ventricular tachycardia [and] resembled the anomalous ventricular complexes present when the heart action was slow and under sinoatrial control."[162]

ducted beats can appear next to wide QRS complexes, and this combination should suggest the correct diagnosis. Atrial fibrillation may reveal the presence of accessory pathways in patients whose QRS complexes are preexcited during the arrhythmia and not in sinus rhythm.[631]

ST and T waves

Atrial fibrillation does not directly affect the ST and T waves. They can, of course, be abnormal when acute or chronic myocardial disease is present or drugs have been administered.

QT Interval

The QT interval shortens with faster rates and lengthens with slower rates of atrial fibrillation, as it does during sinus rhythm.[632] However, the average QT interval seems longer during atrial fibrillation than in sinus rhythm.[632]

ELECTROCARDIOGRAM IN SINUS RHYTHM

When patients with paroxysmal atrial fibrillation are in sinus rhythm, their electrocardiograms may show signs of the cardiac diseases that produce fibrillation. For example, if coronary or hypertensive heart disease is present, signs of myocardial infarction, myocardial fibrosis, or left ventricular hypertrophy can be seen. Patients with thyrotoxicosis characteristically have sinus tachycardia.

P Waves

Although patients with lone atrial fibrillation usually have normal electrocardiograms during sinus rhythm, slight abnormalities in the form and duration of the P waves frequently appear,[633–637] whether or not structural heart disease is present. In mitral valvular disease, left or right atrial enlargement is frequently present.

The duration of the P waves and the size of the P terminal force in lead V_1 are greater in patients with, than in patients without, paroxysmal atrial fibrillation associated with sick sinus syndrome.[638] The form of the P waves is abnormal in patients with atrioventricular block who can be electrically induced into atrial fibrillation.[507]

PR Interval

The PR interval may be slightly prolonged in patients with paroxysmal atrial fibrillation.[236] Elevation or depression of PR segments corresponds with the development of paroxysmal atrial fibrillation in patients with myocardial infarction, probably because of atrial infarction.[639]

QRS Complex

In patients with the Wolff-Parkinson-White syndrome and ventricular preexcitation, short PR intervals and abnormal QRS patterns ("delta waves") can be seen, indicating antegrade conduction through accessory pathways.

DIFFERENTIAL DIAGNOSIS

Atrial Flutter

"Sawtooth" atrial activity occurs at a rate of about 250 to 400 beats per minute in this arrhythmia. The ventricular rate may either be regular or irregular, depending on the degree of atrioventricular block.

Atrial Tachycardia

Atrial reentrant and ectopic tachycardias are relatively uncommon arrhythmias. Each arrhythmia is characterized by usually abnormal P waves preceding all QRS complexes, and the rhythm is regular.

Multifocal Atrial Tachycardia

Multifocal atrial tachycardia has multiform P waves that precede most of the QRS complexes. Some P waves may be blocked from conduction to the ventricles. Multifocal atrial tachycardia is an irregular arrhythmia and is probably the tachycardia most frequently confused with atrial fibrillation. The diagnosis depends on observing whether the atrial activity consists of P waves or F waves.

Reentrant Supraventricular Tachycardia

Reentrant supraventricular tachycardia, whether sustained within the atrioventricular node or through bypass tracks, is usually regular. Although careful measurement reveals slight irregularities in the rhythm of atrial fibrillation, the rate may be similar to that of atrial fibrillation in untreated patients. Furthermore, confusion may arise because the F waves of atrial fibrillation when the ventricular response is rapid and the P waves in supraventricular tachycardia may not be visible.

Sinus Tachycardia

The rhythm of sinus tachycardia is relatively regular, and P waves precede each QRS complex.

Ventricular Tachycardia

Confusion with ventricular tachycardia arises when bundle branch block or antegrade conduction through bypass tracks coexists with atrial fibrillation. Ventricular tachycardia is, in general, more regular than atrial fibrillation. The form of the QRS complexes can guide the observer in recognizing which arrhythmia is present.[640]

Ventricular Flutter and Fibrillation

Ventricular flutter and fibrillation may be simulated during antegrade conduction through accessory pathways when the atria are either in atrial fibrillation or atrial flutter. The diagnosis is usually made by the history and the clinical appearance of the patient during the arrhythmia.

Bradyarrhythmias

When the ventricular rate is slow and regular in patients with atrial fibrillation, either from atrioventricular block or by administration of digitalis and other drugs, atrioventricular dissociation may be present and the ventricles may be driven by an ectopic pacemaker in the His bundle or ventricles. The presence of fibrillation in the atria can usually be discerned from the F waves.

OTHER ELECTROCARDIOGRAPHIC STUDIES

Exercise Testing

In patients with atrial fibrillation, the ventricular rate is faster as exercise progresses,[641–644] and at the peak of exercise than in the same patients during sinus rhythm,[641, 644, 645] or it is faster than the rate predicted for patients the same age.[646] This occurs because the atrioventricular node functions less efficiently as a regulator of ventricular rate than does the sinus node.[647, bbbb] Because patients with atrial fibrillation reach rapid heart rates after relatively small amounts of exercise, chest pain or dyspnea from coronary disease or myocardial dysfunction may occur sooner than in patients in sinus rhythm. Even patients whose resting ventricular rate is reduced from partial atrioventricular block have an abnormally rapid chronotropic response to exercise.[648]

Monitoring. Monitoring of the electrocardiogram during exercise reveals that other arrhythmias can develop in patients with atrial fibrillation.[649] Ventricular beats and regularization of the ventricular response appear in some patients when the ventricular response to atrial fibrillation is rapid. These arrhythmias may indicate the presence of intrinsic heart disease or latent digitalis intoxication.

Atrial fibrillation does not diminish exercise capacity when atrial fibrillation complicates the course of patients with mild or moderate congestive heart failure.[478] The response to exercise in patients with atrial fibrillation depends more on the severity of any associated structural heart disease than on the arrhythmia itself.[650] Transesophageal pacing can induce atrial fibrillation in athletes when they are exercising but not at rest.[651]

Wolff-Parkinson-White syndrome. When patients with Wolff-Parkinson-White syndrome in sinus rhythm or atrial fibrillation exercise, the ventricular rate increases, but fewer beats are preexcited.[652, 653] This finding indicates preferential conduction through the atrioventricular node–His-Purkinje system rather than through accessory pathways. Presumably, the reduction in vagal tone and increase in sympathetic tone affect the atrioventricular node more than accessory pathways. However, upright exercise can increase the maximum rate of conduction over accessory pathways.[654]

Treadmill exercise rarely induces atrial fibrillation in patients with Wolff-Parkinson-White syndrome;[649, 652] paroxysms that develop are brief and terminate spontaneously.[649] The test, therefore, is not useful for provoking the arrhythmia or determining the susceptibility to rapid ventricular rates.[655] However, the risk of cardiac arrest rises when continuous preexcitation persists during exercise.[165]

Ambulatory Electrocardiographic Recordings[656]

Twenty-four-hour ambulatory electrocardiographic recordings show that paroxysms of atrial fibrillation, often asymptomatic,[108] occur in some patients with sinus rhythm and such organic heart diseases as mitral stenosis[108] and hypertrophic cardiomyopathy.[244] Extended monitoring also reveals that paroxysmal atrial fibrillation in patients in sinus rhythm,[529] paroxysmal atrioventricular block in patients with chronic atrial fibrillation,[529, 657, 658] and atrial fibrillation with a rapid ventricular response can cause dizziness and syncope.[659] Paroxysmal atrial fibrillation often begins after an increasing number of atrial premature beats,[660] but when the arrhythmia starts does not usually relate to the heart rate at that moment.[660]

Ambulatory monitoring reveals the following:

- When paroxysms are most likely to start.[395, 397]
- That many patients with paroxysmal atrial fibrillation are unaware when episodes occur.[531]
- Information about the frequency of paroxysmal atrial fibrillation in elderly patients.[81]
- The ventricular response in patients with paroxysmal[584] and chronic atrial fibrillation.[661]
- How atrial arrhythmias respond to digitalis and quinidine.[662]
- How physicians can best use and investigate drugs to control heart rate.[661]

Transtelephonic monitoring has been used to study the following:

- The natural history of atrial fibrillation.[663]
- The recognition of symptoms with the presence of paroxysmal arrhythmias.[664]
- The association of atrial flutter[479] and supraventricular tachycardia with atrial fibrillation.[501, 665]
- The efficacy of drugs for treating ambulatory patients with the arrhythmia.[666, 667]

Heart Rate Variability

The variability of the ventricular response in patients with chronic mitral regurgitation is reduced in patients who require mitral valve surgery[668] or who have a re-

---

bbbb The results from treadmill exercise tests are usually, but not always, reproducible when the same patient with atrial fibrillation exercises several times.[647]

duced prognosis,[668] particularly those with severe congestive heart failure.[669] Vagal tone is an important factor regulating heart rate variability in patients with atrial fibrillation.[670]

Signal-Averaged Electrocardiogram of P Waves[671–673]

High-speed, high-gain recordings of the orthogonal XYZ leads reveal that the P waves have a longer duration in patients with paroxysmal atrial fibrillation than in those without the arrhythmia.[635, 674] Amplified signal-averaged techniques show that abnormalities of the P waves can help to identify those patients who have, or are likely to develop, paroxysmal atrial fibrillation,[674–689] even in the absence of atrial enlargement on the standard electrocardiogram.[677] Information from processed signal can, furthermore, predict which patients with paroxysmal atrial fibrillation will develop the arrhythmia on a long-term basis.[690, 691, cccc] Atrial fibrillation, unlike atrial flutter, rarely interferes with analysis of the signal-averaged electrocardiogram.[692]

Vectorcardiography

The spatial magnitude of the P waves in the vectorcardiogram is significantly greater in patients with paroxysmal atrial fibrillation than in those with sinus rhythm.[635] The P loops in many patients with paroxysmal atrial fibrillation also have abnormal shapes.

ECHOCARDIOGRAPHY

Echocardiographic[693] and Doppler[694] studies are frequently employed to define the origin and severity of intrinsic heart disease found in patients with atrial fibrillation and to confirm the diagnosis of lone fibrillation.[374, 695, dddd] Echocardiography can identify the arrhythmia in human fetuses.[44–46]

Atrial Size

Atrial fibrillation more likely develops in patients whose left atria are enlarged.[41, 241, 440, 460, 696–701] However, factors other than left atrial enlargement must influence the development of atrial fibrillation, because of the following:

- Some patients with atrial fibrillation, including those with lone atrial fibrillation in particular,[702] have normal left atrial dimensions.[703, eeee]
- Few patients in sinus rhythm with a left atrium of at least 45 mm develop atrial fibrillation within 1 to 2 years.[704]

- Many patients with idiopathic congestive cardiomyopathy maintain sinus rhythm despite enlarged left atria.[705]

Effects of atrial fibrillation on enlargement and vice versa

- Atrial fibrillation itself may cause the left[699, 706, 707] and the right[699] atria to enlarge progressively, and sinus rhythm may prevent this process.[707]
- Left atrial enlargement of more than 40 mm predisposes to development of atrial fibrillation in older patients with thyrotoxicosis.[188, ffff]

Paroxysmal atrial fibrillation. The left atrium in patients with paroxysmal atrial fibrillation is slightly dilated, but the size does not relate to the frequency or duration of the paroxysms.[708] The left atrium gradually and progressively enlarges in patients with both paroxysmal and chronic lone atrial fibrillation regardless of changes in left ventricular size or function.[709]

Duration. Left atrial size does not correlate with the duration of atrial fibrillation[710] or with large F waves on the electrocardiogram.[587, 591]

Treatment

- Left atrial size decreases after sinus rhythm has been reestablished in patients with long-standing, chronic atrial fibrillation,[706, 711] but not in those who have had atrial fibrillation for less than 6 weeks.[711]
- Antiarrhythmic drugs are more likely to convert patients with smaller atria from atrial fibrillation to sinus rhythm;[712–714] amiodarone may,[715, 716] or may not,[717] more effectively treat patients with smaller atria, but the drug can sustain sinus rhythm in patients with relatively large atria.[716]
- Echocardiographically measured left atrial size does, according to one study,[718] but not, according to older work,[696, 719] determine which patients can be successfully electrically cardioverted from atrial fibrillation to sinus rhythm.
- Patients whose left atria are large by echocardiographic measurement may,[378, 696, 720, 721] or may not,[710, 719, 722] revert to atrial fibrillation relatively soon after cardioversion.[gggg]

Ventricular Size and Function

- Left ventricular mass,[41] end-diastolic dimension,[41] and wall thickness[701] are increased and left ventricular fractional shortening is decreased in patients with chronic atrial fibrillation when compared with those in sinus rhythm.
- Patients with an increased atrial filling fraction and left ventricular dysfunction are often clinically unstable when atrial fibrillation develops.[532]
- After cardioversion, left ventricular end-diastolic

---

cccc The most satisfactory results are obtained by triggering the recordings from P waves,[676, 678] rather than from QRS complexes. Recording from esophageal leads provides signals of greater amplitude than from surface leads and thereby facilitates identification of patients predisposed to paroxysmal atrial fibrillation.[681, 691]

dddd However, structural heart disease can usually be established or excluded by clinical examination.[374, 695]

eeee Thirty-seven ± six millimeters in 25 patients with lone atrial fibrillation.[477]

ffff In patients with thyrotoxicosis, the left atrium was enlarged in only 2% of those without atrial fibrillation younger than 40 years and in 94% of those with atrial fibrillation older than 40 years.[188]

gggg The pre-echocardiographic data suggested that larger left atria predict shorter maintenance of sinus rhythm after cardioversion.

dimension and stroke volume increase in patients with coronary heart disease and cardiomyopathy.[723] Fractional shortening in patients without these forms of heart disease increases as early as 4 hours after cardioversion.[724]

- His bundle ablation for persistently rapid atrial fibrillation increases ventricular ejection fraction[725] and decreases left ventricular end-systolic, end-diastolic, and left atrial dimensions in some patients with lone atrial fibrillation.[726] The procedure also can increase fractional shortening.[727]

Thromboembolism[728–731]

Transthoracic and transesophageal echocardiography can identify intra-atrial clots that may produce emboli.[439, 452, 732, 733] In addition, certain other echocardiographic findings and measurements predict which patients with atrial fibrillation will most likely have thromboembolism:

- The presence of *spontaneous echo contrast* in the left atrium, smoke-like echoes with a characteristic swirling motion[734–744] in association with atrial dysfunction after cardioversion;[736, 738] conversion to sinus rhythm, regardless of the method employed, decreases left atrial appendage Doppler velocities and formation or intensification of spontaneous contrast echocardiograms.[745, 746, hhhh]
- Thrombus in the left atrial appendage.[742]
- Irregular, low, peak filling and emptying waves associated with almost no visible contraction of the left atrial appendage.[747]
- Abnormal opacification patterns in the left atrial appendage observed with use of an albumin contrast agent.[748]
- Stasis in the posterior portion of the left atrium.[749]
- Low forward and backward peak velocity in the left atrial appendage.[737]
- Size[454] of the left atrium and length and width of the left atrial appendage.[439]
- Left ventricular dysfunction.[454]
- Aortic plaque.[742, 744]

Atrial Function After Cardioversion [iiii]

Echocardiography shows less left ventricular hypertrophy and no obstruction to left ventricular outflow in patients with hypertrophic cardiomyopathy and chronic atrial fibrillation when compared with those in sinus rhythm.[243] Ultrasonography reveals stenosis of at least 50% in the carotid arteries in about 12% of patients older than 70 years of age with atrial fibrillation.[750] However, the presence of this finding in such patients does not add significantly to the risk of stroke.[750]

The peak emptying velocity of the left atrial appendage does not predict in patients with nonvalvular atrial fibrillation of recent onset whether cardioversion will succeed or how long sinus rhythm will persist if the treatment is successful. However, reduced echocardiographically determined peak emptying velocity of the left atrial appendage does seem to predict that atrial fibrillation will recur after internal cardioversion.[751] Doppler echocardiography shows that when the Maze procedure reestablishes sinus rhythm, right atrial contraction is restored and left atrial contraction improves in most patients.[752]

EXTERNAL PULSE RECORDINGS AND PHONOCARDIOGRAPHY

In the venous pulse, the A waves of atrial contraction disappear during atrial fibrillation and are replaced by irregular, undulating activity, which is superimposed on all parts of the tracing[753] (see Fig. 4.1). The arterial pulse is irregular, and its amplitude varies. Left ventricular ejection times increase after conversion to sinus rhythm.[754] A waves from left atrial contraction appear in the apexcardiogram of most patients within 8 hours of conversion to sinus rhythm.[755]

The phonocardiogram confirms the physical findings of atrial fibrillation by demonstrating variations in the following:[756]

- The intensity of the first sound, except in patients with mitral stenosis.
- The interval from the beginning of the QRS complex to the first sound.
- The interval between the second heart sound and the opening snap of the mitral valve.

HEMATOLOGY AND CHEMISTRY
Hematocrit

The hematocrit rises during paroxysmal atrial fibrillation in most patients, possibly from contraction of plasma volume produced by tachycardia-induced polyuria.[757] The mortality of patients with atrial fibrillation and acute stroke increases when the hematocrit is 50% or more.[433]

Thyroid Studies

Because symptoms and findings of hyperthyroidism may easily be missed,[185, 758] laboratory evaluation for the endocrinopathy should be performed in everyone presenting with atrial fibrillation. The values of serum triiodothyronine and thyroxine are higher in patients with thyrotoxicosis over 40 years of age who have atrial fibrillation compared with those in sinus rhythm.[188]

Although thyroxine levels may not adequately detect masked or occult hyperthyroidism, abnormal thyroid scans[759] and unresponsiveness of thyrotropin (thyroid-stimulating hormone) to thyrotropin-releasing hormone can establish the diagnosis.[195, 372, 759–766, jjjj] The

---

hhhh Neither warfarin nor aspirin effectively suppresses left atrial spontaneous echo contrast in patients with nonrheumatic atrial fibrillation.[746]

iiii See section on hemodynamics later.

jjjj Two reports question the significance of abnormal responses of thyroid-stimulating to thyrotropin-releasing hormone for recognizing occult thyrotoxicosis in patients with atrial fibrillation.[372, 765] Nevertheless, endocrinologists accept the importance of subclinical thyrotoxicosis as a cause of atrial fibrillation.[766]

chemiluminescent immunometric assay, which permits measuring exceedingly low thyrotropin levels, provides the most accurate method at this time for recognizing subclinical hyperthyroidism. Thyrotropin-releasing hormone stimulation tests seldom need to be performed because thyroid-stimulating hormone values of less than 0.01 mU/L always correlate with the absence of thyrotropin-releasing hormone–mediated stimulation of thyroid-stimulating hormone.[766] Low serum thyrotropin concentrations in euthyroid subjects 60 years of age or older is associated with a threefold higher risk of developing atrial fibrillation in the subsequent decade.[767, 768]

Magnesium

Hypomagnesemia occurs frequently in patients with symptomatic atrial fibrillation.[769] When the serum magnesium level is low, more digoxin may be needed to control the ventricular rate than when the level is normal.[769]

Coagulation

Several constituents of the blood associated with coagulation rise during atrial fibrillation.[770] Plasma levels of D-dimers (cross-linked fibrin degradation products),[771] increasing amounts of which correlate with a greater tendency toward intravascular clotting, fibrinogen,[772] and von Willebrand factor[772] are higher in patients with atrial fibrillation than in those with sinus rhythm. Consequently, D-dimer levels decrease in some patients after cardioversion to sinus rhythm.[773] These data suggest that atrial fibrillation itself increases the tendency to form clots, because D-dimer levels are not affected by the type or severity of heart disease.

Furthermore, plasma levels of thrombin-antithrombin complex,[774] fibrinogen,[775] and fibrinopeptide[774] rise in patients who develop paroxysmal atrial fibrillation. The levels of fibrinogen are intermediate between those of patients in sinus rhythm and in chronic atrial fibrillation.[775]

Atrial fibrillation also enhances the aggregation and coagulation of platelets and accelerates their activity and coagulability.[776] These changes can be observed within 12 hours after the onset of the arrhythmia.[776]

Atrial Natriuretic Peptide

The concentration in the plasma of atrial natriuretic peptide is higher in patients with atrial fibrillation than in those in sinus rhythm,[777, 778] and it decreases after cardioversion to sinus rhythm,[436, 779–782] probably from recovery of atrial mechanical function.[781] Elevations of atrial pressure, rather than rapid heart rate, probably induce the higher levels of the polypeptide during atrial fibrillation.[783–786]

The release of atrial natriuretic peptide also depends on coordinated atrial contraction, but not on the ventricular rate.[777] Among patients whose ventricular rate is fixed because of atrioventricular block, levels of atrial natriuretic peptide rise during exercise in patients who have intact atrial contraction but not in those with atrial fibrillation.[777]

Miscellaneous Studies

Erythrocyte sedimentation rate, low-shear blood velocity, and anticardiolipin antibody are raised in patients with atrial fibrillation and spontaneous echo contrast.[739] Atrial fibrillation raises the levels of plasma endothelin in patients with congestive heart failure compared with levels during sinus rhythm.[778] Antibodies against cardiac myosin heavy-chain isophorms are higher in the sera of patients with paroxysmal atrial fibrillation than of patients without the arrhythmia.[787, 788]

RADIOLOGY AND NUCLEAR MEDICINE

Radionuclear ventriculography reveals that right ventricular ejection fractions are lower in patients with inferior myocardial infarction who develop atrial fibrillation than in those who remain in sinus rhythm.[155] The left ventricular ejection fraction, measured with radionuclide angiography, rises when patients with idiopathic cardiomyopathy convert to sinus rhythm and persists a year later if sinus rhythm is maintained.[789] Study with a nuclear probe of left ventricular function in patients with nonvalvular atrial fibrillation reveals that longer preceding cycle lengths increase left ventricular ejection fraction and end-diastolic volume.[790]

Computed tomography shows a relatively high frequency of cerebral low-density areas from previous infarctions in patients with chronic atrial fibrillation and no history of cerebrovascular disease.[791] These findings, however, occur no more frequently in patients with paroxysmal atrial fibrillation than in healthy control subjects.[428]

HEMODYNAMICS

Atrial fibrillation reduces cardiac function in many patients.[792–795] In patients with congestive heart failure, the arrhythmia does the following:[796]

- Worsens New York Heart Association class.
- Decreases peak exercise oxygen consumption.
- Lowers cardiac index.
- Increases mitral and tricuspid regurgitation.

Abnormal values of the principal intracardiac hemodynamic measurements during atrial fibrillation approach normal after conversion to sinus rhythm:

- Venous[797] and right atrial mean pressure.[797, 798]
- Right and left ventricular end-diastolic pressure.[798]
- Pulmonary[798] and systemic[797, 798] vascular resistance.
- Pulmonary blood volume.[797]

Cardiac Output and Stroke Volume

Three characteristics of atrial fibrillation reduce the cardiac output of patients with the condition:

- Excessively rapid ventricular rate.[799]
- Loss of coordinated atrial contraction.
- Irregularity of the rhythm.[800–803]

The cardiac output and cardiac index, usually depressed in atrial fibrillation associated with significant structural heart disease,[796] rise after conversion to sinus rhythm.[508, 558, 722, 723, 797, 798, 804–817] Left ventricular ejection fraction,[789, 818] stroke volume,[806, 813, 814] stroke index,[815, 819] stroke work,[819] and peak oxygen consumption[818] also improve when patients convert to sinus rhythm.

Beat-to-beat variation in preload in patients with atrial fibrillation partially explains the observation that the shorter the RR interval, the less the stroke volume.[790] Changing left ventricular performance is influenced by post-extrasystolic potentiation and preload, among other factors.[790]

The cardiac output increases more with exercise when patients are in sinus rhythm than when they are in atrial fibrillation.[558, 806–809, 814, 816, 819] The irregular ventricular rhythm characteristic of atrial fibrillation decreases cardiac output and increases pulmonary wedge and right atrial pressures when compared with a regular (paced) rhythm during atrial fibrillation at approximately the same rate.[803]

Oxygen Uptake

Maximal oxygen uptake and peak oxygen consumption, which decrease when atrial fibrillation develops in patients with heart failure,[796] rise,[820] and efficiency of ventilation improves during exercise after conversion to sinus rhythm,[644] although the changes may not be measurable until weeks after conversion.[818, 821] Similarly, the maximal oxygen uptake on exercise is lower in male patients with chronic heart failure when compared with others with similar degrees of heart failure in sinus rhythm[822] and in patients with lone atrial fibrillation compared with healthy subjects in sinus rhythm.[823] Cardiopulmonary performance in patients with chronic atrial fibrillation improves when pacing regularizes the ventricular rate.[824]

Mitral Stenosis

Atrial contraction contributes less to ventricular filling in patients with mitral stenosis than in those with normal hearts.[825] Consequently, the rapid heart rate, which is more important than the loss of atrial systole in causing decompensation when atrial fibrillation develops,[825] raises pulmonary artery and pulmonary wedge pressures.[826] Atrial fibrillation worsens further the depressed left ventricular ejection fraction and altered geometry of the left ventricle in many patients with mitral stenosis.[827] Exercise performance improves less after surgery for severe mitral stenosis in patients who had atrial fibrillation compared with those who had sinus rhythm before the operation.[825]

Autonomic Influences

Syncope, often ascribed to rapid ventricular rates or poor ventricular function in patients with paroxysmal atrial fibrillation, is frequently produced by neurogenic responses in patients with vasovagal reactions.[527]

Hypertrophic Cardiomyopathy

Cardiac output decreases markedly when patients with hypertrophic cardiomyopathy develop atrial fibrillation because of the loss of the atrial contribution to the filling of left ventricles with poor compliance and because of the varying amounts of outflow obstruction produced by the irregular rhythm.[241] The development of atrial fibrillation in patients with hypertrophic cardiomyopathy is not related to the severity of the left ventricular outflow obstruction or the amount of associated mitral regurgitation.[241]

Atrial Function After Conversion from Atrial Fibrillation to Sinus Rhythm

Apexcardiographic,[553, 755, 828, 829] kinetocardiographic,[830] echocardiographic Doppler,[553, 736, 821, 831–836] nuclear stethoscopic,[818] and hemodynamic[553, 755, 819, 837–839] studies demonstrate that left, and in some cases right, atrial hemodynamic activity may be depressed after transthoracic[834] and internal[836] electrical or pharmacologic conversion from atrial fibrillation to sinus rhythm. Useful atrial contractions[811, 819, 840–842] can appear at once,[736] in minutes,[755] and often within a day, particularly in patients with nonvalvular atrial fibrillation.[843] The atria of most patients that remain in sinus rhythm regain effective mechanical atrial function by no more than 1 week after conversion,[835, 844] but some can take as long as 3 weeks to a month,[817, 828, 832, 845, 846, kkkk] and although most eventually achieve normal function regardless of the duration of the arrhythmia, the process may take several months.[711] The mechanical function of the left atrial appendage after cardioversion tracks that of the body of the left atrium.[847]

The right atrium can regain the ability to contract sooner than the left.[819, 845] Transient increases in left atrial and pulmonary artery pressures that could then be produced may account for the occasional case of pulmonary edema that occurs after cardioversion.[814, 819, 845, 848–850]

Patients who never regain useful atrial contractions[819] seldom remain in sinus rhythm for long.[723, 819] Conversely, sinus rhythm more often persists when atrial contractile function improves quickly after cardioversion.[710] Atrial function returns earlier in patients without structural heart disease or with hypertension than in those with ischemic cardiomyopathy.[834, 851]

Duration of atrial fibrillation. Left atrial contractile function, which is greater in patients with small atria,[710] decreases in the left atrium[711, 831, 832] and in the left atrial appendage[852] as the duration of atrial fibrillation lengthens. Only if the fibrillation lasts no more than 2 weeks does atrial function return fully within 24 hours after cardioversion.[711]

---

kkkk This observation may explain why some investigators reported finding little improvement in cardiac function soon after conversion.[811, 817, 819, 840]

Does electric shock reduce atrial function? Atrial mechanical activity returns sooner when drugs convert atrial fibrillation to sinus rhythm than after electrical cardioversion,[835] although the amount of electrical energy used in the cardioversion does not affect the rate of recovery.[844] This finding has been taken to support the contention that electrical conversion temporarily damages the atria.[853]

However, other investigators argue that the electric shock is unlikely to produce the depression because spontaneous conversion to sinus rhythm produces similar reduction of function in the left atrial appendage.[854] Furthermore, transesophageal echocardiography demonstrates that shocks to patients in sinus rhythm from transthoracic defibrillators and implantable cardioverter-defibrillators do not reduce mechanical function in the left atrium or its appendage.[855] Alternatively, an atrial myopathy produced by the arrhythmia, with similar effects on the atria as prolonged tachycardia on the ventricles, may account for at least some of the depression of atrial contractility in patients with atrial fibrillation.[856]

Lone Atrial Fibrillation

Atrial fibrillation induced in patients with paroxysmal atrial fibrillation and no structural heart disease does not greatly affect cardiac function, but it does significantly

- Decrease stroke volume.[857, llll]
- Decrease systemic systolic pressure.[858]
- Raise systemic diastolic pressure.[857]
- Raise mean wedge pressure.[857, 858]
- Raise pulmonary artery pressures.[857, 858]
- Decrease right and left ventricular end-diastolic pressures.[857]

Consequently, hemodynamic function does not significantly improve when patients with lone atrial fibrillation convert to sinus rhythm.[812, 814]

Polyuria During Tachycardia[859]

As many as half the patients with paroxysmal tachycardia,[860, mmmm] including atrial fibrillation, report polyuria during or after the episode.[386, 861–863] Patients with brief paroxysms of tachycardia were formerly thought not to develop polyuria, but from more recent studies, cardiologists now recognize that even patients with short-lived tachycardias produce some additional urine that may not be enough to attract their attention.[786] When their bladders are catheterized, all patients who develop atrial tachyarrhythmias demonstrate polyuria, natriuresis, and kaliuresis.[757, 786, nnnn]

Polyuria during atrial tachyarrhythmias is most likely caused by decreased secretion of arginine vasopressin, the antidiuretic hormone.[783, 864, 865] Atrial natriuretic polypeptide, blood levels of which increase during tachycardia,[862, 866–869] produce natriuresis. Increased release of renal prostaglandin E_2 also contributes to the natriuresis.[865]

Cerebral Circulation

Regional cerebral blood flow, evaluated by inhalation of xenon-133, in patients without symptoms of heart failure or neurological diseases is reduced in the presence of chronic atrial fibrillation compared with sinus rhythm, even when no acute neurological abnormalities develop.[870]

PATHOLOGY[871–875]

General Features

Fibrosis increasingly replaces functioning muscle tissue as atrial fibrillation develops and becomes chronic.[553, 586, 698, 876] The sinoatrial node[877] and internodal tracts[871] may be severely damaged and replaced by fibrosis.[871]

Patients who die of myocardial infarction and atrial fibrillation usually have occlusions of coronary arteries proximal to the origin of the sinus node artery and infarction of the sinus node itself.[878] Occlusion of the sinoatrial nodal artery can be the only lesion producing atrial fibrillation.[879]

Degeneration of atrial cells, observed with electron microscopy and characteristically severe in patients with atrial fibrillation, is more marked in patients with mitral regurgitation, with or without mitral stenosis, than in those with pure mitral stenosis.[880] The heart of a patient with Wolff-Parkinson-White syndrome and atrial fibrillation who died in ventricular fibrillation was characterized by multiple pathways and replacement of the sinoatrial node with collagen-elastic tissue and degeneration of much of the normal atrial architecture.[516]

Patients with atrial fibrillation and emboli have more mural thrombi than those without emboli.[429] Atrial thrombosis appears with greater frequency in patients who have had atrial fibrillation for a long time and less often in paroxysmal fibrillators.[871] Almost complete separation of the atrioventricular node from the atria and fibrosis of the atrioventricular node, the approaches to it, and the bundle of His characterized the pathological features of a patient with atrial fibrillation treated with atrioventricular nodal ablation.[881]

Lone Atrial Fibrillation

Although patients with lone atrial fibrillation have, by definition, no clinical heart disease, pathological abnormalities[882] were found in the myocardial biopsies

---

llll The most significant change. After induction of atrial fibrillation, the mean stroke volume decreased from 78 milliliters during sinus rhythm to 48 milliliters and the mean heart rate rose from 73 beats per minute during sinus rhythm to 128 beats per minute in 15 patients with paroxysmal atrial fibrillation and no structural heart disease.[857]

mmmm Paul Wood's report on "Polyuria in Paroxysmal Tachycardia and Paroxysmal Atrial Flutter and Fibrillation," edited after Wood's death by Maurice Campbell, was the last paper written by the Australian-born British cardiologist, who died in July 1962.[860]

nnnn The rise in hematocrit usually produced by atrial fibrillation may be caused by the polyuria.[757]

of each of 12 patients with atrial fibrillation and no previously recognized structural heart disease.[883] The findings included severe hypertrophy with vacuolar degeneration of the atrial myocytes, lymphomononuclear infiltrates with necrosis of the adjacent myocytes, or nonspecific fibrosis.[883] Furthermore, coronary heart disease may be demonstrated unexpectedly in patients thought to have lone atrial fibrillation.[373]

CLINICAL ELECTROPHYSIOLOGY[494, 884–890]

Electrophysiological Recognition of Atrial Fibrillation

During sinus rhythm, the A wave, a relatively large signal, can be recorded from atrial activation through catheter electrodes placed in the atria or near the atrioventricular junction.[891] The small H wave then appears from conduction through the bundle of His. Depolarization from the ventricles produces the large-amplitude V wave, which follows the A and H waves.

Atrial activity. In atrial fibrillation, A waves are replaced by rapid, disorganized, irregular deflections from the same electrical activity that produces the F waves on the surface electrocardiogram (Fig. 4.8).[596, 892–901] The amplitude of these signals tends to be smaller than that produced by the atria during sinus rhythm.[902, 903] Drugs such as procainamide decrease the amplitude and the frequency of the atrial signals.[904]

Characteristics of the signals detected from intra-atrial electrodes during atrial fibrillation are similar to

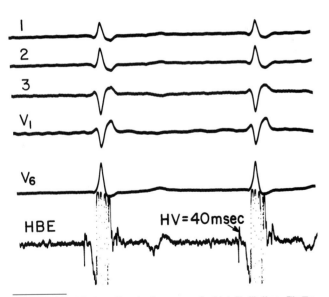

FIGURE 4.8 His bundle electrogram of atrial fibrillation. Fibrillation produces the rapid low-amplitude electrical activity in the His bundle electrogram (HBE). H deflections precede each of the two ventricular complexes, confirming the supraventricular origin of the beats. The *arrow* points to the second H deflection. The HV interval of 40 milliseconds indicates that conduction from the bundle of His to the ventricles is normal. (Electrocardiographic leads shown are I, II, III, V₁, and V₆.)

those recorded from the ventricles during ventricular fibrillation.[905] The morphology of unipolar-recorded intra-atrial signals from patients with atrial fibrillation has been categorized into four types of potentials: single, short-double, long-double, and fragmented.[899] This classification may correspond to the different appearances of atrial fibrillation on the surface electrocardiogram and to the mechanisms of the arrhythmia. The more disorganized the activation of the right atrium, the "finer" the F waves on the electrocardiogram; the more organized the "coarser" the F waves.[596] A few patients with what appears to be atrial fibrillation on the surface electrocardiogram have discrete foci of rapidly discharging impulses that seem more organized than is usually the case.[906–908]

Occasionally, patients with long-standing chronic atrial fibrillation spontaneously convert to sinus rhythm.[553] In one case, when fibrillation disappeared, no atrial activity was seen on the electrocardiogram.[829] Electrophysiological study revealed only left atrial depolarizations with A waves on the His bundle electrogram, but no P waves on the surface electrocardiogram. No electrical activity could be recorded from catheters in the body of the right atrium, nor could electrical stimulation capture that chamber.[829]

Supraventricular versus ventricular beats. Clinicians can usually distinguish supraventricular beats with aberrancy from ventricular premature beats by examining the electrogram. Occasionally, when this is not possible, an electrophysiological study may be necessary to make the diagnosis and to prescribe treatment correctly.

Aberrantly conducted beats in atrial fibrillation produce normal H and V waves, as they course down the bundle of His and through the ventricular conducting system to the myocardium. Beats originating in the ventricles, however, in retrograde manner activate the bundle of His. The H deflection then occurs during or slightly after, but not before, the V wave.[611, 892]

Concealed Conduction[909]

Concealed conduction refers to the ability of a beat to affect subsequent conduction and impulse formation.[606, 617, 910] The activity that produces the change is *concealed* from view on the electrocardiogram. In patients with atrial fibrillation, concealed conduction occurs continuously, usually from the atria but sometimes from the ventricles.[606]

Antegrade concealed conduction. Many more electrical signals are formed in the fibrillating atria than can be transmitted to the ventricles for the production of QRS complexes. Atrial signals that do not reach the ventricles penetrate the atrioventricular node in varying physiological, and probably anatomical, degrees.[606] These partially conducted signals decrease the conduction of subsequent signals, thereby slowing the ventricular rate.

Because of concealed conduction, the more rapid the atrial rate, the slower the ventricular response. For example, when the atrial rate suddenly decreases as atrial fibrillation changes to atrial flutter, the ventricular rate increases because fewer signals from the atria enter the atrioventricular node to delay conduction. Conversely, the ventricular rate decreases when atrial fibrillation replaces atrial flutter or atrial tachycardia.[606, 911, 912] In patients with dual atrioventricular nodal pathways—an important substrate for the development of reentrant supraventricular tachycardia—concealed conduction from one pathway to another does not determine the rate of the ventricular response.[913]

Retrograde concealed conduction. Retrograde concealed conduction occurs when ventricular ectopic beats develop during atrial fibrillation. They may penetrate the His-Purkinje conducting system or the atrioventricular node and may block antegrade conduction from the atria or delay the discharge of a junctional pacemaker.[911] This phenomenon produces the compensatory-like pause that usually follows the ventricular premature beats when they occur in atrial fibrillation or sinus rhythm.[606, 914–916, oooo] Beats conducted down the atrioventricular nodal His-Purkinje system in retrograde manner penetrate and decrease antegrade conduction in the accessory pathways of patients with atrial fibrillation and preexcitation.

Rhythm and Rate of the Ventricular Response to Atrial Fibrillation

Cardiologists still do not know exactly why the ventricular rate is usually irregular in atrial fibrillation despite much thought and study with, among other techniques, computerized analysis of RR intervals.[555, 917–933] The irregularity of the atrial activity, however, must be an important factor.[934] Analysis of the fibrillatory activity in the atria reveals a single peak in the frequency spectrum of many patients.[935] This peak frequency is slower in patients who have had the arrhythmia for shorter periods of time.[935]

The rate of the ventricular response in atrial fibrillation is determined within the atrioventricular node[936, pppp] by its refractoriness, by the direction, summation, and concealed conduction of the atrial impulses within it, and by the effects of autonomic forces on it.[920, 932, 937, 938] Slower ventricular rates at night attest to a circadian fluctuation of atrioventricular nodal conduction.[938, 939] Congestive heart failure appears to reduce this circadian variation.[939] Respiration seldom affects the rate of the ventricular response. However,

in a few patients, the RR intervals are longest at the end of respiration.[940]

Atrial Electrophysiological Abnormalities

Certain electrophysiological features of human atria characterize patients who develop atrial fibrillation.[941]

Vulnerability and induction. Atrial fibrillation begins when an atrial premature beat appears in the atrial vulnerable period, a short segment of time during the QRS complex and ST segment of the electrocardiogram.[qqqq] In the atrial vulnerable period, a single spontaneous or paced beat may disorganize atrial electrical activity so that fibrillation develops[660, 942–944] (Figs. 4.9 and 4.10). It follows, then, that atrial fibrillation will more likely develop in a susceptible patient when the atrial premature beat occurs soon after the previous sinus beat.[942, 945, 946, rrrr]

Introduction of a single, properly timed, atrial stimulus can induce *sustained* atrial fibrillation in patients with a history of the arrhythmia but seldom in patients without clinical atrial fibrillation.[947, 948] Stimulation in the vulnerable period produces *transient* bursts of atrial fibrillation in some patients who do not have the clinical arrhythmia.[943] Pacing in the coronary sinus prevents induction of atrial fibrillation by extrastimuli from the high right atrium.[949]

Surface electrocardiogram and intra-atrial recordings show that a rapid, regular atrial rhythm, like atrial tachycardia or flutter, often briefly precedes the onset of atrial fibrillation.[942, 944] This sequence may occur in reverse when atrial fibrillation changes to sinus rhythm.[944] Deflections in the atrial electrogram become more regular, and in the surface electrocardiogram, the F waves become larger and slower.[944]

Conduction delays. Conduction within the atria, particularly after premature atrial stimuli, takes longer than normal in patients with atrial fibrillation.[383, 636, 638, 948, 950–960, ssss] A wider than normal P wave on the electrocardiogram, which indicates atrial conduction delay, identifies patients likely to have atrial fibrillation after cardiac surgery[634] but it does not discriminate all

---

oooo Studies of retrograde conduction in patients with atrial fibrillation have suggested that the atrioventricular node itself may behave as a pacemaker in such patients[915] and that electrotonically mediated propagation in the junctional area may explain some features of atrioventricular transmission in atrial fibrillation.[916] When heart block and atrial fibrillation coexist, a ventricular beat may echo within the atrioventricular junction and produce an unexpectedly early subsequent ventricular beat.[914]

pppp As observed by Sir Thomas Lewis in 1910: "Auricular fibrillation in man may be accompanied by heart-block of all grades, and the heart-block may or may not result from digitalis administration."[936]

qqqq The *atrial* vulnerable period occurs earlier in the cardiac cycle than the *ventricular* vulnerable period.

rrrr A spontaneous ventricular premature beat may rarely induce atrial fibrillation from ventriculoatrial conduction in an accessory pathway.[945]

ssss In the electrophysiology laboratory, intra-atrial conduction is measured from the PA interval (the time from beginning of the P wave on the electrocardiogram to the A wave of atrial activation taken from the intra-atrial electrode) or from the difference in time of activation measured from electrodes in two or more sites in the atria.[950] To demonstrate abnormal conduction delays, premature beats may be introduced at one of the sites, the conduction of which will be progressively delayed as the premature beat is delivered sooner after the sinus or paced regular atrial beats. Fragmented, prolonged atrial electrograms recorded from intra-atrial electrodes and corresponding to local delayed conduction[959] are found in patients with paroxysmal atrial fibrillation and particularly in those with paroxysmal atrial fibrillation and sick sinus syndrome.[954, 958, 959] These abnormal electrograms, when present, may predict the future occurrence of clinical atrial fibrillation in patients currently in sinus rhythm.[954]

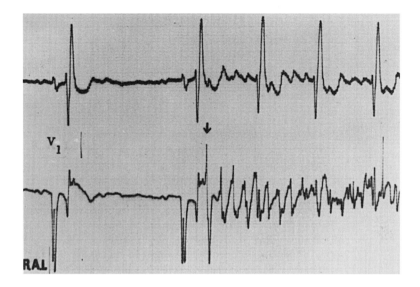

FIGURE 4.9 **An atrial premature beat during the atrial vulnerable period starts a paroxysm of atrial fibrillation.** The first two beats are sinus beats (*upper panel,* lead V₁). Then an atrial premature beat *(arrow)* appears during the atrial vulnerable period, and fibrillation begins. The rapid fibrillatory waves are easily seen in recording from an intra-atrial lead *(lower panel)*. R.A.L., right atrial lead. (From Bennett MA, Pentecost BL. The pattern of onset and spontaneous cessation of atrial fibrillation in man. Circulation 1970; 41:981–988, by permission of the American Heart Association, Inc.)[944]

patients with paroxysmal atrial fibrillation from those without the arrhythmia.[948] Intra-atrial conduction is delayed more frequently in older patients with organic heart disease and atrial fibrillation than in younger patients whose fibrillation is associated with the Wolff-Parkinson-White syndrome and no structural heart disease.[961, 962]

Atrial excitability and refractoriness. Atrial excitability and refractoriness are often abnormal in patients with atrial fibrillation and other atrial arrhythmias such as atrial flutter.[636, 951–953, 956, 959, 963–968, tttt] Atrial fibrillation shortens the refractory period of the atria,[969] and as the arrhythmia spontaneously terminates, the functional refractory period is prolonged, whereas shortening of refractoriness is associated with persistence of the arrhythmia.[900] Atrial premature beats lengthen the dispersion of atrial refractory periods in patients with paroxysmal atrial fibrillation, but they shorten the dis-

---

tttt Investigators have obtained different results while studying human atrial electrophysiological properties, and the interested reader should consult the references for specific information.

persion in subjects free of atrial arrhythmias.[970] Several minutes of induced atrial fibrillation shorten the refractory period of the atria.[971] One cannot capture the entire atrium while it is fibrillating with electrical stimulation. However, atrial pacing can capture small regions[972] of up to 15 millimeters from the pacing site.[973]

Activation.[974] Computerized mapping during open-heart surgery of the left atria of patients with atrial fibrillation demonstrates multiple wave fronts, nonuniform conduction, bidirectional block, and large macroreentrant circuits but no microreentrant circuits or atrial automaticity.[975] The left atrium acts as the "electrical driving chamber" in the majority of patients with atrial fibrillation and isolated mitral value disease.[976] Recordings from electrocatheters reveal significantly various levels of disorganization in different locations within the atria.[977]

Sinus node disease. Electrophysiological abnormalities of sinus function are present more often in pa-

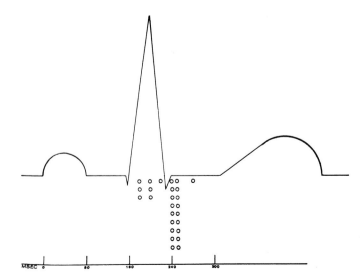

FIGURE 4.10 **Paced atrial premature beats that induce atrial fibrillation** *(circles)* **activate the atria during or soon after the QRS complex while the atria are being repolarized ("atrial vulnerable period").** Stimulation at other times does not induce the arrhythmia. MSEC, time in milliseconds after the beginning of the P waves. (Adapted from Haft JI, Lau SH, Stein E, Kosowsky BD, Damato AN. Atrial fibrillation produced by atrial stimulation. Circulation 1968; 37:70–74, by permission of the American Heart Association, Inc.)[943]

tients with chronic lone atrial fibrillation than in patients without the arrhythmia.[636]

Vagal stimulation. Those patients with lone atrial fibrillation that appears when vagal tone is high have prolonged PA intervals, a finding suggesting intra-atrial conduction defects, but no other abnormalities on electrophysiological evaluation.[383] The arrhythmia characteristically appears when the atria are paced sufficiently *slowly.* Administration of a vagotonic agent such as adenosine can produce vagally mediated atrial fibrillation.[383]

Wolff-Parkinson-White Syndrome

Atrial fibrillation, when it occurs in patients with the Wolff-Parkinson-White syndrome, has special electrophysiological characteristics related to the accessory pathways that are the unique attributes of the syndrome[978–980] (Fig. 4.11).

Importance of supraventricular tachycardia. In many patients with preexcitation, atrial fibrillation develops from the effects on the atria of rapid supraventricular tachycardia, the characteristic arrhythmia of patients with accessory pathways.[163, 164, 501, 517, 665, 981–987] The average rate of supraventricular tachycardia is, according to one group,[979] but may not be, according to another,[164] faster in patients with atrial fibrillation than in those without atrial fibrillation. As atrial rates rise from rapid supraventricular tachycardia, atrial vulnerability increases.[963, 983] In patients without organic heart disease, abnormal atrial vulnerability may facilitate the institution of atrial fibrillation by reentrant supraventricular tachycardia.[983]

Atrial pacing induces atrial fibrillation more readily in patients with supraventricular tachycardia, whether sustained within the atrioventricular node or in accessory pathways, than in patients without the tachycardia.[988] Conversely, supraventricular tachycardia can be induced in more patients with Wolff-Parkinson-White syndrome with atrial fibrillation than in those without atrial fibrillation. Premature beats delivered during supraventricular tachycardia may induce atrial fibrillation,[163, 501, 983, 989] which can also be started by supraventricular tachycardia sustained through concealed accessory pathways that do not produce the electrocardiographic signs of preexcitation in sinus rhythm.[983]

Atrial fibrillation more likely develops in those patients with and without the Wolff-Parkinson-White syndrome who have structural heart disease, particularly when it affects the left atrium. As one would expect, rapid supraventricular tachycardia changes easily to atrial fibrillation in such patients.[164] Patients with preexcitation, atrial fibrillation, and no inducible supraventricular tachycardia usually have structural heart disease.[163] Thus, in those with lone atrial fibrillation, reentrant supraventricular tachycardia is seldom the inciting arrhythmia.[375] Retrograde multiple or multifiber accessory pathways sustain clinical and inducible atrial fibrillation more often than single accessory pathways.[990]

Spontaneous atrial fibrillation occurs infrequently after accessory pathways—essential for sustaining most supraventricular tachycardias in patients with the Wolff-Parkinson-White syndrome—are ablated.[979, 989, 991, 992] Atrial fibrillation, however, can still be induced after accessory pathway ablation, although it subsides spontaneously.[992] This finding suggests that intrinsic atrial abnormalities necessary to sustain atrial fibrillation are still present, but supraventricular tachycardia, the trigger for atrial fibrillation in these patients, has been eliminated.[992]

Electrophysiological characteristics of the atria. Pa-

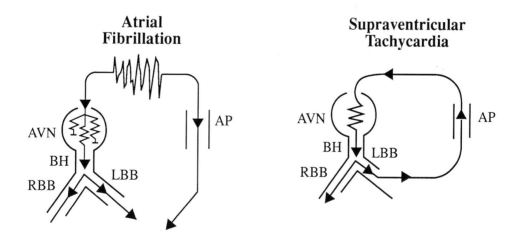

FIGURE 4.11 **Atrial fibrillation and reentrant supraventricular tachycardia in Wolff-Parkinson-White syndrome.** When the atria fibrillate (*intra-atrial electrogram at top,* **left diagram**), signals conduct to the ventricles through the atrioventricular node (AVN) and accessory pathway (AP). The atrioventricular node blocks some signals and slowly transmits others, whereas the signals travel rapidly and with little delay through the accessory pathway. Hence, the ventricular rate will be faster when conduction in the accessory pathway dominates. In supraventricular tachycardia **(right diagram),** the electrical activity usually courses down the atrioventricular node through the bundle of His (BH) and right and left bundle branches (RBB, LBB), into the ventricles, up the accessory pathway, and through the atria to reenter the circuit at the atrioventricular node.

tients with atrial fibrillation and preexcitation often demonstrate the following:

- Delayed intra-atrial conduction.[978, 989, 991, 993–995, uuuu]
- Shorter atrial functional refractoriness.[978, 993, 996]
- Greater atrial irritability.[983, 987, 989, 997]
- Repetitive atrial firing.[994, 996]
- Fragmented atrial activity.[994, 996, 997]

Thus, the atria tend to be similarly abnormal in patients with atrial fibrillation, whether or not these patients have the Wolff-Parkinson-White syndrome. A sufficiently premature atrial[163, 983, 989] or ventricular[945, 981, 998] beat, which reaches the atria via retrograde conduction, can institute atrial fibrillation during the atrial vulnerable period.

Electrophysiological characteristics of accessory pathways. Certain features of accessory pathways affect the frequency with which atrial fibrillation appears[981] in patients with the Wolff-Parkinson-White syndrome.

Refractoriness determines the ease with which the accessory pathway can conduct. When refractoriness is long, relatively few atrial signals can traverse the accessory pathway. When refractoriness is short, more signals reach the ventricles, producing a rapid ventricular response and occasionally ventricular fibrillation. In patients with the Wolff-Parkinson-White syndrome and atrial fibrillation but no organic heart disease, refractoriness of the accessory pathways tends to be short.[166, 978, 989, 991] Increased *sympathetic tone* from anxiety, hypotension, or congestive failure produced by the rapid heart action may predispose patients to maintenance of atrial fibrillation and may produce faster ventricular rates.[991]

Determinants of the ventricular rate and width of the QRS complexes. Ventricular rates in patients with atrial fibrillation and the Wolff-Parkinson-White syndrome can be faster than in patients without preexcitation because accessory pathways may conduct more atrial impulses per minute than can the atrioventricular node. However, the amount of block in accessory pathways can vary widely in individual patients at different times.[999]

Three electrophysiological measurements indicate the rate the ventricles can reach from conduction in accessory pathways during atrial fibrillation:[163, 983, 987, 1000–1002, vvvv]

- The *shortest RR interval* produced by conduction down either the accessory pathways or the atrioventricular node during spontaneous or induced atrial fibrillation. The shorter the shortest

interval, the faster the mean ventricular rate.[937, 997, 1003, 1004] The accessory pathways of patients with RR intervals of less than 250 milliseconds conduct rapidly and predispose such patients to ventricular fibrillation. The effects of drugs on accessory pathways may be evaluated by measuring RR intervals from patients with induced atrial fibrillation.[986] Exercise does not decrease the RR intervals of preexcited beats.[653] The shortest preexcited RR interval of less than 220 milliseconds predicts sudden death more sensitively than the clinical history.[1005]
- The *antegrade refractory period of the accessory pathway.* Shorter refractory periods allow conduction of more beats and produce wider QRS complexes, shorter RR intervals, and faster ventricular rates.[166, 997, 1003, 1004, 1006, 1007] Faster atrial rates often, but not always, shorten refractoriness in the accessory pathway. Consequently, atrial fibrillation and flutter can, by themselves, accelerate conduction in the accessory pathway by their effect on the refractory period.[1003, 1004]
- The *antegrade refractory period of the atrioventricular node.* Atrial impulses enter the atrioventricular node as well as the accessory pathways of patients with the Wolff-Parkinson-White syndrome. If the ventricles are activated via the accessory pathway, the rate is usually faster and the QRS complex is abnormal; rates are slower and the QRS complex is more normal if atrioventricular nodal conduction predominates. Which pathway is favored depends on the refractory periods and extent of concealed conduction[928, 1006, 1008, 1009] in each pathway and the effects of autonomic tone mostly on the atrioventricular node.

When the refractory periods of the atrioventricular node and accessory pathways are similar, ventricular rates are also similar whether activation occurs through the accessory pathway or the atrioventricular node.[1010] This applies even when the conduction of the node is enhanced as in patients with short PR intervals and normal QRS complexes (Lown-Ganong-Levine syndrome).[1010]

Ventricular fibrillation. Patients with the Wolff-Parkinson-White syndrome who sustain cardiac arrest[514] usually have had episodes of clinical atrial fibrillation[515, 516] or have sustained atrial fibrillation that can be produced in the electrophysiology laboratory. The arrhythmia that kills is ventricular fibrillation produced by atrial fibrillation or atrial flutter, transmitted to the ventricles over accessory pathways that conduct rapidly and block relatively few atrial impulses. Human ventricles fibrillate when they are stimulated rapidly enough, and particularly when they are also subjected to strong catecholamine drive.[985] That isoproterenol can speed conduction in accessory pathways and shorten RR intervals[985, 1011] further supports evidence that sympathetic stimulation can increase the risk of ventricular fibrillation.

Patients resuscitated from cardiac arrest and most

uuuu Although not all investigators agree.[989]

vvvv To determine which patients with preexcitation have the highest risk of developing a fatal arrhythmia, electrophysiologists often induce atrial fibrillation by rapidly pacing the atria through electrode catheters in the atria[163, 983] or esophagus.[1000, 1001] The ventricular response to atrial fibrillation induced in the electrophysiology laboratory correlates well with the rate of the clinical arrhythmia in individual patients.[987] Furthermore, rapid pacing frequently produces sustained atrial fibrillation in patients with spontaneous atrial fibrillation and seldom does so in those who are asymptomatic.[526, 1002]

likely to develop ventricular fibrillation have the following:

- Short refractory periods of their accessory pathways,[517] and short RR intervals,[516] usually of less than 250 milliseconds.[517]
- More episodes of supraventricular tachycardia, which may initiate atrial fibrillation.[517]
- A history of atrial fibrillation.
- The combination of atrial fibrillation, supraventricular tachycardia, and multiple accessory pathways.[517, 982, wwww]

Patients with the Wolff-Parkinson-White syndrome and atrial fibrillation may occasionally develop ventricular tachyarrhythmias that cause syncope[530, xxxx] and cardiac arrest from primary, intrinsic ventricular tachycardia, rather than from rapid conduction down accessory pathways. Electrophysiological studies may be needed to establish this diagnosis.[989, 1012] Inducible and spontaneous intrinsic ventricular arrhythmias in patients with the Wolff-Parkinson-White syndrome and atrial fibrillation may decrease after successful ablation of accessory pathways.[989] The reasons are unknown.

Intermittent preexcitation. Intermittent preexcitation in which some beats have short PR intervals and delta waves and others are normal indicates that the accessory pathway conducts poorly. Patients with this finding have long refractory periods of their accessory pathways and shortest RR intervals greater than 250 milliseconds during induced atrial fibrillation.[1013] This electrocardiographic finding in asymptomatic patients predicts a relatively slow ventricular response should atrial fibrillation develop and a favorable prognosis.

Eventually, the accessory pathways of many patients with the Wolff-Parkinson-White syndrome spontaneously lose the ability to conduct and sustain clinical arrhythmias.[1010, 1014] Such patients tend to be older,[1014, yyyy] and as one could expect, had longer effective refractory periods of their accessory pathways when they were able to conduct.[1014] This progression to what has been called "non–Wolff-Parkinson-White" helps to account for the low mortality among asymptomatic patients with preexcitation.[1014]

Other Advances

Clinical investigators have devoted much work, in particular recently, to better understand the electrophysiology of atrial fibrillation in humans.[596, 901, 973, 1015–1023] Detailed discussion of these interesting and important advances is beyond the scope of this book.

TREATMENT[15, 1024–1037]
General Therapy

When atrial fibrillation first develops and the ventricular rate is rapid, patients may present to their physi-

cians with congestive heart failure, angina, and hypotension. Many symptoms resolve when drugs have reduced the ventricular rate. Patients who are acutely ill and in whom further dangerous deterioration seems likely may require early cardioversion. However, the procedure is usually conducted electively when the patient's cardiovascular condition has stabilized. Cardiologists and other trained personnel, transported in mobile cardiac care units, can safely and expeditiously treat paroxysms of atrial fibrillation in patients' homes.[1038, zzzz]

Two large clinical trials in the United States[1039, aaaaa] and Europe[1040, bbbbb] seek to establish whether patients benefit more from maintenance of sinus rhythm with cardioversion and antiarrhythmic drugs or from control of the ventricular rate with the patient remaining in atrial fibrillation.[1041, 1042] Perhaps the results from these studies will help to improve how many physicians treat atrial fibrillation[1043] and will reduce the considerable variation between how cardiologists and other physicians manage patients with the arrhythmia.[1044]

Physical Maneuvers

Carotid sinus pressure,[1045] which increases the vagal influence on the atrioventricular node, decreases the ventricular rate in patients with atrial fibrillation.[1046–1048, ccccc] Carotid sinus pressure occasionally converts the arrhythmia to sinus rhythm.[350, 1047, 1049]

The response to carotid sinus pressure can help physicians to diagnose tachyarrhythmias (Table 4.4). As the rate of the ventricular response to atrial fibrillation decreases, the rhythm's irregularity becomes obvious, and the F waves, which may not be visible at rapid ventricular rates, appear. Atrial fibrillation rarely becomes regular when carotid sinus pressure decreases the ventricular rate, except in the unusual circumstance when the maneuver produces sinus rhythm.

Drugs[1050–1066]

The primary treatment of atrial fibrillation has been, and continues to be, pharmacological. Drugs are given to reduce the ventricular rate and to convert and sustain sinus rhythm. Testing in the electrophysiological laboratory can identify which drug will most effectively sustain sinus rhythm for as long as possible.[1067]

Because most patients with chronic atrial fibrillation cannot be kept in regular rhythm indefinitely, rate control remains the principal use for drugs. An average rate of 90 beats per minute controls the ventricular rate with the least compromise of the cardiac out-

---

[wwww] Hypoxia and hypotension from prolonged periods of atrial fibrillation can also predispose ventricles to fibrillate.[982]

[xxxx] Syncope by itself, however, does not affect the prognosis of patients with the Wolff-Parkinson-White syndrome.[530]

[yyyy] Average of 50 years in 1 series of 9 patients.[1014]

[zzzz] A group in Florence, Italy reported that treating patients with supraventricular tachycardias at home reduced hospitalizations by 50%.[1038]

[aaaaa] Atrial Fibrillation Follow-Up Investigation of Rhythm Management (the AFFIRM study).[1039]

[bbbbb] Pharmacological Intervention in Atrial Fibrillation (the PIAF trial).[1040]

[ccccc] Electrical stimulation of the carotid sinuses greatly slows the ventricular response to atrial fibrillation.[1048]

Table 4.4 EFFECTS OF CORRECTLY PERFORMED CAROTID SINUS PRESSURE ON DIFFERENT ARRHYTHMIAS

Arrhythmia	Ventricular Rhythm	Effects of Carotid Sinus Pressure	After Carotid Sinus Pressure
Sinus tachycardia	Regular	Gradual slowing	Gradual speeding
Reentrant supraventricular tachycardia sustained in atrioventricular node, acccessory pathway, or atria	Regular	Sudden conversion to sinus rhythm	Maintenance in sinus rhythm
Atrial flutter, automatic atrial tachycardia	Regular	Slowing to regular or irregular rhythm	Return to regular tachycardia
Atrial fibrillation, atrial flutter, multifocal atrial tachycardia, automatic atrial tachycardia	Irregular	Slowing, remaining irregular	Return to irregular tachycardia
Ventricular tachycardia	Slightly irregular	No effect	No change

put.[931, ddddd] Because cardiac adverse events occur when antiarrhythmic drugs are started for atrial fibrillation, electrocardiographic monitoring for 24 to 48 hours in the hospital seems wise, particularly for elderly patients and for those who have had myocardial infarction.[1068]

Physicians should recognize when further attempts to produce and sustain sinus rhythm are likely to fail and should select medicines that will permit the patient to live comfortably with his or her arrhythmia.[1069] The protracted search for a safe,[1070] effective pharmacological method of suppressing paroxysmal atrial fibrillation may not contribute as much to a patient's well-being as acceptance of chronic atrial fibrillation and a well-controlled ventricular rate.[1071, 1072] One must also consider the risk of pro-arrhythmia, the property of many antiarrhythmic drugs to *produce* potentially fatal arrhythmias,[1050, 1070, 1073–1076] and that bundle of His modification or ablation and atrial surgery are available for those with persistent symptoms from atrial fibrillation.

Adenosine. Intravenous adenosine briefly produces high-grade atrioventricular nodal block in patients with atrial fibrillation.[1077, 1078] This effect may reveal F waves in patients with rapid responses to atrial fibrillation and may help to confirm the diagnosis. The drug does not affect the atrial rhythm itself.[1077]

Adenosine can induce atrial fibrillation, including that influenced by vagal stimuli,[383] by its ability to shorten atrial refractoriness.[1079] The drug transiently decreases the minimum, but does not affect the average, RR intervals produced by conduction down accessory pathways in patients with preexcitation and atrial fibrillation.[1080] In a patient with orthodromic supraventricular tachycardia, adenosine appeared to produce atrial fibrillation that, while conducting rapidly down the accessory pathway, compromised hemodynamic function.[1081]

Ajmaline. This short-acting, intravenously administered reserpine derivative can help to identify those patients with the Wolff-Parkinson-White syndrome and atrial flutter or atrial fibrillation who are at highest risk of developing ventricular fibrillation.[1082–1084] Ajmaline prolongs the effective refractory period of the acces-

sory pathway and produces high degrees of antegrade block in the accessory pathways of those patients whose refractory periods are relatively long. The drug has little effect on the accessory pathways of patients with short refractory periods, and these are the patients most likely to develop ventricular fibrillation. Ajmaline has no effect on atrioventricular nodal refractoriness or conduction, but it does slow infranodal function and can prolong the HV interval.[1085]

Amiodarone.[1086, 1087] This drug reduces recurrences of atrial fibrillation in many patients.[384, 715–717, 721, 1088–1112, eeeee]

General effects. Amiodarone has the following effects:

- It converts or maintains sinus rhythm well in most patients with paroxysmal or sustained atrial fibrillation, many of whom have failed treatment with other antiarrhythmic drugs such as quinidine.[715–717, 1093, 1098, 1101, 1102, fffff]
- It converts many patients with recent-onset atrial fibrillation to sinus rhythm with a single oral dose.[1113]
- When given intravenously, it decreases the ventricular rate[537, 1114, 1115] and converts some patients, including those with acute myocardial infarction,[1103] to sinus rhythm relatively quickly.[1116–1122]
- It maintains sinus rhythm at an average maintenance dose of 200 milligrams per day with few serious side effects.[1107]
- It maintains sinus rhythm better than sotalol.[1123]
- Given prophylactically, it reduces the incidence of atrial fibrillation after elective cardiac surgery and thereby also reduces the duration and cost of hospitalization.[1111]
- It abolishes atrial fibrillation and restores sinus rhythm in patients with hypertrophic cardiomyopathy who have had the arrhythmia for years.[1094, 1106]
- It helps to reduce the number of paroxysms in about half of patients with vagal-induced atrial

---

ddddd According to a study of 60 patients with atrial fibrillation evaluated by Doppler ultrasound.

eeeee The Canadian Trial of Atrial Fibrillation (CTAF), now under way (1998), compares the value of amiodarone versus sotalol and propafenone in maintaining sinus rhythm in patients with atrial fibrillation.[1112]

fffff Amiodarone produced good (partial) or excellent results in 219 (79%) of 277 patients with atrial fibrillation from 7 of the largest series.[715–717, 1093, 1098, 1101, 1102]

fibrillation, despite the drug's characteristic slowing of the sinus rate.[383, 385]

- Like digitalis and beta-blocking and calcium-channel–blocking drugs, it slows the ventricular response in those patients in whom fibrillation persists.[981, 1083, 1092, 1100, 1105, 1116, 1124, *ggggg*]
- When given concurrently with flecainide,[1125] it reduces the amount of flecainide needed to maintain sinus rhythm and to reduce the number of premature beats that may give rise to atrial fibrillation.
- It has helped those children with atrial flutter and fibrillation who have been treated with the drug.[1126]

Despite receiving prolonged treatment with amiodarone for atrial fibrillation, few patients develop side effects that require the drug to be discontinued.[715–717, 1101, *hhhhh*]

Wolff-Parkinson-White syndrome. Amiodarone decreases the ventricular rate[1090] by blocking conduction in the accessory pathway and thereby lengthening the shortest RR intervals[1100] of many, but not all,[1100, 1127] patients with the Wolff-Parkinson-White syndrome and atrial fibrillation.[1128, 1129, *iiiii*] Therefore, amiodarone has the following effects:

- It reduces the likelihood that some patients with short refractory periods in their accessory pathways will develop ventricular fibrillation.[981, 1100]
- It reduces the number of episodes of paroxysmal atrial fibrillation by decreasing the development of reentrant supraventricular tachycardia and exerting atrial stabilizing effects in patients with the Wolff-Parkinson-White syndrome.[1092, 1100]
- It makes more difficult the induction of atrial fibrillation during electrophysiological testing by rapid atrial stimulation.[1092]
- When given intravenously, it converts and provides up to 48 hours of sinus rhythm in 80% of patients.[1118]
- It has prevented recurrences of atrial and ventricular fibrillation for an average of 30 months in each of 10 patients with the Wolff-Parkinson-White syndrome and a history of spontaneous atrial fibrillation and rapid ventricular response.[1105]

Aprindine. Aprindine prolongs conduction in the accessory pathway of patients with the Wolff-Parkinson-White syndrome and can slow the ventricular rate.[1130] However, too few patients with atrial fibrillation have been studied for conclusions about aprindine's therapeutic value to be drawn.[1067]

Atropine. This vagolytic drug increases the ventricular rate in those patients with atrial fibrillation whose ventricular response is mediated by vagotonia in the atrioventricular node.[1131–1133] However, atropine has not proved useful for treating patients with atrial fibrillation and the tachycardia-bradycardia syndrome even when the abnormal atrial rhythms and bradycardia are due to increased vagal tone.[1134] By maintaining a more rapid sinus rhythm, atropine can suppress vagal-induced atrial fibrillation.[365, 385] However, administration of atropine parenterally and continuously for this purpose is impractical.

Beta-adrenergic–blocking drugs. These drugs are most frequently used in patients with atrial fibrillation to reduce the ventricular rate.[1135]

Reducing ventricular rate. Each of the drugs in this class decreases the ventricular rate in patients with atrial fibrillation,[391, 1136–1161] by blocking beta-adrenergic influences on the atrioventricular node and thereby increasing its refractoriness. The greatest slowing occurs in patients with the fastest rates.[1142] In the clinical electrophysiology laboratory, this property is recognized by lengthening of the AH interval of patients in sinus rhythm.[1162–1164]

Beta-blocking drugs, such as propranolol, control ventricular rates more effectively than digitalis alone, probably because the drugs act in different ways. Digitalis increases vagal tone, and propranolol blocks beta-adrenergic influences on the atrioventricular node.[1165] The combination decreases the maximal heart rate that patients with atrial fibrillation may develop both at rest[1166, *jjjjj*] and on exertion.[1157, 1166–1174]

Although patients may perceive better effort tolerance and reduction or disappearance of palpitations,[1166] their measurable exercise ability is not usually increased by beta blockers.[1169, 1172, 1173, 1175] Even though the heart rate slows, the beta-blocking drug propranolol can occasionally induce congestive failure, particularly in patients with valvular heart disease, even if they have also received digitalis.[1145, 1176]

When beta-blocking drugs decrease the ventricular rate so much that a pacemaker is being considered or the frequency of vagal-induced paroxysmal atrial fibrillation increases, pindolol[1177, 1178] or xamoterol[1179] can be used; they also have intrinsic sympathomimetic activity. Used with digoxin, pindolol controls daytime tachycardia,[1177] prevents nocturnal bradycardia,[1177] reduces the length of nocturnal ventricular pauses,[1177] and produces no clinically expressed negative inotropic effect.[1180] Beta-adrenergic–blocking drugs are particularly effective when the arrhythmia depends on adrenergic drive,[391] but they can aggravate vagal-induced atrial fibrillation.[391]

Conversion. Beta blockers, even when given intravenously, convert few patients with chronic or paroxysmal atrial fibrillation to sinus rhythm.[1138, 1139, 1141, 1150,

---

ggggg Amiodarone prolongs refractory periods and slows conduction in most cardiac tissues,[1124] including the atrioventricular node, bundle of His, accessory pathways,[981, 1083, 1100, 1105] and atrial and ventricular myocardium.

hhhhh Twenty (14%) of 141 patients in 4 series.[715–717, 1101]

iiiii Occasionally, the ventricular rate may temporarily increase after intravenous administration of amiodarone,[1128] and, in one reported case, ventricular fibrillation was produced.[1129]

---

jjjjj The beta blocker timolol has little effect when the resting heart rate is slower than 90 beats per minute.[1166]

[1151, 1156, 1161, 1176, 1181, kkkkk] The combination of quinidine and propranolol does not convert patients more successfully than quinidine alone.[1147, 1148, 1182, 1183]

After cardioversion. Propranolol, when given with other antiarrhythmic drugs before cardioversion, may reduce the incidence of arrhythmias afterward.[1184] Sotalol, a beta-blocking drug with class III antiarrhythmic properties, preserves sinus rhythm after cardioversion as successfully as quinidine[1185] and propafenone,[1186] and, in addition, it controls the ventricular rate if the patient develops atrial fibrillation again.[1185]

Cardiac surgery. Beta blockers administered prophylactically decrease the incidence of supraventricular tachyarrhythmias, including atrial fibrillation, in patients after cardiac surgery,[71, 261, 262, 267, 272, 276, 1187–1208] probably,[267, 1191] but not definitely,[1209, 1210] in low doses and even when the patients had been taking the drugs before surgery.[1192, 1211, lllll] Propranolol,[1144] sotalol,[1212] and esmolol[1213] have been reported to convert patients who developed atrial fibrillation after cardiac surgery to sinus rhythm. Sotalol prevents supraventricular tachyarrhythmias, including atrial fibrillation, from developing after cardiac surgery more effectively than metoprolol.[1201] It is as effective as the combination of digoxin and disopyramide and acts faster.[1212]

Myocardial infarction. Metoprolol reduces the incidence of atrial fibrillation developing during myocardial infarction.[1214]

Wolff-Parkinson-White syndrome. Except for sotalol,[1215] which can prevent excessively short RR intervals by its class III characteristics, beta-blocking drugs have little effect on refractoriness or conduction in accessory pathways.[984, 1216, 1217] Hence, most of the drugs do not significantly reduce the ventricular response in patients with atrial fibrillation and antegrade conduction in the accessory pathway. Propranolol, however, may decrease the ventricular rate during atrial fibrillation by reducing the effects of adrenergic stimulation on accessory pathways.[1217] Propranolol may even increase the ventricular rate when most of the QRS complexes are narrow, possibly by eliminating concealed retrograde conduction in the accessory pathway.[1217]

Specific drugs. Beta-adrenergic–blocking drugs whose function and clinical usefulness have been evaluated in patients with atrial fibrillation include acebutolol,[1199, 1200] alprenolol,[1218] atenolol,[1204, 1205] celiprolol,[1175] esmolol,[1151–1154, 1156, 1213, 1219] labetalol,[1174] metoprolol,[1164, 1214] nadolol,[391, 1150, 1170, 1172, 1203, 1220] pindolol,[1177, 1180, 1221, 1222] propranolol,[242, 267, 271, 391, 1067, 1138, 1139, 1141, 1143–1145, 1147, 1148, 1162, 1167, 1168, 1176, 1181–1183, 1188–1196, 1206, 1209,]

sotalol,[1211, 1223] [1157, 1159–1161, 1185, 1206, 1207, 1212, 1224] timolol,[1166, 1198, 1202] and xamoterol.[1173, 1179]

Calcium-channel–blocking agents. Like beta-adrenergic blockers, these drugs are usually employed in patients with atrial fibrillation to slow the ventricular rate.

Decreasing ventricular rate. Administered orally, with or without digitalis, verapamil decreases the resting heart rate and reduces the excessive increase in heart rate on exertion that is characteristic of patients with atrial fibrillation.[1155, 1158, 1225–1236] Diltiazem has a similar effect.[1237–1243] The combination of verapamil and digoxin causes less nighttime bradycardia, shorter daytime ventricular pauses, and fewer palpitations than does an increased dose of digoxin alone.[1244]

When given intravenously, verapamil[1156, 1227, 1228, 1245–1253] and diltiazem[1254–1259] decrease the ventricular rate rapidly, more quickly than intravenous digoxin.[1260] Intravenous verapamil reliably reduces ventricular rates when atrial fibrillation develops after cardiac surgery,[1250, 1251] and diltiazem maintains ventricular rate control for hours during constant infusion.[1256]

Verapamil[1231, 1261] and diltiazem[1261] increase exercise capacity,[1231] although probably no better than digoxin alone.[1235] Calcium-channel–blocking drugs provide rate control without improvement in exercise capacity. Diltiazem slows the ventricular response without worsening the hemodynamic condition of patients with congestive heart failure, and it may improve function in some patients.[1257]

Conversion. Verapamil seldom converts atrial fibrillation to sinus rhythm.[630, 1120, 1246, 1250, 1251, 1262–1264] Verapamil does not prevent the development of atrial fibrillation after coronary artery bypass surgery,[1208, 1265, 1266] and, according to one report, it is associated with a high incidence of unacceptable hemodynamic side effects when given for this purpose.[1267]

Verapamil[1268] and diltiazem[1269] may prolong the duration of paroxysms of the arrhythmia whether the drug is given orally or intravenously or if the arrhythmia is produced by rapid atrial pacing.[1268] Verapamil occasionally induces the arrhythmia.[1270]

Regularization, F waves. When given intravenously, verapamil makes the ventricular rhythm more regular,[1229, 1245, 1246, 1248] particularly in patients whose ventricular response in the untreated condition is fast.[1246] The cause is not known. Intravenous verapamil decreases the size of the F waves in almost half of patients who receive the drug,[1246] but diltiazem does not.[1254]

Wolff-Parkinson-White syndrome. Verapamil[630, 1271] and diltiazem[1269] can adversely affect the clinical condition of patients with the Wolff-Parkinson-White syndrome and atrial fibrillation by increasing the ventricular rate. This occurs because of the drug's ability to shorten the refractory period of accessory pathways[1272–1274] and thereby to facilitate conduction of atrial impulses to the ventricles through accessory pathways in

kkkkk In one report, about 50% of patients with paroxysmal atrial fibrillation converted to sinus rhythm during intravenous treatment with esmolol, the ultrashort-acting beta blocker.[1156] Whether the drug or nature produced the conversion is not known.

lllll One study, however, found that arrhythmias were not suppressed in patients given propranolol preoperatively who continued taking the drug after operation.[1211]

some,[1269, 1273–1275] but not all,[1247] patients. Intravenous administration of verapamil can induce ventricular fibrillation in patients with preexcitation and atrial fibrillation.[1271, 1276, 1277]

Verapamil and diltiazem[1269] should not be administered intravenously to patients with atrial fibrillation and the Wolff-Parkinson-White syndrome and should probably be avoided for long-term use in all patients with preexcitation whose refractory periods of the accessory pathways are relatively short or unknown.

Digoxin level. Verapamil increases the digoxin level in patients receiving both drugs, but toxicity infrequently develops.[1229, 1230, 1278] However, physicians should consider decreasing the dose of digoxin slightly when verapamil is added and should increase the amount of verapamil rather than digoxin if additional rate control is required.

Clonidine. Clonidine is a selective alpha-2-adrenergic agonist usually employed to treat hypertension. It decreases the ventricular response in patients with atrial fibrillation and may help to convert them to sinus rhythm.[1279]

Digitalis.[1280–1283] Except for its use in congestive heart failure, digitalis is prescribed most frequently to treat atrial fibrillation.[97]

Reducing ventricular rate.[1158] Most physicians order digitalis for patients with atrial fibrillation to reduce the ventricular rate.[1284, 1285] The drug produces this effect by prolonging atrioventricular nodal conduction and refractoriness mostly through vagal stimulation,[1286, 1287] but also, to a lesser degree, by direct action on the atrioventricular node.[1288, 1289] Furthermore, digitalis increases the rate at which the atria discharge and thereby the amount of concealed conduction in the atrioventricular node.[1290]

The ventricular rate during atrial fibrillation may be difficult to control with digitalis in severe cases of mitral regurgitation and in other hyperkinetic circulatory states such as thyrotoxicosis and atrial septal defect. Digitalis can satisfactorily control the ventricular rate in many patients at rest, but on mild or moderate exertion, the ventricular rate often rises quickly to unacceptably high levels.[48, 641, 1166, 1291–1294] Exercise testing frequently reveals that the dose of digoxin may be safely increased to control the ventricular response better.[1294] However, usual therapeutic doses would not be expected to decrease the ventricular rate to less than 100 beats per minute at rest when serious complicating illnesses are present.[1295] Physicians who then administer extra digitalis may intoxicate patients[302, 1295] whose ventricular rates do not need to be 100 beats per minute or less. One should seek a ventricular rate similar to that expected if the patient were in sinus rhythm.[1296]

The ventricular rate in patients with atrial fibrillation corresponds poorly with digoxin dosage,[922, 1295] and with the serum digoxin concentration,[661, 1297–1299] although the heart rate in individual patients decreases

with increasing digoxin concentration. Beta-adrenergic[1166–1169, 1172–1175, 1222] and calcium-channel–blocking drugs[1226, 1231, 1233, 1239, 1300] help digitalis to control the ventricular response at rest and during exercise more effectively.[1233, 1242, 1301] Despite these problems controlling the rate, digitalis usually produces improvement in patients' subjective well-being and physical capacity,[1294] although their measurable increase in work capacity may be less impressive.[1291]

When paroxysmal atrial fibrillation develops, the ventricular rate of patients taking digitalis is no slower than the rate of patients who are not taking the drug.[1302] Patients with hypomagnesemia require additional digoxin to achieve adequate control of the ventricular rate,[769] and the administration of magnesium itself appears to augment the ventricular slowing effects of digoxin.[1303] Investigators now question, on the basis of both clinical efficacy[1158, 1304] and expense,[1304] the use of digoxin to control the ventricular rate[mmmmm] and convert to sinus rhythm when atrial fibrillation develops, and they suggest more efficient methods of treating paroxysmal atrial fibrillation with other drugs available for this purpose.[1304]

Conversion.[1283] Digitalis does not convert established atrial fibrillation to sinus rhythm and probably does not revert paroxysms of atrial fibrillation either.[1284–1285, 1305–1309, nnnnn] Because paroxysmal atrial fibrillation, by definition, occurs for limited periods, the arrhythmia eventually reverts by itself, and the assistance of digitalis in this process may be coincidental. The ventricular rate may not have decreased by the time paroxysmal atrial fibrillation converts after administration of digitalis intravenously; hence, one result may not depend on the other.[1310] Investigators have argued that digitalis should promote conversion because the drug relieves congestive heart failure and reduces left atrial pressure and enlargement. This thesis has not been proved.

"The effects of digitalis [on paroxysmal atrial fibrillation] are complicated and even paradoxical," John Parkinson and Maurice Campbell wrote in 1941.[534] The same can be said for the electrophysiological effects of the drug on the atria.[1289] Although its action on atrial vulnerability favors the ability of digitalis to sustain sinus rhythm,[1311] its vagotonic power should increase rather than relieve the tendency toward fibrillation.[1312]

Production of atrial fibrillation. Digitalis occasionally produces atrial fibrillation,[47, 534, 1313–1315] probably be-

---

[mmmmm] Although even recent studies confirm that the drug decreases the rate,[1285] albeit relatively slowly compared with beta-adrenergic and calcium-channel–blocking drugs.

[nnnnn] Charles K. Friedberg observed in 1966: "There is a surprising number of experienced and even distinguished cardiologists who support the misconception that digitalis is itself capable of converting atrial fibrillation to sinus rhythm."[1305] More recently, other writers have questioned: "How can one be certain that the eventual slowing and/or reversion to sinus rhythm are indeed causally related to digitalis? No double blind controlled study has ever been performed to answer this question; nor will it probably ever be performed, since other, quicker and more effective means now exist to control rapid atrial fibrillation."[1306]

cause of its vagotonic effects in patients with bradycardia-dependent paroxysmal atrial fibrillation.[383, 1315, *ooooo*]

Wolff-Parkinson-White syndrome. By shortening the refractory period of the accessory pathway in some patients with the Wolff-Parkinson-White syndrome, digitalis may encourage rapid and more frequent transmission of atrial impulses to the ventricles.[172, 982, 1316–1318] Consequently, digitalis must not be given to patients with the Wolff-Parkinson-White syndrome if one knows or suspects that they may have atrial fibrillation or flutter.[1319, *ppppp*]

Cardiothoracic surgery.[261, 262, 1187, 1296, 1320] Digitalis probably does not protect patients from developing atrial fibrillation after cardiothoracic surgery,[71, 266, 271, 272, 276, 302, 1189, 1208, 1321, 1322] and it may even predispose patients to supraventricular tachyarrhythmias.[266, 1321] Some workers, however, have concluded that the drug, given either by itself or with other cardioactive drugs, is effective.[265, 269, 282, 313, 1195, 1323–1325]

Intoxication.[1326] Digitalis intoxication in patients with atrial fibrillation produces unique disturbances of cardiac rhythm in addition to the usual systemic manifestations.[503, 1327–1328] The arrhythmias are due to atrioventricular block and acceleration of usually quiescent, intrinsic pacemakers in the bundle of His and the ventricles.[1329–1331, *qqqqq*] The first sign of overdosage, most useful in patients with rapid rates, is unexpectedly slow ventricular response from the effects of digitalis. Many patients with atrial fibrillation have spontaneously slow rates from intrinsic abnormalities of the atrioventricular node or vagotonia.

When the ventricular rate becomes excessively slow, escape beats, which terminate the longest pauses produced by block in patients with atrial fibrillation, appear to protect the ventricles from asystole.[502] Some of the escape beats that arise from the fascicles of the bundle branches produce QRS complexes that may have the appearance of incomplete right bundle branch block.[503, 608, 1332–1340, *rrrrr*]

Digitalis may then accelerate the rate of the escape foci. If the process continues, the subsidiary pacemakers can dominate the rhythm of the heart because atrioventricular block, also produced by the digitalis,

prevents atrial impulses from reaching the ventricles. The result is a regular His bundle[1341–1344, *sssss*] or fascicular tachycardia (Fig. 4.12). *Regularization of the ventricular rate in patients with chronic atrial fibrillation should always suggest digitalis intoxication, because the drug rarely converts such patients to sinus rhythm* (see Fig. 4.12).

Rarely, the arrhythmia known as "atrioventricular junctional tachycardia with exit block" may appear.[1345, 1346, *ttttt*] The ventricular rate then becomes irregular because some impulses from the His bundle or fascicular pacemaker cannot reach the ventricles. The unwary may conclude that atrial fibrillation with a rapid ventricular response is present and that the patient requires additional digitalis.

If digitalis intoxication remains unrecognized, ventricular tachycardia and ultimately ventricular fibrillation may follow. Bidirectional tachycardia is a variant of ventricular tachycardia characteristically produced in patients with severe cardiac disease and digitalis intoxication (Fig. 4.13). This arrhythmia is recognized by alternation of right and left axis duration among QRS complexes with the form of right bundle branch block.[1347–1351, *uuuuu*]

Treatment depends first on recognizing the presence of intoxication and confirming the diagnosis by measuring the digitalis concentration in the blood.[1352, *vvvvv*] Digitalis must be discontinued, and electrolyte abnormalities should be corrected. No further treatment is required for most patients with atrial fibrillation who develop digitalis intoxication. However, if the arrhythmias produce hemodynamic dysfunction or angina or appear otherwise particularly dangerous, digoxin-specific antibodies, now the specific treatment for advanced digitalis intoxication, should be administered.[1353, 1354] When this antidote is not available, antiarrhythmic drugs may be given to suppress ectopic activity. Patients with slow responses to atrial fibrillation resulting from digitalis intoxication may respond to atropine or to careful administration of a catecholamine drug. A ventricular pacemaker is occasionally required. Cardioversion should be avoided whenever possible.

Disopyramide. Disopyramide, a class Ia antiarrhythmic agent like procainamide and quinidine, has the following effects:

• It converts patients in atrial fibrillation to sinus

---

ooooo That digitalis can induce atrial fibrillation has been suspected since the work of Mackenzie more than 80 years ago.[1313]

ppppp In 1948, 18 years after the condition was first described,[1319] Wolff and White reported the ineffectiveness of digitalis in slowing the ventricular rate in patients with atrial fibrillation and Wolff-Parkinson-White syndrome.[161]

qqqqq Paroxysmal (automatic) atrial tachycardia (PAT) with block, a characteristic supraventricular arrhythmia of digitalis intoxication that usually appears in patients in sinus rhythm, occasionally develops when atrial fibrillation is the underlying arrhythmia.[1329–1331] See Chapter 6 for further discussion of PAT with block.

rrrrr Formerly, fascicular beats were thought to start in the atrioventricular node or "junction" with aberrant conduction to the ventricles.[503, 608, 1332–1334] Intracardiac recordings have shown them to start in the ventricles, presumably in fascicles of the bundle branches.[1338–1340] Their characteristic appearance of incomplete right bundle branch block suggests origin in left ventricular tissue, where digitalis-induced ventricular arrhythmias preferentially develop in dogs.[1335–1337]

sssss This arrhythmia was formerly called "nonparoxysmal A-V junctional tachycardia"[1341, 1343, 1344] because it develops and disappears gradually and not paroxysmally and was thought to arise in the atrioventricular node or junction.

ttttt Electrophysiological studies have not yet established the existence of this arrhythmia.

uuuuu Before the 1970s, investigators suggested that bidirectional tachycardia was a supraventricular arrhythmia with varying aberrant conduction to the ventricles.[1347] Intracardiac recordings of patients with this arrhythmia, both associated with[1348, 1350] and unrelated to digitalis,[1349, 1351] have established its origin to be ventricular.[1348–1350] See Chapter 13 for further discussion of bidirectional tachycardia.

vvvvv Digitalis concentrations are usually lower when the toxic arrhythmia is atrioventricular block, rather than ectopic beats.[1352]

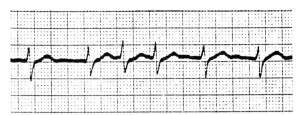

4/23/66 Digoxin 0/25 b.i.d.
started previous day

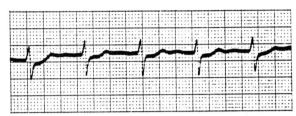

5/3/66 Regular rate = 88

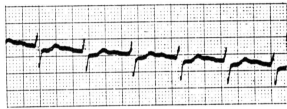

5/5/66 Regular rate = 107;
digoxin stopped

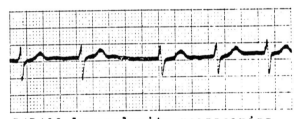

5/7/66 Irregularity reappearing

FIGURE 4.12 Digoxin toxicity during atrial fibrillation. Digoxin had been started recently to decrease this patient's ventricular rate **(top panel)**. The ventricular rhythm becomes regular **(second panel)**, a sign of digitalis intoxication. Toxicity was not recognized, the digoxin was continued, and the ventricular rate increased **(third panel)**. Then the digoxin was stopped, and 2 days later, irregularity reappeared **(bottom panel)**. The toxic effects of digoxin had simultaneously increased atrioventricular nodal block and accelerated a His bundle pacemaker to discharge abnormally rapidly. (From Kastor JA, Yurchak PM. Recognition of digitalis intoxication in the presence of atrial fibrillation. Ann Intern Med 1967; 67:1045–1054, with permission.)[503]

rhythm,[519, 1355–1360] most often those whose arrhythmia is relatively short-lived.[1361]

- It maintains sinus rhythm in patients prone to paroxysmal atrial fibrillation.[1362–1364]
- It maintains sinus rhythm after electrical cardioversion,[1365, 1366] as successfully as quinidine.[1362]
- It often prevents, but occasionally facilitates,

induction of paroxysmal atrial fibrillation in the electrophysiology laboratory.[1363, 1364]

- It favors antegrade conduction of relatively slow, narrow QRS complexes through the atrioventricular node in patients with atrial fibrillation and the Wolff-Parkinson-White syndrome[1367] by prolonging the refractory period of accessory pathways[1358, 1368] and lengthening the shortest RR intervals.[519, 1358, 1367]

Edrophonium.[1369] This cholinergic agent briefly slows the ventricular response to atrial fibrillation. The agent is seldom used for this purpose today.

Flecainide.[1370] Another class Ic antiarrhythmic drug,[1371] Flecainide converts most patients with atrial fibrillation of recent onset to sinus rhythm after intravenous administration[537, 1074, 1264, 1372–1382, *wwwww*] more successfully than procainamide[1380] or sotalol[1383] and after a single oral dose.[1384] Patients with vagal-induced paroxysmal atrial fibrillation also respond favorably.[1125] Patients more likely to convert have smaller left atrial diameters by echocardiography[1385] and have fibrillated for shorter periods of time.[1373, 1385]

Flecainide also has the following effects:

- It restores sinus rhythm after cardiac surgery faster than the combination of digoxin and disopyramide.[1386]
- It suppresses recurrences of paroxysmal atrial fibrillation.[1125, 1375, 1387–1392]
- It permits the amount of amiodarone administered to maintain sinus rhythm to be decreased.[1125, 1388]
- Only slightly,[666, 1378] if at all,[1393] it slows the ventricular response to atrial fibrillation in those patients who do not convert.
- It decreases the ventricular rate in patients with the Wolff-Parkinson-White syndrome and atrial

---

wwwww One hundred twenty-nine (74%) of 175 patients in 6 series. A comprehensive review of the medical literature in English and foreign languages revealed that 211 (62%) of 341 patients converted from atrial flutter or fibrillation to sinus rhythm after intravenous administration of flecainide and 137 (61%) of 235 converted after oral therapy.[1375]

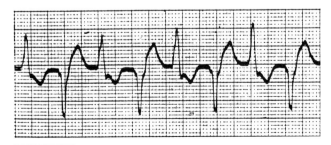

FIGURE 4.13 Bidirectional ventricular tachycardia produced by digitalis intoxication in a patient with atrial fibrillation. The alternating morphology of the ventricular beats is characteristic of bidirectional tachycardia. The form of each beat is different from that of the conducted beats. Electrophysiological studies have shown that this arrhythmia usually originates in the ventricles. (From Kastor JA, Yurchak PM. Recognition of digitalis intoxication in the presence of atrial fibrillation. Ann Intern Med 1967; 67:1045–1054, with permission.)[503]

fibrillation by prolonging the refractory period of the accessory pathway and the shortest RR intervals.[1374, 1394–1397] The drug also reduces the likelihood that atrial fibrillation will be produced by rapid atrial stimulation[1398] in patients with,[1394–1396] and without,[1378] preexcitation.

- It can induce atrial flutter with rapid ventricular response,[1399] ventricular tachycardia,[1400] and ventricular flutter in patients with atrial fibrillation,[1400] but it probably does not increase mortality in patients with supraventricular tachyarrhythmias.[1401]

Ibutilide.[1402] This newly approved class III antiarrhythmic drug for intravenous use converts many paroxysms of atrial fibrillation of recent onset to sinus rhythm,[935, 1403–1404] more successfully than does procainamide.[1405]

Isoproterenol. Isoproterenol simulates the effects of exercise or fright and thereby exposes patients with Wolff-Parkinson-White syndrome and atrial fibrillation to the risk of ventricular fibrillation. The drug itself may even produce atrial fibrillation.[1406] Isoproterenol shortens the refractory period of accessory pathways[653, 985, 1011, 1407, 1408] and increases the ventricular rate as more atrial impulses are transmitted to the ventricles. In asymptomatic patients with the Wolff-Parkinson-White syndrome, isoproterenol increases conduction in the atrioventricular node and the accessory pathway and accelerates the ventricular response, primarily by enhancing atrioventricular nodal conduction.[1408] Infusion of isoproterenol will probably not select those patients at high risk of sudden death. Testing with isoproterenol provides more useful information than exercise, which is not considered adequate to determine which patients may develop extremely rapid ventricular rates.[653] The therapeutic effects of amiodarone on accessory pathways may be partially overcome by isoproterenol.[1011]

Lidocaine. Lidocaine does not convert atrial fibrillation to sinus rhythm, but it may decrease, or occasionally increase, the ventricular response. In patients with the Wolff-Parkinson-White syndrome and atrial fibrillation, lidocaine may decrease the ventricular rate by inhibiting conduction through bypass tracks.[1216, 1409] However, the drug does not always exhibit this effect[1410, 1411] and may shorten the refractory period of the accessory pathway and accelerate the ventricular response during atrial fibrillation.[1411]

Magnesium. Magnesium may,[1412] or may not,[1413] reduce the incidence of atrial fibrillation after coronary artery bypass graft surgery.

Procainamide.[1414] This class Ia antiarrhythmic drug, like quinidine and disopyramide, converts atrial fibrillation to sinus rhythm when given orally[1415–1419] or intravenously.[712, 713, 1415–1418, 1420–1422, xxxxx] Patients are more likely to convert to sinus rhythm if their left atria are small[712] or they have fibrillation that is paroxysmal or of relatively short duration.[713, 1415, 1417, 1419–1422, yyyyy] Procainamide in doses adequate to produce therapeutic blood levels reduces the incidence of paroxysmal atrial fibrillation after coronary bypass surgery.[1423]

In patients with the Wolff-Parkinson-White syndrome and many preexcited beats, procainamide favors conduction through the atrioventricular node and thereby decreases the ventricular rate by prolonging the refractory period of accessory pathways.[1082, 1085, 1424, 1425] Procainamide fails to block conduction in those accessory pathways with short refractory periods and thereby helps to identify patients at risk of rapid responses to atrial fibrillation and possible ventricular fibrillation.[1426–1428, zzzzz]

Procainamide, like quinidine, can "paradoxically" increase the ventricular rate[1415, 1418] by slowing the atrial rate,[1415, 1417, 1418, 1420] thereby reducing concealed conduction, and by decreasing vagal tone in the atrioventricular node.[1165] Intra-atrial recordings have confirmed procainamide's ability to decrease the atrial rate during atrial fibrillation.[904] In patients treated with procainamide, atrial flutter may develop transiently before sinus rhythm appears.[1415, 1416, 1418]

Propafenone. This class Ic antiarrhythmic drug has the following properties:[1371]

- It converts to sinus rhythm many patients, particularly those without structural heart disease,[1429] who have atrial fibrillation that is paroxysmal or of recent onset but seldom when the arrhythmia is chronic.[1430] The drug is effective for this purpose when given intravenously,[714, 1206, 1431, aaaaaa] or orally,[1429, 1432, 1433] even after a single oral dose.[1433–1435] Propafenone, however, converts patients to sinus rhythm less successfully than quinidine.[1436]
- It helps to maintain patients in sinus rhythm,[1186, 1224, 1437–1443] and when given before cardioversion decreases the recurrence of the arrhythmia after the shock.[1444]
- It decreases the ventricular rate during atrial fibrillation.[1430, 1440, 1445]
- It slows the ventricular rate in patients with the Wolff-Parkinson-White syndrome by increasing block in accessory pathways.[1396, 1397, 1428, 1446, 1447]
- It prevents induction of sustained atrial fibrillation by rapid atrial pacing.[1396, 1447]

Atrial flutter with a rapid ventricular response may develop in patients being treated for recurrent atrial fibrillation with propafenone.[1399, 1448] Rapid, regular tachycardias with wide or narrow QRS complexes occasionally develop in patients with paroxysmal atrial fibrillation being treated with propafenone.[667] The nature of these arrhythmias has not been defined, but some may be ventricular tachycardia.

---

xxxxx In 51% of 47 patients.[712, 713]

yyyyy Only 21% of 155 patients with atrial fibrillation of longer than 2 weeks' duration.[1414]

zzzzz Although not all workers agree that the procainamide infusion test consistently identifies such patients.[1427]

aaaaaa In 60% of 88 patients.[714, 1206]

Quinidine.[1449] This quintessential and first generally available class Ia antiarrhythmic drug converts

- About half of patients with atrial fibrillation to sinus rhythm.[1449–1453, bbbbbb] Success is greater when patients have had atrial fibrillation for shorter periods of time and when severe congestive heart failure is absent.[225, 1453] Conversion depends more on the level of the drug in the blood than to the dosing schedule.[1454]
- Patients who have recently had surgical repair of the mitral valve.[1455]
- Patients with lone atrial fibrillation particularly effectively.[92, 236, 350]
- More successfully than flecainide,[1373] propafenone,[1436] or sotalol.[1456, 1457]
- More successfully for postoperative atrial fibrillation than intravenous amiodarone.[1458]

Quinidine helps to maintain sinus rhythm in patients with paroxysmal atrial fibrillation[1459] after electrical cardioversion and reduces the incidence of postoperative atrial fibrillation after thoracic surgery,[1460] although not after mitral valvotomy.[1461] Quinidine maintains sinus rhythm more successfully than does verapamil.[1462]

Ventricular rate. Quinidine, like procainamide, reduces the frequency of atrial signals and may temporarily convert patients to atrial flutter.[1450] The rate of the ventricles may then increase because of less antegrade concealed conduction into the atrioventricular node and quinidine's vagolytic effects.[1463] This characteristic development has led physicians for decades to administer concurrently drugs that block atrioventricular conduction, such as digitalis or calcium-channel– or beta-adrenergic–blocking agents.

Wolff-Parkinson-White syndrome. By blocking conduction in accessory pathways, quinidine reduces the likelihood that a dangerously rapid ventricular response will develop in patients with atrial fibrillation and the Wolff-Parkinson-White syndrome. This effect can be partially reversed by epinephrine[1464] and, therefore, by clinical states in which high levels of catecholamines are circulating. Quinidine prolongs the refractory period of accessory pathways,[982, 1082, 1085, 1464] particularly in those patients whose refractory periods were relatively long before treatment.[1082]

Reserpine. This drug decreases the ventricular rate in patients with atrial fibrillation.[1465]

Sotalol (d, l).[1466, 1467] This class III antiarrhythmic drug with beta-adrenergic–blocking properties slows the ventricular response to atrial fibrillation.[1468, 1469] The drug is relatively ineffective in converting atrial fibrillation to sinus rhythm[1456, 1469]—certainly less effective than quinidine[1456, 1457]—although it has been found

to produce sinus rhythm in patients who develop atrial fibrillation after cardiac surgery.[1212] Sotalol preserves sinus rhythm[1157, 1470] as effectively as quinidine after conversion from atrial fibrillation,[1185] and it may be slightly better tolerated,[1185] but not as well as amiodarone.[1123]

The arrhythmia recurs more frequently after cardioversion in patients taking sotalol who have the following features:[1470]

- Age more than 65 years.
- Atrial fibrillation for more than 2 months before conversion.
- Coronary heart disease.[ccccc]
- Left atrial diameter greater than 60 millimeters.

Sotalol reduces the incidence of supraventricular tachyarrhythmias, including atrial fibrillation, from developing after cardiac surgery[1471] more effectively than metoprolol.[1201] It is as effective as the combination of digoxin and disopyramide and acts faster.[1212]

Sotalol (d). This dextrarotatory isomer of racemic sotalol, is a class III antiarrhythmic agent without beta-blocking properties.[1472] The drug decreases the ventricular response to atrial fibrillation and may reduce the ability of rapid pacing to induce the arrhythmia.[1473, dddddd]

Theophylline. By enhancing conduction through the atrioventricular node, theophylline increases the ventricular rate in patients with atrial fibrillation and a slow ventricular response and relieves asthenia and easy fatigability.[1474]

Anticoagulation.[403, 405, 408, 424, 728] Anticoagulation to prevent stroke should be prescribed for suitable patients with *chronic* atrial fibrillation who have:[1475–1496, eeeee, ffffff]

- Rheumatic mitral valve disease.[415, 417, 431, 445, 1503–1506]
- Nonrheumatic heart disease.[431, 464, 467, 1497, 1499–1501, 1507, 1508]
- Congestive cardiomyopathy.[233]

[ccccc] Atrial fibrillation recurred in 26% with lone atrial fibrillation and 51% with structural heart disease.[1470]

[dddddd] Because of its pro-arrhythmic effects, *d*-sotalol is no longer available.[1472]

[eeeee] Large studies, cited in the test, establish that anticoagulation reduces the incidence of stroke in patients with atrial fibrillation; a study with relatively few subjects did not.[1491]

[ffffff] In a survey reported from Great Britain in 1986, most physicians would not anticoagulate patients with atrial fibrillation and nonvalvular heart disease.[1497] Physicians in the United States

- Underuse anticoagulation in office practice[1914] and in teaching hospitals.[1500]
- Anticoagulate 75% of patients with nonvalvular atrial fibrillation in Baltimore City, Baltimore County, and Prince George's County, Maryland.[1501]
- Anticoagulate elderly patients with atrial fibrillation less often and less intensively than younger patients.[1499, 1915] (Anticoagulation is also underprescribed for atrial fibrillation in elderly patients in the United Kingdom.[1502])
- In one staff-model health maintenance organization, prescribe anticoagulants for most, but not all, patients with atrial fibrillation who have no contraindications.[1498]

[bbbbbb] Three hundred thirty-nine (53%) patients from 636 in 4 series from 1952 to 1963.[1450–1453]

Those at the highest risk of stroke have congestive heart failure, history of hypertension, or previous arterial thromboembolism.[467] Physicians tend to underuse anticoagulation in elderly patients with atrial fibrillation,[718] and they frequently overlook, or do not recognize, the presence of chronic atrial fibrillation in patients whose ventricles are being paced and, consequently, fail to anticoagulate them.[523] Patients with relatively frequent episodes of *paroxysmal* atrial fibrillation and nonvalvular heart disease should be anticoagulated.[431, 464, 467] What constitutes "frequent" is not established.

Anticoagulation has been advised for, but not established as effective for, patients with the following:

- Paroxysmal atrial fibrillation when of recent onset.[427]
- Atrial fibrillation resulting from thyrotoxicosis.[450, 451, 1479, 1509, 1510]
- Atrial fibrillation and obstructive cardiomyopathy.[241, 1479]
- Lone atrial fibrillation and less than 60 years of age.[371]

Warfarin. This is the preferred drug for most patients with atrial fibrillation who require anticoagulation.[742, 1511–1513] The dose favored by most authorities for such patients, including those with nonrheumatic atrial fibrillation and recent cerebral ischemia,[1514] maintains an international normalized ratio (INR) between 2.0 and 3.0,[431, 467, 1507, 1515–1518] even though lower-dose programs with an INR of 1.2 to 1.5[1519] or 1.5 to 2.7[405, 464] reduce stroke in many patients with atrial fibrillation.

Treatment for 3 weeks with warfarin causes clots in the left atrium and its appendage[452] to disappear on transesophageal echocardiography in most, but not all,[1520] patients. Acute anticoagulation after cardioembolic stroke is safe, but its value in preventing early recurrent stroke has yet to be established.[1521] With proper training, patients can adjust their anticoagulation with warfarin themselves.[1522]

Aspirin. This drug slightly reduces the incidence of stroke in patients with atrial fibrillation,[1511, 1523, gggggg] but it is more effective when the stroke is due to noncardiac causes.[1524] Although individual studies show some reduction in strokes in patients with nonrheumatic atrial fibrillation who have had transient ischemic attacks or minor strokes,[1525] the value of aspirin to prevent stroke in all patients with nonrheumatic atrial fibrillation is uncertain.[467, 1514, 1515, 1526, hhhhhh]

Full-dose warfarin is preferable,[1513, 1526, 1527] although it is riskier than aspirin.[1517, 1518] Therefore, when the risk of bleeding is high, low-dose warfarin or aspirin may be employed.[1525] Seventy-five milligrams per day of aspirin, however, is not useful.[467]

Sulfinpyrazone. This platelet-suppressing drug reduces the incidence of thromboemboli in patients with rheumatic heart disease, atrial fibrillation, and shortened platelet survival time.[1528, 1529]

Cost-effectiveness. Prophylaxis for stroke with warfarin is cost-effective in patients with nonvalvular atrial fibrillation and one or more risk factors for stroke.[1512] Anticoagulation with warfarin or aspirin, if contraindications to warfarin exist, is cost-effective, provided the risk of hemorrhage from the anticoagulation is kept low.[1530]

Pacing

Patients with atrial fibrillation may require pacing to sustain an adequately rapid ventricular rate during bradycardia, to regularize the ventricular rate during hemodynamic studies to induce atrial fibrillation, and to reduce the frequency of paroxysms.[1030, 1531–1535]

Bradycardia. Ventricular pacing is the treatment of choice when high-grade atrioventricular block develops in patients with atrial fibrillation and produces symptoms.[506, 657] One must be certain, however, that bradycardia is producing the complaints. Two-second pauses on Holter monitoring in patients with atrial fibrillation and intermittent atrioventricular block do not usually correlate with cerebral symptoms, and in such patients, a ventricular pacemaker may not relieve the complaints.[658] Because the fibrillating atrium cannot trigger synchronous pacemakers, a rate-sensitive unit, which increases the ventricular rate in response to physical activity or other physiological changes, should be employed.

Pacemaking may be required to sustain an adequately rapid heart rate in patients with the tachycardia-bradycardia feature of the sick sinus syndrome in whom paroxysmal atrial fibrillation is the rapid heart rhythm. Most cardiologists favor the use of atrioventricular (DDD) units that can sense or pace from the atria and the ventricles.[1536, iiiii] If atrial fibrillation becomes chronic, the pacemaker may not be needed.[1072]

Because patients with the tachycardia-bradycardia syndrome may develop slow rhythms after electrical conversion of atrial fibrillation, temporary transvenous pacing may occasionally be required.[1537] Prophylactic external pacing can relieve bradycardia while the patient is still unconscious from the anesthesia.[1538]

Regularizing the ventricular rate. A regular ventricular rhythm can simplify the measurement of hemodynamic function.[1539] To accomplish this in atrial fibrillation, the ventricles may be temporarily paced at rates faster than, and, in many cases, slightly slower than, the average ventricular rate.[1540] Retrograde concealed penetration of the conduction system from the paced ventricular beat prevents conduction of atrial activity into the ventricles.

---

gggggg At 75,300 and 325 milligrams in three randomized trials.[1523]

hhhhhh One authority argues: "Warfarin is strikingly more effective than aspirin in preventing strokes in nonrheumatic atrial fibrillation."[1526]

iiiii However, DDD pacemakers may require sophisticated programming to obtain the most satisfactory effects when used in certain patients with atrial fibrillation.[1536]

A similar effect can be achieved by coupled ventricular pacing in which ventricular beats are introduced soon after the refractory period of the supraventricular beats.[1541] Because the paced beat occurs early in the diastolic cycle, little, if any, blood is ejected. This method, which has been called "intercalated" pacing, can cause systolic arterial pressure to rise and diastolic arterial pressure, left ventricular filling pressure, and pulmonary artery pressure to fall.[1541] Pacing with an experimental "rate-smoothing" algorithm also reduces the irregularity of the ventricular rhythm.[1542]

Inducing atrial fibrillation. Rapid atrial pacing induces atrial fibrillation at least briefly in all patients. The arrhythmia reverts quickly to sinus rhythm in subjects without the substrate for fibrillation. Because drugs can usually control the ventricular rate more easily in chronic atrial fibrillation than when paroxysmal atrial fibrillation or resistant atrial tachycardia is present, pacing was employed to produce permanent atrial fibrillation.[1543–1546] There seems little indication for this treatment now.

Rapid atrial pacing through epicardial wires is frequently employed after cardiac surgery to treat patients with postoperative atrial flutter or atrial tachycardia.[1547, 1548] Sinus rhythm often follows as soon as the pacemaker is turned off; not infrequently, however, atrial fibrillation may be produced. Occasionally, atrial fibrillation may be inadvertently produced by atrioventricular sequential pacing, particularly when an atrial stimulus discharges in the atrial vulnerable period.[1549]

Preventing atrial fibrillation. Ventricular (VVI) pacing encourages the development of chronic atrial fibrillation.[499] Atrial or bifocal pacing of patients, many of whom have sick sinus syndrome, decreases the incidence and recurrence of persistent and paroxysmal atrial fibrillation better than does ventricular pacing.[495–497, 1550–1553] Atrioventricular pacing with DDD units is probably more effective than with other models.[1554]

Long-term atrial pacing reduces the number of episodes of vagal-induced atrial fibrillation in some patients with paroxysms despite taking antiarrhythmic drugs.[385] A bifocal pacemaker has been developed for patients with paroxysmal atrial fibrillation that automatically stops sensing the atria when the arrhythmia develops, so the ventricular rate will not become too fast.[1555] Pacing both the right and left atria may reduce the frequency of recurrence of paroxysmal atrial fibrillation.[1556]

External Cardioversion

Synchronized electrical cardioversion, the safest and most effective means of converting chronic atrial fibrillation, produces sinus rhythm in 87% of patients with the arrhythmia.[35, 353, 509, 719, 770, 1455, 1557–1588, jjjjj] Cardio-

version is at least twice as likely to convert atrial fibrillation as is quinidine, the antiarrhythmic drug usually employed for this purpose before cardioversion became the standard method.[1455] Although cardioversion is usually performed in hospitals, patients can be safely treated in properly equipped outpatient clinics or private offices.[1589, 1590, kkkkkk]

When will cardioversion successfully produce sinus rhythm?

Duration, electrocardiographic appearance, and cardiac size. Cardioversion (Table 4.5) more likely succeeds when

- Atrial fibrillation has been present for a shorter rather than a longer period of time.[35, 719, 720, 1565, 1573, 1575, 1576, 1579, 1580, 1583, 1585, 1591–1593, lllll]
- The fibrillatory waves recorded on the electrocardiogram are coarse or large.[35, 720, 1570, 1573, 1583, 1591]
- Radiography shows the left atrium to be small.[35, 720, 1572, 1575, 1576, 1579, 1594] Some,[1573, 1576, 1594] but not all,[719, 1570, 1583] investigators add that cardiomegaly on the chest radiograph identifies patients who are more difficult to convert to sinus rhythm.[1570] The larger that echocardiography finds the left atrium, the less likely will cardioversion produce sinus rhythm, at least according to one study.[718, mmmmmm]

Structural heart disease. The lower the left ventricular ejection fraction, the less likely will cardioversion be to produce sinus rhythm in patients with atrial fibrillation.[718] The cardiac cause and lesions also influence success of treatment. Conversion is probably most successful in patients whose atrial fibrillation is associated with treated thyrotoxicosis.[1360, 1573, 1582, 1595, 1596] About two-thirds of patients convert spontaneously to sinus rhythm after thyrotoxicosis is treated, and three-fourths of those convert to sinus rhythm within 3 weeks.[1596] Elective cardioversion therefore is probably best performed at about the sixteenth week after the euthyroid state has been attained.[1596] Even patients whose atrial fibrillation has lasted for a long time may have a successful result.[1360]

Patients whose mitral lesions are stenotic are easier to convert than when regurgitation predominates.[35, 1573, 1576, 1579, 1594] Cardioversion was successful in each of 16 patients with hypertrophic cardiomyopathy,[241] but most patients with this lesion seldom maintain sinus rhythm for long.[241] Atrial fibrillation is relatively difficult to convert in patients with alcoholic cardiomyopathy,[719] pulmonary disease,[719] and lone atrial fibrillation despite the absence of cardiomegaly.[1594]

---

jjjjj In 2,911 patients from 21 series. Some authors present their results as the number of *episodes* of atrial fibrillation that were successfully converted. By this computation, 84% of 887 conversions produced sinus rhythm.[353, 1455, 1565, 1574, 1577, 1586]

kkkkkk "In about 90% of all cases without change in primary success rate or increased risks," according to one study from Göteborg, Sweden.[1589]

lllll Not all investigators have been able to establish that previous duration of fibrillation determines the success of conversion.[719, 1565, 1579]

mmmmmm Some patients with very large hearts can be converted: "We have been surprised at the ease and safety with which an enormous heart can be converted to sinus rhythm when the atria are known to have been fibrillating for 20 years and more."[1570]

Table 4.5	**FACTORS THAT ARE LIKELY TO MAKE CARDIOVERSION OF ATRIAL FIBRILLATION MORE SUCCESSFUL, REQUIRE LESS POWER, OR SECURE LONGER MAINTENANCE OF SINUS RHYTHM**		
	Successful Conversion	**Less Power**	**Longer Maintenance**
Heart size	Small	—	Small
Left atrial size	Small	—	Small
F waves	Coarse	No effect	No effect
Duration of atrial fibrillation	Short time	Short time	Short time
Diagnosis	Treated thyrotoxicosis, mitral stenosis	Rheumatic valve disease	Treated thyrotoxicosis, mitral stenosis
Drugs	—	Taking quinidine or amiodarone	—
Functional classification	—	—	Healthier

Cardiac surgery. Cardioversion is less likely to succeed in patients who have recently had mitral valvotomy or valve replacement than in unoperated patients with atrial fibrillation,[35, 1579, 1597, 1598] possibly because of the atrial injury and fibrosis produced by cardiac surgery.[35] Postoperative patients are more likely to convert to sinus rhythm successfully in the following circumstances:

- The atrial fibrillation has been present for relatively few years.[1597–1600]
- The left atrium is small.[720, 1597–1599]
- The lesion is mitral stenosis rather than mitral regurgitation.[1597]
- The patient obtained a good operative result.[1597]
- Left atrial disease, determined from study of left atrial appendages removed at operation, is minimal.[876]

The amount of time that elapses between the operation and the cardioversion does not affect the likelihood of successful conversion.[1597–1599]

Miscellaneous factors. Age[719, 1572, 1573, 1583, 1585, 1594, 1601] and sex[719, 1573, 1583, 1594] do not appear to influence the success of conversion.[1593, nnnnnn] Cardioversion of atrial fibrillation in the mother has been performed successfully during pregnancy without complications for mother or fetus.[1602, 1603] Applying manual pressure to the electrodes can facilitate conversion.[1604] Administering flecainide before the procedure improves the likelihood of successful cardioversion.[1605]

How much power is required to convert atrial fibrillation to sinus rhythm? Most patients can be converted to sinus rhythm with 100 to 200 joules (wattseconds),[35, 1570] and almost half can be converted with 50 joules or less (see Table 2.3).[35] Patients who require 400 joules seldom stay in sinus rhythm long;[1455] one group was unable to convert any patients for significant periods of time who required this much power.[1570] However, cardioversion requiring very large amounts of power has succeeded with two defibrillators discharging simultaneously.[1606]

Two hundred joules is usually employed for the first

shock. If the operator is particularly concerned that the cardioversion may produce arrhythmias, 25 to 50 joules should be used, because the amount of power rather than the number of shocks determines the incidence of postconversion arrhythmias.[1607]

Larger amounts of power are usually required for conversion in the following situations:

- When atrial fibrillation is long-standing.[35]
- For patients with lone atrial fibrillation,[1587] ventricular preexcitation, cardiomyopathy, and congestive heart failure.[1608]
- For patients taking flecainide.[1609, 1610]

Patients taking quinidine[510] or amiodarone[1611] may require less power for conversion to sinus rhythm. Only 10 to 20 joules are needed when atrial fibrillation is cardioverted in the operating room with the paddles applied directly to the heart.[1612] Procainamide, however, given before the first cardioversion, does not increase the likelihood of securing sinus rhythm.[1613]

The amount of power required to convert patients externally who have had mitral or aortic valve replacement to sinus rhythm is no greater than that required to convert those who have had valvotomy or no operation.[1600] Body weight, age, sex, and the size of fibrillatory waves on the electrocardiogram do not significantly affect the amount of power required to convert to sinus rhythm successfully.[35] Similar amounts of power are equally effective in successfully converting atrial arrhythmias, whether the paddles are placed in anterolateral or anteroposterior positions.[1614]

Delayed conversion. Rarely, patients with atrial fibrillation do not convert to sinus rhythm immediately after the shock.[1615, 1616] In two cases, 6.8 and 14.6 seconds elapsed before sinus rhythm appeared.[1616] P waves may appear small on the electrocardiogram immediately after conversion, leading to the belief that cardioversion has failed to produce sinus rhythm.[1608]

Esophageal cardioversion. Electrical conversion of atrial fibrillation may be conducted successfully without anesthesia with the use of an electrode in the esophagus behind the left atrium. Shocks of 40 to 60 joules are effective.[1617] This technique has not achieved general acceptance.

Is synchronization necessary? Cardioversion of atrial fibrillation is almost always conducted with equipment

---

nnnnnn The authors of two series, however, suggest that younger patients,[1593] particularly when younger than the age of 50 years,[1573] can be converted to sinus rhythm more easily than older patients.

that synchronizes the shock to a predetermined time in the cardiac cycle and avoids the "vulnerable period" early in the T wave of the electrocardiogram. Most physicians assume that shocking during this vulnerable period may induce ventricular fibrillation. Experience in the 1960s with nonsynchronized conversion suggests that vulnerable phase–induced ventricular fibrillation may be more a theoretical than clinical problem. Nonsynchronized cardioversion appears to convert as effectively and to produce no more arrhythmias than does synchronized conversion.[1574, 1618–1621]

Anatomical effects of successful cardioversion. After cardioversion, left[1622] and right atrial[1622] size decreases in patients with[723] and without[1623] coronary disease and cardiomyopathy. Restoring sinus rhythm also reduces the likelihood of progressive atrial enlargement in patients with chronic atrial fibrillation and mitral valve disease.[1622]

Maintenance of sinus rhythm. Most patients with atrial fibrillation who have been successfully cardioverted to sinus rhythm redevelop their arrhythmia within 1 year (see Table 4.5). The rate of reversion is highest soon after cardioversion.[1624, oooooo] Then, progressively fewer patients sustain sinus rhythm:[pppppp]

- Ninety percent for a few minutes after the shock.[35]
- Seventy percent for 24 hours.[1593]
- Sixty percent for 1 month.[719, 1576, 1577, 1582]
- Fifty percent for 3 months.[1569, 1577, 1579, 1582]
- Twenty percent to 35% for 12 months.[35, 509, 1567, 1576, 1579, 1582, 1584, 1585, 1597, 1598, 1625]

The factors favoring maintenance of sinus rhythm are similar to those favoring successful conversion. Sinus rhythm is more likely to persist when the cardiac disease is due to thyrotoxicosis[1582, 1584, 1588, 1596] or mitral stenosis rather than to mitral regurgitation.[35, 509] Patients whose atrial fibrillation is associated with arteriosclerotic or hypertensive cardiovascular disease probably maintain sinus rhythm poorly after cardioversion,[509, 1579, 1584] as do those with lone atrial fibrillation[719, 1570, 1579, 1582, 1584, 1587, qqqqqq] and hypertrophic cardiomyopathy.[241]

The less power required for cardioversion, the greater the probability that patients will maintain sinus rhythm.[719, 1582, 1598] The worse the functional classification, the more quickly patients revert to atrial fibrillation.[509] The longer atrial fibrillation is present before cardioversion, the shorter the time that sinus rhythm will be maintained.[35, 509, 710, 711, 719, 721, 1571, 1575, 1576, 1578, 1582, 1588, 1625, rrrrrr]

When cardiomegaly or, specifically, large left atria are seen on a chest radiograph[35, 509, 1576, 1579, 1588, 1598, 1626] or echocardiogram, less satisfactory results after cardioversion may be expected, although one study found that left atrial dimension does not determine the length of time that sinus rhythm will continue.[711] Patients with higher left atrial pressure revert to atrial fibrillation sooner than those with normal pressures.[1626]

The size of the F waves on the electrocardiogram does not correlate with the likelihood of maintaining sinus rhythm.[509, 1583, 1598] Age less than 50 years may be advantageous,[1588] and men may sustain sinus rhythm after cardioversion for a slightly longer period than women.[719]

After electrical or pharmacological conversion, paroxysms of atrial fibrillation recur more often in

- Women than in men.
- Those patients with previous episodes of paroxysmal atrial fibrillation.
- Patients with coronary, pulmonary, or valvular disease.[1627]

Cardiac surgery. When cardioversion is performed after cardiac surgery, sinus rhythm is more likely to be maintained in the following circumstances:

- The lesion operated on was mitral stenosis rather than mitral regurgitation.[1597]
- Atrial fibrillation was present less than 3 years before operation.[1597]
- The results of the operation were excellent.[1597]
- Only one valve has undergone operation.[1598]

According to one study, half the patients retain sinus rhythm for up to 7 years after cardioversion performed when they are hemodynamically stable after open mitral commissurotomy even if they reverted to atrial fibrillation from cardioversion performed soon after the operation.[1628] Consequently, one should not be discouraged from attempting to establish sinus rhythm for most of these patients despite their having left atrial enlargement or the arrhythmia for long periods of time.[1628] Patients who have had mitral valve surgery maintain sinus rhythm better when they are cardioverted after, rather than before, the operation.[1625] Patients with atrial septal defects and atrial fibrillation tend to maintain sinus rhythm well when conversion is performed after operative closure.[1582]

Drugs to maintain sinus rhythm. Amiodarone is particularly effective in maintaining sinus rhythm after cardioversion.[716, 1629, 1630]

---

oooooo Atrial fibrillation recurred after external cardioversion in 35 (57%) of 61 patients during the first month following the procedure. The arrhythmia restarted within the first 5 days in 22 (63%) of the 35 who reverted within 1 month.[1624]

pppppp The rate of success of maintaining sinus rhythm after cardioversion is difficult to quantify when one compares the results from the many series published on this subject, mostly during the 1960s. Confounding features among the different series include whether antiarrhythmic drugs, usually quinidine, were given after cardioversion; whether cardiac surgery was performed before conversion; whether the patients who reverted to sinus rhythm were cardioverted again; the different types of heart disease and valve lesions present; and the effects of death and loss of follow-up. In several series, one figure for maintaining sinus rhythm is given for patients followed for different periods of time after cardioversion.[35, 509, 1567, 1597, 1598]

qqqqqq In one series, however, patients with lone atrial fibrillation maintained sinus rhythm satisfactorily.[1584]

---

rrrrrr What constitutes a period of atrial fibrillation that is long enough to decrease the likelihood of maintaining sinus rhythm varies among the different reports: more than 1 year probably; more than 2 to 3 years, almost certainly; and more than 5 years, without question.

Quinidine, administered before or after cardioversion, helps to keep patients in sinus rhythm[1625, 1631–1636] and may reduce the number of shocks required for successful cardioversion.[510, 1573, 1576, 1583, 1588, 1625, 1632, sssss] Long-acting quinidine[1637] and disopyramide[1362, 1365, 1366] also help to maintain sinus rhythm.

Sotalol preserves sinus rhythm as effectively as quinidine after conversion from atrial fibrillation.[1185] Sotalol may be slightly better tolerated than quinidine, and patients are less symptomatic when they relapse into atrial fibrillation because the ventricular response is slower.[1185] Sotalol decreases atrial function immediately after cardioversion.[1638]

Verapamil taken when the patient has atrial fibrillation reduces the likelihood that the arrhythmia will recur after cardioversion.[1624] Administering different antiarrhythmic drugs sequentially can increase the rate of retaining sinus rhythm.[1630]

Repeated cardioversions. Cardioversion of atrial fibrillation is almost always successful when the procedure must be repeated in patients who have reverted to fibrillation.[1567, 1584, 1594] However, when atrial fibrillation recurs within a few weeks or months after cardioversion, maintenance of sinus rhythm after subsequent conversions is unlikely to last longer,[1583, 1584, ttttt] unless antiarrhythmic therapy is added.[1639]

In the 1960s, some workers recommended reconverting the arrhythmia as often as necessary in all patients who seemed to benefit hemodynamically from the procedure.[1579, 1640] The wisdom of this approach is currently being reevaluated.[1039, 1040]

Emboli and anticoagulation[729, 1537, 1641]

Risk for emboli. Symptoms and findings suggesting the development of systemic, and occasionally pulmonary, emboli after cardioversion occur in a few patients, most of whom were not anticoagulated when they were cardioverted.[35, 447, 509, 1565, 1570–1573, 1579, 1580, 1585, 1639, 1644–1646, uuuuuu] Patients at higher risk probably include

those who have had previous emboli or have rheumatic valvular disease.[35, 1646]

The average duration of atrial fibrillation among 13 patients who developed emboli after cardioversion was 12 months, with a range of 1 to 48 months.[1646] Although several investigators report that no emboli developed in patients fibrillating for less than 1 month before cardioversion,[1642, 1643, 1646] 6 patients who had been in atrial fibrillation for less than 1 week had emboli, according to 2 reports.[1647, 1648]

Who should be anticoagulated? [1641, 1649, 1650] Anticoagulation for up to 3 weeks before elective cardioversion reduces the incidence of emboli,[35, 1646] probably by inducing resolution of the thrombi.[452, vvvvvv] No studies, however, indicate how long patients should be anticoagulated before or after conversion to sinus rhythm, but a common practice includes anticoagulation for 3 weeks before conversion and for at least a week after cardioversion.[1651, wwwwww] All the embolic episodes in one series, for example, occurred within 7 days after the shock.[1646] Many physicians, however, do not follow traditional protocols.[1652]

Some physicians make the case that all patients with atrial fibrillation and no specific contraindications should be anticoagulated for elective cardioversion.[811, 1653] However, by identifying intra-atrial clots, transesophageal echocardiography can help to select which patients most need anticoagulation and which can be converted without prolonged anticoagulation.[738, 741, 1654–1659] In one series, none of 186 patients whose transesophageal echocardiography showed no left atrial thrombi and who did not have prolonged anticoagulation suffered embolic events after cardioversion. Uneventful cardioversion was conducted in 18 other patients with atrial thrombi after prolonged anticoagulation.[1657] However, not all cardiologists agree with this approach,[738, 1660–1662] because emboli may still occur in patients whose transesophageal echocardiogram suggests that no emboli will develop.[1663]

One proposal for the rapid elective conversion of patients with atrial fibrillation of unknown or prolonged duration, which seems particularly reasonable, prescribes heparin and warfarin for all subjects. If transthoracic and then transesophageal echocardiograms show no intra-atrial thrombi, pharmacological or electrical conversion is conducted without further delay. Patients are then given warfarin for 3 weeks if

---

sssss According to controlled studies in which patients received either quinidine or placebo. The data from most,[1573, 1576, 1583, 1588] but not all,[1625] uncontrolled series do not show that quinidine helps to maintain sinus rhythm. Because some patients maintain sinus rhythm without an antiarrhythmic drug, the authors of one report advise that quinidine be given only after recardioverting patients who resumed atrial fibrillation when taking no drugs.[1632] According to a meta-analysis, the mortality rate of quinidine-treated patients (2.9%) is about three times that of patients not taking the drug (0.8%).

ttttt Only 1 (4%) of 27 patients who were reconverted remained in sinus rhythm at 1 year, and none who were converted three times maintained sinus rhythm for more than 3 months.[1584]

uuuuuu In 47 (1.7%) of 2,704 patients. Emboli were reported in 0% to 6% of the patients in these series. This relatively wide range probably reflects the different types of heart diseases present—patients with mitral disease have a greater likelihood of emboli—and the specific care that was applied to detect the presence of emboli. Nevertheless, the association of cardioversion with emboli is low. In one autopsy series of 693 patients with atrial fibrillation, which included patients who had converted to sinus rhythm spontaneously, by drugs, or by countershock, H. Aberg concluded (1969): "There was no significant difference in any of the groups comparing patients with recurrent conversions and those with permanent AF [atrial fibrillation]."[447]

vvvvvv In 2 uncontrolled series, 2.7% of 559 patients taking no anticoagulants had emboli, whereas 0.7% of 286 anticoagulated patients had emboli after cardioversion.[35, 1646] Because the anticoagulated patients tended to be those with a higher risk of emboli, the comparison makes an even stronger case for such treatment than the data suggest.[1646]

wwwwww Unable to find the origin for the "rules" about length of anticoagulation before and after cardioversion, I wrote to Dr. Bernard Lown who replied: "I must confess that I started the three- and one-week rule for anticoagulation for cardioversion based on clinical intuition rather than factual evidence. It may be that two weeks prior to cardioversion would be adequate. I knew enough, at least from information available at the time—the early 60's, that atrial activity might not resume for at least one week. Therefore, thromboembolism could postdate the restoration of a sinus mechanism."[1651]

the drug is not contraindicated.[1657] At this writing, how best to prevent emboli produced by converting atrial fibrillation to sinus rhythm remains controversial.[1664, xxxxxx]

Arrhythmias. Cardiac arrhythmias develop in 25% to more than 90% of patients soon after the shock of cardioversion is delivered.[510, 1571, 1573, 1579] Atrial[353, 1571, 1573, 1579, 1644] and ventricular[510, 1573, 1579, 1582] occur most frequently. Nodal rhythms,[510, 1573, 1582, 1665] atrial flutter,[353, 1573, 1579] supraventricular tachycardias,[1573] accelerated intraventricular rhythms,[1666] and ventricular tachycardias[1579, 1582, 1642, 1644, 1666] have been reported less often, each in less than 10% of cases.

Cardioversion occasionally is followed immediately by ventricular fibrillation, which is often short-lived and self-reverting.[509, 1570, 1580, 1582, 1644, 1666] Ventricular fibrillation has also been observed in a few patients minutes to hours after cardioversion and may have been due to the shock alone, to intrinsic heart disease, or to drug toxicity.

Postcardioversion arrhythmias occur most often in patients with acute myocardial infarction, active ischemia, or electrolyte disturbances, particularly hypokalemia. The procedure, when elective, should be postponed in such patients.[35, 1667] More arrhythmias occur after shocks of higher energy,[35, 1580, 1666] but whether this is caused by the energy itself or characteristics of the heart that require more power for conversion is unknown.

Patients who are taking quinidine during cardioversion probably,[353, 510, 1583] but not definitely,[1184, 1635, 1668] have fewer postconversion arrhythmias than patients who are not taking antiarrhythmic drugs. Quinidine, however, has been implicated in causing such dangerous arrhythmias as multifocal ventricular premature beats and ventricular tachycardia, flutter, and fibrillation either soon after cardioversion[1184, 1665, 1669] or later.[35, 510, 1607, yyyyy] Of course, if the ventricular fibrillation persists, additional shocks with appropriate resuscitative measures must be administered.[1670] Propranolol and procainamide, given together before conversion to sinus rhythm, reduce the incidence of postconversion arrhythmias more successfully than procainamide or quinidine given alone.[1184]

Digitalis and postconversion arrhythmias. Stable patients with normal digoxin levels,[1671] and without electrolyte disorders, acute illnesses, or electrocardiographic or clinical findings of digitalis intoxication,[1607, 1667, 1672] rarely, if ever, develop dangerous postconversion arrhythmias. Consequently, one can continue giving digitalis to patients before conversion and thereby maintain control of the ventricular rate. Even in patients taking digitalis, the ventricular rate may increase slightly in the 15 minutes before conversion to sinus rhythm.[1673]

The risk of developing dangerous arrhythmias after cardioversion increases in patients with digitalis intoxication.[1571, 1586, 1607, 1671, 1672, 1674, 1675, zzzzz] Hence, cardioversion should be postponed, if possible, in patients suspected of overdosage with digitalis. Overdigitalized patients with atrial fibrillation require more energy to restore sinus rhythm,[1607, 1675] and they develop more ventricular arrhythmias as the amount of power is raised.[1607] By using small amounts of power initially,[1676] such as 25 joules, and then increasing the power in small increments, one can expose digitalis-induced arrhythmias and avoid complications by stopping the cardioversion[1582] in patients with atrial fibrillation and other supraventricular tachyarrhythmias of uncertain mechanism.[1677]

Atrioventricular block. More patients have prolonged PR intervals in the sinus rhythm that follows conversion from atrial fibrillation than do patients without the arrhythmia.[35, 509, 510, 1573] Prolonged PR intervals are found less often in young patients and in those with large F waves and brief duration of atrial fibrillation.[510] Consequently, one suspects that large left atria and long-standing atrial fibrillation prolong atrioventricular conduction by either pathophysiological or anatomical means. Patients with digitalis toxicity are more likely to have first-degree atrioventricular block after cardioversion than those without toxicity.[1607]

Sick sinus syndrome. Adequate sinus function may not return following cardioversion of patients whose atria have fibrillated for many years[35] and in those with a slow ventricular response in atrial fibrillation.[1640] In such cases, junctional escape beats or accelerated rhythms may appear after the shock.[353, 1579, 1582, 1607]

Most patients in whom normal sinus function does not appear usually revert quickly to atrial fibrillation. Such patients may have the sick sinus syndrome and should be left in atrial fibrillation and not reconverted unless the disorder has been caused or exacerbated by acute illness or drugs like digitalis, quinidine, or amiodarone. Extremely slow heart rates or cardiac asystole occurs so seldom in properly selected patients after cardioversion that insertion of a prophylactic transvenous pacemaker is rarely indicated. Temporary external pacing can be effective in such cases.[1538]

Myocardial damage. Cardioversion seldom significantly damages the human heart despite release of enzymes produced by myocardial tissues.[1580, 1644, 1678–1685] Serial electrocardiographic records[1679] and nuclear

---

xxxxxx The Assessment of Cardioversion Using Transesophageal Echocardiography (ACUTE) Multicenter Study should help to resolve the controversy about what treatment is needed to prevent emboli associated with cardioversion.[1664]

yyyyy Many patients receiving quinidine also take digitalis. Because digoxin levels were not available when these reports were published, and in view of quinidine's ability to increase digoxin levels, some of the arrhythmias thought to be induced by quinidine may have been caused by digitalis intoxication.

zzzzz In the early 1960s, before physicians knew that patients with arrhythmias due to digitalis intoxication should not be cardioverted, ventricular fibrillation and death soon after cardioversion did occur.[1571, 1674] Some investigators then concluded that digitalis intoxication may appear after conversion even "when no indication of digitalis intoxication was present prior to conversion."[1674] More recent clinical studies suggest that this concern is exaggerated.[1671, 1672]

studies[1684, 1686] show no myocardial damage from cardioversion. Creatine phosphokinase, serum glutamic-oxaloacetic transaminase, and lactic dehydrogenase rise in a minority of patients after cardioversion, particularly when 2 or more shocks[1682, 1687, aaaaaaa] or large amounts of power are required for conversion.[1580, 1688] Most of the elevated enzymatic fractions originate from tissues other than the heart—particularly from skeletal muscle, which produces the particular isoenzymes of creatine phosphokinase and lactic dehydrogenase.[1680, 1681] Postmortem examination reveals damage to anterior chest wall muscles in some patients who have had external shocks.[1689]

Nevertheless, cardioversion can produce modest elevations of myocardial-specific (MB) isoenzyme of creatine phosphokinase.[1688, 1690, bbbbbbb] Cardiac troponin I remains normal or rises minimally after elective cardioversion.[1685] When substantial elevations occur, one should suspect myocardial injury from causes unrelated to the procedure.[1685]

ST segment elevations. These features develop in fewer than 20% of patients after cardioversion.[1570, 1573, 1644, 1665, 1684, 1691–1693] These abnormalities, which may last from seconds to a few minutes, develop more frequently in patients who[1693]

• Are older.
• Have recently had operations that include pericardiotomy.
• Are less likely to have been successfully cardioverted to sinus rhythm.
• Maintain regular rhythm for only brief periods after cardioversion.

Most workers believe that the ST segment elevations originate from the effects of shocks on skeletal muscle, although the mechanism has never been established. T-wave changes seldom occur.

Pulmonary edema. A few patients develop pulmonary edema soon after cardioversion.[35, 1580, 1644, 1694–1697] Most have required large amounts of power, such as 350 to 400 joules, for conversion.[1594] Although the cause has not been established, it is possible that the return of contraction in the right, before the left, atrium may contribute to the complication.[819, 845, 848–850, 1580]

Death. None of 2,872 patients with atrial fibrillation died during or soon after cardioversion.[35, 509, 719, 848, 1073, 1567, 1569–1573, 1576, 1578–1580, 1582–1585, 1587, 1588] Quinidine or digitalis was thought to contribute to the sudden deaths of a few patients several hours to days after the procedure.[302, 1570, 1578, 1582, 1584, 1587, 1588, 1674]

Internal Atrial Defibrillation[1030, 1534, 1563, 1698–1708]

Sinus rhythm can also be restored with direct-current shocks introduced through intra-atrial electrode catheters, even in patients who cannot be successfully cardioverted externally.[751, 946, 1709–1738, ccccccc] Sedation or anesthesia is usually administered.

Atrial fibrillation, always initiated by closely coupled atrial premature beats, returns immediately after internal defibrillation in some patients.[946, 1739, ddddddd] However, whether the cardioversion is external or internal does not seem to affect the likelihood that patients will maintain sinus rhythm or will revert to atrial fibrillation.[1470]

Low cardiac output and transient atrioventricular block have been reported as occasional complications of intra-atrial cardioversion.[1740] However, the shocks seldom induce serious ventricular arrhythmias even in patients with a history of ventricular tachycardia.[1736] Permanently implanted atrial defibrillators are being evaluated for the treatment of atrial fibrillation.[1698, 1703, 1715]

Ablation[1030, 1062, 1534, 1741–1748]

Atrioventricular junction.[1749, 1750] When standard methods fail to control the ventricular rate, ablating conduction in the atrioventricular node or bundle of His permanently relieves many of the uncomfortable effects of persistent or paroxysmal supraventricular tachyarrhythmias, including atrial fibrillation, atrial flutter, atrial tachycardia, supraventricular tachycardia, and junctional ectopic tachycardia.

Formerly, ablation was performed with direct-current shock transmitted through electrode catheters.[726, 1751–1772] Radiofrequency current,[725, 727, 801, 802, 1555, 1773–1798] now the preferred method, provides a safer and more successful result, and general anesthesia is not required.[1785, 1786] Catheter ablation is as effective as surgical ablation and avoids the disadvantages of a major operation.[1799] Rarely, other methods may be necessary when catheter ablation is unsuccessful.[1800, eeeeeee]

When atrioventricular conduction is totally or nearly totally interrupted, a ventricular pacemaker must be inserted because the intrinsic escape foci seldom produce an adequately rapid and reliable rhythm.[1796]

---

aaaaaaa However, postmortem examination of the heart of a patient who received at least 140 direct-current countershocks each of about 200 joules for ventricular fibrillation showed no myocardial injury.[1687]

bbbbbbb Although total creatine phosphokinase increased in 15 of 30 cardioverted patients, the MB fraction rose slightly in only 2. The values of myocardial-specific creatine phosphokinase were lower than usually seen in patients with myocardial infarction and comparably elevated total creatine phosphokinase activity.[1690]

ccccccc Intra-atrial cardioversion established sinus rhythm in 22 (88%) of 25 patients with atrial fibrillation who failed to convert with external shock.[1720] Sinus rhythm persisted in 12 (55%) of 22 patients, each of whom took sotalol, for an average of 15 months (range, 0.2 to 33 months).[1720] In a multicenter trial of 141 patients, internal shock restored sinus rhythm in 115 (82%). The average amount of energy administered ranged from 2.0 joules for the patients with paroxysmal atrial fibrillation to 3.6 joules for those with chronic fibrillation. The voltage required for conversion related directly to the duration of atrial fibrillation and the size of the left atrium. No complications, including ventricular arrhythmias, were produced by 1,779 synchronized shocks.[1730]

ddddddd In 5 (13%) of 38 patients.[946]

eeeeeee Ethanol infused into the right coronary artery ablated the atrioventricular node in a young woman with tricuspid atresia and disabling reentrant atrial tachycardia in whom catheter ablation could not be successfully performed.[1800]

About one-third of patients remain dependent on their pacemakers to prevent more than 5 seconds of asystole.[1801] Pacemaker dependence tends to persist in those patients whose escape foci immediately after ablation are too slow.[1801]

For patients with paroxysmal atrial fibrillation, use of dual-chamber pacers seems justified because only about half of patients with the paroxysmal arrhythmia progress to chronic atrial fibrillation within 3 years after atrioventricular junctional ablation and pacing.[1036] For patients in chronic atrial fibrillation, the rate-dependent models allow the ventricular rate to respond to physical activity.

When compared with pharmacological control alone, ablating the bundle of His and inserting a rate-adaptive or dual-chamber pacemaker can decrease[725–727, 802, 1791, 1802–1805]

- Asthenia.
- Dyspnea on effort.
- Mitral regurgitation.
- Palpitations.

Ablation can decrease

- Exercise tolerance and duration.
- Left ventricular function.[fffff]
- New York Heart Association class.
- Quality of life.

The procedure should not be expected to reduce the risk of emboli if the atria continue to fibrillate.[1757, 1764] In patients with hypertrophic cardiomyopathy, radiofrequency ablation of the atrioventricular node with insertion of a rate-responsive ventricular pacemaker improves symptoms and may decrease the left ventricular outflow tract gradient.[1788] Radiofrequency current ablation of the atrioventricular node does not disrupt the normal function of an implanted pacemaker.[1788]

Partial ablation. Partial ablation (modification or modulation) of conduction in the atrioventricular node slows the ventricular response in patients with atrial fibrillation and atrial flutter. If the procedure successfully permits the ventricular rate to be sufficiently rapid, ventricular pacing is not required,[1793, 1806–1821] and, consequently, modification costs less than ablation.[1819]

However, compared with modification, ablation of the atrioventricular junction with permanent pacing in patients with atrial fibrillation

- Improves quality of life.[1822]
- Decreases the symptoms of atrial fibrillation more effectively.[1822]
- In many patients with congestive heart failure, improves cardiac performance more successfully.[1823]

Source of arrhythmia. Radiofrequency catheter ablation of rapidly discharging foci of electrical activity may cure a few patients of what appears on the surface electrocardiogram to be atrial fibrillation.[907, 908, 1824, ggggggg] Each patient successfully treated by this technique has repetitive paroxysms of atrial fibrillation associated with bursts of irregular atrial tachycardia and monomorphic atrial premature beats.[908] None has structural heart disease.[908] Preliminary data suggest that linear lesions in the right atrium produced with catheters transmitting radiofrequency current can suppress idiopathic paroxysmal atrial fibrillation.[1824, 1825]

Effects of ablating other arrhythmias on atrial fibrillation. Ablation of accessory or dual pathways to prevent supraventricular tachycardia in patients who also have paroxysmal atrial fibrillation preceded by episodes of the tachycardia reduces the frequency of,[990, 1826] but does not eliminate recurrences of, atrial fibrillation.[1827]

Antiarrhythmic drugs sometimes change chronic atrial fibrillation into atrial flutter. Early work suggests that ablating the flutter and continued use of antiarrhythmic drugs may suppress both arrhythmias.[1828] Furthermore, in patients with paroxysms of atrial fibrillation preceded by episodes of atrial flutter, ablating the flutter circuit may also abolish the episodes of atrial fibrillation.[489] At electrophysiology study, these patients are identified by documentation of simultaneous flutter of the right atrium and fibrillation of the left atrium.[489]

Complications. Complications that may follow soon after atrioventricular junctional ablation with catheter electrodes delivering direct-current shock or radiofrequency current[1829, hhhhhh] include the following:[1782, 1790]

- Cardiac arrest and sudden death,[1771] resulting from lethal ventricular arrhythmias, which occur most frequently in patients with severe ventricular dysfunction.[1770, 1785]
- Accelerated idioventricular rhythm.[1830]
- Hemodynamic deterioration associated with progression of mitral regurgitation.[1831]
- Cardiac tamponade.[1786]
- Coronary sinus rupture.[1832]
- Pulmonary embolism.[1786]
- Right atrial thrombus formation.[1833]

Surgery[1030, 1534, 1834–1835]

Cardiac surgery increases the likelihood that sinus rhythm will replace atrial fibrillation after operation in the following situations:

[fffff] The ejection fraction increased by an average of 34% when the left ventricular systolic function was depressed by the arrhythmia before ablation.[1916] The worse the function, the greater the recovery.[727]

[ggggggg] In the first reported experience with nine patients, three foci were located in the right atrium—two near the sinus node and one in the ostium of the coronary sinus—and six in the left atrium—five at the ostium of the right pulmonary veins and one at the ostium of the left pulmonary veins.[907, 908]

[hhhhhh] Eleven (5%) of 220 patients with paroxysmal or chronic atrial fibrillation died suddenly out of hospital an average of 15 months after treatment with radiofrequency ablation of their atrioventricular nodes and pacemakers.[1829] Each had depressed left ventricular function. Whether these deaths relate to the procedure or result from the patients' intrinsic heart disease is not known.

- In patients with hypertrophic cardiomyopathy who have left ventriculotomy and myomectomy, particularly if the left atrial size decreases after surgery.[697]
- Not at all in patients with constrictive pericarditis who have successful pericardiectomy.[323]
- To an unknown degree in patients with mitral valve surgery, because many of these patients are cardioverted and then given antiarrhythmic drugs; the specific effects of the operation on the arrhythmia are difficult to quantify.

Emboli. Whether mitral valvotomy by itself reduces the likelihood of patients with atrial fibrillation having emboli has not been proved. When this issue was being studied, mostly in the 1950s and 1960s, some authors thought the operation helped,[64, 412, 456, 1837] whereas others could not establish its value.[415, 1838] Because anticoagulation is advised for most patients with atrial fibrillation, studies to evaluate the value of mitral valvular surgery to prevent emboli would be difficult to perform.

Whether obliteration of the left atrial appendage reduces the incidence of emboli after mitral surgery in patients with atrial fibrillation has long been debated.[412] Workers have reawakened interest in the value of this procedure in preventing stroke in patients with nonrheumatic atrial fibrillation.[1839] Mitral valve surgery can safely be conducted in patients with atrial fibrillation and "massive" left atrial thrombi without late embolic events.[1840]

Maze operation.[1841] In suitable patients, the Maze operation can sustain sinus rhythm in patients with paroxysmal and chronic atrial fibrillation and can reestablish the hemodynamic advantages of a physiologically controlled heart rate and sequential atrioventricular contraction. In this procedure, the surgeon makes several atrial incisions that interrupt the circuits sustaining the arrhythmia.[1836, 1842–1851] The sinus impulse is thereby directed along a specified route from the sinoatrial to the atrioventricular node. Atrial transport is restored in many patients,[752, 1852] even those with giant left atria.[1853]

The Maze procedure can be successfully performed in patients who also receive at the same operation coronary artery bypass grafts, valvular repair or replacement,[1854–1857] repair of congenital heart defects, such as atrial septal defects,[1858, 1859] and other procedures.[1859–1862, iiiiii]

The response to exercise of the reestablished sinus rhythm is blunted soon after the operation, but it may improve within the next 6 months.[1861] This abnormality is thought to be caused by deenervation of the sinus node by the incisions made in the atrial wall during the Maze operation.[1861] The exercise capacity of the patients relates closely to the sinus's response to exercise.[1861] Postoperative factors influencing whether sinus rhythm will be sustained after the operation include the duration of atrial fibrillation, left atrial size,[1863] and cardiothoracic ratio;[1864] left atrial dimension measured after operation is the most potent factor.[1864]

Corridor operation. In this procedure, most of the right and left atria are isolated from the sinus node, the atrioventricular node, and a strip or corridor of atrial tissue between the two.[1865–1869] The sinus node can then control the ventricular rhythm, even though most of the atria are fibrillating.

The operation has limited value because many patients have sick sinus syndrome—either from previous dysfunction of the sinus node or from the surgery itself—and the procedure does not reestablish the hemodynamic advantages of sinus rhythm or reduce the incidence of emboli.[1870] Catheter ablation of the atrioventricular node and insertion of a rate-adaptive pacemaker are preferable.[1870]

Surgical cryoablation. Cryoablation, delivered to sites in the posterior wall of the left atrium during surgery for isolated mitral valve disease, reduces or eliminates chronic atrial fibrillation better than the valvular surgery alone.[1871, 1872, jjjjjj]

Other procedures. Other surgical approaches to the treatment of atrial fibrillation include the "atrial compartment,"[1873–1875] "left atrial isolation,"[1876, 1877] and "right atrial separation"[1878, 1879] procedures.

Surgeons first successfully ablated the human atrioventricular node or bundle of His in patients with atrial tachyarrhythmias at open-heart surgery by dividing, ligating, or cryoablating[1742, 1761, 1772, 1880–1893] the relevant cardiac tissues. Catheter ablation of the atrioventricular junction replaced surgical ablation, which, in turn, has been superseded by direct ablation of the source of many tachyarrhythmias including a few cases of atrial fibrillation.

PROGNOSIS

Although the underlying heart disease determines the prognosis more than the presence of atrial fibrillation itself,[1894] mortality is higher in patients with the arrhythmia,[61, 796, 1895] and it depends, in part, on whether the arrhythmia is chronic or paroxysmal.

Chronic Atrial Fibrillation

Mortality rises when chronic atrial fibrillation develops in older patients,[436] particularly those more than 60 years of age, although the excess risk declines as patients age further.[51]

The prognosis is worse in adults with atrial fibrillation who also have the following:

- Coronary heart disease,[43, 74, 128, 436] in whom the risk

---

iiiiii The investigators who developed the Maze procedure consider the operation to be "the treatment of choice in patients with medically refractory symptomatic atrial fibrillation."[1917]

jjjjjj Cryoablation of the posterior left atrium reduced or eliminated chronic atrial fibrillation in 29 (94%) of 31 patients who had mitral valve surgery, but in only 4 (27%) of 15 patients who had valvular surgery without ablation was the arrhythmia eliminated.[1872]

may be twice as high as for those in sinus rhythm.[67, kkkkkkk]

- Idiopathic congestive cardiomyopathy.[1896]
- Hypertrophic cardiomyopathy, in whom atrial fibrillation before operation increases the risk of dying after myomectomy;[1897] atrial fibrillation, along with congestive heart failure and thromboembolic events, characterizes those patients at higher risk who are members of families with hypertrophic cardiomyopathy.[1898, lllll]
- Sick sinus syndrome.[1899]
- Thyrotoxicosis.[1900]

Congestive Heart Failure

Atrial fibrillation does not worsen the prognosis of patients with mild or moderate congestive heart failure.[478, 1901, mmmmmmm] However, the prognosis is less favorable for patients with heart failure

- And atrial fibrillation, whose left ventricular ejection fraction is reduced.[1902]
- And atrial fibrillation, whose filling pressures are low and who take vasodilator and diuretic drugs.[126, 1903, nnnnnnn]
- Who take antiarrhythmic drugs to prevent symptomatic atrial fibrillation when compared with patients who are similarly ill and not taking such drugs.[1904]

The prognosis for patients with advanced congestive heart failure and atrial fibrillation improved in the period 1990 to 1993 when compared with 1985 to 1989,[1905] a finding probably reflecting greater use of angiotensin-converting enzyme inhibitors and avoidance of class I antiarrhythmic drugs.[1905]

Paroxysmal Atrial Fibrillation

Intermittent atrial fibrillation increases the mortality of patients who have the following:

- Coronary heart disease.[253]
- Mitral stenosis.[253]
- Recent surgical correction of congenital heart disease.[296]
- Recent pneumonectomy.[315]

No Increased Risk

The risk of dying is probably not increased when atrial fibrillation develops in patients with the following conditions:

---

kkkkkkk According to the Coronary Artery Surgery Study (CASS).[67]

lllll The long-term survival of patients with hypertrophic cardiomyopathy, atrial fibrillation, and no other complications is good and is no worse than for those in sinus rhythm.[1106]

mmmmmmm According to the Veterans Affairs Vasodilator–Heart Failure Trial (V-HeFT).[478]

nnnnnnn Although one study questioned whether atrial fibrillation by itself worsens the prognosis of all patients with congestive failure beyond what would be expected if they were in sinus rhythm.[126]

ooooooo From an Israeli study comparing outcomes in 1992, 1994, and 1996 (thrombolytic era) with 1981 to 1983 (prethrombolytic era).[1908]

ppppppp This conclusion was reached before operative repair of mitral valve disease had been developed.

qqqqqqq In one report, the risk in patients with chronic lone fibrillation was slightly greater than in subjects in sinus rhythm.[253]

Acute myocardial infarction. Opinion is divided whether atrial fibrillation during myocardial infarction is,[144, 148, 1906] or is not,[66, 135, 137, 139, 146, 1907, 1908] an independent risk factor for early death. Nevertheless, the prognosis worsens when patients develop atrial fibrillation during myocardial infarction,[1909] particularly when

- The arrhythmia begins later in the course of the infarction.[146]
- The ventricular response immediately after the onset of atrial fibrillation is slower.[146]
- The arrhythmia recurs.[146]

The overall outcome is superior for patients who develop the arrhythmia now, during the thrombolytic era, than it was during the prethrombolytic era.[1908, ooooooo]

Unoperated mitral valve disease. Atrial fibrillation develops in such patients toward the end of their course. The arrhythmia, by itself, does not determine prognosis or life expectancy.[104, ppppppp]

Wolff-Parkinson-White syndrome. The risk is no greater than in those with preexcitation and no atrial fibrillation.[160]

Lone atrial fibrillation. Lone atrial fibrillation,[371, 476, 477] whether chronic or paroxysmal,[253, qqqqqqq] is not associated with an increased risk of dying.

SUMMARY

Atrial fibrillation, the most common sustained cardiac arrhythmia, occurs infrequently in the general population, but it is more common as patients age. Most patients with atrial fibrillation have structural heart disease such as mitral stenosis or regurgitation, acute myocardial infarction, the Wolff-Parkinson-White syndrome, thyrotoxicosis, recent cardiothoracic surgery, cardiomyopathy, myocarditis, or pulmonary disease. Patients with the arrhythmia but no organic heart disease are said to have lone atrial fibrillation. Atrial fibrillation increases the risk of stroke and emboli and the mortality of adults with structural heart disease.

The symptom most frequently reported by patients with atrial fibrillation is rapid, irregular heartbeat. Many also experience chest pain, shortness of breath, lightheadedness, and dizziness. The physical examination reveals an irregular, usually rapid, heartbeat, often with a difference between the rate in the arterial pulse and that at the cardiac apex. Signs of atrial contraction in the neck veins and in the heart examination are absent.

The electrocardiogram of patients with untreated atrial fibrillation usually shows a rapid, irregular ventricular rate in which the P waves are replaced by an undulating baseline. The range of ventricular rates is wide and may exceed 200 beats per minute in patients with preexcitation. The QRS complexes, although usually narrow, may be wide (aberrant) and may simulate ventricular beats and ventricular tachycardia. The left atrium is often enlarged and, after long periods of chronic atrial fibrillation, loses contractile ability when sinus rhythm is reestablished. Cardiac function usually decreases when atrial fibrillation replaces sinus rhythm. Many patients develop polyuria during episodes of paroxysmal atrial fibrillation.

Electrophysiological studies show replacement of organized atrial activity by rapid, irregular electrical activity. Abnormalities of atrial vulnerability, conduction, excitability, and refractoriness characterize patients with atrial fibrillation. The likelihood of extremely rapid ventricular rates and ventricular fibrillation in patients with the Wolff-Parkinson-White syndrome and atrial fibrillation can often be determined in the electrophysiology laboratory.

When the ventricular rate is too rapid, digitalis and beta-adrenergic– or calcium-channel–blocking drugs are administered. Electrical cardioversion is the favorite method of restoring sinus rhythm when it does not return spontaneously. Antiarrhythmic drugs are then employed to preserve regular rhythm in those cases in which this is feasible. In increasing numbers of patients, physicians are ablating the atrioventricular junction and implanting pacemakers to relieve symptoms and to improve cardiac performance in chronic atrial fibrillation. All patients with chronic atrial fibrillation and many patients with paroxysmal atrial fibrillation should be anticoagulated to reduce the occurrence of emboli.

REFERENCES

1. Kulbertus HE, Olsson SB, Schlepper M (eds). Atrial Fibrillation. Molndal, Sweden: AB Hassle, 1982.
2. Benditt DG, Benson DW Jr, Dunnigan A, Gornick CC, Anderson RW. Atrial flutter, atrial fibrillation, and other primary atrial tachycardias. Med Clin North Am 1984; 68:895–918.
3. Selzer A. Atrial fibrillation revisited. N Engl J Med 1982; 306:1044–1045.
4. Alpert JS, Petersen P, Godtfredsen J. Atrial fibrillation: natural history, complications, and management. Annu Rev Med 1988; 39:41–52.
5. Porter CJ. Premature atrial contractions and atrial tachyarrhythmias. In Gillette PC, Garson A Jr (eds). Pediatric Arrhythmias. Electrophysiology and Pacing. Philadelphia: WB Saunders, 1990, pp. 328–359.
6. Touboul P, Waldo AL. Atrial Arrhythmias. Current Concepts and Management. St. Louis: Mosby–Year Book, 1990.
7. Falk RH, Podrid PJ (eds). Atrial Fibrillation. Mechanisms and Management. New York: Raven Press, 1992.
8. Josephson ME. Clinical Cardiac Electrophysiology. Techniques and Interpretations. 2nd ed. Philadelphia, Lea & Febiger, 1993, pp. 275–310.
9. National Heart Lung and Blood Institute Working Group on Atrial Fibrillation. Atrial fibrillation: current understandings and research imperatives. J Am Coll Cardiol 1993; 22:1830–1834.
10. Kerr CR. Atrial fibrillation: the next frontier. Pacing Clin Electrophysiol 1994; 17:1203–1207.
11. Cobbe SM. Incidence and risks associated with atrial fibrillation. Pacing Clin Electrophysiol 1994; 17:1005–1010.
12. Kulbertus HE. Atrial Fibrillation. Facts from Yesterday—Ideas for Tomorrow. Armonk, NY: Futura Publishing Co., 1994.
13. Martin D, Mendelsohn ME, John RM, Loscalzo J. Atrial Fibrillation. Cambridge, MA: Blackwell Scientific Publications, 1994.
14. Olsson SB, Allessie MA, Campbell RWF. Atrial Fibrillation. Mechanisms and Therapeutic Strategies. Armonk, NY: Futura Publishing Co., 1994.
15. Wellens HJJ. Atrial fibrillation: the last big hurdle in treating supraventricular tachycardia. N Engl J Med 1994; 331:944–945.
16. Ryden L. Atrial fibrillation: new aspects of an old problem. Pacing Clin Electrophysiol 1994; 17:1003–1004.
17. DiMarco JP, Prystowsky EN. Atrial Arrhythmias. State of the Art. Armonk, NY: Futura Publishing Co., 1995.
18. Falk RH. Atrial fibrillation. In Podrid PJ, Kowey PR (eds). Cardiac Arrhythmia. Mechanisms, Diagnosis and Management. Baltimore: Williams & Wilkins, 1995, pp. 803–827.
19. Lip GY, Beevers DG, Singh SP, Watson RD. ABC of atrial fibrillation: aetiology, pathophysiology, and clinical features. BMJ 1995; 311:1425–1428.
20. Lip GY, Watson RD. ABC of atrial fibrillation: differential diagnosis of atrial fibrillation. BMJ 1995; 311:1495–1498.
21. Ruffy R. Atrial fibrillation. In Zipes DP, Jalife J (eds). Cardiac Electrophysiology. From Cell to Bedside. 2nd ed. Philadelphia: WB Saunders, 1995, pp. 682–690.
22. Camm AJ, Obel OA. Epidemiology and mechanism of atrial fibrillation and atrial flutter. Am J Cardiol 1996; 78:3–11.
23. Kastor JA. Atrial fibrillation. Adv Intern Med 1996; 41:365–397.
24. Reardon M, Camm AJ. Atrial fibrillation in the elderly. Clin Cardiol 1996; 19:765–775.
25. Allessie MA, Fromer M. Atrial and Ventricular Fibrillation. Mechanisms and Device Therapy. Armonk, NY: Futura Publishing Co., 1997.
26. Murgatroyd FD, Camm AJ. Nonpharmacological Management of Atrial Fibrillation. Armonk, NY: Futura Publishing Co., 1997.
27. Waktare JE, Camm AJ. Atrial fibrillation begets trouble. Heart 1997; 77:393–394.
28. Zipes DP. Atrial fibrillation: from cell to bedside. J Cardiovasc Electrophysiol 1997; 8:927–938.
29. Pritchett ELC. The case for just plain "atrial fibrillation." PACE 1998; 21:637–640.
30. Anonymous. Subject index. Circulation 1984; 70(Suppl II): II-497.
31. Anonymous. Subject index. Circulation 1990; 82(Suppl III):III-837.
32. Anonymous. Subject index. Circulation 1997; 96(Suppl I): I-732–I-733.
33. Zehender M, Meinertz T, Keul J, Just H. ECG variants and cardiac arrhythmias in athletes: clinical relevance and prognostic importance. Am Heart J 1990; 119:1378–1391.
34. Feinberg WM, Blackshear JL, Laupacis A, Kronmal R, Hart RG. Prevalence, age distribution, and gender of patients with atrial fibrillation: analysis and implications. Arch Intern Med 1995; 155:469–473.
35. Lown B. Electrical reversion of cardiac arrhythmias. Br Heart J 1967; 29:469–489.
36. Kannel WB, Wolf PA. Epidemiology and atrial fibrillation. In Falk RH, Podrid PJ (eds). Atrial Fibrillation. Mechanisms and Management. New York: Raven Press, 1992, pp. 81–92.
37. Fosmoe RJ, Averill KH, Lamb LE. Electrocardiographic findings in 67,375 asymptomatic subjects. II. Supraventricular arrhythmias. Am J Cardiol 1960; 6:84–95.
38. Hiss RG, Lamb LE. Electrocardiographic findings in 122,043 individuals. Circulation 1962; 25:947–961.
39. Busby DE, Davis AW. Paroxysmal and chronic atrial fibrillation in airman certification. Aviat Space Environ Med 1976; 47:185–191.
40. Ostrander LD Jr, Brandt RL, Kjelsberg MO, Epstein FH. Electrocardiographic findings among the adult population

of a total natural community, Tecumseh, Michigan. Circulation 1965; 31:888–898.

41. Onundarson PT, Thorgeirsson G, Jonmundsson E, Sigfusson N, Hardarson TH. Chronic atrial fibrillation—epidemiologic features and 14 year follow-up: a case control study. Eur Heart J 1987; 8:521–527.

42. Rose G, Baxter PJ, Reid DD, McCartney P. Prevalence and prognosis of electrocardiographic findings in middle-aged men. Br Heart J 1978; 40:636–643.

43. Kannel WB, Abbott RD, Savage DD, McNamara PM. Epidemiologic features of chronic atrial fibrillation: the Framingham study. N Engl J Med 1982; 306:1018–1022.

44. Belhassen B, Pauzner D, Blieden L, et al. Intrauterine and postnatal atrial fibrillation in the Wolff-Parkinson-White syndrome. Circulation 1982; 66:1124–1128.

45. Bacevice AE, Dierker LJ, Wolfson RN. Intra-uterine atrial fibrillation associated with fetomaternal hemorrhage. Am J Obstet Gynecol 1985; 153:81–82.

46. Chao RC, Ho ES, Hsieh KS. Fetal atrial flutter and fibrillation: prenatal echocardiographic detection and management. Am Heart J 1992; 124:1095–1098.

47. McEachern D, Baker BM. Auricular fibrillation: its etiology, age incidence and production by digitalis therapy. Am J Med 1932; 183:35–48.

48. Lewis T. Auricular fibrillation (irregular tachycardia). In Lewis T (ed). Diseases of the Heart. New York: Macmillan, 1934, pp. 83–84.

49. Goldbloom A, Segall HN. Auricular fibrillation in infancy. Am J Dis Child 1938; 56:587–593.

50. Parkinson J, Papp C, Evans W. The electrocardiogram of the Stokes-Adams attack. Br Heart J 1941; 3:171–199.

51. Edeiken J, Rugel SJ. Auricular fibrillation in infancy. J Pediatr 1946; 28:471–473.

52. Sawyer CG, Bolin LB, Stevens EL, Daniel LB, O'Neil NC, Hayes DM. Atrial fibrillation: its etiology, treatment and association with embolization. South Med J 1958; 51:84–93.

53. Byrum CJ, Wahl RA, Behrendt DM, Dick M. Ventricular fibrillation associated with use of digitalis in a newborn infant with Wolff-Parkinson-White syndrome. J Pediatr 1982; 101:400–403.

54. Porter CJ, Garson A. Incidence and management of dysrhythmias after Fontan procedure. Herz 1993; 18:318–327.

55. Moore EN, Fisher V, Moe GK. The importance of atrial mass in the maintenance of atrial fibrillation. In Tashijan RJ (ed). International Symposium on Comparative Medicine. Philadelphia: Eaton Labs, 1965, pp. 229–238.

56. Bohn FK, Patterson DF, Pyle RL. Atrial fibrillation in dogs. Br Vet J 1971; 127:485–496.

57. Radford DJ, Izukawa T. Atrial fibrillation in children. Pediatrics 1977; 59:250–256.

58. Moore EN, Spear JF. Natural occurrence and experimental initiation of atrial fibrillation in different animal species. In Kulbertus HE, Olsson SP, Schlepper M (eds). Atrial Fibrillation. Molndal, Sweden: AB Hassle, 1982, pp. 33–41.

59. Anonymous. Paul Wood's Diseases of the Heart and Circulation. 3rd ed. Philadelphia: JB Lippincott, 1968, p. 278.

60. Bellet S. Atrial fibrillation in the elderly patient. Geriatrics 1966; 21:239–245.

61. Krahn AD, Manfreda J, Tate RB, Mathewson FA, Cuddy TE. The natural history of atrial fibrillation: incidence, risk factors, and prognosis in the Manitoba follow-up study. Am J Med 1995; 98:476–484.

62. Sandler G, Wilson GM. The nature and prognosis of heart disease in thyrotoxicosis. Q J Med 1959; 28:347–369.

63. Hoffman I, Lowrey RD. The electrocardiogram in thyrotoxicosis. Am J Cardiol 1960; 6:893–904.

64. Coulshed N, Epstein EJ, McKendrick CS, Galloway RW, Walker E. Systemic embolism in mitral valve disease. Br Heart J 1970; 32:26–34.

65. Probst P, Goldschlager N, Selzer A. Left atrial size and atrial fibrillation in mitral stenosis: factors influencing their relationship. Circulation 1973; 48:1282–1287.

66. Sugiura T, Iwasaka T, Ogawa A, et al. Atrial fibrillation in acute myocardial infarction. Am J Cardiol 1985; 56:27–29.

67. Cameron A, Schwartz MJ, Kronmal RA, Kosinski AS. Prevalence and significance of atrial fibrillation in coronary artery disease (CASS registry). Am J Cardiol 1988; 61:714–717.

68. Anonymous. Paul Wood's Diseases of the Heart and Circulation. 3rd ed. Philadelphia: JB Lippincott, 1968, p. 278.

69. Brand FN, Abbott RD, Kannel WB, Wolf PA. Characteristics and prognosis of lone atrial fibrillation. JAMA 1985; 254:3449–3453.

70. Britton M, Gustafsson C. Non-rheumatic atrial fibrillation as a risk factor for stroke. Stroke 1985; 16:182–188.

71. Fuller JA, Adams GG, Buxton B. Atrial fibrillation after coronary artery bypass grafting. J Thorac Cardiovasc Surg 1989; 97:821–825.

72. Leitch JW, Klein GJ, Yee R, Murdock C. Prognostic value of electrophysiology testing in asymptomatic patients with Wolff-Parkinson-White pattern. Circulation 1990; 82:1718–1723.

73. Lake FR, Cullen KJ, de Klerk NH, McCall MG, Rosman DL. Atrial fibrillation and mortality in an elderly population. Aust N Z J Med 1989; 19:321–326.

74. Kitchin AH, Milne JS. Longitudinal survey of ischaemic heart disease in randomly selected sample of older population. Br Heart J 1977; 39:889–893.

75. Hill JD, Mottram EM, Killeen PD. Study of the prevalence of atrial fibrillation in general practice patients over 65 years of age. J R Coll Gen Pract 1987; 37:172–173.

76. Fisch C, Genovese PD, Dyke RW, Laramore W, Marvel RJ. The electrocardiogram in persons over 70. Geriatrics 1957; 12:616–620.

77. Campbell A, Caird FI, Jackson TF. Prevalence of abnormalities of electrocardiogram in old people. Br Heart J 1974; 36:1005–1011.

78. Mihalick MJ, Fisch C. Electrocardiographic findings in the aged. Am Heart J 1974; 87:117–128.

79. Furberg CD, Psaty BM, Manolio TA, Gardin JM, Smith VE, Rautaharju PM. Prevalence of atrial fibrillation in elderly subjects (the cardiovascular health study). Am J Cardiol 1994; 74:236–241.

80. Camm AJ, Evans KE, Ward DE, Martin A. The rhythm of the heart in active elderly subjects. Am Heart J 1980; 99:598–603.

81. Martin A, Benbow LJ, Butrous GS, Leach C, Camm AJ. Five-year follow-up of 101 elderly subjects by means of long-term ambulatory cardiac monitoring. Eur Heart J 1984; 5:592–596.

82. Rajala S, Kaltiala K, Haavisto M, Mattila K. Prevalence of ECG findings in very old people. Eur Heart J 1984; 5:168–174.

83. Golden GS, Golden LH. The "nona" electrocardiogram: findings in 100 patients of the 90 plus age group. J Am Geriatr Soc 1974; 22:329–332.

84. Tikanoja T, Kirkinen P, Nikolajev K, Eresmaa L, Haring P. Familial atrial fibrillation with fetal onset. Heart 1998; 79:195–197.

85. Larsen JA, Kadish AH. Effects of gender on cardiac arrhythmias. J Cardiovasc Electrophysiol 1998; 9:655–664.

86. Rubart M, von der Lohe E. Sex steroids and cardiac arrhythmias: more questions than answers. J Cardiovasc Electrophysiol 1998; 9:665–667.

87. White PD. Heart Disease. New York: Macmillan, 1946.

88. Rodriguez LM, de Chillou C, Schlapfer J, et al. Age at onset and gender of patients with different types of supraventricular tachycardias. Am J Cardiol 1992; 70:1213–1215.

89. Benjamin EJ, Levy D, Vaziri SM, D'Agostino RB, Belanger AJ, Wolf PA. Independent risk factors for atrial fibrillation in a population-based cohort: the Framingham heart study. JAMA 1994; 271:840–844.

90. Allessie MA. Is atrial fibrillation sometimes a genetic disease? N Engl J Med 1997; 336:950–952.

91. Wolff L. Familial auricular fibrillation. N Engl J Med 1943; 229:396–398.

92. Hanson HH, Rutledge DI. Auricular fibrillation in normal hearts. N Engl J Med 1949; 240:947–953.

93. Gould WL. Auricular fibrillation. Arch Intern Med 1957; 100:916–926.

94. Phair WB. Familial atrial fibrillation. Can Med Assoc J 1963; 89:1274–1276.

95. Friedberg CK. Diseases of the Heart. Philadelphia: WB Saunders, 1966.

96. Brugada R, Tapscott T, Czernuszewicz GZ, et al. Identification of a genetic locus for familial atrial fibrillation. N Engl J Med 1997; 336:905–911.

97. Levy S. Factors predisposing to the development of atrial fibrillation. PACE 1997; 20:2670–2674.

98. Gallagher MM, Camm AJ. Classification of atrial fibrillation. Pacing Clin Electrophysiol 1997; 20:1603–1605.

99. Gallagher MM, Camm AJ. Letter to the editor. PACE 1998; 21:776–777.

100. White PD, Jones TD. Heart disease and disorders in New England. Am Heart J 1928; 3:302–318.

101. Horstkotte D. Arrhythmias in the natural history of mitral stenosis. Acta Cardiol 1992; 47:105–113.

102. Rowe JC, Bland EF, Sprague HB, White PD. The course of mitral stenosis without surgery: ten- and twenty-year perspectives. Ann Intern Med 1960; 52:742–749.

103. Anonymous. Paul Wood's Diseases of the Heart and Circulation. 3rd ed. Philadelphia: JB Lippincott, 1968, p. 625.

104. DeGraff AC, Lingg C. The course of rheumatic heart disease in adults. Am Heart J 1935; 10:630–642.

105. Turner RWD, Fraser H. Auricular fibrillation in rheumatic heart disease. Q J Med 1954; 23:454–455.

106. Lowther CP, Turner RWD. Deterioration after mitral valvotomy. BMJ 1962; 1:1102–1107.

107. Riss E, Levine SA. Some clinical notes on patients with mitral valvular disease who have had mitral valvuloplasty. Am Heart J 1958; 56:831–845.

108. Ramsdale DR, Arumugam N, Singh SS, Pearson J, Charles RG. Holter monitoring in patients with mitral stenosis and sinus rhythm. Eur Heart J 1987; 8:164–170.

109. Anonymous. Paul Wood's Diseases of the Heart and Circulation. 3rd ed. Philadelphia: JB Lippincott, 1968, p. 613.

110. Selzer A, Katayama F. Mitral regurgitation: clinical patterns, pathophysiology and natural history. Medicine 1972; 51:337–366.

111. Ellis LB, Ramirez A. The clinical course of patients with severe "rheumatic" mitral insufficiency. Am Heart J 1969; 78:406–418.

112. Brigden W, Leatham A. Mitral incompetence. Br Heart J 1953; 15:55–73.

113. Ross J, Braunwald E, Morrow AG. Clinical and hemodynamic observations in pure mitral insufficiency. Am J Cardiol 1958; 2:11–23.

114. Phillips HR, Levine FH, Carter JE, et al. Mitral valve replacement for isolated mitral regurgitation: analysis of clinical course and late postoperative left ventricular ejection fraction. Am J Cardiol 1981; 48:647–654.

115. Waller BF, Morrow AG, Maron BJ, et al. Etiology of clinically isolated, severe, chronic, pure mitral regurgitation: analysis of 97 patients over 30 years of age having mitral valve replacement. Am Heart J 1982; 104:276–288.

116. Kligfield P, Hochreiter C, Kramer H, et al. Complex arrhythmias in mitral regurgitation with and without mitral valve prolapse: contrast to arrhythmias in mitral valve prolapse without mitral regurgitation. Am J Cardiol 1985; 55:1545–1549.

117. Diker E, Aydogdu S, Ozdemir M, et al. Prevalence and predictors of atrial fibrillation in rheumatic valvular heart disease. Am J Cardiol 1996; 77:96–98.

118. Yahini JH, Vered Z, Atlas P, Neufeld HN. Arrhythmias in the mitral valve prolapse syndrome. In Befeler B, Lazzara K, Scherlag BJ (eds). Selected Topics in Cardiac Arrhythmias. Mount Kisco, NY: Futura Publishing Co., 1980, pp. 323–329.

119. Jhaveri S, Czoniczer G, Reider RB, Massell BF. Relatively benign "pure" mitral regurgitation of rheumatic origin. Circulation 1960; 22:39–48.

120. Korn D, DeSanctis RW, Sell S. Massive calcification of the mitral annulus. N Engl J Med 1962; 267:900–909.

121. Schott CR, Kotler MN, Parry WR, Segal BL. Mitral annular calcification: clinical and echocardiographic correlations. Arch Intern Med 1977; 137:1143–1150.

122. Selzer A, Lombard JT. Clinical findings in adult aortic stenosis: then and now. Eur Heart J 1988; 9:53–55.

123. Myler RK, Sanders CA. Aortic valve disease and atrial fibrillation: report of 122 patients with electrographic, radiographic, and hemodynamic observations. Arch Intern Med 1968; 121:530–533.

124. Lombard JT, Selzer A. Valvular aortic stenosis: a clinical and hemodynamic profile of patients. Ann Intern Med 1987; 106:292–298.

125. Aberg H. Atrial fibrillation: a review of 463 cases from Philadelphia General Hospital from 1955 to 1965. Acta Med Scand 1968; 184:425–431.

126. Godtfredsen J. Atrial fibrillation: course and prognosis—a follow-up study of 1,212 cases. In Kulbertus HE, Olsson SB, Schlepper M (eds). Atrial Fibrillation. Kiruna, Molndal, Sweden: AB Hassle, 1982, pp. 134–147.

127. Davidson E, Weinberger I, Rotenberg Z, Fuchs J, Agmon J. Atrial fibrillation: cause and time of onset. Arch Intern Med 1989; 149:457–459.

128. Kannel WB, Abbott RD, Savage DD, McNamara PM. Coronary heart disease and atrial fibrillation: the Framingham study. Am Heart J 1983; 106:389–396.

129. Aronow WS, Mercando AD, Epstein S. Usefulness of an abnormal signal-averaged electrocardiogram for predicting cardiac death in elderly persons without heart disease. Am J Cardiol 1995; 75:1273–1274.

130. Julian DG, Valentine PA, Miller GG. Disturbances of rate, rhythm and conduction in acute myocardial infarction: a prospective study of 100 consecutive unselected patients with the aid of electrocardiographic monitoring. Am J Med 1964; 37:915–927.

131. Fluck DC, Olsen E, Pentecost BL, et al. Natural history and clinical significance of arrhythmias after acute cardiac infarction. Br Heart J 1967; 29:170–189.

132. Jewitt DE, Balcon R, Raftery EB, Oram S. Incidence and management of supraventricular arrhythmias after acute myocardial infarction. Lancet 1967; 2:734–738.

133. Lown B, Vasaux C, Hood WB Jr, Fakhro AM, Kaplinsky E, Roberge G. Unresolved problems in coronary care. Am J Cardiol 1967; 20:494–508.

134. Restieaux N, Bray C, Bullard H, et al. 150 patients with cardiac infarction treated in a coronary unit. Lancet 1967; 1:1285–1289.

135. Stannard M, Sloman JG. Atrial fibrillation in acute myocardial infarction. Med J Aust 1967; 1:1250–1252.

136. Stock E, Goble A, Sloman G. Assessment of arrhythmias in myocardial infarction. BMJ 1967; 2:719–723.

137. Klass M, Haywood LJ. Atrial fibrillation associated with acute myocardial infarction: a study of 34 cases. Am Heart J 1970; 79:752–760.

138. Helmers C, Lundman T, Mogensen L, Orinius E, Sjogren A, Wester PO. Atrial fibrillation in acute myocardial infarction. Acta Med Scand 1973; 193:39–44.

139. Cristal N, Peterburg I, Szwarcberg J. Atrial fibrillation developing in the acute phase of myocardial infarction: prognostic implications. Chest 1976; 70:8–11.

140. Liberthson RR, Salisbury KW, Hutter AM Jr, DeSanctis RW. Atrial tachyarrhythmias in acute myocardial infarction. Am J Med 1976; 60:956–960.

141. Liem KL, Lie KI, Durrer D, Wellens HJJ. Clinical setting and prognostic significance of atrial fibrillation complicating acute myocardial infarction. Eur J Cardiol 1976; 4:59–62.

142. Hunt D, Sloman G, Penington C. Effects of atrial fibrillation on prognosis of acute myocardial infarction. Br Heart J 1978; 40:303–307.

143. Lofmark R, Orinius E. Supraventricular tachyarrhythmias in acute myocardial infarction. Acta Med Scand 1978; 203:517–520.

144. Sakata K, Kurihara H, Iwamori K, et al. Clinical and prognostic significance of atrial fibrillation in acute myocardial infarction. Am J Cardiol 1997; 80:1522–1527.

145. Hildebrandt P, Jensen G, Kober L, et al. Myocardial infarction 1979–1988 in Denmark: secular trends in age-related incidence, in-hospital mortality and complications. Eur Heart J 1994; 15:877–881.

146. Kobayashi Y, Katoh T, Takano T, Hayakawa H. Paroxysmal atrial fibrillation and flutter associated with acute myocardial infarction: hemodynamic evaluation in relation to the development of arrhythmias and prognosis. Jpn Circ J 1992; 56:1–11.

147. Serrano CV Jr, Ramires JA, Mansur AP, Pileggi F. Importance of the time of onset of supraventricular tachyarrhythmias on prognosis of patients with acute myocardial infarction. Clin Cardiol 1995; 18:84–90.

148. Crenshaw BS, Ward SR, Granger CB, Stebbins AL, Topol EJ, Califf RM. Atrial fibrillation in the setting of acute myocardial infarction: the GUSTO-I experience. Global utilization of streptokinase and TPA for occluded coronary arteries. J Am Coll Cardiol 1997; 30:406–413.

149. Sugiura T, Iwasaka T, Takahashi N, et al. Factors associated with atrial fibrillation in Q wave anterior myocardial infarction. Am Heart J 1991; 121:1409–1412.

150. Nielsen BL. ST-segment elevation in acute myocardial infarction: prognostic importance. Circulation 1973; 48:338–345.

151. Behar S, Goldbourt U, Reicher-Reiss H, Kaplinsky E. Prognosis of acute myocardial infarction complicated by primary ventricular fibrillation: principal investigators of the SPRINT study. Am J Cardiol 1990; 66:1208–1211.

152. Sugiura T, Iwasaka T, Takahashi N, et al. Atrial fibrillation in inferior wall Q-wave acute myocardial infarction. Am J Cardiol 1991; 67:1135–1136.

153. Kyriakidis M, Barbetseas J, Antonopoulos A, Skouros C, Tentolouris C, Toutouzas P. Early atrial arrhythmias in acute myocardial infarction: role of the sinus node artery. Chest 1992; 101:944–947.

154. O'Doherty M, Tayler DI, Quinn E, Vincent R, Chamberlain DA. Five hundred patients with myocardial infarction monitored within one hour of symptoms. Br Med J Clin Res Ed 1994; 1983:1405–1408.

155. Rechavia E, Strasberg B, Mager A, et al. The incidence of atrial arrhythmias during inferior wall myocardial infarction with and without right ventricular involvement. Am Heart J 1992; 124:387–391.

156. Hod H, Lew AS, Keltai M, et al. Early atrial fibrillation during evolving myocardial infarction: a consequence of impaired left atrial perfusion. Circulation 1987; 75:146–150.

157. Friedman HZ, Weber-Bornstein N, Deboe SF, Mancini GB. Cardiac care unit admission criteria for suspected acute myocardial infarction in new-onset atrial fibrillation. Am J Cardiol 1987; 59:866–869.

158. Newman BJ, Donoso E, Friedberg CK. Arrhythmias in the Wolff-Parkinson-White syndrome. Prog Cardiovasc Dis 1966; 9:147–165.

159. Poveda J, Pajaron A, de Micheli A. Atrial fibrillation and flutter in preexcitation syndrome (an analysis of 28 cases). Acta Cardiol 1974; 29:455–468.

160. Pietersen AH, Andersen ED, Sandoe E. Atrial fibrillation in the Wolff-Parkinson-White syndrome. Am J Cardiol 1992; 70:38A–43A.

161. Wolff L, White PD. Syndrome of short P-R interval with abnormal QRS complexes and paroxysmal tachycardia. Arch Intern Med 1948; 82:446–467.

162. Wolff L. Wolff-Parkinson-White syndrome: historical and clinical features. Prog Cardiovasc Dis 1960; 2:677–690.

163. Campbell RW, Smith RA, Gallagher JJ, Pritchett EL, Wallace AG. Atrial fibrillation in the preexcitation syndrome. Am J Cardiol 1977; 40:514–520.

164. Bauernfeind RA, Wyndham CR, Swiryn SP, et al. Paroxysmal atrial fibrillation in the Wolff-Parkinson-White syndrome. Am J Cardiol 1981; 47:562–569.

165. Sharma AD, Yee R, Guiraudon G, Klein GJ. Sensitivity and specificity of invasive and noninvasive testing for risk of sudden death in Wolff-Parkinson-White syndrome. J Am Coll Cardiol 1987; 10:373–381.

166. Della Bella P, Brugada P, Talajic M, et al. Atrial fibrillation in

167. Robinson K, Rowland E, Krikler DM. Wolff-Parkinson-White syndrome: atrial fibrillation as the presenting arrhythmia. Br Heart J 1988; 59:578–580.

168. Beckman KJ, Gallastegui JL, Bauman JL, Hariman RJ. The predictive value of electrophysiologic studies in untreated patients with Wolff-Parkinson-White syndrome. J Am Coll Cardiol 1990; 15:640–647.

169. Engle MA. Wolff-Parkinson-White syndrome in infants and children. Am J Dis Child 1952; 84:692–705.

170. Swiderski J, Lees MH, Nadas AS. The Wolff-Parkinson-White syndrome in infancy and childhood. Br Heart J 1962; 24:561–580.

171. Mantakas ME, McCue CM, Miller WW. Natural history of Wolff-Parkinson-White syndrome discovered in infancy. Am J Cardiol 1978; 41:1097–1103.

172. Gillette PC, Garson A Jr, Kugler JD. Wolff-Parkinson-White syndrome in children: electrophysiologic and pharmacologic characteristics. Circulation 1979; 60:1487–1495.

173. Mehta AV, Pickoff AS, Raptoulis A, et al. Atrial flutter and atrial fibrillation associated with Wolff-Parkinson-White syndrome in childhood. Pediatr Cardiol 1980; 1:197–202.

174. Gillette PC. Pediatric Cardiac Dysrhythmias. New York: Grune & Stratton, 1981.

175. Losekoot TG, Lubbers WL. The Wolff-Parkinson-White syndrome in childhood. Int J Cardiol 1990; 27:293–309.

176. Sung RJ, Gelband H, Castellanos A, Aranda JM, Myerburg RJ. Clinical and electrophysiologic observations in patients with concealed accessory atrioventricular bypass tracts. Am J Cardiol 1977; 40:839–847.

177. Hurwitz JL, German LD, Packer DL, et al. Occurrence of atrial fibrillation in patients with paroxysmal supraventricular tachycardia due to atrioventricular nodal reentry. Pacing Clin Electrophysiol 1990; 13:705–710.

178. Woeber KA. Thyrotoxicosis and the heart. N Engl J Med 1992; 327:94–98.

179. Forfar JC. Atrial fibrillation and the pituitary-thyroid axis: a re-evaluation. Heart 1997; 77:3–4.

180. Kerr C, Boone J, Connolly S, et al. Follow-up of atrial fibrillation: the initial experience of the Canadian registry of atrial fibrillation. Eur Heart J 1996; 17:48–51.

181. Bar-Sela S, Ehrenfeld M, Eliakim M. Arterial embolism in thyrotoxicosis with atrial fibrillation. Arch Intern Med 1981; 141:1191–1192.

182. Olshausen KV, Bischoff S, Kahaly G, et al. Cardiac arrhythmias and heart rate in hyperthyroidism. Am J Cardiol 1989; 63:930–933.

183. Staffurth JS, Gibberd MC, Ng Tang Fui S. Arterial embolism in thyrotoxicosis with atrial fibrillation. BMJ 1977; 2:688–690.

184. Hellman E. Auricular fibrillation following prolonged use of thyroid extract. JAMA 1955; 159:25–26.

185. Brancart M, Hennen G. Atrial fibrillation and thyroid disease. In Kulbertus HE, Olsson SB, Schlepper M (eds). Atrial Fibrillation. Kiruna, Molndal, Sweden: AB Hassle, 1982, pp. 220–230.

186. Daly JG, Greenwood RM, Himsworth RL. Thyrotoxic atrial fibrillation. BMJ 1982; 285:1574.

187. Tibaldi JM, Barzel US, Albin J, Surks M. Thyrotoxicosis in the very old. Am J Med 1986; 81:619–622.

188. Iwasaki T, Naka M, Hiramatsu K, et al. Echocardiographic studies on the relationship between atrial fibrillation and atrial enlargement in patients with hyperthyroidism of Graves' disease. Cardiology 1989; 76:10–17.

189. Davis PJ, Davis FB. Hyperthyroidism in patients over the age of 60 years: clinical features in 85 patients. Medicine 1974; 53:161–181.

190. McClintock JC, Frawley TF, Holden JHP. Hyperthyroidism in children: observations in 50 treated cases, including an evaluation of endocrine factors. J Endocrinol 1956; 16:62–85.

191. Pilapil VR, Watson DG. Electrocardiogram in hyperthyroid children. Am J Dis Child 1970; 119:245–248.

192. Perry LW, Hung W. Atrial fibrillation and hyperthyroidism in a 14-year-old boy. J Pediatr 1971; 79:668–671.

193. Cavallo A, Joseph CJ, Casta A. Cardiac complications in juvenile hyperthyroidism. Am J Dis Child 1984; 138:479–482.
194. Cobler JL, Williams ME, Greenland P. Thyrotoxicosis in institutionalized elderly patients with atrial fibrillation. Arch Intern Med 1984; 144:1758–1760.
195. Tajiri J, Hamasaki S, Shimada T, et al. Masked thyroid dysfunction among elderly patients with atrial fibrillation. Jpn Heart J 1986; 27:183–190.
196. Yinnon AM, Rosenmann D, Zion MM. Hypoglycemia: a rare cause of atrial fibrillation. Isr J Med Sci 1989; 25:346–347.
197. Perloff JK, Natterson PD. Atrial arrhythmias in adults after repair of tetralogy of Fallot. Circulation 1995; 91:2118–2119.
198. Novack P, Segal B, Kasparian H, Likoff W. Atrial septal defect in patients over 40. Geriatrics 1963; 18:421–428.
199. Kuzman WJ, Yuskis AS. Atrial septal defects in the older patient simulating acquired valvular heart disease. Am J Cardiol 1965; 15:303–309.
200. Markman P, Howitt G, Wade EG. Atrial septal defect in the middle-aged and elderly. Q J Med 1965; 34:409–426.
201. Aldridge HE, Yao J. Secundum atrial septal defect in the adult: repair using cardiopulmonary bypass in 133 patients. Can Med Assoc J 1967; 97:269–274.
202. Daicoff GF, Brandenburg RO, Kirklin JW. Results of operation for atrial septal defect in patients forty-five years of age and older. Circulation 1967; 35–36(Suppl I):I-143–I-147.
203. Gault JH, Morrow AG, Gay WA, Ross J. Atrial septal defect in patients over the age of forty years. Circulation 1968; 37:261–272.
204. Tikoff G, Schmidt AM, Hecht HH. Atrial fibrillation in atrial septal defect. Arch Intern Med 1968; 121:402–405.
205. Wolf PS, Vogel JH, Pryor R, Blount SG Jr. Atrial septal defect in patients over 45 years of age: merits of surgical versus medical therapy. Br Heart J 1968; 30:115–124.
206. Hawe A, Rastelli GC, Brandenburg RO, McGoon DC. Embolic complications following repair of atrial septal defects. Circulation 1969; 39(Suppl I):I-185–I-191.
207. Saksena FB, Aldridge HE. Atrial septal defect in the older patient: a clinical and hemodynamic study in patients operated on after age 35. Circulation 1970; 42:1009–1020.
208. Dave KS, Pakrashi BC, Wooler GH, Ionescu MI. Atrial septal defect in adults: clinical and hemodynamic results of surgery. Am J Cardiol 1973; 31:7–13.
209. Kelly JJ, Lyons HA. Atrial septal defect in the aged. Ann Intern Med 1958; 48:267–283.
210. Rodstein M, Zeman FD, Gerber IE. Atrial septal defect in the aged. Circulation 1961; 23:665–674.
211. Sommer LS, Voudoukis IJ. Atrial septal defect in older age groups; with special reference to atypical clinical and electrocardiographic manifestations. Am J Cardiol 1961; 8:198–202.
212. Murphy JG, Gersh BJ, McGoon MD, et al. Long-term outcome after surgical repair of isolated atrial septal defect: follow-up at 27 to 32 years. N Engl J Med 1990; 323:1645–1650.
213. St. John Sutton MG, Tajik AJ, McGoon DC. Atrial septal defect in patients ages 60 years or older: postoperative results and long-term postoperative follow-up. Circulation 1981; 64:402–409.
214. Sakakibara S, Yokoyama M, Takao A, Nogi M, Gomi H. Coronary arteriovenous fistula. Am Heart J 1966; 72:307–314.
215. Giuliani ER, Fuster V, Brandenburg RO, Mair DD. Ebstein's anomaly: the clinical features and natural history of Ebstein's anomaly of the tricuspid valve. Mayo Clin Proc 1979; 54:163–173.
216. Smith WM, Gallagher JJ, Kerr CR, et al. The electrophysiologic basis and management of symptomatic recurrent tachycardia in patients with Ebstein's anomaly of the tricuspid valve. Am J Cardiol 1982; 49:1223–1233.
217. Pressley JC, Wharton JM, Tang AS, Lowe JE, Gallagher JJ, Prystowsky EN. Effect of Ebstein's anomaly on short- and long-term outcome of surgically treated patients with Wolff-Parkinson-White syndrome. Circulation 1992; 86:1147–1155.
218. Wood P. The Eisenmenger syndrome. BMJ 1958; 2:701–709.
219. Brammell HL, Vogel JH, Pryor R, Blount SG Jr. The Eisenmenger syndrome: a clinical and physiologic reappraisal. Am J Cardiol 1971; 28:679–692.
220. Perloff JD. The Clinical Recognition of Congenital Heart Disease. Philadelphia: WB Saunders, 1987.
221. Rokseth R. Congenital heart disease in middle-aged adults. Acta Med Scand 1968; 183:131–138.
222. Burch GE, DePasquale NP. Alcoholic cardiomyopathy. Am J Cardiol 1969; 23:723–731.
223. Wenger NK, Abelmann WH, Roberts WC. Cardiomyopathy and specific heart muscle disease. In Hurst JW, Schlant RC, Rackley CE, Sonnenblick EH, Wenger NK (eds). The Heart. New York: McGraw-Hill, 1990, p. 1285.
224. Evans W. The electrocardiogram of alcoholic cardiomyopathy. Br Heart J 1958; 21:445–456.
225. Brigden W, Robinson J. Alcoholic heart disease. BMJ 1964; 2:1283–1289.
226. Alexander CS. Idiopathic heart disease. Am J Med 1966; 41:213–228.
227. Demakis JG, Proskey A, Rahimtoola SH, et al. The natural course of alcoholic cardiomyopathy. Ann Intern Med 1974; 80:293–297.
228. Tobin JR Jr, Driscoll JF, Lim MT, Sutton GC, Szanto PB, Gunnar RM. Primary myocardial disease and alcoholism: the clinical manifestations and course of the disease in a selected population of patients observed for three or more years. Circulation 1967; 35:754–764.
229. James TN. Pathology of the cardiac conduction system in amyloidosis. Ann Intern Med 1966; 65:28–36.
230. Eriksson P, Karp K, Bjerle P, Olofsson BO. Disturbances of cardiac rhythm and conduction in familial amyloidosis with polyneuropathy. Br Heart J 1984; 51:658–662.
231. Falk RH, Rubinow A, Cohen AS. Cardiac arrhythmias in systemic amyloidosis: correlation with echocardiographic abnormalities. J Am Coll Cardiol 1984; 3:107–113.
232. Hollister RM, Goodwin JF. The electrocardiogram in cardiomyopathy. Br Heart J 1963; 25:357–374.
233. Fuster V, Gersh BJ, Giuliani ER, Tajik AJ, Brandenburg RO, Frye RL. The natural history of idiopathic dilated cardiomyopathy. Am J Cardiol 1981; 47:525–531.
234. Roberts WC, Siegel RJ, McManus BM. Idiopathic dilated cardiomyopathy: analysis of 152 necropsy patients. Am J Cardiol 1987; 60:1340–1355.
235. Kessler G, Rosenblatt S, Friedman J, Kaplinsky E. Recurrent dilated cardiomyopathy reversed with conversion of atrial fibrillation. Am Heart J 1997; 133:384–386.
236. Phillips E, Levine S. Auricular fibrillation without other evidence of heart disease. Am J Med 1949; 7:478–489.
237. Lemery R, Brugada P, Cheriex E, Wellens HJJ. Reversibility of tachycardia-induced left ventricular dysfunction after closed-chest catheter ablation of the atrioventricular junction for intractable atrial fibrillation. Am J Cardiol 1987; 60:1406–1408.
238. Peters KG, Kienzle MG. Severe cardiomyopathy due to chronic rapidly conducted atrial fibrillation: complete recovery after restoration of sinus rhythm. Am J Med 1988; 85:242–244.
239. Grogan M, Smith HC, Gersh BJ, Wood DL. Left ventricular dysfunction due to atrial fibrillation in patients initially believed to have idiopathic dilated cardiomyopathy. Am J Cardiol 1992; 69:1570–1573.
240. Stewart JT, McKenna WJ. Arrhythmias in hypertrophic cardiomyopathy. J Cardiovasc Electrophysiol 1991; 2:516–524.
241. Glancy DL, O'Brien KP, Gold HK, Epstein SE. Atrial fibrillation in patients with idiopathic hypertrophic subaortic stenosis. Br Heart J 1970; 32:652–659.
242. Canedo MI, Frank MJ, Abdulla AM. Rhythm disturbances in hypertrophic cardiomyopathy: prevalence, relation to symptoms and management. Am J Cardiol 1980; 45:848–855.
243. Spirito P, Lakatos E, Maron BJ. Degree of left ventricular hypertrophy in patients with hypertrophic cardiomyopathy and chronic atrial fibrillation. Am J Cardiol 1992; 69:1217–1222.
244. Savage DD, Seides SF, Maron BJ, Myers DJ, Epstein SE. Prevalence of arrhythmias during 24-hour

electrocardiographic monitoring and exercise testing in patients with obstructive and nonobstructive hypertrophic cardiomyopathy. Circulation 1979; 59:866–875.

245. McKenna WJ, Chetty S, Oakley CM, Goodwin JF. Arrhythmia in hypertrophic cardiomyopathy: exercise and 48 hour ambulatory electrocardiographic assessment with and without beta adrenergic blocking therapy. Am J Cardiol 1980; 45:1–5.

246. Bjarnason I, Hardarson T, Jonsson S. Cardiac arrhythmias in hypertrophic cardiomyopathy. Br Heart J 1982; 48:198–203.

247. Levander-Lindgren M. Studies in myocarditis. II. Electrocardiographic changes. Cardiologia 1965; 47:73–95.

248. Reid JM, Kennedy JR, McArthur J. Unusual cause of atrial fibrillation. BMJ 1982; 284:237–238.

249. Walsh JJ, Burch GE, Black WC, Ferrans VJ, Hibbs RG. Idiopathic myocardiopathy of the puerperium (postpartal heart disease). Circulation 1965; 32:19–31.

250. Demakis JG, Rahimtoola SH, Sutton GC, et al. Natural course of peripartum cardiomyopathy. Circulation 1971; 44:1053–1061.

251. Roberts WC, McAllister HA Jr, Ferrans VJ. Sarcoidosis of the heart: a clinicopathologic study of 35 necropsy patients (group I) and review of 78 previously described necropsy patients (group II). Am J Med 1977; 63:86–108.

252. Kanemoto N, Sasamoto H. Arrhythmias in primary pulmonary hypertension. Jpn Heart J 1979; 20:765–775.

253. Gajewski J, Singer RB. Mortality in an insured population with atrial fibrillation. JAMA 1981; 245:1540–1544.

254. Shih HT, Webb CR, Conway WA, Peterson E, Tilley B, Goldstein S. Frequency and significance of cardiac arrhythmias in chronic obstructive lung disease. Chest 1988; 94:44–48.

255. Corazza LJ, Pastor BH. Cardiac arrhythmias in chronic cor pulmonale. N Engl J Med 1958; 259:862–865.

256. Thomas AJ, Valabhji P. Arrhythmia and tachycardia in pulmonary heart disease. Br Heart J 1969; 31:491–495.

257. Hudson LD, Kurt TL, Petty TL, Genton E. Arrhythmias associated with acute respiratory failure in patients with chronic airway obstruction. Chest 1973; 63:661–665.

258. Lowenstein SR, Gabow PA, Cramer J, Oliva PB, Ratner K. The role of alcohol in new-onset atrial fibrillation. Arch Intern Med 1983; 143:1882–1885.

259. Angelini P, Feldman MI, Lufschanowski R, Leachman RD. Cardiac arrhythmias during and after heart surgery: diagnosis and management. Prog Cardiovasc Dis 1974; 16:469–495.

260. Ommen SR, Odell JA, Stanton MS. Atrial arrhythmias after cardiothoracic surgery. N Engl J Med 1997; 336:1429–1434.

261. Lauer MS, Eagle KA, Buckley MJ, DeSanctis RW. Atrial fibrillation following coronary artery bypass surgery. Prog Cardiovasc Dis 1989; 31:367–378.

262. Lauer MS, Eagle KA. Atrial fibrillation following cardiac surgery. In Falk RH, Podrid PJ (eds). Atrial Fibrillation. Mechanisms and Management. New York: Raven Press, 1992, pp. 127–143.

263. Pires LA, Wagshal AB, Lancey R, Huang SK. Arrhythmias and conduction disturbances after coronary artery bypass graft surgery: epidemiology, management, and prognosis. Am Heart J 1995; 129:799–808.

264. Rose MR, Glassman E, Spencer FC. Arrhythmias following cardiac surgery: relation to serum digoxin levels. Am Heart J 1975; 89:288–294.

265. Johnson LW, Dickstein RA, Fruehan CT, et al. Prophylactic digitalization for coronary artery bypass surgery. Circulation 1976; 53:819–822.

266. Tyras DH, Stothert JC Jr, Kaiser GC, Barner HB, Codd JE, Willman VL. Supraventricular tachyarrhythmias after myocardial revascularization: a randomized trial of prophylactic digitalization. J Thorac Cardiovasc Surg 1979; 77:310–314.

267. Matangi MF, Neutze JM, Graham KJ, Hill DG, Kerr AR, Barratt-Boyes BG. Arrhythmia prophylaxis after aorta-coronary bypass: the effect of minidose propranolol. J Thorac Cardiovasc Surg 1985; 89:439–443.

268. Michelson EL, Morganroth J. Spontaneous variability in arrhythmia frequency. Am Heart J 1979; 97:815.

269. Csicsko JF, Schatzlein MH, King RD. Immediate postoperative digitalization in the prophylaxis of supraventricular arrhythmias following coronary artery bypass. J Thorac Cardiovasc Surg 1981; 81:419–422.

270. Parker FB Jr, Greiner-Hayes C, Bove EL, Marvasti MA, Johnson LW, Eich RH. Supraventricular arrhythmias following coronary artery bypass: the effect of preoperative digitalis. J Thorac Cardiovasc Surg 1983; 86:594–600.

271. Ormerod OJ, McGregor CG, Stone DL, Wisbey C, Petch MC. Arrhythmias after coronary bypass surgery. Br Heart J 1984; 51:618–621.

272. Rubin DA, Nieminski KE, Reed GE, Herman MV. Predictors, prevention, and long-term prognosis of atrial fibrillation after coronary artery bypass graft operations. J Thorac Cardiovasc Surg 1987; 94:331–335.

273. Crosby LH, Pifalo WB, Woll KR, Burkholder JA. Risk factors for atrial fibrillation after coronary artery bypass grafting. Am J Cardiol 1990; 66:1520–1522.

274. Aranki SF, Shaw DP, Adams DH, et al. Predictors of atrial fibrillation after coronary artery surgery: current trends and impact on hospital resources. Circulation 1996; 94:390–397.

275. Mathew JP, Parks R, Savino JS, et al. Atrial fibrillation following coronary artery bypass graft surgery: predictors, outcomes, and resource utilization. Multicenter study of perioperative ischemia research group. JAMA 1996; 276:300–306.

276. Roffman JA, Fieldman A. Digoxin and propranolol in the prophylaxis of supraventricular tachydysrhythmias after coronary artery bypass surgery. Ann Thorac Surg 1981; 31:496–501.

277. Dixon FE, Genton E, Vacek JL, Moore CB, Landry J. Factors predisposing to supraventricular tachyarrhythmias after coronary artery bypass grafting. Am J Cardiol 1986; 58:476–478.

278. Leitch JW, Thomson D, Baird DK, Harris PJ. The importance of age as a predictor of atrial fibrillation and flutter after coronary artery bypass grafting. J Thorac Cardiovasc Surg 1990; 100:338–342.

279. Frost L, Molgaard H, Christiansen EH, Jacobsen CJ, Allermand H, Thomsen PE. Low vagal tone and supraventricular ectopic activity predict atrial fibrillation and flutter after coronary artery bypass grafting. Eur Heart J 1995; 16:825–831.

280. Dimmer C, Tavernier R, Gjorgov N, Van Nooten G, Clement DL, Jordaens L. Variations of autonomic tone preceding onset of atrial fibrillation after coronary artery grafting. Am J Cardiol 1998; 82:22–25.

281. Yousif H, Davies G, Oakley CM. Peri-operative supraventricular arrhythmias in coronary bypass surgery. Int J Cardiol 1990; 26:313–318.

282. Chee TP, Prakash NS, Desser KB, Benchimol A. Postoperative supraventricular arrhythmias and the role of prophylactic digoxin in cardiac surgery. Am Heart J 1982; 104:974–977.

283. Mendes LA, Connelly GP, McKenney PA, et al. Right coronary artery stenosis: an independent predictor of atrial fibrillation after coronary artery bypass surgery. J Am Coll Cardiol 1995; 25:198–202.

284. Mullen JC, Khan N, Weisel RD, et al. Atrial activity during cardioplegia and postoperative arrhythmias. J Thorac Cardiovasc Surg 1987; 94:558–565.

285. Tchervenkov CI, Wynands JE, Symes JF, Malcolm ID, Dobell AR, Morin JE. Persistent atrial activity during cardioplegic arrest: a possible factor in the etiology of postoperative supraventricular tachyarrhythmias. Ann Thorac Surg 1983; 36:437–443.

286. Lowe JE, Hendry PJ, Hendrickson SC, Wells R. Intraoperative identification of cardiac patients at risk to develop postoperative atrial fibrillation. Ann Surg 1991; 213:388–391.

287. Rousou JA, Meeran MK, Engelman RM, Breyer RH, Lemeshow S. Does the type of venous drainage or cardioplegia affect postoperative conduction and atrial arrhythmias? Circulation 1985; 72:259–263.

288. Flack JE III, Hafer J, Engelman RM, Rousou JA, Deaton DW,

Pekow P. Effect of normothermic blood cardioplegia on postoperative conduction abnormalities and supraventricular arrhythmias. Circulation 1992; 86(Suppl II):II-385–II-392.

289. Taylor GJ, Malik SA, Colliver JA, et al. Usefulness of atrial fibrillation as a predictor of stroke after isolated coronary artery bypass grafting. Am J Cardiol 1987; 60:905–907.

290. Perloff JK. Surgical closure of atrial septal defect in adults. N Engl J Med 1995; 333:513–514.

291. Popper RW, Knott JM, Selzer A, Gerbode F. Arrhythmias after cardiac surgery. I. Uncomplicated atrial septal defect. Am Heart J 1962; 64:455–461.

292. Reid JM, Stevenson JC. Cardiac arrhythmias following successful surgical closure of atrial septal defect. Br Heart J 1967; 29:742–747.

293. Konstantinides S, Geibel A, Olschewski M, et al. A comparison of surgical and medical therapy for atrial septal defect in adults. N Engl J Med 1995; 333:469–473.

294. Brandenburg RO Jr, Holmes DR Jr, Brandenburg RO, McGoon DC. Clinical follow-up study of paroxysmal supraventricular tachyarrhythmias after operative repair of a secundum type atrial septal defect in adults. Am J Cardiol 1983; 51:273–276.

295. Magilligan DJ Jr, Lam CR, Lewis JW Jr, Davila JC. Late results of atrial septal defect repair in adults. Arch Surg 1978; 113:1245–1247.

296. Bink-Boelkens MT, Velvis H, van der Heide JJ, Eygelaar A, Hardjowijono RA. Dysrhythmias after atrial surgery in children. Am Heart J 1983; 106:125–130.

297. Peters NS, Somerville J. Arrhythmias after the Fontan procedure. Br Heart J 1992; 68:199–204.

298. Roos-Hesselink J, Perlroth MG, McGhie J, Spitaels S. Atrial arrhythmias in adults after repair of tetralogy of Fallot: correlations with clinical, exercise, and echocardiographic findings. Circulation 1995; 91:2214–2219.

299. Heinz R, Hultgren H. Atrial fibrillation following mitral valvulotomy. Arch Intern Med 1957; 99:896–904.

300. Black H, Lown B, Bartholomay AF. The value of quinidine in the prevention of atrial fibrillation after mitral valvuloplasty. Circulation 1961; 23:519–524.

301. Smith R, Grossman W, Johnson L, Segal H, Collins J, Dalen J. Arrhythmias following cardiac valve replacement. Circulation 1972; 45:1018–1023.

302. Selzer A, Walter RM. Adequacy of preoperative digitalis therapy in controlling ventricular rate in postoperative atrial fibrillation. Circulation 1966; 34:119–122.

303. Hoie J, Forfang K. Arrhythmias and conduction disturbances following aortic valve implantation. Scand J Thorac Cardiovasc Surg 1980; 14:177–183.

304. Jacquet L, Ziady G, Stein K, et al. Cardiac rhythm disturbances early after orthotopic heart transplantation: prevalence and clinical importance of the observed abnormalities. J Am Coll Cardiol 1990; 16:832–837.

305. Ong JJ, Hsu PC, Lin L, et al. Arrhythmias after cardioverter-defibrillator implantation: comparison of epicardial and transvenous systems. Am J Cardiol 1995; 75:137–140.

306. Bailey CC, Betts RH. Cardiac arrhythmias following pneumonectomy. N Engl J Med 1943; 229:356–359.

307. Currens JH, White PD, Churchill ED. Cardiac arrhythmias following thoracic surgery. N Engl J Med 1943; 229:360–364.

308. Krosnick A. Cardiac arrhythmias in the older age group following thoracic surgery. Am J Med Sci 1955; 23:541–550.

309. Cerney CI. The prophylaxis of cardiac arrhythmias complicating pulmonary surgery. J Thorac Surg 1957; 34:105–110.

310. Cohen MG, Pastor BH. Delayed cardiac arrhythmias following noncardiac thoracic surgery. Dis Chest 1957; 32:435–440.

311. Calatayud JB, Kelser GA, Caceres CA. Incidence of cardiac arrhythmias following noncardiac thoracic surgery. J Thorac Cardiovasc Surg 1961; 41:498–502.

312. Mowry FM, Reynolds EW. Cardiac rhythm disturbances complicating resectional surgery of the lung. Ann Intern Med 1964; 61:688–695.

313. Shields TW, Ujiki GT. Digitalization for prevention of arrhythmias following pulmonary surgery. Surg Gynecol Obstet 1968; 126:743–746.

314. Ghosh P, Pakrashi BC. Cardiac dysrhythmias after thoracotomy. Br Heart J 1972; 34:374–376.

315. Krowka MJ, Pairolero PC, Trastek VF, Payne WS, Bernatz PE. Cardiac dysrhythmia following pneumonectomy: clinical correlates and prognostic significance. Chest 1987; 91:490–495.

316. Goldman L. Supraventricular tachyarrhythmias in hospitalized adults after surgery. Chest 1978; 73:450–454.

317. Solomon AJ, Kouretas PC, Hopkins RA, Katz NM, Wallace RB, Hannan RL. Early discharge of patients with new-onset atrial fibrillation after cardiovascular surgery. Am Heart J 1998; 135:557–563.

318. Rabinovich S, Evans J, Smith IM, January LE. A long-term view of bacterial endocarditis. Ann Intern Med 1965; 63:185–198.

319. Libman E. The clinical features of subacute streptococcus (and influenzal) endocarditis in the bacterial stage. Med Clin North Am 1918; 2:117–151.

320. Rothschild MA, Sacks B, Libman E. The disturbances of the cardiac mechanism in subacute endocarditis and rheumatic fever. Am Heart J 1927; 2:356–374.

321. McDonald RK. The coincidence of auricular fibrillation and bacterial endocarditis. Am Heart J 1946; 31:308–313.

322. Anonymous. Paul Wood's Diseases of the Heart and Circulation. 3rd ed. Philadelphia: JB Lippincott, 1968, p. 278.

323. Evans W, Jackson F. Constrictive pericarditis. Br Heart J 1952; 14:53–69.

324. Dalton JC, Pearson RJ, White PD. Constrictive pericarditis: a review and long-term follow-up of 78 cases. Ann Intern Med 1956; 45:445–458.

325. Wood P. Chronic constrictive pericarditis. Am J Cardiol 1961; 7:48–61.

326. Lazarides DP, Avgoustakis DG, Lekos D, Michaelides GB. Evaluation of radical pericardiectomy for constrictive pericarditis: a clinical, hemodynamic and electrocardiographic study of twenty cases. J Thorac Cardiovasc Surg 1966; 51:821–833.

327. Levine HD. Myocardial fibrosis in constrictive pericarditis: electrocardiographic and pathologic observations. Circulation 1973; 48:1268–1281.

328. Anonymous. Paul Wood's Diseases of the Heart and Circulation. 3rd ed. Philadelphia: JB Lippincott, 1968, p 278.

329. Robinson J, Brigden W. Recurrent pericarditis. BMJ 1968; 2:272–275.

330. Spodick DH. Arrhythmias during acute pericarditis: a prospective study of 100 consecutive cases. JAMA 1976; 235:39–41.

331. Prichard RW. Tumors of the heart. Arch Pathol 1951; 51:98–128.

332. Friedberg CK. Diseases of the Heart. Philadelphia: WB Saunders, 1966.

333. Goodwin JF. The spectrum of cardiac tumors. Am J Cardiol 1968; 21:307–314.

334. Harvey WP. Clinical aspects of cardiac tumors. Am J Cardiol 1968; 21:328–343.

335. Bellet S. Clinical Disorders of the Heart Beat. Philadelphia: Lea & Febiger, 1971.

336. Rosenthal DS, Braunwald E. Hematological-oncological disorders and heart disease. In Braunwald E (ed). Heart Disease. A Textbook of Cardiovascular Medicine. 4th ed. Philadelphia: WB Saunders, 1992, pp. 1742–1766.

337. Davies MJ, Pomerance A. Pathology of atrial fibrillation in man. Br Heart J 1972; 34:520–525.

338. Goodwin JF. Diagnosis of left atrial myxoma. Lancet 1963; 1:464–467.

339. Bulkley BH, Hutchins GM. Atrial myxomas: a fifty year review. Am Heart J 1979; 97:639–643.

340. St. John Sutton MG, Mercier LA, Giuliani ER, Lie JT. Atrial myxomas: a review of clinical experience in 40 patients. Mayo Clin Proc 1980; 55:371–376.

341. Fallon JT, Dec GW. Cardiac tumors. In Eagle KA, Haber E, DeSanctis RW, Austen WG (eds). The Practice of Cardiology. 2nd ed. Boston: Little, Brown, 1989, p. 1015.

342. Ridker PM, Gibson CM, Lopez R. Atrial fibrillation induced by breath spray. N Engl J Med 1989; 320:124.

343. Katz LN, Pick A. Clinical Electrocardiography. Part I. The Arrhythmias. Philadelphia: Lea & Febiger, 1956.

344. Cohen EJ, Klatsky AL, Armstrong MA. Alcohol use and supraventricular arrhythmia. Am J Cardiol 1988; 62:971–973.

345. Ettinger PO, Wu CF, De La Cruz C Jr, Weisse AB, Ahmed SS, Regan TJ. Arrhythmias and the "holiday heart": alcohol-associated cardiac rhythm disorders. Am Heart J 1978; 95:555–562.

346. Koskinen P, Kupari M, Leinonen H. Role of alcohol in recurrences of atrial fibrillation in persons less than 65 years of age. Am J Cardiol 1990; 66:954–958.

347. Rich EC, Siebold C, Campion B. Alcohol-related acute atrial fibrillation: a case-control study and review of 40 patients. Arch Intern Med 1985; 145:830–833.

348. Ettinger PO. Holiday heart arrhythmias. Int J Cardiol 1984; 5:540–542.

349. Thornton JR. Atrial fibrillation in healthy non-alcoholic people after an alcoholic binge. Lancet 1984; 2:1013–1015.

350. Peter RH, Gracey JG, Beach TB. A clinical profile of idiopathic atrial fibrillation: a functional disorder of atrial rhythm. Ann Intern Med 1968; 68:1288–1295.

351. Kupari M, Koskinen P. Time of onset of supraventricular tachyarrhythmia in relation to alcohol consumption. Am J Cardiol 1991; 67:718–722.

352. Greenspon AJ, Schaal SF. The "holiday heart": electrophysiologic studies of alcohol effects in alcoholics. Ann Intern Med 1983; 98:135–139.

353. Lemberg L, Castellanos A, Swenson J, Gosselin A. Arrhythmias related to cardioversion. Circulation 1964; 30:163–170.

354. DeSilva RA, Graboys TB, Podrid PJ, Lown B. Cardioversion and defibrillation. Am Heart J 1980; 100:881–895.

355. Waldecker B, Brugada P, Zehender M, Stevenson W, Wellens HJJ. Dysrhythmias after direct-current cardioversion. Am J Cardiol 1986; 57:120–123.

356. Ciccone JM, Saksena S, Shah Y, Pantopoulos D. A prospective randomized study of the clinical efficacy and safety of transvenous cardioversion for termination of ventricular tachycardia. Circulation 1985; 71:571–578.

357. Mirowski M. The automatic implantable cardioverter-defibrillator: an overview. J Am Coll Cardiol 1985; 6:461–466.

358. Kelly PA, Cannom DS, Garan H, et al. The automatic implantable cardioverter-defibrillator: efficacy, complications and survival in patients with malignant ventricular arrhythmias. J Am Coll Cardiol 1988; 11:1278–1286.

359. Winkle RA, Mead RH, Ruder MA, et al. Long-term outcome with the automatic implantable cardioverter-defibrillator. J Am Coll Cardiol 1989; 13:1353–1361.

360. Florin TJ, Weiss DN, Peters RW, Shorofsky SR, Gold MR. Induction of atrial fibrillation with low-energy defibrillator shocks in patients with implantable cardioverter defibrillators. Am J Cardiol 1997; 80:960–962.

361. Katz A, Evans JJ, Fogel RI, et al. Atrial fibrillation/flutter induced by implantable ventricular defibrillator shocks: difference between epicardial and endocardial energy delivery. J Cardiovasc Electrophysiol 1997; 8:35–41.

362. Kirkorian G, Moncada E, Chevalier P, et al. Radiofrequency ablation of atrial flutter: efficacy of an anatomically guided approach. Circulation 1994; 90:2804–2814.

363. Philippon F, Plumb VJ, Epstein AE, Kay GN. The risk of atrial fibrillation following radiofrequency catheter ablation of atrial flutter. Circulation 1995; 92:430–435.

364. Bussan R, Reid ER, Sherf D. Conversion of atrial flutter into atrial fibrillation by carotid pressure. Ann Intern Med 1957; 46:814–818.

365. Cannata D, Narbone NB. Clinical observations on the role of the vegetative nervous system in the pathogenesis of atrial fibrillation. Cardiologia 1958; 32:329–345.

366. Heron JR, Anderson EG, Noble EM. Cardiac abnormalities associated with carotid-sinus syndrome. Lancet 1965; 1:214–216.

367. Scherf D, Bornemann C. Appearance of ventricular ectopic rhythm during carotid sinus pressure. Dis Chest 1966; 50:530–532.

368. Anbe DT, Rubenfire M, Drake EH. Conversion of atrial flutter to atrial fibrillation with carotid sinus pressure. J Electrocardiol 1969; 2:377–380.

369. Leather RA, Kerr CR. Atrial fibrillation in the absence of overt cardiac disease. In Falk RH, Podrid PJ (eds). Atrial Fibrillation. Mechanisms and Management. New York: Raven Press, 1992, pp. 93–108.

370. Evans W, Swann P. Lone auricular fibrillation. Br Heart J 1954; 16:189–194.

371. Kopecky SL, Gersh BJ, McGoon MD, et al. The natural history of lone atrial fibrillation. N Engl J Med 1987; 317:669–674.

372. Davies AB, Williams I, John R, Hall R, Scanlon MF. Diagnostic value of thyrotrophin releasing hormone tests in elderly patients with atrial fibrillation. Br Med J Clin Res Ed 1994; 1985:773–776.

373. Neufeld HN, Wagenvoort CA, Burchell HB, Edwards JE. Idiopathic atrial fibrillation. Am J Cardiol 1961; 8:193–197.

374. Godtfredsen J, Egeblad H, Berning J. Echocardiography in lone atrial fibrillation. Acta Med Scand 1983; 213:111–113.

375. Wolfe K, Klein GJ, Yee R. Prevalence of reciprocating tachycardia in patients aged <50 years with apparent lone atrial fibrillation. Am J Cardiol 1993; 71:1232–1233.

376. Zaldivar N, Gelband H, Tamer D, Garcia O. Atrial fibrillation in infancy. J Pediatrics 1973; 83:821–822.

377. Friedlander RD, Levine SA. Auricular fibrillation and auricular flutter without evidence of organic heart disease. N Engl J Med 1934; 211:624–629.

378. Hoglund C, Rosenhamer G. Echocardiographic left atrial dimension as a predictor of maintaining sinus rhythm after conversion of atrial fibrillation. Acta Med Scand 1985; 217:411–415.

379. Coumel P. Paroxysmal atrial fibrillation: a disorder of autonomic tone? Eur Heart J 1994; 15(Suppl A):9–16.

380. Coumel P. Autonomic influences in atrial tachyarrhythmias. J Cardiovasc Electrophysiol 1996; 7:999–1007.

381. Coumel P. Neural aspects of paroxysmal atrial fibrillation. In Falk RH, Podrid PJ (eds). Atrial Fibrillation. Mechanisms and Management. New York: Raven Press, 1992, pp. 109–125.

382. Coumel P. Cardiac arrhythmias and the autonomic nervous system. J Cardiovasc Electrophysiol 1993; 4:338–355.

383. Coumel P, Leclercq JF, Attuel P, Lavallee JP, Flammang D. Autonomic influences in the genesis of atrial arrhythmias: atrial flutter and fibrillation of vagal origin. In Narula OS (ed). Cardiac Arrhythmias. Electrophysiology, Diagnosis and Management. Baltimore: Williams & Wilkins, 1980, pp. 243–255.

384. Coumel P, Leclercq JF, Attuel P. Paroxysmal atrial fibrillation. In Kulbertus HE, Olsson SB, Schlepper M (eds). Atrial Fibrillation. Kiruna, Molndal, Sweden: AB Hassle, 1982, pp. 158–178.

385. Coumel P, Friocourt P, Mugica J, Attuel P, Leclercq JF. Long-term prevention of vagal atrial arrhythmias by atrial pacing at 90/minute: experience with 6 cases. Pacing Clin Electrophysiol 1983; 6:552–560.

386. Coumel P. Atrial fibrillation. In Surawicz B, Reddy CP, Prystowsky EN (eds). Tachycardias. Boston: Martinus Nijhoff, 1984, pp. 231–244.

387. Coumel P. Neurogenic and humoral influences of the autonomic nervous system in the determination of paroxysmal atrial fibrillation. In Attuel P, Coumel P, Janse MJ (eds). The Atrium in Health and Disease. New York: Futura Publishing Co., 1989, pp. 213–232.

388. Coumel P. Role of the autonomic nervous system in paroxysmal atrial fibrillation. In Touboul P, Waldo AL (eds). Atrial Arrhythmias: Current Concepts and Management. St. Louis: Mosby–Year Book, 1990, pp. 248–261.

389. Leitch J, Klein G, Tee R, Murdock C, Teo WS. Neurally mediated syncope and atrial fibrillation. N Engl J Med 1991; 324:495–496.

390. Weitzman S, Margulis G, Lehmann E. Uncommon cardiovascular manifestations and high catecholamine levels die to "black widow" bite. Am Heart J 1977; 93:89–90.

391. Coumel P, Escoubet B, Attuel P. Beta-blocking therapy in

atrial and ventricular tachyarrhythmias: experience with nadolol. Am Heart J 1984; 108:1098–1108.

392. Wong TC, Cooper ES. Atrial fibrillation with ventricular slowing in a patient with spontaneous subarachnoid hemorrhage. Am J Cardiol 1969; 23:473–477.

393. Davies MJ, Pomerance A. Quantitative study of ageing changes in the human sinoatrial node and internodal tracts. Br Heart J 1972; 34:150–152.

394. Kupari M, Koskinen P, Leinonen H. Double-peaking circadian variation in the occurrence of sustained supraventricular tachyarrhythmias. Am Heart J 1990; 120:1364–1369.

395. Yamashita T, Murakawa Y, Sezaki K, et al. Circadian variation of paroxysmal atrial fibrillation. Circulation 1997; 96:1537–1541.

396. Rostagno C, Taddei T, Paladini B, Modesti PA, Utari P, Bertini G. The onset of symptomatic atrial fibrillation and paroxysmal supraventricular tachycardia is characterized by different circadian rhythms. Am J Cardiol 1993; 71:453–455.

397. Clair WK, Wilkinson WE, McCarthy EA, Page RL, Pritchett EL. Spontaneous occurrence of symptomatic paroxysmal atrial fibrillation and paroxysmal supraventricular tachycardia in untreated patients. Circulation 1993; 87:1114–1122.

398. Perloff JK. Neurological disorders and heart disease. In Braunwald E (ed). Heart Disease. A Textbook of Cardiovascular Medicine. Philadelphia: WB Saunders, 1992, pp. 1810–1819.

399. Cooper MJ, deLorimier AA, Higgins CB, Van Hare GF, Enderlein MA. Atrial flutter-fibrillation resulting from left atrial compression by an intrapericardial lipoma. Am Heart J 1994; 127:950–951.

400. Balsaver AM, Morales AR, Whitehouse FW. Fat infiltration of myocardium as a cause of cardiac conduction defect. Am J Cardiol 1967; 19:261–265.

401. Kupari M, Koskinen P. Seasonal variation in occurrence of acute atrial fibrillation and relation to air temperature and sale of alcohol. Am J Cardiol 1990; 66:1519–1520.

402. Brodsky MA, Orlov MV, Allen BJ, Selvan A. Frozen yogurt near deep-freeze. Am J Cardiol 1994; 73:617–618.

403. Andersson B, Abdon NJ, Hammarsten J. Arterial embolism and atrial arrhythmias. Eur J Vasc Surg 1989; 3:261–266.

404. Hart RG, Halperin JL. Atrial fibrillation and stroke: revisiting the dilemmas. Stroke 1994; 25:1337–1341.

405. Atrial Fibrillation Investigators. Risk factors for stroke and efficacy of antithrombotic therapy in atrial fibrillation. Analysis of pooled data from five randomized controlled trials. Arch Intern Med 1994; 154:1449–1457.

406. Alt E, Lehmann G. Stroke and atrial fibrillation in sick sinus syndrome. Heart 1997; 77:495–497.

407. Capucci A, Villani GQ, Aschieri D. Risk of complications of atrial fibrillation. PACE 1997; 20:2684–2691.

408. Gershlick AH. Treating the non-electrical risks of atrial fibrillation. Eur Heart J 1997; 18:C19–C26.

409. Giardina EG. Atrial fibrillation and stroke: elucidating a newly discovered risk factor. Am J Cardiol 1997; 80:11D–18D.

410. Cerebral Embolism Task Force. Cardiogenic brain embolism. Arch Neurol 1989; 46:727–743.

411. Petersen P. Thromboembolic complications in atrial fibrillation. Stroke 1990; 21:4–13.

412. Belcher JR, Somerville W. Systemic embolism and left auricular thrombosis in relation to mitral valvotomy. BMJ 1955; 2:1000–1003.

413. Bannister RG. The risks of deferring valvotomy in patients with moderate mitral stenosis. Lancet 1960; 2:329–333.

414. Casella L, Abelmann WH, Ellis LB. Patients with mitral stenosis and systemic emboli. Arch Intern Med 1964; 114:773–781.

415. Szekely P. Systemic embolism and anticoagulant prophylaxis in rheumatic heart disease. BMJ 1964; 1:1209–1212.

416. Friedman GD, Loveland DB, Ehrlich SP Jr. Relationship of stroke to other cardiovascular disease. Circulation 1968; 38:533–541.

417. Fleming HA, Bailey SM. Mitral valve disease, systemic embolism and anticoagulants. Postgrad Med J 1971; 47:599–604.

418. Abbott WM, Maloney RD, McCabe CC, Lee CE, Wirthlin LS. Arterial embolism: a 44 year perspective. Am J Surg 1982; 143:460–464.

419. Fisher CM. Embolism in atrial fibrillation. In Kulbertus HE, Olsson SB, Schlepper M (eds). Atrial Fibrillation. Kiruna, Molndal, Sweden: AB Hassle, 1982, pp. 192–210.

420. Kogure S, Yamamoto Y, Tomono S, Hasegawa A, Suzuki T, Murata K. High risk of systemic embolism in hypertrophic cardiomyopathy. Jpn Heart J 1986; 27:475–480.

421. Wiener I. Clinical and echocardiographic correlates of systemic embolization in nonrheumatic atrial fibrillation. Am J Cardiol 1987; 59:177.

422. Boysen G, Nyboe J, Appleyard M, et al. Stroke incidence and risk factors for stroke in Copenhagen, Denmark. Stroke 1988; 19:1345–1353.

423. Shimomura K, Ohe T, Uehara S, Matsuhisa M, Kamakura S, Sato I. Significance of atrial fibrillation as a precursor of embolism. Am J Cardiol 1989; 63:1405–1407.

424. Chesebro JH, Fuster V, Halperin JL. Atrial fibrillation—risk marker for stroke. N Engl J Med 1990; 323:1556–1558.

425. Wolf PA, Abbott RD, Kannel WB. Atrial fibrillation as an independent risk factor for stroke: the Framingham study. Stroke 1991; 22:983–988.

426. Cioffi G, Pozzoli M, Forni G, et al. Systemic thromboembolism in chronic heart failure: a prospective study in 406 patients. Eur Heart J 1996; 17:1381–1389.

427. Petersen P, Godtfredsen J. Embolic complications in paroxysmal atrial fibrillation. Stroke 1986; 17:622–626.

428. Petersen P, Pedersen F, Johnsen A, et al. Cerebral computed tomography in paroxysmal atrial fibrillation. Acta Neurol Scand 1989; 79:482–486.

429. Hinton RC, Kistler JP, Fallon JT, Friedlich AL, Fisher CM. Influence of etiology of atrial fibrillation on incidence of systemic embolism. Am J Cardiol 1977; 40:509–513.

430. Sherman DG, Goldman L, Whiting RB, Jurgensen K, Kaste M, Easton JD. Thromboembolism in patients with atrial fibrillation. Arch Neurol 1984; 41:708–710.

431. Roy D, Marchand E, Gagne P, Chabot M, Cartier R. Usefulness of anticoagulant therapy in the prevention of embolic complications of atrial fibrillation. Am Heart J 1986; 112:1039–1043.

432. Bogousslavsky J, Van Melle G, Regli F, Kappenberger L. Pathogenesis of anterior circulation stroke in patients with nonvalvular atrial fibrillation: the Lausanne stroke registry. Neurology 1990; 40:1046–1050.

433. Lowe GD, Jaap AJ, Forbes CD. Relation of atrial fibrillation and high haematocrit to mortality in acute stroke. Lancet 1983; 1:784–786.

434. Wolf PA, Kannel WB, McGee DL, Meeks SL, Bharucha NE, McNamara PM. Duration of atrial fibrillation and imminence of stroke: the Framingham study. Stroke 1983; 14:664–667.

435. Darling RC, Austen WG, Linton RR. Arterial embolism. Surg Gynecol Obstet 1967; 124:106–114.

436. Petersen P, Godtfredsen J. Risk factors for stroke in chronic atrial fibrillation. Eur Heart J 1988; 9:291–294.

437. Ezekowitz MD, James KE, Nazarian SM, et al. Silent cerebral infarction in patients with nonrheumatic atrial fibrillation: the Veterans Affairs stroke prevention in nonrheumatic atrial fibrillation investigators. Circulation 1995; 92:2178–2182.

438. Aronow WS, Ahn C, Kronzon I, Gutstein H. Risk factors for new thromboembolic stroke in patients 62 years of age with chronic atrial fibrillation. Am J Cardiol 1998; 82:119–121.

439. Stollberger C, Chnupa P, Kronik G, et al. Transesophageal echocardiography to assess embolic risk in patients with atrial fibrillation. Ann Intern Med 1998; 128:630–638.

440. Cabin HS, Clubb KS, Hall C, Perlmutter RA, Feinstein AR. Risk for systemic embolization of atrial fibrillation without mitral stenosis. Am J Cardiol 1990; 65:1112–1116.

441. Dewar HA, Weightman D. A study of embolism in mitral valve disease and atrial fibrillation. Br Heart J 1983; 49:133–140.

442. Wolf PA, Abbott RD, Kannel WB. Atrial fibrillation: a major

contributor to stroke in the elderly. The Framingham study. Arch Intern Med 1987; 147:1561–1564.

443. Ratcliffe PJ, Wilcock GK. Cerebrovascular disease in dementia: the importance of atrial fibrillation. Postgrad Med J 1985; 61:201–204.

444. Hart RG, Coull BM, Hart D. Early recurrent embolism associated with nonvalvular atrial fibrillation: a retrospective study. Stroke 1983; 14:688–693.

445. Kelley RE, Berger JR, Alter M, Kovacs AG. Cerebral ischemia and atrial fibrillation: prospective study. Neurology 1984; 34:1285–1291.

446. Kempster PA, Gerraty RP, Gates PC. Asymptomatic cerebral infarction in patients with chronic atrial fibrillation. Stroke 1988; 19:955–957.

447. Aberg H. Atrial fibrillation. I. A study of atrial thrombosis and systemic embolism in a necropsy material. Acta Med Scand 1969; 185:373–379.

448. Vingerhoets F, Bogousslavsky J, Regli F, Van Melle G. Atrial fibrillation after acute stroke. Stroke 1993; 24:26–30.

449. Giddings HB, Surks MI. Cerebral embolization in atrial fibrillation complicating hyperthyroidism. JAMA 1978; 240:2567.

450. Yuen RW, Gutteridge DH, Thompson PL, Robinson JS. Embolism in thyrotoxic atrial fibrillation. Med J Aust 1979; 1:630–631.

451. Hurley DM, Hunter AN, Hewett MJ, Stockigt JR. Atrial fibrillation and arterial embolism in hyperthyroidism. Aust N Z J Med 1981; 11:391–393.

452. Collins LJ, Silverman DI, Douglas PS, Manning WJ. Cardioversion of nonrheumatic atrial fibrillation: reduced thromboembolic complications with 4 weeks of precardioversion anticoagulation are related to atrial thrombus resolution. Circulation 1995; 92:160–163.

453. Somerville W, Chambers RJ. Systemic embolism in mitral stenosis: relation to size of the left atrial appendix. BMJ 1964; 2:1167–1169.

454. Stroke Prevention in Atrial Fibrillation Investigators. Predictors of thromboembolism in atrial fibrillation. II. Echocardiographic features of patients at risk. Ann Intern Med 1992; 116:6–12.

455. Wolf PA, Dawber TR, Thomas HE Jr, Kannel WB. Epidemiologic assessment of chronic atrial fibrillation and risk of stroke: the Framingham study. Neurology 1978; 28:973–977.

456. Ellis LB, Harken DE. Arterial embolization in relation to mitral valvuloplasty. Am Heart J 1961; 62:611–620.

457. Blackshear JL, Pearce LA, Asinger RW, et al. Mitral regurgitation associated with reduced thromboembolic events in high-risk patients with nonrheumatic atrial fibrillation: Stroke Prevention in Atrial Fibrillation Investigators. Am J Cardiol 1993; 72:840–843.

458. Fukazawa H, Yamamoto K, Ikeda U, Shimada K. Effect of mitral regurgitation on coagulation activity in atrial fibrillation. Am J Cardiol 1998; 81:93–96.

459. Benjamin EJ, Plehn JF, D'Agostino RB, et al. Mitral annular calcification and the risk of stroke in an elderly cohort. N Engl J Med 1992; 327:374–379.

460. Aronow WS, Gutstein H, Hsieh FY. Risk factors for thromboembolic stroke in elderly patients with chronic atrial fibrillation. Am J Cardiol 1989; 63:366–367.

461. Flegel KM, Shipley MJ, Rose G. Risk of stroke in non-rheumatic atrial fibrillation. Lancet 1987; 1:526–529.

462. Flegel KM, Hanley J. Risk factors for stroke and other embolic events in patients with nonrheumatic atrial fibrillation. Stroke 1989; 20:1000–1004.

463. Moulton AW, Singer DE, Haas JS. Risk factors for stroke in patients with nonrheumatic atrial fibrillation: a case-control study. Am J Med 1991; 91:156–161.

464. Boston Area Anticoagulation Trial for Atrial Fibrillation Investigators. The effect of low-dose warfarin on the risk of stroke in patients with nonrheumatic atrial fibrillation. N Engl J Med 1990; 323:1505–1511.

465. Sage JI, Van Uitert RL. Risk of recurrent stroke in patients with atrial fibrillation and non-valvular heart disease. Stroke 1983; 14:537–540.

466. Yamanouchi H, Tomonaga M, Shimada H, Matsushita S, Kuramoto K, Toyokura Y. Nonvalvular atrial fibrillation as a cause of fatal massive cerebral infarction in the elderly. Stroke 1989; 20:1653–1656.

467. Stroke Prevention in Atrial Fibrillation Investigators. Predictors of thromboembolism in atrial fibrillation. I. Clinical features of patients at risk. Ann Intern Med 1992; 116:1–5.

468. Petersen P, Kastrup J, Helweg-Larsen S, Boysen G, Godtfredsen J. Risk factors for thromboembolic complications in chronic atrial fibrillation: the Copenhagen AFASAK study. Arch Intern Med 1990; 150:819–821.

469. Rodstein M, Moise S, Neufeld R, Wolloch L, Mulvihill M. Nonvalvular atrial fibrillation and strokes in the aged. J Insurance Med 1989; 21:192–194.

470. Caplan LR, Hier DB, D'Cruz I. Cerebral embolism in the Michael Reese stroke registry. Stroke 1983; 14:530–536.

471. Feinberg WM, Seeger JF, Carmody RF, Anderson DC, Hart RG, Pearce LA. Epidemiologic features of asymptomatic cerebral infarction in patients with nonvalvular atrial fibrillation. Arch Intern Med 1990; 150:2340–2344.

472. Corbalan R, Arriagada D, Braun S, et al. Risk factors for systemic embolism in patients with paroxysmal atrial fibrillation. Am Heart J 1992; 124:149–153.

473. Lovett JL, Sandok BA, Giuliani ER, Nasser FN. Two-dimensional echocardiography in patients with focal cerebral ischemia. Ann Intern Med 1981; 95:1–4.

474. Anonymous. Is lone atrial fibrillation really benign? Lancet 1989; 1:305–306.

475. Weintraub G, Specage G. Paroxysmal atrial fibrillation and cerebral embolism with apparently normal heart. N Engl J Med 1958; 259:875–876.

476. Close JB, Evans DW, Bailey SM. Persistent lone atrial fibrillation: its prognosis after clinical diagnosis. J R Coll Gen Pract 1979; 29:547–549.

477. Rostagno C, Bacci F, Martelli M, Naldoni A, Bertini G, Gensini G. Clinical course of lone atrial fibrillation since first symptomatic arrhythmic episode. Am J Cardiol 1995; 76:837–839.

478. Carson PE, Johnson GR, Dunkman WB, Fletcher RD, Farrell L, Cohn JN. The influence of atrial fibrillation on prognosis in mild to moderate heart failure: the V-HeFT studies. The V-HeFT AA cooperative studies group. Circulation 1993; 87(Suppl VI):VI-102–VI-110.

479. Tunick PA, McElhinney L, Mitchell T, Kronzon I. The alternation between atrial flutter and atrial fibrillation. Chest 1992; 101:34–36.

480. Deitz GW, Marriott HJL, Fletcher E, Bellet S. Atrial dissociation and uniatrial fibrillation. Circulation 1957; 15:883–888.

481. Cohen J, Scherf D. Complete interatrial and intraatrial block (atrial dissociation). Am Heart J 1965; 70:23–34.

482. Higgins TG, Phillips JH Jr, Sumner RG. Atrial dissociation: an electrocardiographic artifact produced by the accessory muscles of respiration. Am J Cardiol 1966; 18:132–139.

483. Chung EK. Atrial dissociation due to unilateral atrial fibrillation. J Electrocardiol 1969; 2:373–376.

484. Zipes DP, DeJoseph RL. Dissimilar atrial rhythms in man and dog. Am J Cardiol 1973; 32:618–628.

485. Soler-Soler J, Angel-Ferrer J. Complete atrial dissociation versus diaphragmatic action potentials. Br Heart J 1974; 36:452–456.

486. Suarez LD, Kretz A, Alvarez JA, Martinez JA, Perosio AM. Dissimilar atrial rhythms: a patient with triple right atrial rhythm. Am Heart J 1980; 100:678–682.

487. Gomes JA, Kang PS, Matheson M, Gough WB Jr, el-Sherif N. Coexistence of sick sinus rhythm and atrial flutter-fibrillation. Circulation 1981; 63:80–86.

488. Rakovec P, Horvat M, Jakopin J, Kenda MF, Kranjec I, Jagodic A. Induced concealed dissimilar atrial rhythms. Pacing Clin Electrophysiol 1982; 5:523–528.

489. Katritsis D, Iliodromitis E, Fragakis N, Adamopoulos S, Kremastinos D. Ablation therapy of type I atrial flutter may eradicate paroxysmal atrial fibrillation. Am J Cardiol 1996; 78:345–347.

490. Bhagwat AR, Markel ML, Abdalla IS. Dissimilar right atrial rhythms: a case report. Pacing Clin Electrophysiol 1997; 20:1363–1364.

491. Li YH, Lo HM, Lin FY, Lin JL, Lien WP. Atrial dissociation after atrial compartment operation for chronic atrial fibrillation in mitral valve disease. PACE 1998; 21:756–759.

492. Chung EK. A reappraisal of atrial dissociation. Am J Cardiol 1971; 28:111–117.

493. Leier CV, Schaal SF. Biatrial electrograms during coarse atrial fibrillation and flutter-fibrillation. Am Heart J 1980; 99:331–341.

494. Page PL. Sinus node during atrial fibrillation: to beat or not to beat? Circulation 1992; 86:334–336.

495. Sutton R, Kenny RA. The natural history of sick sinus syndrome. Pacing Clin Electrophysiol 1986; 9:1110–1114.

496. Rosenqvist M, Vallin H, Edhag O. Clinical and electrophysiologic course of sinus node disease: five-year follow-up study. Am Heart J 1985; 109:513–522.

497. Rosenqvist M, Brandt J, Schuller H. Long-term pacing in sinus node disease: effects of stimulation mode on cardiovascular morbidity and mortality. Am Heart J 1988; 116:16–22.

498. Brandt J, Anderson H, Fahraeus T, Schuller H. Natural history of sinus node disease treated with atrial pacing in 213 patients: implications for selection of stimulation mode. J Am Coll Cardiol 1992; 20:633–639.

499. Langenfeld H, Grimm W, Maisch B, Kochsiek K. Atrial fibrillation and embolic complications in paced patients. Pacing Clin Electrophysiol 1988; 11:1667–1672.

500. Hamer ME, Wilkinson WE, Clair WK, Page RL, McCarthy EA, Pritchett EL. Incidence of symptomatic atrial fibrillation in patients with paroxysmal supraventricular tachycardia. J Am Coll Cardiol 1995; 25:984–988.

501. Roark SF, McCarthy EA, Lee KL, Pritchett EL. Observations on the occurrence of atrial fibrillation in paroxysmal supraventricular tachycardia. Am J Cardiol 1986; 57:571–575.

502. Hwang W, Langendorf R. Auriculoventricular nodal escape in the presence of auricular fibrillation. Circulation 1950; 1:930–935.

503. Kastor JA, Yurchak PM. Recognition of digitalis intoxication in the presence of atrial fibrillation. Ann Intern Med 1967; 67:1045–1054.

504. Urbach JR, Grauman JJ, Straus SH. Quantitative methods for the recognition of atrioventricular junctional rhythms in atrial fibrillation. Circulation 1969; 39:803–817.

505. Urbach JR, Grauman JJ, Straus SH. Effects of inspiration, expiration, and apnea upon pacemaking and block in atrial fibrillation. Circulation 1970; 42:261–269.

506. Reid DS, Jachuck SJ, Henderson CB. Cardiac pacing in incomplete atrioventricular block with atrial fibrillation. Br Heart J 1973; 35:1154–1160.

507. Yamashita T, Murakawa Y, Ajiki K, Omata M. Incidence of induced atrial fibrillation/flutter in complete atrioventricular block: a concept of "atrial-malfunctioning" atrio-Hisian block. Circulation 1997; 95:650–654.

508. Halmos PB, Patterson GC. Effect of atrial fibrillation on cardiac output. Br Heart J 1965; 27:719–723.

509. Morris JJ, Peter RH, McIntosh HD. Electrical conversion of atrial fibrillation. Ann Intern Med 1966; 65:216–231.

510. Rossi M, Lown B. The use of quinidine in cardioversion. Am J Cardiol 1967; 19:234–238.

511. Klainer MJ, Altschule MD. Prolongation of the P-R interval in patients with paroxysmal auricular fibrillation and flutter following myocardial infarction. Am J Med Sci 1942; 203:215–218.

512. Ide LW. The clinical aspects of complete auriculoventricular heart block: a clinical analysis of 71 cases. Ann Intern Med 1952; 32:510–523.

513. Okel BB. The Wolff-Parkinson-White syndrome: report of a case with fatal arrhythmia and autopsy findings of myocarditis, interatrial lipomatous hypertrophy, and prominent right moderator band. Am Heart J 1968; 75:673–678.

514. Kaplan MA, Cohen KL. Ventricular fibrillation in the Wolff-Parkinson-White syndrome. Am J Cardiol 1969; 24:259–264.

515. Dreifus LS, Haiat R, Watanabe Y, Arriaga J, Reitman N. Ventricular fibrillation: a possible mechanism of sudden death in patients and Wolff-Parkinson-White syndrome. Circulation 1971; 43:520–527.

516. Dreifus LS, Wellens HJJ, Watanabe Y, Kimbiris D, Truex R. Sinus bradycardia and atrial fibrillation associated with the Wolff-Parkinson-White syndrome. Am J Cardiol 1976; 38:149–156.

517. Klein GJ, Bashore TM, Sellers TD, Pritchett EL, Smith WM, Gallagher JJ. Ventricular fibrillation in the Wolff-Parkinson-White syndrome. N Engl J Med 1979; 301:1080–1085.

518. Stafford WJ, Trohman RG, Bilsker M, Zaman L, Castellanos A, Myerburg RJ. Cardiac arrest in an adolescent with atrial fibrillation and hypertrophic cardiomyopathy. J Am Coll Cardiol 1986; 7:701–704.

519. Fujimura O, Klein GJ, Sharma AD, Yee R, Szabo T. Acute effect of disopyramide on atrial fibrillation in the Wolff-Parkinson-White syndrome. J Am Coll Cardiol 1989; 13:1133–1137.

520. Wang YS, Scheinman MM, Chien WW, Cohen TJ, Lesh MD, Griffin JC. Patients with supraventricular tachycardia presenting with aborted sudden death: incidence, mechanism and long-term follow-up. J Am Coll Cardiol 1991; 18:1711–1719.

521. Lown B, Ganong WF, Levine SA. The syndrome of short P-R interval, normal QRS complex and paroxysmal heart action. Circulation 1952; 5:693–706.

522. Myerburg RJ, Sung RJ, Castellanos A. Ventricular tachycardia and ventricular fibrillation in patients with short P-R intervals and narrow QRS complexes. Pacing Clin Electrophysiol 1979; 2:568–578.

523. Sparks PB, Mond HG, Kalman JM, Jayaprakash S, Lewis MA, Grigg LE. Atrial fibrillation and anticoagulation in patients with permanent pacemakers: implications for stroke prevention. PACE 1998; 21:1258–1267.

524. Jenkins LS, Bubien RS. Quality of life in patients with atrial fibrillation. Cardiol Clin 1996; 14:597–606.

525. Leitch JW, Klein GJ, Yee R. Can patients discriminate between atrial fibrillation and regular supraventricular tachycardia? Am J Cardiol 1991; 68:964–966.

526. Paul T, Guccione P, Garson A Jr. Relation of syncope in young patients with Wolff-Parkinson-White syndrome to rapid ventricular response during atrial fibrillation. Am J Cardiol 1990; 65:318–321.

527. Brignole M, Gianfranchi L, Menozzi C, et al. Role of autonomic reflexes in syncope associated with paroxysmal atrial fibrillation. J Am Coll Cardiol 1993; 22:1123–1129.

528. Hamer ME, Blumenthal JA, McCarthy EA, Phillips BG, Pritchett EL. Quality-of-life assessment in patients with paroxysmal atrial fibrillation or paroxysmal supraventricular tachycardia. Am J Cardiol 1994; 74:826–829.

529. Van Durme JP. Tachyarrhythmias and transient cerebral ischemic attacks. Am Heart J 1975; 89:538–540.

530. Auricchio A, Klein H, Trappe HJ, Wenzlaff P. Lack of prognostic value of syncope in patients with Wolff-Parkinson-White syndrome. J Am Coll Cardiol 1991; 17:152–158.

531. Page RL, Wilkinson WE, Clair WK, McCarthy EA, Pritchett EL. Asymptomatic arrhythmias in patients with symptomatic paroxysmal atrial fibrillation and paroxysmal supraventricular tachycardia. Circulation 1994; 89:224–227.

532. Tischler MD, Lee TH, McAndrew KA, Sax PE, Sutton MS, Lee RT. Clinical, echocardiographic and Doppler correlates of clinical instability with onset of atrial fibrillation. Am J Cardiol 1990; 66:721–724.

533. Takahashi N, Seki A, Imataka K, Fujii J. Clinical features of paroxysmal atrial fibrillation: an observation of 94 patients. Jpn Heart J 1981; 22:143–149.

534. Parkinson J, Campbell M. Paroxysmal auricular fibrillation: a record of 200 patients. Q J Med 1941; 24:67–100.

535. Campbell M. The paroxysmal tachycardias. Lancet 1947; 1:641–647.

536. Danias PG, Caulfield TA, Weigner MJ, Silverman DI, Manning WJ. Likelihood of spontaneous conversion of atrial fibrillation to sinus rhythm. J Am Coll Cardiol 1998; 31:588–592.

537. Donovan KD, Power BM, Hockings BE, Dobb GJ, Lee KY. Intravenous flecainide versus amiodarone for recent-onset atrial fibrillation. Am J Cardiol 1995; 75:693–697.

538. Cohen L, Larson DW, Strandjord N. Swallowing-induced atrial fibrillation. Circulation 1970; 51–52(Suppl III):III-145.

539. Sakamoto H, Okamoto E, Imataka K, Ieki K, Fujii J. Prediction of early development of chronic nonrheumatic atrial fibrillation. Jpn Heart J 1995; 36:191–199.

540. Curtis AB. How to approach classification of paroxysmal atrial fibrillation. J Cardiovasc Electrophysiol 1995; 6:75–77.

541. Levy S, Novella P, Ricard P, Paganelli F. Paroxysmal atrial fibrillation: a need for classification. J Cardiovasc Electrophysiol 1995; 6:69–74.

542. Burch GE. Auricular fibrillation of twenty-two months duration, with return to normal sinus mechanism without the aid of quinidine. Am Heart J 1939; 18:102–107.

543. Fogel M. Auricular fibrillation of long standing, with spontaneous return to normal sinus rhythm. Am Heart J 1943; 25:700–705.

544. Vaisrub S. Spontaneous reversion to normal sinus rhythm in a case of auricular fibrillation of long standing. Can Med Assoc J 1950; 63:599–600.

545. Lewis JK. Auricular fibrillation for many years with spontaneous reversion to sinus rhythm. Stanford Med Bull 1955; 13:131–137.

546. Halpern MM. Spontaneous sinus rhythm after several years of persistent atrial fibrillation in rheumatic valvular disease. Postgrad Med J 1956; 20:564–567.

547. Eichler BB. Spontaneous reversion of "permanent" atrial fibrillation to regular sinus rhythm. Angiologia 1961; 18:476–483.

548. Holzmann M. Exhaustion of atrial fibrillation in aneurysmatic dilatation of the left atrium. Cardiology 1966; 48:92–101.

549. Hanson R, Tuna N. Spontaneous conversion of chronic atrial fibrillation of twenty-two years' duration to sinus rhythm. Minn Med 1971; 54:543–546.

550. Zimmerman TJ, Basta LL, January LE. Spontaneous return of sinus rhythm in older patients with chronic atrial fibrillation and rheumatic mitral valve disease: Description of three patients. Am Heart J 1973; 86:676–680.

551. Reeve R, Galbraith GT, Reeve FJ, Lin TK. Letter: sinus rhythm after prolonged atrial fibrillation complicated by sinus arrest and syncope. Am Heart J 1975; 90:127.

552. Chevalier H. Spontaneous resumption of sinus rhythm in an elderly patient after 13 years of permanent atrial fibrillation. Am Heart J 1979; 98:361–365.

553. Olsson SB, Orndahl G, Ernestrom S, et al. Spontaneous reversion from long-lasting atrial fibrillation to sinus rhythm. Acta Med Scand 1980; 207:5–20.

554. Gardner JD, Dunn M. Spontaneous conversion of long-standing atrial fibrillation. Chest 1982; 81:429–432.

555. Meijler FL. The pulse in atrial fibrillation. Br Heart J 1986; 56:1–3.

556. Hardman SM, Noble MI, Seed WA. Postextrasystolic potentiation and its contribution to the beat-to-beat variation of the pulse during atrial fibrillation. Circulation 1992; 86:1223–1232.

557. Einthoven W, Korteweg AJ. On the variability of the size of the pulse in cases of auricular fibrillation. Heart 1915; 6:107–120.

558. Ferrer MI, Harvey RM. Some hemodynamic aspects of cardiac arrhythmias in man: a clinico-physiologic correlation. Am Heart J 1964; 68:153–165.

559. Lewis T. Observations upon disorders of the heart's action. Heart 1912; 3:279–310.

560. Brachman DS. Auricular fibrillation. Lancet 1921; 1:374–377.

561. Rodbard S, Margolis J. The significance of the intensity and time of appearance of the Korotkoff sounds in auricular fibrillation. Circulation 1956; 13:510–514.

562. Gibson DG, Broder G, Sowton E. Effect of varying pulse interval in atrial fibrillation on left ventricular function in man. Br Heart J 1971; 33:388–393.

563. Lip GYH, Zarifis J, Beevers M, Beevers DG. Ambulatory blood pressure monitoring in atrial fibrillation. Am J Cardiol 1996; 78:350–353.

564. Constant J. Bedside Cardiology. 3rd ed. Boston: Little, Brown, 1985.

565. Sanders CA, Harthorne JW, DeSanctis RW, Austen WE. Tricuspid stenosis, a difficult diagnosis in the presence of atrial fibrillation. Circulation 1966; 33:26–33.

566. Harvey WP, Ronan JA Jr. Bedside diagnosis of arrhythmias. Prog Cardiovasc Dis 1966; 8:419–445.

567. Rytand DA. The variable loudness of the first heart sound in auricular fibrillation. Am Heart J 1949; 37:187–204.

568. Ravin A, Bershof E. The intensity of the first heart sound in auricular fibrillation with mitral stenosis. Am Heart J 1951; 41:539–548.

569. Neporent LM. Atrial heart sounds in atrial fibrillation and flutter. Circulation 1964; 30:893–896.

570. Shaver JA, Salerni R. Auscultation of the heart. In Hurst JW, Schlant RC, Rackley CE, Sonnenblick EH, Wenger NK (eds). The Heart. 7th ed. New York: McGraw-Hill, 1985, p. 201.

571. Shaver JA, Salerni R. Auscultation of the heart. In Hurst JW, Schlant RC, Rackley CE, Sonnenblick EH, Wenger NK (eds). The Heart. 7th ed. New York: McGraw-Hill, 1985, p. 204.

572. Perloff JK, Harvey WP. Auscultatory and phonocardiographic manifestations of pure mitral regurgitation. Prog Cardiovasc Dis 1962; 5:172–194.

573. Karliner JS, O'Rourke RA, Kearney DJ, Shabetai R. Haemodynamic explanation of why the murmur of mitral regurgitation is independent of cycle length. Br Heart J 1973; 35:397–401.

574. Ongley PA, Sprague HB, Rappaport MB. The diastolic murmur of mitral stenosis. N Engl J Med 1955; 253:1049–1057.

575. Criley JM, Hermer AJ. The crescendo presystolic murmur of mitral stenosis with atrial fibrillation. N Engl J Med 1971; 285:1284–1287.

576. Lakier JB, Pocock WA, Gale GE, Barlow JB. Haemodynamic and sound events preceding first heart sound in mitral stenosis. Br Heart J 1972; 34:1152–1155.

577. Shaver JA, Salerni R. Auscultation of the heart. In Hurst JW, Schlant RC, Rackley CE, Sonnenblick EH, Wenger NK (eds). The Heart. 7th ed. New York: McGraw-Hill, 1985, pp. 229–230.

578. Bonner AJ Jr, Stewart J, Tavel ME. "Presystolic" augmentation of diastolic heart sounds in atrial fibrillation. Am J Cardiol 1976; 37:427–431.

579. Friedberg CK. Diseases of the Heart. 3rd ed. Philadelphia, WB Saunders, 1966, p. 536.

580. Atwood JE, Myers J, Sandhu S, et al. Optimal sampling interval to estimate heart rate at rest and during exercise in atrial fibrillation. Am J Cardiol 1989; 63:45–48.

581. Yurchak PM, McGovern BA. Supraventricular arrhythmias. In Eagle KA, Haber E, DeSanctis RW, Austen WG (eds). The Practice of Cardiology. 2nd ed. Boston: Little, Brown, 1989, pp. 158–162.

582. Zipes DP. Specific arrhythmias: diagnosis and treatment. In Braunwald E (ed). Heart Disease. A Textbook of Cardiovascular Medicine. 5th ed. Philadelphia: WB Saunders, 1997, pp. 675–677.

583. Godtfredsen J. Atrial Fibrillation. Etiology, Course and Prognosis: A Follow-up Study of 1212 Cases. Thesis, Copenhagen, 1975.

584. Kawakubo K, Murayama M, Itai T, et al. Heart rate at onset and termination of paroxysmal atrial fibrillation in apparently healthy subjects. Jpn Heart J 1986; 27:645–651.

585. Friedberg CK. Diseases of the Heart. 3rd ed. Philadelphia: WB Saunders, 1966, p. 538.

586. Inoue H, Ohkawa S, Ueyama C, Abe H, Ueda K, Sugiura M. Clinicopathologic study on determinants of the amplitude of atrial fibrillation waves in the geriatric population. Am Heart J 1982; 104:1382–1384.

587. Garber EB, Morgan MG, Glasser SP. Left atrial size in patients with atrial fibrillation: an echocardiographic study. Am J Med Sci 1976; 272:57–64.

588. Skoulas A, Horlick L. The atrial F wave in various types of heart disease and its response to treatment. Am J Cardiol 1964; 14:174–177.

589. Aberg H. Atrial fibrillation. II. A study of fibrillatory wave

size on the regular scalar electrocardiogram. Acta Med Scand 1969; 185:381–385.

590. Thurmann M. Coarse atrial fibrillation in congenital heart disease. Circulation 1965; 32:290–292.

591. Morganroth J, Horowitz LN, Josephson ME, Kastor JA. Relationship of atrial fibrillatory wave amplitude to left atrial size and etiology of heart disease: an old generalization re-examined. Am Heart J 1979; 97:184–186.

592. Thurmann M, Janney JG. The diagnostic importance of fibrillatory wave size. Circulation 1962; 25:991–994.

593. Peter RH, Morris JJ, McIntosh HD. Relationship of fibrillatory waves and P waves in the electrocardiogram. Circulation 1966; 33:599–606.

594. Culler MR, Boone JA, Gazes PC. Fibrillatory wave as a clue to etiological diagnosis. Am Heart J 1963; 66:435–436.

595. de Silva P. Fibrillatory wave size in the diagnosis of heart disease. Can Med Assoc J 1966; 95:684–685.

596. Roithinger FX, SippensGroenewegen A, Karch MR, Steiner PR, Ellis WS, Lesh MD. Organized activation during atrial fibrillation in man: endocardial and electrocardiographic manifestations. J Cardiovasc Electrophysiol 1998; 9:451–461.

597. Mandel WJ, Danzig R, Hayakawa H. Lown-Ganong-Levine syndrome: a study using His bundle electrograms. Circulation 1971; 44:696–708.

598. Bissett JK, Thompson AJ, de Soyza N, Murphy ML. Atrioventricular conduction in patients with short PR intervals and normal QRS complexes. Br Heart J 1973; 35:123–127.

599. Bissett JK, de Soyza N, Kane JJ, Murphy ML. Altered refractory periods in patients with short P-R intervals and normal QRS complex. Am J Cardiol 1975; 35:487–491.

600. Caracta AR, Damato AN, Gallagher JJ, et al. Electrophysiologic studies in the syndrome of short P-R interval, normal QRS complex. Am J Cardiol 1973; 31:245–253.

601. Benditt DG, Pritchett LC, Smith WM, Wallace AG, Gallagher JJ. Characteristics of atrioventricular conduction and the spectrum of arrhythmias in Lown-Ganong-Levine syndrome. Circulation 1978; 57:454–465.

602. Castellanos A, Zaman L, Luceri RM, Myerburg RJ. Arrhythmias in patients with short PR intervals and narrow QRS complexes. In Josephson ME, Wellens HJJ (eds). Tachycardias. Mechanisms, Diagnosis, Treatment. Philadelphia: Lea & Febiger, 1984, pp. 171–190.

603. Altschule MD. The relation between prolonged P-R interval and auricular fibrillation in patients with rheumatic heart disease. Am Heart J 1939; 18:1–7.

604. Ashman R, Byer E. Aberration in the conduction of premature supraventricular impulses. J La State Univ Sch Med 1946; 8:62–65.

605. Gouaux JL, Ashman R. Auricular fibrillation with aberration simulating ventricular paroxysmal tachycardia. Am Heart J 1947; 34:366–373.

606. Langendorf R, Pick A, Katz LN. Ventricular response in atrial fibrillation. Circulation 1965; 32:69–75.

607. Chaudry II, Ramsaran EK, Spodick DH. Observations on the reliability of the Ashman phenomenon. Am Heart J 1994; 128:205–209.

608. Marriott HJL, Sandler IA. Criteria, old and new, for differentiating between ectopic ventricular beats and aberrant ventricular conduction in the presence of atrial fibrillation. Prog Cardiovasc Dis 1966; 9:18–28.

609. Sandler IA, Marriott HJL. The differential morphology of anomalous ventricular complexes of RBBB-type in lead V1: ventricular ectopy versus aberration. Circulation 1965; 31:551–556.

610. Marriott HJ. Simulation of ectopic ventricular rhythms by aberrant conduction. JAMA 1966; 196:787.

611. Gulamhusein S, Yee R, Ko PT, Klein GJ. Electro-cardiographic criteria for differentiating aberrancy and ventricular extrasystole in chronic atrial fibrillation: validation by intracardiac recordings. J Electrocardiol 1985; 18:41–50.

612. Drew BJ, Scheinman MM. Value of electrocardiographic leads MCL1, MCL6 and other selected leads in the diagnosis

of wide QRS complex tachycardia. J Am Coll Cardiol 1991; 18:1025–1033.

613. Schamroth L, Chesler E. Phasic aberrant ventricular conduction. Br Heart J 1963; 25:219–226.

614. Sheiner LB, Stock RJ. Coupled pacing and coupled pacing with concealed conduction. Circulation 1966; 34:759–766.

615. Pritchett EL, Smith WM, Klein GJ, Hammill SC, Gallagher JJ. The "compensatory pause" of atrial fibrillation. Circulation 1980; 62:1021–1025.

616. Morady F, DiCarlo LA Jr, Krol RB, de Buitleir M, Baerman JM. An analysis of post-pacing R-R intervals during atrial fibrillation. Pacing Clin Electrophysiol 1986; 9:411–416.

617. Langendorf R. Concealed A-V conduction: the effect of blocked impulses on the formation and conduction of subsequent impulses. Am Heart J 1948; 35:542–552.

618. Langendorf R. Aberrant ventricular conduction. Am Heart J 1951; 41:700–707.

619. Langendorf R, Pick A, Winternitz M. Mechanisms of intermittent ventricular bigeminy. I. Appearance of ectopic beats dependent upon length of the ventricular cycle, the "rule of bigeminy." Circulation 1955; 11:422–430.

620. Wellens HJJ, Bar FWHM, Lie KI. The value of the electrocardiogram in the differential diagnosis of a tachycardia with a widened QRS complex. Am J Med 1978; 64:27–33.

621. Young RL, Mower MM, Ramapuram GM, Tabatznik B. Atrial fibrillation with ventricular tachycardia showing "Dressler" beats. Chest 1973; 63:96–97.

622. Brugada P, Wylick AR, Abdollah H, Stappers J, Wellens HJJ. Identical QRS complexes during atrial fibrillation with aberrant conduction and ventricular tachycardia: the value of a His bundle recording. Pacing Clin Electrophysiol 1983; 6:1057–1061.

623. Suyama AC, Sunagawa K, Sugimachi M, Anan T, Egashira K, Takeshita A. Differentiation between aberrant ventricular conduction and ventricular ectopy in atrial fibrillation using RR interval scattergram. Circulation 1993; 88:2307–2314.

624. Raev D. Carotid sinus pressure: a new application of an old maneuver: a preliminary report. Int J Cardiol 1996; 57:241–244.

625. Langendorf R, Lev M, Pick R. Auricular fibrillation with anomalous A-V excitation (WPW syndrome) imitating ventricular paroxysmal tachycardia. Acta Cardiol 1952; 7:241–260.

626. Katz LN, Pick A. Clinical Electrocardiography. Part I. The Arrhythmias. Philadelphia: Lea & Febiger, 1956, p. 695.

627. Herrmann GR, Oates JR, Runge TM, Hejtmancik MR. Paroxysmal pseudoventricular tachycardia and pseudoventricular fibrillation in patients with accelerated A-V conduction. Am Heart J 1957; 53:254–264.

628. Yahini JH, Zahavi I, Neufeld HN. Paroxysmal atrial fibrillation in Wolff-Parkinson-White syndrome simulating ventricular tachycardia. Am J Cardiol 1964; 14:248–254.

629. Gatzoulis K, Carlson MD, Johnson NJ, Biblo LA, Waldo AL. Regular wide QRS complex tachycardia during atrial fibrillation in a patient with preexcitation syndrome: a case report. J Cardiovasc Electrophysiol 1995; 6:493–497.

630. Garratt C, Antoniou A, Ward D, Camm AJ. Misuse of verapamil in pre-excited atrial fibrillation. Lancet 1989; 1:367–369.

631. Robinson K, Rowland E, Krikler DM. Latent pre-excitation: exposure of anterograde accessory pathway conduction during atrial fibrillation. Br Heart J 1988; 59:53–55.

632. Pai GR, Rawles JM. The QT interval in atrial fibrillation. Br Heart J 1989; 61:510–513.

633. Robitaille GA, Phillips JH. An analysis of the P wave in patients with transient benign atrial fibrillation. Dis Chest 1967; 52:806–812.

634. Buxton AE, Josephson ME. The role of P wave duration as a predictor of postoperative atrial arrhythmias. Chest 1981; 80:68–73.

635. Kawano S, Hiraoka M, Sawanobori T. Electrocardiographic features of P waves from patients with transient atrial fibrillation. Jpn Heart J 1988; 29:57–67.

636. Kumagai K, Akimitsu S, Kawahira K, et al.

Electrophysiological properties in chronic lone atrial fibrillation. Circulation 1991; 84:1662–1668.

637. Dilaveris PE, Gialafos EJ, Sideris SK, et al. Simple electrocardiographic markers for the prediction of paroxysmal idiopathic atrial fibrillation. Am Heart J 1998; 135:733–738.

638. Liu Z, Hayano M, Hirata T, et al. Abnormalities of electrocardiographic P wave morphology and their relation to electrophysiological parameters of the atrium in patients with sick sinus syndrome. PACE 1998; 21:79–86.

639. Nielsen FE, Andersen HH, Gram-Hansen P, Sorensen HT, Klausen IC. The relationship between ECG signs of atrial infarction and the development of supraventricular arrhythmias in patients with acute myocardial infarction. Am Heart J 1992; 123:69–72.

640. Wellens HJJ, Bar FW, Vanagt EJ, Brugada P, Farre J. The differentiation between ventricular tachycardia and supraventricular tachycardia and supraventricular tachycardia with aberrant conduction: the value of the 12-lead electrocardiogram. In Wellens HJJ, Kulbertus HE (eds). What's New in Electrocardiography. The Hague: Martinus Nijhoff, 1981, pp. 184–199.

641. Blumgart H. The reaction to exercise of the heart affected by auricular fibrillation. Heart 1924; 11:49–56.

642. Knox JAC. The heart rate with exercise of the heart affected by auricular fibrillation. Br Heart J 1949; 11:119–125.

643. Hornsten TR, Bruce RA. Effects of atrial fibrillation on exercise performance in patients with cardiac disease. Circulation 1968; 37:543–548.

644. Atwood JE, Myers J, Sullivan M, et al. Maximal exercise testing and gas exchange in patients with chronic atrial fibrillation. J Am Coll Cardiol 1988; 11:508–513.

645. Wetherbee DG, Brown MG, Holzman D. Ventricular rate response following exercise during auricular fibrillation and after conversion to normal sinus rhythm. Am J Med Sci 1952; 223:667–670.

646. Ueshima K, Myers J, Graettinger WF, et al. Exercise and morphologic comparison of chronic atrial fibrillation and normal sinus rhythm. Am Heart J 1993; 126:260–261.

647. Aberg H, Strom G, Werner I. On the reproducibility of exercise tests in patients with atrial fibrillation. Upsala J Med Sci 1977; 82:27–30.

648. Corbelli R, Masterson M, Wilkoff BL. Chronotropic response to exercise in patients with atrial fibrillation. Pacing Clin Electrophysiol 1990; 13:179–187.

649. Gooch AS, Natarajan G, Goldberg H. Influence of exercise on arrhythmias induced by digitalis-diuretic therapy in patients with atrial fibrillation. Am J Cardiol 1974; 33:230–237.

650. Ueshima K, Myers J, Ribisl PM, et al. Hemodynamic determinants of exercise capacity in chronic atrial fibrillation. Am Heart J 1993; 125:1301–1305.

651. Biffi A, Ammirati F, Caselli G, et al. Usefulness of transesophageal pacing during exercise for evaluating palpitations in top-level athletes. Am J Cardiol 1993; 72:922–926.

652. Strasberg B, Ashley WW, Wyndham CR, et al. Treadmill exercise testing in the Wolff-Parkinson-White syndrome. Am J Cardiol 1980; 45:742–748.

653. German LD, Gallagher JJ, Broughton A, Guarnieri T, Trantham JL. Effects of exercise and isoproterenol during atrial fibrillation in patients with Wolff-Parkinson-White syndrome. Am J Cardiol 1983; 51:1203–1206.

654. Crick JC, Davies DW, Holt P, Curry PV, Sowton E. Effect of exercise on ventricular response to atrial fibrillation in Wolff-Parkinson-White syndrome. Br Heart J 1985; 54:80–85.

655. Critelli G, Gallagher JJ, Perticone F, Coltorti F, Monda V, Condorelli M. Evaluation of noninvasive tests for identifying patients with preexcitation syndrome at risk of rapid ventricular response. Am Heart J 1984; 108:905–909.

656. Romero CA Jr. Holter monitoring in the diagnosis and management of cardiac rhythm disturbances. Med Clin North Am 1976; 60:299–313.

657. Rebello R, Brownlee WC. Intermittent ventricular standstill during chronic atrial fibrillation in patients with dizziness or syncope. Pacing Clin Electrophysiol 1987; 10:1271–1276.

658. Saxon LA, Albert BH, Uretz EF, Denes P. Permanent pacemaker placement in chronic atrial fibrillation associated with intermittent AV block and cerebral symptoms. Pacing Clin Electrophysiol 1990; 13:724–729.

659. Aronow WS, Mercando AD, Epstein S. Prevalence of arrhythmias detected by 24-hour ambulatory electrocardiography and value of antiarrhythmic therapy in elderly patients with unexplained syncope. Am J Cardiol 1992; 70:408–410.

660. Hnatkova K, Waktare JEP, Murgatroyd FD, et al. Analysis of the cardiac rhythm preceding episodes of paroxysmal atrial fibrillation. Am Heart J 1998; 135:1010–1019.

661. Pitcher D, Papouchado M, James MA, Rees JR. Twenty-four hour ambulatory electrocardiography in patients with chronic atrial fibrillation. BMJ 1986; 292:594.

662. Reynolds EW Jr, MacDonald WJ, Greenfield BM, Semion AA. Mechanisms of onset and termination of abnormal cardiac rhythm studied by constant monitoring. Am Heart J 1967; 74:473–481.

663. Greer GS, Wilkinson WE, McCarthy EA, Pritchett EL. Random and nonrandom behavior of symptomatic paroxysmal atrial fibrillation. Am J Cardiol 1989; 64:339–342.

664. Bhandari AK, Anderson JL, Gilbert EM, et al. Correlation of symptoms with occurrence of paroxysmal supraventricular tachycardia or atrial fibrillation: a transtelephonic monitoring study. The flecainide supraventricular tachycardia study group. Am Heart J 1992; 124:381–386.

665. Bauernfeind RA, Swiryn SP, Wyndham CR, Palileo E, Rosen KM. Telephonic documentation of paroxysmal atrioventricular reentrant tachycardia in preexcitation with recurrent paroxysmal atrial fibrillation. Chest 1980; 78:771–773.

666. Anderson JL, Gilbert EM, Alpert BL, et al: Prevention of symptomatic recurrences of paroxysmal atrial fibrillation in patients initially tolerating antiarrhythmic therapy: a multicenter, double-blind, crossover study of flecainide and placebo with transtelephonic monitoring. Flecainide supraventricular tachycardia study group. Circulation 1989; 80:1557–1570.

667. Weiner HL, McCarthy EA, Pritchett EL. Regular ventricular rhythms in patients with symptomatic paroxysmal atrial fibrillation. J Am Coll Cardiol 1991; 17:1283–1287.

668. Stein KM, Borer JS, Hochreiter C, Devereux RB, Kligfield P. Variability of the ventricular response in atrial fibrillation and prognosis in chronic nonischemic mitral regurgitation. Am J Cardiol 1994; 74:906–911.

669. Frey B, Heinz G, Binder T, et al. Diurnal variation of ventricular response to atrial fibrillation in patients with advanced heart failure. Am Heart J 1995; 129:58–65.

670. Van Den Berg MP, Haaksma J, Brouwer J, Tieleman RG, Mulder G, Crijns HJ. Heart rate variability in patients with atrial fibrillation is related to vagal tone. Circulation 1997; 96:1209–1216.

671. Seifert M, Josephson ME. P-wave signal averaging: high tech or an expensive alternative to the standard ECG? Circulation 1993; 88:2980–2982.

672. Hofmann M, Goedel-Meinen L, Beckhoff A, Rehbach K, Schomig A. Analysis of the P wave in the signal-averaged electrocardiogram: normal values and reproducibility. Pacing Clin Electrophysiol 1996; 19:1928–1932.

673. Rosenheck S. Signal-averaged P wave in patients with paroxysmal atrial fibrillation. PACE 1997; 20:2577–2586.

674. Steinberg JS, Zelenkofske S, Wong SC, Gelernt M, Sciacca R, Menchavez E. Value of the P-wave signal-averaged ECG for predicting atrial fibrillation after cardiac surgery. Circulation 1993; 88:2618–2622.

675. Engel TR, Vallone N, Windle J. Signal-averaged electrocardiograms in patients with atrial fibrillation or flutter. Am Heart J 1988; 115:592–597.

676. Fukunami M, Yamada T, Ohmori M, et al. Detection of patients at risk for paroxysmal atrial fibrillation during sinus rhythm by P wave-triggered signal-averaged electrocardiogram. Circulation 1991; 83:162–169.

677. Opolski G, Stanislawska J, Slomka K, Kraska T. Value of the atrial signal-averaged electrocardiogram in identifying

patients with paroxysmal atrial fibrillation. Int J Cardiol 1991; 30:315–319.

678. Pollak A, Falk RH. Predictive value of P wave-triggered signal averaging of the electrocardiogram. Circulation 1991; 84:2606–2607.

679. Stafford PJ, Turner I, Vincent R. Quantitative analysis of signal-averaged P waves in idiopathic paroxysmal atrial fibrillation. Am J Cardiol 1991; 68:751–755.

680. Guidera SA, Steinberg JS. The signal-averaged P wave duration: a rapid and noninvasive marker of risk of atrial fibrillation. J Am Coll Cardiol 1993; 21:1645–1651.

681. Villani GQ, Piepoli M, Cripps T, Rosi A, Gazzola U. Atrial late potentials in patients with paroxysmal atrial fibrillation detected using a high gain, signal-averaged esophageal lead. Pacing Clin Electrophysiol 1994; 17:1118–1123.

682. Gondo N, Kumagai K, Matsuo K, et al. The best criterion for discrimination between patients with and without paroxysmal atrial fibrillation on signal-averaged electrocardiogram. Am J Cardiol 1995; 75:93–95.

683. Klein M, Evans SJ, Blumberg S, Cataldo L, Bodenheimer MM. Use of P-wave-triggered, P-wave signal-averaged electrocardiogram to predict atrial fibrillation after coronary artery bypass surgery. Am Heart J 1995; 129:895–901.

684. Stafford PJ, Robinson D, Vincent R. Optimal analysis of the signal averaged P wave in patients with paroxysmal atrial fibrillation. Br Heart J 1995; 74:413–418.

685. Cecchi F, Montereggi A, Olivotto I, Marconi P, Dolara A, Maron BJ. Risk for atrial fibrillation in patients with hypertrophic cardiomyopathy assessed by signal averaged P wave duration. Heart 1997; 78:44–49.

686. Ehlert FA, Korenstein D, Steinberg JS. Evaluation of P wave signal-averaged electrocardiographic filtering and analysis methods. Am Heart J 1997; 134:985–993.

687. Stafford PJ, Kolvekar S, Cooper J, et al. Signal averaged P wave compared with standard electrocardiography or echocardiography for prediction of atrial fibrillation after coronary bypass grafting. Heart 1997; 77:417–422.

688. Zaman AG, Alamgir F, Richens T, Williams R, Rothman MT, Mills PG. The role of signal averaged P wave duration and serum magnesium as a combined predictor of atrial fibrillation after elective coronary artery bypass surgery. Heart 1997; 77:527–531.

689. Hiraki T, Ikeda H, Ohga M, et al. Frequency- and time-domain analysis of P wave in patients with paroxysmal atrial fibrillation. PACE 1998; 21:56–64.

690. Abe Y, Fukunami M, Yamada T, et al. Prediction of transition of chronic atrial fibrillation in patients with paroxysmal atrial fibrillation by signal-averaged electrocardiography: a prospective study. Circulation 1997; 96:2612–2616.

691. Valverde ER, Quinteiro RA, Bertran GC, Arini PD, Glenny P, Biagetti MO. Influence of filtering techniques on the time-domain analysis of signal-averaged P wave electrocardiogram. J Cardiovasc Electrophysiol 1998; 9:253–260.

692. Fitzgerald DM, Hawthorne HR, Crossley GH, Simmons TW, Haisty WK Jr. Effects of atrial fibrillation and atrial flutter on the signal-averaged electrocardiogram. Am J Cardiol 1996; 77:205–209.

693. Pollick C. Echocardiography in atrial fibrillation. In Falk RH, Podrid PJ (eds). Atrial Fibrillation. Mechanisms and Management. New York: Raven Press, 1992, pp. 165–180.

694. Benchimol A, Maia IG, Gartlan JL, Franklin D. Telemetry of arterial flow in man with a Doppler ultrasonic flowmeter. Am J Cardiol 1968; 22:75–84.

695. Kupari M, Leinonen H, Koskinen P. Value of routine echocardiography in new-onset atrial fibrillation. Int J Cardiol 1987; 16:106–108.

696. Henry WL, Morganroth J, Pearlman AS, et al. Relation between echocardiographically determined left atrial size and atrial fibrillation. Circulation 1976; 53:273–279.

697. Watson DC, Henry WL, Epstein SE, Morrow AG. Effects of operation on left atrial size and the occurrence of atrial fibrillation in patients with hypertrophic subaortic stenosis. Circulation 1977; 55:178–181.

698. Unverferth DV, Fertel RH, Unverferth BJ, Leier CV. Atrial fibrillation in mitral stenosis: histologic, hemodynamic and metabolic factors. Int J Cardiol 1984; 5:143–154.

699. Keren G, Etzion T, Sherez J, et al. Atrial fibrillation and atrial enlargement in patients with mitral stenosis. Am Heart J 1987; 114:1146–1155.

700. Santos-Ocampo CD, Sadaniantz A, Elion JL, Garber CE, Malone LL, Parisi AF. Echocardiographic assessment of the cardiac anatomy in patients with multifocal atrial tachycardia: a comparison with atrial fibrillation. Am J Med Sci 1994; 307:264–268.

701. Vaziri SM, Larson MG, Benjamin EJ, Levy D. Echocardiographic predictors of nonrheumatic atrial fibrillation: the Framingham heart study. Circulation 1994; 89:724–730.

702. Davidson E, Rotenberg Z, Weinberger I, Fuchs J, Agmon J. Diagnosis and characteristics of lone atrial fibrillation. Chest 1989; 95:1048–1050.

703. Ewy GA, Ulfers L, Hager WD, Rosenfeld AR, Roeske WR, Goldman S. Response of atrial fibrillation to therapy: role of etiology and left atrial diameter. J Electrocardiol 1980; 13:119–123.

704. Andersen JS, Egeblad H, Abildgaard U, Aldershvile J, Godtfredsen J. Atrial fibrillation and left atrial enlargement: cause or effect? J Int Med 1991; 229:253–256.

705. Mann B, Ray R, Goldberger AL, Shabetai R, Green C, Kelley M. Atrial fibrillation in congestive cardiomyopathy: echocardiographic and hemodynamic correlates. Cathet Cardiovasc Diagn 1981; 7:387–395.

706. Petersen P, Kastrup J, Brinch K, Godtfredsen J, Boysen G. Relation between left atrial dimension and duration of atrial fibrillation. Am J Cardiol 1987; 60:382–384.

707. Sanfilippo AJ, Abascal VM, Sheehan M, et al. Atrial enlargement as a consequence of atrial fibrillation: a prospective echocardiographic study. Circulation 1990; 82:792–797.

708. Takahashi N, Imataka K, Seki A, Fujii J. Left atrial enlargement in patients with paroxysmal atrial fibrillation. Jpn Heart J 1982; 23:677–683.

709. Suarez GS, Lampert S, Ravid S, Lown B. Changes in left atrial size in patients with lone atrial fibrillation. Clin Cardiol 1991; 14:652–656.

710. Dethy M, Chassat C, Roy D, Mercier LA. Doppler echocardiographic predictors of recurrence of atrial fibrillation after cardioversion. Am J Cardiol 1988; 62:723–726.

711. Manning WJ, Silverman DI, Katz SE, et al. Impaired left atrial mechanical function after cardioversion: relation to the duration of atrial fibrillation. J Am Coll Cardiol 1994; 23:1535–1540.

712. Halpern SW, Ellrodt G, Singh BN, Mandel WJ. Efficacy of intravenous procainamide infusion in converting atrial fibrillation to sinus rhythm: relation to left atrial size. Br Heart J 1980; 44:589–595.

713. Fenster PE, Comess KA, Marsh R, Katzenberg C, Hager WD. Conversion of atrial fibrillation to sinus rhythm by acute intravenous procainamide infusion. Am Heart J 1983; 106:501–504.

714. Bianconi L, Boccadamo R, Pappalardo A, Gentili C, Pistolese M. Effectiveness of intravenous propafenone for conversion of atrial fibrillation and flutter of recent onset. Am J Cardiol 1989; 64:335–338.

715. Horowitz LN, Spielman SR, Greenspan AM, et al. Use of amiodarone in the treatment of persistent and paroxysmal atrial fibrillation resistant to quinidine therapy. J Am Coll Cardiol 1985; 6:1402–1407.

716. Brodsky MA, Allen BJ, Walker CJ III, Casey TP, Luckett CR, Henry WL. Amiodarone for maintenance of sinus rhythm after conversion of atrial fibrillation in the setting of a dilated left atrium. Am J Cardiol 1987; 60:572–575.

717. Gold RL, Haffajee CI, Charos G, Sloan K, Baker S, Alpert JS. Amiodarone for refractory atrial fibrillation. Am J Cardiol 1986; 57:124–127.

718. Carlsson J, Tebbe U, Rox J, et al. Cardioversion of atrial fibrillation in the elderly: ALKK-study group. Arbeitsgemeinschaft Leitender Kardiologischer Krankenhausaerzte. Am J Cardiol 1996; 78:1380–1384.

719. Dittrich HC, Erickson JS, Schneiderman T, Blacky AR,

Savides T, Nicod PH. Echocardiographic and clinical predictors for outcome of elective cardioversion of atrial fibrillation. Am J Cardiol 1989; 63:193–197.

720. Flugelman MY, Hasin Y, Katznelson N, Kriwisky M, Shefer A, Gotsman MS. Restoration and maintenance of sinus rhythm after mitral valve surgery for mitral stenosis. Am J Cardiol 1984; 54:617–619.

721. Skoularigis J, Rothlisberger C, Skudicky D, Essop MR, Wisenbaugh T, Sareli P. Effectiveness of amiodarone and electrical cardioversion for chronic rheumatic atrial fibrillation after mitral valve surgery. Am J Cardiol 1993; 72:423–427.

722. Orlando JR, van Herick R, Aronow WS, Olson HG. Hemodynamics and echocardiograms before and after cardioversion of atrial fibrillation to normal sinus rhythm. Chest 1979; 76:521–526.

723. DeMaria AN, Lies JE, King JF, Miller RR, Amsterdam EA, Mason DT. Echographic assessment of atrial transport, mitral movement, and ventricular performance following electroversion of supraventricular arrhythmias. Circulation 1975; 51:273–282.

724. Alam M, Thorstrand C. Left ventricular function in patients with atrial fibrillation before and after cardioversion. Am J Cardiol 1992; 69:694–696.

725. Twidale N, Sutton K, Bartlett L, et al. Effects on cardiac performance of atrioventricular node catheter ablation using radiofrequency current for drug-refractory atrial arrhythmias. Pacing Clin Electrophysiol 1993; 16:1275–1284.

726. Rodriguez LM, Smeets JL, Xie B, et al. Improvement in left ventricular function by ablation of atrioventricular nodal conduction in selected patients with lone atrial fibrillation. Am J Cardiol 1993; 72:1137–1141.

727. Heinz G, Siostrzonek P, Kreiner G, Gossinger H. Improvement in left ventricular systolic function after successful radiofrequency His bundle ablation for drug refractory, chronic atrial fibrillation and recurrent atrial flutter. Am J Cardiol 1992; 69:489–492.

728. Petersen P. Thromboembolic complications of atrial fibrillation and their prevention: a review. Am J Cardiol 1990; 65:24C–28C.

729. Leung DY, Grimm RA, Klein AL. Transesophageal echocardiography-guided approach to cardioversion of atrial fibrillation. Prog Cardiovasc Dis 1996; 39:21–32.

730. Manning WJ. Role of transesophageal echocardiography in the management of thromboembolic stroke. Am J Cardiol 1997; 80:19D–28D.

731. Manning WJ, Douglas PS. Transesophageal echocardiography and atrial fibrillation: added value or expensive toy? Ann Intern Med 1998; 128:685–687.

732. de Belder MA, Lovat LB, Tourikis L, Leech G, Camm A. Left atrial spontaneous contrast echoes: markers of thromboembolic risk in patients with atrial fibrillation. Eur Heart J 1993; 14:326–335.

733. Orsinelli DA, Pearson AC. Usefulness of transesophageal echocardiography to screen for left atrial thrombus before elective cardioversion for atrial fibrillation. Am J Cardiol 1993; 72:1337–1339.

734. Obarski TP, Salcedo EE, Castle LW, Stewart WJ. Spontaneous echo contrast in the left atrium during paroxysmal atrial fibrillation. Am Heart J 1990; 120:988–990.

735. Black IW, Chesterman CN, Hopkins AP, Lee LC, Chong BH, Walsh WF. Hematologic correlates of left atrial spontaneous echo contrast and thromboembolism in nonvalvular atrial fibrillation. J Am Coll Cardiol 1993; 21:451–457.

736. Grimm RA, Stewart WJ, Maloney JD, et al. Impact of electrical cardioversion for atrial fibrillation on left atrial appendage function and spontaneous echo contrast: characterization by simultaneous transesophageal echocardiography. J Am Coll Cardiol 1993; 22:1359–1366.

737. Verhorst PM, Kamp O, Visser CA, Verheugt FW. Left atrial appendage flow velocity assessment using transesophageal echocardiography in nonrheumatic atrial fibrillation and systemic embolism. Am J Cardiol 1993; 71:192–196.

738. Fatkin D, Kuchar DL, Thorburn CW, Feneley MP.

Transesophageal echocardiography before and during direct current cardioversion of atrial fibrillation: evidence for "atrial stunning" as a mechanism of thromboembolic complications. J Am Coll Cardiol 1994; 23:307–316.

739. Fatkin D, Herbert E, Feneley MP. Hematologic correlates of spontaneous echo contrast in patients with atrial fibrillation and implications for thromboembolic risk. Am J Cardiol 1994; 73:672–676.

740. Leung DY, Black IW, Cranney GB, Hopkins AP, Walsh WF. Prognostic implications of left atrial spontaneous echo contrast in nonvalvular atrial fibrillation. J Am Coll Cardiol 1994; 24:755–762.

741. Stoddard MF, Dawkins PR, Prince CR, Longaker RA. Transesophageal echocardiographic guidance of cardioversion in patients with atrial fibrillation. Am Heart J 1995; 129:1204–1215.

742. Stroke Prevention in Atrial Fibrillation Investigators Committee on Echocardiography. Transesophageal echocardiographic correlates of thromboembolism in high-risk patients with nonvalvular atrial fibrillation. Ann Intern Med 1998; 128:639–647.

743. Tsai LM, Chen JH, Tsao CJ. Relation of left atrial spontaneous echo contrast with prethrombotic state in atrial fibrillation associated with systemic hypertension, idiopathic dilated cardiomyopathy, or no identifiable cause (lone). Am J Cardiol 1998; 81:1249–1252.

744. Zabalgoitia M, Halperin JL, Pearce LA, Blackshear JL, Asinger RW, Hart RG. Transesophageal echocardiographic correlates of clinical risk of thromboembolism in nonvalvular atrial fibrillation. J Am Coll Cardiol 1998; 31:1622–1626.

745. Falcone RA, Morady F, Armstrong WF. Transesophageal echocardiographic evaluation of left atrial appendage function and spontaneous contrast formation after chemical or electrical cardioversion of atrial fibrillation. Am J Cardiol 1996; 78:435–439.

746. Tsai LM, Chen JH, Lin LJ, Teng JK. Natural history of left atrial spontaneous echo contrast in nonrheumatic atrial fibrillation. Am J Cardiol 1997; 80:897–900.

747. Mugge A, Kuhn H, Nikutta P, Grote J, Lopez JA, Daniel WG. Assessment of left atrial appendage function by biplane transesophageal echocardiography in patients with nonrheumatic atrial fibrillation: identification of a subgroup of patients at increased embolic risk. J Am Coll Cardiol 1994; 23:599–607.

748. Kato H, Nakanishi M, Maekawa N, Ohnishi T, Yamamoto M. Evaluation of left atrial appendage stasis in patients with atrial fibrillation using transesophageal echocardiography with an intravenous albumin-contrast agent. Am J Cardiol 1996; 78:365–369.

749. Shively BK, Gelgand EA, Crawford MH. Regional left atrial stasis during atrial fibrillation and flutter: determinants and relation to stroke. J Am Coll Cardiol 1996; 27:1722–1729.

750. Kanter MC, Tegeler CH, Pearce LA, et al. Carotid stenosis in patients with atrial fibrillation: prevalence, risk factors, and relationship to stroke in the stroke prevention in atrial fibrillation study. Arch Intern Med 1994; 154:1372–1377.

751. Omran H, Jung W, Schimpf R, et al. Echocardiographic parameters for predicting maintenance of sinus rhythm after internal atrial defibrillation. Am J Cardiol 1998; 81:1446–1449.

752. Feinberg MS, Waggoner AD, Kater KM, Cox JL, Lindsay BD, Perez JE. Restoration of atrial function after the Maze procedure for patients with atrial fibrillation: assessment by Doppler echocardiography. Circulation 1994; 90(Suppl I): I-1285–I-1292.

753. Tavel ME. Clinical Phonocardiography and External Pulse Recording. 2nd ed. Chicago: Year Book Medical Publishers, 1973, pp. 211–225.

754. Krohn BG, Magidson O. Left ventricular ejection time following cardioversion. Am J Cardiol 1966; 18:729–737.

755. Grover DN, Mathur VS, Shrivastava S, Roy SB. Electromechanical correlation of left atrial function after cardioversion. Br Heart J 1971; 33:226–232.

756. Tavel ME. Clinical Phonocardiography and External Pulse

Recording. 2nd ed. Chicago: Year Book Medical Publishers, 1973, pp. 62, 67, 93, 94.

757. Imataka K, Nakaoka H, Kitahara Y, Fujii J, Ishibashi M, Yamaji T. Blood hematocrit changes during paroxysmal atrial fibrillation. Am J Cardiol 1987; 59:172–173.

758. Forfar JC, Toft AD. Thyrotoxic atrial fibrillation: an underdiagnosed condition? BMJ 1982; 2:909–910.

759. Bruce SA, Rangedara DC, Lewis RR, Corless D. Hyperthyroidism in elderly patients with atrial fibrillation and normal thyroid hormone measurements. J R Soc Med 1987; 80:74–76.

760. Forfar JC, Miller HC, Toft AD. Occult thyrotoxicosis: a correctable cause of "idiopathic" atrial fibrillation. Am J Cardiol 1979; 44:9–12.

761. Symons C, Myers A, Kingstone D, Boss M. Response to thyrotrophin-releasing hormone in atrial dysrhythmias. Postgrad Med J 1978; 54:658–662.

762. Forfar JC, Feek CM, Miller HC, Toft AD. Atrial fibrillation and isolated suppression of the pituitary-thyroid axis: response to specific antithyroid therapy. Int J Cardiol 1981; 1:43–48.

763. Ciaccheri M, Cecchi F, Arcangeli C, Dolara A, Zuppiroli A, Pieroni C. Occult thyrotoxicosis in patients with chronic and paroxysmal isolated atrial fibrillation. Clin Cardiol 1984; 7:413–416.

764. Sulimani RA. Diagnostic algorithm for atrial fibrillation caused by occult hyperthyroidism. Geriatrics 1989; 44:61–64.

765. Giladi M, Aderka D, Zeligman-Melatzki L, Finkelstein A, Ayalon D, Levo Y. Is idiopathic atrial fibrillation caused by occult thyrotoxicosis? A study of one hundred consecutive patients with atrial fibrillation. Int J Cardiol 1991; 30:309–313.

766. Wilber JK. Personal communication, 1998.

767. Sawin CT, Geller A, Wolf PA, et al. Low serum thyrotropin concentrations as a risk factor for atrial fibrillation in older persons. N Engl J Med 1994; 331:1249–1252.

768. Utiger RD. Subclinical hyperthyroidism: just a low serum thyrotropin concentration, or something more? N Engl J Med 1994; 331:1302–1303.

769. DeCarli C, Sprouse G, LaRosa JC. Serum magnesium levels in symptomatic atrial fibrillation and their relation to rhythm control by intravenous digoxin. Am J Cardiol 1986; 57:956–959.

770. Lip GY. Cardioversion of atrial fibrillation. Postgrad Med J 1995; 71:457–465.

771. Kumagai K, Fukunami M, Ohmori M, Kitabatake A, Kamada T, Hoki N. Increased intracardiovascular clotting in patients with chronic atrial fibrillation. J Am Coll Cardiol 1990; 16:377–380.

772. Lip GY, Lowe GD, Rumley A, Dunn FG. Increased markers of thrombogenesis in chronic atrial fibrillation: effects of warfarin treatment. Br Heart J 1995; 73:527–533.

773. Lip GY, Rumley A, Dunn FG, Lowe GD. Plasma fibrinogen and fibrin d-dimer in patients with atrial fibrillation: effects of cardioversion to sinus rhythm. Int J Cardiol 1995; 51:245–251.

774. Oltrona L, Broccolino M, Merlini PA, Spinola A, Pezzano A, Mannucci PM. Activation of the hemostatic mechanism after pharmacological cardioversion of acute nonvalvular atrial fibrillation. Circulation 1997; 95:2003–2006.

775. Lip GY, Lowe GD, Rumley A, Dunn FG. Fibrinogen and fibrin d-dimer levels in paroxysmal atrial fibrillation: evidence for intermediate elevated levels of intravascular thrombogenesis. Am Heart J 1996; 131:724–730.

776. Sohara H, Amitani S, Kurose M, Miyahara K. Atrial fibrillation activates platelets and coagulation in a time-dependent manner: a study in patients with paroxysmal atrial fibrillation. J Am Coll Cardiol 1997; 29:106–112.

777. Kelly PA, MacAulay-Hunter E, Astridge PS, Lowry PJ, Perrins EJ, Kaye GC. Failure of plasma atrial natriuretic peptide levels to increase during exercise in patients with chronic atrial fibrillation. Pacing Clin Electrophysiol 1997; 20:10–16.

778. Tuinenburg AE, van Veldhuisen DJ, Boomsma F, Van Den Berg MP, de Kam PJ, Crijns HJGM. Comparison of plasma neurohormones in congestive heart failure patients with atrial fibrillation versus patients with sinus rhythm. Am J Cardiol 1998; 81:1207–1209.

779. Mookherjee S, Anderson G Jr, Smulyan H, Vardan S. Atrial natriuretic peptide response to cardioversion of atrial flutter and fibrillation and role of associated heart failure. Am J Cardiol 1991; 67:377–380.

780. Arakawa M, Miwa H, Kambara K, et al. Changes in plasma concentrations of atrial natriuretic peptides after cardioversion of chronic atrial fibrillation. Am J Cardiol 1992; 70:550–552.

781. Fujiwara H, Ishikura F, Nagata S, Beppu S, Miyatake K. Plasma atrial natriuretic peptide response to direct current cardioversion of atrial fibrillation in patients with mitral stenosis. J Am Coll Cardiol 1993; 22:575–580.

782. Arakawa M, Miwa H, Noda T, et al. Alternations in atrial natriuretic peptide release after DC cardioversion of non-valvular chronic atrial fibrillation. Eur Heart J 1995; 16:977–985.

783. Nicklas JM, DiCarlo LA, Koller PT, et al. Plasma levels of immunoreactive atrial natriuretic factor increase during supraventricular tachycardia. Am Heart J 1986; 112:923–928.

784. Crozier IG, Ikram H, Nicholls MG, Espiner EA, Yandle TG. Atrial natriuretic peptide in spontaneous tachycardias. Br Heart J 1987; 58:96–100.

785. Hirata Y, Nozaki A, Toda I, et al. Plasma concentration of atrial natriuretic polypeptide in patients with atrial tachycardia. Jpn Heart J 1987; 28:53–61.

786. Tsai RC, Yamaji T, Ishibashi M, et al. Atrial natriuretic peptide during supraventricular tachycardia and relation to hemodynamic changes and renal function. Am J Cardiol 1988; 61:1260–1264.

787. Field LJ. Lone atrial fibrillation and autoantibodies: cause versus effect. J Cardiovasc Electrophysiol 1998; 9:618–619.

788. Maixent JM, Paganelli F, Scaglione J, Levy S. Antibodies against myosin in sera of patients with idiopathic paroxysmal atrial fibrillation. J Cardiovasc Electrophysiol 1998; 9:612–617.

789. Kieny JR, Sacrez A, Facello A, et al. Increase in radionuclide left ventricular ejection fraction after cardioversion of chronic atrial fibrillation in idiopathic dilated cardiomyopathy. Eur Heart J 1992; 13:1290–1295.

790. Gosselink AT, Blanksma PK, Crijns HJ, et al. Left ventricular beat-to-beat performance in atrial fibrillation: contribution of Frank-Starling mechanism after short rather than long RR intervals. J Am Coll Cardiol 1995; 26:1516–1521.

791. Petersen P, Madsen EB, Brun B, Pedersen F, Gyldensted C, Boysen G. Silent cerebral infarction in chronic atrial fibrillation. Stroke 1987; 18:1098–1100.

792. McIntosh HD, Kong Y, Morris JJ Jr. Hemodynamic effects of supraventricular tachycardia. Am J Med 1964; 37:712–727.

793. Mitchell JH, Shapiro W. Atrial function and the hemodynamic consequences of atrial fibrillation in man. Am J Cardiol 1969; 23:556–567.

794. Edmands RE, Greenspan K. Hemodynamic consequences of atrial fibrillation. Geriatrics 1971; 26:99–107.

795. Atwood JE. Exercise hemodynamics of atrial fibrillation. In Falk RH, Podrid PJ (eds). Atrial Fibrillation. Mechanisms and Management. New York: Raven Press, 1992, pp. 145–163.

796. Pozzoli M, Cioffi G, Traversi E, Pinna GD, Cobelli F, Tavazzi L. Predictors of primary atrial fibrillation and concomitant clinical and hemodynamic changes in patients with chronic heart failure: a prospective study in 344 patients with baseline sinus rhythm. J Am Coll Cardiol 1998; 32:197–204.

797. Hansen WR, McClendon RL, Kinsman JM. Auricular fibrillation; hemodynamic studies before and after conversion with quinidine. Am Heart J 1952; 44:499–516.

798. Reale A. Acute effects of countershock conversion of atrial fibrillation upon right and left heart hemodynamics. Circulation 1965; 32:214–222.

799. Herbert WH. Cardiac output and the varying R-R interval of atrial fibrillation. J Electrocardiol 1973; 6:131–135.

800. Gibson DG, Chamberlain DA, Coltart DJ, Mercer J. Effect of changes in ventricular activation on cardiac haemodynamics in man: comparison of right ventricular, left ventricular, and

simultaneous pacing of both ventricles. Br Heart J 1971; 33:397–400.

801. Daoud EG, Weiss R, Bahu M, et al. Effect of an irregular ventricular rhythm on cardiac output. Am J Cardiol 1996; 78:1433–1436.

802. Natale A, Zimerman L, Tomassoni G, et al. Impact on ventricular function and quality of life of transcatheter ablation of the atrioventricular junction in chronic atrial fibrillation with a normal ventricular response. Am J Cardiol 1996; 78:1431–1433.

803. Clark DM, Plumb VJ, Epstein AE, Kay GN. Hemodynamic effects of an irregular sequence of ventricular cycle lengths during atrial fibrillation. J Am Coll Cardiol 1997; 30:1039–1045.

804. Broch OJ, Muller O. Haemodynamic studies during auricular fibrillation and after restoration of sinus rhythm. Br Heart J 1957; 19:222–226.

805. Selzer A. Effects of atrial fibrillation upon the circulation in patients with mitral stenosis. Am Heart J 1960; 59:518–526.

806. Gilbert R, Eich RH, Smulyan H, Keighley J, Chir B, Auchincloss H. Effect on circulation of conversion of atrial fibrillation to sinus rhythm. Circulation 1963; 27:1079–1085.

807. Kahn DR, Wilson WS, Weber W, Sloan H. Hemodynamic studies before and after cardioversion. J Thorac Cardiovasc Surg 1964; 48:898–905.

808. Benchimol A, Ellis JG, Dimond EG, Wu T-L. Hemodynamic consequences of atrial and ventricular arrhythmias in man. Am Heart J 1965; 70:775–788.

809. Benchimol A, Lowe HM, Akre PR. Cardiovascular response to exercise during atrial fibrillation and after conversion to sinus rhythm. Am J Cardiol 1965; 16:31–41.

810. Morris JJ, Entman M, North WC, Kong Y, McIntosh H. The changes in cardiac output with reversion of atrial fibrillation to sinus rhythm. Circulation 1965; 31:670–678.

811. Duchelle RA. Indications for conversion of atrial fibrillation to normal sinus rhythm. Med Clin North Am 1966; 50:117–125.

812. Killip T, Baer RA. Hemodynamic effects after reversion from atrial fibrillation to sinus rhythm by precordial shock. J Clin Invest 1966; 45:658–671.

813. Rodman T, Pastor BH, Figueroa W. Effect on cardiac output of conversion from atrial fibrillation to normal sinus mechanism. Am J Med 1966; 41:249–258.

814. Resnekov L. Haemodynamic studies before and after electrical conversion of atrial fibrillation and flutter to sinus rhythm. Br Heart J 1967; 29:700–708.

815. Kaplan MA, Gray RE, Iseri LT. Metabolic and hemodynamic responses to exercise during atrial fibrillation and sinus rhythm. Am J Cardiol 1968; 22:543–549.

816. Shapiro W, Klein G. Alterations in cardiac function immediately following electrical conversion of atrial fibrillation to normal sinus rhythm. Circulation 1968; 38:1074–1084.

817. Scott ME, Patterson GC. Cardiac output after direct current conversion of atrial fibrillation. Br Heart J 1969; 31:87–90.

818. Van Gelder IC, Crijns HJ, Blanksma PK, et al. Time course of hemodynamic changes and improvement of exercise tolerance after cardioversion of chronic atrial fibrillation unassociated with cardiac valve disease. Am J Cardiol 1993; 72:560–566.

819. Khaja F, Parker JO. Hemodynamic effects of cardioversion in chronic atrial fibrillation: special reference to coronary artery disease. Arch Intern Med 1972; 129:433–440.

820. Gosselink AT, Crijns HJ, Van Den Berg MP, et al. Functional capacity before and after cardioversion of atrial fibrillation: a controlled study. Br Heart J 1994; 72:161–166.

821. Lipkin DP, Frenneaux M, Stewart R, Joshi J, Lowe T, McKenna WJ. Delayed improvement in exercise capacity after cardioversion of atrial fibrillation to sinus rhythm. Br Heart J 1988; 59:572–577.

822. Pardaens K, Van Cleemput J, Vanhaecke J, Fagard RH. Atrial fibrillation is associated with a lower exercise capacity in male chronic heart failure patients. Heart 1997; 78:564–568.

823. Ueshima K, Myers J, Morris CK, Atwood JE, Kawaguchi T, Froelicher VF. The effect of cardioversion on exercise

capacity in patients with atrial fibrillation. Am Heart J 1993; 126:1021–1024.

824. Lau CP, Jiang ZY, Tang MO. Efficacy of ventricular rate stabilization by right ventricular pacing during atrial fibrillation. PACE 1998; 21:542–548.

825. Meisner JS, Keren G, Pajaro OE, et al. Atrial contribution to ventricular filling in mitral stenosis. Circulation 1991; 84:1469–1480.

826. Arani DT, Carleton RA. The deleterious role of tachycardia in mitral stenosis. Circulation 1967; 36:511–516.

827. Mohan JC, Arora R. Effects of atrial fibrillation on left ventricular function and geometry in mitral stenosis. Am J Cardiol 1997; 80:1618–1620.

828. Ikram H, Nixon PG, Arcan T. Left atrial function after electrical conversion to sinus rhythm. Br Heart J 1968; 30:80–83.

829. Friedman HS, Gomes JA, Tardio A, Levites R, Haft JI. Appearance of atrial rhythm with absent P wave in longstanding atrial fibrillation. Chest 1974; 66:172–175.

830. Mahlich J, Schweizer W, Burkart F. Atrial function after cardioversion for atrial fibrillation. Br Heart J 1973; 35:24–27.

831. Shapiro EP, Effron MB, Lima S, Ouyang P, Siu CO, Bush D. Transient atrial dysfunction after conversion of chronic atrial fibrillation to sinus rhythm. Am J Cardiol 1988; 62:1202–1207.

832. Manning WJ, Leeman DE, Gotch PJ, Come PC. Pulsed Doppler evaluation of atrial mechanical function after electrical cardioversion of atrial fibrillation. J Am Coll Cardiol 1989; 13:617–623.

833. O'Neill PG, Puleo PR, Bolli R, Rokey R. Return of atrial mechanical function following electrical conversion of atrial dysrhythmias. Am Heart J 1990; 120:353–359.

834. Iuchi A, Oki T, Fukuda N, et al. Changes in transmitral and pulmonary venous flow velocity patterns after cardioversion of atrial fibrillation. Am Heart J 1996; 131:270–275.

835. Harjai KJ, Mobarek SK, Cheirif J, Boulos LM, Murgo JP, Abi-Samra F. Clinical variables affecting recovery of left atrial mechanical function after cardioversion from atrial fibrillation. J Am Coll Cardiol 1997; 30:481–486.

836. Omran H, Jung W, Rabahieh R, et al. Left atrial chamber and appendage function after internal atrial defibrillation: a prospective and serial transesophageal echocardiographic study. J Am Coll Cardiol 1997; 29:131–138.

837. Braunwald E. Symposium on cardiac arrhythmias. Am J Med 1964; 37:665–669.

838. Logan WFWE, Rowlands DJ, Howitt G, Holmes AM. Left atrial activity following cardioversion. Lancet 1965; 2:471–473.

839. Thompson ME, Metzger CC, Shaver JA, Heidenreich FP, Martin CE, Leonard JJ. Assessment of left atrial transport function immediately after cardioversion. Am J Cardiol 1972; 29:481–489.

840. Graettinger JS, Carleton RA, Muenster JJ. Circulatory consequences of changes in cardiac rhythm produced in patients by transthoracic direct-current shock. J Clin Invest 1964; 43:2290–2302.

841. Scott ME, Geddes JS, Patterson GC. The long term prognosis of atrial fibrillation following direct current conversion. Ulster Med J 1968; 37:155–161.

842. Jovic A, Troskot R. Recovery of atrial systolic function after pharmacological conversion of chronic atrial fibrillation to sinus rhythm: a Doppler echocardiographic study. Heart 1997; 77:46–49.

843. Bellotti P, Spirito P, Lupi G, Vecchio C. Left atrial appendage function assessed by transesophageal echocardiography before and on the day after elective cardioversion for nonvalvular atrial fibrillation. Am J Cardiol 1998; 81:1199–1202.

844. Harjai K, Mobarek S, Abi-Samra F, et al. Mechanical dysfunction of the left atrium and the left atrial appendage following cardioversion of atrial fibrillation and its relation to total electrical energy used for cardioversion. Am J Cardiol 1998; 81:1125–1129.

845. Rowlands DJ, Logan WFWE, Howitt G. Atrial function after cardioversion. Am Heart J 1967; 74:149–160.

846. Shite J, Yokota Y, Yokoyama M. Heterogeneity and time course of improvement in cardiac function after cardioversion of chronic atrial fibrillation: assessment of serial echocardiographic indices. Br Heart J 1993; 70:154–159.

847. Ito T, Suwa M, Otake Y, et al. Assessment of left atrial appendage function after cardioversion of atrial fibrillation: relation to left atrial mechanical function. Am Heart J 1998; 135:1020–1026.

848. Bell HE. Direct-current shock for atrial fibrillation. Lancet 1966; 2:911.

849. Ikram H, Nixon PGF, Arcan T. Direct-current shock for atrial fibrillation. Lancet 1966; 2:911.

850. Lindsay J. Pulmonary edema following cardioversion. Am Heart J 1967; 74:434–435.

851. Mattioli AV, Tarabini Castellani E, Vivoli D, Molinari R, Mattioli G. Restoration of atrial function after atrial fibrillation of different etiological origins. Cardiology 1996; 87:205–211.

852. Mitusch R, Garbe M, Schmucker G, Schwabe K, Stierle U, Sheikhzadeh A. Relation of left atrial appendage function to the duration and reversibility of nonvalvular atrial fibrillation. Am J Cardiol 1995; 75:944–947.

853. Manning WJ, Silverman DI, Katz SE, et al. Temporal dependence of the return of atrial mechanical function on the mode of cardioversion of atrial fibrillation to sinus rhythm. Am J Cardiol 1995; 75:624–626.

854. Grimm RA, Leung DY, Black IW, Stewart WJ, Thomas JD, Klein AL. Left atrial appendage "stunning" after spontaneous conversion of atrial fibrillation demonstrated by transesophageal Doppler echocardiography. Am Heart J 1995; 130:174–176.

855. Sparks PB, Kulkarni R, Vohra JK, et al. Effect of direct current shocks on left atrial mechanical function in patients with structural heart disease. J Am Coll Cardiol 1998; 31:1395–1399.

856. Gallagher MM, Obel OA, Camm JA. Tachycardia-induced atrial myopathy: an important mechanism in the pathophysiology of atrial fibrillation? J Cardiovasc Electrophysiol 1997; 8:1065–1074.

857. Alboni P, Scarfo S, Fuca G, Paparella N, Yannacopulu P. Hemodynamics of idiopathic paroxysmal atrial fibrillation. Pacing Clin Electrophysiol 1995; 18:980–985.

858. Lau CP, Leung WH, Wong CK, Cheng CH. Haemodynamics of induced atrial fibrillation: a comparative assessment with sinus rhythm, atrial and ventricular pacing. Eur Heart J 1990; 11:219–224.

859. Kaye GC, Nathan AW, Camm AJ. Polyuria associated with paroxysmal tachycardia. Clin Prog Pacing Electrophysiol 1984; 2:349–359.

860. Wood P. Polyuria in paroxysmal tachycardia and paroxysmal atrial flutter and fibrillation. Br Heart J 1963; 25:273–282.

861. Flensted-Jensen E. Wolff-Parkinson-White syndrome. A long-term follow-up of 47 cases. Acta Med Scand 1969; 186:65–74.

862. Nilsson G, Pettersson A, Hedner J, Hedner T. Increased plasma levels of atrial natriuretic peptide (ANP) in patients with paroxysmal supraventricular tachyarrhythmias. Acta Med Scand 1987; 221:15–21.

863. Tsai RC, Yamaji T, Ishibashi M, et al. Mechanism of polyuria and natriuresis associated with paroxysmal supraventricular tachycardia. Jpn Heart J 1987; 28:203–209.

864. Canepa-Anson R, Williams M, Marshall J, Mitsuoka T, Lightman S, Sutton R. Mechanism of polyuria and natriuresis in atrioventricular nodal tachycardia. Br Med J Clin Res Ed 1984; 289:861–868.

865. Fujii T, Kojima S, Imanishi M, Ohe T, Omae T. Different mechanisms of polyuria and natriuresis associated with paroxysmal supraventricular tachycardia. Am J Cardiol 1991; 68:343–348.

866. Schiffrin EL, Gutkowska J, Kuchel O, Cantin M, Genest J. Plasma concentration of atrial natriuretic factor in a patient with paroxysmal atrial tachycardia. N Engl J Med 1985; 312:1196–1197.

867. Yamaji T, Ishibashi M, Nakaoka H, Imataka K, Amano M, Fujii J. Possible role for atrial natriuretic peptide in polyuria associated with paroxysmal atrial arrhythmias. Lancet 1985; 1:1211.

868. Roy D, Paillard F, Cassidy D, et al. Atrial natriuretic factor during atrial fibrillation and supraventricular tachycardia. J Am Coll Cardiol 1987; 9:509–514.

869. Kojima S, Fujii T, Ohe T, et al. Physiologic changes during supraventricular tachycardia and release of atrial natriuretic peptide. Am J Cardiol 1988; 62:576–579.

870. Lavy S, Stern S, Melamed E, Cooper G, Keren A, Levy P. Effect of chronic atrial fibrillation on regional cerebral blood flow. Stroke 1980; 11:35–38.

871. Davies MJ. Pathology of Conducting Tissue of the Heart. New York: Appleton-Century-Crofts, 1971.

872. James TN. Diversity of histopathologic correlates of atrial fibrillation. In Kulbertus HE, Olsson SB, Schlepper M (eds). Atrial Fibrillation. Kiruna, Molndal, Sweden: AB Hassle, 1982, pp. 13–32.

873. Rossi L. Histopathologic correlates of atrial arrhythmias. In Touboul P, Waldo AL (eds). Atrial Arrhythmias. Current Concepts and Management. St. Louis: Mosby–Year Book, 1990, pp. 27–40.

874. Bharati S, Lev M. Histology of the normal and diseased atrium. In Falk RH, Podrid PJ (eds). Atrial Fibrillation. Mechanisms and Management. New York: Raven Press, 1992, pp. 15–39.

875. Lie JT, Falk RH. Pathology of atrial fibrillation: insights from autopsy studies. In Falk RH, Podrid PJ (eds). Atrial Fibrillation. Mechanisms and Management. New York: Raven Press, 1992, pp. 1–14.

876. Bailey GW, Braniff BA, Hancock EW, Cohn KE. Relation of left atrial pathology to atrial fibrillation in mitral valvular disease. Ann Intern Med 1968; 69:13–20.

877. Hudson REB. The human pacemaker and its pathology. Br Heart J 1960; 22:153–167.

878. James TN. Myocardial infarction and atrial arrhythmias. Circulation 1961; 24:761–776.

879. Cancilla PA, Nicklaus TM. Atrial fibrillation with occlusion of the sinus node artery. Arch Intern Med 1966; 117:422–424.

880. Thiedemann KU, Ferrans VJ. Left atrial ultrastructure in mitral valvular disease. Am J Pathol 1977; 89:575–604.

881. Bharati S, Scheinman M, Lev M. Histologic findings of the heart and the conduction system in the first patient who underwent catheter ablation. Pacing Clin Electrophysiol 1992; 15:1291–1299.

882. Frustaci A, Caldarulo M, Buffon A, Bellocci F, Fenici R, Melina D. Cardiac biopsy in patients with "primary" atrial fibrillation: histologic evidence of occult myocardial diseases. Chest 1991; 100:303–306.

883. Frustaci A, Chimenti C, Bellocci F, Morgante E, Russo MA, Maseri A. Histological substrate of atrial biopsies in patients with lone atrial fibrillation. Circulation 1997; 96:1180–1184.

884. Waldo AL. Mechanisms of atrial fibrillation, atrial flutter, and ectopic atrial tachycardia: a brief review. Circulation 1987; 75(Suppl III):III-37–III-40.

885. Cox JL, Schuessler RB, Boineau JP. The surgical treatment of atrial fibrillation. I. Summary of the current concepts of the mechanisms of atrial flutter and atrial fibrillation. J Thorac Cardiovasc Surg 1991; 101:402–405.

886. Josephson ME. Clinical Cardiac Electrophysiology. Techniques and Interpretations. 2nd ed. Philadelphia: Lea & Febiger, 1993, pp. 5–21.

887. Allessie MA, Konings K, Kirchhof CJ, Wijffels M. Electrophysiologic mechanisms of perpetuation of atrial fibrillation. Am J Cardiol 1996; 77:10A–23A.

888. Hashiba K, Centurion OA, Shimizu A. Electrophysiologic characteristics of human atrial muscle in paroxysmal atrial fibrillation. Am Heart J 1996; 131:778–789.

889. Janse MJ. Why does atrial fibrillation occur? Eur Heart J 1997; 18:C12–C18.

890. Zipes DP. Atrial fibrillation: a tachycardia-induced atrial cardiomyopathy. Circulation 1997; 95:562–564.

891. Scherlag BJ, Lau SH, Helfant RH, Berkowitz WD, Stein E, Damato AN. Catheter technique for recording His bundle activity in man. Circulation 1969; 39:13–18.

892. Lau SH, Damato AN, Berkowitz WD, Patton RD. A study of

atrioventricular conduction in atrial fibrillation and flutter in man using His bundle recordings. Circulation 1969; 40:71–78.

893. Waldo AL, MacLean WA, Cooper TB, Kouchoukos NT, Karp RB. Use of temporarily placed epicardial atrial wire electrodes for the diagnosis and treatment of cardiac arrhythmias following open-heart surgery. J Thorac Cardiovasc Surg 1978; 76:500–505.

894. Waldo AL, Henthorn RW, Plumb VJ. Temporary epicardial wire electrodes in the diagnosis and treatment of arrhythmias after open heart surgery. Am J Surg 1984; 148:275–283.

895. Wells JL Jr, Karp RB, Kouchoukos NT, MacLean WA, James TN, Waldo AL. Characterization of atrial fibrillation in man: studies following open heart surgery. Pacing Clin Electrophysiol 1978; 1:426–438.

896. Puech P, Grolleau R, Rebuffat G. Intra-atrial mapping of atrial fibrillation in man. In Kulbertus HE, Olsson SB, Schlepper M (eds). Atrial Fibrillation. Kiruna, Molndal, Sweden: AB Hassle, 1982, pp. 94–109.

897. Waldo AL, Henthorn RW, Plumb VJ. Relevance of electrograms and transient entrainment for antitachycardia devices. PACE 1984; 7:588–600.

898. Tanigawa M, Fukatani M, Konoe A, Isomoto S, Kadena M, Hashiba K. Prolonged and fractionated right atrial electrograms during sinus rhythm in patients with paroxysmal atrial fibrillation and sick sinus node syndrome. J Am Coll Cardiol 1991; 17:403–408.

899. Konings KT, Smeets JL, Penn OC, Wellens HJJ, Allessie MA. Configuration of unipolar atrial electrograms during electrically induced atrial fibrillation in humans. Circulation 1997; 95:1231–1241.

900. Capucci A, Biffi M, Boriani G, et al. Dynamic electrophysiological behavior of human atria during paroxysmal atrial fibrillation. Circulation 1995; 92:1193–1202.

901. Hoekstra BP, Diks CG, Allessie MA, DeGoede J. Nonlinear analysis of epicardial atrial electrograms of electrically induced atrial fibrillation in man. J Cardiovasc Electrophysiol 1995; 6:419–440.

902. Kerr CR, Mason MA. Amplitude of atrial electrical activity during sinus rhythm and during atrial flutter-fibrillation. Pacing Clin Electrophysiol 1985; 8:348–355.

903. Wood MA, Moskovljevic P, Stambler BS, Ellenbogen KA. Comparison of bipolar atrial electrogram amplitude in sinus rhythm, atrial fibrillation, and atrial flutter. Pacing Clin Electrophysiol 1996; 19:150–156.

904. Ropella KM, Sahakian AV, Baerman JM, Swiryn S. Effects of procainamide on intra-atrial (corrected) electrograms during atrial fibrillation: implications (corrected) for detection algorithms. Circulation 1988; 77:1047–1054.

905. Slocum J, Sahakian A, Swiryn S. Computer discrimination of atrial fibrillation and regular atrial rhythms from intra-atrial electrograms. Pacing Clin Electrophysiol 1988; 11:610–621.

906. Haissaguerre M, Gencel L, Fischer B, et al. Successful catheter ablation of atrial fibrillation. J Cardiovasc Electrophysiol 1994; 5:1045–1052.

907. Haissaguerre M, Marcus FI, Fischer B, Clementy J. Radiofrequency catheter ablation in unusual mechanisms of atrial fibrillation: report of three cases. J Cardiovasc Electrophysiol 1994; 5:743–751.

908. Jais P, Haissaguerre M, Shah DC, et al. A focal source of atrial fibrillation treated by discrete radiofrequency ablation. Circulation 1997; 95:572–576.

909. Langendorf R. How everything started in clinical electrophysiology. In Brugada P, Wellens HJJ (eds). Cardiac Arrhythmias. Where to Go from Here? Mount Kisco, NY: Futura Publishing Co., 1987, pp. 715–722.

910. Langendorf R, Pick A. Concealed conduction: further evaluation of a fundamental aspect of propagation of the cardiac impulse. Circulation 1956; 13:381–399.

911. Langendorf R, Pick A, Edelist A, Katz LN. Experimental demonstration of concealed AV conduction in the human heart. Circulation 1965; 32:386–393.

912. Cohen SI, Lau SH, Berkowitz WD, Damato AN. Concealed

conduction during atrial fibrillation. Am J Cardiol 1970; 25:416–419.

913. Brugada P, Roy D, Weiss J, Dassen WR, Wellens HJJ. Dual atrio-ventricular nodal pathways and atrial fibrillation. Pacing Clin Electrophysiol 1984; 7:240–247.

914. Schamroth L. Reciprocal rhythm of ventricular origin during atrial fibrillation with complete AV block. Br Heart J 1970; 32:564–567.

915. Wittkampf FHM, de Jongste MJL, Meijler FL. Competitive anterograde and retrograde atrioventricular junctional activation in atrial fibrillation. J Cardiovasc Electrophysiol 1990; 1:448–456.

916. Wittkampf FHM, de Jongste MJL, Meijler FL. Atrioventricular nodal response to retrograde activation in atrial fibrillation. J Cardiovasc Electrophysiol 1990; 1:437–447.

917. Soderstrom N. What is the reason for the ventricular arrhythmia in cases of auricular fibrillation? Am Heart J 1950; 40:212–223.

918. Horan LG, Kistler JC. Study of ventricular response in atrial fibrillation. Circ Res 1961; 9:305–311.

919. Goldstein RE, Barnett GO. A statistical study of the ventricular irregularity of atrial fibrillation. Comput Biomed Res 1967; 1:146–161.

920. Bootsma BK, Hoelsen AJ, Strackee J, Meijler FL. Analysis of R-R intervals in patients with atrial fibrillation at rest and during exercise. Circulation 1970; 41:783–794.

921. Brody DA. Ventricular rate patterns in atrial fibrillation. Circulation 1970; 41:733–735.

922. Redfors A. Digoxin dosage and ventricular rate at rest and exercise in patients with atrial fibrillation. Acta Med Scand 1971; 190:321–333.

923. Ware JH, Tecklenberg PL, Miller M, Raff MS, Grauer L, Goldstein RE. A new method for quantifying ventricular regularization during atrial fibrillation. J Electrocardiol 1977; 10:149–155.

924. Hashida E, Yoshitani N, Tasaki T. A study on the irregularity of the sequence of R-R intervals in chronic atrial fibrillation in man based on the time series analysis and the information theory. Jpn Heart J 1978; 19:839–851.

925. Meijler FL. Atrial fibrillation: a new look at an old arrhythmia. J Am Coll Cardiol 1983; 2:391–393.

926. Hashida E, Tasaki T. Considerations on the nature of irregularity of the sequence of RR intervals and the function of the atrioventricular node in atrial fibrillation in man based on time series analysis. Jpn Heart J 1984; 25:669–687.

927. Watt JH, Donner AP, McKinney CM, Klein GJ. Atrial fibrillation: minimal sampling interval to estimate average rate. J Electrocardiol 1984; 17:153–156.

928. Meijler FL, van der Tweel I, Herbschleb JN, Hauer RN, Robles de Medina EO. Role of atrial fibrillation and atrioventricular conduction (including Wolff-Parkinson-White syndrome) in sudden death. J Am Coll Cardiol 1985; 5:17B–22B.

929. Olsson SB, Cai N, Edvardsson N, Talwar KK. Prediction of terminal atrial myocardial repolarisation from incomplete phase 3 data. Cardiovasc Res 1989; 23:53–59.

930. Fujiki A, Tani M, Mizumaki K, Yoshida S, Sasayama S. Quantification of human concealed atrioventricular nodal conduction: relation to ventricular response during atrial fibrillation. Am Heart J 1990; 120:598–603.

931. Rawles JM. What is meant by a "controlled" ventricular rate in atrial fibrillation? Br Heart J 1990; 63:157–161.

932. Toivonen L, Kadish A, Kou W, Morady F. Determinants of the ventricular rate during atrial fibrillation. J Am Coll Cardiol 1990; 16:1194–1200.

933. Meijler FL, Wittkampf FHM. Role of the atrioventricular node in atrial fibrillation. In Falk RH, Podrid PJ (eds). Atrial Fibrillation. Mechanisms and Management. New York: Raven Press, 1992, pp. 59–80.

934. Kirsh JA, Sahakian AV, Baerman JM, Swiryn S. Ventricular response to atrial fibrillation: role of atrioventricular conduction pathways. J Am Coll Cardiol 1988; 12:1265–1272.

935. Bollmann A, Kanuru NK, McTeague KK, Walter PF, DeLurgio DB, Langberg JJ. Frequency analysis of human

atrial fibrillation using the surface electrocardiogram and its response to ibutilide. Am J Cardiol 1998; 81:1439–1445.

936. Lewis T. Auricular fibrillation and its relationship to clinical irregularity of the heart. Heart 1910; 1:368.

937. Rowland E, Curry P, Fox K, Krikler D. Relation between atrioventricular pathways and ventricular response during atrial fibrillation and flutter. Br Heart J 1981; 45:83–87.

938. Raeder EA. Circadian fluctuations in ventricular response to atrial fibrillation. Am J Cardiol 1990; 66:1013–1016.

939. Hayano J, Sakata S, Okada A, Mukai S, Fujinami T. Circadian rhythms of atrioventricular conduction properties in chronic atrial fibrillation with and without heart failure. J Am Coll Cardiol 1998; 31:158–166.

940. Rawles JM, Pai GR, Reid SR. Paradoxical effect of respiration on ventricular rate in atrial fibrillation. Clin Sci 1989; 76:109–112.

941. Simpson RJ Jr, Foster JR, Mulrow JP, Gettes LS. The electrophysiological substrate of atrial fibrillation. Pacing Clin Electrophysiol 1983; 6:1166–1170.

942. Killip T, Gault JH. Model of onset of atrial fibrillation in man. Am Heart J 1965; 70:172–179.

943. Haft JI, Lau SH, Stein E, Kosowsky BD, Damato AN. Atrial fibrillation produced by atrial stimulation. Circulation 1968; 37:70–74.

944. Bennett MA, Pentecost BL. The pattern of onset and spontaneous cessation of atrial fibrillation in man. Circulation 1970; 41:981–988.

945. Shen EN, Sung RJ. Initiation of atrial fibrillation by spontaneous ventricular premature beats in concealed Wolff-Parkinson-White syndrome. Am Heart J 1982; 103:911–912.

946. Timmermans C, Rodriguez LM, Smeets JLRM, Wellens HJJ. Immediate reinitiation of atrial fibrillation following internal atrial defibrillation. J Cardiovasc Electrophysiol 1998; 9:122–128.

947. Watson RM, Josephson ME. Atrial flutter. I. Electrophysiologic substrates and modes of initiation and termination. Am J Cardiol 1980; 45:732–741.

948. Kuhlkamp V, Haasis R, Seipel L. Atrial vulnerability and electrophysiology determined in patients with and without paroxysmal atrial fibrillation. Pacing Clin Electrophysiol 1992; 15:71–80.

949. Papageorgiou P, Anselme F, Kirchhof CJ, et al. Coronary sinus pacing prevents induction of atrial fibrillation. Circulation 1997; 96:1893–1898.

950. Josephson ME, Scharf DL, Kastor JA, Kitchen JG. Atrial endocardial activation in man: electrode catheter technique of endocardial mapping. Am J Cardiol 1977; 39:972–981.

951. Michelucci A, Padeletti L, Fradella GA. Atrial refractoriness and spontaneous or induced atrial fibrillation. Acta Cardiol 1982; 37:333–344.

952. Simpson RJ Jr, Foster JR, Gettes LS. Atrial excitability and conduction in patients with interatrial conduction defects. Am J Cardiol 1982; 50:1331–1337.

953. Cosio FG, Palacios J, Vidal JM, Cocina EG, Gomez-Sanchez MA, Tamargo L. Electrophysiologic studies in atrial fibrillation: slow conduction of premature impulses: a possible manifestation of the background for reentry. Am J Cardiol 1983; 51:122–130.

954. Ohe T, Matsuhisa M, Kamakura S, et al. Relation between the widening of the fragmented atrial activity zone and atrial fibrillation. Am J Cardiol 1983; 52:1219–1222.

955. Buxton AE, Waxman HL, Marchlinski FE, Josephson ME. Atrial conduction: effects of extrastimuli with and without atrial dysrhythmias. Am J Cardiol 1984; 54:755–761.

956. Simpson RJ Jr, Amara I, Foster JR, Woelfel A, Gettes LS. Thresholds, refractory periods, and conduction times of the normal and diseased human atrium. Am Heart J 1988; 116:1080–1090.

957. Aizawa Y, Miyajima S, Niwano S, Tamura M, Shibata A. Augmented fragmentation of atrial activity upon premature electrical stimuli by verapamil. Angiology 1989; 40:94–100.

958. Shimizu A, Fukatani M, Tanigawa M, Mori M, Hashiba K. Intra-atrial conduction delay and fragmented atrial activity in patients with paroxysmal atrial fibrillation. Jpn Circul J 1989; 53:1023–1030.

959. Niwano S, Aizawa Y. Fragmented atrial activity in patients with transient atrial fibrillation. Am Heart J 1991; 121:62–67.

960. Simpson RJ. Clinical electrophysiology of the normal and diseased human atria. In Falk RH, Podrid PJ (eds). Atrial Fibrillation. Mechanisms and Management. New York: Raven Press, 1992, pp. 321–332.

961. Gaita F, Giustetto C, Riccardi R, Mangiardi L, Rosettani E, Brusca A. A Wolff-Parkinson-White syndrome: atrial vulnerability and electrophysiologic features in patients with and without atrial fibrillation. In Attuel P, Coumel P, Janse MJ (eds). The Atrium in Health and Disease. Mount Kisco, NY: Futura Publishing Co., 1989, pp. 203–212.

962. Gaita F, Giustetto C, Riccardi R, et al. Relation between spontaneous atrial fibrillation and atrial vulnerability in patients with Wolff-Parkinson-White pattern. Pacing Clin Electrophysiol 1990; 13:1249–1253.

963. Wyndham CRC, Amat-y-Leon F, Wu D, et al. Effects of cycle length on atrial vulnerability. Circulation 1977; 55:260–267.

964. Luck JC, Engel TR. Dispersion of atrial refractoriness in patients with sinus node dysfunction. Circulation 1979; 60:404–412.

965. Attuel P, Childers R, Cauchemez B, Poveda J, Mugica J, Coumel P. Failure in the rate adaptation of the atrial refractory period: its relationship to vulnerability. Int J Cardiol 1982; 2:179–197.

966. Fujiki A, Yoshida S, Sasayama S. Paroxysmal atrial fibrillation with and without primary atrial vulnerability: clinical and electrophysiological differences. J Electrocardiol 1989; 22:153–158.

967. Misier AR, Opthof T, van Hemel NM, et al. Increased dispersion of "refractoriness" in patients with idiopathic paroxysmal atrial fibrillation. J Am Coll Cardiol 1992; 19:1531–1535.

968. Franz MR, Karasik PL, Li C, Moubarak J, Chavez M. Electrical remodeling of the human atrium: similar effects in patients with chronic atrial fibrillation and atrial flutter. J Am Coll Cardiol 1997; 30:1785–1792.

969. Yu WC, Chen SA, Lee SH, et al. Tachycardia-induced change of atrial refractory period in humans. Rate dependency and effects of antiarrhythmic drugs. Circulation 1998; 97:2331–2337.

970. Chauvin M, Brechenmacher C. Atrial refractory periods after atrial premature beats in patients with paroxysmal atrial fibrillation. Pacing Clin Electrophysiol 1989; 12:1018–1026.

971. Daoud EG, Bogun F, Goyal R, et al. Effect of atrial fibrillation on atrial refractoriness in humans. Circulation 1996; 94:1600–1606.

972. Daoud EG, Pariseau B, Niebauer M, et al. Response of type I atrial fibrillation to atrial pacing in humans. Circulation 1996; 94:1036–1040.

973. Pandozi C, Bianconi L, Villani M, et al. Local capture by atrial pacing in spontaneous chronic atrial fibrillation. Circulation 1997; 95:2416–2422.

974. Brembilla-Perrot B. Activation of atria in chronic atrial fibrillation is not a random phenomenon in man. Eur Heart J 1997; 18:186–187.

975. Cox JL, Canavan TE, Schuessler RB, et al. The surgical treatment of atrial fibrillation. II. Intraoperative electrophysiologic mapping and description of the electrophysiologic basis of atrial flutter and atrial fibrillation. J Thorac Cardiovasc Surg 1991; 101:406–426.

976. Harada A, Sasaki K, Fukushima T, et al. Atrial activation during chronic atrial fibrillation in patients with isolated mitral valve disease. Ann Thorac Surg 1996; 61:104–111.

977. Jais P, Haissaguerre M, Shah DC, Chouairi S, Clementy J. Regional disparities of endocardial atrial activation in paroxysmal atrial fibrillation. Pacing Clin Electrophysiol 1996; 19:1998–2003.

978. Fujimura O, Klein GJ, Yee R, Sharma AD, Boahene KA. Atrial fibrillation in the Wolff-Parkinson-White syndrome. In Touboul P, Waldo AL (eds). Atrial Arrhythmias. Current Concepts and Management. St. Louis: Mosby–Year Book, 1990, pp. 262–269.

979. Chen PS, Pressley JC, Tang AS, Packer DL, Gallagher JJ, Prystowsky EN. New observations on atrial fibrillation before

and after surgical treatment in patients with the Wolff-Parkinson-White syndrome. J Am Coll Cardiol 1992; 19:974–981.

980. Wellens HJJ, Smeets JLRM, Rodriguez LM, Gorgels APM. Atrial fibrillation in Wolff-Parkinson-White syndrome. In Falk RH, Podrid PJ (eds). Atrial Fibrillation. Mechanisms and Management. New York: Raven Press, 1992, pp. 333–344.

981. Wellens HJJ. The electrophysiologic properties of the accessory pathway in the Wolff-Parkinson-White syndrome. In Wellens HJJ, Lie KI, Janse KI (eds). The Conduction System of the Heart. Philadelphia: Lea & Febiger, 1976, pp. 578–581.

982. Sellers TD Jr, Bashore TM, Gallagher JJ. Digitalis in the pre-excitation syndrome: analysis during atrial fibrillation. Circulation 1977; 56:260–267.

983. Sung RJ, Castellanos A, Mallon SM, Bloom MG, Gelband H, Myerburg RJ. Mechanisms of spontaneous alternation between reciprocating tachycardia and atrial flutter-fibrillation in the Wolff-Parkinson-White syndrome. Circulation 1977; 56:409–416.

984. Denes P, Cummings JM, Simpson R, et al. Effects of propranolol on anomalous pathway refractoriness and circus movement tachycardias in patients with preexcitation. Am J Cardiol 1978; 41:1061–1067.

985. Cosio FG, Benson DW, Anderson RW, et al. Onset of atrial fibrillation during antidromic tachycardia: association with sudden cardiac arrest and ventricular fibrillation in a patient with Wolff-Parkinson-White syndrome. Am J Cardiol 1982; 50:353–359.

986. Morady F, Sledge C, Shen E, Sung RJ, Gonzales R, Scheinman MM. Electrophysiologic testing in the management of patients with the Wolff-Parkinson-White syndrome and atrial fibrillation. Am J Cardiol 1983; 51:1623–1628.

987. Rinne C, Klein GJ, Sharma AD, Yee R, Milstein S, Rattes MF. Relation between clinical presentation and induced arrhythmias in the Wolff-Parkinson-White syndrome. Am J Cardiol 1987; 60:576–579.

988. D'Este D, Pasqual A, Bertaglia M, et al. Evaluation of atrial vulnerability with transoesophageal stimulation in patients with atrioventricular junctional reentrant tachycardia: comparison with patients with ventricular pre-excitation and with normal subjects. Eur Heart J 1995; 16:1632–1636.

989. Waspe LE, Brodman R, Kim SG, Fisher JD. Susceptibility to atrial fibrillation and ventricular tachyarrhythmia in the Wolff-Parkinson-White syndrome: role of the accessory pathway. Am Heart J 1986; 112:1141–1152.

990. Iesaka Y, Yamane T, Takahashi A, et al. Retrograde multiple and multifiber accessory pathway conduction in the Wolff-Parkinson-White syndrome: potential precipitating factor of atrial fibrillation. J Cardiovasc Electrophysiol 1998; 9:141–151.

991. Sharma AD, Klein GJ, Guiraudon GM, Milstein S. Atrial fibrillation in patients with Wolff-Parkinson-White syndrome: incidence after surgical ablation of the accessory pathway. Circulation 1985; 72:161–169.

992. Wathen M, Natale A, Wolfe K, Yee R, Klein G. Initiation of atrial fibrillation in the Wolff-Parkinson-White syndrome: the importance of the accessory pathway. Am Heart J 1993; 125:753–759.

993. Fujimura O, Klein GJ, Yee R, Sharma AD. Mode of onset of atrial fibrillation in the Wolff-Parkinson-White syndrome: how important is the accessory pathway? J Am Coll Cardiol 1990; 15:1082–1086.

994. Konoe A, Fukatani M, Tanigawa M, et al. Electro-physiological abnormalities of the atrial muscle in patients with manifest Wolff-Parkinson-White syndrome associated with paroxysmal atrial fibrillation. Pacing Clin Electrophysiol 1992; 15:1040–1052.

995. Riccardi R, Gaita F, Giustetto C, Gardiol S. Atrial electrophysiological features in patients with Wolff-Parkinson-White and atrial fibrillation: absence of rate adaptation of intraatrial conduction time parameters. Pacing Clin Electrophysiol 1997; 20:1318–1327.

996. Muraoka Y, Karakawa S, Yamagata T, Matsuura H, Kajiyama

G. Dependency on atrial electrophysiological properties of appearance of paroxysmal atrial fibrillation in patients with Wolff-Parkinson-White syndrome: evidence from atrial vulnerability before and after radiofrequency catheter ablation and surgical cryoablation. PACE 1998; 21:438–446.

997. Fukatani M, Tanigawa M, Mori M, et al. Prediction of a fatal atrial fibrillation in patients with asymptomatic Wolff-Parkinson-White pattern. Jpn Circ J 1990; 54:1331–1339.

998. Gallagher JJ, Pritchett EL, Sealy WC, Kasell J, Wallace AG. The preexcitation syndromes (review). Prog Cardiovasc Dis 1978; 20:285–327.

999. Peters RW, Alikhan M, Morady F, Carliner N, Scheinman MM. Unusual features of bypass conduction in Wolff-Parkinson-White syndrome and atrial fibrillation. Am J Cardiol 1983; 52:1357–1359.

1000. Critelli G, Grassi G, Perticone F, Coltorti F, Monda V, Condorelli M. Transesophageal pacing for prognostic evaluation of preexcitation syndrome and assessment of protective therapy. Am J Cardiol 1983; 51:513–518.

1001. Kerr CR, Gallagher JJ, Smith WM, et al. The induction of atrial flutter and fibrillation and the termination of atrial flutter by esophageal pacing. Pacing Clin Electrophysiol 1983; 6:60–72.

1002. Milstein S, Sharma AD, Klein GJ. Electrophysiologic profile of asymptomatic Wolff-Parkinson-White pattern. Am J Cardiol 1986; 57:1097–1100.

1003. Wellens HJJ, Durrer D. Wolff-Parkinson-White syndrome and atrial fibrillation: relation between refractory period of accessory pathway and ventricular rate during atrial fibrillation. Am J Cardiol 1974; 34:777–782.

1004. Tonkin AM, Miller HC, Svenson RH, Wallace AG, Gallagher JJ. Refractory periods of the accessory pathway in the Wolff-Parkinson-White syndrome. Circulation 1975; 52:563–569.

1005. Bromberg BI, Lindsay BD, Cain ME, Cox JL. Impact of clinical history and electrophysiologic characterization of accessory pathways on management strategies to reduce sudden death among children with Wolff-Parkinson-White syndrome. J Am Coll Cardiol 1996; 27:690–695.

1006. Castellanos A Jr, Myerburg RJ, Craparo K, Befeler B, Agha AS. Factors regulating ventricular rates during atrial flutter and fibrillation in preexcitation (Wolff-Parkinson-White) syndrome. Br Heart J 1973; 35:811–816.

1007. Rakovec P, Cijan A, Kenda MF, Rode P, Jakopin J, Turk J. Failure of the refractory period of the accessory pathway to predict the ventricular rate during atrial fibrillation in Wolff-Parkinson-White syndrome. Int J Cardiol 1982; 1:329–330.

1008. Klein GJ, Yee R, Sharma AD. Concealed conduction in accessory atrioventricular pathways: an important determinant of the expression of arrhythmias in patients with Wolff-Parkinson-White syndrome. Circulation 1984; 70:402–411.

1009. Fujimura O, Kuo CS, Smith BA. Pre-excited RR intervals during atrial fibrillation in the Wolff-Parkinson-White syndrome: influence of the atrioventricular node refractory period. J Am Coll Cardiol 1991; 18:1722–1726.

1010. Milstein S, Klein GJ, Rattes MF, Sharma AD, Yee R. Comparison of the ventricular response during atrial fibrillation in patients with enhanced atrioventricular node conduction and Wolff-Parkinson-White syndrome. J Am Coll Cardiol 1987; 10:1244–1248.

1011. Wellens HJJ, Brugada P, Roy D, Weiss J, Bar FW. Effect of isoproterenol on the anterograde refractory period of the accessory pathway in patients with the Wolff-Parkinson-White syndrome. Am J Cardiol 1982; 50:180–184.

1012. Lloyd EA, Hauer RN, Zipes DP, Heger JJ, Prystowsky EN. Syncope and ventricular tachycardia in patients with ventricular preexcitation. Am J Cardiol 1983; 52:79–82.

1013. Klein GJ, Gulamhusein SS. Intermittent preexcitation in the Wolff-Parkinson-White syndrome. Am J Cardiol 1983; 52:292–296.

1014. Klein GJ, Yee R, Sharma AD. Longitudinal electrophysiologic assessment of asymptomatic patients with the Wolff-Parkinson-White electrocardiographic pattern. N Engl J Med 1989; 320:1229–1233.

1015. Gerstenfeld EP, Sahakian AV, Swiryn S. Evidence for

transient linking of atrial excitation during atrial fibrillation in humans. Circulation 1992; 86:375–382.

1016. Konings KT, Kirchhof CJ, Smeets JR, Wellens HJJ, Penn OC, Allessie MA. High-density mapping of electrically induced atrial fibrillation in humans. Circulation 1994; 89:1665–1680.

1017. Botteron GW, Smith JM. Quantitative assessment of the spatial organization of atrial fibrillation in the intact human heart. Circulation 1996; 93:513–518.

1018. Holm M, Johansson R, Brandt J, Luhrs C, Olsson SB. Epicardial right atrial free wall mapping in chronic atrial fibrillation: documentation of repetitive activation with a focal spread—a hitherto unrecognised phenomenon in man. Eur Heart J 1997; 18:290–310.

1019. Kalman JM, Olgin JE, Saxon LA, Lee RJ, Scheinman MM, Lesh MD. Electrocardiographic and electrophysiologic characterization of atypical atrial flutter in man: use of activation and entrainment mapping and implications for catheter ablation. J Cardiovasc Electrophysiol 1997; 8:121–144.

1020. Ong JJ, Kriett JM, Feld GK, Chen PS. Prevalence of retrograde accessory pathway conduction during atrial fibrillation. J Cardiovasc Electrophysiol 1997; 8:377–387.

1021. Roithinger FX, Karch MR, Steiner PR, SippensGroenewegen A, Lesh MD. Relationship between atrial fibrillation and typical atrial flutter in humans: activation sequence changes during spontaneous conversion. Circulation 1997; 96:3484–3491.

1022. Matsuo K, Shimizu W, Kurita T, et al. Increased dispersion of repolarization time determined by monophasic action potentials in two patients with familial idiopathic ventricular fibrillation. J Cardiovasc Electrophysiol 1998; 9:74–83.

1023. Schoenwald AT, Sahakian AV, Sih HJ, Swiryn S. Further observations of "linking" of atrial excitation during clinical atrial fibrillation. PACE 1998; 21:25–34.

1024. Pritchett EL. Management of atrial fibrillation. N Engl J Med 1992; 326:1264–1271.

1025. Naglie IG, Detsky AS. Treatment of chronic nonvalvular atrial fibrillation in the elderly: a decision analysis. Med Decis Making 1992; 12:239–249.

1026. Repique LJ, Shah SN, Marais GE. Atrial fibrillation 1992. Management strategies in flux. Chest 1992; 101:1095–1103.

1027. Lip GY, Singh SP, Watson RD. Abc of atrial fibrillation. Investigation and non-drug management of atrial fibrillation. BMJ 1995; 311:1562–1565.

1028. Nattel S. Newer developments in the management of atrial fibrillation. Am Heart J 1995; 130:1094–1106.

1029. Gilligan DM, Ellenbogen KA, Epstein AE. The management of atrial fibrillation. Am J Med 1996; 101:413–421.

1030. Luderitz B, Pfeiffer D, Tebbenjohanns J, Jung W. Nonpharmacologic strategies for treating atrial fibrillation. Am J Cardiol 1996; 77:45A–52A.

1031. Prystowsky EN, Benson DW, Fuster V, et al. Management of patients with atrial fibrillation: a statement for healthcare professionals. From the subcommittee on electrocardiography and electrophysiology, American Heart Association. Circulation 1996; 93:1262–1277.

1032. Gallagher MM, Camm AJ. Long-term management of atrial fibrillation. Clin Cardiol 1997; 20:381–390.

1033. Prystowsky EN. Management of atrial fibrillation: simplicity surrounded by controversy. Ann Intern Med 1997; 126:244–246.

1034. Jung F, DiMarco JP. Treatment strategies for atrial fibrillation. Am J Med 1998; 104:272–286.

1035. Kowey PR, Marinchak RA, Rials SJ, Filart RA. Acute treatment of atrial fibrillation. Am J Cardiol 1998; 81:16C–22C.

1036. Pratt CM. Impact of managed care on the treatment of atrial fibrillation. Am J Cardiol 1998; 81:30C–34C.

1037. Waktare JEP, Camm AJ. Acute treatment of atrial fibrillation: why and when to maintain sinus rhythm. Am J Cardiol 1998; 81:3C–15C.

1038. Rostagno C, Paladini B, Pini C, et al. Feasibility of out-of-hospital treatment of supraventricular tachycardias. Am J Cardiol 1991; 68:119–122.

1039. Planning and steering committees of the AFFIRM study for the NHLBI AFFIRM investigators: atrial fibrillation follow-up investigation of rhythm management—the AFFIRM study design. Am J Cardiol 1997; 79:1198–1202.

1040. Hohnloser SH, Kuck KH. Atrial fibrillation: maintaining stability of sinus rhythm or ventricular rate control? The need for prospective data: the PIAF trial. Pacing Clin Electrophysiol 1997; 20:1989–1992.

1041. Sopher SM, Camm AJ. Atrial fibrillation: maintenance of sinus rhythm versus rate control. Am J Cardiol 1996; 77:24A–37A.

1042. Sager PT. Atrial fibrillation: antiarrhythmic therapy versus rate control with antithrombotic therapy. Am J Cardiol 1997; 80:74G–81G.

1043. Lip GY, Tean KN, Dunn FG. Treatment of atrial fibrillation in a district general hospital. Br Heart J 1994; 71:92–95.

1044. Lip GY, Zarifis J, Watson RD, Beevers DG. Physician variation in the management of patients with atrial fibrillation. Heart 1996; 75:200–205.

1045. Anonymous. Hazard of carotid-sinus stimulation. N Engl J Med 1966; 275:165–166.

1046. Linenthal AJ. Effects of carotid sinus reflex on cardiac impulse formation and conduction. Circulation 1959; 20:595–601.

1047. Lown B, Levine SA. The carotid sinus: clinical value of its stimulation. Circulation 1961; 23:766–789.

1048. Borst C, Meijler FL. Baroreflex modulation of ventricular rhythm in atrial fibrillation. Eur Heart J 1984; 5:870–875.

1049. Kirchhof CJHJ, Gorgels APM, Wellens HJJ. Carotid sinus massage as a diagnostic and therapeutic tool for atrial flutter-fibrillation. PACE 1998; 21:1319–1321.

1050. Falk RH. Proarrhythmia in patients treated for atrial fibrillation or flutter. Ann Intern Med 1992; 117:141–150.

1051. Anonymous. Treatment of atrial fibrillation. Recommendations from a workshop arranged by the medical products agency (Uppsala, Sweden) and the Swedish society of cardiology. Eur Heart J 1993; 14:1427–1433.

1052. Cowan JC. Antiarrhythmic drugs in the management of atrial fibrillation. Br Heart J 1993; 70:304–306.

1053. Edvardsson N. Comparison of class I and class III action in atrial fibrillation. Eur Heart J 1993; 14:H62–H66.

1054. Crijns HJ, Van Gelder IC, Lie KI. Benefits and risks of antiarrhythmic drug therapy after DC electrical cardioversion of atrial fibrillation or flutter. Eur Heart J 1994; 15:A17–A21.

1055. Fromer MA. Indications and limitations of class I drugs in atrial fibrillation. Pacing Clin Electrophysiol 1994; 17:1016–1018.

1056. Hohnloser SH. Indications and limitations of class II and III antiarrhythmic drugs in atrial fibrillation. Pacing Clin Electrophysiol 1994; 17:1019–1025.

1057. Lip GY, Watson RD, Singh SP. ABC of atrial fibrillation: drugs for atrial fibrillation. BMJ 1995; 311:1631–1634.

1058. Reimold SC. Clinical challenge. I: control of recurrent symptomatic atrial fibrillation. Eur Heart J 1996; 17:C35–C40.

1059. Cobbe SM. Using the right drug. A treatment algorithm for atrial fibrillation. Eur Heart J 1997; 18:C33–C39.

1060. Riley RD, Pritchett EL. Pharmacologic management of atrial fibrillation. J Cardiovasc Electrophysiol 1997; 8:818–829.

1061. Ganz LI, Antman EM. Antiarrhythmic drug therapy in the management of atrial fibrillation. J Cardiovasc Electrophysiol 1997; 8:1175–1189.

1062. Saxon LA. Atrial fibrillation and dilated cardiomyopathy: therapeutic strategies when sinus rhythm cannot be maintained. Pacing Clin Electrophysiol 1997; 20:720–725.

1063. Blitzer M, Costeas C, Kassotis J, Reiffel JA. Rhythm management in atrial fibrillation: with a primary emphasis on pharmacological therapy. Part I. PACE 1998; 21:590–602.

1064. Costeas C, Kassotis J, Blitzer M, Reiffel JA. Rhythm management in atrial fibrillation: with a primary emphasis on pharmacological therapy. Part 2. PACE 1998; 21:742–752.

1065. Kassotis J, Costeas C, Blitzer M, Reiffel JA. Rhythm management in atrial fibrillation: with a primary emphasis on pharmacologic therapy. Part 3. PACE 1998; 21:1133–1145.

1066. Waldo AL, Prystowsky EN. Drug treatment of atrial fibrillation in the managed care era. Am J Cardiol 1998; 81:23C–29C.

1067. Bauernfeind RA, Swiryn SP, Strasberg B, Palileo E, Scagliotti D, Rosen KM. Electrophysiologic drug testing in prophylaxis of sporadic paroxysmal atrial fibrillation: technique, application, and efficacy in severely symptomatic preexcitation patients. Am Heart J 1982; 103:941–949.

1068. Maisel WH, Kuntz KM, Reimold SC, et al. Risk of initiating antiarrhythmic drug therapy for atrial fibrillation in patients admitted to a university hospital. Ann Intern Med 1997; 127:281–284.

1069. Chevalier H. A plea for atrial fibrillation. Am Heart J 1966; 72:423–425.

1070. Feld GK. Atrial fibrillation: is there a safe and highly effective pharmacological treatment? Circulation 1990; 82:2248–2250.

1071. White PD, Griffith GC. Invalidism abolished by transforming paroxysmal to permanent atrial fibrillation. JAMA 1959; 169:596–597.

1072. Vera Z, Mason DT, Awan NA, et al. Improvement of symptoms in patients with sick sinus syndrome by spontaneous development of stable atrial fibrillation. Br Heart J 1977; 39:160–167.

1073. Coplen SE, Antman EM, Berlin JA, Hewitt P, Chalmers TC. Efficacy and safety of quinidine therapy for maintenance of sinus rhythm after cardioversion: a meta-analysis of randomized control trials. Circulation 1990; 82:1106–1116.

1074. Sihm I, Hansen FA, Rasmussen J, Pedersen AK, Thygesen K. Flecainide acetate in atrial flutter and fibrillation: the arrhythmogenic effects. Eur Heart J 1990; 11:145–148.

1075. Reimold SC, Chalmers TC, Berlin JA, Antman EM. Assessment of the efficacy and safety of antiarrhythmic therapy for chronic atrial fibrillation: observations on the role of trial design and implications of drug-related mortality. Am Heart J 1992; 124:924–932.

1076. Kerin NZ, Somberg J. Proarrhythmia: definition, risk factors, causes, treatment, and controversies. Am Heart J 1994; 128:575–585.

1077. DiMarco JP, Sellers TD, Lerman BB, Greenberg ML, Berne RM, Belardinelli L. Diagnostic and therapeutic use of adenosine in patients with supraventricular tachyarrhythmias. J Am Coll Cardiol 1985; 6:417–425.

1078. DiMarco JP, Miles W, Akhtar M, et al. Adenosine for paroxysmal supraventricular tachycardia: dose ranging and comparison with verapamil. Assessment in placebo-controlled, multicenter trials: the adenosine for PSVT study group. Ann Intern Med 1990; 113:104–110.

1079. Botteron GW, Smith JM. Spatial and temporal inhomogeneity of adenosine's effect on atrial refractoriness in humans: using atrial fibrillation to probe atrial refractoriness. J Cardiovasc Electrophysiol 1994; 5:477–484.

1080. Garratt CJ, Griffith MJ, O'Nunain S, Ward DE, Camm AJ. Effects of intravenous adenosine on antegrade refractoriness of accessory atrioventricular connections. Circulation 1991; 84:1962–1968.

1081. Tebbenjohanns J, Pfeiffer D, Schumacher B, Jung W, Manz M, Luderitz B. Intravenous adenosine during atrioventricular reentrant tachycardia: induction of atrial fibrillation with rapid conduction over an accessory pathway. Pacing Clin Electrophysiol 1995; 18:743–746.

1082. Wellens HJJ, Bar FW, Dassen WR, Brugada P, Vanagt EJ, Farre J. Effect of drugs in the Wolff-Parkinson-White syndrome: importance of initial length of effective refractory period of the accessory pathway. Am J Cardiol 1980; 46:665–669.

1083. Wellens HJJ, Bar FW, Gorgels AP, Vanagt EJ. Use of ajmaline in patients with the Wolff-Parkinson-White syndrome to disclose short refractory period of the accessory pathway. Am J Cardiol 1980; 45:130–133.

1084. Eshchar Y, Belhassen B, Laniado S. Comparison of exercise and ajmaline tests with electrophysiologic study in the Wolff-Parkinson-White syndrome. Am J Cardiol 1986; 57:782–786.

1085. Wellens HJJ, Durrer D. Effect of procaine amide, quinidine, and ajmaline in the Wolff-Parkinson-White syndrome. Circulation 1974; 50:114–120.

1086. Podrid PJ. Amiodarone: reevaluation of an old drug. Ann Intern Med 1995; 122:689–700.

1087. Desai AD, Chun S, Sung RJ. The role of intravenous amiodarone in the management of cardiac arrhythmias. Ann Intern Med 1997; 127:294–303.

1088. Olsson SB, Brorson L, Varnauskas E. Class 3 antiarrhythmic action in man: observations from monophasic action potential recordings and amiodarone treatment. Br Heart J 1973; 35:1255–1259.

1089. Rosenbaum MB, Chiale PA, Ryba D, Elizari MV. Control of tachyarrhythmias associated with Wolff-Parkinson-White syndrome by amiodarone hydrochloride. Am J Cardiol 1974; 34:215–223.

1090. Chamberlain DA, Clark AN. Atrial fibrillation complicating Wolff-Parkinson-White syndrome treated with amiodarone. Br Med J 1977; 2:1519–1520.

1091. Wheeler PJ, Puritz R, Ingram DV, Chamberlain DA. Amiodarone in the treatment of refractory supraventricular and ventricular arrhythmias. Postgrad Med J 1979; 55:1–9.

1092. Rowland E, Krikler DM. Electrophysiological assessment of amiodarone in treatment of resistant supraventricular arrhythmias. Br Heart J 1980; 44:82–90.

1093. Ward DE, Camm AJ, Spurrell RA. Clinical antiarrhythmic effects of amiodarone in patients with resistant paroxysmal tachycardias. Br Heart J 1980; 44:91–95.

1094. McKenna WJ, Harris L, Perez G, Krikler DM, Oakley C, Goodwin JF. Arrhythmia in hypertrophic cardiomyopathy. II. Comparison of amiodarone and verapamil in treatment. Br Heart J 1981; 46:173–178.

1095. Podrid PJ, Lown B. Amiodarone therapy in symptomatic, sustained refractory atrial and ventricular tachyarrhythmias. Am Heart J 1981; 101:374–379.

1096. Rowland E, McKenna WJ, Harris L, Holt DW, Krikler DM. Amiodarone in the prophylaxis of atrial fibrillation. In Kulbertus H, Olsson SB, Schlepper M (eds). Atrial Fibrillation. Kiruna, Molndal, Sweden: AB Hassle, 1982, pp. 262–273.

1097. Fogoros RN, Anderson KP, Winkle RA, Swerdlow CD, Mason JW. Amiodarone: clinical efficacy and toxicity in 96 patients with recurrent, drug-refractory arrhythmias. Circulation 1983; 68:88–94.

1098. Graboys TB, Podrid PJ, Lown B. Efficacy of amiodarone for refractory supraventricular tachyarrhythmias. Am Heart J 1983; 106:870–876.

1099. Haffajee CI, Love JC, Canada AT, Lesko LJ, Asdourian G, Alpert JS. Clinical pharmacokinetics and efficacy of amiodarone for refractory tachyarrhythmias. Circulation 1983; 67:1347–1355.

1100. Wellens HJJ, Brugada P, Abdollah H. Effect of amiodarone in paroxysmal supraventricular tachycardia with or without Wolff-Parkinson-White syndrome. Am Heart J 1983; 106:876–880.

1101. Blomstrom P, Edvardsson N, Olsson SB. Amiodarone in atrial fibrillation. Acta Med Scand 1984; 216:517–524.

1102. McKenna WJ, Harris L, Rowland E, et al. Amiodarone for long-term management of patients with hypertrophic cardiomyopathy. Am J Cardiol 1984; 54:802–810.

1103. Cowan JC, Gardiner P, Reid DS, Newell DJ, Campbell RW. A comparison of amiodarone and digoxin in the treatment of atrial fibrillation complicating suspected acute myocardial infarction. J Cardiovasc Pharmacol 1986; 8:252–256.

1104. Blevins RD, Kerin NZ, Benaderet D, et al. Amiodarone in the management of refractory atrial fibrillation. Arch Intern Med 1987; 147:1401–1404.

1105. Feld GK, Nademanee K, Stevenson W, Weiss J, Klitzner T, Singh BN. Clinical and electrophysiologic effects of amiodarone in patients with atrial fibrillation complicating the Wolff-Parkinson-White syndrome. Am Heart J 1988; 115:102–107.

1106. Robinson K, Frenneaux MP, Stockins B, Karatasakis G, Poloniecki JD, McKenna WJ. Atrial fibrillation in hypertrophic cardiomyopathy: a longitudinal study. J Am Coll Cardiol 1990; 15:1279–1285.

1107. Gosselink AT, Crijns HJ, Van Gelder IC, Hillige H, Wiesfeld AC, Lie KI. Low-dose amiodarone for maintenance of sinus rhythm after cardioversion of atrial fibrillation or flutter. JAMA 1992; 267:3289–3293.

1108. Zehender M, Hohnloser S, Muller B, Meinertz T, Just H. Effects of amiodarone versus quinidine and verapamil in patients with chronic atrial fibrillation: results of a comparative study and a 2-year follow-up. J Am Coll Cardiol 1992; 19:1054–1059.

1109. Disch DL, Greenberg ML, Holzberger PT, Malenka DJ, Birkmeyer JD. Managing chronic atrial fibrillation: a Markov decision analysis comparing warfarin, quinidine, and low-dose amiodarone. Ann Intern Med 1994; 120:449–457.

1110. Chun SH, Sager PT, Stevenson WG, Nademanee K, Middlekauff HR, Singh BN. Long-term efficacy of amiodarone for the maintenance of normal sinus rhythm in patients with refractory atrial fibrillation or flutter. Am J Cardiol 1995; 76:47–50.

1111. Daoud EG, Strickberger SA, Man KC, et al. Preoperative amiodarone as prophylaxis against atrial fibrillation after heart surgery. N Engl J Med 1997; 337:1785–1791.

1112. Roy D, Talajic M, Thibault B, et al. Pilot study and protocol of the Canadian Trial of Atrial Fibrillation (CTAF). Am J Cardiol 1997; 80:464–468.

1113. Andrivet P, Boubakri E, Dove PJ, Mach V, Vu Ngoc C. A clinical study of amiodarone as a single oral dose in patients with recent-onset atrial tachyarrhythmia. Eur Heart J 1994; 15:1396–1402.

1114. Hou ZY, Chang MS, Chen CY, et al. Acute treatment of recent-onset atrial fibrillation and flutter with a tailored dosing regimen of intravenous amiodarone: a randomized, digoxin-controlled study. Eur Heart J 1995; 16:521–528.

1115. Clemo HF, Wood MA, Gilligan DM, Ellenbogen KA. Intravenous amiodarone for acute heart rate control in the critically ill patient with atrial tachyarrhythmias. Am J Cardiol 1998; 81:594–598.

1116. Installe E, Schoevaerdts JC, Gadisseux P, Charles S, Tremouroux J. Intravenous amiodarone in the treatment of various arrhythmias following cardiac operations. J Thorac Cardiovasc Surg 1981; 81:302–308.

1117. Blandford RL, Crampton J, Kudlac H. Intravenous amiodarone in atrial fibrillation complicating myocardial infarction. Br Med J Clin Res Ed 1982; 284:16–17.

1118. Faniel R, Schoenfeld P. Efficacy of I. V. amiodarone in converting rapid atrial fibrillation and flutter to sinus rhythm in intensive care patients. Eur Heart J 1983; 4:180–185.

1119. Strasberg B, Arditti A, Sclarovsky S, Lewin RF, Buimovici B, Agmon J. Efficacy of intravenous amiodarone in the management of paroxysmal or new atrial fibrillation with fast ventricular response. Int J Cardiol 1985; 7:47–58.

1120. Noc M, Stajer D, Horvat M. Intravenous amiodarone versus verapamil for acute conversion of paroxysmal atrial fibrillation to sinus rhythm. Am J Cardiol 1990; 65:679–680.

1121. Cybulski J, Kulakowski P, Makowska E, Czepiel A, Sikora-Frac M, Ceremuzynski L. Intravenous amiodarone is safe and seems to be effective in termination of paroxysmal supraventricular tachyarrhythmias. Clin Cardiol 1996; 19:563–566.

1122. Galve E, Rius T, Ballester R, et al. Intravenous amiodarone in treatment of recent-onset atrial fibrillation: results of a randomized, controlled study. J Am Coll Cardiol 1996; 27:1079–1082.

1123. Kochiadakis GE, Igoumenidis NE, Marketou ME, Solomou MC, Kanoupakis EM, Vardas PE. Low-dose amiodarone versus sotalol for suppression of recurrent symptomatic atrial fibrillation. Am J Cardiol 1998; 81:995–998.

1124. Wellens HJJ, Lie KI, Bar FW, et al. Effect of amiodarone in the Wolff-Parkinson-White syndrome. Am J Cardiol 1976; 38:189–194.

1125. Chouty F, Coumel P. Oral flecainide for prophylaxis of paroxysmal atrial fibrillation. Am J Cardiol 1988; 62:35D–37D.

1126. Coumel P, Lucet V, Do Ngoc D. The use of amiodarone in children. Pacing Clin Electrophysiol 1983; 6:930–939.

1127. Kappenberger LJ, Fromer MA, Steinbrunn W, Shenasa M. Efficacy of amiodarone in the Wolff-Parkinson-White

syndrome with rapid ventricular response via accessory pathway during atrial fibrillation. Am J Cardiol 1984; 54:330–335.

1128. Schutzenberger W, Leisch F, Gmeiner R. Enhanced accessory pathway conduction following intravenous amiodarone in atrial fibrillation: a case report. Int J Cardiol 1987; 16:93–95.

1129. Boriani G, Biffi M, Frabetti L, et al. Ventricular fibrillation after intravenous amiodarone in Wolff-Parkinson-White syndrome with atrial fibrillation. Am Heart J 1996; 131:1214–1216.

1130. Zipes DP, Gaum WE, Foster PR, et al. Aprindine for treatment of supraventricular tachycardias: with particular application to Wolff-Parkinson-White syndrome. Am J Cardiol 1977; 40:586–596.

1131. Gold H, Kwit NT, Otto H, Fox T. Physiological adaptations in cardiac slowing by digitalis and their bearing on problems of digitalization in patients with auricular fibrillation. J Pharmacol Exp Ther 1939; 67:224–238.

1132. Cooper JA, Frieden J. Atropine in the treatment of cardiac disease. Am Heart J 1969; 78:124–127.

1133. Brown JH. Atropine, scopolamine and related antimuscarinic drugs. In Gilman AG, Rall TW, Nies AS, Taylor P (eds). Goodman and Gilman's The Pharmacological Basis of Therapeutics. New York: Pergamon Press, 1990, p. 155.

1134. Anonymous. Paul Wood's Diseases of the Heart and Circulation. Philadelphia: JB Lippincott, 1968, p. 283.

1135. Gibson D, Sowton E. The use of beta-adrenergic receptor blocking drugs in dysrhythmias. Prog Cardiovasc Dis 1969; 12:16–39.

1136. Harrison DC, Griffin JR, Fiene TJ. Effects of beta-adrenergic blockade with propranolol in patients with atrial arrhythmias. N Engl J Med 1965; 273:410–415.

1137. Rowlands DJ, Howitt G, Markman P. Propranolol (Inderal) in disturbances of cardiac rhythm. BMJ 1965; 1:891–894.

1138. Luria MH, Adelson EI, Miller AJ. Acute and chronic effects of an adrenergic beta-receptor blocking agent (propranolol) in treatment of cardiac arrhythmias. Circulation 1966; 34:767–773.

1139. Schamroth L. Immediate effects of intravenous propranolol on various cardiac arrhythmias. Am J Cardiol 1966; 18:438–443.

1140. Turner JRB. Propranolol in the treatment of digitalis-induced and digitalis-resistant tachycardia. Am J Cardiol 1966; 18:450–457.

1141. Wolfson S, Robbins SI, Krasnow N. Treatment of cardiac arrhythmias with beta-adrenergic blocking agents: clinical and experimental studies. Am Heart J 1966; 72:176–187.

1142. Gianelly R, Griffin JR, Harrison DC. Propranolol in the treatment and prevention of cardiac arrhythmias. Ann Intern Med 1967; 66:667–676.

1143. Sloman G, Stannard M. Beta-adrenergic blockade and cardiac arrhythmias. BMJ 1967; 4:508–512.

1144. Wolfson S, Herman MV, Sullivan JM, Gorlin R. Conversion of atrial fibrillation and flutter by propranolol. Br Heart J 1967; 29:305–309.

1145. Conway N, Seymour J, Gelson A. Cardiac failure in patients with valvar heart disease after use of propranolol to control atrial fibrillation. BMJ 1968; 2:213–214.

1146. Frieden J, Rosenblum R, Enselberg CD, Rosenberg A. Propranolol treatment of chronic intractable supraventricular arrhythmias. Am J Cardiol 1968; 22:711–717.

1147. Levi GF, Proto C. Combined treatment of atrial fibrillation with propranolol and quinidine. Cardiology 1970; 55:249–254.

1148. Fors WJ Jr, VanderArk CR, Reynolds EW Jr. Evaluation of propranolol and quinidine in the treatment of quinidine-resistant arrhythmias. Am J Cardiol 1971; 27:190–194.

1149. Yahalom J, Klein HO, Kaplinsky E. Beta-adrenergic blockade as adjunctive oral therapy in patients with chronic atrial fibrillation. Chest 1977; 71:592–596.

1150. Frishman W, Davis R, Strom J, et al. Clinical pharmacology of the new beta-adrenergic blocking drugs. Part 5. Pindolol (lb-46) therapy for supraventricular arrhythmia: a viable alternative to propranolol in patients with bronchospasm. Am Heart J 1979; 98:393–398.

1151. Byrd RC, Sung RJ, Marks J, Parmley WW. Safety and efficacy of esmolol (ASL-8052: an ultrashort-acting beta-adrenergic blocking agent) for control of ventricular rate in supraventricular tachycardias. J Am Coll Cardiol 1984; 3:394–399.

1152. Abrams J, Allen J, Allin D, et al. Efficacy and safety of esmolol vs propranolol in the treatment of supraventricular tachyarrhythmias: a multicenter double-blind clinical trial. Am Heart J 1985; 110:913–922.

1153. Das G, Ferris J. Esmolol in the treatment of supraventricular tachyarrhythmias. Can J Cardiol 1988; 4:177–180.

1154. Schwartz M, Michelson EL, Sawin HS, MacVaugh H III. Esmolol: safety and efficacy in postoperative cardiothoracic patients with supraventricular tachyarrhythmias. Chest 1988; 93:705–711.

1155. Ahuja RC, Sinha N, Saran RK, Jain AK, Hasan M. Digoxin or verapamil or metoprolol for heart rate control in patients with mitral stenosis—a randomised cross-over study. Int J Cardiol 1989; 25:325–331.

1156. Platia EV, Michelson EL, Porterfield JK, Das G. Esmolol versus verapamil in the acute treatment of atrial fibrillation or atrial flutter. Am J Cardiol 1989; 63:925–929.

1157. Singh S, Saini RK, DiMarco J, Kluger J, Gold R, Chen YW. Efficacy and safety of sotalol in digitalized patients with chronic atrial fibrillation: the sotalol study group. Am J Cardiol 1991; 68:1227–1230.

1158. Falk RH. Control of the ventricular rate in atrial fibrillation. In Falk RH, Podrid PJ (eds). Atrial Fibrillation. Mechanisms and Management. New York: Raven Press, 1992, pp. 255–282.

1159. Alboni P, Razzolini R, Scarfo S, et al. Hemodynamic effects of oral sotalol during both sinus rhythm and atrial fibrillation. J Am Coll Cardiol 1993; 22:1373–1377.

1160. Brodsky M, Saini R, Bellinger R, Zoble R, Weiss R, Powers L. Comparative effects of the combination of digoxin and dl-sotalol therapy versus digoxin monotherapy for control of ventricular response in chronic atrial fibrillation: dl-sotalol atrial fibrillation study group. Am Heart J 1994; 127:572–577.

1161. Sung RJ, Tan HL, Karagounis L, et al. Intravenous sotalol for the termination of supraventricular tachycardia and atrial fibrillation and flutter: a multicenter, randomized, double-blind, placebo-controlled study. Sotalol Multicenter Study Group. Am Heart J 1995; 129:739–748.

1162. Berkowitz WD, Wit AL, Lau SH, Steiner C, Damato AN. The effects of propranolol on cardiac conduction. Circulation 1969; 40:855–862.

1163. Seides SF, Josephson ME, Batsford WP, Weisfogel GM, Lau SH, Damato AN. The electrophysiology of propranolol in man. Am Heart J 1974; 88:733–741.

1164. Marchlinski FE, Buxton AE, Waxman HL, Josephson ME. Electrophysiologic effects of intravenous metoprolol. Am Heart J 1984; 107:1125–1131.

1165. Bigger JT, Hoffman BF. Antiarrhythmic drugs. In Gilman AG, Rall TW, Nies AS, Taylor P (eds). The Pharmacological Basis of Therapeutics. 8th ed. New York: Pergamon Press, 1990, pp. 840–873.

1166. David D, Segni ED, Klein HO, Kaplinsky E. Inefficacy of digitalis in the control of heart rate in patients with chronic atrial fibrillation: beneficial effect of an added beta adrenergic blocking agent. Am J Cardiol 1979; 44:1378–1382.

1167. Szekely P, Jackson F, Wynne NA, Vohra JK, Batson GA, Dow WI. Clinical observations on the use of propranolol in disorders of cardiac rhythm. Am J Cardiol 1966; 18:426–430.

1168. Stock JP. Beta adrenergic blocking drugs in the clinical management of cardiac arrhythmias. Am J Cardiol 1966; 18:444–449.

1169. Brown RW, Goble AJ. Effect of propranolol on exercise tolerance of patients with atrial fibrillation. BMJ 1969; 2:279–280.

1170. Zoble RG, Brewington J, Olukotun AY, Gore R. Comparative effects of nadolol-digoxin combination therapy and digoxin monotherapy for chronic atrial fibrillation. Am J Cardiol 1987; 60:39D–45D.

1171. Atwood JE, Myers J, Sullivan M, et al. The effect of cardioversion on maximal exercise capacity in patients with chronic atrial fibrillation. Am Heart J 1989; 118:913–918.

1172. DiBianco R, Morganroth J, Freitag JA, et al. Effects of nadolol on the spontaneous and exercise-provoked heart rate of patients with chronic atrial fibrillation receiving stable dosages of digoxin. Am Heart J 1984; 108:1121–1127.

1173. Molajo AO, Coupe MO, Bennett DH. Effect of Corwin (ICI 118587) on resting and exercise heart rate and exercise tolerance in digitalised patients with chronic atrial fibrillation. Br Heart J 1984; 52:392–395.

1174. Wong CK, Lau CP, Leung WH, Cheng CH. Usefulness of labetalol in chronic atrial fibrillation. Am J Cardiol 1990; 66:1212–1215.

1175. Atwood JE, Sullivan M, Forbes S, et al. Effect of beta-adrenergic blockade on exercise performance in patients with chronic atrial fibrillation. J Am Coll Cardiol 1987; 10:314–320.

1176. Bath JCJL. Treatment of cardiac arrhythmias in unanesthetized patients. Am J Cardiol 1966; 18:415–425.

1177. James MA, Channer KS, Papouchado M, Rees JR. Improved control of atrial fibrillation with combined pindolol and digoxin therapy. Eur Heart J 1989; 10:83–90.

1178. Reiffel JA. Improved rate control in atrial fibrillation. Am Heart J 1992; 123:1094–1098.

1179. Ang EL, Chan WL, Cleland JG, et al. Placebo controlled trial of xamoterol versus digoxin in chronic atrial fibrillation. Br Heart J 1990; 64:256–260.

1180. Cristodorescu R, Rosu D, Deutsch G, Verdes A, Luca C. The heart rate slowing effect of pindolol in patients with digitalis resistant atrial fibrillation and heart failure. Med Interna 1986; 24:207–215.

1181. Tsolakas TC, Davies JPH, Oram S. Propranolol in attempted maintenance of sinus rhythm after electrical defibrillation. Lancet 1964; 2:1064.

1182. Stern S. Conversion of chronic atrial fibrillation to sinus rhythm with combined propranolol and quinidine treatment. Am Heart J 1967; 74:170–172.

1183. Hillestad L, Storstein O. Conversion of chronic atrial fibrillation to sinus rhythm with combined propranolol and quinidine treatment. Am Heart J 1969; 77:137–139.

1184. Szekely P, Wynne NA, Pearson DT, Batson GA, Sideris DA. Direct current shock and antidysrhythmic drugs. Br Heart J 1970; 32:209–218.

1185. Juul-Moller S, Edvardsson N, Rehnqvist-Ahlberg N. Sotalol versus quinidine for the maintenance of sinus rhythm after direct current conversion of atrial fibrillation. Circulation 1990; 82:1932–1939.

1186. Reimold SC, Cantillon CO, Friedman PL, Antman EM. Propafenone versus sotalol for suppression of recurrent symptomatic atrial fibrillation. Am J Cardiol 1993; 71:558–563.

1187. Kowey PR, Taylor JE, Rials SJ, Marinchak RA. Meta-analysis of the effectiveness of prophylactic drug therapy in preventing supraventricular arrhythmia early after coronary artery bypass grafting. Am J Cardiol 1992; 69:963–965.

1188. Boudoulas H, Lewis RP, Snyder GL, Karayannacos P, Vasko JS. Beneficial effect of continuation of propranolol through coronary bypass surgery. Clin Cardiol 1979; 2:87–91.

1189. Salazar C, Frishman W, Friedman S, et al. Beta-blockade therapy for supraventricular tachyarrhythmias after coronary surgery: a propranolol withdrawal syndrome? Angiology 1979; 30:816–819.

1190. Oka Y, Frishman W, Becker RM, et al. Clinical pharmacology of the new beta-adrenergic blocking drugs. Part 10. Beta-adrenoceptor blockade and coronary artery surgery. Am Heart J 1980; 99:255–269.

1191. Stephenson LW, MacVaugh H III, Tomasello DN, Josephson ME. Propranolol for prevention of postoperative cardiac arrhythmias: a randomized study. Ann Thorac Surg 1980; 29:113–116.

1192. Mohr R, Smolinsky A, Goor DA. Prevention of supraventricular tachyarrhythmia with low-dose propranolol after coronary bypass. J Thorac Cardiovasc Surg 1981; 81:840–845.

1193. Silverman NA, Wright R, Levitsky S. Efficacy of low-dose propranolol in preventing postoperative supraventricular tachyarrhythmias: a prospective, randomized study. Ann Surg 1982; 196:194–197.

1194. Abel RM, van Gelder HM, Pores IH, Liguori J, Gielchinsky I, Parsonnet V. Continued propranolol administration following coronary bypass surgery: antiarrhythmic effects. Arch Surg 1983; 118:727–731.

1195. Mills SA, Poole GV Jr, Breyer RH, et al. Digoxin and propranolol in the prophylaxis of dysrhythmias after coronary artery bypass grafting. Circulation 1983; 68(Suppl II):II-222–II-225.

1196. Hammon JW Jr, Wood AJ, Prager RL, Wood M, Muirhead J, Bender HW Jr. Perioperative beta blockade with propranolol: reduction in myocardial oxygen demands and incidence of atrial and ventricular arrhythmias. Ann Thorac Surg 1984; 38:363–367.

1197. Myhre ES, Sorlie D, Aarbakke J, Hals PA, Straume B. Effects of low dose propranolol after coronary bypass surgery. J Cardiovasc Surg 1984; 25:348–352.

1198. White HD, Antman EM, Glynn MA, et al. Efficacy and safety of timolol for prevention of supraventricular tachyarrhythmias after coronary artery bypass surgery. Circulation 1984; 70:479–484.

1199. Materne P, Larbuisson R, Collignon P, Limet R, Kulbertus H. Prevention by acebutolol of rhythm disorders following coronary bypass surgery. Int J Cardiol 1985; 8:275–286.

1200. Daudon P, Corcos T, Gandjbakhch I, Levasseur JP, Cabrol A, Cabrol C. Prevention of atrial fibrillation or flutter by acebutolol after coronary bypass grafting. Am J Cardiol 1986; 58:933–936.

1201. Janssen J, Loomans L, Harink J, et al. Prevention and treatment of supraventricular tachycardia shortly after coronary artery bypass grafting: a randomized open trial. Angiology 1986; 37:601–609.

1202. Vecht RJ, Nicolaides EP, Ikweuke JK, Liassides C, Cleary J, Cooper WB. Incidence and prevention of supraventricular tachyarrhythmias after coronary bypass surgery. Int J Cardiol 1986; 13:125–134.

1203. Khuri SF, Okike ON, Josa M, et al. Efficacy of nadolol in preventing supraventricular tachycardia after coronary artery bypass grafting. Am J Cardiol 1987; 60:51D–58D.

1204. Lamb RK, Prabhakar G, Thorpe JA, Smith S, Norton R, Dyde JA. The use of atenolol in the prevention of supraventricular arrhythmias following coronary artery surgery. Eur Heart J 1988; 9:32–36.

1205. Matangi MF, Strickland J, Garbe GJ, et al. Atenolol for the prevention of arrhythmias following coronary artery bypass grafting. Can J Cardiol 1989; 5:229–234.

1206. Suttorp MJ, Kingma JH, Tjon Joe Gin RM, et al. Efficacy and safety of low- and high-dose sotalol versus propranolol in the prevention of supraventricular tachyarrhythmias early after coronary artery bypass operations. J Thorac Cardiovasc Surg 1990; 100:921–926.

1207. Suttorp MJ, Kingma JH, Peels HO, et al. Effectiveness of sotalol in preventing supraventricular tachyarrhythmias shortly after coronary artery bypass grafting. Am J Cardiol 1991; 68:1163–1169.

1208. Andrews TC, Reimold SC, Berlin JA, Antman EM. Prevention of supraventricular arrhythmias after coronary artery bypass surgery: a meta-analysis of randomized control trials. Circulation 1991; 84:236–244.

1209. Martinussen HJ, Lolk A, Szczepanski C, Alstrup P. Supraventricular tachyarrhythmias after coronary artery bypass surgery: a double blind randomized trial of prophylactic low dose propranolol. Thorac Cardiovasc Surg 1988; 36:206–207.

1210. Shafei H, Nashef SA, Turner MA, Bain WH. Does low-dose propranolol reduce the incidence of supraventricular tachyarrhythmias following myocardial revascularisation? A clinical study. Thorac Cardiovasc Surg 1988; 36:202–205.

1211. Ivey MF, Ivey TD, Bailey WW, Williams DB, Hessel EA II, Miller DW Jr. Influence of propranolol on supraventricular

tachycardia early after coronary artery revascularization: a randomized trial. J Thorac Cardiovasc Surg 1983; 85:214–218.

1212. Campbell TJ, Gavaghan TP, Morgan JJ. Intravenous sotalol for the treatment of atrial fibrillation and flutter after cardiopulmonary bypass: comparison with disopyramide and digoxin in a randomised trial. Br Heart J 1985; 54:86–90.

1213. Gray RJ, Bateman TM, Czer LS, Conklin CM, Matloff JM. Esmolol: a new ultrashort-acting beta-adrenergic blocking agent for rapid control of heart rate in postoperative supraventricular tachyarrhythmias. J Am Coll Cardiol 1985; 5:1451–1456.

1214. Miami Trial Research Group. Metoprolol in acute myocardial infarction. Arrhythmias. Am J Cardiol 1985; 56:35G–38G.

1215. Mitchell LB, Wyse DG, Duff HJ. Electropharmacology of sotalol in patients with Wolff-Parkinson-White syndrome. Circulation 1987; 76:810–818.

1216. Rosen KM, Barwolf C, Ehsani A, Rahimtoola SH. Effects of lidocaine and propranolol on the normal and anomalous pathways in patients with preexcitation. Am J Cardiol 1972; 30:801–809.

1217. Morady F, DiCarlo LA Jr, Baerman JM, de Buitleir M. Effect of propranolol on ventricular rate during atrial fibrillation in the Wolff-Parkinson-White syndrome. Pacing Clin Electrophysiol 1987; 10:492–496.

1218. Kerber RE, Goldman RH, Gianelly RE, Harrison DC. Treatment of atrial arrhythmias with alprenolol. JAMA 1970; 214:1849–1854.

1219. Anderson S, Blanski L, Byrd RC, et al. Comparison of the efficacy and safety of esmolol, a short-acting beta blocker, with placebo in the treatment of supraventricular tachyarrhythmias: the esmolol vs placebo multicenter study group. Am Heart J 1986; 111:42–48.

1220. Saksena S, Klein GJ, Kowey PR, et al. Electrophysiologic effects, clinical efficacy and safety of intravenous and oral nadolol in refractory supraventricular tachyarrhythmias. Am J Cardiol 1987; 59:307–312.

1221. Aronow WS, Uyeyama RR. Treatment of arrhythmias with pindolol. Clin Pharmacol Ther 1972; 13:15–22.

1222. Wang R, Camm J, Ward D, Washington H, Martin A. Treatment of chronic atrial fibrillation in the elderly, assessed by ambulatory electrocardiographic monitoring. J Am Geriatr Soc 1980; 28:529–534.

1223. Harris A. Long term treatment of paroxysmal cardiac arrhythmias with propranolol. Am J Cardiol 1966; 18:431–436.

1224. Antman EM, Beamer AD, Cantillon C, McGowan N, Friedman PL. Therapy of refractory symptomatic atrial fibrillation and atrial flutter: a staged care approach with new antiarrhythmic drugs. J Am Coll Cardiol 1990; 15:698–707.

1225. Dominic J, McAllister RG Jr, Kuo CS, Reddy CP, Surawicz B. Verapamil plasma levels and ventricular rate response in patients with atrial fibrillation and flutter. Clin Pharmacol Ther 1979; 26:710–714.

1226. Klein HO, Pauzner H, Di Segni E, David D, Kaplinsky E. The beneficial effects of verapamil in chronic atrial fibrillation. Arch Intern Med 1979; 139:747–749.

1227. Follath F, Fromer M, Meier P, Vozeh S. Pharmacodynamic comparison of oral and intravenous verapamil in atrial fibrillation. Clin Invest Med 1980; 3:49–52.

1228. Gonzalez R, Scheinman MM. Treatment of supraventricular arrhythmias with intravenous and oral verapamil. Chest 1981; 80:465–470.

1229. Schwartz JB, Keefe D, Kates RE, Kirsten E, Harrison DC. Acute and chronic pharmacodynamic interaction of verapamil and digoxin in atrial fibrillation. Circulation 1982; 65:1163–1170.

1230. Stern EH, Pitchon R, King BD, Guerrero J, Schneider RR, Wiener I. Clinical use of oral verapamil in chronic and paroxysmal atrial fibrillation. Chest 1982; 81:308–311.

1231. Lang R, Klein HO, Di Segni E, et al. Verapamil improves exercise capacity in chronic atrial fibrillation: double-blind crossover study. Am Heart J 1983; 105:820–825.

1232. Lang R, Klein HO, Weiss E, et al. Superiority of oral verapamil therapy to digoxin in treatment of chronic atrial fibrillation. Chest 1983; 83:491–499.

1233. Panidis IP, Morganroth J, Baessler C. Effectiveness and safety of oral verapamil to control exercise-induced tachycardia in patients with atrial fibrillation receiving digitalis. Am J Cardiol 1983; 52:1197–1201.

1234. Haft JI, Habbab MA. Treatment of atrial arrhythmias. Effectiveness of verapamil when preceded by calcium infusion. Arch Intern Med 1986; 146:1085–1089.

1235. Lewis R, Lakhani M, Moreland TA, McDevitt DG. A comparison of verapamil and digoxin in the treatment of atrial fibrillation. Eur Heart J 1987; 8:148–153.

1236. Pomfret SM, Beasley CR, Challenor V, Holgate ST. Relative efficacy of oral verapamil and digoxin alone and in combination for the treatment of patients with chronic atrial fibrillation. Clin Sci 1988; 74:351–357.

1237. Theisen K, Haufe M, Peters J, Theisen F, Jahrmarker H. Effect of the calcium antagonist diltiazem on atrioventricular conduction in chronic atrial fibrillation. Am J Cardiol 1985; 55:98–102.

1238. Roth A, Harrison E, Mitani G, Cohen J, Rahimtoola SH, Elkayam U. Efficacy and safety of medium- and high-dose diltiazem alone and in combination with digoxin for control of heart rate at rest and during exercise in patients with chronic atrial fibrillation. Circulation 1986; 73:316–324.

1239. Steinberg JS, Katz RJ, Bren GB, Buff LA, Varghese PJ. Efficacy of oral diltiazem to control ventricular response in chronic atrial fibrillation at rest and during exercise. J Am Coll Cardiol 1987; 9:405–411.

1240. Atwood JE, Myers JN, Sullivan MJ, Forbes SM, Pewen WF, Froelicher VF. Diltiazem and exercise performance in patients with chronic atrial fibrillation. Chest 1988; 93:20–25.

1241. Lewis RV, Irvine N, McDevitt DG. Relationships between heart rate, exercise tolerance and cardiac output in atrial fibrillation: the effects of treatment with digoxin, verapamil and diltiazem. Eur Heart J 1988; 9:777–781.

1242. Maragno I, Santostasi G, Gaion RM, et al. Low- and medium-dose diltiazem in chronic atrial fibrillation: comparison with digoxin and correlation with drug plasma levels. Am Heart J 1988; 116:385–392.

1243. Koh KK, Song JH, Kwon KS, et al. Comparative study of efficacy and safety of low-dose diltiazem or betaxolol in combination with digoxin to control ventricular rate in chronic atrial fibrillation: randomized crossover study. Int J Cardiol 1995; 52:167–174.

1244. Channer KS, Papouchado M, James MA, Pitcher DW, Rees JR. Towards improved control of atrial fibrillation. Eur Heart J 1987; 8:141–147.

1245. Schamroth L. Immediate effects of intravenous verapamil on atrial fibrillation. Cardiovasc Res 1971; 5:419–424.

1246. Schamroth L, Krikler DM, Garrett C. Immediate effects of intravenous verapamil in cardiac arrhythmias. BMJ 1972; 1:660–662.

1247. Heng MK, Singh BN, Roche AH, Norris RM, Mercer CJ. Effects of intravenous verapamil on cardiac arrhythmias and on the electrocardiogram. Am Heart J 1975; 90:487–498.

1248. Khalsa A, Olsson B, Henriksson BA. Effect of oral verapamil on ventricular irregularity in long-standing atrial fibrillation. Acta Med Scand 1979; 205:39–47.

1249. Rinkenberger RL, Prystowsky EN, Heger JJ, Troup PJ, Jackman WM, Zipes DP. Effects of intravenous and chronic oral verapamil administration in patients with supraventricular tachyarrhythmias. Circulation 1980; 62:996–1010.

1250. Gray RJ, Conklin CM, Sethna DH, Mandel WJ, Matloff JM. Role of intravenous verapamil in supraventricular tachyarrhythmias after open-heart surgery. Am Heart J 1982; 104:799–802.

1251. Plumb VJ, Karp RB, Kouchoukos NT, Zorn GL Jr, James TN, Waldo AL. Verapamil therapy of atrial fibrillation and atrial flutter following cardiac operation. J Thorac Cardiovasc Surg 1982; 83:590–596.

1252. Tommaso C, McDonough T, Parker M, Talano JV. Atrial fibrillation and flutter: immediate control and conversion with intravenously administered verapamil. Arch Intern Med 1983; 143:877–881.

1253. Buxton AE, Waxman HL, Marchlinski FE, Josephson ME. Electropharmacology of nonsustained ventricular tachycardia: effects of class I antiarrhythmic agents, verapamil and propranolol. Am J Cardiol 1984; 53:738–744.

1254. Betriu A, Chaitman BR, Bourassa MG, et al. Beneficial effect of intravenous diltiazem in the acute management of paroxysmal supraventricular tachyarrhythmias. Circulation 1983; 67:88–94.

1255. Salerno DM, Dias VC, Kleiger RE, et al. Efficacy and safety of intravenous diltiazem for treatment of atrial fibrillation and atrial flutter: the diltiazem-atrial fibrillation/flutter study group. Am J Cardiol 1989; 63:1046–1051.

1256. Ellenbogen KA, Dias VC, Plumb VJ, Heywood JT, Mirvis DM. A placebo-controlled trial of continuous intravenous diltiazem infusion for 24-hour heart rate control during atrial fibrillation and atrial flutter: a multicenter study. J Am Coll Cardiol 1991; 18:891–897.

1257. Heywood JT, Graham B, Marais GE, Jutzy KR. Effects of intravenous diltiazem on rapid atrial fibrillation accompanied by congestive heart failure. Am J Cardiol 1991; 67:1150–1152.

1258. Goldenberg IF, Lewis WR, Dias VC, Heywood JT, Pedersen WR. Intravenous diltiazem for the treatment of patients with atrial fibrillation or flutter and moderate to severe congestive heart failure. Am J Cardiol 1994; 74:884–889.

1259. Boudonas G, Lefkos N, Efthymiadis AP, Styliadis IG, Tsapas G. Intravenous administration of diltiazem in the treatment of supraventricular tachyarrhythmias. Acta Cardiol 1995; 50:125–134.

1260. Tisdale JE, Padhi ID, Goldberg AD, et al. A randomized, double-blind comparison of intravenous diltiazem and digoxin for atrial fibrillation after coronary artery bypass surgery. Am Heart J 1998; 135:739–747.

1261. Lundstrom T, Ryden L. Ventricular rate control and exercise performance in chronic atrial fibrillation: effects of diltiazem and verapamil. J Am Coll Cardiol 1990; 16:86–90.

1262. Hagemeijer F. Verapamil in the management of supraventricular tachyarrhythmias occurring after a recent myocardial infarction. Circulation 1978; 57:751–755.

1263. Waxman HL, Myerburg RJ, Appel R, Sung RJ. Verapamil for control of ventricular rate in paroxysmal supraventricular tachycardia and atrial fibrillation or flutter: a double-blind randomized cross-over study. Ann Intern Med 1981; 94:1–6.

1264. Suttorp MJ, Kingma JH, Lie-A-Huen L, Mast EG. Intravenous flecainide versus verapamil for acute conversion of paroxysmal atrial fibrillation or flutter to sinus rhythm. Am J Cardiol 1989; 63:693–696.

1265. Smith EE, Shore DF, Monro JL, Ross JK. Oral verapamil fails to prevent supraventricular tachycardia following coronary artery surgery. Int J Cardiol 1985; 9:37–44.

1266. Williams DB, Misbach GA, Kruse AP, Ivey TD. Oral verapamil for prophylaxis of supraventricular tachycardia after myocardial revascularization: a randomized trial. J Thorac Cardiovasc Surg 1985; 90:592–596.

1267. Davison R, Hartz R, Kaplan K, Parker M, Feiereisel P, Michaelis L. Prophylaxis of supraventricular tachyarrhythmia after coronary bypass surgery with oral verapamil: a randomized, double-blind trial. Ann Thorac Surg 1985; 39:336–339.

1268. Shenasa M, Kus T, Fromer M, Leblanc RA, Dubuc M, Nadeau R. Effect of intravenous and oral calcium antagonists (diltiazem and verapamil) on sustenance of atrial fibrillation. Am J Cardiol 1988; 62:403–407.

1269. Shenasa M, Fromer M, Faugere G, et al. Efficacy and safety of intravenous and oral diltiazem for Wolff-Parkinson-White syndrome. Am J Cardiol 1987; 59:301–306.

1270. Falk RH, Knowlton AA, Manaker S. Verapamil-induced atrial fibrillation. N Engl J Med 1988; 318:640–641.

1271. McGovern B, Garan H, Ruskin JN. Precipitation of cardiac arrest by verapamil in patients with Wolff-Parkinson-White syndrome. Ann Intern Med 1986; 104:791–794.

1272. Spurrell RA, Krikler DM, Sowton E. Effects of verapamil on electrophysiological properties of anomalous atrioventricular connexion in Wolff-Parkinson-White syndrome. Br Heart J 1974; 36:256–264.

1273. Gulamhusein S, Ko P, Carruthers SG, Klein GJ. Acceleration of the ventricular response during atrial fibrillation in the Wolff-Parkinson-White syndrome after verapamil. Circulation 1982; 65:348–354.

1274. Harper RW, Whitford E, Middlebrook K, Federman J, Anderson S, Pitt A. Effects of verapamil on the electrophysiologic properties of the accessory pathway in patients with the Wolff-Parkinson-White syndrome. Am J Cardiol 1982; 50:1323–1330.

1275. Rowland TW. Augmented ventricular rate following verapamil treatment for atrial fibrillation with Wolff-Parkinson-White syndrome. Pediatrics 1983; 72:245–246.

1276. Gulamhusein S, Ko P, Klein GJ. Ventricular fibrillation following verapamil in the Wolff-Parkinson-White syndrome. Am Heart J 1983; 106:145–147.

1277. Jacob AS, Nielsen DH, Gianelly RE. Fatal ventricular fibrillation following verapamil in Wolff-Parkinson-White syndrome with atrial fibrillation. Ann Emerg Med 1985; 14:159–160.

1278. Klein HO, Kaplinsky E. Verapamil and digoxin: their respective effects on atrial fibrillation and their interaction. Am J Cardiol 1982; 50:894–902.

1279. Roth A, Kaluski E, Felner S, Heller K, Laniado S. Clonidine for patients with rapid atrial fibrillation. Ann Intern Med 1992; 116:388–390.

1280. Vanagt EJ, Wellens HJJ. The electrocardiogram in digitalis intoxication. In Wellens HJJ, Kulbertus HE (eds). What's New in Electrocardiography. Boston: Martinus Nijhoff, 1981, pp. 315–343.

1281. Simpson RJ Jr, Foster JR, Woelfel AK, Gettes LS. Management of atrial fibrillation and flutter: a reappraisal of digitalis therapy. Postgrad Med 1986; 79:241–253.

1282. Sarter BH, Marchlinski FE. Redefining the role of digoxin in the treatment of atrial fibrillation. Am J Cardiol 1992; 69:71G–78G.

1283. Levy S. Intravenous digoxin: still the drug of choice for acute termination of atrial fibrillation? Eur Heart J 1997; 18:546–547.

1284. Jordaens L, Trouerbach J, Calle P, et al. Conversion of atrial fibrillation to sinus rhythm and rate control by digoxin in comparison to placebo. Eur Heart J 1997; 18:643–648.

1285. Digitalis in Acute Atrial Fibrillation (DAAF) Trial Group. Intravenous digoxin in acute atrial fibrillation: results of a randomized, placebo-controlled multicentre trial in 239 patients. Eur Heart J 1997; 18:649–654.

1286. Gold H, Kwit NT, Otto H, Fox T. On vagal and extravagal factors in cardiac slowing by digitalis in patients with auricular fibrillation. J Clin Invest 1939; 18:429–437.

1287. Goodman DJ, Rossen RM, Cannom DS, Rider AK, Harrison DC. Effect of digoxin on atrioventricular conduction: studies in patients with and without cardiac autonomic innervation. Circulation 1975; 51:251–256.

1288. Ricci DR, Orlick AE, Reitz BA, Mason JW, Stinson EB, Harrison DC. Depressant effect of digoxin on atrioventricular conduction in man. Circulation 1978; 57:898–903.

1289. Hoffman BF, Bigger JT. Digitalis and allied cardiac glycosides. In Gilman AG, Rall TW, Nies AS, Taylor P (eds). Goodman and Gilman's The Pharmacological Basis of Therapeutics. 8th ed. New York: Pergamon Press, 1990, pp. 814–839.

1290. Meijler FL. An "account" of digitalis and atrial fibrillation. J Am Coll Cardiol 1985; 5:60A–68A.

1291. Redfors A. The effect of different digoxin doses on subjective symptoms and physical working capacity in patients with atrial fibrillation. Acta Med Scand 1971; 190:307–320.

1292. Aberg H, Strom G, Werner I. The effect of digitalis on the heart rate during exercise in patients with atrial fibrillation. Acta Med Scand 1972; 191:441–445.

1293. Aberg H, Strom G, Werner I. Heart rate during exercise in patients with atrial fibrillation. Acta Med Scand 1972; 191:315–320.

1294. Davidson DM, Hagan AD. Role of exercise stress testing in assessing digoxin dosage in chronic atrial fibrillation. Cardiovasc Med 1979; June:671–678.

1295. Goldman S, Probst P, Selzer A, Cohn K. Inefficacy of "therapeutic" serum levels of digoxin in controlling the ventricular rate in atrial fibrillation. Am J Cardiol 1975; 35:651–655.

1296. Bristow JD, Griswold HE. The use of digitalis in cardiovascular surgery. Prog Cardiovasc Dis 1965; 7:387–397.

1297. Chamberlain DA, White RJ, Howard MR, Smith TW. Plasma digoxin concentrations in patients with atrial fibrillation. BMJ 1970; 3:429–432.

1298. Redfors A. Plasma digoxin concentration—its relation to digoxin dosage and clinical effects in patients with atrial fibrillation. Br Heart J 1972; 34:383–391.

1299. Zener JC, Anggard EE, Harrison DC, Kalman SM. Persistence of digoxin effect in atrial fibrillation. JAMA 1973; 224:239–241.

1300. Schwartz JB. Verapamil in atrial fibrillation: the expected, the unexpected, and the unknown. Am Heart J 1983; 106:173–176.

1301. Zarowitz BJ, Gheorghiade M. Optimal heart rate control for patients with chronic atrial fibrillation: are pharmacologic choices truly changing? Am Heart J 1992; 123:1401–1403.

1302. Galun E, Flugelman MY, Glickson M, Eliakim M. Failure of long-term digitalization to prevent rapid ventricular response in patients with paroxysmal atrial fibrillation. Chest 1991; 99:1038–1040.

1303. Brodsky MA, Orlov MV, Capparelli EV, et al. Magnesium therapy in new-onset atrial fibrillation. Am J Cardiol 1994; 73:1227–1229.

1304. Roberts SA, Diaz C, Nolan PE, et al. Effectiveness and costs of digoxin treatment for atrial fibrillation and flutter. Am J Cardiol 1993; 72:567–573.

1305. Friedberg CK. Diseases of the Heart. Philadelphia: WB Saunders, 1966, p. 545.

1306. Klein HO, Kaplinsky E. Digitalis and verapamil in atrial fibrillation and flutter: is verapamil now the preferred agent? Drugs 1986; 31:185–197.

1307. Falk RH, Knowlton AA, Bernard SA, Gotlieb NE, Battinelli NJ. Digoxin for converting recent-onset atrial fibrillation to sinus rhythm: a randomized, double-blinded trial. Ann Intern Med 1987; 106:503–506.

1308. Rawles JM, Metcalfe MJ, Jennings K. Time of occurrence, duration, and ventricular rate of paroxysmal atrial fibrillation: the effect of digoxin. Br Heart J 1990; 63:225–227.

1309. Falk RH, Leavitt JI. Digoxin for atrial fibrillation: a drug whose time has gone? Ann Intern Med 1991; 114:573–575.

1310. Weiner P, Bassan MM, Jarchovsky J, Iusim S, Plavnick L. Clinical course of acute atrial fibrillation treated with rapid digitalization. Am Heart J 1983; 105:223–227.

1311. Engel TR, Gonzalez AD. Effects of digitalis on atrial vulnerability. Am J Cardiol 1978; 42:570–576.

1312. Rosen MR, Wit AL, Hoffman BF. Electrophysiology and pharmacology of cardiac arrhythmias. IV. Cardiac antiarrhythmic and toxic effects of digitalis. Am Heart J 1975; 89:391–399.

1313. Mackenzie J. Digitalis. Heart 1910; 2:335–339.

1314. Resnick WH. Transient auricular fibrillation following digitalis therapy with observations upon the reaction to atropine. J Clin Invest 1924; 1:181–195.

1315. Coumel P, Leclercq JF. Cardiac arrhythmias and autonomic nervous system. In Levy S, Scheinman MM (eds). Cardiac Arrhythmias. From Diagnosis to Therapy. Mount Kisco, NY: Futura Publishing Co., 1984, pp. 37–55.

1316. Wellens HJJ, Durrer D. Effect of digitalis on atrioventricular conduction and circus-movement tachycardias in patients with Wolff-Parkinson-White syndrome. Circulation 1973; 47:1229–1233.

1317. Dhingra RC, Palileo EV, Strasberg B, et al. Electrophysiologic effects of ouabain in patients with preexcitation and circus movement tachycardia. Am J Cardiol 1981; 47:139–144.

1318. Jedeikin R, Gillette PC, Garson A Jr, et al. Effect of ouabain on the anterograde effective refractory period of accessory atrioventricular connections in children. J Am Coll Cardiol 1983; 1:869–872.

1319. Wolff L, Parkinson J, White PD. Bundle-branch block with short P-R interval in healthy young people prone to paroxysmal tachycardia. Am Heart J 1930; 5:685–704.

1320. Deutsch S, Dalen JE. Indications for prophylactic digitalization. Anesthesiology 1969; 30:648–656.

1321. Juler GL, Stemmer EA, Connolly JE. Complications of prophylactic digitalization in thoracic surgical patients. J Thorac Cardiovasc Surg 1969; 58:352–360.

1322. Selzer A, Cohn KE. Some thoughts concerning the prophylactic use of digitalis. Am J Cardiol 1970; 26:215–217.

1323. Wheat MW, Burford TH. Digitalis in surgery: extension of classical indications. J Thorac Cardiovasc Surg 1961; 41:162–168.

1324. Burman SO. Digitalis and thoracic surgery. J Thorac Cardiovasc Surg 1965; 50:873–881.

1325. Burman SO. The prophylactic use of digitalis before thoracotomy. Ann Thorac Surg 1972; 14:359–368.

1326. Moorman JR, Pritchett EL. The arrhythmias of digitalis intoxication. Arch Intern Med 1985; 145:1289–1292.

1327. Chung EK, Dean HM. A recognition of digitalis intoxication in the presence of atrial fibrillation. Cardiology 1970; 55:22–27.

1328. Moorman JR. Digitalis toxicity at Duke Hospital, 1973 to 1984. South Med J 1985; 78:561–564.

1329. Lown B, Wyatt NF, Crocker AT, Goodale WT, Levine S. Interrelationship of digitalis and potassium in auricular tachycardia with block. Am Heart J 1953; 45:589–601.

1330. Lown B, Marcus F, Levine HD. Digitalis and atrial tachycardia with block. N Engl J Med 1959; 260:301–309.

1331. Taguchi JT, Ryan JM. Spontaneous conversion of established atrial fibrillation: clinical significance of a change to atrial flutter or to paroxysmal atrial tachycardia with AV block. Arch Intern Med 1969; 124:468–476.

1332. Pick A. Aberrant ventricular conduction of escaped beats. Circulation 1956; 13:702–711.

1333. Walsh TJ. Ventricular aberration of A-V nodal escape beats. Am J Cardiol 1962; 10:217–222.

1334. Kistin AD. Problems in the differentiation of ventricular arrhythmia from supraventricular arrhythmia with abnormal QRS. Prog Cardiovasc Dis 1966; 9:1–17.

1335. Damato AN, Lau SH, Bobb GA. Digitalis-induced bundle-branch ventricular tachycardia studied by electrode catheter recordings of the specialized conducting tissues of the dog. Circ Res 1971; 28:16–22.

1336. Kastor JA, Spear JF, Moore EN. Localization of ventricular irritability by epicardial mapping: origin of digitalis-induced unifocal tachycardia from left ventricular Purkinje tissue. Circulation 1972; 45:952–964.

1337. Reiser J, Anderson GJ. Preferential sensitivity of the left canine Purkinje system to cardiac glycosides. Circ Res 1981; 49:1043–1054.

1338. Massumi RA, Ertem GE, Vera Z. Aberrancy of junctional escape beats: evidence for origin in the fascicles of the left bundle branch. Am J Cardiol 1972; 29:351–359.

1339. Wieland JM, Marchlinski FE. Electrocardiographic response of digoxin-toxic fascicular tachycardia to Fab fragments: implications for tachycardia mechanism. Pacing Clin Electrophysiol 1986; 9:727–738.

1340. Josephson ME, Seides SF. Clinical Cardiac Electrophysiology. Techniques and Interpretations. Philadelphia: Lea & Febiger, 1979.

1341. Pick A, Dominguez P. Nonparoxysmal A-V nodal tachycardia. Circulation 1957; 16:1022–1032.

1342. Damato AN, Lau SH. His bundle rhythm. Circulation 1969; 40:527–534.

1343. Fisch C, Knoebel SB. Junctional rhythms. Prog Cardiovasc Dis 1970; 13:141–158.

1344. Pick A, Langendorf R. The dual function of the A-V junction. Am Heart J 1974; 88:790–797.

1345. Pick A, Langendorf R, Katz LN. A-V nodal tachycardia with block. Circulation 1961; 24:12–22.

1346. Castellanos A, Lemberg L. The relationship between digitalis and A-V nodal tachycardia with block. Am Heart J 1963; 66:605–613.

1347. Rosenbaum MB, Elizari MV, Lazzari JO. The mechanism of bidirectional tachycardia. Am Heart J 1969; 78:4–12.

1348. Cohen SI, Deisseroth A, Hecht HS. Infra-His bundle origin of bidirectional tachycardia. Circulation 1973; 47:1260–1266.

1349. Kastor JA, Goldreyer BN. Ventricular origin of bidirectional tachycardia: case report of a patient not toxic from digitalis. Circulation 1973; 48:897–903.

1350. Morris SN, Zipes DP. His bundle electrocardiography during bidirectional tachycardia. Circulation 1973; 48:32–36.

1351. Reid DS, Tynan M, Braidwood L, Fitzgerald GR. Bidirectional tachycardia in a child: a study using His bundle electrography. Br Heart J 1975; 37:339–344.

1352. Smith TW, Haber E. Digoxin intoxication: the relationship of clinical presentation to serum digoxin concentration. J Clin Invest 1970; 49:2377–2386.

1353. Smith TW, Butler VP Jr, Haber E, et al. Treatment of life-threatening digitalis intoxication with digoxin-specific Fab antibody fragments. N Engl J Med 1982; 307:1357–1400.

1354. Wenger TL, Butler VP Jr, Haber E, Smith TW. Treatment of 63 severely digitalis-toxic patients with digoxin-specific antibody fragments. J Am Coll Cardiol 1985; 5:118A–123A.

1355. Deano DA, Wu D, Mautner RK, Sherman RH, Ehsani AI, Rosen KM. The antiarrhythmic efficacy of intravenous therapy with disopyramide phosphate. Chest 1977; 71:597–606.

1356. Campbell TJ, Morgan JJ. Treatment of atrial arrhythmias after cardiac surgery with intravenous disopyramide. Aust N Z J Med 1980; 10:644–649.

1357. DeBacker M, Stoupel E, Kahn RJ. Efficacy of intravenous disopyramide in acute cardiac arrhythmias. Eur J Clin Pharmacol 1981; 19:11–18.

1358. Kerr CR, Prystowsky EN, Smith WM, Cook L, Gallagher JJ. Electrophysiologic effects of disopyramide phosphate in patients with Wolff-Parkinson-White syndrome. Circulation 1982; 65:869–878.

1359. Gavaghan TP, Feneley MP, Campbell TJ, Morgan JJ. Atrial tachyarrhythmias after cardiac surgery: results of disopyramide therapy. Aust N Z J Med 1985; 15:27–32.

1360. Nakazawa HK, Handa S, Nakamura Y, et al. High maintenance rate of sinus rhythm after cardioversion in post-thyrotoxic chronic atrial fibrillation. Int J Cardiol 1987; 16:47–55.

1361. Luoma PV, Kujala PA, Juustila HJ, Takkunen JT. Efficacy of intravenous disopyramide in the termination of supraventricular arrhythmias. J Clin Pharmacol 1978; 18:293–301.

1362. Kimura E, Mashima S, Tanaka T. Clinical evaluation of antiarrhythmic effects of disopyramide by multiclinical controlled double-blind methods. Int J Clin Pharmacol Ther Toxicol 1980; 18:338–343.

1363. Bauernfeind RA, Strasberg B, Rosen KM. Slowing of paroxysmal tachycardia with loss of functional bundle-branch block. Br Heart J 1982; 48:75–77.

1364. Ito M, Onodera S, Hashimoto J, et al. Effect of disopyramide on initiation of atrial fibrillation and relation to effective refractory period. Am J Cardiol 1989; 63:561–566.

1365. Hartel G, Louhija A, Konttinen A. Disopyramide in the prevention of recurrence of atrial fibrillation after electroconversion. Clin Pharmacol Ther 1974; 15:551–555.

1366. Karlson BW, Torstensson I, Abjorn C, Jansson SO, Peterson LE. Disopyramide in the maintenance of sinus rhythm after electroconversion of atrial fibrillation: a placebo-controlled one-year follow-up study. Eur Heart J 1988; 9:284–290.

1367. Bennett DH. Disopyramide in patients with the Wolff-Parkinson-White syndrome and atrial fibrillation. Chest 1978; 74:624–628.

1368. Spurrell RA, Thorburn CW, Camm J, Sowton E, Deuchar DC. Effects of disopyramide on electrophysiological properties of specialized conduction system in man and on accessory atrioventricular pathway in Wolff-Parkinson-White syndrome. Br Heart J 1975; 37:861–867.

1369. Moss AJ, Aledort LM. Use of edrophonium (Tensilon) in the evaluation of supraventricular tachycardias. Am J Cardiol 1966; 17:58–62.

1370. Goy JJ, Kappenberger L. Flecainide acetate in supraventricular arrhythmias. J Electrophysiol 1987; 1:113–119.
1371. Marcus FI. The hazards of using type IC antiarrhythmic drugs for the treatment of paroxysmal atrial fibrillation. Am J Cardiol 1990; 66:366–367.
1372. Goy JJ, Grbic M, Hurni M, et al. Conversion of supraventricular arrhythmias to sinus rhythm using flecainide. Eur Heart J 1985; 6:518–524.
1373. Borgeat A, Goy JJ, Maendly R, Kaufmann U, Grbic M, Sigwart U. Flecainide versus quinidine for conversion of atrial fibrillation to sinus rhythm. Am J Cardiol 1986; 58:496–498.
1374. Crozier IG, Ikram H, Kenealy M, Levy L. Flecainide acetate for conversion of acute supraventricular tachycardia to sinus rhythm. Am J Cardiol 1987; 59:607–609.
1375. Anderson JL, Jolivette DM, Fredell PA. Summary of efficacy and safety of flecainide for supraventricular arrhythmias. Am J Cardiol 1988; 62:62D–66D.
1376. Crijns HJ, van Wijk LM, van Gilst WH, Kingma JH, Van Gelder IC, Lie KI. Acute conversion of atrial fibrillation to sinus rhythm: clinical efficacy of flecainide acetate. Comparison of two regimens. Eur Heart J 1988; 9:634–638.
1377. Goy JJ, Kaufmann U, Kappenberger L, Sigwart U. Restoration of sinus rhythm with flecainide in patients with atrial fibrillation. Am J Cardiol 1988; 62:38D–40D.
1378. Hellestrand KJ. Intravenous flecainide acetate for supraventricular tachycardias. Am J Cardiol 1988; 62:16D–22D.
1379. Suttorp MJ, Kingma JH, Jessurun ER, Lie-A-Huen L, van Hemel NM, Lie KI. The value of class IC antiarrhythmic drugs for acute conversion of paroxysmal atrial fibrillation or flutter to sinus rhythm. J Am Coll Cardiol 1990; 16:1722–1727.
1380. Madrid AH, Moro C, Marin-Huerta E, Mestre JL, Novo L, Costa A. Comparison of flecainide and procainamide in cardioversion of atrial fibrillation. Eur Heart J 1993; 14:1127–1131.
1381. Barranco F, Sanchez M, Rodriguez J, Guerrero M. Efficacy of flecainide in patients with supraventricular arrhythmias and respiratory insufficiency. Intensive Care Med 1994; 20:42–44.
1382. Hohnloser SH, Zabel M. Short- and long-term efficacy and safety of flecainide acetate for supraventricular arrhythmias. Am J Cardiol 1992; 70:3A–9A.
1383. Reisinger J, Gatterer E, Heinze G, et al. Prospective comparison of flecainide versus sotalol for immediate cardioversion of atrial fibrillation. Am J Cardiol 1998; 81:1450–1454.
1384. Capucci A, Lenzi T, Boriani G, et al. Effectiveness of loading oral flecainide for converting recent-onset atrial fibrillation to sinus rhythm in patients without organic heart disease or with only systemic hypertension. Am J Cardiol 1992; 70:69–72.
1385. Crijns HJ, den Heijer P, van Wijk LM, Lie KI. Successful use of flecainide in atrial fibrillation with rapid ventricular rate in the Wolff-Parkinson-White syndrome. Am Heart J 1988; 115:1317–1321.
1386. Gavaghan TP, Koegh AM, Kelly RP, Campbell TJ, Thorburn C, Morgan JJ. Flecainide compared with a combination of digoxin and disopyramide for acute atrial arrhythmias after cardiopulmonary bypass. Br Heart J 1988; 60:497–501.
1387. Berns E, Rinkenberger RL, Jeang MK, Dougherty AH, Jenkins M, Naccarelli GV. Efficacy and safety of flecainide acetate for atrial tachycardia or fibrillation. Am J Cardiol 1987; 59:1337–1341.
1388. Mary-Rabine L, Telerman M. Long term evaluation of flecainide acetate in supraventricular tachyarrhythmias. Acta Cardiol 1988; 43:37–48.
1389. Sonnhag C, Kallryd A, Nylander E, Ryden L. Long-term efficacy of flecainide in paroxysmal atrial fibrillation. Acta Med Scand 1988; 224:563–569.
1390. Wiseman MN, Elstob JE, Camm AJ, Nathan AW. A study of the use of flecainide acetate in the long-term management of cardiac arrhythmias. Pacing Clin Electrophysiol 1990; 13:767–775.
1391. Pietersen AH, Hellemann H. Usefulness of flecainide for prevention of paroxysmal atrial fibrillation and flutter: Danish-Norwegian flecainide multicenter study group. Am J Cardiol 1991; 67:713–717.
1392. Pritchett EL, DaTorre SD, Platt ML, McCarville SE, Hougham AJ. Flecainide acetate treatment of paroxysmal supraventricular tachycardia and paroxysmal atrial fibrillation: dose-response studies. The flecainide supraventricular tachycardia study group. J Am Coll Cardiol 1991; 17:297–303.
1393. Katritsis D, Rowland E, O'Nunain S, Shakespeare CF, Poloniecki J, Camm AJ. Effect of flecainide on atrial and ventricular refractoriness and conduction in patients with normal left ventricle: implications for possible antiarrhythmic and proarrhythmic mechanisms. Eur Heart J 1995; 16:1930–1935.
1394. Kappenberger LJ, Fromer MA, Shenasa M, Gloor HO. Evaluation of flecainide acetate in rapid atrial fibrillation complicating Wolff-Parkinson-White syndrome. Clin Cardiol 1985; 8:321–326.
1395. Kim SS, Smith P, Ruffy R. Treatment of atrial tachy-arrhythmias and preexcitation syndrome with flecainide acetate. Am J Cardiol 1988; 62:29D–34D.
1396. O'Nunain S, Garratt CJ, Linker NJ, Gill J, Ward DE, Camm AJ. A comparison of intravenous propafenone and flecainide in the treatment of tachycardias associated with the Wolff-Parkinson-White syndrome. Pacing Clin Electrophysiol 1991; 14:2028–2034.
1397. Auricchio A. Reversible protective effect of propafenone or flecainide during atrial fibrillation in patients with an accessory atrioventricular connection. Am Heart J 1992; 124:932–937.
1398. van Wijk LM, Crijns HJ, van Gilst WH, Wesseling H, Lie KI. Flecainide acetate in the treatment of supraventricular tachycardias: value of programmed electrical stimulation for long-term prognosis. Am Heart J 1989; 117:365–369.
1399. Capucci A, Boriani G, Botto GL, et al. Conversion of recent-onset atrial fibrillation by a single oral loading dose of propafenone or flecainide. Am J Cardiol 1994; 74:503–505.
1400. Falk RH. Flecainide-induced ventricular tachycardia and fibrillation in patients treated for atrial fibrillation. Ann Intern Med 1989; 111:107–111.
1401. Pritchett ELC, Wilkinson WE. Mortality in patients treated with flecainide and encainide for supraventricular arrhythmias. Am J Cardiol 1991; 67:976–980.
1402. Murray KT. Ibutilide. Circulation 1998; 97:493–497.
1403. Ellenbogen KA, Stambler BS, Wood MA, et al. Efficacy of intravenous ibutilide for rapid termination of atrial fibrillation and atrial flutter: a dose-response study. J Am Coll Cardiol 1996; 28:130–136.
1404. Stambler BS, Wood MA, Ellenbogen KA. Antiarrhythmic actions of intravenous ibutilide compared with procainamide during human atrial flutter and fibrillation: electro-physiological determinants of enhanced conversion efficacy. Circulation 1997; 96:4298–4306.
1405. Volgman AS, Carberry PA, Stambler B, et al. Conversion efficacy and safety of intravenous ibutilide compared with intravenous procainamide in patients with atrial flutter or fibrillation. J Am Coll Cardiol 1998; 31:1414–1419.
1406. Schwartz SP, Schwartz LS. The Adams-Stokes syndrome during normal sinus rhythm and transient heart block. I. The effects of isuprel on patients with the Adams-Stokes syndrome during normal sinus rhythm and transient heart block. Am Heart J 1959; 57:849–861.
1407. Yamamoto T, Yeh SJ, Lin FC, Wu DL. Effects of isoproterenol on accessory pathway conduction in intermittent or concealed Wolff-Parkinson-White syndrome. Am J Cardiol 1990; 65:1438–1442.
1408. Szabo TS, Klein GJ, Sharma AD, Yee R, Milstein S. Usefulness of isoproterenol during atrial fibrillation in evaluation of asymptomatic Wolff-Parkinson-White pattern. Am J Cardiol 1989; 63:187–192.
1409. Josephson ME, Kastor JA, Kitchen JG III. Lidocaine in Wolff-Parkinson-White syndrome with atrial fibrillation. Ann Intern Med 1976; 84:44–45.

1410. Barrett PA, Laks MM, Mandel WJ, Yamaguchi I. The electrophysiologic effects of intravenous lidocaine in the Wolff-Parkinson-White syndrome. Am Heart J 1980; 100:23–33.

1411. Akhtar M, Gilbert CJ, Shenasa M. Effect of lidocaine on atrioventricular response via the accessory pathway in patients with Wolff-Parkinson-White syndrome. Circulation 1981; 63:435–441.

1412. Fanning WJ, Thomas CS Jr, Roach A, Tomichek R, Alford WC, Stoney WS Jr. Prophylaxis of atrial fibrillation with magnesium sulfate after coronary artery bypass grafting. Ann Thorac Surg 1991; 52:529–533.

1413. Parikka H, Toivonen L, Pellinen T, Verkkala K, Jarvinen A, Nieminen MS. The influence of intravenous magnesium sulphate on the occurrence of atrial fibrillation after coronary artery by-pass operation. Eur Heart J 1993; 14:251–258.

1414. Kayden HJ, Brodie BB, Steele JM. Procaine amide: a review. Circulation 1957; 25:118–126.

1415. McCord MC, Taguchi JT. A study of the effect of procaine amide hydrochloride in supraventricular arrhythmias. Circulation 1951; 4:387–393.

1416. Schaffer AI, Blumenfeld S, Pitman ER, Dix JH. Procaine amide: its effect on auricular arrhythmias. Am Heart J 1951; 42:115–123.

1417. Lucas BGB, Short DS. Procaine amide in the control of cardiac arrhythmias. Br Heart J 1952; 14:470–474.

1418. Miller G, Weinberg SL, Pick A. The effect of procaine amide (Pronestyl) in clinical auricular fibrillation and flutter. Circulation 1952; 6:41–50.

1419. Schack JA, Hoffman I, Vesell H. The response of arrhythmias and tachycardias of supraventricular origin to oral procaine amide. Br Heart J 1952; 14:465–469.

1420. Kayden HJ, Steele JM, Mark LC, Brodie BB. The use of procaine amide in cardiac arrhythmias. Circulation 1951; 4:13–22.

1421. Kinsman JM, Hansen WR, McClendon RL. Procaine amide (Pronestyl) in the treatment of cardiac arrhythmias. Am J Med Sci 1951; 222:365–374.

1422. Miller H, Nathanson MH, Griffith GC. The action of procaine amide in cardiac arrhythmias. JAMA 1951; 146:1004–1007.

1423. Gold MR, Ungaro MA, Ory DS, O'Gara PT, Buckley MJ, DeSanctis RW. Procainamide prevents arrhythmias following coronary bypass surgery. Circulation 1991; 83(Suppl II): II-285.

1424. Mandel WJ, Laks MM, Obayashi K, Hayakawa H, Daley W. The Wolff-Parkinson-White syndrome: pharmacologic effects of procaine amide. Am Heart J 1975; 90:744–754.

1425. Sellers TD Jr, Campbell RW, Bashore TM, Gallagher JJ. Effects of procainamide and quinidine sulfate in the Wolff-Parkinson-White syndrome. Circulation 1977; 55:15–22.

1426. Wellens HJJ, Braat S, Brugada P, Gorgels AP, Bar FW. Use of procainamide in patients with the Wolff-Parkinson-White syndrome to disclose a short refractory period of the accessory pathway. Am J Cardiol 1982; 50:1087–1089.

1427. Fananapazir L, Packer DL, German LD, et al. Procainamide infusion test: inability to identify patients with Wolff-Parkinson-White syndrome who are potentially at risk of sudden death. Circulation 1988; 77:1291–1296.

1428. Gaita F, Giustetto C, Riccardi R, Mangiardi L, Brusca A. Stress and pharmacologic tests as methods to identify patients with Wolff-Parkinson-White syndrome at risk of sudden death. Am J Cardiol 1989; 64:487–490.

1429. Boriani G, Biffi M, Capucci A, et al. Oral propafenone to convert recent-onset atrial fibrillation in patients with and without underlying heart disease: a randomized, controlled trial. Ann Intern Med 1997; 126:621–625.

1430. Vita JA, Friedman PL, Cantillon C, Antman EM. Efficacy of intravenous propafenone for the acute management of atrial fibrillation. Am J Cardiol 1989; 63:1275–1278.

1431. Connolly SJ, Mulji AS, Hoffert DL, Davis C, Shragge BW. Randomized placebo-controlled trial of propafenone for treatment of atrial tachyarrhythmias after cardiac surgery. J Am Coll Cardiol 1987; 10:1145–1148.

1432. Weiner P, Ganam R, Ganem R, Zidan F, Rabner M. Clinical course of recent-onset atrial fibrillation treated with oral propafenone. Chest 1994; 105:1013–1016.

1433. Azpitarte J, Alvarez M, Baun O, et al. Value of single oral loading dose of propafenone in converting recent-onset atrial fibrillation: results of a randomized, double-blind, controlled study. Eur Heart J 1997; 18:1649–1654.

1434. Capucci A, Boriani G, Rubino I, Della Casa S, Sanguinetti M, Magnani B. A controlled study on oral propafenone versus digoxin plus quinidine in converting recent onset atrial fibrillation to sinus rhythm. Int J Cardiol 1994; 43:305–313.

1435. Boriani G, Capucci A, Lenzi T, Sanguinetti M, Magnani B. Propafenone for conversion of recent-onset atrial fibrillation: a controlled comparison between oral loading dose and intravenous administration. Chest 1995; 108:355–358.

1436. Di Benedetto S. Quinidine versus propafenone for conversion of atrial fibrillation to sinus rhythm. Am J Cardiol 1997; 80:518–519.

1437. Antman EM, Beamer AD, Cantillon C, McGowan N, Goldman L, Friedman PL. Long-term oral propafenone therapy for suppression of refractory symptomatic atrial fibrillation and atrial flutter. J Am Coll Cardiol 1988; 12:1005–1011.

1438. Hammill SC, Wood DL, Gersh BJ, Osborn MJ, Holmes DR Jr. Propafenone for paroxysmal atrial fibrillation. Am J Cardiol 1988; 61:473–474.

1439. Kerr CR, Klein GJ, Axelson JE, Cooper JC. Propafenone for prevention of recurrent atrial fibrillation. Am J Cardiol 1988; 61:914–916.

1440. Connolly SJ, Hoffert DL. Usefulness of propafenone for recurrent paroxysmal atrial fibrillation. Am J Cardiol 1989; 63:817–819.

1441. Porterfield JG, Porterfield LM. Therapeutic efficacy and safety of oral propafenone for atrial fibrillation. Am J Cardiol 1989; 63:114–116.

1442. Pritchett EL, McCarthy EA, Wilkinson WE. Propafenone treatment of symptomatic paroxysmal supraventricular arrhythmias: a randomized, placebo-controlled, crossover trial in patients tolerating oral therapy. Ann Intern Med 1991; 114:539–544.

1443. UK Propafenone PSVT Study Group. A randomized, placebo-controlled trial of propafenone in the prophylaxis of paroxysmal supraventricular tachycardia and paroxysmal atrial fibrillation. Circulation 1995; 92:2550–2557.

1444. Bianconi L, Mennuni M, Lukic V, Castro A, Chieffi M, Santini M. Effects of oral propafenone administration before electrical cardioversion of chronic atrial fibrillation: a placebo-controlled study. J Am Coll Cardiol 1996; 28:700–706.

1445. Alboni P, Scarfo S, Fuca G, Paparella N, Pedini I, Mele D. Hemodynamic effects of oral propafenone during both sinus rhythm and atrial fibrillation. Am J Cardiol 1995; 75:91–93.

1446. Breithardt G, Borggrefe M, Wiebringhaus E, Seipel L. Effect of propafenone in the Wolff-Parkinson-White syndrome: electrophysiologic findings and long-term follow-up. Am J Cardiol 1984; 54:29D–39D.

1447. Ludmer PL, McGowan NE, Antman EM, Friedman PL. Efficacy of propafenone in Wolff-Parkinson-White syndrome: electrophysiologic findings and long-term follow-up. J Am Coll Cardiol 1987; 9:1357–1363.

1448. Murdock CJ, Kyles AE, Yeung-Lai-Wah JA, Qi A, Vorderbrugge S, Kerr CR. Atrial flutter in patients treated for atrial fibrillation with propafenone. Am J Cardiol 1990; 66:755–757.

1449. Grace AA, Camm AJ. Quinidine. N Engl J Med 1998; 338:35–45.

1450. Yount EH, Rosenblum M, McMillan RL. Use of quinidine in treatment of chronic auricular fibrillation. Arch Intern Med 1952; 89:63–69.

1451. Storstein O, Tveten H. Quinidine treatment of established auricular fibrillation. Acta Med Scand 1955; 153:57–66.

1452. Friedberg R, Sjoestroem B. Quinidine therapy of chronic auricular fibrillation. Acta Med Scand 1956; 155:293–305.

1453. Rokseth R, Storstein O. Quinidine therapy of chronic auricular fibrillation. Arch Intern Med 1963; 111:184–189.

1454. Sokolow M, Ball RE. Factors influencing conversion of chronic atrial fibrillation with special reference to serum quinidine concentration. Circulation 1956; 14:568–583.

1455. Selzer A, Kelly JJ, Gerbode F, et al. Treatment of atrial fibrillation after surgical repair of the mitral valve. Ann Intern Med 1965; 62:1213–1222.

1456. Halinen MO, Huttunen M, Paakkinen S, Tarssanen L. Comparison of sotalol with digoxin-quinidine for conversion of acute atrial fibrillation to sinus rhythm (the sotalol-digoxin-quinidine trial). Am J Cardiol 1995; 76:495–498.

1457. Hohnloser SH, van de Loo A, Baedeker F. Efficacy and proarrhythmic hazards of pharmacologic cardioversion of atrial fibrillation: prospective comparison of sotalol versus quinidine. J Am Coll Cardiol 1995; 26:852–858.

1458. McAlister HF, Luke RA, Whitlock RM, Smith WM. Intravenous amiodarone bolus versus oral quinidine for atrial flutter and fibrillation after cardiac operations. J Thorac Cardiovasc Surg 1990; 99:911–918.

1459. Lau CP, Leung WH, Wong CK. A randomized double-blind crossover study comparing the efficacy and tolerability of flecainide and quinidine in the control of patients with symptomatic paroxysmal atrial fibrillation. Am Heart J 1992; 124:645–650.

1460. Hurt RL, Bates M. The value of quinidine in the prevention of cardiac arrhythmias after pulmonary resection. Thorax 1958; 13:39–41.

1461. McCarty RJ, Jahnke EJ, Walker WJ. Ineffectiveness of quinidine in preventing atrial fibrillation following mitral valvotomy. Circulation 1966; 34:792–794.

1462. Rasmussen K, Wang H, Fausa D. Comparative efficiency of quinidine and verapamil in the maintenance of sinus rhythm after DC conversion of atrial fibrillation: a controlled clinical trial. Acta Med Scand Suppl 1981; 645:23–28.

1463. Bigger JT, Hoffman BF. Antiarrhythmic drugs. In Gilman AG, Rall TW, Nies AS, Taylor P (eds). Goodman and Gilman's The Pharmacological Basis of Therapeutics. 8th ed. New York: Pergamon Press, 1990, p. 855.

1464. Morady F, Kou WH, Kadish AH, Toivonen LK, Kushner JA, Schmaltz S. Effects of epinephrine in patients with an accessory atrioventricular connection treated with quinidine. Am J Cardiol 1988; 62:580–584.

1465. Modell W, Hussar AE. Effect of reserpine on atrial and ventricular rates in atrial fibrillation in man. Nature 1965; 205:1019.

1466. Soyka LF, Wirtz C, Spangenberg RB. Clinical safety profile of sotalol in patients with arrhythmias. Am J Cardiol 1990; 65:74A–81A.

1467. Hohnloser SH, Woosley RL. Sotalol. N Engl J Med 1994; 331:31–38.

1468. Prakash R, Parmley WW, Allen HN, Matloff JM. Effect of sotalol on clinical arrhythmias. Am J Cardiol 1972; 29:397–400.

1469. Gallik DM, Kim SG, Ferrick KJ, Roth JA, Fisher JD. Efficacy and safety of sotalol in patients with refractory atrial fibrillation or flutter. Am Heart J 1997; 134:155–160.

1470. Alt E, Ammer R, Lehmann G, et al. Patient characteristics and underlying heart disease as predictors of recurrent atrial fibrillation after internal and external cardioversion in patients treated with oral sotalol. Am Heart J 1997; 134:419–425.

1471. Nystrom U, Edvardsson N, Berggren H, Pizzarelli GP, Radegran K. Oral sotalol reduces the incidence of atrial fibrillation after coronary artery bypass surgery. Thorac Cardiovasc Surg 1993; 41:34–37.

1472. Waldo AL, Camm AJ, deRuyter H, et al. Effect of d-sotalol on mortality in patients with left ventricular dysfunction after recent and remote myocardial infarction, the SWORD Investigators. Survival with oral d-sotalol. Lancet 1996; 348:7–12.

1473. Sahar DI, Reiffel JA, Bigger JT Jr, Squatrito A, Kidwell GA. Efficacy, safety, and tolerance of d-sotalol in patients with refractory supraventricular tachyarrhythmias. Am Heart J 1989; 117:562–568.

1474. Alboni P, Paparella N, Cappato R, Pirani R, Yiannacopulu P, Antonioli GE. Long-term effects of theophylline in atrial fibrillation with a slow ventricular response. Am J Cardiol 1993; 72:1142–1145.

1475. Wilson DB. Chronic atrial fibrillation in the elderly: risks vs. benefits of long-term anticoagulation. J Am Geriatr Soc 1985; 33:298–302.

1476. Sandercock P, Warlow C, Bamford J, Peto R, Starkey I. Is a controlled trial of long-term oral anticoagulants in patients with stroke and non-rheumatic atrial fibrillation worthwhile? Lancet 1986; 1:788–792.

1477. Sherman DG, Hart RG, Easton JD. The secondary prevention of stroke in patients with atrial fibrillation. Arch Neurol 1986; 43:68–70.

1478. Halperin JL, Hart RG. Atrial fibrillation and stroke: new ideas, persisting dilemmas. Stroke 1988; 19:937–941.

1479. Dunn M, Alexander J, de Silva R, Hildner F. Antithrombotic therapy in atrial fibrillation. Chest 1989; 95:118S–127S.

1480. Wipf JE, Lipsky BA. Atrial fibrillation: thromboembolic risk and indications for anticoagulation. Arch Intern Med 1990; 150:1598–1603.

1481. Albers GW, Atwood JE, Hirsh J, Sherman DG, Hughes RA, Connolly SJ. Stroke prevention in nonvalvular atrial fibrillation. Ann Intern Med 1991; 115:727–736.

1482. Albers GW, Sherman DG, Gress DR, Paulseth JE, Petersen P. Stroke prevention in nonvalvular atrial fibrillation: a review of prospective randomized trials. Ann Neurol 1991; 30:511–518.

1483. Cairns JA. Stroke prevention in atrial fibrillation trial. Circulation 1991; 84:933–935.

1484. Cairns JA, Connolly SJ. Nonrheumatic atrial fibrillation: risk of stroke and role of antithrombotic therapy. Circulation 1991; 84:469–481.

1485. Flegel KM, Hutchinson TA, Groome PA, Tousignant P. Factors relevant to preventing embolic stroke in patients with non-rheumatic atrial fibrillation. J Clin Epidemiol 1991; 44:551–560.

1486. Nolan J, Bloomfield P. Non-rheumatic atrial fibrillation: warfarin or aspirin for all? Br Heart J 1992; 68:544–547.

1487. Petersen P. Anticoagulation therapy for atrial fibrillation. In Falk RH, Podrid PJ (eds). Atrial Fibrillation. Mechanisms and Management. New York: Raven Press, 1992, pp. 307–319.

1488. Singer DE. Randomized trials of warfarin for atrial fibrillation. N Engl J Med 1992; 327:1451–1453.

1489. Caro JJ, Groome PA, Flegel KM. Atrial fibrillation and anticoagulation: from randomised trials to practice. Lancet 1993; 341:1381–1384.

1490. Albers GW. Atrial fibrillation and stroke: three new studies, three remaining questions. Arch Intern Med 1994; 154:1443–1448.

1491. Lodder J, Dennis MS, Van Raak L, Jones LN, Warlow CP. Cooperative study on the value of long term anticoagulation in patients with stroke and non-rheumatic atrial fibrillation. Br Med J Clin Res Ed 1994; 1988:1435–1438.

1492. Theiss W. Anticoagulants: when and how? Pacing Clin Electrophysiol 1994; 17:1011–1015.

1493. Laupacis A, Albers G, Dalen J, Dunn M, Feinberg W, Jacobson A. Antithrombotic therapy in atrial fibrillation. Chest 1995; 108:352S–359S.

1494. Wheeldon NM. Atrial fibrillation and anticoagulant therapy. Eur Heart J 1995; 16:302–312.

1495. Cleland JG, Cowburn PJ, Falk RH. Should all patients with atrial fibrillation receive warfarin? Evidence from randomized clinical trials. Eur Heart J 1996; 17:674–681.

1496. Rosendaal FR. The scylla and charybdis of oral anticoagulant treatment. N Engl J Med 1996; 335:587–589.

1497. Bucknall CA, Morris GK, Mitchell JR. Physicians' attitudes to four common problems: hypertension, atrial fibrillation, transient ischaemic attacks, and angina pectoris. Br Med J Clin Res Ed 1986; 293:739–742.

1498. Gottlieb LK, Salem-Schatz S. Anticoagulation in atrial fibrillation: does efficacy in clinical trials translate into effectiveness in practice? Arch Intern Med 1994; 154:1945–1953.

1499. McCrory DC, Matchar DB, Samsa G, Sanders LL, Pritchett EL. Physician attitudes about anticoagulation for nonvalvular atrial fibrillation in the elderly. Arch Intern Med 1995; 155:277–281.

1500. Albers GW, Yim JM, Belew KM, et al. Status of antithrombotic therapy for patients with atrial fibrillation in university hospitals. Arch Intern Med 1996; 156:2311–2316.

1501. Bush D, Tayback M. Anticoagulation for nonvalvular atrial fibrillation: effects of type of practice on physicians' self-reported behavior. Am J Med 1998; 104:148–151.

1502. Wheeldon NM, Tayler DI, Anagnostou E, Cook D, Wales C, Oakley GD. Screening for atrial fibrillation in primary care. Heart 1998; 79:50–55.

1503. Askey JM, Cherry CB. Thromboembolism associated with auricular fibrillation. JAMA 1950; 144:97–100.

1504. Wood JC, Conn HL. Prevention of systemic arterial embolism in chronic rheumatic heart disease by means of protracted anticoagulant therapy. Circulation 1954; 10:517–523.

1505. Adams GF, Merrett JD, Hutchinson WM, Pollock AM. Cerebral embolism and mitral stenosis: survival with and without anticoagulants. J Neurol Neurosurg Psychiatry 1974; 37:378–383.

1506. Cosgriff SW. Chronic anticoagulant therapy in recurrent embolism of cardiac origin. Ann Intern Med 1981; 38:278–287.

1507. Connolly SJ, Laupacis A, Gent M, Roberts RS, Cairns JA, Joyner C. Canadian Atrial Fibrillation Anticoagulation (CAFA) study. J Am Coll Cardiol 1991; 18:349–355.

1508. Stroke Prevention in Atrial Fibrillation Investigators. Stroke prevention in atrial fibrillation study: final results. Circulation 1991; 84:527–539.

1509. Petersen P, Hansen JM. Stroke in thyrotoxicosis with atrial fibrillation. Stroke 1988; 19:15–18.

1510. Presti CF, Hart RG. Thyrotoxicosis, atrial fibrillation, and embolism, revisited. Am Heart J 1989; 117:976–977.

1511. Stroke Prevention in Atrial Fibrillation Investigators. Warfarin versus aspirin for prevention of thromboembolism in atrial fibrillation: stroke prevention in fibrillation II study. Lancet 1994; 343:687–691.

1512. Gage BF, Cardinalli AB, Albers GW, Owens DK. Cost-effectiveness of warfarin and aspirin for prophylaxis of stroke in patients with nonvalvular atrial fibrillation. JAMA 1995; 274:1839–1845.

1513. Miller VT, Pearce LA, Feinberg WM, Rothrock JF, Anderson DC, Hart RG. Differential effect of aspirin versus warfarin on clinical stroke types in patients with atrial fibrillation. Stroke prevention in atrial fibrillation investigators. Neurology 1996; 46:238–240.

1514. European Atrial Fibrillation Trial Study Group. Optimal oral anticoagulant therapy in patients with nonrheumatic atrial fibrillation and recent cerebral ischemia. N Engl J Med 1995; 333:5–10.

1515. Petersen P, Boysen G, Godtfredsen J, Andersen ED, Andersen B. Placebo-controlled, randomised trial of warfarin and aspirin for prevention of thromboembolic complications in chronic atrial fibrillation: the Copenhagen AFASAK study. Lancet 1989; 1:175–179.

1516. Hylek EM, Skates SJ, Sheehan MA, Singer DE. An analysis of the lowest effective intensity of prophylactic anticoagulation for patients with nonrheumatic atrial fibrillation. N Engl J Med 1996; 335:540–546.

1517. Stroke Prevention in Atrial Fibrillation Investigators. Bleeding during antithrombotic therapy in patients with atrial fibrillation. Arch Intern Med 1996; 156:409–416.

1518. Stroke Prevention in Atrial Fibrillation Investigators. Adjusted-dose warfarin versus low-intensity, fixed-dose warfarin plus aspirin for high-risk patients with atrial fibrillation. Lancet 1996; 348:633–638.

1519. Ezekowitz MD, Bridgers SL, James KE, et al. Warfarin in the prevention of stroke associated with nonrheumatic atrial fibrillation: Veterans Affairs Stroke Prevention in Nonrheumatic Atrial Fibrillation Investigators. N Engl J Med 1992; 327:1406–1412.

1520. Archer SL, James KE, Kvernen LR, Cohen IS, Ezekowitz MD, Gornick CC. Role of transesophageal echocardiography in the detection of left atrial thrombus in patients with chronic nonrheumatic atrial fibrillation. Am Heart J 1995; 130:287–295.

1521. Rothrock JF, Dittrich HC, McAllen S, Taft BJ, Lyden PD. Acute anticoagulation following cardioembolic stroke. Stroke 1989; 20:730–734.

1522. Ansell JE, Patel N, Ostrovsky D, Nozzolillo E, Peterson AM. Long-term patient self-management of oral anticoagulation. Arch Intern Med 1995; 155:2185–2189.

1523. Atrial Fibrillation Investigators. The efficacy of aspirin in patients with atrial fibrillation: analysis of pooled data from 3 randomized trials. The Atrial Fibrillation Investigators. Arch Intern Med 1997; 157:1237–1240.

1524. Miller VT, Rothrock JF, Pearce LA, Feinberg WM, Hart RG, Anderson DC. Ischemic stroke in patients with atrial fibrillation: effect of aspirin according to stroke mechanism. Stroke Prevention in Atrial Fibrillation Investigators. Neurology 1993; 43:32–36.

1525. European Atrial Fibrillation Trial Study Group. Secondary prevention in non-rheumatic atrial fibrillation after transient ischaemic attack or minor stroke. Lancet 1993; 342:1255–1262.

1526. Singer DE, Hughes RA, Gress DR, et al. The effect of aspirin on the risk of stroke in patients with nonrheumatic atrial fibrillation: the BAATAF study. Am Heart J 1992; 124:1567–1573.

1527. Yamamoto K, Ikeda U, Fukazawa H, Shimada K. Effects of aspirin on status of thrombin generation in atrial fibrillation. Am J Cardiol 1996; 77:528–530.

1528. Goodnight SH. Antiplatelet therapy for mitral stenosis. Circulation 1980; 62:466–468.

1529. Steele P, Rainwater J. Favorable effect of sulfinpyrazone on thromboembolism in patients with rheumatic heart disease. Circulation 1980; 62:462–465.

1530. Gustafsson C, Asplund K, Britton M, Norrving B, Olsson B, Marke LA. Cost effectiveness of primary stroke prevention in atrial fibrillation: Swedish national perspective. BMJ 1992; 305:1457–1460.

1531. Pollak A, Falk RH. Pacemaker therapy in patients with atrial fibrillation. Am Heart J 1993; 125:824–830.

1532. Sgarbossa EB, Pinski SL. Pacemaker therapies for atrial fibrillation. Primary Cardiology 1994; 20:16–20.

1533. Glikson M, Hayes DL, Nishimura RA. Newer clinical applications of pacing. J Cardiovasc Electrophysiol 1997; 8:1190–1203.

1534. Keane D, Zou L, Ruskin J. Nonpharmacologic therapies for atrial fibrillation. Am J Cardiol 1998; 81:41C–45C.

1535. Pollak A, Falk RH. The use of pacemakers in atrial fibrillation. In Falk RH, Podrid PJ (eds). Atrial Fibrillation. Mechanisms and Management. New York: Raven Press, 1992, pp. 345–358.

1536. Levine PA, Seltzer JP. AV universal (DDD) pacing and atrial fibrillation. Clin Prog Pacing Electrophysiol 1983; 1:275–281.

1537. Mancini GB, Goldberger AL. Cardioversion of atrial fibrillation: consideration of embolization, anticoagulation, prophylactic pacemaker, and long-term success. Am Heart J 1982; 104:617–621.

1538. Sharkey SW, Chaffee V, Kapsner S. Prophylactic external pacing during cardioversion of atrial tachyarrhythmias. Am J Cardiol 1985; 55:1632–1634.

1539. Miller PH, Carleton RA. Hemodynamic assessment during atrial fibrillation. Value of ventricular pacing. Am J Cardiol 1968; 22:568–571.

1540. Wittkampf FHM, de Jongste MJL, Lie HI, Meijler FL. Effect of right ventricular pacing on ventricular rhythm during atrial fibrillation. J Am Coll Cardiol 1988; 11:539–545.

1541. Lau CP, Leung WH, Wong CK, Tai YT, Cheng CH. A new pacing method for rapid regularization and rate control in atrial fibrillation. Am J Cardiol 1990; 65:1198–1203.

1542. Duckers HJ, van Hemel NM, Kelder JC, Bakema H, Yee R. Effective use of a novel rate-smoothing algorithm in atrial fibrillation by ventricular pacing. Eur Heart J 1997; 18:1951–1955.

1543. Cohen HE, Meltzer LE, Lattimer G, Linares H, Agrin R. Treatment of refractory supraventricular arrhythmias with induced permanent atrial fibrillation. Am J Cardiol 1971; 28:472–474.

1544. Wiener L, Dwyer EM Jr. Electrical induction of atrial fibrillation: an approach to intractable atrial tachycardia. Am J Cardiol 1968; 21:731–734.

1545. Moreira DA, Shepard RB, Waldo AL. Chronic rapid atrial pacing to maintain atrial fibrillation: use to permit control of ventricular rate in order to treat tachycardia induced cardiomyopathy. Pacing Clin Electrophysiol 1989; 12:761–775.

1546. Saksena S, Prakash A, Hill M, et al. Prevention of recurrent atrial fibrillation with chronic dual-site right atrial pacing. J Am Coll Cardiol 1996; 28:687–694.

1547. Waldo AL, MacLean WA, Karp RB, Kouchoukos NT, James TN. Continuous rapid atrial pacing to control recurrent or sustained supraventricular tachycardias following open heart surgery. Circulation 1976; 54:245–250.

1548. Waldo AL, MacLean WAH. Diagnosis and Treatment of Cardiac Arrhythmias Following Open Heart Surgery. Emphasis on the Use of Atrial and Ventricular Epicardial Wire Electrodes. Mount Kisco, NY: Futura Publishing Co., 1980.

1549. Furman S, Cooper JA. Atrial fibrillation during A-V sequential pacing. Pacing Clin Electrophysiol 1982; 5:133–135.

1550. Markewitz A, Schad N, Hemmer W, Bernheim C, Ciavolella M, Weinhold C. What is the most appropriate stimulation mode in patients with sinus node dysfunction? Pacing Clin Electrophysiol 1986; 9:1115–1120.

1551. Sgarbossa EB, Pinski SL, Maloney JD, et al. Chronic atrial fibrillation and stroke in paced patients with sick sinus syndrome: relevance of clinical characteristics and pacing modalities. Circulation 1993; 88:1045–1053.

1552. Andersen HR, Thuesen L, Bagger JP, Vesterlund T, Thomsen PE. Prospective randomised trial of atrial versus ventricular pacing in sick-sinus syndrome. Lancet 1994; 344:1523–1528.

1553. Reimold SC, Lamas GA, Cantillon CO, Antman EM. Risk factors for the development of recurrent atrial fibrillation: role of pacing and clinical variables. Am Heart J 1995; 129:1127–1132.

1554. Feuer JM, Shandling AH, Messenger JC. Influence of cardiac pacing mode on the long-term development of atrial fibrillation. Am J Cardiol 1989; 64:1376–1379.

1555. Brignole M, Gianfranchi L, Menozzi C, et al. A new pacemaker for paroxysmal atrial fibrillation treated with radiofrequency ablation of the AV junction. Pacing Clin Electrophysiol 1994; 17:1889–1894.

1556. Yu WC, Chen SA, Tai CT, Feng AN, Chang MS. Effects of different atrial pacing modes on atrial electrophysiology: implicating the mechanism of biatrial pacing in prevention of atrial fibrillation. Circulation 1997; 96:2992–2996.

1557. Killip T, Lambrew CT. Electrical control of cardiac rhythm. Annu Rev Med 1966; 17:447–462.

1558. Selzer A, Kelly JJ, Johnson RB, Kerth WJ. Immediate and long-term results of electrical conversion of arrhythmias. Prog Cardiovasc Dis 1966; 9:90–104.

1559. Resnekov L. Cardiac arrhythmias. VI. Present status of electroversion in the management of cardiac dysrhythmias. Circulation 1973; 47:1356–1363.

1560. DeSilva RA, Graboys TB, Podrid PJ, Lown B. Cardioversion and defibrillation. Am Heart J 1980; 100:881–895.

1561. Falk RH, Podrid PJ. Electrical cardioversion of atrial fibrillation. In Falk RH, Podrid PJ (eds). Atrial Fibrillation. Mechanisms and Management. New York: Raven Press, 1992, pp. 181–195.

1562. Yurchak PM, Williams SV, Achord JL, et al. Clinical competence in elective direct current (DC) cardioversion: a statement for physicians from the AHA/ACC/ACP task force on clinical privileges in cardiology. Circulation 1993; 88:342–345.

1563. Van Gelder IC, Crijns HJGM. Cardioversion of atrial fibrillation and subsequent maintenance of sinus rhythm. PACE 1997; 20:2675–2683.

1564. Lown B, Amarasingham R, Neuman J. New method for terminating cardiac arrhythmias: use of synchronized capacitor discharge. JAMA 1962; 182:548–555.

1565. Killip T. Synchronized DC precordial shock for arrhythmias: safe new technique to establish normal rhythm may be utilized on an elective or an emergency basis. JAMA 1963; 186:107–113.

1566. Lown B, Bey SK, Perlroth MG, Abe T. Cardioversion of ectopic tachycardias. Am J Med Sci 1963; 246:35/257–42/264.

1567. Hurst JW, Paulk EA, Proctor HD, Schlant RC. Management of patients with atrial fibrillation. Am J Med 1964; 37:728–741.

1568. McDonald L, Resnekov L, O'Brien K. Direct-current shock in treatment of drug-resistant cardiac arrhythmias. BMJ 1965; 1:1468–1470.

1569. Miller HS. Synchronized precordial electroshock for control of cardiac arrhythmias. JAMA 1964; 189:549–552.

1570. Oram S, Davies JPH. Further experience of electrical conversion of atrial fibrillation to sinus rhythm: analysis of 100 patients. Lancet 1964; 1:1294–1298.

1571. Rabbino MD, Likoff W, Dreifus LS. Complications and limitations of direct-current countershock. JAMA 1964; 190:417–420.

1572. Meltzer LE, Aytan N, Yun DD, Ural ME, Palmon FP, Kitchell JR. Atrial fibrillation treated with direct current countershock. Arch Intern Med 1965; 115:537–541.

1573. Halmos PB. Direct current conversion of atrial fibrillation. Br Heart J 1966; 28:302–308.

1574. Kreus KE, Salokannel SJ, Waris EK. Non-synchronised and synchronised direct-current countershock in cardiac arrhythmias. Lancet 1966; 2:405–408.

1575. Bell H, Pugh D, Dunn M. Failure of cardioversion in mitral valve disease. Arch Intern Med 1967; 119:257–280.

1576. Coelho E, Pinto LS, Luiz AS, Coelho EM, Pereira AL, Barreiros R. Long-term results of conversion of atrial fibrillation by direct current countershock. Cardiology 1967; 50:147–155.

1577. Eberdt EC, Brill IC, Rogers WR. Value of cardioversion in chronic atrial fibrillation. Arch Intern Med 1967; 119:253–256.

1578. Futral AA, McGuire LB. Reversion of chronic atrial fibrillation. JAMA 1967; 199:885–888.

1579. Kastor JA, DeSanctis RW. The electrical conversion of atrial fibrillation. Am J Med Sci 1967; 253:511–519.

1580. Resnekov L, McDonald L. Complications in 220 patients with cardiac dysrhythmias treated by phased direct current shock, and indications for electroconversion. Br Heart J 1967; 29:926–936.

1581. Wikland B, Edhag O, Eliasch H. Atrial fibrillation and flutter treated with synchronized DC shock: a study on immediate and long-term results. Acta Med Scand 1967; 182:665–671.

1582. Bjerkelund C, Orning OM. An evaluation of DC shock treatment of atrial arrhythmias. Acta Med Scand 1968; 184:481–491.

1583. Hall JI, Wood DR. Factors affecting cardioversion of atrial arrhythmias with special reference to quinidine. Br Heart J 1968; 30:84–90.

1584. Radford MD, Evans DW. Long-term results of DC reversion of atrial fibrillation. Br Heart J 1968; 30:91–96.

1585. McCarthy C, Varghese PJ, Barritt DW. Prognosis of atrial arrhythmias treated by electrical counter shock therapy: a three-year follow-up. Br Heart J 1969; 31:496–500.

1586. Szekely P, Wynne NA, Pearson DT, Batson GA, Sideris DA. Direct current shock and digitalis: a clinical and experimental study. Br Heart J 1969; 31:91–96.

1587. Resnekov L, McDonald L. Electroversion of lone atrial fibrillation and flutter including haemodynamic studies at rest and on exercise. Br Heart J 1971; 33:339–350.

1588. Waris E, Kreus KE, Salokannel J. Factors influencing persistence of sinus rhythm after DC shock treatment of atrial fibrillation. Acta Med Scand 1971; 189:161–166.

1589. Edvardsson B, Olsson SB. Outpatient electroconversion of chronic atrial fibrillation. In Kulbertus HE, Olsson SB, Schlepper M (eds). Atrial Fibrillation. Kiruna, Molndal, Sweden: AB Hassle, 1982, pp. 242–249.

1590. Lesser MF. Safety and efficacy of in-office cardioversion for treatment of supraventricular arrhythmias. Am J Cardiol 1990; 66:1267–1268.

1591. Upton AR, Honey M. Electroconversion of atrial fibrillation after mitral valvotomy. Br Heart J 1971; 33:732–738.

1592. Dalzell GW, Anderson J, Adgey AA. Factors determining success and energy requirements for cardioversion of atrial fibrillation. Q J Med 1990; 76:903–913.

1593. Van Gelder IC, Crijns HJ, van Gilst WH, Verwer R, Lie KI. Prediction of uneventful cardioversion and maintenance of sinus rhythm from direct-current electrical cardioversion of chronic atrial fibrillation and flutter. Am J Cardiol 1991; 68:41–46.

1594. Resnekov L, McDonald L. Appraisal of electroconversion in treatment of cardiac dysrhythmias. Br Heart J 1968; 30:786–811.

1595. Emery P, Staffurth JS. Electrical cardioversion for persistent atrial fibrillation after treatment of thyrotoxicosis. Postgrad Med J 1982; 58:746–748.

1596. Nakazawa HK, Sakurai K, Hamada N, Momotani N, Ito K. Management of atrial fibrillation in the post-thyrotoxic state. Am J Med 1982; 72:903–906.

1597. Kahn DR, Kirsh MM, Ferguson PW, Sloan H. Cardioversion after mitral valve operations. Circulation 1967; 35(Suppl I): I-82–I-85.

1598. Semer H, Hultgren H, Kleiger R, Braniff B. Cardioversion following prosthetic mitral valve replacement. Circulation 1967; 35:523–529.

1599. Yang SS, Maranhao V, Monheit R, Ablaza SGG, Goldberg H. Cardioversion following open-heart valvular surgery. Br Heart J 1966; 28:309–315.

1600. Jenzer H, Lown B. Cardioversion of atrial fibrillation after valve replacement. Am Heart J 1972; 84:840–842.

1601. Brodsky MA, Allen BJ, Luckett CR, Capparelli EV, Wolff LJ, Henry WL. Antiarrhythmic efficacy of solitary beta-adrenergic blockade for patients with sustained ventricular tachyarrhythmias. Am Heart J 1989; 118:272–280.

1602. Vogel JHK, Pryor R, Blount SG. Direct-current defibrillation during pregnancy. JAMA 1965; 193:970–971.

1603. Cullhed I. Cardioversion during pregnancy: a case report. Acta Med Scand 1983; 214:169–172.

1604. Cohen TJ, Ibrahim B, Denier D, Haji A, Quan W. Active compression cardioversion for refractory atrial fibrillation. Am J Cardiol 1997; 80:354–355.

1605. Leclercq JF, Bizot J, Attuel P, Coumel P. Direct-current cardioversion of atrial tachyarrhythmias under oral flecainide therapy. Am J Cardiol 1997; 80:645–648.

1606. Bleyer FL, Quattromani A, Caracciolo EA, Bjerregaard P. An aggressive approach in converting resistant atrial fibrillation. Am Heart J 1996; 132:1304–1306.

1607. Kleiger R, Lown B. Cardioversion and digitalis. II. Clinical studies. Circulation 1966; 33:878–887.

1608. Lown B, DeSilva RA. Cardioversion and defibrillation. In Hurst JW (ed). The Heart. New York: McGraw-Hill, 1990, pp. 2095–2100.

1609. Van Gelder IC, Crijns HJ, van Gilst WH, de Langen CD, van Wijk LM, Lie KI. Effects of flecainide on the atrial defibrillation threshold. Am J Cardiol 1989; 63:112–114.

1610. Guarnieri T, Tomaselli G, Griffith LS, Brinker J. The interaction of antiarrhythmic drugs and the energy for cardioversion of chronic atrial fibrillation. Pacing Clin Electrophysiol 1991; 14:1007–1012.

1611. Sagrista-Sauleda J, Permanyer-Miralda G, Soler-Soler J. Electrical cardioversion after amiodarone administration. Am Heart J 1992; 123:1536–1542.

1612. Kerth WJ, Selzer A, Keyani K, Gerbode F. The electrical conversion of cardiac arrhythmias. J Cardiovasc Surg 1964; 25:212–222.

1613. Jacobs LO, Andrews TC, Pederson DN, Donovan DJ. Effect of intravenous procainamide on direct-current cardioversion of atrial fibrillation. Am J Cardiol 1998; 82:241–242.

1614. Kerber RE, Jensen SR, Grayzel J, Kennedy J, Hoyt R. Elective cardioversion: influence of paddle-electrode location and size on success rates and energy requirements. N Engl J Med 1981; 305:658–662.

1615. Mower MM, Mirowski M. Phenomenon of delayed reversion following atrial cardioversion. Circulation 1974; 49(Suppl III):III-194.

1616. Duvernoy WF, Anbe DT. Delayed conversion to sinus rhythm after direct-current countershock. Heart Lung 1976; 5:465–470.

1617. McNally EM, Meyer EC, Langendorf R. Elective countershock in unanesthetized patients with use of an esophageal electrode. Circulation 1966; 33:124–127.

1618. Jensen JB, Humphries JO, Kouwenhoven WB, Jude JR. Electroshock for atrial flutter and atrial fibrillation. JAMA 1965; 194:123–126.

1619. Waris EK, Scheinin TM, Kreus KE, Salokannel J, Scheinin BM. Non-synchronized direct current countershock: conversion of atrial fibrillation and subsequent electrocardiographic findings. Acta Med Scand 1965; 178:309–320.

1620. Kavanagh-Gray D. Non-synchronized direct-current countershock in cardiac arrhythmias. Can Med Assoc J 1967; 96:1460–1462.

1621. Kreus KE, Waris EK, Salokannel SJ. Nonsynchronized direct-current countershock. Am Heart J 1967; 74:286–287.

1622. Gosselink AT, Crijns HJ, Hamer HP, Hillege H, Lie KI. Changes in left and right atrial size after cardioversion of atrial fibrillation: role of mitral valve disease. J Am Coll Cardiol 1993; 22:1666–1672.

1623. Alam M, Sun I. Transesophageal echocardiographic evaluation of left atrial mass lesions. J Am Soc Echocardiogr 1991; 4:323–330.

1624. Tieleman RG, Van Gelder IC, Crijns HJGM, et al. Early recurrences of atrial fibrillation after electrical cardioversion: a result of fibrillation-induced electrical remodeling of the atria? J Am Coll Cardiol 1998; 31:167–173.

1625. Szekely P, Sideris DA, Batson GA. Maintenance of sinus rhythm after atrial defibrillation. Br Heart J 1970; 32:741–746.

1626. Fisher RD, Mason DT, Morrow AG. Restoration of sinus rhythm after mitral valve replacement: correlations with left atrial pressure and size. Circulation 1968; 37–38(Suppl II): II-173–II-177.

1627. Suttorp MJ, Kingma JH, Koomen EM, van 't Hof A, Tijssen JG, Lie KI. Recurrence of paroxysmal atrial fibrillation or flutter after successful cardioversion in patients with normal left ventricular function. Am J Cardiol 1993; 71:710–713.

1628. Sato S, Kawashima Y, Hirose H, Nakano S, Matsuda H, Shirakura R. Long-term results of direct-current cardioversion after open commissurotomy for mitral stenosis. Am J Cardiol 1986; 57:629–633.

1629. Vitolo E, Tronci M, Larovere MT, Rumolo R, Morabito A. Amiodarone versus quinidine in the prophylaxis of atrial fibrillation. Acta Cardiol 1981; 36:431–444.

1630. Crijns HJ, Van Gelder IC, van Gilst WH, Hillege H, Gosselink AM, Lie KI. Serial antiarrhythmic drug treatment to maintain sinus rhythm after electrical cardioversion for chronic atrial fibrillation or atrial flutter. Am J Cardiol 1991; 68:335–341.

1631. Byrne-Quinn E, Wing AJ. Maintenance of sinus rhythm after DC reversion of atrial fibrillation: a double-blind controlled trial of long-acting quinidine bisulphate. Br Heart J 1970; 32:370–376.

1632. Hartel G, Louhija A, Konttinen A, Halonen PI. Value of quinidine in maintenance of sinus rhythm after electric conversion of atrial fibrillation. Br Heart J 1970; 32:57–60.

1633. Hillestad L, Bjerkelund C, Dale J, Maltau J, Storstein O. Quinidine in maintenance of sinus rhythm after electroconversion of chronic atrial fibrillation: a controlled clinical study. Br Heart J 1971; 33:518–521.

1634. Resnekov L, Gibson D, Waich S, Muir J, McDonald L. Sustained-release quinidine (kinidin durules) in maintaining sinus rhythm after electroversion of atrial dysrhythmias. Br Heart J 1971; 33:220–225.

1635. Sodermark T, Jonsson B, Olsson A, et al. Effect of quinidine on maintaining sinus rhythm after conversion of atrial fibrillation or flutter: a multicentre study from Stockholm. Br Heart J 1975; 37:486–492.

1636. Boissel JP, Wolf E, Gillet J, et al. Controlled trial of a long-acting quinidine for maintenance of sinus rhythm after conversion of sustained atrial fibrillation. Eur Heart J 1981; 2:49–55.

1637. Normand JP, Legendre M, Kahn JC, Bourdarias JP, Mathivat A. Comparative efficacy of short-acting and long-acting quinidine for maintenance of sinus rhythm after electrical conversion of atrial fibrillation. Br Heart J 1976; 38:381–387.

1638. Pollak A, Falk RH. Aggravation of postcardioversion atrial dysfunction by sotalol. J Am Coll Cardiol 1995; 25:665–671.

1639. Lundstrom T, Ryden L. Chronic atrial fibrillation: long-term results of direct current conversion. Acta Med Scand 1988; 223:53–59.

1640. Paulk EA Jr, Hurst JW. Clinical problems of cardioversion. Am Heart J 1965; 70:248–274.

1641. Lown B, Lampert S. Do you give anticoagulants to your patients undergoing cardioversion? J Cardiovasc Med 1981; 6:871–876.

1642. Graf WS, Etkins P. Ventricular tachycardia after synchronized direct-current countershock. JAMA 1964; 190:470–471.

1643. Navab A, LaDue JS. Postconversion systemic arterial embolism. Am J Cardiol 1965; 16:452–453.

1644. Turner JRB, Towers JRH. Complications of cardioversion. Lancet 1965; 2:612–614.

1645. Szekely P, Batson GA, Stark DC. Direct current shock therapy of cardiac arrhythmias. Br Heart J 1966; 28:366–373.

1646. Bjerkelund CJ, Orning OM. The efficacy of anticoagulant therapy in preventing embolism related to DC electrical conversion of atrial fibrillation. Am J Cardiol 1969; 23:208–216.

1647. Yapa RS, Green GJ. Embolic stroke following cardioversion of atrial fibrillation to sinus rhythm with oral amiodarone therapy. Postgrad Med J 1990; 66:410.

1648. Arnold AZ, Mick MJ, Mazurek RP, Loop FD, Trohman RG. Role of prophylactic anticoagulation for direct current cardioversion in patients with atrial fibrillation or atrial flutter. J Am Coll Cardiol 1992; 19:851–855.

1649. Conti CR. Atrial fibrillation, transesophageal echo, electrical cardioversion, and anticoagulation. Clin Cardiol 1994; 17:639–640.

1650. Stein B, Halperin JL, Fuster V. Should patients with atrial fibrillation be anticoagulated prior to and chronically following cardioversion? Cardiovasc Clin 1990; 21:231–247.

1651. Lown B. Personal communication, 1997.

1652. Schlicht JR, Davis RC, Naqi K, Cooper W, Rao BV. Physician practices regarding anticoagulation and cardioversion of atrial fibrillation. Arch Intern Med 1996; 156:290–294.

1653. Weinberg DM, Mancini J. Anticoagulation for cardioversion of atrial fibrillation. Am J Cardiol 1989; 63:745–746.

1654. Daniel WG. Should transesophageal echocardiography be used to guide cardioversion? N Engl J Med 1993; 328:803–804.

1655. Manning WJ, Silverman DI, Gordon SP, Krumholz HM, Douglas PS. Cardioversion from atrial fibrillation without prolonged anticoagulation with use of transesophageal echocardiography to exclude the presence of atrial thrombi. N Engl J Med 1993; 328:750–755.

1656. Grimm RA, Stewart WJ, Black IW, Thomas JD, Klein AL. Should all patients undergo transesophageal echocardiography before electrical cardioversion of atrial fibrillation? J Am Coll Cardiol 1994; 23:533–541.

1657. Manning WJ, Silverman DI, Keighley CS, Oettgen P, Douglas PS. Transesophageal echocardiographically facilitated early cardioversion from atrial fibrillation using short-term anticoagulation: final results of a prospective 4.5-year study. J Am Coll Cardiol 1995; 25:1354–1361.

1658. Pearson AC. Transesophageal echocardiographic screening for atrial thrombus before cardioversion of atrial fibrillation: when should we look before we leap? J Am Coll Cardiol 1995; 25:1362–1364.

1659. Klein AL, Grimm RA, Black IW, et al. Cardioversion guided by transesophageal echocardiography: the acute PILOT study. A randomized, controlled trial: assessment of cardioversion using transesophageal echocardiography. Ann Intern Med 1997; 126:200–209.

1660. Salka S, Saeian K, Sagar KB. Cerebral thromboembolization after cardioversion of atrial fibrillation in patients without transesophageal echocardiographic findings of left atrial thrombus. Am Heart J 1993; 126:722–724.

1661. Black IW, Fatkin D, Sagar KB, et al. Exclusion of atrial thrombus by transesophageal echocardiography does not preclude embolism after cardioversion of atrial fibrillation. A multicenter study. Circulation 1994; 89:2509–2513.

1662. Moreyra E, Finkelhor RS, Cebul RD. Limitations of transesophageal echocardiography in the risk assessment of patients before nonanticoagulated cardioversion from atrial fibrillation and flutter: an analysis of pooled trials. Am Heart J 1995; 129:71–75.

1663. Missault L, Jordaens L, Gheeraert P, Adang L, Clement D. Embolic stroke after unanticoagulated cardioversion despite prior exclusion of atrial thrombi by transesophageal echocardiography. Eur Heart J 1994; 15:1279–1280.

1664. Steering and Publications Committees of the ACUTE Study for the study investigators. Design of a clinical trial for the assessment of cardioversion using transesophageal echocardiography (the ACUTE Multicenter Study). Am J Cardiol 1998; 81:877–883.

1665. Aberg H, Cullhed I. Direct current countershock complications. Acta Med Scand 1968; 183:415–421.

1666. Castellanos A, Lemberg L, Fonseca EJ. Significance of ventricular and pseudoventricular arrhythmias appearing after DC countershock. Am Heart J 1965; 70:583–594.

1667. Thind GS, Blakemore WS, Zinsser HF. Direct current cardioversion in digitalized patients with mitral valve disease. Arch Intern Med 1969; 123:156–159.

1668. Hillestad L, Dale J, Storstein O. Quinidine before direct current countershock: a controlled study. Br Heart J 1972; 34:139–142.

1669. Castellanos A, Lemberg L, Gilmore H, Johnson D. Countershock exposed quinidine syncope. Am J Med Sci 1965; 250:254–260.

1670. Morris JJ, Kong Y, North WC, McIntosh HD. Experience with "cardioversion" of atrial fibrillation and flutter. Am J Cardiol 1964; 14:94–100.

1671. Mann DL, Maisel AS, Atwood JE, Engler RL, LeWinter MM. Absence of cardioversion-induced ventricular arrhythmias in patients with therapeutic digoxin levels. J Am Coll Cardiol 1985; 5:882–890.

1672. Ditchey RV, Karliner JS. Safety of electrical cardioversion in patients without digitalis toxicity. Ann Intern Med 1981; 95:676–679.

1673. Knowlton AA, Falk RH. Paradoxical increase in heart rate before conversion to sinus rhythm in patients with recent-onset atrial fibrillation. Am J Cardiol 1990; 65:930–932.

1674. Gilbert R, Cuddy RP. Digitalis intoxication following conversion to sinus rhythm. Circulation 1965; 32:58–64.

1675. Stern S. The effect of maintenance doses of digitalis on the rate of success of cardioversion. Am J Med Sci 1965; 250:509–512.

1676. Castellanos A, Lemberg L, Brown JP, Berkovits BV. An electrical digitalis tolerance test. Am J Med Sci 1967; 254:159/717–168/726.

1677. Vassaux C, Lown B. Cardioversion of supraventricular tachycardias. Circulation 1969; 39:791–802.

1678. Slodki SJ, Falicov RE, Katz MJ, West M, Zimmerman HJ. Serum enzyme changes following external direct current shock therapy for cardiac arrhythmias. Am J Cardiol 1966; 17:792–797.

1679. Hunt D, Bailie MJ. Enzyme changes following direct current countershock. Am Heart J 1968; 76:340–344.

1680. Warbasse JR, Wesley JE, Connolly V, Galluzzi NJ. Lactic dehydrogenase isoenzymes after electroshock treatment of cardiac arrhythmias. Am J Cardiol 1968; 21:496–503.

1681. Konttinen A, Hupli V, Louhija A, Hartel G. Origin of elevated serum enzyme activities after direct-current countershock. N Engl J Med 1969; 281:231–234.

1682. Mandecki T, Giec L, Kargul W. Serum enzyme activities after cardioversion. Br Heart J 1970; 32:600–602.

1683. Reiffel JA, Gambino SR, McCarthy DM, Leahey EB Jr. Direct current cardioversion: effect on creatine kinase, lactic dehydrogenase and myocardial isoenzymes. JAMA 1978; 239:122–124.

1684. Chun PK, Davia JE, Donohue DJ. ST-segment elevation with elective DC cardioversion. Circulation 1981; 63:220–224.

1685. Allan JJ, Feld RD, Russell AA, et al. Cardiac troponin I levels are normal or minimally elevated after transthoracic cardioversion. J Am Coll Cardiol 1997; 30:1052–1056.
1686. Metcalfe MJ, Smith F, Jennings K, Paterson N. Does cardioversion of atrial fibrillation result in myocardial damage? Br Med J Clin Res Ed 1988; 296:1364.
1687. Kong TQ, Proudfit WL. Repeated direct-current countershock without myocardial injury. JAMA 1964; 187:60–61.
1688. Jakobsson J, Odmansson I, Nordlander R. Enzyme release after elective cardioversion. Eur Heart J 1990; 11:749–752.
1689. Corbitt JD Jr, Sybers J, Levin JM. Muscle changes of the anterior chest wall secondary to electrical countershock. Am J Clin Pathol 1969; 51:107–112.
1690. Ehsani A, Ewy GA, Sobel BE. Effects of electrical countershock on serum creatine phosphokinase (CPK) isoenzyme activity. Am J Cardiol 1976; 37:12–18.
1691. Sussman RM, Woldenberg DH, Cohen M. Myocardial changes after direct current electroshock. JAMA 1964; 189:739–742.
1692. Ovsyshcher IA, Ilia R, Wanderman KL. Conduction disturbance and ST elevation following cardioversion. Isr J Med Sci 1984; 20:736–738.
1693. Van Gelder IC, Crijns HJ, van der Laarse A, van Gilst WH, Lie KI. Incidence and clinical significance of ST segment elevation after electrical cardioversion of atrial fibrillation and atrial flutter. Am Heart J 1991; 121:51–56.
1694. Paloheimo JA. Pulmonary edema after defibrillation. Lancet 1965; 2:439.
1695. Resnekov L, McDonald L. Pulmonary edema following treatment of arrhythmias by direct-current shock. Lancet 1965; 1:506–508.
1696. Hollman A, Nicholson H. Direct-current shock for atrial fibrillation. Lancet 1966; 2:801.
1697. Sutton RB, Tsagaris TJ. Pulmonary edema following direct current cardioversion. Chest 1970; 57:191–194.
1698. Levy S, Morady F. A randomized comparison of external and internal cardioversion of chronic atrial fibrillation. Circulation 1993; 87:1052.
1699. Levy S, Camm J. An implantable atrial defibrillator: an impossible dream? Circulation 1993; 87:1769–1771.
1700. Ideker RE, Cooper RA, Walcott KT. Comparison of atrial ventricular fibrillation and defibrillation. Pacing Clin Electrophysiol 1994; 17:1034–1042.
1701. Keane D. Impact of pulse characteristics on atrial defibrillation energy requirements. Pacing Clin Electrophysiol 1994; 17:1048–1057.
1702. Levy S, Richard P. Is there any indication for an intracardiac defibrillator for the treatment of atrial fibrillation? J Cardiovasc Electrophysiol 1994; 5:982–985.
1703. Wharton JM, Johnson EE. Catheter based atrial defibrillation. Pacing Clin Electrophysiol 1994; 17:1058–1066.
1704. Hillsley RE, Wharton JM. Implantable atrial defibrillators. J Cardiovasc Electrophysiol 1995; 6:634–648.
1705. Griffin JC, Ayers GM, Adams J, et al. Is the automatic atrial defibrillator a promising approach? J Cardiovasc Electrophysiol 1996; 7:1217–1224.
1706. Jung W, Luderitz B. Implantable atrial defibrillator: quo vadis? PACE 1997; 20:2141–2145.
1707. Kulbertus HE. Low energy intracardiac cardioversion of atrial fibrillation. Eur Heart J 1997; 18:1693–1695.
1708. Olgin JE, Sih HJ. Ablation of atrial fibrillation. J Cardiovasc Electrophysiol 1997; 8:1266–1268.
1709. Jain SC, Bhatnagar VM, Azami RU, Awasthey P. Elective countershock in atrial fibrillation with an intracardiac electrode: a preliminary report. J Assoc Physicians India 1970; 18:821–824.
1710. Levy S, Lacombe P, Cointe R, Bru P. High energy transcatheter cardioversion of chronic atrial fibrillation. J Am Coll Cardiol 1988; 12:514–518.
1711. Cooper RA, Johnson EE, Kanter RJ, Merrill JJ, Sorentino RA, Wharton JM. Internal cardioversion in two patients with atrial fibrillation refractory to external cardioversion. Pacing Clin Electrophysiol 1996; 19:872–875.
1712. Kumagai K, Yamanouchi Y, Hiroki T, Arakawa K. Effects of transcatheter cardioversion on chronic lone atrial fibrillation. Pacing Clin Electrophysiol 1991; 14:1571–1575.
1713. Levy S, Lauribe P, Dolla E, et al. A randomized comparison of external and internal cardioversion of chronic atrial fibrillation. Circulation 1992; 86:1415–1420.
1714. Alferness C, Ayers GM, Cooper RA, Ideker RE. Lead systems for atrial defibrillation. Pacing Clin Electrophysiol 1994; 17:1043–1047.
1715. Alt E, Schmitt C, Ammer R, et al. Initial experience with intracardiac atrial defibrillation in patients with chronic atrial fibrillation. Pacing Clin Electrophysiol 1994; 17:1067–1078.
1716. Baker BM, Botteron GW, Smith JM. Low-energy internal cardioversion for atrial fibrillation resistant to external cardioversion. J Cardiovasc Electrophysiol 1995; 6:44–47.
1717. Murgatroyd FD, Slade AK, Sopher SM, Rowland E, Ward DE, Camm AJ. Efficacy and tolerability of transvenous low energy cardioversion of paroxysmal atrial fibrillation in humans. J Am Coll Cardiol 1995; 25:1347–1353.
1718. Saksena S, Prakash A, Mangeon L, et al. Clinical efficacy and safety of atrial defibrillation using biphasic shocks and current nonthoracotomy endocardial lead configurations. Am J Cardiol 1995; 76:913–921.
1719. Forgione NF, Acquati F, Caico SI, et al. High energy transcatheter cardioversion for chronic, poorly tolerated atrial fibrillation. Pacing Clin Electrophysiol 1996; 19:1049–1052.
1720. Schmitt C, Alt E, Plewan A, et al. Low energy intracardiac cardioversion after failed conventional external cardioversion of atrial fibrillation. J Am Coll Cardiol 1996; 28:994–999.
1721. Sopher SM, Murgatroyd FD, Slade AK, et al. Low energy internal cardioversion of atrial fibrillation resistant to transthoracic shocks. Heart 1996; 75:635–638.
1722. Sra JS, Maglio C, Dhala A, et al. Feasibility of atrial fibrillation detection and use of a preceding synchronization interval as a criterion for shock delivery in humans with atrial fibrillation. J Am Coll Cardiol 1996; 28:1532–1538.
1723. Tomassoni G, Newby KH, Kearney MM, Brandon MJ, Barold H, Natale A. Testing different biphasic waveforms and capacitances: effect on atrial defibrillation threshold and pain perception. J Am Coll Cardiol 1996; 28:695–699.
1724. Alt E, Ammer R, Schmitt C, et al. A comparison of treatment of atrial fibrillation with low-energy intracardiac cardioversion and conventional external cardioversion. Eur Heart J 1997; 18:1796–1804.
1725. Ammer R, Alt E, Ayers G, et al. Pain threshold for low energy intracardiac cardioversion of atrial fibrillation with low or no sedation. Pacing Clin Electrophysiol 1997; 20:230–236.
1726. Cooper RA, Johnson EE, Wharton JM. Internal atrial defibrillation in humans: improved efficacy of biphasic waveforms and the importance of phase duration. Circulation 1997; 95:1487–1496.
1727. Gjorgov N, Provenier F, Jordaens L. Low-energy intracardiac shocks during atrial fibrillation: effects on cardiac rhythm. Am Heart J 1997; 133:101–107.
1728. Heisel A, Jung J, Fries R, et al. Low energy transvenous cardioversion of short duration atrial tachyarrhythmias in humans using a single lead system. Pacing Clin Electrophysiol 1997; 20:65–71.
1729. Lau CP, Lok NS. A comparison of transvenous atrial defibrillation of acute and chronic atrial fibrillation and the effect of intravenous sotalol on human atrial defibrillation threshold. PACE 1997; 20:2442–2452.
1730. Levy S, Ricard P, Lau CP, et al. Multicenter low energy transvenous atrial defibrillation (XAD) trial results in different subsets of atrial fibrillation. J Am Coll Cardiol 1997; 29:750–755.
1731. Levy S, Ricard P, Gueunoun M, et al. Low-energy cardioversion of spontaneous atrial fibrillation: immediate and long-term results. Circulation 1997; 96:253–259.
1732. Lok NS, Lau CP, Ho DS, Tang YW. Hemodynamic effects and clinical determinants of defibrillation threshold for

transvenous atrial defibrillation using biatrial biphasic shocks in patients with chronic atrial fibrillation. Pacing Clin Electrophysiol 1997; 20:899–908.

1733. Neri R, Palermo P, Cesario AS, Baragli D, Amici E, Gambelli G. Internal cardioversion of chronic atrial fibrillation in patients. Pacing Clin Electrophysiol 1997; 20:2237–2242.

1734. Prakash A, Saksena S, Mathew P, Krol RB. Internal atrial defibrillation: effect on sinus and atrioventricular nodal function and implanted cardiac pacemakers. PACE 1997; 20:2434–2441.

1735. Boriani G, Biffi M, Bronzetti G, et al. Efficacy and tolerability in fully conscious patients of transvenous low-energy internal atrial cardioversion for atrial fibrillation. Am J Cardiol 1998; 81:241–244.

1736. Simons GR, Newby KH, Kearney MM, Brandon MJ, Natale A. Safety of transvenous low energy cardioversion of atrial fibrillation in patients with a history of ventricular tachycardia: effects of rate and repolarization time on proarrhythmic risk. PACE 1998; 21:430–437.

1737. Cooper RAS, Plumb VJ, Epstein AE, Kay GN, Ideker RE. Marked reduction in internal atrial defibrillation thresholds with dual-current pathways and sequential shocks in humans. Circulation 1998; 97:2527–2535.

1738. Stafford PJ, Kamalvand K, Tan K, Vincent R, Sulke N. Prediction of maintenance of sinus rhythm after cardioversion of atrial fibrillation by analysis of serial signal-averaged P waves. PACE 1998; 21:1387–1395.

1739. Sra J, Biehl M, Blanck Z, et al. Spontaneous reinitiation of atrial fibrillation following transvenous atrial defibrillation. PACE 1998; 21:1105–1110.

1740. Mansourati J, Larlet JM, Salaun G, Maheu B, Blanc JJ. Safety of high energy internal cardioversion for atrial fibrillation. Pacing Clin Electrophysiol 1997; 20:1919–1923.

1741. Borggrefe M, Hindricks G, Haverkamp W, Breithardt G. Catheter ablation using radiofrequency energy. Clin Cardiol 1990; 13:127–131.

1742. Camm AJ, Sneddon JF. High-energy His bundle ablation: a treatment of last resort. Circulation 1991; 84:2187–2189.

1743. American College of Cardiology Cardiovascular Technology Assessment Committee. Catheter ablation for cardiac arrhythmias: clinical applications, personnel and facilities: American College of Cardiology Cardiovascular Technology Assessment Committee. J Am Coll Cardiol 1994; 24:828–833.

1744. Manolis AS, Wang PJ, Estes NA III. Radiofrequency catheter ablation for cardiac tachyarrhythmias. Ann Intern Med 1994; 121:452–461.

1745. Feld GK. Radiofrequency catheter ablation versus modification of the AV node for control of rapid ventricular response in atrial fibrillation. J Cardiovasc Electrophysiol 1995; 6:217–228.

1746. Scheinman MM. NASPE survey on catheter ablation. Pacing Clin Electrophysiol 1995; 18:1474–1478.

1747. Brignole M, Menozzi C. Control of rapid heart rate in patients with atrial fibrillation: drugs or ablation? Pacing Clin Electrophysiol 1996; 19:348–356.

1748. Stevenson WG, Ellison KE, Lefroy DC, Friedman PL. Ablation therapy for cardiac arrhythmias. Am J Cardiol 1997; 80:56G–66G.

1749. Surawicz B. A tactic of last resort. N Engl J Med 1982; 306:234–236.

1750. Josephson ME. Catheter ablation of arrhythmias. Ann Intern Med 1984; 101:234–237.

1751. Gallagher JJ, Svenson RH, Kasell JH, et al. Catheter technique for closed-chest ablation of the atrioventricular conduction system. N Engl J Med 1982; 306:194–200.

1752. Scheinman MM, Morady F, Hess DS, Gonzalez R. Catheter-induced ablation of the atrioventricular junction to control refractory supraventricular arrhythmias. JAMA 1982; 248:851–855.

1753. Critelli G, Perticone F, Coltorti F, Monda V, Gallagher J. Closed chest modification of atrioventricular conduction system in man for treatment of refractory supraventricular tachycardia. Br Heart J 1983; 49:544–549.

1754. Gillette PC, Garson A Jr, Porter CJ, et al. Junctional automatic ectopic tachycardia: new proposed treatment by

transcatheter His bundle ablation. Am Heart J 1983; 106:619–623.

1755. Wood DL, Hammill SC, Holmes DR Jr, Osborn MJ, Gersh BJ. Catheter ablation of the atrioventricular conduction system in patients with supraventricular tachycardia. Mayo Clin Proc 1983; 58:791–796.

1756. Nathan AW, Bennett DH, Ward DE, Bexton RS, Camm AJ. Catheter ablation of atrioventricular conduction. Lancet 1984; 1:1280–1284.

1757. Scheinman MM, Evans-Bell T. Catheter ablation of the atrioventricular junction: a report of the percutaneous mapping and ablation registry. Circulation 1984; 70:1024–1029.

1758. Ward DE, Jones S, Gibson RV. Emergency transvenous ablation of atrioventricular conduction to control refractory atrial tachycardia. Eur Heart J 1984; 5:126–129.

1759. Ellenbogen KA, O'Callaghan WG, Colavita PG, Packer DL, Gilbert MR, German LD. Catheter atrioventricular junction ablation for recurrent supraventricular tachycardia with nodoventricular fibers. Am J Cardiol 1985; 55:1227–1229.

1760. Davis J, Scheinman MM, Ruder MA, et al. Ablation of cardiac tissues by an electrode catheter technique for treatment of ectopic supraventricular tachycardia in adults. Circulation 1986; 74:1044–1053.

1761. Packer DL, Bardy GH, Worley SJ, et al. Tachycardia-induced cardiomyopathy: a reversible form of left ventricular dysfunction. Am J Cardiol 1986; 57:563–570.

1762. Ruder MA, Davis JC, Eldar M, et al. Clinical and electrophysiologic characterization of automatic junctional tachycardia in adults. Circulation 1986; 73:930–937.

1763. Schofield PM, Bowes RJ, Brooks N, Bennett DH. Exercise capacity and spontaneous heart rhythm after transvenous fulguration of atrioventricular conduction. Br Heart J 1986; 56:358–365.

1764. Evans GT Jr, Scheinman MM, Zipes DP, et al. The percutaneous cardiac mapping and ablation registry: summary of results. Pacing Clin Electrophysiol 1987; 10:1395–1399.

1765. Evans GT Jr, Scheinman MM, Zipes DP, et al. The percutaneous cardiac mapping and ablation registry: final summary of results. Pacing Clin Electrophysiol 1988; 11:1621–1626.

1766. Levy S, Bru P, Aliot E, et al. Long-term follow-up of atrioventricular junctional transcatheter electrical ablation. Pacing Clin Electrophysiol 1988; 11:1149–1153.

1767. Lemery R, Brugada P, Della Bella P, et al. Predictors of long-term success during closed-chest catheter ablation of the atrioventricular junction. Eur Heart J 1989; 10:826–832.

1768. Rowland E, Cunningham D, Ahsan A, Rickards A. Transvenous ablation of atrioventricular conduction with a low energy power source. Br Heart J 1989; 62:361–366.

1769. Rosenqvist M, Lee MA, Moulinier L, et al. Long-term follow-up of patients after transcatheter direct current ablation of the atrioventricular junction. J Am Coll Cardiol 1990; 16:1467–1474.

1770. Evans GT Jr, Scheinman MM, Bardy G, et al. Predictors of in-hospital mortality after DC catheter ablation of atrioventricular junction: results of a prospective, international, multicenter study. Circulation 1991; 84:1924–1937.

1771. Perry JC, Kearney DL, Friedman RA, Moak JP, Garson A Jr. Late ventricular arrhythmia and sudden death following direct-current catheter ablation of the atrioventricular junction. Am J Cardiol 1992; 70:765–768.

1772. Rodriguez LM. Improvement in left heart function by ablation of AV nodal conduction in selected patients with lone atrial fibrillation. In Rodriguez LM (ed). New Observations on Cardiac Arrhythmias. Maastricht, Netherlands: Universitaire Pers Maastricht, 1994, pp. 55–66.

1773. Langberg JJ, Chin MC, Rosenqvist M, et al. Catheter ablation of the atrioventricular junction with radiofrequency energy. Circulation 1989; 80:1527–1535.

1774. Denes P. Radiofrequency catheter ablation of the AV node. J Am Coll Cardiol 1991; 18:1759–1760.

1775. Jackman WM, Wang XZ, Friday KJ, et al. Catheter ablation of atrioventricular junction using radiofrequency current in 17 patients: comparison of standard and large-tip catheter electrodes. Circulation 1991; 83:1562–1576.

1776. Langberg JJ, Chin M, Schamp DJ, et al. Ablation of the atrioventricular junction with radiofrequency energy using a new electrode catheter. Am J Cardiol 1991; 67:142–147.

1777. Scheinman MM, Laks MM, DiMarco J, Plumb V. Current role of catheter ablative procedures in patients with cardiac arrhythmias: a report for health professionals from the subcommittee on electrocardiography and electrophysiology, American Heart Association. Circulation 1991; 83:2146–2153.

1778. Sousa J, el-Atassi R, Rosenheck S, Calkins H, Langberg J, Morady F. Radiofrequency catheter ablation of the atrioventricular junction from the left ventricle. Circulation 1991; 84:567–571.

1779. Yeung-Lai-Wah JA, Alison JF, Lonergan L, Mohama R, Leather R, Kerr CR. High success rate of atrioventricular node ablation with radiofrequency energy. J Am Coll Cardiol 1991; 18:1753–1758.

1780. Souza O, Gursoy S, Simonis F, Steurer G, Andries E, Brugada P. Right-sided versus left-sided radiofrequency ablation of the His bundle. Pacing Clin Electrophysiol 1992; 15:1454–1459.

1781. Trohman RG, Simmons TW, Moore SL, Firstenberg MS, Williams D, Maloney JD. Catheter ablation of the atrioventricular junction using radiofrequency energy and a bilateral cardiac approach. Am J Cardiol 1992; 70:1438–1443.

1782. Hindricks G. The Multicentre European Radiofrequency Survey (MERFS): complications of radiofrequency catheter ablation of arrhythmias. The Multicentre European Radiofrequency Survey (MERFS) investigators of the working group on arrhythmias of the European Society of Cardiology. Eur Heart J 1993; 14:1644–1653.

1783. Hoffmann E, Mattke S, Dorwarth U, Muller D, Haberl R, Steinbeck G. Temperature-controlled radiofrequency catheter ablation of AV conduction: first clinical experience. Eur Heart J 1993; 14:57–64.

1784. Kalbfleisch SJ, Williamson B, Man KC, et al. A randomized comparison of the right- and left-sided approaches to ablation of the atrioventricular junction. Am J Cardiol 1993; 72:1406–1410.

1785. Morady F, Calkins H, Langberg JJ, et al. A prospective randomized comparison of direct current and radiofrequency ablation of the atrioventricular junction. J Am Coll Cardiol 1993; 21:102–109.

1786. Olgin JE, Scheinman MM. Comparison of high energy direct current and radiofrequency catheter ablation of the atrioventricular junction. J Am Coll Cardiol 1993; 21:557–564.

1787. Urcelay G, Dick M II, Bove EL, et al. Intraoperative mapping and radiofrequency ablation of the His bundle in a patient with complex congenital heart disease and intractable atrial arrhythmias following the Fontan operation. Pacing Clin Electrophysiol 1993; 16:1437–1440.

1788. Chang AC, McAreavey D, Tripodi D, Fananapazir L. Radiofrequency catheter atrioventricular node ablation in patients with permanent cardiac pacing systems. Pacing Clin Electrophysiol 1994; 17:65–69.

1789. Cuello C, Huang SK, Wagshal AB, Pires LA, Mittleman RS, Bonavita GJ. Radiofrequency catheter ablation of the atrioventricular junction by a supravalvular noncoronary aortic cusp approach. Pacing Clin Electrophysiol 1994; 17:1182–1185.

1790. Greene TO, Huang SK, Wagshal AB, et al. Cardiovascular complications after radiofrequency catheter ablation of supraventricular tachyarrhythmias. Am J Cardiol 1994; 74:615–617.

1791. Edner M, Caidahl K, Bergfeldt L, Darpo B, Edvardsson N, Rosenqvist M. Prospective study of left ventricular function after radiofrequency ablation of atrioventricular junction in patients with atrial fibrillation. Br Heart J 1995; 74:261–267.

1792. Erickson CC, Carr D, Greer GS, Kiel EA, Tryka AF. Emergent radiofrequency ablation of the AV node in a neonate with unstable, refractory supraventricular tachycardia. Pacing Clin Electrophysiol 1995; 18:1959–1962.

1793. Jensen SM, Bergfeldt L, Rosenqvist M. Long-term follow-up of patients treated by radiofrequency ablation of the atrioventricular junction. Pacing Clin Electrophysiol 1995; 18:1609–1614.

1794. Nath S, DiMarco JP, Mounsey JP, Lobban JH, Haines DE. Correlation of temperature and pathophysiological effect during radiofrequency catheter ablation of the AV junction. Circulation 1995; 92:1188–1192.

1795. Anza C, Kourouyan HD, Siu A, et al. Quality of life and outcomes after radiofrequency His-bundle catheter ablation and permanent pacemaker implantation: impact of treatment in paroxysmal and established atrial fibrillation. Am Heart J 1996; 131:499–507.

1796. Piot O, Sebag C, Lavergne T, et al. Initial and long-term evaluation of escape rhythm after radiofrequency ablation of the AV junction in 50 patients. Pacing Clin Electrophysiol 1996; 19:1988–1992.

1797. Vaksmann G, Lacroix D, Klug D. Radiofrequency ablation of the His bundle for malignant atrial flutter after Mustard procedure for transposition of the great arteries. Am J Cardiol 1996; 77:669–670.

1798. Fenrich AL, Friedman RA, Cecchin FC, Kearney D. Left-sided atrioventricular nodal ablation using the transseptal approach: clinico-histopathologic correlation. J Cardiovasc Electrophysiol 1998; 9:757–760.

1799. Marchese AC, Pressley JC, Sintetos AL, Gilbert MR, German LD. Cryosurgical versus catheter ablation of the atrioventricular junction. Am J Cardiol 1987; 59:870–873.

1800. Costeas XF, Berul CI, Foote CB, et al. Transcoronary ethanol ablation of the atrioventricular node in a young patient with tricuspid atresia. PACE 1998; 21:620–623.

1801. Deharo JC, Mansourati J, Graux P, et al. Long-term pacemaker dependency after radiofrequency ablation of the atrioventricular junction. Am Heart J 1997; 133:580–584.

1802. Brignole M, Gianfranchi L, Menozzi C, et al. Influence of atrioventricular junction radiofrequency ablation in patients with chronic atrial fibrillation and flutter on quality of life and cardiac performance. Am J Cardiol 1994; 74:242–246.

1803. Brown CS, Mills RM, Conti JB, Curtis AB. Clinical improvement after atrioventricular nodal ablation for atrial fibrillation does not correlate with improved ejection fraction. Am J Cardiol 1997; 80:1090–1091.

1804. Buys EM, van Hemel NM, Kelder JC, et al. Exercise capacity after His bundle ablation and rate response ventricular pacing for drug refractory chronic atrial fibrillation. Heart 1997; 77:238–241.

1805. Geelen P, Goethals M, de Bruyne B, Brugada P. A prospective hemodynamic evaluation of patients with chronic atrial fibrillation undergoing radiofrequency catheter ablation of the atrioventricular junction. Am J Cardiol 1997; 80:1606–1609.

1806. Kunze KP, Schluter M, Geiger M, Kuck KH. Modulation of atrioventricular nodal conduction using radiofrequency current. Am J Cardiol 1988; 61:657–658.

1807. Fleck RP, Chen PS, Boyce K, Ross R, Dittrich HC, Feld GK. Radiofrequency modification of atrioventricular conduction by selective ablation of the low posterior septal right atrium in a patient with atrial fibrillation and a rapid ventricular response. Pacing Clin Electrophysiol 1993; 16:377–381.

1808. Duckeck W, Engelstein ED, Kuck KH. Radiofrequency current therapy in atrial tachyarrhythmias: modulation versus ablation of atrioventricular nodal conduction. Pacing Clin Electrophysiol 1993; 16:629–636.

1809. Menozzi C, Brignole M, Gianfranchi L, et al. Radiofrequency catheter ablation and modulation of atrioventricular conduction in patients with atrial fibrillation. Pacing Clin Electrophysiol 1994; 17:2143–2149.

1810. Feld GK, Fleck RP, Fujimura O, Prothro DL, Bahnson TD, Ibarra M. Control of rapid ventricular response by radiofrequency catheter modification of the atrioventricular node in patients with medically refractory atrial fibrillation. Circulation 1994; 90:2299–2307.

1811. Williamson BD, Man KC, Daoud E, Niebauer M, Strickberger SA, Morady F. Radiofrequency catheter modification of atrioventricular conduction to control the ventricular rate during atrial fibrillation. N Engl J Med 1994; 331:910–917.

1812. Blanck Z, Dhala AA, Sra J, et al. Characterization of atrioventricular nodal behavior and ventricular response during atrial fibrillation before and after a selective slow-pathway ablation. Circulation 1995; 91:1086–1094.

1813. Della Bella P, Maslowsky F, Tondo C, Riva S. Modulation of atrioventricular conduction by ablation of the "slow" atrioventricular node pathway in patients with drug-refractory atrial fibrillation or flutter. J Am Coll Cardiol 1995; 25:39–46.

1814. Tebbenjohanns J, Pfeiffer D, Schumacher B, Jung W, Manz M, Luderitz B. Slowing of the ventricular rate during atrial fibrillation by ablation of the slow pathway of AV nodal reentrant tachycardia. J Cardiovasc Electrophysiol 1995; 6:711–715.

1815. Canby RC, Roman CA, Kessler DJ, Horton RP, Page RL. Selective radiofrequency ablation of the "slow" atrioventricular nodal pathway for control of the ventricular response to atrial fibrillation. Am J Cardiol 1996; 77:1358–1361.

1816. Chen SA, Lee SH, Chiang CE, et al. Electrophysiological mechanisms in successful radiofrequency catheter modification of atrioventricular junction for patients with medically refractory paroxysmal atrial fibrillation. Circulation 1996; 93:1690–1701.

1817. Kreiner G, Heinz G, Siostrzonek P, Gossinger HD. Effect of slow pathway ablation on ventricular rate during atrial fibrillation: dependence on electrophysiological properties of the fast pathway. Circulation 1996; 93:277–283.

1818. Markowitz SM, Stein KM, Lerman BB. Mechanism of ventricular rate control after radiofrequency modification of atrioventricular conduction in patients with atrial fibrillation. Circulation 1996; 94:2856–2864.

1819. Knight BP, Weiss R, Bahu M, et al. Cost comparison of radiofrequency modification and ablation of the atrioventricular junction in patients with chronic atrial fibrillation. Circulation 1997; 96:1532–1536.

1820. Krahn AD, Klein GJ, Yee R, Basta MN, Lee JK. Progressive anterior ablation in the coronary sinus region: evidence to support the presence of a 'slow pathway' input in normal patients? Circulation 1997; 96:3477–3483.

1821. Stabile G, Turco P, De Simone A, Coltorti F, De Matteis C. Radiofrequency modification of the atrioventricular node in patients with chronic atrial fibrillation: comparison between anterior and posterior approaches. J Cardiovasc Electrophysiol 1998; 9:709–717.

1822. Lee SH, Chen SA, Tai CT, et al. Comparisons of quality of life and cardiac performance after complete atrioventricular junction ablation and atrioventricular junction modification in patients with medically refractory atrial fibrillation. J Am Coll Cardiol 1998; 31:637–644.

1823. Twidale N, McDonald T, Nave K, Seal A. Comparison of the effects of AV nodal ablation versus AV nodal modification in patients with congestive heart failure and uncontrolled atrial fibrillation. PACE 1998; 21:641–651.

1824. Haissaguerre M, Jais P, Shah DC, et al. Right and left atrial radiofrequency catheter therapy of paroxysmal atrial fibrillation. J Cardiovasc Electrophysiol 1996; 7:1132–1144.

1825. Gaita F, Riccardi R, Calo L, et al. Atrial mapping and radiofrequency catheter ablation in patients with idiopathic atrial fibrillation: electrophysiological findings and ablation results. Circulation 1998; 97:2136–2145.

1826. Haissaguerre M, Fischer B, Labbe T, et al. Frequency of recurrent atrial fibrillation after catheter ablation of overt accessory pathways. Am J Cardiol 1992; 69:493–497.

1827. Weiss R, Knight BP, Bahu M, et al. Long-term follow-up after radiofrequency ablation of paroxysmal supraventricular tachycardia in patients with tachycardia-induced atrial fibrillation. Am J Cardiol 1997; 80:1609–1610.

1828. Huang DT, Monahan KM, Zimetbaum P, Papageorgiou P, Epstein LM, Josephson ME. Hybrid pharmacologic and ablative therapy: a novel and effective approach for the management of atrial fibrillation. J Cardiovasc Electrophysiol 1998; 9:462–469.

1829. Darpo B, Walfridsson H, Aunes M, et al. Incidence of sudden death after radiofrequency ablation of the atrioventricular junction for atrial fibrillation. Am J Cardiol 1997; 80:1174–1177.

1830. Goldstein M, Dunnigan A, Staley NA, Benditt DG, Benson DW, Milstein S. Accelerated idioventricular rhythm complicating atrioventricular junction ablation for automatic atrial tachycardia. Int J Cardiol 1989; 25:81–86.

1831. Vanderheyden M, Goethals M, Anguera I, et al. Hemodynamic deterioration following radiofrequency ablation of the atrioventricular conduction system. PACE 1997; 20:2422–2428.

1832. Feld M, Fisher J, Brodman R, Golier F. Coronary sinus rupture complicating catheter ablation of the atrioventricular junction. J Electrophysiol 1987; 1:257–260.

1833. Kunze KP, Schluter M, Costard A, Nienaber CA, Kuck KH. Right atrial thrombus formation after transvenous catheter ablation of the atrioventricular node. J Am Coll Cardiol 1985; 6:1428–1430.

1834. Cox JL, Boineau JP, Schuessler RB, et al. Operations for atrial fibrillation. Clin Cardiol 1991; 14:827–834.

1835. McComb JM. Surgery for atrial fibrillation. Br Heart J 1994; 71:501–503.

1836. Cox JL, Schuessler RB, Lappas DG, Boineau JP. An 8½-year clinical experience with surgery for atrial fibrillation. Ann Surg 1996; 224:267–273.

1837. Greenwood WF, Aldridge HE, McKelvey AD. Effect of mitral commissurotomy on duration of life, functional capacity, hemoptysis and systemic embolism. Am J Cardiol 1963; 11:348–356.

1838. Kellogg F, Liu CK, Fishman IW, Larson R. Systemic and pulmonary emboli before and after mitral commissurotomy. Circulation 1961; 24:263–266.

1839. Blackshear JL, Odell JA. Appendage obliteration to reduce stroke in cardiac surgical patients with atrial fibrillation. Ann Thorac Surg 1996; 61:755–759.

1840. John S, Muralidharan S, Jairaj PS, Krishnaswamy S, Sukumar IP, Cherian G. Massive left atrial thrombus complicating mitral stenosis with atrial fibrillation: results of surgical treatment. Ann Thorac Surg 1976; 21:103–106.

1841. Darpo B, Ryden L. Restoration of atrial function after the Maze procedure. Eur Heart J 1997; 18:360–361.

1842. Cox JL, Boineau JP, Schuessler RB, et al. Successful surgical treatment of atrial fibrillation: review and clinical update. JAMA 1991; 266:1976–1980.

1843. Cox JL. The surgical treatment of atrial fibrillation. IV. Surgical technique. J Thorac Cardiovasc Surg 1991; 101:584–592.

1844. Cox JL, Schuessler RB, D'Agostino HJ Jr, et al. The surgical treatment of atrial fibrillation. III. Development of a definitive surgical procedure. J Thorac Cardiovasc Surg 1991; 101:569–583.

1845. Cox JL, Boineau JP, Schuessler RB, et al. A review of surgery for atrial fibrillation. J Cardiovasc Electrophysiol 1991; 2:541–561.

1846. Defauw JJ, Guiraudon GM, van Hemel NM, Vermeulen FE, Kingma JH, de Bakker JM. Surgical therapy of paroxysmal atrial fibrillation with the "corridor" operation. Ann Thorac Surg 1992; 53:564–570.

1847. McCarthy PM, Castle LW, Maloney JD, et al. Initial experience with the Maze procedure for atrial fibrillation. J Thorac Cardiovasc Surg 1993; 105:1077–1087.

1848. Tsui SS, Grace AA, Ludman PF, et al. Maze 3 for atrial fibrillation: two cuts too few? Pacing Clin Electrophysiol 1994; 17:2163–2166.

1849. Cox JL, Jaquiss RD, Schuessler RB, Boineau JP. Modification of the Maze procedure for atrial flutter and atrial fibrillation. II. Surgical technique of the Maze III procedure. J Thorac Cardiovasc Surg 1995; 110:485–495.

1850. Cox JL, Boineau JP, Schuessler RB, Jaquiss RD, Lappas DG. Modification of the Maze procedure for atrial flutter and atrial fibrillation. I. Rationale and surgical results. J Thorac Cardiovasc Surg 1995; 110:473–484.

1851. Ueshima K, Hashimoto K, Chiba M, et al. Recovery of atrial function after combined treatment with surgical repair for organic heart disease and Maze procedure for atrial fibrillation. J Thorac Cardiovasc Surg 1997; 113:214–215.

1852. Cox JL, Boineau JP, Schuessler RB, Kater KM, Lappas DG. From fisherman to fibrillation: an unbroken line of progress. Ann Thorac Surg 1994; 58:1269–1273.

1853. Yuda S, Nakatani S, Isobe F, Kosakai Y, Miyatake K. Comparative efficacy of the Maze procedure for restoration of atrial contraction in patients with and without giant left atrium associated with mitral valve disease. J Am Coll Cardiol 1998; 31:1097–1102.

1854. Hioki M, Ikeshita M, Iedokoro Y, et al. Successful combined operation for mitral stenosis and atrial fibrillation. Ann Thorac Surg 1993; 55:776–778.

1855. McCarthy PM, Cosgrove DM III, Castle LW, White RD, Klein AL. Combined treatment of mitral regurgitation and atrial fibrillation with valvuloplasty and the Maze procedure. Am J Cardiol 1993; 71:483–486.

1856. Chua YL, Schaff HV, Orszulak TA, Morris JJ. Outcome of mitral valve repair in patients with preoperative atrial fibrillation: should the Maze procedure be combined with mitral valvuloplasty? J Thorac Cardiovasc Surg 1994; 107:408–415.

1857. Kosakai Y, Kawaguchi AT, Isobe F, et al. Cox Maze procedure for chronic atrial fibrillation associated with mitral valve disease. J Thorac Cardiovasc Surg 1994; 108:1049–1054.

1858. Bonchek LI, Burlingame MW, Worley SJ, Vazales BE, Lundy EF. Cox/Maze procedure for atrial septal defect with atrial fibrillation: management strategies. Ann Thorac Surg 1993; 55:607–610.

1859. Sandoval N, Velasco VM, Orjuela H, et al. Concomitant mitral valve or atrial septal defect surgery and the modified Cox-Maze procedure. Am J Cardiol 1996; 77:591–596.

1860. Kosakai Y, Kawaguchi AT, Isobe F, et al. Modified Maze procedure for patients with atrial fibrillation undergoing simultaneous open heart surgery. Circulation 1995; 92(Suppl II):II-359–II-364.

1861. Tamai J, Kosakai Y, Yoshioka T, et al. Delayed improvement in exercise capacity with restoration of sinoatrial node response in patients after combined treatment with surgical repair for organic heart disease and the Maze procedure for atrial fibrillation. Circulation 1995; 91:2392–2399.

1862. Kawaguchi AT, Kosakai Y, Sasako Y, Eishi K, Nakano K, Kawashima Y. Risks and benefits of combined Maze procedure for atrial fibrillation associated with organic heart disease. J Am Coll Cardiol 1996; 28:985–990.

1863. Kamata J, Nakai K, Chiba N, et al. Electrocardiographic nature of restored sinus rhythm after Cox Maze procedure in patients with chronic atrial fibrillation who also had other cardiac surgery. Heart 1997; 77:50–55.

1864. Kawaguchi AT, Kosakai Y, Isobe F, et al. Factors affecting rhythm after the Maze procedure for atrial fibrillation. Circulation 1996; 94(Suppl II):II-139–II-142.

1865. Guiraudon GM, Klein GJ, Yee R, Leitch JW, Kaushik RR, McLellan DG. Surgery for atrial tachycardia. Pacing Clin Electrophysiol 1990; 13:1996–1999.

1866. Leitch JW, Klein G, Yee R, Guiraudon G. Sinus node-atrioventricular node isolation: long-term results with the "corridor" operation for atrial fibrillation. J Am Coll Cardiol 1991; 17:970–975.

1867. Leitch JW, Guiraudon GM, Klein GJ, Yee R. Surgical management of symptomatic atrial fibrillation. In Falk RH, Podrid PJ (eds). Atrial Fibrillation. Mechanisms and Management. New York: Raven Press, 1992, pp. 375–387.

1868. van Hemel NM, Defauw JJ, Kingma JH, et al. Long-term results of the corridor operation for atrial fibrillation. Br Heart J 1994; 71:170–176.

1869. van Hemel NM, Defauw JJ, Guiraudon GM, Kelder JC, Jessurun ER, Ernst JM. Long-term follow-up of corridor operation for lone atrial fibrillation: evidence for progression of disease? J Cardiovasc Electrophysiol 1997; 8:967–973.

1870. DiMarco JP. Surgical therapy for atrial fibrillation: a first step on what may be a long road. J Am Coll Cardiol 1991; 17:976–977.

1871. Sueda T, Nagata H, Shikata H, et al. Simple left atrial

procedure for chronic atrial fibrillation associated with mitral valve disease. Ann Thorac Surg 1996; 62:1796–1800.

1872. Sueda T, Nagata H, Orihashi K, et al. Efficacy of a simple left atrial procedure for chronic atrial fibrillation in mitral valve operations. Ann Thorac Surg 1997; 63:1070–1075.

1873. Shyu KG, Cheng JJ, Chen JJ, et al. Recovery of atrial function after atrial compartment operation for chronic atrial fibrillation in mitral valve disease. J Am Coll Cardiol 1994; 24:392–398.

1874. Lin FY, Huang JH, Lin JL, Chen WJ, Lo HM, Chu SH. Atrial compartment surgery for chronic atrial fibrillation associated with congenital heart defects. J Thorac Cardiovasc Surg 1996; 111:231–237.

1875. Lo HM, Lin FY, Lin JL, et al. Electrophysiological properties in patients undergoing atrial compartment operation for chronic atrial fibrillation with mitral valve disease. Eur Heart J 1997; 18:1805–1815.

1876. Williams JM, Ungerleider RM, Lofland GK, Cox JL. Left atrial isolation: new technique for the treatment of supraventricular arrhythmias. J Thorac Cardiovasc Surg 1980; 80:373–380.

1877. Graffigna A, Pagani F, Minzioni G, Salerno J, Vigano M. Left atrial isolation associated with mitral valve operations. Ann Thorac Surg 1992; 54:1093–1097.

1878. Sueda T, Nagata H, Okada K, et al. Right atrial separation procedure for eliminating chronic atrial fibrillation associated with atrial septal defect. Pacing Clin Electrophysiol 1997; 20:1870–1873.

1879. Sueda T, Okada K, Hirai S, Orihashi K, Nagata H, Matsuura Y. Right atrial separation for chronic atrial fibrillation with atrial septal defects. Ann Thorac Surg 1997; 64:541–542.

1880. Giannelli S Jr, Ayres SM, Gomprecht RF, Conklin EF, Kennedy RJ. Therapeutic surgical division of the human conduction system. JAMA 1967; 199:155–160.

1881. Dreifus LS, Nichols H, Morse D, Watanabe Y, Truex R. Control of recurrent tachycardia of Wolff-Parkinson-White syndrome by surgical ligature of the A-V bundle. Circulation 1968; 38:1030–1036.

1882. Edmonds JH Jr, Ellison RG, Crews TL. Surgically induced atrioventricular block as treatment for recurrent atrial tachycardia in Wolff-Parkinson-White syndrome. Circulation 1969; 39(Suppl I):I-105–I-111.

1883. Coumel P, Waynberger M, Fabiato A, Slama R, Aigueperse J, Bouvrain Y. Wolff-Parkinson-White syndrome: problems in evaluation of multiple accessory pathways and surgical therapy. Circulation 1972; 45:1216–1230.

1884. Gooch AS, Jan MA, Fernandez J, Fertig H, Morse D, Maranhao V. Uncontrolled tachycardia in atrial fibrillation: management by surgical ligature of A-V bundle and pacemaker. Ann Thorac Surg 1974; 17:181–185.

1885. Harrison L, Gallagher JJ, Kasell J, et al. Cryosurgical ablation of the A-V node-His bundle: a new method for producing A-V block. Circulation 1977; 55:463–470.

1886. Sealy WC, Anderson RW, Gallagher JJ. Surgical treatment of supraventricular tachyarrhythmias. J Thorac Cardiovasc Surg 1977; 73:511–522.

1887. Gallagher JJ, Sealy WC. The permanent form of junctional reciprocating tachycardia: further elucidation of the underlying mechanism. Eur J Cardiol 1978; 8:413–430.

1888. Sealy WC, Hackel DB, Seaber AV. A study of methods for surgical interruption of the His bundle. J Thorac Cardiovasc Surg 1977; 73:424–430.

1889. Klein GJ, Sealy WC, Pritchett EL, et al. Cryosurgical ablation of the atrioventricular node-His bundle: long-term follow-up and properties of the junctional pacemaker. Circulation 1980; 61:8–15.

1890. Sealy WC. His bundle interruption for reentry tachycardia in Wolff-Parkinson-White syndrome. Ann Thorac Surg 1983; 36:345–352.

1891. Johnson DC, Nunn GR, Richards DA, Uther JB, Ross DL. Surgical therapy for supraventricular tachycardia, a potentially curable disorder. J Thorac Cardiovasc Surg 1987; 93:913–918.

1892. Lawrie GM, Lin HT, Wyndham CR, DeBakey ME. Surgical treatment of supraventricular arrhythmias: results in 67 patients. Ann Surg 1987; 205:700–711.

1893. McGuire MA, Johnson DC, Nunn GR, Yung T, Uther JB, Ross DL. Surgical therapy for atrial tachycardia in adults. J Am Coll Cardiol 1989; 14:1777–1782.

1894. Ueshima K, Myers J, Ribisl PM, et al. Exercise capacity and prognosis in patients with chronic atrial fibrillation. Cardiology 1995; 86:108–113.

1895. Nunain SO, Debbas NMG, Camm AJ. Determinants of the course and prognosis of atrial fibrillation. In Touboul P, Waldo AL (eds). Atrial Arrhythmias. Current Concepts and Management. St. Louis: Mosby–Year Book, 1990, pp. 350–358.

1896. Hofmann T, Meinertz T, Kasper W, et al. Mode of death in idiopathic dilated cardiomyopathy: a multivariate analysis of prognostic determinants. Am Heart J 1988; 116:1455–1463.

1897. Maron BJ, Merrill WH, Freier PA, Kent KM, Epstein SE, Morrow AG. Long-term clinical course and symptomatic status of patients after operation for hypertrophic subaortic stenosis. Circulation 1978; 57:1205–1213.

1898. Maron BJ, Lipson LC, Roberts WC, Savage DD, Epstein SE. "Malignant" hypertrophic cardiomyopathy: identification of a subgroup of families with unusually frequent premature death. Am J Cardiol 1978; 41:1133–1140.

1899. Alt E, Volker R, Wirtzfeld A, Ulm K. Survival and follow-up after pacemaker implantation: a comparison of patients with sick sinus syndrome, complete heart block, and atrial fibrillation. Pacing Clin Electrophysiol 1985; 8:849–855.

1900. Parker JLW, Lawson DH. Death from thyrotoxicosis. Lancet 1973; 2:894–895.

1901. Carson P, Johnson G, Fletcher R, Dunkman B, VHeFT investigators. Atrial fibrillation does not affect prognosis in mild-moderate heart failure. Circulation 1992; 86(Suppl I): I-664.

1902. Fitzpatrick AP, Kourouyan HD, Siu A, et al. Quality of life and outcomes after radiofrequency His-bundle catheter ablation and permanent pacemaker implantation: impact of treatment in paroxysmal and established atrial fibrillation. Am Heart J 1996; 131:499–507.

1903. Middlekauff HR, Stevenson WG, Stevenson LW. Prognostic significance of atrial fibrillation in advanced heart failure: a study of 390 patients. Circulation 1991; 84:40–48.

1904. Flaker GC, Blackshear JL, McBride R, Kronmal RA, Halperin JL, Hart RG. Antiarrhythmic drug therapy and cardiac mortality in atrial fibrillation: the Stroke Prevention in Atrial Fibrillation Investigators. J Am Coll Cardiol 1992; 20:527–532.

1905. Stevenson WG, Stevenson LW, Middlekauff HR, et al. Improving survival for patients with atrial fibrillation and advanced heart failure. J Am Coll Cardiol 1996; 28:1458–1463.

1906. Behar S, Zahavi Z, Goldbourt U, Reicher-Reiss H. Long-term prognosis of patients with paroxysmal atrial fibrillation complicating acute myocardial infarction. SPRINT study group. Eur Heart J 1992; 13:45–50.

1907. Goldberg RJ, Seeley D, Becker RC, et al. Impact of atrial fibrillation on the in-hospital and long-term survival of patients with acute myocardial infarction: a community-wide perspective. Am Heart J 1990; 119:996–1001.

1908. Eldar M, Canetti M, Rotstein Z, et al. Significance of paroxysmal atrial fibrillation complicating acute myocardial infarction in the thrombolytic era. Circulation 1998; 97:965–970.

1909. Widdershoven JW, Gorgels AP, Vermeer F, et al. Changing characteristics and in-hospital outcome in patients admitted with acute myocardial infarction: observations from 1982 to 1994. Eur Heart J 1997; 18:1073–1080.

1910. Anonymous. Paul Wood's Diseases of the Heart and Circulation. Philadelphia: JB Lippincott, 1968, p. 613.

1911. Orndahl G, Thulesius O, Hood B. Incidence of persistent atrial fibrillation and conduction defects in coronary heart disease. Am Heart J 1972; 84:120–131.

1912. Anonymous. Paul Wood's Diseases of the Heart and Circulation. Philadelphia: JB Lippincott, 1968, p. 752.

1913. Spodick DH. Frequency of arrhythmias in acute pericarditis determined by Holter monitoring. Am J Cardiol 1984; 53:842–845.

1914. Stafford RS, Singer DE. Recent national patterns of warfarin use in atrial fibrillation. Circulation 1998; 97:1231–1233.

1915. Kutner M, Nixon G, Silverstone F. Physicians' attitudes toward oral anticoagulants and antiplatelet agents for stroke prevention in elderly patients with atrial fibrillation. Arch Intern Med 1991; 151:1950–1953.

1916. Brignole M, Menozzi C, Sartore B, Barra M, Monducci I. The use of atrial pacing to induce atrial fibrillation and flutter. Int J Cardiol 1986; 12:45–54.

1917. Cox JL. A perspective of postoperative atrial fibrillation in cardiac operations. Ann Thorac Surg 1993; 56:405–409.

Atrial Flutter[1-8a]

Atrial flutter has finally yielded to the skills of the clinical electrophysiologist and can now be cured with radiofrequency ablation—not perfectly, of course, but more effectively than by any previously developed technique. More often than its more prevalent cousin, atrial fibrillation, atrial flutter taxes the patience of the patient and physician. Usually paroxysmal, difficult to control with medicines despite its ease in conversion, atrial flutter seriously complicates the lives of some men and women, many of whom are afflicted with serious cardiopulmonary disease.

SOME ADVANCES SINCE THE FIRST EDITION OF THIS BOOK

- Understanding that atrial flutter occurs more frequently than previously thought in patients without structural heart disease.
- Documentation of the frequency of clots in the left atrium of patients with flutter.
- More complete understanding of the clinical electrophysiology of flutter.
- Refinement of catheter ablation with radiofrequency current.
- Application of intravascular echocardiography to assist ablation.

PREVALENCE

Atrial flutter occurs rarely in the general population and infrequently in patients with cardiac disease, less than one-tenth as often as atrial fibrillation[9-14] (Table 5.1).[b] Using standard electrocardiograms, short rhythm

strips and ambulatory electrocardiography, investigators have found atrial flutter in only:

- One of 125,043 men in the Air Force.[15-17c]
- None of 5,129 members of the adult population of Tecumseh, Michigan.[18]
- None of 18,403 presumably healthy British male civil servants aged 40 to 64 years.[19]
- None of 1,404 subjects without heart disease from newborns to adults aged 60 years.[20-27d]

Among patients specifically examined for the presence of heart disease, atrial flutter appeared in the following:[e]

- One hundred four (1%) of 10,000 patients examined with electrocardiograms at the Massachusetts General Hospital in Boston from 1914 to 1931.[11]
- Two hundred seventy (0.5%) of 50,000 consecutive electrocardiograms at the Michael Reese Hospital in Chicago.[12]
- Forty-five (0.8%) of 5,396 consecutive new patients studied in Augusta, Georgia from 1967 to 1970.[28]
- Sixteen (0.2%) of 9,458 patients in Manchester, England observed from 1942 to 1947.[10]

---

[c]From three series: two from the U.S. Air Force of 122,043[17] and 1,000[16] men and one from the Royal Canadian Air Force of 2,000 men.[15]
[d]From eight series.[20-27]
[e]These studies were performed several decades ago, and whether the same incidence of atrial flutter applies today is unknown.

---

[a]This chapter has been adapted from Chapter 3, "Atrial Flutter," by Albert L. Waldo and me, in the first edition of this book.[1]
[b]"It is a relatively uncommon but capricious rhythm, and may occur when least expected" (Paul Wood, 1968).[13] "Atrial flutter is largely a nuisance arrhythmia" (Albert Waldo, 1995).[6] Its infrequency is an old story. In a report published in 1928 about 3,000 patients with heart disease seen by Dr. Paul Dudley White at the Massachusetts General Hospital and by "thirteen reliable and representative general practitioners throughout New England," only six patients had "auricular flutter."[9]

Table 5.1	ATRIAL FLUTTER OCCURS MUCH LESS OFTEN THAN ATRIAL FIBRILLATION		
Authors	Subjects or Electrocardiograms	Atrial Flutter (%)	Atrial Fibrillation (%)
Doliopoulos and Marousis[14]	3,780	0.7	24.6
Makinson and Wade[10]	9,458	0.2	7.6
White[11]	10,000	1.0	14.2
Katz and Pick[12]	50,000	0.5	11.7

• Twenty-six (0.7%) of 3,780 cardiac cases in the Piraeus (Greece) General Hospital in the 1960s.[14]

Atrial flutter develops occasionally in infants and children,[29, 30] including those with heart disease,[23, 24, 31–34] but it occurs less frequently than supraventricular tachycardia,[31, 34] although probably more often than atrial fibrillation.[f] Fetuses may rarely have atrial flutter.[35–38]

AGE AND GENDER

Atrial flutter devlops more frequently as patients age and acquire more cardiac and pulmonary disease.[10, 39] Even so, atrial flutter is infrequently present in older ambulatory subjects. The arrhythmia was observed in only two of 4,011 men and women 60 years of age or older.[40–46g]

Most observers[h] report that atrial flutter occurs more often in men than in women,[11, 14, 39, 47–51] as much as 4.7 times as frequently according to a report.[49] The average age was 10.3 years among 380 cases[i] of atrial flutter in infants, children, and young adults from 12 months to 25 years of age,[33] and the arrhythmia occurred more frequently in the older children.[33]

CLINICAL SETTING

Atrial flutter frequently appears in patients with significant heart or lung disease.

Heart Disease

Atrial flutter is more often associated with diseases of the right side of the heart than is atrial fibrillation, which tends to develop in patients with left-sided heart disease.

Coronary Heart Disease. Patients with atrial flutter are more likely to have coronary heart disease, sometimes complicated by hypertension, than any other affliction.[49, 50, 52] Nevertheless, they seldom develop paroxysmal atrial flutter during acute myocardial infarction[53–69j] and very infrequently after the infarction.[70]

Rheumatic Heart Disease. Investigators have reported that rheumatic heart disease frequently causes atrial flutter but less often than does coronary heart

disease.[10, 49, 50] The arrhythmia is "curiously rare" in mitral stenosis[k] and tricuspid stenosis, wrote Paul Wood in 1968.[13] Atrial flutter occasionally occurs in patients with mitral valve prolapse.[71]

Congenital Heart Disease. A few adults may develop atrial flutter from uncorrected congenital heart disease such as atrial septal defect.[72] However, children with atrial flutter frequently have congenital heart disease. In the series of 380 young patients aged 1 to 25 years with atrial flutter,[33] the cardiac diagnoses were as follows:

• Repaired congenital heart disease, 60%.
• Palliated congenital heart disease, 13%.
• Unoperated congenital heart disease, 8%.
• Cardiomyopathy, 6%.
• Rheumatic heart disease, 4%.
• Other lesions, 2%.
• Otherwise normal heart, 8%.

The most common congenital cardiac abnormalities were the following:[33]

• D-transposition of the great arteries, 20.5%.
• Complex congenital lesions, 17.8%.
• Atrial septal defect, 12.1%.
• Tetralogy of Fallot, 7.9%.
• Atrioventricular canal, 5.0%.
• Total anomalous pulmonary venous return, 4.7%.

Cardiomyopathy. Atrial flutter uncommonly develops in patients with cardiomyopathy.[6, 73–77l] Persistent atrial flutter at rapid ventricular rates may occasionally *produce* cardiomyopathy.[78m]

Pericardial Disease. As with atrial fibrillation, flutter appears in patients with chronic constrictive pericarditis,[79–81] but rarely in acute pericarditis.[82, 83n]

Lung Disease[84]

Many patients with severe pulmonary disease develop atrial flutter.[14, 50, 52, 85–88] When specifically examined for arrhythmias, 10% to 30% of such patients have flutter.[o] In 21 patients with atrial flutter, pulmonary disease was the precipitating factor in 53%.[39]

When patients develop atrial flutter with no clear etiologic basis, covert pulmonary embolus should be considered. Twenty-five of 45 (56%) patients with flut-

---

[f]The incidence in children and particularly in infants may be understated unless one uses specialized methods of detection such as esophageal electrocardiography.[32] Another confounding factor when studying the incidence of atrial flutter in children is that some authorities call intra-atrial reentrant tachycardia[520] the arrhythmia that others would consider to be flutter.

[g]From seven series.[40–46]

[h]Although not all.[14]

[i]Collected from 19 institutions.

[j]In 3.1% of 2,646 patients whose electrocardiograms were continuously monitored (12 series).[53–60, 62–64, 66] When computers are employed to analyze the electrocardiographic data, the incidence of flutter varies from none[62] to 5.3%.[59] For comparison, 11% of patients developed atrial fibrillation during the course of myocardial infarction.[68]

[k]In a consecutive series of 1,000 cases of mitral stenosis, flutter was present or paroxysmal in only five patients, whereas atrial fibrillation was found in 502 patients.[13]

[l]Only one patient from six series of 453 cases of congestive cardiomyopathy and primary myocardial disease had atrial flutter.[6, 73–77]

[m]The ejection fraction of 30% in a patient with at least 18 months of atrial flutter and 12 months of congestive heart failure became normal three months after ablation of the flutter produced sinus rhythm.[78]

[n]Atrial flutter developed in 6% of 118 English[80] and American[79] patients with chronic constrictive pericarditis.

[o]Lower incidences have been reported, but, I suspect, what was diagnosed as "atrial tachycardia" in some cases may have been flutter.[14, 85–87]

ter in one series had definite evidence of pulmonary embolism.[28]

Surgery[89–91]

Atrial flutter occurs relatively frequently after cardiac surgery but seldom after general and noncardiac thoracic operations.[92–99] The arrhythmia developed in the following:

- One hundred sixty-one (8%) of 1,996 patients after coronary artery bypass grafting and valve replacements.[6, 100–104p]
- Fifteen (9%) of 165 patients after cardiac transplantation.[105]
- Seventeen (2%) of 900 patients after noncardiac thoracic surgery.[106–110q]
- Five (1%) of 916 patients (1%) who underwent major operations.[111]

Many children develop flutter after atrial surgery.[112–126] Twenty-seven percent of 50 children developed the arrhythmia in the postoperative period after the Mustard procedure[r] and 18% after closure of atrial septal defects.[118s] After recovery from the Mustard operation, the arrhythmia develops in 8% by 5 years, in 17% by 20 years,[126] and more frequently in those with the following:[126]

- Perioperative bradyarrhythmia.
- Loss of sinus rhythm during follow-up.
- Reoperation.

Atrial flutter also appears after the Fontan procedure[125, 127] and after repair of other congenital lesions, including tetralogy of Fallot.[128]

Drugs

Digitalis[129] can cause atrial flutter,[49, 130–136] but the infrequency with which flutter is discussed in the literature on digitalis intoxication suggests that this complication is unusual. Many antiarrhythmic agents may convert atrial fibrillation into flutter, sometimes in the course of establishing sinus rhythm.

Miscellaneous

Intoxication with alcohol produces atrial flutter approximately half as often as it does atrial fibrillation ("holiday heart syndrome").[137–139] Paroxysms of atrial flutter may, like atrial fibrillation, develop when vagal tone is high.[140, 141] Atrial flutter rarely occurs during endocarditis, acute rheumatic fever, or other febrile illnesses.[10] Other medical conditions have occasionally been associated with atrial flutter (Table 5.2).[142–153]

Lone Atrial Flutter. Clinical studies formerly reported that atrial flutter was only occasionally found in

Table 5.2 **MISCELLANEOUS, UNCOMMON CAUSES OF ATRIAL FLUTTER**
Cardiac lymphoma (in a patient with AIDS)[152]
Chest trauma[142]
Hypertrophic cardiomyopathy[149]
Hypokalemia[151]
Hypothyroidism[146, 147a]
Marfan syndrome[144, 145]
Myotonic dystrophy[143]
Paraesophageal hernia[153]
Stroke[148]
Swallowing[150]

[a]Flutter was seen in none of 85 patients with *hyper*thyroidism over the age of 60 years; 33, however, had atrial fibrillation.[146]

otherwise healthy persons.[13, 14, 47, 154, 155] We now know, however, that about half of patients with atrial flutter have no clinically evident structural heart disease.[156–160t] These patients may be referred to as having lone atrial flutter.

Thrombi and Emboli. About one-fourth of patients with flutter have left atrial thrombi,[161, 162u] which are more likely to develop when the patients are male,[162] have had recent or remote emboli,[162] and have left ventricular ejection fractions of less than 40%.[162] The incidence of thromboemboli in patients with atrial flutter is not known.

OTHER ARRHYTHMIAS

Atrial Fibrillation. Patients with atrial flutter may also have atrial fibrillation.[163, 164] This association is seen particularly often after cardiac surgery.[163] Treating one arrhythmia may sometimes eliminate the other.

Atrial Tachycardia. Atrial stimulation of a patient with reentrant atrial tachycardia has transformed the arrhythmia into both types of atrial flutter.[165]

Atrioventricular Block. The atrial rhythm in some patients with complete atrioventricular block is flutter.[166, 167]

Ventricular Tachycardia. Atrial flutter may coexist with ventricular tachycardia.[168]

PATIENT HISTORY

The usual symptoms, present in varying degrees in patients who develop atrial flutter, are characteristic of all tachycardias. These include the following:

- Palpitations, probably the most frequent symptom of all,[169] and perception of rapid heart action.
- Dyspnea and breathlessness.[170]

---

[p]From six series.[6, 100–104]

[q]From five series.[106–110]

[r]From two series.[118, 122]

[s]Distinguishing flutter from atrial tachycardia in some of these patients can be complicated,[124] a long-standing dilemma for electrocardiographers.[112]

---

[t]One hundred eighty-five (49%) of 377 patients from five series.[52, 157–160] In older patients, lone atrial flutter may be an early manifestation of the sick sinus syndrome.[160]

[u]Left atrial thrombi, detected by transesophageal echocardiography, were present in five (21%) of 24 patients with flutter and in six (3%) of 184 patients in sinus rhythm.[162]

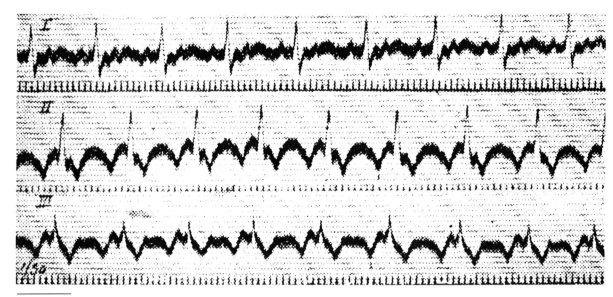

FIGURE 5.1 **An early recording of atrial flutter** from a clergyman when first seen by Thomas Lewis in 1912. The patient's flutter persisted for at least 26 years. (From Lewis T. Auricular flutter continuing for 24 years. BMJ 1937; 6/19, 1248, with permission.)[172]

- Chest pain.[170]
- Weakness and faintness, although syncope is uncommon.[48]
- "Disinclination for effort."[v]

Symptoms are more likely and disturbing when the ventricular rate is rapid, when the arrhythmia is paroxysmal rather than chronic, and when heart disease is advanced.[2]

The first episode of flutter may be either paroxysmal or the initiation of the chronic form.[171w] Unless specific measures are taken to convert or ablate the arrhythmia, paroxysms of atrial flutter tend to last longer than those of atrial fibrillation.[49] Individual cases of apparently chronic atrial flutter have been documented for as long as 24[172x] and 43 years (Fig. 5.1).[y] As one may suspect, paroxysmal flutter tends to become chronic or established as structural heart disease worsens.[52]

Atrial Flutter in Children

Thirty percent of children are asymptomatic at the onset of flutter.[33] In the others, the following symptoms appear:

- Dyspnea or other symptoms of congestive heart failure, 28%.
- Palpitations, 24%.
- Syncope, 9%, occurring more frequently in those with normal hearts (29%) or with the Wolff-Parkinson-White syndrome (50%).
- "Presyncope" with dizziness, 8%.
- "Sudden death" from which resuscitation was attempted, 1%.

The average duration of flutter in 357 children, many of whom had congenital heart disease, was at least 2.5 years.[33] In 33% of these patients, flutter occurred only once, and in an additional 21%, the duration of atrial flutter was one year or less.[z]

PHYSICAL EXAMINATION AND PULSE RECORDINGS

Physical examination of patients with atrial flutter reveals the pulse to be rapid and more often regular than irregular. The patient's blood pressure may be lower than during sinus rhythm. The venous pressure is normal unless congestive heart failure is present, but normal A waves in the neck veins from right atrial contraction are absent. The amplitude of the carotid pulses reflects the rapid ventricular rate and the stroke volume.

Sometimes small, rapid waves may be seen in the jugular pulse[173–175] (Fig. 5.2). They are produced by contraction of the fluttering right atrium and are

---

[v]From a series of 52 patients with flutter observed by John Parkinson and D. Evan Bedford, "between the years 1913 and 1926, of whom 2 only were seen during the War (1914–1919)."[170]

[w]In Campbell's series (1947), flutter persisted for more than 72 hours in 51 (62%) of 82 patients.[48] Katz and Pick (1956) observed that, compared with atrial fibrillation, flutter is more often paroxysmal than chronic.[2] White (1951) summarized his experience as follows: "Generally atrial flutter lasts for hours, days, or weeks, rarely for minutes, months, or years."[11] Waldo, who has intensively studied patients with atrial flutter for more than 20 years, more recently (1995) wrote: "Atrial flutter infrequently is a persistent rhythm. . . . It is primarily paroxysmal, lasting for variable periods of time, usually seconds to hours, but on occasion even 1 day or more. Persistent atrial flutter . . . is unusual, as atrial flutter usually reverts to sinus rhythm or atrial fibrillation, either spontaneously or as a result of therapy."[6]

[x]In an English clergyman, reported by Thomas Lewis, who was able to lead a reasonably active life although "unable to walk more than a mile without undue fatigue" (1937).[172]

[y]In a woman described to be "in constant good health" (P. D. White and H. Donovan 1967).[606]

[z]From those patients in the collaborative series of 364 patients from whom historical information could be obtained.[33]

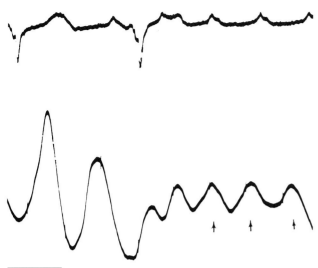

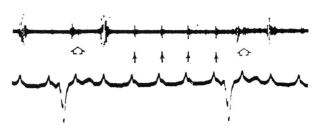

FIGURE 5.4 **Sounds produced by atrial flutter** recorded (40–100 cycles/sec) from the third right parasternal space (*solid arrows,* **top**) and the electrocardiogram **(bottom)** confirming the coincidence of the flutter waves with the sounds. (Adapted from Massumi RA, Hernandez T, Just G, Tawakkol AA. The audible sounds of atrial tachyarrhythmia (flutter?). Circulation 1966; 33:607–612, with permission.)[175]

FIGURE 5.2 **Flutter waves in the jugular vein (bottom) produced by contractions of the right atrium during atrial flutter (top)**. (Adapted from Massumi RA, Hernandez T, Just G, Tawakkol AA. The audible sounds of atrial tachyarrhythmia (flutter?). Circulation 1966; 33:607–612, with permission.)[175]

larger when right atrial hypertrophy is present.[173] They may be missed in obese patients or when the head of the bed is incorrectly elevated.[173] Pulse waves produced by flutter in the left atrium can be detected in the left ventricle by apexcardiography[175] (Fig. 5.3).

The auscultatory examination of the heart reveals, first of all, the rapid heart action. The intensity of the first heart sound is constant when the ventricular rate is regular[174] and association between atrial and ventricular signals is sustained, but it varies in intensity when the ventricular rate is irregular.[176] Abnormal sounds,

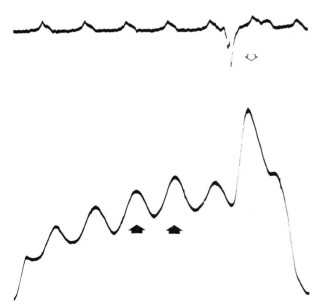

FIGURE 5.3 **Flutter waves in the apexcardiogram (bottom) produced by contractions of the left atrium during atrial flutter (top)**. (Adapted from Massumi RA, Hernandez T, Just G, Tawakkol AA. The audible sounds of atrial tachyarrhythmia (flutter?). Circulation 1966; 33:607–612, with permission.)[175]

sometimes soft and low pitched, sometimes clicking, have been heard and recorded during atrial flutter, particularly when the ventricular rate is relatively slow[173, 175, 177–181] (Fig. 5.4).

ELECTROCARDIOGRAPHY

Atrial Activity and Flutter Waves

Rapid, regular, continuous, undulating deflections of low amplitude and broad width characterize the electrocardiogram of the patient with atrial flutter[182] (Figs. 5.5 to 5.7).[aa] In most cases, each cycle consists of a downstroke with a slow, relatively prolonged portion followed by a shorter, more rapid upstroke.[183, 184bb] Usually, leads II, III, aVF, and V_1 best reveal flutter waves, and lead I reveals them least well.[185] The words "sawtooth" and "picket fence" have traditionally been applied to the appearance of flutter waves. Clonic contractions of an extremity[186] and the discharging of a transcutaneous electrical nerve stimulator[187] may produce waves similar to those produced by flutter ("pseudoatrial flutter").

Finding the Flutter Waves. Two methods reveal the presence of flutter waves when these waves cannot be seen:

- Increasing atrioventricular block with carotid sinus pressure (Fig. 5.8) or with drugs that slow atrioventricular conduction such as digitalis and beta-adrenergic– or calcium-channel–blocking drugs. This method reduces the frequency of QRS complexes and T waves that may obscure the flutter waves.
- Recording from epicardial leads inserted during cardiac surgery[188, 189] or from intracardiac or esophageal[32] electrodes or echocardiograms,[190–192]

[aa]The electrocardiographic deflections of the atrial activity during flutter are so specific that I prefer to call them "flutter waves" rather than "abnormal P waves." Atrial activity with similar appearance can be produced by pacing at flutter rates in the coronary sinus.[182]

[bb]Formerly, the "first," usually the positive portion of the flutter wave, was thought to represent atrial depolarization, and the "second," usually negative portion or "Ta wave," atrial repolarization.[3] Now we know that all parts of the flutter waves are produced by activation of different parts of the atria.

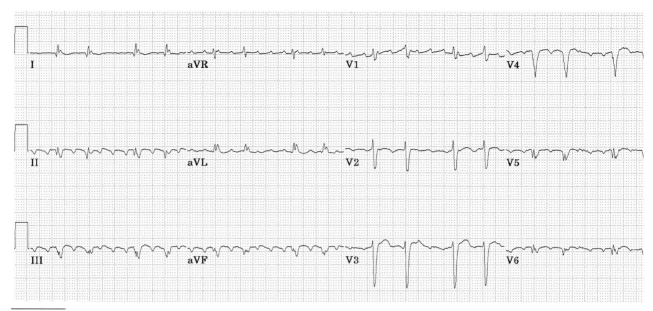

FIGURE 5.5 Typical electrocardiographic example of type I atrial flutter. The atrial rate is 300 beats per minute, and the average ventricular rate is 125 beats per minute. Atrioventricular block varies from 2:1 to 4:1. Notice how the atrial activity is best seen in leads II, III, aVF, and V₁ and is barely perceptible in lead I. (The electrophysiological mechanism sustaining this example is clockwise reentry in the right atrium.)

each of which shows atrial activity not easily seen in the surface electrocardiogram.

Predicting Flutter. During sinus rhythm, the P waves of patients with paroxysmal atrial flutter are often abnormally wide.[cc] This finding can predict the development of atrial flutter and atrial fibrillation after cardiac bypass surgery.[193]

[cc]The width of the P waves during sinus rhythm was 110 milliseconds or longer in 27 (66%) and 120 milliseconds or longer in 21 (51%) of 41 patients with clinical episodes of flutter.[297] In another series, the mean P wave duration was 132 milliseconds.[312]

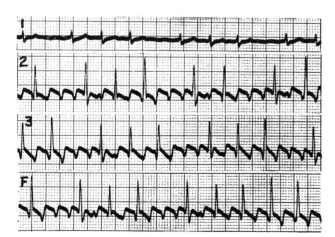

FIGURE 5.6 Atrial flutter with atrioventricular block varying between 2:1 and 4:1. Again, notice that the flutter waves are best seen in the inferior leads and barely visible in lead I. (Adapted from Marriott HJL. Practical Electrocardiography. 4th ed. Baltimore: Williams & Wilkins, 1968; and Waldo AL. Atrial flutter. In Kastor JA, ed. Arrhythmias. Philadelphia: WB Saunders, 1994, with permission.)[604]

Atrial Dissociation. In the infrequently encountered arrhythmia, atrial dissociation, each of the atria sustains different rhythms. Occasionally in this condition, the rhythm in one of the chambers is flutter.[194–197]

Types of Atrial Flutter[198]

Two types of atrial flutter are seen in the electrocardiogram[188, 199–201] (Fig. 5.9 and Table 5.3).

Type I or "classic" flutter occurs more often,[202dd] is slower than type II flutter, and appears in two forms, both of which can occur in the same patient:[200, 203–206ee]

• Common (counterclockwise) form—the flutter

[dd]In the series of 25 patients studied after cardiac surgery in which the distinction between the two types of flutter was first described in English, 18 had type I and seven had type II flutter.[202]

[ee]In one series of 33 patients with type I flutter, 24 (73%) had the common (typical) and nine the uncommon (atypical) form.[205] In another group of 38 patients, the arrhythmia in 20 (53%) was typical and in eight (21%) atypical. Ten (26%) had both forms.[200] Vectorcardiographic studies demonstrate characteristic differences between the two forms of type I flutter.[204]

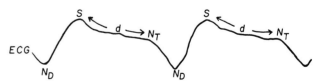

FIGURE 5.7 Flutter waves. In this enlarged diagram of two flutter waves (ECG lead II), we see how most of the principal motion of the wave is downward. (d, downsweep; N_D, nadir; N_T, notch; S, summit.) (Adapted from Alderman EL, Rytand DA, Crow RS, Finegan RE, Harrison DC. Normal and prosthetic atrioventricular valve motion in atrial flutter: correlation of ultrasound, vectorcardiographic, and phonocardiographic findings. Circulation 1972; 45:1206–1215, with permission.)[183]

Continuous ECG Monitor

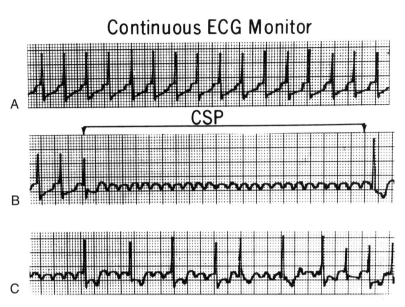

FIGURE 5.8 Carotid sinus pressure revealing atrial flutter by increasing atrioventricular block. The arrhythmia is a rapid regular tachycardia at a rate of about 175 beats per minute **(A)**. What is the mechanism? Carotid sinus pressure (CSP) increased (rather impressively*) atrioventricular block, revealing the atrial flutter waves **(B)**. On stopping carotid pressure, flutter with varying block appears **(C)**. (From Waldo AL. Atrial flutter. In Kastor JA, ed. Arrhythmias. Philadelphia: WB Saunders, 1994, with permission.)

Table 5.3 **CHARACTERISTICS OF TYPES I AND II ATRIAL FLUTTER**

Types of Atrial Flutter	Two Forms of Type I Flutter	Rate (beats/min) of Flutter Waves	Form of Flutter Waves in Leads II, III, and aVF	Form of Flutter Waves in Lead V_1	Mechanism	Can be Entrained or Converted by Rapid Pacing
I "classic"	Common	240–350	Negative	Positive	Counterclockwise reentry	Yes
I "classic"	Uncommon	240–350	Positive	Negative	Clockwise reentry	Yes
II atypical		Faster than 350	Variable	Variable	Not known	No

FIGURE 5.9 Types I and II atrial flutter confirmed with atrial electrograms (A_{EG}). In this example of type I flutter (*top,* **A** with lead III and the atrial electrogram), the atrial rate is 296 beats per minute. The atrial rate in type II flutter is typically faster, 420 beats per minute in this case (*bottom,* **B**). In each example, the constant beat-to-beat cycle length, polarity, morphology, and amplitude of the atrial electrogram are characteristic of atrial flutter. (From Waldo AL. Atrial flutter. In Kastor JA, ed. Arrhythmias. Philadelphia: WB Saunders, 1994, with permission.)

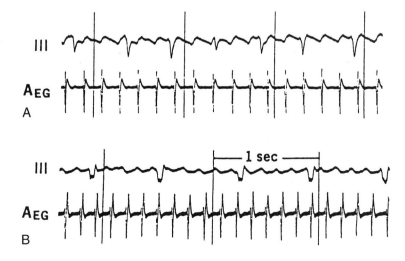

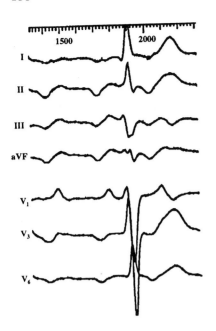 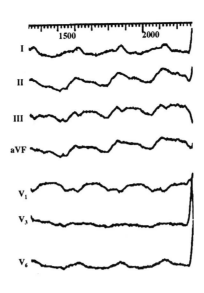

FIGURE 5.10 **Counterclockwise (left) and clockwise (right) atrial flutter.** The flutter waves are characteristically negative in leads II, III and aVF and are positive in lead V_1 when atrial flutter is sustained in a counterclockwise reentrant pattern in the right atrium **(left)**. They are predominantly upright in the inferior leads and negative in lead V_1 when the circuit takes a clockwise course **(right)**. (Adapted from Saoudi N, Nair M, Abdelazziz A, Poty H, Daou A, Anselme F, et al. Electrocardiographic patterns and results of radiofrequency catheter ablation of clockwise type I atrial flutter. J Cardiovasc Electrophysiol 1996; 7:931–942, with permission.)[200]

waves are predominantly negative in the inferior electrocardiographic leads, biphasic in lead I, and upright in lead V_1 (Fig. 5.10).

• Uncommon (clockwise) form—the motion of the flutter waves is predominantly positive in the inferior leads and inverted in lead V_1, and the rate is somewhat slower in the uncommon form of type I flutter. In addition, the plateau phase is shorter and the negative component of the flutter waves is wide, as seen in the inferior electrocardiographic leads[200ff] (see Fig. 5.10).

Type I flutter does not begin immediately after a single premature atrial beat, as characterizes the onset of reentrant supraventricular tachycardia sustained in the atrioventricular node or accessory pathways.[207] At least among patients recovering from open-heart surgery, in whom atrial flutter frequently occurs, the onset of the flutter is usually preceded by a "transitional" arrhythmia, usually atrial fibrillation, which may itself be precipitated by type II flutter.[207]

Type II or atypical flutter, characteristically produced during rapid pacing to interrupt type I flutter, is transient and usually leads to atrial fibrillation or returns to type I flutter in a few minutes.[208, 209]

Atrial Rate and Rhythm

Atrial Rate. Most authorities define the average rate of the atrial signals in adults as 300 beats per minute, whereas they assign different upper and lower limits[2, 6, 11, 210–212] (Table 5.4), depending, in part, on whether they include type II flutter, which has a faster atrial rate (see Table 5.3):

• In 50 patients with electrophysiological studies, the mean atrial rate was 299 beats per minute.[213]

• In 16 infants from two series,[31, 32] the atrial rate ranged from 280 to 460 flutter waves per minute and averaged 403 in eight of them.

• In 17 children with Mustard repair of complete transposition of the great arteries and clinical episodes of atrial flutter, the mean atrial rate, when the arrhythmia was induced by electrophysiological study, was 249 beats per minute, with a range of 171 to 333 beats per minute.[122]

Several factors, including the length of time that chronic and paroxysmal flutter persists, can influence the atrial rate[147, 214–219] (Table 5.5). Exit block may account for the rare instance of sudden halving (2:1 block)[220] or other relatively large and sudden changes[221] in the atrial rate. Block between the atria can also occur.[197]

Periodic Patterns. Small variations commonly present in the atrial cycle length (the time between the atrial beats) have a periodic pattern that is modulated on a beat-to-beat basis from interactions among the following:[222]

• Autonomic nervous system.

Table 5.4	**RATES OF FLUTTER WAVES AS DESCRIBED IN TEXTBOOKS OF CARDIOLOGY DURING THE PAST 50 YEARS[a]**	
Authors	**Minimum (beats/min)**	**Maximum (beats/min)**
White 1951[11]	200 (or slightly less)	400 (or slightly more)
Katz and Pick 1956[2]	250	350
Friedberg 1966[210]	250	350
Yurchak and McGovern 1980[211]	250	350
Zipes 1997[212]	250	450
Waldo, in Podrid[6]	240	340

ff Electrophysiologists often call common type I flutter "counterclockwise flutter" and uncommon type I flutter "clockwise flutter" in reference to the direction of the arrhythmia's reentrant circuit in the right atrium.

[a] The standard texts in the past 50 years list average rates and ranges for the atrial activity of flutter without reference to specific studies.

Table 5.5 FACTORS THAT CHANGE THE RATE OF FLUTTER WAVES

Increase	Decrease
Digitalis[216]	Antiarrhythmic drugs[216]
Exercise[217a]	Exercise[249b]
Expiration[218, 219c]	Inspiration[218, 219c]
Fever[214d]	—
Nitrates[219]	—
Thyrotoxicosis[147, 214c]	—
Tilting head up[218, 219c]	Tilting head down[219]
Decrease in right atrial size[219]	Right atrial enlargement[214, 219e]
Valsalva maneuver[218, 219]	
—	More time in flutter[214]

[a]The atrial rate did not change in 18 of 22 patients during exercise and rose 10 to 60 beats per minute in 4.[217]

[b]The average atrial cycle lengths increased (the rate slowed) during exercise from 245 to 256 milliseconds.[249]

[c]Changes in atrial rate from inspiration, expiration, raising the head 60 degrees, and the Valsalva maneuver develop despite beta-adrenergic and muscarinic blockade and, consequently, do not depend on autonomic tone.[218]

[d]To an average of 341 flutter waves per minute in 13 patients with fever or thyrotoxicosis.[214]

[e]To an average of 224 flutter waves per minute in eight patients and as low as 176 per minute in one patient.[214] Patients with the largest atria have the slowest rates although "very appreciable dilatation of the right atrium is required" (David A. Rytand et al., 1958).[214] When flutter develops because of left atrial disease, which is rare,[214] enlargement of that chamber seldom affects the atrial rate and usually changes the flutter to fibrillation.

- Respiratory system.
- Ventricular rate.

The periodic variation in flutter may take the form of slight alternation in the atrial cycle length ("flutter interval alternans"),[202, 223, 224] a finding established with special recordings and not easily detected in the standard electrocardiogram.

Ventricular Rate and Rhythm

The ventricular rate and rhythm in patients with atrial flutter depend primarily on the amount of block produced by the atrioventricular node and secondarily on the atrial rate. In most untreated patients, the node blocks transmission of every other impulse and produces a ventricular rate of about 150 beats per minute.[gg] The greater the block, the slower the ventricular rate, and vice versa.

The ventricular rhythm is regular in atrial flutter when the block is constant; the ratio of atrial to ventricular beats is usually 2:1 or 4:1. Persistent ratios of odd numbers such as 3:1 or 5:1 are "extremely rare."[2] Similarly, 1:1 conduction is also infrequent, and this is fortunate because the rapid ventricular rate usually produces severe symptoms and even death.[225–236] The effects of 1:1 conduction can be simulated even when

[gg]The block was 2:1 in the preadmission electrocardiograms of each of 50 patients with atrial flutter[213] and in each of eight infants with flutter.[32] In another series, 80% of 39 patients with flutter who were not taking digitalis had 2:1 block when first examined,[52] and the first electrocardiograms taken in 21 untreated patients with atrial flutter showed 2:1 block in 10, an irregular but predominantly 2:1 ventricular response in five, a totally irregular response in five, and 1:1 conduction in one.[237] As John Parkinson observed in 1927: "A regular tachycardia with a fixed rate between 120 and 160 per minute which persists for over a fortnight is almost certainly flutter."[170]

2:1 block is present if the atrial rate is sufficiently rapid, as in a patient with thyrotoxicosis.[147]

As the amount of block increases, the ventricular response becomes irregular, often producing Wenckebach periodicity of the QRS complexes.[237, 238] Such complex numerical relationships between atrial and ventricular activation are thought to be caused by block at several levels within the atrioventricular node.[237–239hh] As block increases further, atrioventricular dissociation may develop. When no atrial impulses are transmitted, complete heart block results, with the expected slow ventricular rate.[167]

Paradoxically, when the atrial rate decreases, the ventricular rate may *increase*. This is due to reduction in concealed conduction within the atrioventricular node. The fewer the atrial impulses, the fewer beats are concealed within the node. Transmission of subsequent beats is less impeded, and the intervals between ventricular responses shorten. Conversely, faster atrial rates may increase concealed conduction and may produce a slower ventricular response.

During sinus rhythm, the heart rate increases slightly for several minutes in many patients before paroxysms of atrial flutter begin, suggesting that increasing sympathetic or decreasing parasympathetic tone may facilitate the initiation of flutter.[240]

Wolff-Parkinson-White Syndrome[241ii]

Patients with ventricular preexcitation resulting from accessory pathways may conduct many or every flutter beat and thereby may sustain dangerously rapid ventricular rates similar to those in patients with atrial fibrillation and preexcitation.[242–246] Flutter was the most frequent supraventricular arrhythmia with wide QRS complexes producing rapid ventricular rates in 26 patients studied in an electrophysiological laboratory.[244] The ventricular rate was at least 240 beats per minute in 12 of the 15 patients with flutter.[244]

Lown-Ganong-Levine Syndrome

In the first report of this condition—short PR intervals, normal QRS complexes, and paroxysmal heart action—flutter was the tachyarrhythmia in four (12%) of 34 patients.[247]

Exercise Electrocardiography

Exercise can induce paroxysmal atrial flutter in patients with sinus rhythm or atrial fibrillation at rest.[217, 248] Exercising patients with flutter may reduce the amount of atrioventricular block, so that, occasionally, 1:1 conduction and a very rapid ventricular rate can develop,[217, 249] as are more likely to occur under the following conditions:[217]

- Atrial rates of 250 beats per minute or less.
- Inadequate doses of atrioventricular blocking drugs.

[hh]A concept known as "complexity theory" may apply to the progression of 2:1 to 4:1 conduction.[238]

[ii]See Chapter 4 for additional information about this topic.

- Administration of drugs with vagolytic effects such as quinidine.

Signal-Averaged Electrocardiogram

Atrial activation in flutter can produce "pseudo late potentials" in the signal-averaged electrocardiogram that may be incorrectly interpreted to indicate abnormal ventricular activation.[250, 251]

ECHOCARDIOGRAPHY

The echocardiogram of patients with atrial flutter demonstrates, coincident with each flutter wave, regular, undulating movement of the posterior left atrial wall and upper left interventricular septum.[252] The echocardiogram also shows mechanical motion[183] and slight reopening of the mitral valve,[252] even when no flutter waves appear on the electrocardiogram.[192] The left atrial appendage is smaller and contracts better in patients with atrial flutter than in those with atrial fibrillation or "flutter-fibrillation."[253]

Dual echocardiography shows that the left atrium contracts before the right atrium during atrial flutter,[254] even though the arrhythmia originates in the right atrium. Intracardiac echocardiography can visualize anatomic landmarks, ensure stable endocardial contact, and guide transseptal puncture during activation mapping[255] and ablation of the atrial circuit sustaining flutter.[256] Echocardiography measures the changes in ventricular function produced by atrioventricular junctional ablation and ventricular pacing.[257, 258] Atrial flutter can be demonstrated in fetuses by echocardiography.[36, 38]

Atrial Size

Echocardiography demonstrates the relationships among right atrial size, intracardiac volume, and cycle length.[219]

The size of the left atrium determined echocardiographically

- Relates directly to the duration of the atrial flutter waves, but not to the maximum amplitude of the waves seen in leads II and V_1.[259]
- Is often enlarged in children with atrial flutter, many of whom have congenital heart disease.[jj]

Function of the Left Atrium After Cardioversion

Transthoracic and transesophageal echocardiography, which can demonstrate the changes in atrial function produced by cardioversion,[260] shows that the left atrial appendage regains its contractile function better (is less "stunned") after cardioversion from atrial flutter than from atrial fibrillation.[261] Even though no atrial

mechanical activity may appear immediately after cardioversion from flutter,[262, 263] contractile function returns quickly in most patients,[262] a finding helping to explain why thromboembolism occurs less often after conversion from atrial flutter than from fibrillation.

Atrial Thrombi and Spontaneous Echo Contrast

Transesophageal echocardiography reveals that as many as one-third of patients with atrial flutter have thrombi or spontaneous echo contrast in their left atria.[161, 162, 263, 264kk] Intra-atrial thrombi and spontaneous echo contrast are found less frequently in patients with atrial flutter than those in flutter-fibrillation.[253] Furthermore, patients with flutter and intermittent atrial fibrillation have more spontaneous echo contrast than those with flutter alone.[265]

Effects of Ablation

Restoration of sinus rhythm by ablating the circuit that sustains chronic atrial flutter with radiofrequency current improves left ventricular function in patients with dilated cardiomyopathy, which may, in some cases, have been induced by the tachyarrhythmia.[266]

HEMODYNAMICS[267, 268]

The development of atrial flutter often decreases hemodynamic function. This can be seen in the drop of 14 mm Hg in average systolic blood pressure of patients recovering from noncardiac surgery when flutter replaces sinus rhythm.[269] Accordingly, the cardiac output often rises,[270] ejection fraction increases[271ll] and, occasionally, wall motion abnormalities improve[271] when patients in atrial flutter are cardioverted to sinus rhythm. Ablating the atrioventricular junction and pacing the ventricles of patients with flutter often improve depressed ventricular function.[258]

Some patients, however, tolerate the development of flutter with little disruptive hemodynamic effect. Although slight tricuspid and mitral insufficiency developed in a patient with mitral stenosis, the cardiac output and blood pressure did not change when flutter replaced sinus rhythm.[272] In another patient, the cardiac output and oxygen consumption were the same when exercise produced 1:1 conduction with a ventricular rate of 260 beats per minute and during a slower rate in flutter or sinus rhythm.[273]

Flutter Rate

The atrial rate in flutter is inversely related to the volume of blood in the right atrium and to the right

---

jjThe left atrial dimension exceeds the upper limit of normal for age in 64% of such children and is greater than 150% of the upper limit of normal in 24%.[33]

kkOf 19 patients with congenital heart disease and nonfibrillatory atrial arrhythmias, six had solitary thrombi in the right atrium, and two had such thrombi in the left atrium.[264]

llIn 11 men, the mean ejection fraction increased in six, did not change in four, and was unchanged in one, as measured with gate-synchronized equilibrium blood pool radionuclide angiograms. The changes did not relate to the age of the patients.[271]

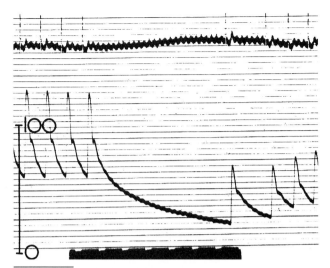

FIGURE 5.11 Flutter waves recorded from the brachial artery in a patient with atrial flutter. Carotid sinus pressure has increased atrioventricular block producing a pause between ventricular contractions that reveals the low-amplitude arterial deflections **(bottom)** coincident with the electrocardiographic flutter waves **(top)**. The cause of this finding has never been established. (Adapted from Howarth S. Atrial waves on arterial pressure records in normal rhythm, heart block, and auricular flutter. Br Heart J 1954; 16:171–176, with permission.)[275]

atrial size. Accordingly, when the size of the right atrium increases to accommodate a greater volume of blood induced by tilting down the head of the body, the rate of the flutter waves decreases, and vice versa.[218, 219]

Hemodynamic Counterpart of Flutter Waves

Small fluctuations in pressure at the rate of the flutter waves can be recorded through catheters in the right atrium,[173, 274] right ventricle,[268, 274] pulmonary artery,[268, 274] and systemic arteries[275] (Fig. 5.11). Unlike in atrial fibrillation, tricuspid regurgitation is seldom recorded in atrial flutter.[274]

Polyuria

Diuresis frequently accompanies paroxysms of supraventricular tachyarrhythmias including atrial flutter.[276–278]

Atrial Natriuretic Peptide

The concentration of atrial natriuretic peptide rises in patients with atrial flutter, whether or not congestive heart failure is present, and it falls promptly after return of sinus rhythm.[279]

CLINICAL ELECTROPHYSIOLOGY[5, 89, 184, 280–292]
Mechanisms and Types

Clinical electrophysiological studies have established that most cases of atrial flutter are caused by reentry in tissues of the right atrium,[293–311] a finding that sup-

ports the long-held clinical maxim that atrial flutter is predominantly a disease of the right atrium.[mm] Both forms of type I ("classic") atrial flutter are due to reentry. Type II flutter, the mechanism of which has not been established, may constitute a heterogeneous group of arrhythmias transitional to atrial fibrillation.[201]

Widespread Electrophysiological Disease

The concurrent presence of electrophysiological abnormalities of the sinus node and of ventricular conduction in patients with atrial flutter suggests that many patients with flutter also suffer from a generalized electrophysiological abnormality involving more than just the atria.[312] Severe electrophysiological dysfunction of the sinus node appears in patients who develop flutter after corrective surgery on the atria for congenital heart disease.[122]

Recognition

A Waves. The characteristic feature of the electrophysiological record of patients with atrial flutter is frequent A waves with uniform morphology, polarity, amplitude, and beat-to-beat cycle length.[202] Slight variations in the intervals between the flutter waves, including alternation, sometimes appear.[202, 223, 311] In type I flutter, the intervals between the flutter waves, when irregular, are slightly prolonged after a ventricular beat, possibly from stretch of the atria produced by the ventricular contraction.[311] In the more rapid type II flutter, the atrial cycle length decreases and then increases.[311nn]

The A waves, produced by the rapidly discharging atria, frequently have two or more deflections ("double" or "split" A waves), which are assumed to indicate slow conduction and the reentrant character of the arrhythmia.[255, 301, 302, 305] Their amplitude, however, is similar to that recorded during sinus rhythm.[313] Continuous and fragmented activity, which also suggests abnormally delayed conduction, may be recorded in the atria during flutter.[301]

HV Complexes. The A waves are followed at varying intervals by the HV complexes, recorded from the bundle of His and the ventricles.[314] When 2:1 block is present, the HV complexes occur regularly and follow every other A wave. The beat is dropped between the inscription of the A and the H wave, an indication that the block is in the atrioventricular node. When the block varies from, for example, 2:1 to 4:1 the HV complexes appear irregularly, sometimes in the rhythm of a Wenckebach cycle.

[mm]These studies put to rest the long-standing controversy over whether flutter is predominantly due to an automatically discharging focus or to reentry.[291, 293–296]

[nn]One cannot help but note the similarity of this phenomenon to ventriculophasic sinus arrhythmia in complete atrioventricular block in which the PP intervals of sinus rhythm that encompass a QRS complex are shorter than those that do not.

Atrial Conduction and Refractoriness

When patients with flutter are studied during sinus rhythm the following are noted:

- Conduction from right to left atrium is prolonged[254, 312, 315] in most[oo] and within the right atrium[315] in some[pp] patients. The PA interval is prolonged.[297, 316qq]
- Conduction is abnormally prolonged when extrastimuli are introduced at certain coupling intervals and paced rates.[5, 297, 316, 317]

The normal shortening of refractoriness in the high right atrium as it is paced more rapidly does not occur.[5, 297] The velocity of the action potential, not the duration of the action potential, determines the cycle length of the flutter waves.[318] Monophasic action potentials recorded from catheters in the right atrium reveal that sinus rhythm returns to patients with atrial flutter when the duration of refractoriness becomes sufficiently long.[319]

Induction

One can usually[rr] start atrial flutter in susceptible patients by pacing the atria rapidly or by stimulating the chambers with up to two extra beats at several paced rates.[5, 297] Induced atrial flutter begins with delayed intra-atrial conduction and fragmentation and oscillations of the atrial electrograms.[297] When fragmentation does not appear, attempting induction of the arrhythmia usually fails. Flutter can also be induced with esophageal pacing.[320]

Sustained flutter can seldom be induced in patients who have not had clinical episodes of atrial flutter or fibrillation[5ss] or at least a history of symptoms such as palpitations, tachycardia, syncope, or chest pain not typical of angina.[315] This observation is supported by the experience of some children who, after atrial surgery, can be induced into flutter and subsequently develop the arrhythmia spontaneously.[122] The substrate for the flutter, presumably, was produced by the surgery. Transient, but not sustained, flutter can occasionally be established in subjects without a clinical history of arrhythmia or of electrocardiographic or electrophysiological abnormalities.[tt]

[oo]In 55 of 71 patients.[5]

[pp]In 16 of 71 patients.[5]

[qq]PA interval, the time that elapses from the onset of the P wave in the electrocardiogram to the inscription of atrial depolarization recorded from an intra-atrial lead.

[rr]In more than 95% of patients with typical type I atrial flutter (negative flutter waves in the inferior electrocardiographic leads) and about 75% with atypical type I flutter (positive flutter waves in the inferior leads).[5] The arrhythmia is started more easily by introducing extrastimuli in the high right atrium than in the coronary sinus, but rapid pacing is probably the most consistently reliable method.

[ss]However, by rapidly pacing at very short cycle lengths such as 100 milliseconds (600 beats per minute), one group was able to induce flutter in one-third of patients with no clinical history of the arrhythmia.[309] The arrhythmia induced by this method may bear no relation to the patients' spontaneous arrhythmia.

[tt]As was the case in six of 137 children studied before surgery for congenital heart disease. The episodes lasted from 0.4 to 60 seconds.[607]

The best sites for inducing the two forms of type I flutter differ slightly. In the more common counterclockwise variety, induction is most likely from the trabeculated right atrium, whereas the less frequent clockwise variety is best started from the smooth right atrium.[321]

Patients with atrioventricular nodal reentrant supraventricular tachycardia may have an increased susceptibility to atrial flutter.[322] In some subjects with the holiday heart syndrome flutter can be induced after they drink alcohol.[323]

Activation and Site of Origin and Block[208, 324–326]

Recording from several sites within the atria during intracardiac electrophysiological studies or from the surface of the heart during cardiac operations reveals the sequence of atrial activation during flutter.[105, 157, 200, 255, 295, 299, 303, 304, 306, 313, 327–331] The reentrant circuit that sustains flutter is located in the right atrium, as predicted from earlier clinical reports.[39]

In the common form of type I flutter (negative flutter waves in the inferior leads of the electrocardiogram), the electrical activity travels *counterclockwise*, up (caudocranially) the interatrial septum and down (craniocaudally) the lateral wall of the chamber[329] (see Fig. 5.10; Fig. 5.12). In the uncommon form (positive flutter waves in the inferior leads) of type I flutter, activation spreads *clockwise* in the right atrium, up the anterior and lateral walls and down the septum and posterior wall.[201, 304] The size of the reentrant center is

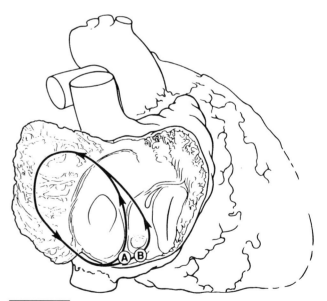

FIGURE 5.12　Circuit sustaining atrial flutter. In this schematic cutaway view of the interior of the right atrium, the *black ovals* indicate the path of the reentrant circuit that sustains the flutter, and the arrows show the more common counterclockwise route. Radiofrequency current applied posterior (*A*) or anterior (*B*) to the os of the coronary sinus usually cures the patient of the arrhythmia. (Adapted from Feld GK, Fleck RP, Chen PS, Boyce K, Bahnson TD, Stein JB, et al. Radiofrequency catheter ablation for the treatment of human type I atrial flutter: identification of a critical zone in the reentrant circuit by endocardial mapping techniques. Circulation 1992; 86:1233–1240, with permission.)[563]

controversial, and some investigators believe it to be relatively large.[310]

The tricuspid annulus constitutes a continuous anterior barrier constraining the reentrant wave front in type I flutter.[328] The site of unidirectional block with its slow conduction, essential to sustaining the arrhythmia, is probably a relatively small area in the isthmus between the tricuspid valve, coronary sinus, and inferior vena cava.[5, 295, 299, 304, 306, 307, 321]

Left Atrial Activation. The left atrium, although important, and probably the more important chamber in forming the electrocardiographic appearance of the flutter waves,[5] is activated secondarily from the circuit in the right atrium[301] along the coronary sinus from the os to the high lateral wall.[5, 157] Activation of the left atrium produces most of the predominantly negative appearance of the flutter waves in the electrocardiogram.[5] Occasionally, electrophysiological findings suggest that the arrhythmia originates in a left atrial reentrant circuit.[208, 332uu] The route of the flutter in these cases is always clockwise.

Supraventricular Tachycardia. Because atrial flutter can frequently be induced in patients with atrioventricular nodal reentrant supraventricular tachycardia, the two arrhythmias may share an area in the lower right atrium in their reentrant pathways. Ablation in the tricuspid annulus above the coronary sinus can cure the patient of supraventricular tachycardia and may prevent induction of either arrhythmia.[333] However, ablation of the atrioventricular nodal slow pathway does not influence the inducibility of atrial flutter.[309]

Entrainment[5, 7, 208, 292]

One can transiently capture or entrain the reentrant circuit in patients with type I flutter by pacing the atria at rates that slightly exceed those of the clinical arrhythmia.[205, 255, 310, 330, 334–338] The rate of the reentry then increases to the pacing rate, but when pacing stops, flutter at the intrinsic, slower rate returns. Entrainment has been taken as further proof of the reentrant nature of flutter. Both the common and uncommon forms of type I flutter can be transiently entrained,[205] but certain characteristics of the entrainment suggest that each has a different origin.[205]

Other Advances

Sophisticated studies have provided additional information, beyond the scope of this book to discuss, that has advanced further our understanding of the electrophysiology of atrial flutter.[339–345]

TREATMENT[288, 346]

Modifying some of the ordinary or unusual features of daily living[11vv] has long been advocated, but never proven, to prevent paroxysms of atrial flutter.

Physical Maneuvers

Carotid Sinus Pressure.[174, 346–349] Applying carotid sinus pressure to patients with atrial flutter increases atrioventricular block and temporarily decreases the ventricular rate, which then gradually returns, in a "jerky" manner, to the original rate and rhythm. This pattern contrasts with the more gradual and smooth return after carotid sinus pressure is applied to patients with sinus rhythm. By slowing conduction in the atrioventricular node and increasing the interval between the QRS complexes, carotid sinus pressure can uncover the flutter waves and may reveal the correct diagnosis.

Carotid sinus pressure may also

- Induce atrial flutter,[350, 351] a change prevented by atropine.[351]
- Convert atrial flutter to atrial fibrillation.[352]
- Convert atrial fibrillation to atrial flutter.[353]

Valsalva Maneuver.[174, 218] By increasing vagal tone, the straining phase of the Valsalva maneuver produces effects similar to those of carotid sinus pressure.

Drugs[354, 355]

Drugs have three purposes in the treatment of patients with atrial flutter (Table 5.6):

- Increase atrioventricular block and decrease the ventricular rate.
- Convert the arrhythmia to sinus rhythm, an often lengthy, frustrating and, at times, dangerous enterprise.
- Maintain sinus rhythm and prevent recurrences of flutter, a variably effective treatment that requires patients' frequently accepting troublesome and occasionally dangerous side effects. When used for this purpose, all drugs are more likely to succeed when the flutter is relatively short-lived.

Adenosine.[356, 357] By transiently slowing the ventricular rate, this intravenously administered short-acting drug can reveal flutter waves and thereby may facilitate recognition of the arrhythmia. Adenosine does not, however, convert atrial flutter or affect the atrial rate in adults[358] or in children.[359, 360]

By increasing atrioventricular block, adenosine may dangerously slow the ventricular rate in a few patients with atrial flutter, thereby producing ventricular bradycardia, temporary asystole, ventricular tachycardia, and hypotension.[361] Conversely, probably from sympathetic

---

uu"Michel Mirowski, the developer of the implantable cardioverter-defibrillator, thought the left atrium was always the source of flutter.[332] We now know that he was partially correct.

vv"Such as fatigue, physical or mental, sudden exertion, overeating, excessive use of tobacco, alcohol, tea, or coffee, infections, focal or general, unnecessary surgical operations, and congestive heart failure" (Paul D. White 1951).[11]

Table 5.6 CARDIAC EFFECTS OF DRUGS USED IN TREATING PATIENTS WITH ATRIAL FLUTTER

	Amiodarone	Beta-Adrenergic–Blocking Drugs	Calcium-Channel–Blocking Drugs	Digitalis	Disopyramide, Procainamide, and Quinidine	Flecainide	Propafenone
Atrial rate	—	—	—	↑	↓	↓	↓
Ventricular rate	↓	↓	↓	↑	May ↑	—	↓
Converts to sinus rhythm	Yes	No	No	?	Yes	No	Sometimes
Suppresses after cardiac surgery[a]	—	Yes	No	No	—	—	—

[a]According to studies of individual drugs[610] or classes of drugs and a meta-analysis[434] of the ability of beta-adrenergic–blocking drugs, verapamil, and digoxin to suppress supraventricular arrhythmias developing after coronary bypass surgery.

stimulation,[362] adenosine may speed the ventricular rate[363] by decreasing the amount of atrioventricular block[361] or by facilitating conduction in accessory pathways.[364]

Aminophylline. This drug can produce 1:1 conduction and a very rapid ventricular rate.[365]

Amiodarone.[356, 357] By prolonging conduction in the atrioventricular node, amiodarone decreases the ventricular rate in patients with atrial flutter.[368] The drug also converts some patients from flutter and helps to maintain them in sinus rhythm,[369–380] even at the relatively low dose of about 200 milligrams per day.[379] Amiodarone effectively suppresses flutter after cardiac surgery,[381, 382ww] including atrial surgery to correct congenital lesions.[383]

Beta-Adrenergic–Blocking Drugs.[384] As in atrial fibrillation, this class of drugs decreases the ventricular rate by increasing atrioventricular block in patients with flutter,[385–395] but it exerts less of this effect if the ventricular rate is relatively slow before treatment begins.[386] Beta blockers reduce the rise in ventricular rate that occurs with exercise and thereby diminish the palpitations[386] that may then develop. These agents do not affect the atrial rate of flutter.[386xx]

Despite occasional successful conversions,[396] beta-adrenergic–blocking drugs seldom change paroxysmal or chronic flutter to sinus rhythm.[386, 388–391, 393, 397, 398] However, their prophylactic administration can reduce the development of atrial flutter after open-heart surgery.[394, 399–403] The effects of the beta-adrenergic–blocking drugs acebutolol,[401] alprenolol,[389] esmolol,[391–395, 397, 398, 404] pindolol,[405] propranolol,[385–388, 391, 393, 400, 406–408] and sotalol[403, 409, 410] have been studied in patients with atrial flutter.

Calcium-Channel Antagonists. Like beta-adrenergic–blocking drugs, the calcium-channel antagonists verapamil[395, 411–422] and diltiazem[423–427] slow atrioventricular conduction and decrease the ventricular rate in patients with atrial flutter. This effect, which most consistently occurs when the drugs are administered intra-

venously, often appears within 5 minutes, but it may not follow oral administration in all cases.[428] Prolonged infusion of diltiazem provides continuing control of the ventricular rate.[425]

Calcium-channel antagonists occasionally, but infrequently, convert atrial flutter to sinus rhythm.[355, 411, 412, 414, 422, 423, 426, 429] Occasionally, atrial fibrillation may replace the flutter, but whether the drugs produce this effect is uncertain.[419, 430] Verapamil, given prophylactically, does not inhibit the development of supraventricular arrhythmias, including atrial flutter, after cardiac surgery[428, 431] or affect the ventricular rate when these arrhythmias do appear.[431]

The principal side effect of the calcium-channel antagonists is hypotension, which may occasionally have clinical significance. Previous administration of calcium reduces this amount of hypotension.[421] Because calcium-channel–blocking drugs may exacerbate congestive heart failure, diltiazem and verapamil should be administered intravenously with great caution, if at all, to patients with atrial flutter and moderately or severely reduced ventricular function.

Digitalis.[432] Digitalis slows the ventricular rate in flutter by increasing atrioventricular block but has distinct disadvantages when used for this purpose:

- Relatively large amounts of digitalis, which may approach toxic doses, are often required to achieve adequate control of the rate.[433yy]
- Even when given intravenously, digitalis achieves its effect more slowly than the beta-adrenergic– and calcium-channel–blocking agents.[zz]

Digitalis increases the atrial rate in flutter and can promote conversion to atrial fibrillation[346] (see Tables 5.5 and 5.6). Given alone or more commonly with verapamil, digoxin effectively treats atrial flutter in fetuses.[34] Digitalis does not prevent the development of supraventricular arrhythmias, including flutter, after cardiac surgery.[434]

---

wwAmiodarone eliminated episodes of atrial flutter in 15 (94%) of 16 children and young adults after cardiac surgery.[382] The ages of the patients were six weeks to 30 years, nine of them younger than two years.[382]

xxAt least when measured with the electrocardiogram.

---

yyAdequate amounts of digitalis can, however, prevent 1:1 conduction from developing during exercise.[217] The greater success of digitalis in controlling the ventricular rate in atrial fibrillation is due to the more rapid atrial rate in fibrillation, which produces more impulses to be concealed within the atrioventricular node that reduce the transmission of subsequent signals to the ventricles.

zzAn average of 12.3 hours was required for digitalis to reduce the ventricular rate of six patients with atrial flutter to less than 120 beats per minute.[433]

Digitalis has long been given with the hope that it will convert flutter to sinus rhythm and sustain normal rhythm. Although uncontrolled reports suggest that digitalis has this property,[52, 346aaa] and despite being used for this purpose for decades, its ability to convert flutter has not been unequivocally established. Furthermore, the use of digoxin to control the ventricular rate and to convert atrial flutter to sinus rhythm has been questioned, not only for its clinical efficacy,[433, 435] but also because of the expense of such treatment.[433]

Disopyramide. When given intravenously, in some patients disopyramide converts atrial flutter of recent onset to sinus rhythm.[436–438bbb] The drug's atrial slowing[439] and vagolytic actions may speed atrioventricular conduction and ventricular rates,[45] and may even produce 1:1 conduction.[236] The oral preparation helps to suppress flutter after spontaneous or induced conversion.

Edrophonium.[440] This drug, which temporarily increases atrioventricular block and may thereby reveal flutter waves, in one patient converted flutter to sinus rhythm.[441]

Flecainide.[442] Although this class Ic antiarrhythmic drug may postpone recurrence of flutter after conversion,[443] the drug has limited value in treating the arrhythmia.[444] It seldom converts flutter to sinus rhythm,[445, 446ccc] and only slightly increases atrioventricular block.[422, 447–451] Furthermore, flecainide may decrease the atrial rate, promote 1:1 conduction, and accelerate the ventricular rate.[449]

Ibutilide.[452] This type III agent, recently approved for intravenous use, slows the ventricular rate in patients with flutter[453] and converts flutter of recent onset to sinus rhythm[454, 455] more successfully than amiodarone,[455] procainamide,[456, 457] or propafenone.[455] Irregularity of the intervals between the flutter waves increases as conversion approaches.[453]

Lidocaine. This drug slows the atrial rate and may increase, decrease, or not affect the ventricular rate of patients with atrial flutter.[458] The drug has no particular value for flutter itself, although it may be used to treat other, usually ventricular, arrhythmias in patients with flutter.

Procainamide.[459] This familiar type Ia antiarrhythmic agent, usually given intravenously, converts many patients with flutter of recent onset to sinus rhythm, but it is seldom effective when the arrhythmia is chronic.[173, 460–463ddd] The drug also helps to maintain sinus rhythm. By slowing the atrial rate and speeding atrioventricular conduction, through its vagolytic action, procainamide may produce a rapid ventricular rate[225] (Fig. 5.13).[eee]

Propafenone. This class Ic antiarrhythmic agent converts some patients,[450, 464] including children,[465, 466] with atrial flutter to sinus rhythm.[fff] The drug slows the atrial and ventricular rate and can produce 1:1 conduction.[467]

Quinidine. One of cardiology's oldest drugs, quinidine is seldom employed now to convert atrial flutter, although, formerly, this was a common use for patients with the arrhythmia.[346] Like procainamide, this Ia agent slows the atrial rate, increases atrioventricular conduction, and may speed the ventricular response.[225] Quinidine was also prescribed, although seldom now, to maintain sinus rhythm in patients with paroxysmal flutter.

Sotalol *(d,l).*[468] This type III antiarrhythmic drug with beta-adrenergic–blocking properties decreases the ventricular response to atrial flutter, but it does not usually convert it to sinus rhythm.[410ggg] The drug, however, does appear to convert atrial flutter in children who develop the arrhythmia after surgery for congenital heart disease[469, 470] and to help to keep them in sinus rhythm.[470]

Anticoagulation. Although transesophageal echocardiography has shown that patients with atrial flutter have more thrombi in their left atria than patients in sinus rhythm,[162] the incidence of thromboembolic events and the value of anticoagulation have not as yet been established as they have for patients with atrial fibrillation. Consequently, we do not know which patients with paroxysmal or chronic atrial flutter, other than those with previous thromboembolic events, to anticoagulate. Ablation of the arrhythmia in most patients may make the question moot in the future.

Cardioversion[471hhh]

External, direct-current, synchronized shock converts most patients with atrial flutter to sinus

---

[aaa]In a review published in the early 1950s when digitalis and quinidine were the principal drugs available to treat flutter, digitalis often converted flutter to atrial fibrillation. Sinus rhythm then followed when the digitalis was stopped and quinidine begun (if the quinidine did not reinduce flutter⁻).[346] Used with a type I antiarrhythmic drug such as procainamide or quinidine, digoxin was the most effective regimen in eliminating atrial flutter in 347 children with the arrhythmia, and when given alone, it was successful in 44% of the patients to whom it was administered.[33]
[bbb]In 14 of 16 episodes in 11 patients.[438]
[ccc]Flutter converted to sinus rhythm in only 28% of 36 patients, collected from 15 series, when given flecainide intravenously.[446]

[ddd]Procainamide converted only 7 of 53 patients with atrial flutter to sinus rhythm according to a review published in 1957, toward the end of the decade when the drug was first introduced into clinical medicine.[459] Many of the patients appeared to have had flutter for months or years, and the amount administered varied.
[eee]This is why we were taught in our pharmacology courses also to give an atrioventricular nodal blocking agent such as digitalis in the past and beta-adrenergic–blocking drugs or calcium-channel antagonists now. The same advice applies when disopyramide and quinidine are used to convert atrial flutter.
[fff]Seven of 20 patients in two series.[450, 464]
[ggg]At a dose of 1.5 milligrams per kilogram.[410]
[hhh]For more details, see the discussion on cardioversion in Chapter 4.

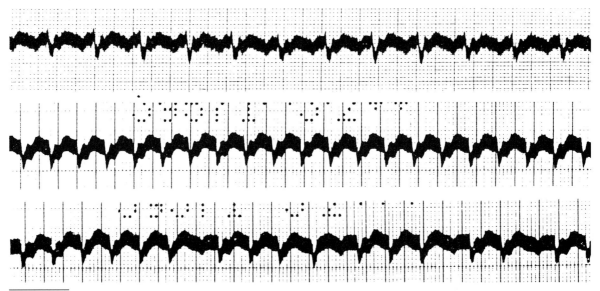

FIGURE 5.13   Atrial flutter with 1:1 conduction produced by procainamide. The patient developed atrial flutter with 2:1 block **(top)**. Procainamide administration decreased the atrial rate from 250 to 218 beats per minute **(middle)**. Because of the vagolytic properties of procainamide improving atrioventricular nodal conduction and the decrease in concealed conduction into the node from a slower atrial rate, every atrial beat could now be transmitted through the atrioventricular node, producing 1:1 conduction and a very rapid ventricular rate **(middle)**. That the rhythm is still flutter is shown by the appearance of flutter waves during Wenckebach periods **(bottom)**. (Adapted from Katz LN, Pick A. Clinical Electrocardiography. Part I: The Arrhythmias. Philadelphia: Lea & Febiger, 1956, with permission.)[605]

rhythm.[51, 156, 472–489][iii] Elective cardioversion of hemodynamically stable patients with atrial flutter can be safely performed in properly equipped outpatient offices.[160, 490] One group has found that an experienced respiratory therapist trained in intubation can provide safe airway management.[160]

Power. Fifty watt-seconds or less may often be sufficient to convert patients with atrial flutter,[51][jjj] in keeping with the principle that reentrant arrhythmias can be converted with less power than fibrillation. However, some patients with lone atrial flutter require 150 to 200 watt-seconds.[156]

The larger amount of power employed, the greater the likelihood of successful conversion from the first shock. For example, in a series of patients with atrial flutter:[160]

- Fifty-seven percent converted to sinus rhythm from shocks of less than 100 joules.
- Seventy-five percent converted from shocks of 100 to less than 200 joules.
- Eighty-five percent converted from shocks of 200 or more joules.

Therefore, because 200 watt-seconds will usually secure conversion,[160] many workers simply start with this dose and thereby avoid using a second shock.[160] When many shocks are required, the possibility that the arrhythmia cannot be converted increases; for example, when more than three shocks were required in one series, four of seven episodes did not result in conversion to sinus rhythm.[160]

Recurrence.[316, 479, 485, 491] This is more likely in the first 8 weeks after conversion to sinus rhythm than later (Table 5.7). Patients converted from atrial flutter more likely remain in sinus rhythm if the arrhythmia has been present for a relatively short time[485, 489] and when ventricular function is preserved.[489] Age, heart size, and cardiac diagnosis do not determine how long sinus rhythm will be maintained.[485] Patients cardioverted from flutter tend to be free of the arrhythmia longer than those converted from chronic atrial fibrillation,[487] but not longer than those converted from paroxysmal fibrillation.[492]

Atrial Fibrillation. Cardioversion replaces atrial flutter with atrial fibrillation in about 15% of cases and

---

[iii]Four hundred eighty-four (98%) of 495 patients or episodes of atrial flutter collected from 10 series.[51, 160, 238, 478, 479, 482, 484, 485, 487, 608]

[jjj]Bernard Lown, who developed the technique, converted flutter with an "average requirement of 15 watt-seconds in over 200 patients studied with this arrhythmia. Usually, only a single discharge is necessary."[471]

Table 5.7	**WHICH FINDINGS REDUCE THE LIKELIHOOD OF MAINTAINING SINUS RHYTHM AFTER CARDIOVERSION OR PACING IN PATIENTS WITH ATRIAL FLUTTER?**		
Finding		**Cardioversion**	**Pacing**
Age		No[485]	Yes[316]
Length of time of flutter		Yes[485]	—
Previous flutter		—	Yes[316]
Cardiac diagnosis		Maybe[479, 485]	—
Structural heart disease		—	Yes[316]
More severe congestive failure		—	Yes[316]
Heart size		No[485]	—
Left atrial size		—	No[316]
Delayed intra-atrial conduction		—	Yes[316]

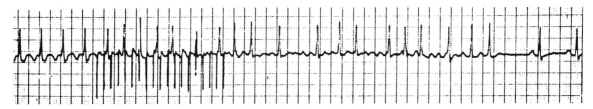

FIGURE 5.14 Atrial pacing converting atrial flutter. A short burst of pacing from the right atrium in a patient with atrial flutter and 2:1 block produces atrial fibrillation, which then converts spontaneously to sinus rhythm (lead II).

is most likely to occur when smaller amounts of power are used.[160, 486] The rate of the flutter waves may increase after a shock, which is subsequently followed by atrial fibrillation.[493] The timing of the shock does not seem to affect whether or not fibrillation will appear.[486]

Low-power shocks may be used to *produce* atrial fibrillation when flutter cannot be successfully suppressed and fibrillation seems a preferable rhythm.[51] This treatment is seldom used today.

Anticoagulation. The infrequency with which emboli complicate cardioversion of atrial flutter[160, 263, 494] suggests to some that prophylactic anticoagulation specifically given before the procedure is not needed, except, of course, for patients who have had previous emboli. One report, however, warns that not anticoagulating is dangerous when the flutter is chronic.[495][kkk] Furthermore, some physicians prefer to anticoagulate because results of transesophageal echocardiography have demonstrated that some patients with flutter have clots in their left atria.[161, 162, 263, 264] In summary, whether to anticoagulate patients being converted from flutter remains controversial.

Pacing[189, 282, 496–501]

Type I, both common and uncommon, but not type II, atrial flutter may frequently, but far from always,[502] be converted to sinus rhythm by rapidly stimulating the atria through wires attached to the atrial epicardium during cardiac surgery[188, 334, 503–505] or with electrode catheters in the right atrium[45, 297, 298, 316, 491, 502, 506–521] or esophagus.[32, 520, 522–528][lll] Care must be taken that the atria and not the ventricles are paced, but this can easily be determined by pacing at a slow rate and observing the electrocardiogram.

To convert the arrhythmia, the atria must be paced

at rates that exceed both the flutter rate and the rate that entrains the arrhythmia[6, 334, 499, 529] (Fig. 5.14).[mmm] When the high right atrium is paced at increasingly faster rates, the flutter waves become upright as the source of atrial activation shifts from the origin of the arrhythmia in the lower part of the chamber to the site of the electrodes.[nnn] Pacing at 120% to 130% of the flutter's rate usually converts the arrhythmia. The operator can choose such rates at the beginning of treatment rather than gradually increasing the rate toward this range.[ooo] Occasionally, pacing at or exceeding 400 beats per minute is required.

The duration of pacing must also be adequate, but this requirement for successful conversion varies greatly. An average of 10 seconds (range, 2–22 sec) is necessary with epicardial pacing. The amplitude of the signal needed varies according to the various reports.

At this point, the arrhythmia has usually been interrupted, and the pacing can either be abruptly stopped or the rate gradually decreased and then stopped as the rate of sinus rhythm is approached. Progressively slowing the rate can avoid prolonged asystole if the sinus mechanism has been suppressed by the flutter, rapid pacing, or disease of the sinus node. Pacing at the septal or posterior right atrial region, close to the region of primary reentry, gives the highest rate of conversion,[307] whereas pacing in the coronary sinus or left atrium is rarely successful.[307]

Procainamide, given before pacing, increases the likelihood,[521] whereas age and a history of congestive heart failure reduce the likelihood,[491] that pacing will convert flutter. Pacemakers that rapidly discharge the atria automatically or by instruction may also be implanted permanently to convert paroxysms of flutter.[500, 520, 530–537] This technique is seldom employed now.

Esophageal Pacing. Conversion with esophageal pacing is best conducted with the electrodes located where the largest and most rapid atrial deflections are recorded.[522–524, 538] The pacing rate needed to convert is often as much as 150% of the atrial flutter rate, somewhat faster than the rate required for successful atrial pacing.[524]

Esophageal pacing converts atrial flutter in children very effectively.[539] The efficacy of the technique is unaf-

---

[kkk]Among 110 patients converted from flutter that they had had from 6 months to 5 years, 6 who were not or were inadequately anticoagulated and none who were properly anticoagulated suffered a thromboembolic event.[495]

[lll]Fifty-one (89%) of 57 patients with atrial pacing,[491] and 163 (90%) of 181 episodes of flutter by esophageal pacing.[524] The success in another series of 124 procedures in 101 inpatients was less striking with sinus rhythm achieved in only 60% of attempts.[502] The patients in this series were older and had had more episodes of flutter. Earlier attempts with pacing failed to convert atrial flutter probably because the pacing rates were too slow, the duration of pacing too short, or the atrial electrodes improperly positioned.[609] Premature stimuli introduced into the atria do not by themselves convert atrial flutter,[297] but premature stimuli added *after* rapid pacing may improve the likelihood of converting flutter than does rapid pacing alone.[540]

[mmm]This description of the technique of epicardial pacing is based, in particular, on the work of Waldo and his associates.[6, 334, 499, 529]

[nnn]When this change in the form of the flutter waves is difficult to determine, one can record from atrial electrodes not involved in the pacing and more easily document atrial capture.[491]

[ooo]The "ramp" technique.[334]

fected by age, previous drug therapy, cycle length of the flutter, history of prior atrial fibrillation, or concomitant medical illnesses.[517] Left and right atrial enlargement and a greater amount of left ventricular dilatation and dysfunction may,[527] or may not,[517] decrease the probability of successful conversion by esophageal pacing.

Compared with endocardial pacing, esophageal pacing is somewhat less invasive and can be performed without fluoroscopy, but it is slightly less likely to produce sinus rhythm. Endocardial pacing is painless, whereas esophageal pacing routinely produces retrosternal burning or pain of mild to moderate degree.[523, 524]

Atrial Fibrillation. Pacing in patients with atrial flutter may produce transient atrial fibrillation, which usually converts spontaneously to sinus rhythm.[491, 508] In some patients, however, the atrial fibrillation persists.[491ppp]

Atrial fibrillation more likely develops when the rate of pacing is fast.[540] If one paces with adequately rapid rates, all patients with flutter can be forced to develop atrial fibrillation. Thus, in a sense, pacing can eliminate flutter in *every* patient with the arrhythmia,[516] although some are left with persistent atrial fibrillation and require antiarrhythmic drugs or cardioversion to achieve sinus rhythm finally. Occasionally, pacing, like cardioverting with low power,[51] has been used to *produce* atrial fibrillation in patients with persistent atrial flutter in whom sinus rhythm cannot be maintained. The ventricular response in fibrillation is often more easily controlled than in flutter.[89, 505]

Antiarrhythmic Drugs. Administering disopyramide,[45, 514, 541] flecainide,[542] procainamide,[506, 516, 530, 541] or quinidine[506] in association with pacing[6] can

- Increase the likelihood of producing sinus rhythm after atrial pacing.
- Reduce the production of atrial fibrillation after pacing.
- Decrease recurrence of the flutter later.

Recurrence. Atrial flutter frequently recurs.[316qqq] Similar factors influence recurrence differently when flutter is treated with cardioversion compared with pacing (see Table 5.6). Left atrial size does not appear to affect recurrence after pacing,[491] but factors that do reduce maintenance of sinus rhythm include the following:

- Greater age.[491]
- Previous episodes of flutter.[316]
- Organic heart disease,[316] including more severe congestive heart failure.[491]
- More conduction delay within the atria.[316]

Esophageal pacing is equally effective whether applied during the initial episode or for a recurrence.[527]

Pacing Versus Cardioversion.[491] When comparing the virtues of pacing or cardioversion for treating atrial flutter, one notes that with an electrode in the atrium, pacing at normal rates can be instituted immediately after conversion for those with bradycardia due to sick sinus syndrome. However, rapid pacing is

- Slightly less effective.
- Somewhat more technically demanding.
- In the case of esophageal pacing, slightly or moderately painful.
- Inadequate to convert persistent atrial fibrillation when it develops after rapid pacing for atrial flutter. These patients require cardioversion anyway.

Cardioversion[485, 543] is more effective but

- Requires general anesthesia.
- Can leave the patient who also has sick sinus syndrome with deleterious bradycardia or even asystole and no means of intravascular pacing immediately available.
- May arouse other arrhythmias, particularly in patients taking digitalis.

Pacing at Standard Rates. Paroxysms of vagally induced atrial flutter can be suppressed by permanent pacing at 90 beats per minute.[544] External ventricular pacing can be temporarily used to prevent injuriously slow rates after cardioversion.[545] Some DDD pacemakers, implanted for treatment of bradycardia particularly when resulting from the sick sinus syndrome, may sense atrial flutter when it develops and may pace the ventricles at dangerously fast rates.[546, 547]

Ablation[200, 209, 285, 548-560]

Source of the Arrhythmia. Many adults[78, 157-159, 169, 206, 209, 327, 560-579] and children[313, 580-584] with atrial flutter can be cured of the arrhythmia by ablating the reentrant circuit sustaining the arrhythmia with radiofrequency current applied through electrode catheters to the right atrial endocardium between the orifice of the inferior vena cava and the tricuspid valve.[rrr] Ablating the slow pathway for supraventricular tachycardia, which is conducted at a different location than for flutter, does not prevent the induction of atrial flutter in patients who have both arrhythmias.[309]

Most adults referred for the procedure are men[157-159] who have the following:

- Chronic rather than paroxysmal flutter,[158] although patients with paroxysmal flutter may benefit from the procedure.[575]
- No organic heart disease other than the arrhythmia.[157-159]

- Type I or "classic" flutter. Ablation cures both the common (counterclockwise) and the uncommon (clockwise)[157, 158, 200, 206, 585]*sss* forms of type I flutter.

Flutter was formerly ablated with low-energy shocks administered through electrode catheters[561, 586–589] or with cryoablation during surgery.[300, 590] The use of laser catheters to ablate arrhythmias is being investigated.[591]

Site of Ablation. In ablating flutter, the electrophysiologist locates landmarks from fluoroscopic observation and study of the electrograms recorded from electrode catheters.[157, 158, 169, 206, 331, 563, 569, 575, 583, 585, 592] Intravascular echocardiography can help to locate the most suitable site for ablation.[256]

Recurrence. If the flutter recurs,[593] it can often be successfully ablated again,[575] but flutter persists in some patients despite the treatment and particularly in those with the following:

- The uncommon (clockwise) form of type I flutter,[158, 169] although not all agree.[200]
- A nonclinical atrial arrhythmia induced after ablation.[78, 169]
- Persistent conduction at the isthmus of the inferior vena cava and tricuspid annulus.[327]
- Enlarged right atria.[594]
- Atrial fibrillation, which developed or was induced during the procedure.[594]

Characteristics not determining recurrence include the following:[169]

- Age.
- Duration of atrial flutter.
- Prior cardiac surgery.
- Cycle length (rate) of the flutter.

Atrial Fibrillation. Paroxysmal or chronic atrial fibrillation appears in about one-fourth of patients after ablation for atrial flutter[159, 595]*ttt* even when the arrhythmia was absent before the procedure.[157] Those most likely to develop atrial fibrillation after radiofrequency ablation for atrial flutter tend to have the following:

- Structural heart disease,[579] sometimes with left atrial enlargement[596] and mitral regurgitation.[159]
- History of atrial fibrillation.[159]
- Failed suppression of flutter after use of several antiarrhythmic drugs.[159]
- Inducible sustained atrial fibrillation after ablation,[159] the feature that most reliably predicts development of atrial fibrillation after ablation.[159]

Patients without structural heart disease and a history of paroxysmal atrial fibrillation may have atrial flutter in the right atrium and atrial fibrillation in the left atrium. Ablation of the flutter may also cure the fibrillation.[597]

Ablation of Accessory Pathways. For patients with preexcitation and the Wolff-Parkinson-White syndrome, ablating accessory pathways may be essential to prevent dangerously rapid ventricular arrhythmias when atrial flutter develops.*uuu*

Ablation of the Atrioventricular Junction. Before the development of radiofrequency current ablation of the circuit sustaining flutter, physicians and surgeons relieved intractable symptoms by ablating the bundle of His or atrioventricular junction at surgery or through electrode catheters with shock or radiofrequency current. Ventricular pacing, preferably with variable rate capacity, is then required.*vvv* The technique of partial atrioventricular nodal ablation or "modulation" reduces the ventricular rate in flutter, but it maintains some atrioventricular conduction during sinus rhythm.[598, 599] This technique is seldom used today to treat patients with flutter.

Surgery

The circuit sustaining atrial flutter can be interrupted surgically.[300] The Maze procedure, designed primarily for the treatment of atrial fibrillation, has also been applied effectively in a few cases of atrial flutter.[600, 601] Excision of a congenital right atrial aneurysm cured a patient of chronic atrial flutter that was assumed to arise within the aneurysm.[602] "A long reentrant pathway through and around the aneurysm" was taken as the reason that the atrial rate was only 220 beats per minute.[602] Catheter ablation with radiofrequency current has replaced surgical operations for cure of atrial flutter. Surgical repair of a large paraesophageal hernia relieved a patient of atrial flutter.[153]

PROGNOSIS

Atrial flutter has long been assumed to worsen the prognosis of patients who have the arrhythmia, particularly those with structural heart disease.*www* Patients whose myocardial infarction is complicated by atrial flutter are less likely to recover than those without it.[603]

Atrial flutter greatly worsens the prognosis in children.[33] Their chances of "sudden death" are four times greater if they continue to have flutter despite pharmacological therapy than if they maintain sinus rhythm. The effects of the more contemporary pharmacological and electrical treatments on the prognosis in patients with flutter are not yet known.

---

*sss*Each of 11 cases with clockwise flutter in an obviously successful series.[200]

*ttt*Twenty-six percent of patients followed for an average of 13 months according to one study[159] and in 28 (25%) of 110 patients during a mean follow-up study of 20 months according to another.[595] A history of spontaneous atrial fibrillation before the procedure and left ventricular ejection fraction of less than 50% appear to be the most potent factors predicting that atrial fibrillation will appear after ablation for flutter.[595]

*uuu*For further discussion, see Chapter 4.

*vvv*For further discussion, see Chapter 4.

www"Where flutter persists in spite of treatment, there is great incapacity and a higher mortality" (John Parkinson, 1927).[170]

SUMMARY

Atrial flutter is a relatively uncommon supraventricular tachyarrhythmia that develops in adults with various types of heart disease, severe pulmonary disease, after cardiac surgery, and in some with no structural heart disease. Children develop atrial flutter after operations to correct congenital defects involving the atria. Atrial flutter is more often paroxysmal than chronic, but flutter may persist continuously for years.

Patients with atrial flutter complain most frequently of palpitations, but they may also experience—in different degrees of severity—dyspnea, chest pain, weakness, and, rarely, syncope. Symptoms more likely appear when the arrhythmia is rapid or paroxysmal or when heart disease is advanced.

On physical examination, the pulse is rapid and more frequently regular than irregular. Normal atrial waveforms in the neck veins are absent. Auscultation reveals rapid heart action and, if irregular, the signs of partial atrioventricular dissociation such as varying intensity of the first heart sound.

The electrocardiogram shows the characteristic atrial flutter waves at about 250 to 350 beats per minute. These are predominantly negative in the inferior leads in the common or typical form of flutter and are upright in the less frequent uncommon or atypical form. In untreated patients, the atrioventricular ratio is usually 2:1, which produces a ventricular rate of about 150 beats per minute. The atrioventricular ratio is most frequently an even number, such as 2:1 or 4:1, or it may vary between these two to produce an irregular ventricular rhythm. Occasionally, the ventricles beat very rapidly with 1:1 conduction through the normal conducting system or through accessory pathways (Wolff-Parkinson-White syndrome).

There are two types of atrial flutter. Type I is the familiar variety with a maximum atrial rate of about 350 beats per minute. It is sustained by a reentrant circuit, traversing the right atrium most often in a counterclockwise motion, with a region of slow conduction located, in most cases, at the junction of the tricuspid valve, coronary sinus, and inferior vena cava. Type I flutter can be started with premature atrial beats or by rapid pacing of the atria in patients with a clinical history of arrhythmia. Type II flutter is less common, is faster, and cannot be started with electrophysiological techniques as can type I. The mechanism of type II flutter is not known.

Carotid sinus pressure and the Valsalva maneuver, by increasing vagal tone and atrioventricular block, decrease the ventricular rate in many patients with atrial flutter and thereby reveal the flutter waves in the electrocardiogram when they cannot be discerned at rapid ventricular rates.

Drugs are used in patients with flutter to decrease the ventricular rate, to convert to sinus rhythm, or to prevent recurrences of the arrhythmia. Adenosine, amiodarone, beta-adrenergic–blocking agents, calcium-channel antagonists, and digitalis slow the ventricular rate by increasing atrioventricular block. Amiodarone and the type I antiarrhythmic agents (disopyramide, procainamide, and quinidine) convert some patients to sinus rhythm and help to maintain normal rhythm afterward. Because of their atrial slowing and vagolytic effects, atrioventricular nodal blocking drugs should supplement type I agents to prevent unacceptable increases in the ventricular rate during therapy.

Cardioversion produces sinus rhythm in almost all patients with atrial flutter. Similarly, rapid atrial or esophageal pacing converts most with type I flutter, although pacing may produce transient or persistent atrial fibrillation. Administering type I antiarrhythmic drugs with pacing increases the likelihood of conversion and suppresses the appearance of sustained atrial fibrillation. Atrial flutter recurs in many patients, particularly those who are older, who have had previous paroxysms of the arrhythmia, or who have structural heart disease.

Ablation of the reentrant circuit with radiofrequency current produces long-term relief from further paroxysms in many patients with type I and in a few with type II flutter. Recurrence of flutter or conversion to atrial fibrillation limits the results, however. A few patients require ablation of the atrioventricular junction with subsequent ventricular pacing when symptom-producing flutter cannot be controlled or cured. The presence of atrial flutter worsens the prognosis of those patients with the arrhythmia who have structural heart disease.

REFERENCES

1. Waldo AL, Kastor JA. Atrial flutter. In Kastor JA (ed). Arrhythmias. Philadelphia: WB Saunders, 1994, pp. 105–115.
2. Katz LN, Pick A. Clinical Electrocardiography. Part I. The Arrhythmias. Philadelphia: Lea & Febiger, 1956, pp. 382–390.
3. Chung EK. Principles of Cardiac Arrhythmias. Baltimore: Williams & Wilkins, 1971, pp. 121–141.
4. Porter CJ. Premature atrial contractions and atrial tachyarrhythmias. In Gillette PC, Garson A Jr (eds). Pediatric Arrhythmias. Electrophysiology and Pacing. Philadelphia: WB Saunders, 1990, pp. 328–359.
5. Josephson ME. Clinical Cardiac Electrophysiology. Techniques and Interpretations. 2nd ed. Philadelphia: Lea & Febiger, 1993.
6. Waldo AL. Atrial flutter. In Podrid PJ, Kowey PR (eds). Cardiac Arrhythmia. Mechanisms, Diagnosis and Management. Baltimore: Williams & Wilkins, 1995, pp. 790–802.
7. Waldo AL. Atrial flutter: mechanisms, clinical features, and management. In Zipes DP, Jalife J (eds). Cardiac Electrophysiology. From Cell to Bedside. 2nd ed. Philadelphia: WB Saunders Company, 1995, pp. 666–681.
8. Camm AJ, Obel OA. Epidemiology and mechanism of atrial fibrillation and atrial flutter. Am J Cardiol 1996; 78:3–11.
9. White PD, Jones TD. Heart disease and disorders in New England. Am Heart J 1928; 3:302–318.
10. Makinson DH, Wade G. Aetiology and treatment of auricular flutter. Lancet 1950; 1:105–108.
11. White PD. Heart Disease. 4th ed. New York: Macmillan, 1951.
12. Katz LN, Pick A. Clinical Electrocardiography. Part I. The Arrhythmias. Philadelphia: Lea & Febiger, 1956, p. 43.
13. Anonymous. Paul Wood's Diseases of the Heart and Circulation. 3rd ed. Philadelphia: JB Lippincott, 1968, pp. 272–275.
14. Doliopoulos T, Marousis S. Incidence, rhythm, diagnosis and treatment of atrial flutter. Cardiology 1968; 52:113–120.

15. Hall CG, Stewart LC, Manning GW. The electrocardiographic records of 2,000 R. C. A. F. aircrew. Can Med Assoc J 1942; 46:226–230.

16. Graybiel A, McFarland RA, Gates DC, Webster FA. Analysis of the electrocardiograms obtained from 1,000 young healthy aviators. Am Heart J 1944; 27:524–549.

17. Hiss RG, Lamb LE. Electrocardiographic findings in 122,043 individuals. Circulation 1962; 25:947–961.

18. Ostrander LD Jr, Brandt RL, Kjelsberg MO, Epstein FH. Electrocardiographic findings among the adult population of a total natural community, Tecumseh, Michigan. Circulation 1965; 31:888–898.

19. Rose G, Baxter PJ, Reid DD, McCartney P. Prevalence and prognosis of electrocardiographic findings in middle-aged men. Br Heart J 1978; 40:636–643.

20. Clarke JM, Hamer J, Shelton JR, Taylor S, Venning GR. The rhythm of the normal human heart. Lancet 1976; 1:508–512.

21. Raftery EB, Cashman PM. Long-term recording of the electrocardiogram in a normal population. Postgrad Med J 1976; 52:32–38.

22. Brodsky M, Wu D, Denes P, Kanakis C, Rosen KM. Arrhythmias documented by 24-hour continuous electrocardiographic monitoring in 50 male medical students without apparent heart disease. Am J Cardiol 1977; 39:390–395.

23. Scott O, Williams GJ, Fiddler GI. Results of 24-hour ambulatory monitoring of electrocardiogram in 131 healthy boys aged 10 to 13 years. Br Heart J 1980; 44:304–308.

24. Dickinson DF, Scott O. Ambulatory electrocardiographic monitoring in 100 healthy teenage boys. Br Heart J 1984; 51:179–183.

25. Sobotka PA, Mayer JH, Bauernfeind RA, Kanakis C Jr, Rosen KM. Arrhythmias documented by 24-hour continuous ambulatory electrocardiographic monitoring in young women without apparent heart disease. Am Heart J 1981; 101:753–759.

26. Southall DP, Johnston F, Shinebourne EA, Johnston PG. 24-hour electrocardiographic study of heart rate and rhythm patterns in population of healthy children. Br Heart J 1981; 45:281–291.

27. Romhilt DW, Chaffin C, Choi SC, Irby EC. Arrhythmias on ambulatory electrocardiographic monitoring in women without apparent heart disease. Am J Cardiol 1984; 54:582–586.

28. Johnson JC, Flowers NC, Horan LG. Unexplained atrial flutter: a frequent herald of pulmonary embolism. Chest 1971; 60:29–34.

29. Southall DP, Richards J, Mitchell P, Brown DJ, Johnston PG, Shinebourne EA. Study of cardiac rhythm in healthy newborn infants. Br Heart J 1980; 43:14–20.

30. Southall DP, Richards J, Brown DJ, Johnston PG, de Swiet M, Shinebourne EA. 24-hour tape recordings of ECG and respiration in the newborn infant with findings related to sudden death and unexplained brain damage in infancy. Arch Dis Child 1980; 55:7–16.

31. Lubbers WJ, Losekoot TG, Anderson RH, Wellens HJJ. Paroxysmal supraventricular tachycardia in infancy and childhood. Eur J Cardiol 1974; 2:91–99.

32. Dunnigan A, Benson W Jr, Benditt DG. Atrial flutter in infancy: diagnosis, clinical features, and treatment. Pediatrics 1985; 75:725–729.

33. Garson A Jr, Bink-Boelkens M, Hesslein PS, et al. Atrial flutter in the young: a collaborative study of 380 cases. J Am Coll Cardiol 1985; 6:871–878.

34. Maxwell DJ, Crawford DC, Curry PV, Tynan MJ, Allan LD. Obstetric importance, diagnosis, and management of fetal tachycardias. BMJ 1988; 297:107–110.

35. Blumenthal S, Jacobs JC, Steer CM, Williamson SW. Congenital atrial flutter: report of a case documented by intra-uterine electrocardiogram. Pediatrics 1968; 41:659–661.

36. Johnson WH Jr, Dunnigan A, Fehr P, Benson DW. Association of atrial flutter with orthodromic reciprocating fetal tachycardia. Am J Cardiol 1987; 59:374–375.

37. Chao RC, Ho ES, Hsieh KS. Fetal atrial flutter and fibrillation: prenatal echocardiographic detection and management. Am Heart J 1992; 124:1095–1098.

38. Soyeur DJ. Atrial flutter in the human fetus: diagnosis, hemodynamic consequences, and therapy. J Cardiovasc Electrophysiol 1996; 7:989–998.

39. Cosby RS, Herman LM. Atrial flutter and pulmonary disease. Geriatrics 1966; 21:140–144.

40. Fox TT, Weaver JC, Francis RL. Further studies on electrocardiographic changes in old age. Geriatrics 1948; 3:35–41.

41. Wosika PH, Feldman E, Chesrow EJ, Myers GB. Unipolar precordial and limb lead electrocardiograms in the aged. Geriatrics 1950; 5:131–141.

42. Fisch C, Genovese PD, Dyke RW, Laramore W, Marvel RJ. The electrocardiogram in persons over 70. Geriatrics 1957; 12:616–620.

43. Campbell A, Caird FI, Jackson TF. Prevalence of abnormalities of electrocardiogram in old people. Br Heart J 1974; 36:1005–1011.

44. Mihalick MJ, Fisch C. Electrocardiographic findings in the aged. Am Heart J 1974; 87:117–128.

45. Camm J, Ward D, Spurrell R. Response of atrial flutter to overdrive atrial pacing and intravenous disopyramide phosphate, singly and in combination. Br Heart J 1980; 44:240–247.

46. Fleg JL, Kennedy HL. Cardiac arrhythmias in a healthy elderly population: detection by 24-hour ambulatory electrocardiography. Chest 1982; 81:302–307.

47. Bell WN, Strong GF. Auricular flutter (the results of therapy in a general hospital over a 10-year period). Can Med Assoc J 1947; 56:404–406.

48. Campbell M. The paroxysmal tachycardias. Lancet 1947; 1:641–647.

49. Hejtmancik MR, Herrmann GR, Bradfield JV. Atrial flutter. I. Clinical aspects. Am Heart J 1950; 40:884–890.

50. Goldberger E, Baer A. Observations on the etiology and treatment of auricular flutter: an analysis of fifty cases. Am Pract 1951; 2:124–127.

51. Lown B. Electrical reversion of cardiac arrhythmias. Br Heart J 1967; 29:469–489.

52. Lindsay J Jr, Hurst JW. The clinical features of atrial flutter and their therapeutic implications. Chest 1974; 66:114–121.

53. Julian DG, Valentine PA, Miller GG. Disturbances of rate, rhythm and conduction in acute myocardial infarction: a prospective study of 100 consecutive unselected patients with the aid of electrocardiographic monitoring. Am J Med 1964; 37:915–927.

54. Robinson JS, Sloman G, McRae C. Continuous electrocardiographic monitoring in the early stages after acute myocardial infarction. Med J Aust 1964; 1:427–432.

55. Kurland GS, Pressman D. The incidence of arrhythmias in acute myocardial infarction studies with a constant monitoring system. Circulation 1965; 31:834–841.

56. Meltzer LE, Kitchell JB. The incidence of arrhythmias associated with acute myocardial infarction. Prog Cardiovasc Dis 1966; 9:50–63.

57. Langhorne WH. The coronary care unit: a year's experience in a community hospital. JAMA 1967; 201:92–95.

58. Lawrie DM, Goddard M, Greenwood TW, et al. A coronary care unit in the routine management of acute myocardial infarction. Lancet 1967; 2:109–114.

59. Lown B, Vasaux C, Hood WB Jr, Fakhro AM, Kaplinsky E, Roberge G. Unresolved problems in coronary care. Am J Cardiol 1967; 20:494–508.

60. Norris RM. Acute coronary care. N Z Med J 1968; 67:470–476.

61. DeSanctis RW, Block P, Hutter AM Jr. Tachyarrhythmias in myocardial infarction. Circulation 1972; 45:681–702.

62. Romhilt DW, Bloomfield SS, Chou T-C, Fowler NO. Unreliability of conventional electrocardiographic monitoring for arrhythmia detection in coronary care units. Am J Cardiol 1973; 31:457–461.

63. Scheinman MM, Abbott JA. Clinical significance of transmural versus nontransmural electrocardiographic changes in

patients with acute myocardial infarction. Am J Med 1973; 55:602–607.

64. Liberthson RR, Salisbury KW, Hutter AM Jr, DeSanctis RW. Atrial tachyarrhythmias in acute myocardial infarction. Am J Med 1976; 60:956–960.

65. Josephson ME, Horowitz LN, Kastor JA. Supraventricular tachyarrhythmias in acute myocardial infarction. In Donoso E, Lipski J (eds). Acute Myocardial Infarction. New York: Stratton Intercontinental Medical Book Corp. 1977, pp. 99–111.

66. Lofmark R, Orinius E. Supraventricular tachyarrhythmias in acute myocardial infarction. Acta Med Scand 1978; 203:517–520.

67. Kobayashi Y, Katoh T, Takano T, Hayakawa H. Paroxysmal atrial fibrillation and flutter associated with acute myocardial infarction: hemodynamic evaluation in relation to the development of arrhythmias and prognosis. Jpn Circ J 1992; 56:1–11.

68. Kastor JA. Atrial fibrillation. In Kastor JA (ed). Arrhythmias. Philadelphia: WB Saunders, 1994, pp. 25–104.

69. Serrano CV Jr, Ramires JA, Mansur AP, Pileggi F. Importance of the time of onset of supraventricular tachyarrhythmias on prognosis of patients with acute myocardial infarction. Clin Cardiol 1995; 18:84–90.

70. Zoni Berisso M, Carratino L, Ferroni A, Mela GS, Mazzotta G, Vecchio C. Frequency, characteristics and significance of supraventricular tachyarrhythmias detected by 24-hour electrocardiographic recording in the late hospital phase of acute myocardial infarction. Am J Cardiol 1990; 65:1064–1070.

71. Zuppiroli A, Mori F, Favilli S, et al. Arrhythmias in mitral valve prolapse: relation to anterior mitral leaflet thickening, clinical variables, and color Doppler echocardiographic parameters. Am Heart J 1994; 128:919–927.

72. Rodstein M, Zeman FD, Gerber IE. Atrial septal defect in the aged. Circulation 1961; 23:665–674.

73. Evans W. The electrocardiogram of alcoholic cardiomyopathy. Br Heart J 1958; 21:445–456.

74. Hollister RM, Goodwin JF. The electrocardiogram in cardiomyopathy. Br Heart J 1963; 25:357–374.

75. Brigden W, Robinson J. Alcoholic heart disease. BMJ 1964; 2:1283–1289.

76. Demakis JG, Proskey A, Rahimtoola SH, et al. The natural course of alcoholic cardiomyopathy. Ann Intern Med 1974; 80:293–297.

77. Roberts WC, Siegel RJ, McManus BM. Idiopathic dilated cardiomyopathy: analysis of 152 necropsy patients. Am J Cardiol 1987; 60:1340–1355.

78. Steinberg JS, Prasher S, Zelenkofske S, Ehlert FA. Radiofrequency catheter ablation of atrial flutter: procedural success and long-term outcome. Am Heart J 1995; 130:85–92.

79. Dalton JC, Pearson RJ, White PD. Constrictive pericarditis: a review and long-term follow-up of 78 cases. Ann Intern Med 1956; 45:445–458.

80. Wood P. Chronic constrictive pericarditis. Am J Cardiol 1961; 7:48–61.

81. Hirschmann JV. Pericardial constriction. Am Heart J 1978; 96:110–122.

82. Spodick DH. Arrhythmias during acute pericarditis: a prospective study of 100 consecutive cases. JAMA 1976; 235:39–41.

83. Spodick DH. Frequency of arrhythmias in acute pericarditis determined by Holter monitoring. Am J Cardiol 1984; 53:842–845.

84. Biggs FD, Lefrak SS, Kleiger RE, Senior RM, Oliver GC. Disturbances of rhythm in chronic lung disease. Heart Lung 1977; 6:256–261.

85. Corazza LJ, Pastor BH. Cardiac arrhythmias in chronic cor pulmonale. N Engl J Med 1958; 259:862–865.

86. Hejtmancik MR, Herrmann GR, Wright JC. Paroxysmal supraventricular tachycardias complicating organic heart disease. Am Heart J 1958; 56:671–684.

87. Thomas AJ, Valabhji P. Arrhythmia and tachycardia in pulmonary heart disease. Br Heart J 1969; 31:491–495.

88. Hudson LD, Kurt TL, Petty TL, Genton E. Arrhythmias associated with acute respiratory failure in patients with chronic airway obstruction. Chest 1973; 63:661–665.

89. Waldo AL, MacLean WAH. Diagnosis and Treatment of Cardiac Arrhythmias Following Open Heart Surgery. Emphasis on the Use of Atrial and Ventricular Epicardial Wire Electrodes. Mount Kisco, NY: Futura Publishing Co., 1980.

90. Perloff JK. Surgical closure of atrial septal defect in adults. N Engl J Med 1995; 333:513–514.

91. Ommen SR, Odell JA, Stanton MS. Atrial arrhythmias after cardiothoracic surgery. N Engl J Med 1997; 336:1429–1434.

92. Rabbino MD, Dreifus LS, Likoff W. Cardiac arrhythmias following intracardiac surgery. Am J Cardiol 1961; 5:681–689.

93. Reid JM, Stevenson JC. Cardiac arrhythmias following successful surgical closure of atrial septal defect. Br Heart J 1967; 29:742–747.

94. Schroeder JS, Berke DK, Graham AF, Rider AK, Harrison DC. Arrhythmias after cardiac transplantation. Am J Cardiol 1974; 33:604–607.

95. Brandenburg RO Jr, Holmes DR Jr, Brandenburg RO, McGoon DC. Clinical follow-up study of paroxysmal supraventricular tachyarrhythmias after operative repair of a secundum type atrial septal defect in adults. Am J Cardiol 1983; 51:273–276.

96. Little RE, Kay GN, Epstein AE, et al. Arrhythmias after orthotopic cardiac transplantation: prevalence and determinants during initial hospitalization and late follow-up. Circulation 1989; 80:140–146.

97. Jacquet L, Ziady G, Stein K, et al. Cardiac rhythm disturbances early after orthotopic heart transplantation: prevalence and clinical importance of the observed abnormalities. J Am Coll Cardiol 1990; 16:832–837.

98. Scott CD, Dark JH, McComb JM. Arrhythmias after cardiac transplantation. Am J Cardiol 1992; 70:1061–1063.

99. Konstantinides S, Geibel A, Olschewski M, et al. A comparison of surgical and medical therapy for atrial septal defect in adults. N Engl J Med 1995; 333:469–473.

100. Smith R, Grossman W, Johnson L, Segal H, Collins J, Dalen J. Arrhythmias following cardiac valve replacement. Circulation 1972; 45:1018–1023.

101. Rose MR, Glassman E, Spencer FC. Arrhythmias following cardiac surgery: relation to serum digoxin levels. Am Heart J 1975; 89:288–294.

102. Parker FB Jr, Greiner-Hayes C, Bove EL, Marvasti MA, Johnson LW, Eich RH. Supraventricular arrhythmias following coronary artery bypass: the effect of preoperative digitalis. J Thorac Cardiovasc Surg 1983; 86:594–600.

103. Gavaghan TP, Feneley MP, Campbell TJ, Morgan JJ. Atrial tachyarrhythmias after cardiac surgery: results of disopyramide therapy. Aust NZ J Med 1985; 15:27–32.

104. Dixon FE, Genton E, Vacek JL, Moore CB, Landry J. Factors predisposing to supraventricular tachyarrhythmias after coronary artery bypass grafting. Am J Cardiol 1986; 58:476–478.

105. Arenal A, Almendral J, Munoz R, et al. Mechanism and location of atrial flutter in transplanted hearts: observations during transient entrainment from distant sites. J Am Coll Cardiol 1997; 30:539–546.

106. Bailey CC, Betts RH. Cardiac arrhythmias following pneumonectomy. N Engl J Med 1943; 229:356–359.

107. Currens JH, White PD, Churchill ED. Cardiac arrhythmias following thoracic surgery. N Engl J Med 1943; 229:360–364.

108. Cohen MG, Pastor BH. Delayed cardiac arrhythmias following noncardiac thoracic surgery. Dis Chest 1957; 32:435–440.

109. Mowry FM, Reynolds EW. Cardiac rhythm disturbances complicating resectional surgery of the lung. Ann Intern Med 1964; 61:688–695.

110. Ghosh P, Pakrashi BC. Cardiac dysrhythmias after thoracotomy. Br Heart J 1972; 34:374–376.

111. Goldman L. Supraventricular tachyarrhythmias in hospitalized adults after surgery: clinical correlates in patients over 40 years of age after major noncardiac surgery. Chest 1978; 73:450–454.

112. Evans W. The unity of paroxysmal tachycardia and auricular flutter. Br Heart J 1944; 6:221–237.

113. El-Said G, Rosenberg HS, Mullins CE, Hallman GL, Cooley DA, McNamara DG. Dysrhythmias after Mustard's operation for transposition of the great arteries. Am J Cardiol 1972; 30:526–532.

114. Gillette PC, El-Said GM, Sivarajan N, Mullins CE, Williams RL, McNamara DG. Electrophysiological abnormalities after Mustard's operation for transposition of the great arteries. Br Heart J 1974; 36:186–191.

115. Greenwood RD, Rosenthal A, Sloss LJ, LaCorte M, Nadas AS. Sick sinus syndrome after surgery for congenital heart disease. Circulation 1975; 52:208–213.

116. El-Said GM, Gillette PC, Cooley DA, Mullins CE, McNamara DG. Protection of the sinus node in Mustard's operation. Circulation 1976; 53:788–791.

117. Saalouke MG, Rios J, Perry LW, Shapiro SR, Scott LP. Electrophysiologic studies after Mustard's operation for d-transposition of the great vessels. Am J Cardiol 1978; 41:1104–1109.

118. Bink-Boelkens MT, Velvis H, van der Heide JJ, Eygelaar A, Hardjowijono RA. Dysrhythmias after atrial surgery in children. Am Heart J 1983; 106:125–130.

119. Beerman LB, Neches WH, Fricker FJ, et al. Arrhythmias in transposition of the great arteries after the Mustard operation. Am J Cardiol 1983; 51:1530–1534.

120. Flinn CJ, Wolff GS, Dick M II, et al. Cardiac rhythm after the Mustard operation for complete transposition of the great arteries. N Engl J Med 1984; 310:1635–1638.

121. Deanfield J, Camm, J, Macartney F, et al. Arrhythmia and late mortality after Mustard and Senning operation for transposition of the great arteries. J Thorac Cardiovasc Surg 1988; 96:569–576.

122. Vetter VL, Tanner CS, Horowitz LN. Inducible atrial flutter after the Mustard repair of complete transposition of the great arteries. Am J Cardiol 1988; 61:428–435.

123. Gewillig M, Cullen S, Mertens B, Lesaffre E, Deanfield J. Risk factors for arrhythmia and death after Mustard operation for simple transposition of the great arteries. Circulation 1991; 84(Suppl III):III-187–III-192.

124. Muller GI, Deal BJ, Strasburger JF, Benson DW. Electrocardiographic features of atrial tachycardias after operation for congenital heart disease. Am J Cardiol 1993; 71:122–124.

125. Fishberger SB, Wernovsky G, Gentles TL, et al. Factors that influence the development of atrial flutter after the Fontan operation. J Thorac Cardiovasc Surg 1997; 113:80–86.

126. Gelatt M, Hamilton RM, McCrindle BW, et al. Arrhythmia and mortality after the Mustard procedure: a 30-year single-center experience. J Am Coll Cardiol 1997; 29:194–201.

127. Gandhi SK, Bromberg BI, Rodefeld MD, et al. Lateral tunnel suture line variation reduces atrial flutter after the modified Fontan operation. Ann Thorac Surg 1996; 61:1299–1309.

128. Roos-Hesselink J, Perlroth MG, McGhie J, Spitaels S. Atrial arrhythmias in adults after repair of tetralogy of Fallot: correlations with clinical, exercise, and echocardiographic findings. Circulation 1995; 91:2214–2219.

129. Vanagt EJ, Wellens HJJ. The electrocardiogram in digitalis intoxication. In Wellens HJJ, Kulbertus HE (eds). What's New in Electrocardiography. Boston: Martinus Nijhoff, 1981, pp. 315–343.

130. Cole SL. Digitalis intoxication: chronic effects manifested by diarrhea and auricular flutter. Am Heart J 1950; 39:900–903.

131. Aravanis C, Michaelides G. Paroxysmal auricular flutter and right bundle branch block following digitalis therapy. Am J Cardiol 1959; 4:124–127.

132. Coffman JD, Whipple GH. Atrial flutter as a manifestation of digitalis toxicity. Circulation 1959; 19:188–194.

133. Brest AN, Durge NG, Goldberg H. Conversion of atrial fibrillation to atrial flutter as a manifestation of digitalis toxicity. Am J Cardiol 1960; 6:682–684.

134. Delman AJ, Stein E. Atrial flutter secondary to digitalis toxicity: report of 3 cases and review of the literature. Circulation 1964; 29:593–597.

135. Taguchi JT, Ryan JM. Spontaneous conversion of established atrial fibrillation: clinical significance of a change to atrial flutter or to paroxysmal atrial tachycardia with AV block. Arch Intern Med 1969; 124:468–476.

136. Agarwal BL, Agarwal BV, Agarwal RK, Kansal SC. Atrial flutter: a rare manifestation of digitalis intoxication. Br Heart J 1972; 34:392–395.

137. Ettinger PO, Wu CF, De La Cruz C Jr, Weisse AB, Ahmed SS, Regan TJ. Arrhythmias and the "holiday heart": alcohol-associated cardiac rhythm disorders. Am Heart J 1978; 95:555–562.

138. Ettinger PO. Holiday heart arrhythmias. Int J Cardiol 1984; 5:540–542.

139. Cohen EJ, Klatsky AL, Armstrong MA. Alcohol use and supraventricular arrhythmia. Am J Cardiol 1988; 62:971–973.

140. Coumel P, Leclercq JF, Attuel P, Lavallee JP, Flammang D. Autonomic influences in the genesis of atrial arrhythmias: atrial flutter and fibrillation of vagal origin. In Narula OS (ed). Cardiac Arrhythmias. Electrophysiology, Diagnosis and Management. Baltimore: Williams & Wilkins, 1980, pp. 243–255.

141. Coumel P, Escoubet B, Attuel P. Beta-blocking therapy in atrial and ventricular tachyarrhythmias: experience with nadolol. Am Heart J 1984; 108:1098–1108.

142. Weinberg SL, Schoenwetter AH. Auricular flutter and indirect cardiac trauma. Arch Intern Med 1951; 88:252–257.

143. Spurny OM, Wolf JW. Prolonged atrial flutter in myotonic dystrophy. Am J Cardiol 1962; 10:886–889.

144. Cipolloni PB, Shane SR, Marshall RJ. Chronic atrial flutter in brothers with the Marfan syndrome. Circulation 1965; 31:572–574.

145. Sahadevan MG, Raman PT, Hoon RS. Chronic atrial flutter in a case of Marfan's syndrome. Am J Med 1969; 47:965–966.

146. Davis PJ, Davis FB. Hyperthyroidism in patients over the age of 60 years: clinical features in 85 patients. Medicine 1974; 53:161–181.

147. Deutsch PG, Kronzon I, Weiss EC. Unusually rapid atrial rate in a patient with thyrotoxicosis and atrial flutter. Chest 1975; 67:350–351.

148. Norris JW, Froggatt GM, Hachinski VC. Cardiac arrhythmias in acute stroke. Stroke 1978; 9:392–396.

149. Canedo MI, Frank MJ, Abdulla AM. Rhythm disturbances in hypertrophic cardiomyopathy: prevalence, relation to symptoms and management. Am J Cardiol 1980; 45:848–855.

150. Suarez LD, Chiozza MA, Foye R, Mosso H, Perosio AM. Swallowing-dependent atrial tachyarrhythmias: their mechanism. J Electrocardiol 1980; 13:301–305.

151. Varriale P, Kwa RP, Parikh N. Atrial flutter secondary to hypokalemia. Pacing Clin Electrophysiol 1983; 6:8–12.

152. Pousset F, Le Heuzey JY, Pialoux G, et al. Cardiac lymphoma presenting as atrial flutter in an AIDS patient. Eur Heart J 1994; 15:862–864.

153. Schilling RJ, Kaye GC. Paroxysmal atrial flutter suppressed by repair of a large paraesophageal hernia. PACE 1998; 21:1303–1305.

154. Friedlander RD, Levine SA. Auricular fibrillation and auricular flutter without evidence of organic heart disease. N Engl J Med 1934; 211:624–629.

155. Orgain ES, Wolff L, White PD. Uncomplicated auricular fibrillation and auricular flutter: frequent occurrence and good prognosis in patients without other evidence of cardiac disease. Arch Intern Med 1936; 57:493–513.

156. Resnekov L, McDonald L. Electroversion of lone atrial fibrillation and flutter including haemodynamic studies at rest and on exercise. Br Heart J 1971; 33:339–350.

157. Kirkorian G, Moncada E, Chevalier P, et al. Radiofrequency ablation of atrial flutter: efficacy of an anatomically guided approach. Circulation 1994; 90:2804–2814.

158. Fischer B, Haissaguerre M, Garrigues S, et al. Radiofrequency catheter ablation of common atrial flutter in 80 patients. J Am Coll Cardiol 1995; 25:1365–1372.

159. Philippon F, Plumb VJ, Epstein AE, Kay GN. The risk of atrial fibrillation following radiofrequency catheter ablation of atrial flutter. Circulation 1995; 92:430–435.

160. Chalasani P, Cambre S, Silverman ME. Direct-current cardioversion for the conversion of atrial flutter. Am J Cardiol 1996; 77:658–660.

161. Black IW, Hopkins AP, Lee LC, Walsh WF. Evaluation of transesophageal echocardiography before cardioversion of

atrial fibrillation and flutter in nonanticoagulated patients. Am Heart J 1993; 126:375–381.

162. Bikkina M, Alpert MA, Mulekar M, Shakoor A, Massey CV, Covin FA. Prevalence of intraatrial thrombus in patients with atrial flutter. Am J Cardiol 1995; 76:186–189.

163. Tunick PA, McElhinney L, Mitchell T, Kronzon I. The alternation between atrial flutter and atrial fibrillation. Chest 1992; 101:34–36.

164. Roithinger FX, Karch MR, Steiner PR, Sippens-Groenewegen A, Lesh MD. Relationship between atrial fibrillation and typical atrial flutter in humans: activation sequence changes during spontaneous conversion. Circulation 1997; 96:3484–3491.

165. Komatsu C, Ishinaga T, Tateishi O, et al. Shift of atrial reentrant tachycardia with transient entrainment to an uncommon and a common type of atrial flutter. Pacing Clin Electrophysiol 1988; 11:687–695.

166. Hanssen P. The incidence of auricular flutter and auricular fibrillation associated with complete auriculo-ventricular dissociation. Acta Med Scand 1949; 136:112–121.

167. Korst DR, Wasserburger RH. Auricular flutter associated with complete heart block. Am Heart J 1954; 48:383–389.

168. Anderson A, Rubin IL. Simultaneous atrial flutter and ventricular tachycardia. Am Heart J 1958; 56:299–303.

169. Calkins H, Leon AR, Deam AG, Kalbfleisch SJ, Langberg JJ, Morady F. Catheter ablation of atrial flutter using radiofrequency energy. Am J Cardiol 1994; 73:353–356.

170. Parkinson J, Bedford DE. The course and treatment of auricular flutter. Q J Med 1927; 21:21–50.

171. Hoffman JB, Pomerance M. Chronic auricular flutter. Ann Intern Med 1955; 42:885–901.

172. Lewis T. Auricular flutter continuing for 24 years. BMJ 1937; 1:1248.

173. McCord MC, Blount SG. Auricular flutter: a hemodynamic basis of clinical features. Am Heart J 1955; 50:731–741.

174. Harvey WP, Ronan JA Jr. Bedside diagnosis of arrhythmias. Prog Cardiovasc Dis 1966; 8:419–445.

175. Massumi RA, Hernandez T, Just G, Tawakkol AA. The audible sounds of atrial tachyarrhythmia (flutter?). Circulation 1966; 33:607–612.

176. Harvey WP, Levine SA. The changing intensity of the first sound in auricular flutter, an aid to the diagnosis by auscultation. Am Heart J 1948; 35:924–939.

177. Rattigan JP, Byrnes WW, Kraus H, Sise HS. Audible auricular heart sounds in auricular flutter. N Engl J Med 1952; 246:130–131.

178. Neporent LM. Atrial heart sounds in atrial fibrillation and flutter. Circulation 1964; 30:893–896.

179. Penny JL, Gregory JJ, Ayres SM. Audible atrial sounds in a case of atrial flutter. Am J Cardiol 1967; 19:305–307.

180. Neporent LM, Da Silva JA. Heart sounds in atrial flutter-fibrillation. Am J Cardiol 1967; 19:301–304.

181. Dolara A, Tordini B. Atrial flutter sounds: report of a case. Am Heart J 1969; 78:369–372.

182. Rosen KM, Lau SH, Damato AN. Simulation of atrial flutter by rapid coronary sinus pacing. Am Heart J 1969; 78:635–642.

183. Alderman EL, Rytand DA, Crow RS, Finegan RE, Harrison DC. Normal and prosthetic atrioventricular valve motion in atrial flutter: correlation of ultrasound, vectorcardiographic, and phonocardiographic findings. Circulation 1972; 45:1206–1215.

184. Almendral J, Arenal A. Electrophysiology of human atrial flutter. In Josephson ME, Wellens HJJ (eds). Tachycardias. Mechanisms and Management. Mount Kisco, NY: Futura Publishing Co., 1993, pp. 107–119.

185. MacLean D, Emslie-Smith D, Lowe KG. Spatial atrial vectorcardiogram in naturally occurring atrial flutter in man. Br Heart J 1973; 35:817–823.

186. Cheng TO, Efpraxiades J. Electrocardiogram of the month: pseudo-atrial flutter. Chest 1970; 57:290–292.

187. Weitz SH, Tunick PA, McElhinney L, Mitchell T, Kronzon I. Pseudoatrial flutter: artifact simulating atrial flutter caused by a transcutaneous electrical nerve stimulator (TENS). PACE 1997; 20:3010–3011.

188. Waldo AL, MacLean WA, Cooper TB, Kouchoukos NT, Karp RB. Use of temporarily placed epicardial atrial wire electrodes for the diagnosis and treatment of cardiac arrhythmias following open-heart surgery. J Thorac Cardiovasc Surg 1978; 76:500–505.

189. Waldo AL, Henthorn RW, Plumb VJ. Temporary epicardial wire electrodes in the diagnosis and treatment of arrhythmias after open heart surgery. Am J Surg 1984; 148:275–283.

190. Bayes de Luna A, Boada FX, Casellas A, et al. Concealed atrial electrical activity. J Electrocardiol 1978; 11:301–305.

191. Rakovec P, Horvat M, Jakopin J, Kenda MF, Kranjec I, Jagodic A. Induced concealed dissimilar atrial rhythms. Pacing Clin Electrophysiol 1982; 5:523–528.

192. Luca C, Petrescu LP. Atrial flutter with inapparent flutter waves on the surface electrocardiogram. Acta Cardiol 1985; 40:477–483.

193. Buxton AE, Josephson ME. The role of P wave duration as a predictor of postoperative atrial arrhythmias. Chest 1981; 80:68–73.

194. Chung EK. Principles of Cardiac Arrhythmias: Baltimore, Williams & Wilkins, 1971, 378–384.

195. Wu D, Denes P, Leon FA, Chhablani RC, Rosen KM. Limitation of the surface electrocardiogram in diagnosis of atrial arrhythmias: further observations on dissimilar atrial rhythms. Am J Cardiol 1975; 36:91–97.

196. Gomes JA, Kang PS, Matheson M, Gough WB Jr, el-Sherif N. Coexistence of sick sinus rhythm and atrial flutter-fibrillation. Circulation 1981; 63:80–86.

197. Friedman PL, Brugada P, Kuck KH, et al. Inter- and intraatrial dissociation during spontaneous atrial flutter: evidence for a focal origin of the arrhythmia. Am J Cardiol 1982; 50:756–761.

198. Lesh MD, Kalman JM. To fumble flutter or tackle "tach"? Toward updated classifiers for atrial tachyarrhythmias. J Cardiovasc Electrophysiol 1996; 7:460–466.

199. Puech P, Latour H, Grolleau R. Le flutter et ses limites. Arch Mal Coeur Vaiss 1970; 63:116–144.

200. Saoudi N, Nair M, Abdelazziz A, et al. Electrocardiographic patterns and results of radiofrequency catheter ablation of clockwise type I atrial flutter. J Cardiovasc Electrophysiol 1996; 7:931–942.

201. Kalman JM, Olgin JE, Saxon LA, Lee RJ, Scheinman MM, Lesh MD. Electrocardiographic and electrophysiologic characterization of atypical atrial flutter in man: use of activation and entrainment mapping and implications for catheter ablation. J Cardiovasc Electrophysiol 1997; 8:121–144.

202. Wells JL Jr, MacLean WA, James TN, Waldo AL. Characterization of atrial flutter: studies in man after open heart surgery using fixed atrial electrodes. Circulation 1979; 60:665–673.

203. Louvros N, Costeas F. Change in direction of electrical axis of F waves in atrial flutter. Dis Chest 1965; 48:425–426.

204. Cohen SI, Koh D, Lau SH, Rosen KM, Damato AN. P loops during common and uncommon atrial flutter in man. Br Heart J 1977; 39:173–180.

205. Arenal A, Almendral J, San Roman D, Delcan JL, Josephson ME. Frequency and implications of resetting and entrainment with right atrial stimulation in atrial flutter. Am J Cardiol 1992; 70:1292–1298.

206. Tai CT, Chen SA, Chiang CE, et al. Electrophysiologic characteristics and radiofrequency catheter ablation in patients with clockwise atrial flutter. J Cardiovasc Electrophysiol 1997; 8:24–34.

207. Waldo AI, Cooper TB. Spontaneous onset of type I atrial flutter in patients. J Am Coll Cardiol 1996; 28:707–712.

208. Cosio FG, Arribas F, Lopez-Gil M, Palacios J. Atrial flutter mapping and ablation. I. Studying atrial flutter mechanisms by mapping and entrainment. Pacing Clin Electrophysiol 1996; 19:841–853.

209. Cosio FG, Arribas F, Lopez-Gil M, Gonzalez HD. Atrial flutter mapping and ablation. II. Radiofrequency ablation of atrial flutter circuits. Pacing Clin Electrophysiol 1996; 19:965–975.

210. Friedberg CK. Diseases of the Heart. 3rd ed. Philadelphia: WB Saunders, 1966.

211. Yurchak PM, McGovern BA. Supraventricular arrhythmias. In

Eagle KA, Haber E, DeSanctis RW, Austen WG (eds). The Practice of Cardiology. The Medical and Surgical Cardiac Units at the Massachusetts General Hospital. 2nd ed. Boston: Little, Brown, 1980, pp. 154–158.

212. Zipes DP. Specific arrhythmias: diagnosis and treatment. In Braunwald E (ed). Heart Disease. A Textbook of Cardiovascular Medicine. 5th ed. Philadelphia: WB Saunders, 1997, pp. 675–677.

213. Bar FW, Brugada P, Dassen WR, Wellens HJJ. Differential diagnosis of tachycardia with narrow QRS complex (shorter than 0.12 second). Am J Cardiol 1984; 54:555–560.

214. Rytand DA, Onesti SJ, Bruns DL. The atrial rate in patients with flutter: a relationship between atrial enlargement and slow rate. Stanford Med Bull 1958; 16:169–202.

215. Rytand DA, Frank A, Profant GR. Simple optical methods for the recognition of atrial flutter, especially at slow atrial rates. Circulation 1966; 34:111–118.

216. Reynolds EW Jr, MacDonald WJ, Greenfield BM, Semion AA. Mechanisms of onset and termination of abnormal cardiac rhythm studied by constant monitoring. Am Heart J 1967; 74:473–481.

217. Gooch AS, Sumathisena DR. The influence of exercise on atrial flutter. J Electrocardiol 1975; 8:39–48.

218. Waxman MB, Yao L, Cameron DA, Kirsh JA. Effects of posture, Valsalva maneuver and respiration on atrial flutter rate: an effect mediated through cardiac volume. J Am Coll Cardiol 1991; 17:1545–1552.

219. Vulliemin P, Del Bufalo A, Schlaepfer J, Fromer M, Kappenberger L. Relation between cycle length, volume, and pressure in type I atrial flutter. Pacing Clin Electrophysiol 1994; 17:1391–1398.

220. Homcy CJ, Lorell B, Yurchak PM. Atrial flutter with exit block. Circulation 1979; 60:711–714.

221. Javier RP, Narula OS, Samet P. Atrial tachysystole (flutter?) with apparent exit block. Circulation 1969; 40:179–183.

222. Stambler BS, Ellenbogen KA. Elucidating the mechanisms of atrial flutter cycle length variability using power spectral analysis techniques. Circulation 1996; 94:2515–2525.

223. Rozanski JJ, Zaman L, Luceri R, et al. The mechanism of flutter electrical alternans. Pacing Clin Electrophysiol 1981; 4:193–198.

224. Waxman MB, Kirsh JA, Cameron DA, Wald RW. The mechanism of flutter interval alternans. Pacing Clin Electrophysiol 1990; 13:138–143.

225. London F, Howell M. Atrial flutter: 1 to 1 conduction during treatment with quinidine and digitalis. Am Heart J 1954; 48:152–156.

226. Finkelstein D, Gold H, Bellet S. Atrial flutter with 1:1 A-V conduction. Am J Med 1956; 20:65–76.

227. Marks J. Atrial flutter with 1:1 A-V conduction. Arch Intern Med 1959; 100:989–993.

228. Greenwood RJ, Finkelstein D. 1:1 atrial flutter with the Wenckebach phenomenon. Am Heart J 1960; 59:594–599.

229. Jackson A, O'Donnell MJ. Progressive muscular dystrophy with 1:1 atrial flutter. Am Heart J 1960; 59:277–282.

230. Rodensky PL, Wasserman F. Atrial flutter with 1:1 A-V conduction. Dis Chest 1960; 38:563–566.

231. Spivack AP, Sackner MA, Schnabel TG. Atrial flutter with 1:1 A-V conduction associated with pulmonary embolism in the aged. Am Heart J 1960; 59:53–57.

232. Rubeiz GA, Bey SK. Atrial flutter with 1:1 A-V conduction. Am J Cardiol 1961; 7:753–756.

233. Sussman HF, Duque D, Lesser ME. Atrial flutter with 1:1 A-V conduction: report of a case in a pregnant woman successfully treated with DC countershock. Dis Chest 1966; 49:99–103.

234. Patton RD, Helfant RH. Atrial flutter with 1:1 conduction. Dis Chest 1969; 55:250–252.

235. Kennelly BM, Lane GK. Electrophysiological studies in 4 patients with atrial flutter with 1:1 atrioventricular conduction. Am Heart J 1978; 96:723–730.

236. Robertson CE, Miller HC. Extreme tachycardia complicating the use of disopyramide in atrial flutter. Br Heart J 1980; 44:602–603.

237. Besoain-Santander M, Pick A, Langendorf R. A-V conduction in auricular flutter. Circulation 1950; 2:604–616.

238. Castellanos A, Moleiro F, Saoudi N, de la Hera A, Myerburg RJ. Does complexity theory apply to the conduction ratios occurring during progression of stable atrial flutter with 2:1 into 4:1 atrioventricular block? Am J Cardiol 1995; 75:947–949.

239. Slama R, Leclercq JF, Rosengarten M, Coumel P, Bouvrain Y. Multilevel block in the atrioventricular node during atrial tachycardia and flutter alternating with Wenckebach phenomenon. Br Heart J 1979; 42:463–470.

240. Wen ZC, Chen SA, Tai CT, Huang JL, Chang MS. Role of autonomic tone in facilitating spontaneous onset of typical atrial flutter. J Am Coll Cardiol 1998; 31:602–607.

241. Newman BJ, Donoso E, Friedberg CK. Arrhythmias in the Wolff-Parkinson-White syndrome. Prog Cardiovasc Dis 1966; 9:147–165.

242. Castellanos A Jr, Myerburg RJ, Craparo K, Befeler B, Agha AS. Factors regulating ventricular rates during atrial flutter and fibrillation in preexcitation (Wolff-Parkinson-White) syndrome. Br Heart J 1973; 35:811–816.

243. Aranda JM, Moleiro F, Castellanos A, Befeler B. Electrophysiologic studies in a patient with atrial flutter and 1:1 atrioventricular conduction. Chest 1975; 68:200–204.

244. Benditt DG, Pritchett EL, Gallagher JJ. Spectrum of regular tachycardias with wide QRS complexes in patients with accessory atrioventricular pathways. Am J Cardiol 1978; 42:828–838.

245. Rowland E, Curry P, Fox K, Krikler D. Relation between atrioventricular pathways and ventricular response during atrial fibrillation and flutter. Br Heart J 1981; 45:83–87.

246. Blanc JJ, Fontaliran F, Gerbaux A, Boschat J, Penther P. Atrial flutter with 1:1 atrioventricular conduction: electrophysiologic and histologic correlations. Am Heart J 1984; 107:1044–1049.

247. Lown B, Ganong WF, Levine SA. The syndrome of short P-R interval, normal QRS complex and paroxysmal heart action. Circulation 1952; 5:693–706.

248. Panebianco R, Coplan NL. Atrial arrhythmias in athletes. Am Heart J 1994; 127:471–474.

249. Van Den Berg MP, Crijns HJ, Szabo BM, Brouwer J, Lie KI. Effect of exercise on cycle length in atrial flutter. Br Heart J 1995; 73:263–264.

250. Gatzoulis KA, Biblo LA, Waldo AL, Carlson MD. Atrial flutter causes pseudo late potentials on signal-averaged electrocardiogram. Am J Cardiol 1993; 71:251–253.

251. Fitzgerald DM, Hawthorne HR, Crossley GH, Simmons TW, Haisty WK Jr. Effects of atrial fibrillation and atrial flutter on the signal-averaged electrocardiogram. Am J Cardiol 1996; 77:205–209.

252. Zoneraich S, Zoneraich O, Rhee JJ. Echocardiographic findings in atrial flutter. Circulation 1975; 52:455–459.

253. Santiago D, Warshofsky M, Li Mandri G, et al. Left atrial appendage function and thrombus formation in atrial fibrillation-flutter: a transesophageal echocardiographic study. J Am Coll Cardiol 1994; 24:159–164.

254. Fujii J, Foster JR, Mills PG, Moos S, Craige E. Dual echocardiographic determination of atrial contraction sequence in atrial flutter and other related atrial arrhythmias. Circulation 1978; 58:314–321.

255. Olgin JE, Kalman JM, Anza C, Lesh MD. Role of right atrial endocardial structures as barriers to conduction during human type I atrial flutter: activation and entrainment mapping guided by intracardiac echocardiography. Circulation 1995; 92:1839–1848.

256. Chu E, Kalman JM, Kwasman MA, et al. Intracardiac echocardiography during radiofrequency catheter ablation of cardiac arrhythmias in humans. J Am Coll Cardiol 1994; 24:1351–1357.

257. Heinz G, Siostrzonek P, Kreiner G, Gossinger H. Improvement in left ventricular systolic function after successful radiofrequency His bundle ablation for drug refractory, chronic atrial fibrillation and recurrent atrial flutter. Am J Cardiol 1992; 69:489–492.

258. Brignole M, Gianfranchi L, Menozzi C, et al. Influence of atrioventricular junction radiofrequency ablation in patients with chronic atrial fibrillation and flutter on quality of life and cardiac performance. Am J Cardiol 1994; 74:242–246.

259. Zoneraich O, Zoneraich S, Rhee JJ, Jordan D. Atrial flutter: electrocardiographic, vectorcardiographic and echocardiographic correlation. Am Heart J 1978; 96:286–294.

260. O'Neill PG, Puleo PR, Bolli R, Rokey R. Return of atrial mechanical function following electrical conversion of atrial dysrhythmias. Am Heart J 1990; 120:353–359.

261. Grimm RA, Stewart WJ, Arheart K, Thomas JD, Klein AL. Left atrial appendage "stunning" after electrical cardioversion of atrial flutter: an attenuated response compared with atrial fibrillation as the mechanism for lower susceptibility to thromboembolic events. J Am Coll Cardiol 1997; 29:582–589.

262. Jordaens L, Missault L, Germonpre E, et al. Delayed restoration of atrial function after conversion of atrial flutter by pacing or electrical cardioversion. Am J Cardiol 1993; 71:63–67.

263. Irani WN, Grayburn PA, Afridi I. Prevalence of thrombus, spontaneous echo contrast, and atrial stunning in patients undergoing cardioversion of atrial flutter: a prospective study using transesophageal echocardiography. Circulation 1997; 95:962–966.

264. Feltes TF, Friedman RA. Transesophageal echocardiographic detection of atrial thrombi in patients with nonfibrillation atrial tachyarrhythmias and congenital heart disease. J Am Coll Cardiol 1994; 24:1365–1370.

265. Omran H, Jung W, Rabahieh R, et al. Left atrial appendage function in patients with atrial flutter. Heart 1997; 78:250–254.

266. Luchsinger JA, Steinberg JS. Resolution of cardiomyopathy after ablation of atrial flutter. J Am Coll Cardiol 1998; 32:205–210.

267. Ferrer MI. Editorial: atrial flutter. Chest 1974; 66:111–112.

268. McIntosh CL, Greenberg GJ, Maron BJ, Leon MB, Cannon RO III, Clark RE. Clinical and hemodynamic results after mitral valve replacement in patients with obstructive hypertrophic cardiomyopathy. Ann Thorac Surg 1989; 47:236–246.

269. Goldman BS, Chisholm AW, MacGregor DC, Froggatt GM. Permanent transvenous atrial pacing. Can J Surg 1978; 21:138–140.

270. Resnekov L. Haemodynamic studies before and after electrical conversion of atrial fibrillation and flutter to sinus rhythm. Br Heart J 1967; 29:700–708.

271. Karnegis JN, Matoole JJ, Bjorling VG. Immediate improvement in left ventricular function after cardioversion of atrial flutter. Am J Cardiol 1989; 64:1043–1047.

272. Mahrer PR, Killip T, Lukas DS. Hemodynamics in atrial flutter with spontaneous reversion to normal sinus rhythm. Am Heart J 1957; 53:680–686.

273. Astrand I, Cuddy TE, Landegren J, Malmborg RO, Saltin B. Hemodynamic response to exercise during atrial flutter and sinus rhythm. Acta Med Scand 1963; 173:121–127.

274. Harvey RM, Ferrer MI, Cournand A, Richards DW. Cardiocirculatory performance in atrial flutter. Circulation 1955; 12:507–519.

275. Howarth S. Atrial waves on arterial pressure records in normal rhythm, heart block, and auricular flutter. Br Heart J 1954; 16:171–176.

276. Kaye GC, Nathan AW, Camm AJ. Polyuria associated with paroxysmal tachycardia. Clin Prog Pacing Electrophysiol 1984; 2:349–359.

277. Wood P. Polyuria in paroxysmal tachycardia and paroxysmal atrial flutter and fibrillation. Br Heart J 1963; 25:273–282.

278. Luria MH, Adelson EI, Lochaya S. Paroxysmal tachycardia with polyuria. Ann Intern Med 1966; 65:461–470.

279. Mookherjee S, Anderson G Jr, Smulyan H, Vardan S. Atrial natriuretic peptide response to cardioversion of atrial flutter and fibrillation and role of associated heart failure. Am J Cardiol 1991; 67:377–380.

280. Rytand DA. Atrial flutter and the circus movement hypothesis. Circulation 1966; 34:713–714.

281. Wellens HJJ. Value and limitations of programmed electrical stimulation of the heart in the study and treatment of tachycardias. Circulation 1978; 57:845–853.

282. Waldo AL, Henthorn RW, Plumb VJ. Atrial flutter: recent observations in man. In Josephson ME, Wellens HJJ (eds).

Tachycardias. Mechanisms, Diagnosis, Treatment. Philadelphia: Lea & Febiger, 1984, pp. 113–135.

283. Boineau JP. Atrial flutter: a synthesis of concepts. Circulation 1985; 72:249–257.

284. Puech P, Gallay P, Grolleau R. Mechanism of atrial flutter in humans. In Touboul P, Waldo AL (eds). Atrial Arrhythmias. Current Concepts and Management. St. Louis: Mosby–Year Book, 1990, pp. 190–209.

285. Waldo AL. Atrial flutter. New directions in management and mechanism. Circulation 1990; 81:1142–1143.

286. Wellens HJJ. Atrial flutter: progress, but no final answer. J Am Coll Cardiol 1991; 17:1235–1236.

287. Cosio FG, Lopez-Gil M, Goicolea A. Electrophysiologic studies in atrial flutter. Clin Cardiol 1992; 15:667–673.

288. Olshansky B, Wilber DJ, Hariman RJ. Atrial flutter: update on the mechanism and treatment. Pacing Clin Electrophysiol 1992; 15:2308–2335.

289. Shakespeare CF, Anderson M, Camm AJ. Pathophysiology of supraventricular tachycardia. Eur Heart J 1993; 14:2–8.

290. Waldo AL, Wit AL. Mechanisms of cardiac arrhythmias. Lancet 1993; 341:1189–1193.

291. Mary-Rabine L, Mahaux V, Waleffe A, Kulbertus H. Atrial flutter: historical background. J Cardiovasc Electrophysiol 1997; 8:353–358.

292. Waldo AL. Atrial flutter: entrainment characteristics. J Cardiovasc Electrophysiol 1997; 8:337–352.

293. Rytand DA. The circus movement (entrapped circuit wave) hypothesis and atrial flutter. Ann Intern Med 1966; 65:125–159.

294. Scherf D. The mechanism of flutter and fibrillation. Am Heart J 1966; 71:273–280.

295. Kishon Y, Smith RE. Studies in human atrial flutter with the use of proximity electrodes. Circulation 1969; 40:513–525.

296. Wellens HJJ, Janse MJ, Van Dam RT, Durrer D. Epicardial excitation of the atria in a patient with atrial flutter. Br Heart J 1971; 33:233–237.

297. Watson RM, Josephson ME. Atrial flutter. I. Electrophysiologic substrates and modes of initiation and termination. Am J Cardiol 1980; 45:732–741.

298. Disertori M, Molinis G, Inama G, Vergara G, Del Favero A, Furlanello F. Overdrive and programmed atrial electrostimulation in the study of the electrogenetic mechanism of atrial flutter in man. Pacing Clin Electrophysiol 1981; 4:133–147.

299. Disertori M, Inama G, Vergara G, Guarnerio M, Del Favero A, Furlanello F. Evidence of a reentry circuit in the common type of atrial flutter in man. Circulation 1983; 67:434–440.

300. Klein GJ, Guiraudon GM, Sharma AD, Milstein S. Demonstration of macroreentry and feasibility of operative therapy in the common type of atrial flutter. Am J Cardiol 1986; 57:587–591.

301. Cosio FG, Arribas F, Palacios J, Tascon J. Fragmented electrograms and continuous electrical activity in atrial flutter. Am J Cardiol 1986; 57:1309–1314.

302. Cosio FG, Arribas F, Barbero JM, Kallmeyer C, Goicolea A. Validation of double-spike electrograms as markers of conduction delay or block in atrial flutter. Am J Cardiol 1988; 61:775–780.

303. Chang BC, Schuessler RB, Stone CM, et al. Computerized activation sequence mapping of the human atrial septum. Ann Thorac Surg 1990; 49:231–241.

304. Cosio FG, Goicolea A, Lopez-Gil M, Arribas F, Barroso JL, Chicote R. Atrial endocardial mapping in the rare form of atrial flutter. Am J Cardiol 1990; 66:715–720.

305. Olshansky B, Okumura K, Henthorn RW, Waldo AL. Characterization of double potentials in human atrial flutter: studies during transient entrainment. J Am Coll Cardiol 1990; 15:833–841.

306. Olshansky B, Okumura K, Hess PG, Waldo AL. Demonstration of an area of slow conduction in human atrial flutter. J Am Coll Cardiol 1990; 16:1639–1648.

307. Della Bella P, Marenzi G, Tondo C, et al. Usefulness of excitable gap and pattern of resetting in atrial flutter for determining reentry circuit location. Am J Cardiol 1991; 68:492–497.

308. Lammers WJEP, Ravelli F, Disertori M, Antolini R, Furlanello F, Allessie MA. Variations in human atrial flutter cycle length induced by ventricular beats: evidence of a reentrant circuit with a partially excitable gap. J Cardiovasc Electrophysiol 1991; 2:375–387.

309. Kalbfleisch SJ, el-Atassi R, Calkins H, Langberg JJ, Morady F. Association between atrioventricular node reentrant tachycardia and inducible atrial flutter. J Am Coll Cardiol 1993; 22:80–84.

310. Cosio FG, Lopez Gil M, Arribas F, Palacios J, Goicolea A, Nunez A. Mechanisms of entrainment of human common flutter studied with multiple endocardial recordings. Circulation 1994; 89:2117–2125.

311. Ravelli F, Disertori M, Cozzi F, Antolini R, Allessie MA. Ventricular beats induce variations in cycle length of rapid (type II) atrial flutter in humans: evidence of leading circle reentry. Circulation 1994; 89:2107–2116.

312. Leier CV, Meacham JA, Schaal SF. Prolonged atrial conduction: a major predisposing factor for the development of atrial flutter. Circulation 1978; 57:213–216.

313. Nakagawa H, Lazzara R, Khastgir T, et al. Role of the tricuspid annulus and the eustachian valve/ridge on atrial flutter: relevance to catheter ablation of the septal isthmus and a new technique for rapid identification of ablation success. Circulation 1996; 94:407–424.

314. Lau SH, Damato AN, Berkowitz WD, Patton RD. A study of atrioventricular conduction in atrial fibrillation and flutter in man using His bundle recordings. Circulation 1969; 40:71–78.

315. Dobmeyer DJ, Stine RA, Leier CV, Schaal SF. Electrophysiologic mechanisms of provoked atrial flutter in mitral valve prolapse syndrome. Am J Cardiol 1985; 56:602–604.

316. Gossinger HD, Siostrzonek P, Jung M, Wagner L, Mosslacher H. Electrophysiologic determinants of recurrent atrial flutter after successful termination by overdrive pacing. Am J Cardiol 1990; 65:463–466.

317. Buxton AE, Waxman HL, Marchlinski FE, Josephson ME. Atrial conduction: effects of extrastimuli with and without atrial dysrhythmias. Am J Cardiol 1984; 54:755–761.

318. Stambler BS, Wood MA, Ellenbogen KA. Pharmacologic alterations in human type I atrial flutter cycle length and monophasic action potential duration: evidence of a fully excitable gap in the reentrant circuit. J Am Coll Cardiol 1996; 27:453–461.

319. Gavrilescu S, Cotoi S. Monophasic action potential of right human atrium during atrial flutter and after conversion to sinus rhythm: argument for reentry theory. Br Heart J 1972; 34:396–402.

320. Kerr CR, Gallagher JJ, Smith WM, et al. The induction of atrial flutter and fibrillation and the termination of atrial flutter by esophageal pacing. Pacing Clin Electrophysiol 1983; 6:60–72.

321. Olgin JE, Kalman JM, Saxon LA, Lee RJ, Lesh MD. Mechanism of initiation of atrial flutter in humans: site of unidirectional block and direction of rotation. J Am Coll Cardiol 1997; 29:376–384.

322. Kalbfleisch SJ, el-Atassi R, Calkins H, Langberg JJ, Morady F. Inducibility of atrial fibrillation before and after radiofrequency catheter ablation of accessory atrioventricular connections. J Cardiovasc Electrophysiol 1993; 4:499–503.

323. Engel TR, Luck JC. Effect of whiskey on atrial vulnerability and "holiday heart." J Am Coll Cardiol 1983; 1:816–818.

324. Cosio FG. Endocardial mapping of atrial flutter. In Touboul P, Waldo AL (eds). Atrial Arrhythmias. Current Concepts and Management. St. Louis: Mosby–Year Book, 1990, pp. 229–240.

325. Olgin JE, Kalman JM, Lesh MD. Conduction barriers in human atrial flutter: correlation of electrophysiology and anatomy. J Cardiovasc Electrophysiol 1996; 7:1112–1126.

326. Van Hare GF, Waldo AL. The atrial flutter reentrant circuit: additional pieces of the puzzle. Circulation 1996; 94:244–246.

327. Poty H, Saoudi N, Abdel Aziz A, Nair M, Letac B. Radiofrequency catheter ablation of type I atrial flutter: prediction of late success by electrophysiological criteria. Circulation 1995; 92:1389–1392.

328. Kalman JM, Olgin JE, Saxon LA, Fisher WG, Lee RJ, Lesh MD. Activation and entrainment mapping defines the tricuspid annulus as the anterior barrier in typical atrial flutter. Circulation 1996; 94:398–406.

329. Arribas F, Lopez-Gil M, Cosio FG, Nunez A. The upper link of human common atrial flutter circuit: definition by multiple endocardial recordings during entrainment. PACE 1997; 20:2924–2929.

330. Kinder C, Kall J, Kopp D, Rubenstein D, Burke M, Wilber D. Conduction properties of the inferior vena cava-tricuspid annular isthmus in patients with typical atrial flutter. J Cardiovasc Electrophysiol 1997; 8:727–737.

331. Shah DC, Haissaguerre M, Jais P, et al. Simplified electrophysiologically directed catheter ablation of recurrent common atrial flutter. Circulation 1997; 96:2505–2508.

332. Mirowski M, Alkan WJ. Left atrial impulse formation in atrial flutter. Br Heart J 1967; 29:299–304.

333. Interian A Jr, Cox MM, Jimenez RA, et al. A shared pathway in atrioventricular nodal reentrant tachycardia and atrial flutter: implications for pathophysiology and therapy. Am J Cardiol 1993; 71:297–303.

334. Waldo AL, MacLean WA, Karp RB, Kouchoukos NT, James TN. Entrainment and interruption of atrial flutter with atrial pacing: studies in man following open heart surgery. Circulation 1977; 56:737–745.

335. Inoue H, Matsuo H, Takayanagi K, Murao S. Clinical and experimental studies of the effects of atrial extrastimulation and rapid pacing on atrial flutter cycle: evidence of macro-reentry with an excitable gap. Am J Cardiol 1981; 48:623–631.

336. Beckman K, Ta-Lin H, Krafchek J, Wyndham CR. Classic and concealed entrainment of typical and atypical atrial flutter. Pacing Clin Electrophysiol 1986; 9:826–835.

337. Henthorn RW, Okumura K, Olshansky B, Plumb VJ, Hess PG, Waldo AL. A fourth criterion for transient entrainment: the electrogram equivalent of progressive fusion. Circulation 1988; 77:1003–1012.

338. Fujimoto T, Inoue T, Fukuzaki H. Characterization of slow conduction in the common type of atrial flutter: using transient entrainment. Jpn Circ J 1990; 54:21–31.

339. Tanoiri T, Komatsu C, Ishinaga T, et al. Study on the genesis of the double potential recorded in the high right atrium in atrial flutter and its role in the reentry circuit of atrial flutter. Am Heart J 1991; 121:57–61.

340. Callans DJ, Schwartzman D, Gottlieb CD, Dillon SM, Marchlinski FE. Characterization of the excitable gap in human type I atrial flutter. J Am Coll Cardiol 1997; 30:1793–1801.

341. Feld GK, Mollerus M, Birgersdotter-Green U, et al. Conduction velocity in the tricuspid valve-inferior vena cava isthmus is slower in patients with type I atrial flutter compared to those without a history of atrial flutter. J Cardiovasc Electrophysiol 1997; 8:1338–1348.

342. Tai CT, Chen SA, Chiang CE, et al. Characterization of low right atrial isthmus as the slow conduction zone and pharmacological target in typical atrial flutter. Circulation 1997; 96:2601–2611.

343. Jalil E, LeFranc P, LeBeau R, Molin F, Costi P, Kus T. Effects of procainamide on the excitable gap composition in common human atrial flutter. PACE 1998; 21:528–535.

344. Cheng J, Scheinman MM. Acceleration of typical atrial flutter due to double-wave reentry induced by programmed electrical stimulation. Circulation 1998; 97:1589–1596.

345. Cosio FG, Lopez-Gil M, Arribas F, Gonzalez HD. Mechanisms of induction of typical and reversed atrial flutter. J Cardiovasc Electrophysiol 1998; 9:281–291.

346. Herrmann GR, Hejtmancik MR. Atrial flutter. II. Methods of treatment. Am Heart J 1951; 41:182–191.

347. Linenthal AJ. Effects of carotid sinus reflex on cardiac impulse formation and conduction. Circulation 1959; 20:595–601.

348. Lown B, Levine SA. The carotid sinus. Clinical value of its stimulation. Circulation 1961; 23:766–789.

349. Anonymous. Hazard of carotid-sinus stimulation. N Engl J Med 1966; 275:165–166.

350. Scherf D, Cohen J, Rafailzadeh M. Excitatory effects of carotid sinus pressure: enhancement of ectopic impulse

formation and of impulse conduction. Am J Cardiol 1966; 17:240–252.

351. el-Sherif N. Paroxysmal atrial flutter and fibrillation: induction by carotid sinus compression and prevention by atropine. Br Heart J 1972; 34:1024–1028.

352. Anbe DT, Rubenfire M, Drake EH. Conversion of atrial flutter to atrial fibrillation with carotid sinus pressure. J Electrocardiol 1969; 2:377–380.

353. Bussan R, Reid ER, Scherf D. Conversion of atrial flutter into atrial fibrillation by carotid pressure. Ann Intern Med 1957; 46:814–818.

354. Falk RH. Proarrhythmia in patients treated for atrial fibrillation or flutter. Ann Intern Med 1992; 117:141–150.

355. Campbell RW. Pharmacologic therapy of atrial flutter. J Cardiovasc Electrophysiol 1996; 7:1008–1012.

356. Camm AJ, Garratt CJ. Adenosine and supraventricular tachycardia. N Engl J Med 1991; 325:1621–1629.

357. DiMarco JP. Adenosine. In Podrid PJ, Kowey PR (eds). Cardiac Arrhythmia. Mechanisms, Diagnosis, and Management. Baltimore: Williams & Wilkins, 1995, pp. 488–498.

358. DiMarco JP, Sellers TD, Lerman BB, Greenberg ML, Berne RM, Belardinelli L. Diagnostic and therapeutic use of adenosine in patients with supraventricular tachyarrhythmias. J Am Coll Cardiol 1985; 6:417–425.

359. Overholt ED, Rheuban KS, Gutgesell HP, Lerman BB, DiMarco JP. Usefulness of adenosine for arrhythmias in infants and children. Am J Cardiol 1988; 61:336–340.

360. Till J, Shinebourne EA, Rigby ML, Clarke B, Ward DE, Rowland E. Efficacy and safety of adenosine in the treatment of supraventricular tachycardia in infants and children. Br Heart J 1989; 62:204–211.

361. Brodsky MA, Hwang C, Hunter D, et al. Life-threatening alterations in heart rate after the use of adenosine in atrial flutter. Am Heart J 1995; 130:564–571.

362. Slade AK, Garratt CJ. Proarrhythmic effect of adenosine in a patient with atrial flutter. Br Heart J 1993; 70:91–92.

363. Rankin AC, Rae AP, Houston A. Acceleration of ventricular response to atrial flutter after intravenous adenosine. Br Heart J 1993; 69:263–265.

364. Garratt CJ, Griffith MJ, O'Nunain S, Ward DE, Camm AJ. Effects of intravenous adenosine on antegrade refractoriness of accessory atrioventricular connections. Circulation 1991; 84:1962–1968.

365. Greenberg HB, Antin SH. 1:1 conduction in atrial flutter after intravenous injection of aminophylline. J Electrocardiol 1972; 5:391–393.

366. Podrid PJ. Amiodarone: reevaluation of an old drug. Ann Intern Med 1995; 122:689–700.

367. Desai AD, Chun S, Sung RJ. The role of intravenous amiodarone in the management of cardiac arrhythmias. Ann Intern Med 1997; 127:294–303.

368. Hou ZY, Chang MS, Chen CY, et al. Acute treatment of recent-onset atrial fibrillation and flutter with a tailored dosing regimen of intravenous amiodarone: a randomized, digoxin-controlled study. Eur Heart J 1995; 16:521–528.

369. Rosenbaum MB, Chiale PA, Halpern MS, et al. Clinical efficacy of amiodarone as an antiarrhythmic agent. Am J Cardiol 1976; 38:934–944.

370. Wheeler PJ, Puritz R, Ingram DV, Chamberlain DA. Amiodarone in the treatment of refractory supraventricular and ventricular arrhythmias. Postgrad Med J 1979; 55:1–9.

371. Rowland E, Krikler DM. Electrophysiological assessment of amiodarone in treatment of resistant supraventricular arrhythmias. Br Heart J 1980; 44:82–90.

372. Coumel P, Fidelle J, Loges-en-Josas L. Amiodarone in the treatment of cardiac arrhythmias in children: one hundred thirty-five cases. Am Heart J 1980; 100:1063–1069.

373. Ward DE, Camm AJ, Spurrell RA. Clinical antiarrhythmic effects of amiodarone in patients with resistant paroxysmal tachycardias. Br Heart J 1980; 44:91–95.

374. Faniel R, Schoenfeld P. Efficacy of I.V. amiodarone in converting rapid atrial fibrillation and flutter to sinus rhythm in intensive care patients. Eur Heart J 1983; 4:180–185.

375. Graboys TB, Podrid PJ, Lown B. Efficacy of amiodarone for

refractory supraventricular tachyarrhythmias. Am Heart J 1983; 106:870–876.

376. Haffajee CI, Love JC, Alpert JS, Asdourian GK, Sloan KC. Efficacy and safety of long-term amiodarone in treatment of cardiac arrhythmias: dosage experience. Am Heart J 1983; 106:935–943.

377. Peter T, Hamer A, Mandel WJ, Weiss D. Evaluation of amiodarone therapy in the treatment of drug-resistant cardiac arrhythmias: long-term follow-up. Am Heart J 1983; 106:943–950.

378. Mostow ND, Vrobel TR, Noon D, Rakita L. Rapid control of refractory atrial tachyarrhythmias with high-dose oral amiodarone. Am Heart J 1990; 120:1356–1363.

379. Gosselink AT, Crijns HJ, Van Gelder IC, Hillige H, Wiesfeld AC, Lie KI. Low-dose amiodarone for maintenance of sinus rhythm after cardioversion of atrial fibrillation or flutter. JAMA 1992; 267:3289–3293.

380. Chun SH, Sager PT, Stevenson WG, Nademanee K, Middlekauff HR, Singh BN. Long-term efficacy of amiodarone for the maintenance of normal sinus rhythm in patients with refractory atrial fibrillation or flutter. Am J Cardiol 1995; 76:47–50.

381. Installe E, Schoevaerdts JC, Gadisseux P, Charles S, Tremouroux J. Intravenous amiodarone in the treatment of various arrhythmias following cardiac operations. J Thorac Cardiovasc Surg 1981; 81:302–308.

382. Garson A Jr, Gillette PC, McVey P, et al. Amiodarone treatment of critical arrhythmias in children and young adults. J Am Coll Cardiol 1984; 4:749–755.

383. Villain E. Amiodarone as treatment for atrial tachycardias after surgery. Pacing Clin Electrophysiol 1997; 20:2130–2132.

384. Gibson D, Sowton E. The use of beta-adrenergic receptor blocking drugs in dysrhythmias. (review) (140 refs). Prog Cardiovasc Dis 1969; 12:16–39.

385. Harrison DC, Griffin JR, Fiene TJ. Effects of beta-adrenergic blockade with propranolol in patients with atrial arrhythmias. N Engl J Med 1963; 273:410–415.

386. Rowlands DJ, Howitt G, Markman P. Propranolol (Inderal) in disturbances of cardiac rhythm. BMJ 1965; 1:891–894.

387. Stock JP. Beta adrenergic blocking drugs in the clinical management of cardiac arrhythmias. Am J Cardiol 1966; 18:444–449.

388. Gianelly R, Griffin JR, Harrison DC. Propranolol in the treatment and prevention of cardiac arrhythmias. Ann Intern Med 1967; 66:667–676.

389. Kerber RE, Goldman RH, Gianelly RE, Harrison DC. Treatment of atrial arrhythmias with alprenolol. JAMA 1970; 214:1849–1854.

390. Byrd RC, Sung RJ, Marks J, Parmley WW. Safety and efficacy of esmolol (ASL-8052: an ultrashort-acting beta-adrenergic blocking agent) for control of ventricular rate in supraventricular tachycardias. J Am Coll Cardiol 1984; 3:394–399.

391. Abrams J, Allen J, Allin D, et al. Efficacy and safety of esmolol vs propranolol in the treatment of supraventricular tachyarrhythmias: a multicenter double-blind clinical trial. Am Heart J 1985; 110:913–922.

392. Gray RJ, Bateman TM, Czer LS, Conklin CM, Matloff JM. Esmolol: a new ultrashort-acting beta-adrenergic blocking agent for rapid control of heart rate in postoperative supraventricular tachyarrhythmias. J Am Coll Cardiol 1985; 5:1451–1456.

393. Morganroth J, Horowitz LN, Anderson J, Turlapaty P. Comparative efficacy and tolerance of esmolol to propranolol for control of supraventricular tachyarrhythmia. Am J Cardiol 1985; 56:33F–39F.

394. Schwartz M, Michelson EL, Sawin HS, MacVaugh H III. Esmolol: safety and efficacy in postoperative cardiothoracic patients with supraventricular tachyarrhythmias. Chest 1988; 93:705–711.

395. Platia EV, Michelson EL, Porterfield JK, Das G. Esmolol versus verapamil in the acute treatment of atrial fibrillation or atrial flutter. Am J Cardiol 1989; 63:925–929.

396. Watt DA, Livingstone WR, MacKay RK, Obineche EN. Use of propranolol in atrial flutter. Br Heart J 1970; 32:453–457.

397. Anderson S, Blanski L, Byrd RC, et al. Comparison of the efficacy and safety of esmolol, a short-acting beta blocker, with placebo in the treatment of supraventricular tachyarrhythmias: the esmolol vs placebo multicenter study group. Am Heart J 1986; 111:42–48.

398. Das G, Ferris J. Esmolol in the treatment of supraventricular tachyarrhythmias. Can J Cardiol 1988; 4:177–180.

399. Silverman NA, Wright R, Levitsky S. Efficacy of low-dose propranolol in preventing postoperative supraventricular tachyarrhythmias: a prospective, randomized study. Ann Surg 1982; 196:194–197.

400. Hammon JW Jr, Wood AJ, Prager RL, Wood M, Muirhead J, Bender HW Jr. Perioperative beta blockade with propranolol: reduction in myocardial oxygen demands and incidence of atrial and ventricular arrhythmias. Ann Thorac Surg 1984; 38:363–367.

401. Daudon P, Corcos T, Gandjbakhch I, Levasseur JP, Cabrol A, Cabrol C. Prevention of atrial fibrillation or flutter by acebutolol after coronary bypass grafting. Am J Cardiol 1986; 58:933–936.

402. Khuri SF, Okike ON, Josa M, et al. Efficacy of nadolol in preventing supraventricular tachycardia after coronary artery bypass grafting. Am J Cardiol 1987; 60:51D–58D.

403. Suttorp MJ, Kingma JH, Peels HO, et al. Effectiveness of sotalol in preventing supraventricular tachyarrhythmias shortly after coronary artery bypass grafting. Am J Cardiol 1991; 68:1163–1169.

404. Byrd RC, Sung RJ, Marks J, Parmley WW. Safety and efficacy of esmolol (ASL-8052: an ultrashort-acting beta-adrenergic blocking agent) for control of ventricular rate in supraventricular tachycardias. J Am Coll Cardiol 1984; 3:394–399.

405. Aronow WS, Uyeyama RR. Treatment of arrhythmias with pindolol. Clin Pharmacol Ther 1972; 13:15–22.

406. Wolfson S, Robbins SI, Krasnow N. Treatment of cardiac arrhythmias with beta-adrenergic blocking agents: clinical and experimental studies. Am Heart J 1966; 72:176–187.

407. Williams JB, Stephensen LW, Holford FD, Langer T, Dunkman WB, Josephson ME. Arrhythmia prophylaxis using propranolol after coronary artery surgery. Ann Thorac Surg 1982; 34:435–438.

408. Abel RM, van Gelder HM, Pores IH, Liguori J, Gielchinsky I, Parsonnet V. Continued propranolol administration following coronary bypass surgery: antiarrhythmic effects. Arch Surg 1983; 118:727–731.

409. Campbell TJ, Gavaghan TP, Morgan JJ. Intravenous sotalol for the treatment of atrial fibrillation and flutter after cardiopulmonary bypass: comparison with disopyramide and digoxin in a randomised trial. Br Heart J 1985; 54:86–90.

410. Sung RJ, Tan HL, Karagounis L, et al. Intravenous sotalol for the termination of supraventricular tachycardia and atrial fibrillation and flutter: a multicenter, randomized, double-blind, placebo-controlled study. Sotalol multicenter study group. Am Heart J 1995; 129:739–748.

411. Schamroth L, Krikler DM, Garrett C. Immediate effects of intravenous verapamil in cardiac arrhythmias. BMJ 1972; 1:660–662.

412. Heng MK, Singh BN, Roche AH, Norris RM, Mercer CJ. Effects of intravenous verapamil on cardiac arrhythmias and on the electrocardiogram. Am Heart J 1975; 90:487–498.

413. Dominic J, McAllister RG Jr, Kuo CS, Reddy CP, Surawicz B. Verapamil plasma levels and ventricular rate response in patients with atrial fibrillation and flutter. Clin Pharmacol Ther 1979; 26:710–714.

414. Aronow WS, Ferlinz J. Verapamil versus placebo in atrial fibrillation and atrial flutter. Clin Invest Med 1980; 3:35–39.

415. Rinkenberger RL, Prystowsky EN, Heger JJ, Troup PJ, Jackman WM, Zipes DP. Effects of intravenous and chronic oral verapamil administration in patients with supraventricular tachyarrhythmias. Circulation 1980; 62:996–1010.

416. Sung RJ, Waxman HL, Elser B, Juma Z. Treatment of paroxysmal supraventricular tachycardia and atrial flutter-fibrillation with intravenous verapamil: efficacy and mechanism of action. Clin Invest Med 1980; 3:41–47.

417. Gonzalez R, Scheinman MM. Treatment of supraventricular arrhythmias with intravenous and oral verapamil. Chest 1981; 80:465–470.

418. Waxman HL, Myerburg RJ, Appel R, Sung RJ. Verapamil for control of ventricular rate in paroxysmal supraventricular tachycardia and atrial fibrillation or flutter: a double-blind randomized cross-over study. Ann Intern Med 1981; 94:1–6.

419. Plumb VJ, Karp RB, Kouchoukos NT, Zorn GL Jr, James TN, Waldo AL. Verapamil therapy of atrial fibrillation and atrial flutter following cardiac operation. J Thorac Cardiovasc Surg 1982; 83:590–596.

420. Tommaso C, McDonough T, Parker M, Talano JV. Atrial fibrillation and flutter: immediate control and conversion with intravenously administered verapamil. Arch Intern Med 1983; 143:877–881.

421. Haft JI, Habbab MA. Treatment of atrial arrhythmias: effectiveness of verapamil when preceded by calcium infusion. Arch Intern Med 1986; 146:1085–1089.

422. Suttorp MJ, Kingma JH, Lie-A-Huen L, Mast EG. Intravenous flecainide versus verapamil for acute conversion of paroxysmal atrial fibrillation or flutter to sinus rhythm. Am J Cardiol 1989; 63:693–696.

423. Betriu A, Chaitman BR, Bourassa MG, et al. Beneficial effect of intravenous diltiazem in the acute management of paroxysmal supraventricular tachyarrhythmias. Circulation 1983; 67:88–94.

424. Salerno DM, Dias VC, Kleiger RE, et al. Efficacy and safety of intravenous diltiazem for treatment of atrial fibrillation and atrial flutter: the diltiazem-atrial fibrillation/flutter study group. Am J Cardiol 1989; 63:1046–1051.

425. Ellenbogen KA, Dias VC, Plumb VJ, Heywood JT, Mirvis DM. A placebo-controlled trial of continuous intravenous diltiazem infusion for 24-hour heart rate control during atrial fibrillation and atrial flutter: a multicenter study. J Am Coll Cardiol 1991; 18:891–897.

426. Goldenberg IF, Lewis WR, Dias VC, Heywood JT, Pedersen WR. Intravenous diltiazem for the treatment of patients with atrial fibrillation or flutter and moderate to severe congestive heart failure. Am J Cardiol 1994; 74:884–889.

427. Ellenbogen KA, Dias VC, Cardello FP, et al. Safety and efficacy of intravenous diltiazem in atrial fibrillation or atrial flutter. Am J Cardiol 1995; 75:45–49.

428. Williams DB, Misbach GA, Kruse AP, Ivey TD. Oral verapamil for prophylaxis of supraventricular tachycardia after myocardial revascularization: a randomized trial. J Thorac Cardiovasc Surg 1985; 90:592–596.

429. Hagemeijer F. Verapamil in the management of supraventricular tachyarrhythmias occurring after a recent myocardial infarction. Circulation 1978; 57:751–755.

430. Aronow WS, Landa D, Plasencia G, Wong R, Karlsberg RP, Ferlinz J. Verapamil in atrial fibrillation and atrial flutter. Clin Pharmacol Ther 1979; 26:578–583.

431. Smith EE, Shore DF, Monro JL, Ross JK. Oral verapamil fails to prevent supraventricular tachycardia following coronary artery surgery. Int J Cardiol 1985; 9:37–44.

432. Simpson RJ Jr, Foster JR, Woelfel AK, Gettes LS. Management of atrial fibrillation and flutter: a reappraisal of digitalis therapy. Postgrad Med 1986; 79:241–253.

433. Roberts SA, Diaz C, Nolan PE, et al. Effectiveness and costs of digoxin treatment for atrial fibrillation and flutter. Am J Cardiol 1993; 72:567–573.

434. Andrews TC, Reimold SC, Berlin JA, Antman EM. Prevention of supraventricular arrhythmias after coronary artery bypass surgery: a meta-analysis of randomized control trials. Circulation 1991; 84:236–244.

435. Falk RH. Control of the ventricular rate in atrial fibrillation. In Falk RH, Podrid PJ (eds). Atrial Fibrillation. Mechanisms and Management. New York: Raven Press, 1992, pp. 255–282.

436. Deano DA, Wu D, Mautner RK, Sherman RH, Ehsani AI, Rosen KM. The antiarrhythmic efficacy of intravenous therapy with disopyramide phosphate. Chest 1977; 71:597–606.

437. Luoma PV, Kujala PA, Juustila HJ, Takkunen JT. Efficacy of intravenous disopyramide in the termination of supraventricular arrhythmias. J Clin Pharmacol 1978; 18:293–301.

438. De Backer M, Stoupel E, Kahn RJ. Efficacy of intravenous disopyramide in acute cardiac arrhythmias. Eur J Clin Pharmacol 1981; 19:11–18.

439. Della Bella P, Marenzi G, Tondo C, et al. Effects of disopyramide on cycle length, effective refractory period and excitable gap of atrial flutter, and relation to arrhythmia termination by overdrive pacing. Am J Cardiol 1989; 63:812–816.

440. Moss AJ, Aledort LM. Use of edrophonium (Tensilon) in the evaluation of supraventricular tachycardias. Am J Cardiol 1966; 17:58–62.

441. Fleischmann D, Bellet S, Roman LR. Conversion of atrial flutter to normal sinus rhythm after intravenous administration of edrophonium chloride. Chest 1971; 59:113–115.

442. Goy JJ, Kappenberger L. Flecainide acetate in supraventricular arrhythmias. J Electrophysiol 1987; 1:113–119.

443. Van Gelder IC, Crijns HJ, van Gilst WH, van Wijk LM, Hamer HP, Lie KI. Efficacy and safety of flecainide acetate in the maintenance of sinus rhythm after electrical cardioversion of chronic atrial fibrillation or atrial flutter. Am J Cardiol 1989; 64:1317–1321.

444. Sihm I, Hansen FA, Rasmussen J, Pedersen AK, Thygesen K. Flecainide acetate in atrial flutter and fibrillation: the arrhythmogenic effects. Eur Heart J 1990; 11:145–148.

445. Nathan AW, Camm AJ, Bexton RS, Hellestrand KJ. Intravenous flecainide acetate for the clinical management of paroxysmal tachycardias. Clin Cardiol 1987; 10:317–322.

446. Hohnloser SH, Zabel M. Short- and long-term efficacy and safety of flecainide acetate for supraventricular arrhythmias. Am J Cardiol 1992; 70:3A–9A.

447. Hohnloser S, Zeiher A, Hust MH, Wollschlager H, Just H. Flecainide-induced aggravation of ventricular tachycardia. Clin Cardiol 1983; 6:130–135.

448. Goy JJ, Grbic M, Hurni M, et al. Conversion of supraventricular arrhythmias to sinus rhythm using flecainide. Eur Heart J 1985; 6:518–524.

449. Hellestrand KJ. Intravenous flecainide acetate for supraventricular tachycardias. Am J Cardiol 1988; 62:16D–22D.

450. Suttorp MJ, Kingma JH, Jessurun ER, Lie-A-Huen L, van Hemel NM, Lie KI. The value of class IC antiarrhythmic drugs for acute conversion of paroxysmal atrial fibrillation or flutter to sinus rhythm. J Am Coll Cardiol 1990; 16:1722–1727.

451. Kingma JH, Suttorp MJ. Acute pharmacologic conversion of atrial fibrillation and flutter: the role of flecainide, propafenone, and verapamil. Am J Cardiol 1992; 70:56A–60A.

452. Murray KT. Ibutilide. Circulation 1998; 97:493–497.

453. Guo GB, Ellenbogen KA, Wood MA, Stambler BS. Conversion of atrial flutter by ibutilide is associated with increased atrial cycle length variability. J Am Coll Cardiol 1996; 27:1083–1089.

454. Ellenbogen KA, Stambler BS, Wood MA, et al. Efficacy of intravenous ibutilide for rapid termination of atrial fibrillation and atrial flutter: a dose-response study. J Am Coll Cardiol 1996; 28:130–136.

455. Tai CT, Chen SA, Feng AN, Yu WC, Chen YJ, Chang MS. Electropharmacologic effects of class I and class III antiarrhythmic drugs on typical atrial flutter: insights into the mechanism of termination. Circulation 1998; 97:1935–1945.

456. Stambler BS, Wood MA, Ellenbogen KA. Antiarrhythmic actions of intravenous ibutilide compared with procainamide during human atrial flutter and fibrillation: electrophysiological determinants of enhanced conversion efficacy. Circulation 1997; 96:4298–4306.

457. Volgman AS, Carberry PA, Stambler B, et al. Conversion efficacy and safety of intravenous ibutilide compared with intravenous procainamide in patients with atrial flutter or fibrillation. J Am Coll Cardiol 1998; 31:1414–1419.

458. Danahy DT, Aronow WS. Lidocaine-induced cardiac rate changes in atrial fibrillation and atrial flutter. Am Heart J 1978; 95:474–482.

459. Kayden HJ, Brodie BB, Steele JM. Procaine amide: a review. Circulation 1957; 25:118–126.

460. Schack JA, Hoffman I, Vesell H. The response of arrhythmias and tachycardias of supraventricular origin to oral procaine amide. Br Heart J 1952; 14:465–469.

461. Pascale LR, Bernstein LM, Schoolman HM, Foley EF. Intravenous procaine amide in the treatment of cardiac arrhythmias. Am Heart J 1954; 48:110–122.

462. Wu KM, Hoffman BF. Effect of procainamide and N-acetyl-procainamide on atrial flutter: studies in vivo and in vitro. Circulation 1987; 76:1397–1408.

463. Miller CD, Oleshansky MA, Gibson KF, Cantilena LR. Procainamide-induced myasthenia-like weakness and dysphagia. Ther Drug Monit 1993; 15:251–254.

464. Bianconi L, Boccadamo R, Pappalardo A, Gentili C, Pistolese M. Effectiveness of intravenous propafenone for conversion of atrial fibrillation and flutter of recent onset. Am J Cardiol 1989; 64:335–338.

465. Guccione P, Drago F, Di Donato RM, et al. Oral propafenone therapy for children with arrhythmias: efficacy and adverse effects in midterm follow-up. Am Heart J 1991; 122:1022–1027.

466. Herzberg GZ, Rossi AF. Atrial flutter in a pediatric patient in the immediate period after the Fontan procedure: control with oral propafenone. PACE 1997; 20:3002–3003.

467. Murdock CJ, Kyles AE, Yeung-Lai-Wah JA, Qi A, Vorderbrugge S, Kerr CR. Atrial flutter in patients treated for atrial fibrillation with propafenone. Am J Cardiol 1990; 66:755–757.

468. Hohnloser SH, Woosley RL. Sotalol. N Engl J Med 1994; 331:31–38.

469. Beaufort-Krol GC, Bink-Boelkens MT. Effectiveness of sotalol for atrial flutter in children after surgery for congenital heart disease. Am J Cardiol 1997; 79:92–94.

470. Beaufort-Krol GC, Bink-Boelkens MT. Sotalol for atrial tachycardias after surgery for congenital heart disease. Pacing Clin Electrophysiol 1997; 20:2125–2129.

471. DeSilva RA, Graboys TB, Podrid PJ, Lown B. Cardioversion and defibrillation. Am Heart J 1980; 100:881–895.

472. Killip T. Synchronized DC precordial shock for arrhythmias: safe new technique to establish normal rhythm may be utilized on an elective or an emergency basis. JAMA 1963; 186:107–113.

473. Lown B, Bey SK, Perlroth MG, Abe T. Cardioversion of ectopic tachycardias. Am J Med Sci 1963; 246:257–262.

474. Miller DI, Nachlas MM. Electrocardiographic patterns during resuscitation after experimentally induced ventricular fibrillation. Circ Res 1964; 15:199–207.

475. Morris JJ, Kong Y, North WC, McIntosh HD. Experience with "cardioversion" of atrial fibrillation and flutter. Am J Cardiol 1964; 14:94–100.

476. Castellanos A, Lemberg L, Gosselin A, Fonseca EJ. Evaluation of countershock treatment of atrial flutter. Arch Intern Med 1965; 115:426–433.

477. Hassenruck A, Chojnacki B, Barker HJ. Cardioversion of auricular flutter in a newborn infant. Am J Cardiol 1965; 15:726–731.

478. McDonald L, Resnekov L, O'Brien K. Direct-current shock in treatment of drug-resistant cardiac arrhythmias. BMJ 1965; 1:1468–1470.

479. Selzer A, Kelly JJ, Johnson RB, Kerth WJ. Immediate and long-term results of electrical conversion of arrhythmias. Prog Cardiovasc Dis 1966; 9:90–104.

480. Szekely P, Batson GA, Stark DC. Direct current shock therapy of cardiac arrhythmias. Br Heart J 1966; 28:366–373.

481. Jewitt DE, Balcon R, Raftery EB, Oram S. Incidence and management of supraventricular arrhythmias after acute myocardial infarction. Lancet 1967; 2:734–738.

482. Resnekov L, McDonald L. Complications in 220 patients with cardiac dysrhythmias treated by phased direct current shock, and indications for electroconversion. Br Heart J 1967; 29:926–936.

483. Wikland B, Edhag O, Eliasch H. Atrial fibrillation and flutter treated with synchronized DC shock: a study on immediate and long-term results. Acta Med Scand 1967; 182:665–671.

484. Bjerkelund C, Orning OM. An evaluation of DC shock treatment of atrial arrhythmias. Acta Med Scand 1968; 184:481–491.

485. Frithz G, Aberg H. Direct current conversion of atrial flutter. Acta Med Scand 1970; 187:271–274.
486. Guiney TE, Lown B. Electrical conversion of atrial flutter to atrial fibrillation: flutter mechanism in man. Br Heart J 1972; 34:1215–1224.
487. Van Gelder IC, Crijns HJ, van Gilst WH, Verwer R, Lie KI. Prediction of uneventful cardioversion and maintenance of sinus rhythm from direct-current electrical cardioversion of chronic atrial fibrillation and flutter. Am J Cardiol 1991; 68:41–46.
488. Kerber RE. Transthoracic cardioversion of atrial fibrillation and flutter: standard techniques and new advances. Am J Cardiol 1996; 78:22–26.
489. Crijns HJ, Van Gelder IC, Tieleman RG, et al. Long-term outcome of electrical cardioversion in patients with chronic atrial flutter. Heart 1997; 77:56–61.
490. Lesser MF. Safety and efficacy of in-office cardioversion for treatment of supraventricular arrhythmias. Am J Cardiol 1990; 66:1267–1268.
491. Greenberg ML, Kelly TA, Lerman BB, DiMarco JP. Atrial pacing for conversion of atrial flutter. Am J Cardiol 1986; 58:95–99.
492. Suttorp MJ, Kingma JH, Koomen EM, van 't Hof A, Tijssen JG, Lie KI. Recurrence of paroxysmal atrial fibrillation or flutter after successful cardioversion in patients with normal left ventricular function. Am J Cardiol 1993; 71:710–713.
493. Shalan LJ, Lyon AF. Paradoxical acceleration of atrial flutter after "cardioversion." Am Heart J 1965; 69:684–685.
494. Arnold AZ, Mick MJ, Mazurek RP, Loop FD, Trohman RG. Role of prophylactic anticoagulation for direct current cardioversion in patients with atrial fibrillation or atrial flutter. J Am Coll Cardiol 1992; 19:851–855.
495. Lanzarotti CJ, Olshansky B. Thromboembolism in chronic atrial flutter: is the risk underestimated? J Am Coll Cardiol 1997; 30:1506–1511.
496. DeSanctis RW. Diagnostic and therapeutic uses of atrial pacing. Circulation 1971; 43:748–761.
497. Zipes DP. The contribution of artificial pacemaking to understanding the pathogenesis of arrhythmias. Am J Cardiol 1971; 28:211–222.
498. Cooper TB, MacLean WA, Waldo AL. Overdrive pacing for supraventricular tachycardia: a review of theoretical implications and therapeutic techniques. Pacing Clin Electrophysiol 1978; 1:196–221.
499. Waldo AL. Some observations concerning atrial flutter in man. Pacing Clin Electrophysiol 1983; 6:1181–1189.
500. Waldo AL, Olshansky B, Henthorn RW. Use of implanted antitachycardia pacemakers to treat paroxysmal atrial flutter. Ann Intern Med 1987; 107:247–248.
501. Gillette PC. Antitachycardia pacing. Pacing Clin Electrophysiol 1997; 20:2121–2124.
502. Peters RW, Weiss DN, Carliner NH, Feliciano Z, Shorofsky SR, Gold MR. Overdrive pacing for atrial flutter. Am J Cardiol 1994; 74:1021–1023.
503. Pittman DE, Makar JS, Kooros KS, Joyner CR. Rapid atrial stimulation: successful method of conversion of atrial flutter and atrial tachycardia. Am J Cardiol 1973; 32:700–706.
504. Mills NL, Ochsner JL. Experience with atrial pacemaker wires implanted during cardiac operations. J Thorac Cardiovasc Surg 1973; 66:878–886.
505. Waldo AL, MacLean WA, Karp RB, Kouchoukos NT, James TN. Continuous rapid atrial pacing to control recurrent or sustained supraventricular tachycardias following open heart surgery. Circulation 1976; 54:245–250.
506. Haft JI, Kosowsky BD, Lau SH, Stein E, Damato AN. Termination of atrial flutter by rapid electrical pacing of the atrium. Am J Cardiol 1967; 20:239–244.
507. Hunt NC, Cobb FR, Waxman MB, Zeft HJ, Peter RH, Morris JJ Jr. Conversion of supraventricular tachycardias with atrial stimulation: evidence for reentry mechanisms. Circulation 1968; 38:1060–1065.
508. Zeft HJ, Cobb FR, Waxman MB, Hunt NC, Morris JJ Jr. Right atrial stimulation in the treatment of atrial flutter. Ann Intern Med 1969; 70:447–456.
509. Gulotta SJ, Aronson AL. Cardioversion of atrial tachycardia and flutter by atrial stimulation. Am J Cardiol 1970; 26:262–269.
510. Vergara GS, Hildner FJ, Schoenfeld CB, Javier RP, Cohen LS, Samet P. Conversion of supraventricular tachycardias with rapid atrial stimulation. Circulation 1972; 46:788–793.
511. Orlando J, Cassidy J, Aronow WS. High reversion of atrial flutter to sinus rhythm after atrial pacing in patients with pulmonary disease. Chest 1977; 71:580–582.
512. Das G, Anand KM, Ankineedu K, Chinnavaso T, Talmers FN, Weissler AM. Atrial pacing for cardioversion of atrial flutter in digitalized patients. Am J Cardiol 1978; 41:308–312.
513. Henthorn R, Roberts WS, Kelly K, Leier CV. Conversion of atrial flutter: rapid atrial pacing as a bedside technique. Pacing Clin Electrophysiol 1980; 3:202–206.
514. Della Bella P, Tondo C, Marenzi G, et al. Facilitating influence of disopyramide on atrial flutter termination by overdrive pacing. Am J Cardiol 1988; 61:1046–1049.
515. Hassett JA, Elrod PA, Arciniegas JG, MacLean WA, Duncan JL. Noninvasive diagnosis and treatment of atrial flutter utilizing previously implanted dual chamber pacemaker. Pacing Clin Electrophysiol 1988; 11:1662–1666.
516. Olshansky B, Okumura K, Hess PG, Henthorn RW, Waldo AL. Use of procainamide with rapid atrial pacing for successful conversion of atrial flutter to sinus rhythm. J Am Coll Cardiol 1988; 11:359–364.
517. Crawford W, Plumb VJ, Epstein AE, Kay GN. Prospective evaluation of transesophageal pacing for the interruption of atrial flutter. Am J Med 1989; 86:663–667.
518. Cunningham D, Somerville J, Kennedy JA, Rowland E, Rickards AF. Successful intracardiac electrical conversion of atrial flutter in patients with complex congenital heart disease. Br Heart J 1991; 65:349–354.
519. Della Bella P, Marenzi G, Tondo C, et al. Usefulness of excitable gap and pattern of resetting in atrial flutter for determining reentry circuit location. Am J Cardiol 1991; 68:492–497.
520. Gillette PC, Zeigler VL, Case CL, Harold M, Buckles DS. Atrial antitachycardia pacing in children and young adults. Am Heart J 1991; 122:844–849.
521. Heisel A, Jung J, Stopp M, Schieffer H. Facilitating influence of procainamide on conversion of atrial flutter by rapid atrial pacing. Eur Heart J 1997; 18:866–869.
522. Montoyo JV, Angel J, Valle V, Gausi C. Cardioversion of tachycardias by transesophageal atrial pacing. Am J Cardiol 1973; 32:85–90.
523. Chung DC, Kerr CR, Cooper J. Termination of spontaneous atrial flutter by transesophageal pacing. Pacing Clin Electrophysiol 1987; 10:1147–1153.
524. Guarnerio M, Furlanello F, Del Greco M, Vergara G, Inama G, Disertori M. Transesophageal atrial pacing: a first-choice technique in atrial flutter therapy. Am Heart J 1989; 117:1241–1252.
525. Kaneda S, Inoue T, Fukuzaki H. Treatment of atrial flutter and rapid atrial tachycardia with transesophageal atrial pacing. Jpn Heart J 1989; 30:471–478.
526. Tucker KJ, Wilson C. A comparison of transesophageal atrial pacing and direct current cardioversion for the termination of atrial flutter: a prospective, randomised clinical trial. Br Heart J 1993; 69:530–535.
527. Kantharia BK, Mookherjee S. Clinical utility and the predictors of outcome of overdrive transesophageal atrial pacing in the treatment of atrial flutter. Am J Cardiol 1995; 76:144–147.
528. Rhodes LA, Walsh EP, Saul JP. Conversion of atrial flutter in pediatric patients by transesophageal atrial pacing: a safe, effective, minimally invasive procedure. Am Heart J 1995; 130:323–327.
529. Waldo AL, Carlson MD, Biblo LA, Henthorn RW. The role of transient entrainment in atrial flutter. In Touboul P, Waldo AL (eds). Atrial Arrhythmias. Current Concepts and Management. St. Louis: Mosby–Year Book, 1990, pp. 210–228.
530. Wyndham CR, Wu D, Denes P, Sugarman D, Levitsky S, Rosen KM. Self-initiated conversion of paroxysmal atrial flutter utilizing a radiofrequency pacemaker. Am J Cardiol 1978; 41:1119–1122.

531. Luceri RM, Castellanos A, Thurer RJ, Myerburg RJ. Noninvasive conversion of atrial flutter using a multiprogrammable DDD pulse generator. Pacing Clin Electrophysiol 1986; 9:137–140.

532. Fisher JD, Johnston DR, Kim SG, Furman S, Mercando AM. Implantable pacers for tachycardia termination: stimulation techniques and long-term efficacy. Pacing Clin Electrophysiol 1986; 9:1325–1333.

533. Frohlig G, Sen S, Rettig G, Schieffer H, Bette L. Termination of atrial flutter during DDD pacing by rapid overdrive stimulation using the implanted pacemaker lead system. Am J Cardiol 1986; 57:483–485.

534. Barold SS, Wyndham CR, Kappenberger LL, Abinader EG, Griffin JC, Falkoff MD. Implanted atrial pacemakers for paroxysmal atrial flutter. Long-term efficacy. Ann Intern Med 1987; 107:144–149.

535. Case CL, Gillette PC, Zeigler VL, Oslizlok PC. Successful treatment of congenital atrial flutter with antitachycardia pacing. Pacing Clin Electrophysiol 1990; 13:571–573.

536. Li CK, Shandling AH, Nolasco M, Thomas LA, Messenger JC, Warren J. Atrial automatic tachycardia-reversion pacemakers: their economic viability and impact on quality-of-life. Pacing Clin Electrophysiol 1990; 13:639–645.

537. Barold SS, Falkoff MD. Treatment of atrial flutter by antitachycardia pacemaker: a 13-year follow-up. Am Heart J 1995; 130:187–191.

538. Benson DW, Sanford M, Dunnigan A, Benditt DG. Transesophageal atrial pacing threshold: role of interelectrode spacing, pulse width and catheter insertion depth. Am J Cardiol 1984; 53:63–67.

539. Campbell RM, Dick M II, Jenkins JM, et al. Atrial overdrive pacing for conversion of atrial flutter in children. Pediatrics 1985; 75:730–736.

540. Hii JT, Mitchell LB, Duff HJ, Wyse DG, Gillis AM. Comparison of atrial overdrive pacing with and without extrastimuli for termination of atrial flutter. Am J Cardiol 1992; 70:463–467.

541. Fujimoto T, Inoue T, Ogawa S, et al. The effects of class IA antiarrhythmic drug on the common type of atrial flutter in combination with pacing therapy. Jpn Circ J 1989; 53:237–244.

542. Heldal M, Orning OM. Effects of flecainide on termination of atrial flutter by rapid atrial pacing. Eur Heart J 1993; 14:421–424.

543. Castellanos A, Lemberg L, Fonseca EJ. Significance of ventricular and pseudoventricular arrhythmias appearing after DC countershock. Am Heart J 1965; 70:583–594.

544. Coumel P, Friocourt P, Mugica J, Attuel P, Leclercq JF. Long-term prevention of vagal atrial arrhythmias by atrial pacing at 90/minute: experience with 6 cases. Pacing Clin Electrophysiol 1983; 6:552–560.

545. Sharkey SW, Chaffee V, Kapsner S. Prophylactic external pacing during cardioversion of atrial tachyarrhythmias. Am J Cardiol 1985; 55:1632–1634.

546. Greenspon AJ, Greenberg RM, Frankl WS. Tracking of atrial flutter during DDD pacing: another form of pacemaker-mediated tachycardia. Pacing Clin Electrophysiol 1984; 7:955–960.

547. Kerr CR, Mason MA. Amplitude of atrial electrical activity during sinus rhythm and during atrial flutter-fibrillation. Pacing Clin Electrophysiol 1985; 8:348–355.

548. Touboul P, Saoudi N, Atallah G, Kirkorian G. Electrophysiologic basis of catheter ablation in atrial flutter. Am J Cardiol 1989; 64:79J–82J.

549. Saoudi N, Atallah G, Deschamps D, Sun H, Bouzon R, Chevallier JC. Catheter ablation for atrial flutter. In Touboul P, Waldo AL (eds). Atrial Arrhythmias. Current Concepts and Management. St. Louis: Mosby–Year Book, 1990, pp. 462–475.

550. Saoudi N, Derumeaux G, Cribier A, Letac B. The role of catheter ablation techniques in the treatment of classic (type I) atrial flutter. Pacing Clin Electrophysiol 1991; 14:2022–2027.

551. Scheinman MM. Catheter ablation for cardiac arrhythmias, personnel, and facilities: North American Society of Pacing and Electrophysiology ad hoc committee on catheter ablation. Pacing Clin Electrophysiol 1992; 15:715–721.

552. Hindricks G. The Multicentre European Radiofrequency Survey (MERFS): complications of radiofrequency catheter ablation of arrhythmias. The Multicentre European Radiofrequency Survey (MERFS) investigators of the working group on arrhythmias of the European Society of Cardiology. Eur Heart J 1993; 14:1644–1653.

553. American College of Cardiology Cardiovascular Technology Assessment Committee. Catheter ablation for cardiac arrhythmias: clinical applications, personnel and facilities. American College of Cardiology cardiovascular technology assessment committee. J Am Coll Cardiol 1994; 24:828–833.

554. Bashir Y, Ward DE. Radiofrequency catheter ablation: a new frontier in interventional cardiology. Br Heart J 1994; 71:119–124.

555. Kugler JD. Radiofrequency catheter ablation for supraventricular tachycardia: should it be used in infants and small children? Circulation 1994; 90:639–641.

556. Lesh MD, Van Hare GF. Status of ablation in patients with atrial tachycardia and flutter. PACE 1994; 17:1026–1033.

557. Manolis AS, Wang PJ, Estes NA III. Radiofrequency catheter ablation for cardiac tachyarrhythmias. Ann Intern Med 1994; 121:452–461.

558. Scheinman M, Olgin J. Catheter ablation of cardiac arrhythmias of atrial origin. In Zipes DP (ed). Catheter Ablation of Arrhythmias. Armonk, NY: Futura Publishing Co., 1994, pp. 129–149.

559. Scheinman MM. NASPE survey on catheter ablation. Pacing Clin Electrophysiol 1995; 18:1474–1478.

560. Cosio FG, Arribas F, Lopez-Gil M, Gonzalez HD. Radiofrequency ablation of atrial flutter. J Cardiovasc Electrophysiol 1996; 7:60–70.

561. Saoudi N, Atallah G, Kirkorian G, Touboul P. Catheter ablation of the atrial myocardium in human type I atrial flutter. Circulation 1990; 81:762–771.

562. Trohman RG, Simmons TW, Moore SL, Firstenberg MS, Williams D, Maloney JD. Catheter ablation of the atrioventricular junction using radiofrequency energy and a bilateral cardiac approach. Am J Cardiol 1992; 70:1438–1443.

563. Feld GK, Fleck RP, Chen PS, et al. Radiofrequency catheter ablation for the treatment of human type I atrial flutter: identification of a critical zone in the reentrant circuit by endocardial mapping techniques. Circulation 1992; 86:1233–1240.

564. Cosio FG, Lopez GM, Goicolea A, Barroso JL. Radiofrequency ablation of the inferior vena cava–tricuspid valve isthmus in common atrial flutter. Am J Cardiol 1993; 71:705–709.

565. Cosio FG, Goicolea A, Lopez GM, Arribas F. Catheter ablation of atrial flutter circuits. Pacing Clin Electrophysiol 1993; 16:637–642.

566. Kay GN, Epstein AE, Dailey SM, Plumb VJ. Role of radiofrequency ablation in the management of supraventricular arrhythmias: experience in 760 consecutive patients. J Cardiovasc Electrophysiol 1993; 4:371–389.

567. Lesh MD, Van Hare GF, Epstein LM, et al. Radiofrequency catheter ablation of atrial arrhythmias: results and mechanisms. Circulation 1994; 89:1074–1089.

568. Lesh MD, Van Hare GF. Status of ablation in patients with atrial tachycardia and flutter. Pacing Clin Electrophysiol 1994; 17:1026–1033.

569. Poty H, Saoudi N, Nair M, Anselme F, Letac B. Radiofrequency catheter ablation of atrial flutter: further insights into the various types of isthmus block: application to ablation during sinus rhythm. Circulation 1996; 94:3204–3213.

570. Schwartzman D, Callans DJ, Gottlieb CD, Dillon SM, Movsowitz C, Marchlinski FE. Conduction block in the inferior vena caval-tricuspid valve isthmus: association with outcome of radiofrequency ablation of type I atrial flutter. J Am Coll Cardiol 1996; 28:1519–1531.

571. Saxon LA, Kalman JM, Olgin JE, Scheinman MM, Lee RJ, Lesh MD. Results of radiofrequency catheter ablation for atrial flutter. Am J Cardiol 1996; 77:1014–1016.

572. Chen SA, Chiang CE, Wu TJ, et al. Radiofrequency catheter ablation of common atrial flutter: comparison of electrophysiologically guided focal ablation technique and linear ablation technique. J Am Coll Cardiol 1996; 27:860–868.

573. Lesh MD, Kalman JM, Olgin JE. New approaches to treatment of atrial flutter and tachycardia. J Cardiovasc Electrophysiol 1996; 7:368–381.

574. Cauchemez B, Haissaguerre M, Fischer B, Thomas O, Clementy J, Coumel P. Electrophysiological effects of catheter ablation of inferior vena cava–tricuspid annulus isthmus in common atrial flutter. Circulation 1996; 93:284–294.

575. Fischer B, Jais P, Shah D, et al. Radiofrequency catheter ablation of common atrial flutter in 200 patients. J Cardiovasc Electrophysiol 1996; 7:1225–1233.

576. Shah DC, Jais P, Haissaguerre M, et al. Three-dimensional mapping of the common atrial flutter circuit in the right atrium. Circulation 1997; 96:3904–3912.

577. Stevenson WG, Ellison KE, Lefroy DC, Friedman PL. Ablation therapy for cardiac arrhythmias. Am J Cardiol 1997; 80:56G–66G.

578. Rodriguez E, Man DC, Coyne RF, Callans DJ, Gottlieb CD, Marchlinski FE. Type I atrial flutter ablation guided by a basket catheter. J Cardiovasc Electrophysiol 1998; 9:761–766.

579. Tai CT, Chen SA, Chiang CE, et al. Long-term outcome of radiofrequency catheter ablation for typical atrial flutter: risk prediction of recurrent arrhythmias. J Cardiovasc Electrophysiol 1998; 9:115–121.

580. Case CL, Gillette PC, Douglas DE, Liebermann RA. Radiofrequency catheter ablation of atrial flutter in a patient with postoperative congenital heart disease. Am Heart J 1993; 126:715–716.

581. Van Hare GF, Witherell CL, Lesh MD. Follow-up of radiofrequency catheter ablation in children: results in 100 consecutive patients. J Am Coll Cardiol 1994; 23:1651–1659.

582. Triedman JK, Saul JP, Weindling SN, Walsh EP. Radiofrequency ablation of intraatrial reentrant tachycardia after surgical palliation of congenital heart disease. Circulation 1995; 91:707–714.

583. Iesaka Y, Takahashi A, Goya M, et al. High energy radiofrequency catheter ablation for common atrial flutter targeting the isthmus between the inferior vena cava and tricuspid valve annulus using a super long tip electrode. PACE 1998; 21:401–409.

584. Schumacher B, Pfeiffer D, Tebbenjohanns J, LeWalter T, Jung W, Luderitz B. Acute and long-term effects of consecutive radiofrequency applications on conduction properties of the subeustachian isthmus in type I atrial flutter. J Cardiovasc Electrophysiol 1998; 9:152–163.

585. Cosio FG, Lopez Gil M, Arribas F, Goicolea A. Radiofrequency catheter ablation for the treatment of human type I atrial flutter. Circulation 1993; 88:804–805.

586. Chauvin M, Brechenmacher C. Endocardial catheter fulguration for treatment of atrial flutter. Am J Cardiol 1988; 61:471–473.

587. Chauvin M, Brechenmacher C. A clinical study of the application of endocardial fulguration in the treatment of recurrent atrial flutter. Pacing Clin Electrophysiol 1989; 12:219–224.

588. O'Nunain S, Linker NJ, Sneddon JF, Debbas NM, Camm AJ, Ward DE. Catheter ablation by low energy DC shocks for successful management of atrial flutter. Br Heart J 1992; 67:67–71.

589. Xie B, Murgatroyd FD, Heald SC, Camm AJ, Rowland E, Ward DE. Late follow-up of catheter ablation of atrial flutter using low-energy direct current. Am J Cardiol 1994; 74:947–951.

590. Guiraudon GM, Klein GJ, Yee R, Leitch JW, Kaushik RR, McLellan DG. Surgery for atrial tachycardia. Pacing Clin Electrophysiol 1990; 13:1996–1999.

591. Weber HP, Heinze A. Laser catheter ablation of atrial flutter

and of atrioventricular nodal reentrant tachycardia in a single session. Eur Heart J 1994; 15:1147–1149.

592. Nakagawa H, Jackman WM. Use of a three-dimensional, nonfluoroscopic mapping system for catheter ablation of typical atrial flutter. PACE 1998; 21:1279–1286.

593. Cheema AN, Grais IM, Burke JH, Inbar S, Kadish AH, Goldberger JJ. Late recurrence of atrial flutter following radiofrequency catheter ablation. PACE 1997; 20:2998–3001.

594. Nath S, Mounsey JP, Haines DE, DiMarco JP. Predictors of acute and long-term success after radiofrequency catheter ablation of type I atrial flutter. Am J Cardiol 1995; 76:604–606.

595. Paydak H, Kall JG, Burke MC, et al. Atrial fibrillation after radiofrequency ablation of type I atrial flutter: time to onset, determinants, and clinical course. Circulation 1998; 98:315–322.

596. Frey B, Kreiner G, Binder T, Heinz G, Baumgartner H, Gossinger HD. Relation between left atrial size and secondary atrial arrhythmias after successful catheter ablation of common atrial flutter. PACE 1997; 20:2936–2942.

597. Katritsis D, Iliodromitis E, Fragakis N, Adamopoulos S, Kremastinos D. Ablation therapy of type I atrial flutter may eradicate paroxysmal atrial fibrillation. Am J Cardiol 1996; 78:345–347.

598. Duckeck W, Engelstein ED, Kuck KH. Radiofrequency current therapy in atrial tachyarrhythmias: modulation versus ablation of atrioventricular nodal conduction. Pacing Clin Electrophysiol 1993; 16:629–636.

599. Della Bella P, Maslowsky F, Tondo C, Riva S. Modulation of atrioventricular conduction by ablation of the ''slow'' atrioventricular node pathway in patients with drug-refractory atrial fibrillation or flutter. J Am Coll Cardiol 1995; 25:39–46.

600. Cox JL, Jaquiss RD, Schuessler RB, Boineau JP. Modification of the Maze procedure for atrial flutter and atrial fibrillation. II. Surgical technique of the Maze III procedure. J Thorac Cardiovasc Surg 1995; 110:485–495.

601. Cox JL, Boineau JP, Schuessler RB, Jaquiss RD, Lappas DG. Modification of the Maze procedure for atrial flutter and atrial fibrillation. I. Rationale and surgical results. J Thorac Cardiovasc Surg 1995; 110:473–484.

602. Scalia GM, Stafford WJ, Burstow DJ, Carruthers T, Tesar PJ. Successful treatment of incessant atrial flutter with excision of congenital giant right atrial aneurysm diagnosed by transesophageal echocardiography. Am Heart J 1995; 129:834–835.

603. Luria MH, Knoke JD, Wachs JS, Luria MA. Survival after recovery from acute myocardial infarction: two and five year prognostic indices. Am J Med 1979; 67:7–14.

604. Marriott HJL. Practical Electrocardiography. 4th ed. Baltimore: Williams & Wilkins, 1968.

605. Katz LN, Pick A. Clinical Electrocardiography. Part I: The Arrhythmias. Philadelphia: Lea & Febiger, 1956, 446.

606. White PD, Donovan H. Hearts. Their Long Follow-up. Philadelphia: WB Saunders, 1967, pp. 259–267.

607. Casta A, Wolff GS, Mehta AV, Tamer DF, Pickoff AS, Gelband H. Induction of nonsustained atrial flutter by programmed atrial stimulation in children: incidence, mechanisms, and clinical implications. Am Heart J 1984; 107:444–448.

608. Kerber RE, Jensen SR, Grayzel J, Kennedy J, Hoyt R. Elective cardioversion: influence of paddle-electrode location and size on success rates and energy requirements. N Engl J Med 1981; 305:658–662.

609. Rosen KM, Sinno MZ, Gunnar RM, Rahimtoola SH. Failure of rapid atrial pacing in the conversion of atrial flutter. Am J Cardiol 1972; 29:524–528.

610. Daoud EG, Strickberger SA, Man KC, et al. Preoperative amiodarone as prophylaxis against atrial fibrillation after heart surgery. N Engl J Med 1997; 337:1785–1791.

Atrial Tachycardia[1-16a]

In its long life, atrial tachycardia has had many names[17, 18] (Table 6.1). The phrase is specifically applied, in this chapter, to those arrhythmias that originate in the left or right atria, including the sinus node, and have discrete and uniform P waves preceding the QRS complexes. This definition excludes atrial fibrillation, atrial flutter, and multifocal atrial tachycardia. Furthermore, although atrial tachycardia is a supraventricular and not a ventricular tachycardia, it is not what we have come to call *the* supraventricular tachycardia, which activates the atria but is sustained by reentry in the atrioventricular node and accessory pathways.

Despite the different mechanisms that cause atrial tachycardia and the different places within the atria from which it originates, for clinical purposes, this arrhythmia lends itself to description under one heading because of its

- Consistent electrocardiographic appearance.
- Origin within the atria.
- Susceptibility to treatment by catheter ablation with radiofrequency current.

With the different types of these tachycardias consolidated under one title, let us look at the recent history of our understanding of atrial tachycardia as revealed by the techniques of clinical electrophysiology.

ATRIAL TACHYCARDIA DUE TO ATRIAL REENTRY

Although reciprocation in the atria was suggested as possible early in the twentieth century, it was not until the development of electrophysiological techniques in the 1970s that a clinical arrhythmia in the atria due to this mechanism was described. Clinical studies about reentrant atrial tachycardia often include cases thought to be due to "sinoatrial node reentry." The authors, however, are often describing reentry elsewhere in the atria rather than within or near the sinus node itself. Debate continues whether clinical

reentrant tachycardia in humans does occur *within* the sinus node.[13, 19–21] For purposes of this discussion, let us consider sinus node reentry as part of intra-atrial reentry and reserve the niceties of the distinction to the section of this chapter on electrophysiology.

ATRIAL TACHYCARDIA DUE TO ABNORMAL AUTOMATICITY

Although an automatic mechanism for cases of atrial tachycardia had long been suspected, proof awaited the contemporary use of intracardiac recordings and programmed stimulation. This occurred in Staten Island, New York, where a group of young cardiologists in the cardiac laboratory of the United States Public Health Service Hospital were developing clinical cardiac electrophysiology in the United States during the late 1960s and early 1970s. The report in 1973, by Goldreyer, Gallagher, and Damato,[22] consisted of only three cases, but the thoroughness and care of the analysis defined the clinical and electrophysiological characteristics of automatic atrial tachycardia so well that little additional electrophysiological information has been added since then. Although the first patients proven to have atrial tachycardia due to abnormal automaticity were adults,[22] the arrhythmia occurs more frequently in children, in whom it was first reported after electrophysiological studies in 1976.[23]

Atrial tachycardia caused by abnormally enhanced automaticity almost certainly was observed before its contemporary characterization. Authors reporting pa-

Table 6.1 OTHER NAMES FOR ATRIAL TACHYCARDIA
Atrial tachycardia with exit block[17]
Automatic atrial tachycardia
Ectopic atrial tachycardia
Idioatrial tachycardia[18]
Intra-atrial reentrant supraventricular tachycardia
Sinus nodal reentrant supraventricular tachycardia
Paroxysmal atrial tachycardia
Paroxysmal atrial tachycardia with block
Supraventricular tachycardia

---

*a*This chapter contains material from my Chapter 4[1] and from Chapter 12 by Daniel Flammang and Philippe Coumel,[2] in the first edition of this book.

tients, often children, with chronic supraventricular tachycardia were probably describing, in many cases, automatic atrial tachycardia, the mechanism of which could not be established because the patients were evaluated without electrophysiological studies.[24–41]

OTHER MECHANISMS[42]

Investigators have suggested that triggered activity may cause the arrhythmia thought in some cases to be due to reentry.[43–44]

SOME ADVANCES SINCE THE FIRST EDITION OF THIS BOOK

- Description of the circuits sustaining atrial tachycardia when it develops after surgery for congenital heart disease.
- Use of body-surface mapping to locate the origin of atrial tachycardia.
- Catheter ablation with radiofrequency current ablation superseding surgery as the definitive treatment for many patients.
- Application of intracardiac and transesophageal echocardiography to guide ablation of the arrhythmia.

PREVALENCE

Atrial tachycardia accounts for about 15% of cases of regular supraventricular tachyarrhythmias in adults[13b] and 14% to 23% in children.[45, 46c] Reentry is much the more common mechanism of atrial tachycardia among adults—9% versus 2% for automaticity.[13] Even with different definitions for its diagnosis, reentrant atrial tachycardia arising in or near the sinus node ("sino-atrial nodal reentrant tachycardia") is rare.[47, 48d]

Until the 1990s, few cases of adults with automatic atrial tachycardia proven by electrophysiological study had been reported.[22, 49–51] More recently, however, the arrhythmia has been documented more frequently.[44, 52–54e]

Children

Among children with supraventricular tachycardias, reentry and automaticity account for approximately the same proportion—12% from reentry, 11% from automaticity.[45] Automaticity is the most common cause of chronic or persistent supraventricular tachycardias in children,[55] and about 20% of all supraventricular tachycardias in children are chronic.[11, 56]

Digitalis[57–60]

Atrial tachycardia with atrioventricular block, long associated with digitalis overdosage, was a frequently diagnosed arrhythmia several decades ago.[61f] It occurs less often now because of the following:

- Greater awareness of digitalis toxicity, thanks in great measure to the digitalis assay.[58]
- The use of other agents such as beta-adrenergic and calcium-channel–blocking drugs to slow atrioventricular nodal conduction and to decrease ventricular rates in arrhythmias such as atrial fibrillation and atrial flutter.
- The availability of drugs other than digitalis to treat congestive heart failure.

AGE

In general, automatic atrial tachycardia occurs at an earlier age than does the reentrant arrhythmia.[62]

Adults

The mean age of 49 patients presenting with atrial tachycardia for electrophysiologic study was 35 years, with a range of 2 to 73 years.[63] Among 46 adults with reentrant atrial tachycardia, the mean age was 55 years, with a range of 24 to 80 years.[47, 64, 65g] The average age at which 37 adults with automatic atrial tachycardia presented for treatment was 42 years.[22, 49, 51, 54, 66–69]

Children

Among 12 children, the average age of onset of atrial tachycardia due to reentry was 7 to 8 years.[45] The average age of presentation of 54 children from the largest published series of patients with automatic atrial tachycardia was 7.2 years,[11] and the average age of 54 children collected from 10 other reports was 5.5 years.[5, 45, 47, 70–76] Atrial tachycardia has been detected *in utero.*[77, 78]

The average age of *onset* of automatic atrial tachycardia in children is earlier than with most other supraventricular tachycardias. In a series of 11 patients, it was 2 years,[45] and the arrhythmia was observed in no child older than 6 years.[45] The age at which most children first come to medical attention, however, is often later.[45]

GENDER

Males and females, whether adults or children, develop atrial tachycardia in equal proportion.[5, 22, 49, 51, 53, 54, 66–74, 76, 79h]

---

[b]Range is 11% to 19% from two large series from Philadelphia and Maastricht of 663 patients, mostly adults, and each studied with electrophysiological techniques.[13]

[c]Twenty-four (23%) of 103 children in one series[45] and 19 (14%) of 137 in another.[46] Electrophysiological studies established the mechanisms in each case.[45, 46]

[d]It was found in only 1 of 20 patients with reentrant atrial tachycardia[47] and in 3.2% of 343 patients with supraventricular tachycardia referred for electrophysiological evaluation.[48]

[e]Eight patients in one series[44] and 25 in another.[54]

---

[f]Atrial tachycardia due to digitalis was found in 32 (0.4%) of 896 electrocardiograms read at one university teaching hospital during 1957.[61]

[g]From three of the largest series of reentrant atrial tachycardia, including some patients labeled as having sinoatrial reentrant atrial tachycardia.[47, 64, 65]

[h]Of 49 patients with atrial tachycardia, 23 were men and 26 were women.[79] In those reports in which the gender of the patients with atrial tachycardia due to automaticity was given, 18 of 37 adults were male,[22, 49, 51, 54, 66–69] and 14 of 23 children were female.[5, 70–74, 76]

GENETICS

One group reported a family history of supraventricular tachycardias in 50% of children with automatic atrial tachycardia.[45] In another study of 10 children, only 1 had a family history of supraventricular tachycardia.[76] A father and his two sons each presented with atrial tachycardia in the newborn period.[80]

CLINICAL SETTING

Structural Heart Disease

Most adults with atrial tachycardia due to reentry have structural heart disease.[13] Among 73 patients, 71% had, in descending order of occurrence, ischemic cardiomyopathy, valvular heart disease, dilated cardiomyopathy, hypertensive cardiomyopathy, and pulmonary disease.[47, 64, 65, 81–84][i] Those with reentry in or near the sinus node seem less likely to have structural heart disease.[43, 48] About half of adults with automatic atrial tachycardia have no structural heart disease.[54][j]

Except for tachycardia-induced cardiomyopathy, structural heart disease is seldom present in children with atrial tachycardia.[11, 45, 54, 76, 85] Atrial tachycardia, usually reentrant, however, can develop from operations that remodel the atria in treating congenital heart disease, such as the Mustard, Senning, and Fontan procedures,[86–95] and from repair of atrial septal defect.[k] Limiting the number of atrial incisions to those absolutely necessary reduces the incidence of reentrant atrial tachycardia.[96] Rarely, primary skeletal and cardiac myopathy and automatic atrial tachycardia occur in the same patient.[97]

Myocardial Infarction. Seven percent of patients develop atrial and supraventricular tachycardias during acute myocardial infarction.[98–106][l]

Pulmonary Disease and Cor Pulmonale

Several observers reported, before contemporary criteria for the arrhythmia and techniques to confirm its electrophysiology were available, what appear to be paroxysms of atrial tachycardia in patients with severe pulmonary disease.[107, 108]

Valvular Heart Disease

Ambulatory monitoring has documented paroxysms of atrial tachycardia in patients with mitral stenosis.[109]

---

[i]From seven series; range, 40% to 100%.[47, 64, 65, 81–84]

[j]Fourteen of 25 adults in one series. Five of the remaining 11 with structural heart disease had cardiomyopathy.[54]

[k]In some of the literature on pediatric atrial tachycardia, writers confuse the reader by using the terms "atrial tachycardia" and "atrial flutter" almost interchangeably.[21, 87, 90]

[l]One hundred forty of 2,020 in eight series (range 2% to 16% in the series with more than 100 patients).[98–103, 105, 106] The data on this subject were developed from electrocardiographic monitoring without electrophysiological evaluation, so we do not definitely know the mechanisms of these arrhythmias and how many originated in the atria. I suspect, however, that many, if not most, were atrial tachycardias as defined in this chapter.

Secondary Cardiomyopathy[110]

Persistent, usually automatic, atrial tachycardia produces cardiomyopathy,[45, 54, 66, 69, 73–76, 80, 85, 111–120] particularly in children, approximately half of whom when evaluated for chronic atrial tachycardia have cardiomyopathy on initial examination.[11, 55, 76] An enlarged heart on chest radiograph or echocardiographic evidence of chamber enlargement or reduced ventricular function confirms the diagnosis.[11, 116] The persistence of atrial tachycardia for weeks, months, and sometimes years probably accounts for the relatively high incidence of secondary cardiomyopathy found in these patients.[45]

Digitalis Toxicity[121]

Because atrioventricular block often accompanies the tachycardia that results from intoxication with digitalis, the arrhythmia has long been called "paroxysmal atrial tachycardia with block"—paroxysmal because of its relatively short life, with resolution when the drug is withdrawn.

Paroxysmal atrial tachycardia with block usually develops in adults with digitalis overdosage who have severe heart or pulmonary disease and, in many cases, hypokalemia.[61, 122–132] The arrhythmia, however, can develop from causes other than digitalis toxicity.[125, 133–135]

Miscellaneous

Atrial tachycardia has also been associated with the following:

- The combination of "nontoxic" blood levels of theophylline and therapeutic concentrations of digoxin.[136]
- The site of electroshock catheter ablation of an accessory pathway.[137]
- The postoperative period after cardiac transplantation.[138]
- Atrial rhabdomyoma.[117]
- Exercise in a patient taking flecainide.[139]
- Pregnancy.[140, 141]
- Swallowing.[142–144]
- Sitting and standing in a patient whose atrial tachycardia, probably automatic, stopped when supine.[145]

OTHER ARRHYTHMIAS IN PATIENTS WITH ATRIAL TACHYCARDIA

Supraventricular Arrhythmias

Another atrial arrhythmia, particularly atrial flutter or atrial fibrillation, occurs either clinically or during electrophysiological study in about one-fourth of patients with reentrant atrial tachycardia.[47, 146–148][m] Supraventricular tachycardia sustained in the atrioventricular node or accessory pathways may also appear concurrently with reentrant atrial tachycardia.[47, 48, 149–151]

---

[m]In 45 patients from three series.[47, 146, 147]

Ventricular Arrhythmias

Spontaneous polymorphic ventricular tachycardia, which was successfully converted, developed in a 24-year-old woman with automatic atrial tachycardia probably from an associated peripartum cardiomyopathy possibly exacerbated by the tachycardia and from the pro-arrhythmic effect of amiodarone or flecainide.[69]

Atrial Dissociation and Double Tachycardia

Atrial tachycardia in one atrium can coexist with a different arrhythmia in the other[92, 152] in the arrhythmia known as atrial dissociation. In double or simultaneous tachycardia, atrial tachycardia and another arrhythmia in the atrioventricular junction or ventricles coexist.[n]

HISTORY

The symptoms most patients with reentrant atrial tachycardia report are palpitations, dizziness, and occasionally syncope. A few have angina or heart failure.

Paroxysms of the arrhythmia characterize most patients with reentrant atrial tachycardia.[62] They observe the typical symptoms—episodic, transient bursts of regular tachycardia, sometimes lasting only a few seconds, with sudden onset and termination.[44] However, about one-third of patients are unaware when the arrhythmia is present, partly, it is thought, because of the relatively slow rate of the tachycardia in some cases.[47, 48, 64, 81, 146, 153o]

Automatic atrial tachycardia is characteristically a persistent or chronic arrhythmia and is seldom paroxysmal.[62p] Many patients have known of rapid heart action for months and even years. Shortness of breath on exertion, easy fatiguability, and, in young children, failure to thrive are the most commonly reported symptoms.[49, 66, 73, 75, 76] Syncope occasionally occurs.[51, 66, 75] Patients who develop cardiomyopathy from the tachycardia present with the usual symptoms of this condition.

PHYSICAL EXAMINATION

The physical examination of patients with atrial tachycardia has seldom been reported. In a series of 20 patients, examination revealed—except when the arrhythmia was incessant—normal rhythm interrupted by single premature beats, short runs, or sustained episodes of regular tachycardia.[47] Findings of mitral valve disease were observed in four, and findings of aortic valve disease were noted in one patient.[47]

Observers also report diaphoresis and hypotension,[51] augmented pulmonary component of the second heart sound,[72] edema,[154] and hypotension with cyanosis and shock.[112] Patients with cardiomyopathy due to the arrhythmia develop the physical signs of congestive heart failure.

ELECTROCARDIOGRAPHY

Atrial tachycardia when due to reentry usually appears as short bursts of paroxysmal regular supraventricular tachycardia, the onset of which is abrupt and the termination spontaneous and sudden. Automatic atrial tachycardia is more frequently chronic or incessant without a well-defined beginning or end.

Rate

The average rate is about 151 beats per minute, with a range of 95 to 230 beats per minute.[47, 64, 81, 146, 147, 155–158q] Generally, the faster the tachycardia, the longer the spontaneous episodes.[47] Occasionally, the arrhythmia starts when the sinus rate rises to a particular rate (Fig. 6.1).

The fastest average atrial rate—and consequently the fastest ventricular rate because most adults with automatic atrial tachycardia have 1:1 conduction—is about 165 beats per minute (range, 136–280 beats/min).[22, 49, 51, 66–69, 137, 154r] The average slowest rate reported is 135 beats per minute (range, 117–150 beats/min).[49, 51, 67–69, 137, 154]

Digitalis Toxicity.[57] The atrial rate of paroxysmal atrial tachycardia with block usually ranges from 150 to 250 beats per minute.[128] The slowest atrial rate, in a series of 88 patients, was 106 beats per minute, and in three-fourths of 83 episodes, the atrial rate did not exceed 190 beats per minute.[128] Some patients reported to have "paroxysmal atrial tachycardia with block" and faster atrial rates may have had atrial flutter.[159] The ventricular rate is characteristically slower than the atrial rate because atrioventricular block, often in the ratio of 2:1, is usually present when digitalis overdosage produces atrial tachycardia.

Children. In the largest single series of children with atrial tachycardia due to automaticity, the mean rate was 143 beats per minute (range, 90–240 beats/min). In 47 cases, the average rate was 207 beats per minute (range, 110–320 beats/min).[5, 45, 71–76, 112s]

In general, the younger the child with automatic atrial tachycardia is, the faster the rate. For example, in a series of 10 children, the average rate of six patients younger than one year of age was 168 beats per minute, whereas the average rate was 133 beats per minute in the four older children.[76]

---

[n]See Chapter 9 for a discussion of double tachycardia.

[o]From 58 patients in five reports.[47, 64, 81, 146, 153] In a series of 20 patients,[47] palpitations were reported by 12, mild dyspnea by seven, dizziness by three, and fainting by one; eight had no symptoms.

[p]Authors apply different criteria when defining which arrhythmias are persistent or chronic. The group with the largest series of children with automatic atrial tachycardia considers the arrhythmia to be persistent when it is present more than 90% of the time during a 24-hour period.[11]

[q]Among 84 patients in nine series.[47, 64, 81, 146, 147, 155–158]

[r]Among 13 patients with automatic atrial tachycardia collected from nine series.[22, 49, 51, 66–69, 137, 154]

[s]Rate abstracted from 10 other reports.[5, 45, 71–76, 112] The variance in heart rates between the single largest series[11] and the 47 cases abstracted from the other reports may be due to inconsistencies in reporting average rates and fastest rates for individual patients and because of differences in age.

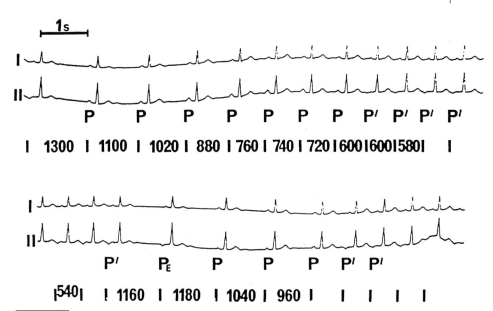

FIGURE 6.1 Spontaneous onset of reentrant atrial tachycardia. The progressive acceleration of the sinus rate initiates an episode of reentrant atrial tachycardia that can be identified by beat P', the first beat with the abnormal P wave **(top)**. An episode of reentrant atrial tachycardia (first three beats, the last one identified as P') terminates with an atrial escape beat (beat P$_E$). Then, sinus rhythm resumes, and progressive acceleration of the sinus rate restarts the reentrant tachycardia (beat P') **(bottom)**. Each panel consists of leads I and II and the intervals or cycle lengths in milliseconds between the P waves. (From Flammang D, Coumel P. Supraventricular tachycardia with reentry in the sinus node or atria. In Kastor JA, ed. Arrhythmias. Philadelphia: WB Saunders, 1994, with permission.)[2]

The rate of the tachycardia determines the likelihood of developing, and the severity of, the secondary cardiomyopathy that many children with automatic atrial tachycardia develop.[11, 112] Left ventricular function is reduced in 94% of children with automatic atrial tachycardia whose heart rate is 130 beats per minute or faster and in 100% of those with heart rates of 150 beats per minute or greater.[11] In infants, rates of 180 to 200 beats per minute are probably necessary to cause cardiomyopathy.[75]

P Wave

As during sinus rhythm, P waves with uniform morphology precede the QRS complexes in patients with both reentrant (Figs. 6.2 and 6.3) and automatic atrial tachycardia[11, 17, 45, 52, 70, 116, 147, 160, 161] (Figs. 6.4 to 6.6). The form of the P waves is usually different from those in sinus rhythm in patients whose arrhythmia is due to reentry.[47, 54, 70, 137, 162t] When the P waves are similar, the arrhythmia arises in or near the sinus node ("sinoatrial nodal reentrant atrial tachycardia") (see Fig. 6.2).

The form of the P waves can often,[52, 54, 70, 137, 152, 162, 163] but not always,[164] predict where in the atria the arrhythmia arises (Table 6.2). For example, the axes

---

tIn one series of reentrant atrial tachycardia, the P waves were slightly or greatly different than during sinus rhythm in 19 of 20 patients (see Fig. 6.2).[47] In only one patient was the form of the P wave the same.

V$_1$

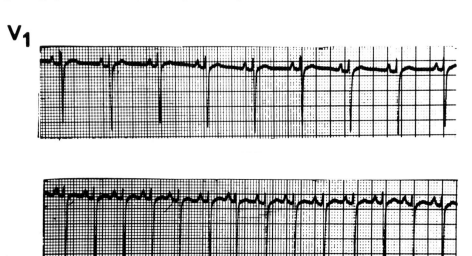

FIGURE 6.2 Reentrant atrial tachycardia. Notice that P waves in lead V$_1$ precede the QRS complexes when the patient is in sinus rhythm at 88 beats per minute **(top)** and in atrial tachycardia at 150 beats per minute **(bottom)**. The arrhythmia probably originates near the sinus node in view of the similar form of the P waves during both the tachycardia and sinus rhythm.

25mm/sec   1 sec

A

B

C

FIGURE 6.3   Paroxysmal reentrant atrial tachycardia originating in or near the sinus node (Lead II). Intermittent 2:1 sinoatrial block **(A)**. An atrial premature beat (beat 3) provokes an episode of reentrant atrial tachycardia at a rate of 125 beats per minute, which spontaneously terminates **(B)**. During another episode, three junctional escape beats appear between spontaneous termination and reinitiation **(C)**. Notice the similar form of the P waves, as best one can tell, during tachycardia and sinus rhythm. First-degree atrioventricular block is present during the arrhythmia. (From Flammang D, Coumel P. Supraventricular tachycardia with reentry in the sinus node or atria. In Kastor JA, ed. Arrhythmias. Philadelphia: WB Saunders, 1994, with permission.)[2]

of the P wave were 0 to +90 degrees in 69% of 64 children with automatic atrial tachycardia from two large series.[11, 76] This is the range of axes for sinus rhythm and suggests that the arrhythmia usually originates in the high right atrium.[52] Axes of 0 to −90 degrees suggested origin in the low right atrium in

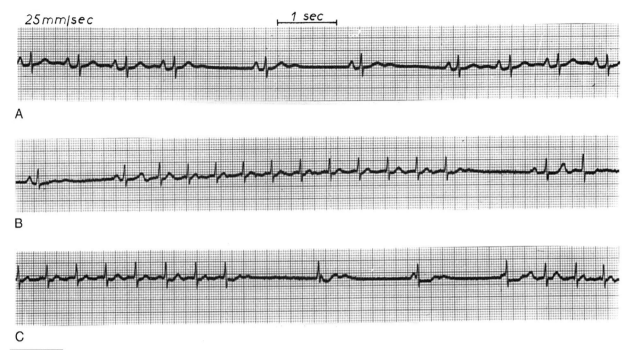

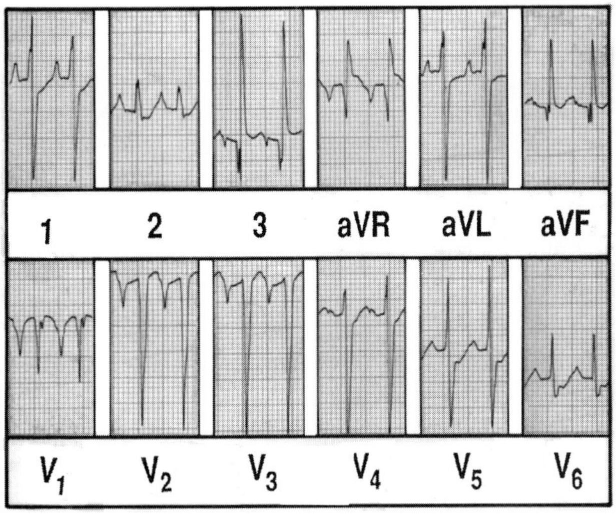

FIGURE 6.4   A child with automatic atrial tachycardia. The heart rate is 180 beats per minute with 1:1 atrioventricular conduction. Notice the unusual form of the P waves, the axis of which in the frontal plane is about +30 degrees. (Courtesy of Dr. Paul C. Gillette, from Kastor JA. Automatic atrial tachycardia. In Kastor JA, ed. Arrhythmias. Philadelphia: WB Saunders, 1994, with permission.)[1]

9%, and axes of +91 to 180 degrees in 22% suggested left atrial origin.

PR Interval

Atrioventricular conduction during atrial tachycardia is either normal or prolonged. The PR interval may be shorter, equal to, or longer than the PR interval during sinus rhythm. Second- or third-degree atrioventricular block[165] may occur at any time during tachycardia without affecting the atrial rhythm (Fig. 6.7).[u] In atrial tachycardia produced by digitalis toxicity, the degree of block is often 2:1 (Fig. 6.8).

Among children with atrial tachycardia due to abnormal automaticity, first-degree atrioventricular block occurs in 20%[166] to 91%,[11, 167] according to the two largest series.[v] As many as 24% develop second-degree atrioventricular block,[11] but third-degree block has not been reported.[168] Individual patients may have differ-

---

[u]Second-degree block within the atrioventricular node was present in 11 of 20 cases of atrial tachycardia due to reentry.[47]

[v]The reasons for the range of incidence of heart block between these two series has not been completely explained. Mehta[166] reported that most of his patients came from primary care practices and were not referred as particularly troublesome cases. He suggested that the cases of Garson and colleagues[11] may have been sicker and referred for tertiary care. Garson[167] observed that first-degree atrioventricular block occurs frequently in children with automatic atrial tachycardia because the acceleration of atrioventricular nodal conduction, expected during sinus tachycardia with its associated autonomic changes, may not develop to the same degree in most children with automatic atrial tachycardia.

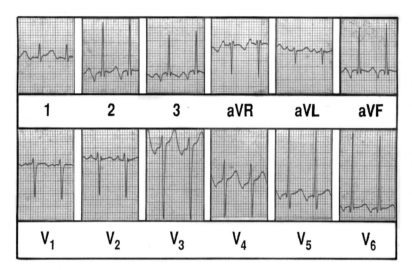

FIGURE 6.5 A child with automatic atrial tachycardia. The heart rate is 140 beats per minute and there is one P wave for every QRS complex. One can easily see the abnormal, usually biphasic appearance of the P waves in most of the leads. (Courtesy of Dr. Paul C. Gillette, from Kastor JA. Automatic atrial tachycardia. In Kastor JA, ed. Arrhythmias. Philadelphia: WB Saunders, 1994, with permission.)[1]

Table 6.2 **SITE OF ORIGIN OF ATRIAL TACHYCARDIA ACCORDING TO THE FORM OF THE P WAVES**

	Electrocardiographic Leads					
Location	I	II, III, aVF	II, III	aVL	V$_1$	V$_4$–V$_6$
Right atrium					Positive	
Appendage or superior lateral		Positive				
Inferior vena cava, coronary sinus ostium, or posteroseptal space		Negative				
Left atrium				Negative	"Dome and dart"	Negative
Appendage or superior pulmonary veins			Positive			
Inferior left lateral			Negative			
Low lateral	Negative					

(Data from references 54, 70, 137, and 162.)

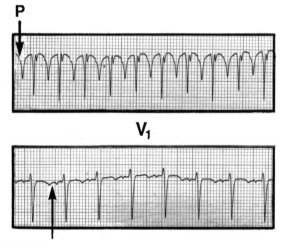

FIGURE 6.6 A child with automatic atrial tachycardia. Rhythm strips of lead V$_1$ of the patients illustrated in Figures 6.4 and 6.5. The ectopic P waves are indicated. (Courtesy of Dr. Paul C. Gillette, from Kastor JA. Automatic atrial tachycardia. In Kastor JA, ed. Arrhythmias. Philadelphia: WB Saunders, 1994, with permission.)[1]

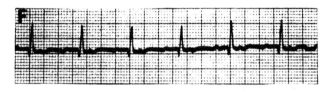
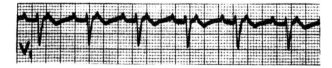

FIGURE 6.7 Automatic atrial tachycardia with 2:1 block. The atrial rate is 176 beats per minute, and the ventricular rate is 88 beats per minute. Ventriculophasic sinus arrhythmia is present; the PP intervals, which include the QRS complexes, are slightly shorter than those which do not. Note that the P waves are better recognized in lead V$_1$ and that a cursory look at aVF may lead to the incorrect diagnosis of sinus rhythm. (Illustration by Dr. Arthur Garson, Jr., from a patient of Dr. Paul C. Gillette, from Kastor JA. Automatic atrial tachycardia. In Kastor JA, ed. Arrhythmias. Philadelphia: WB Saunders, 1994, with permission.)[1]

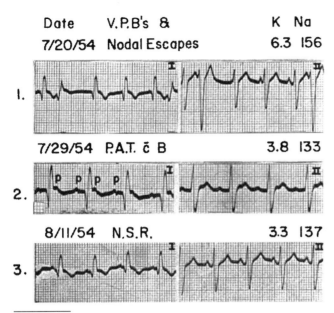

FIGURE 6.8 Automatic atrial tachycardia with atrioventricular block, or "paroxysmal atrial tachycardia (PAT) with block" as it was formerly called, produced in this case by digitalis toxicity (2) in a 45-year-old man with uremia. Sinus rhythm returned when the drug was stopped (3). (Adapted from Lown B, Wyatt NF, Levine HD. Paroxysmal atrial tachycardia with block. Circulation 1960; 21:129–143, with permission. In this article, the arrhythmia when produced by digitalis was first described.)[128]

ent degrees of atrioventricular block at different times.[49, 72, 74]

QRS Complex

The QRS complexes of children with automatic atrial tachycardia are usually normal,[76] although a few have left ventricular hypertrophy with strain[71] and rate-related right bundle branch block.[51] Chronic bundle branch block or other abnormalities of intraventricular conduction present during sinus rhythm usually persist during the tachycardia and do not affect the tachycardia even when they develop for the first time during the arrhythmia.

Alternans. The form of the QRS complexes may alternate in patients with atrial tachycardia as in patients with supraventricular tachycardia.[169–171] The faster the rate, the more likely alternans will develop.[171]

ST and T Wave

Depression of the ST segments of 2 millimeters or more or inverted T waves or both are seldom present in the electrocardiograms of patients with atrial tachycardia compared with patients with supraventricular tachycardia sustained in the atrioventricular node or accessory pathways.[158] This finding presumably relates to the absence of retrograde P waves in the ST segments during atrial tachycardia.[158]

In addition, of course, ST- and T-wave abnormalities may reflect ischemia or metabolic abnormalities. In

patients with coronary heart disease, these abnormalities may worsen when the tachycardia is rapid.

Defining the Mechanism of a Regular Supraventricular Tachycardia from the Electrocardiogram

From careful study of the surface electrocardiogram, one can often decide whether a regular tachyarrhythmia with narrow QRS complexes is sinus rhythm, atrial tachycardia, or supraventricular tachycardia sustained in the atrioventricular node or an accessory pathway and whether the arrhythmia is due to reentry or to abnormal automaticity.[170, 172, 173]

Sinus Tachycardia Versus Atrial Tachycardia. Atrial tachycardia can easily be mistaken for sinus tachycardia because, in most patients, the P waves in both conditions precede the QRS complexes, and the abnormal P waves of atrial tachycardia can easily be misinterpreted to be slightly deformed P waves of sinus rhythm. To complicate matters further, the P waves in sinus rhythm and automatic atrial tachycardia often have similar axes, particularly in children.[11, 76] The absence of a tracing in sinus rhythm adds to the confusion. As a result, patients with cardiomyopathy due to automatic atrial tachycardia may be thought to have primary cardiomyopathy with secondary sinus tachycardia[75, 174] (Fig. 6.9).[w]

Several electrocardiographic[168] and echocardiographic clues (Table 6.3) can help to differentiate

[w]A 12-year-old girl was referred for cardiac transplantation because of congestive heart failure and "sinus tachycardia" of 150 beats per minute.[75] Myocardial biopsies showed slight increase in fibrous tissue and polymorphonuclear leukocytes. She was treated with prednisone until an electrophysiological study demonstrated atrial tachycardia, which was then successfully ablated with cryotherapy producing sinus rhythm and resolution of the cardiomyopathy (see Fig. 6.9).

Table 6.3	**AUTOMATIC ATRIAL TACHYCARDIA FROM THE RIGHT ATRIUM VERSUS SINUS TACHYCARDIA: DIFFERENCES IN THE ELECTROCARDIOGRAM, HOLTER RECORDING, AND ECHOCARDIOGRAM AMONG CHILDREN WITH CARDIOMYOPATHY**	
Finding[a]	**Right Atrial Automatic Tachycardia**	**Sinus Tachycardia**
Atrial rate (%)[b]	148	103
P-wave axis (degrees in the horizontal plane)	31	58
P-wave duration in lead V_1 (msec)	90	78
Maximum rate awake (%)[b]	182	145
Maximum rate asleep (%)[b]	159	127
Left ventricular end-diastolic dimension[c]	101	127
Shortening fraction (%)	30	16

[a]Each comparison is significant at $P<.015$ to $P<.0001$.
[b]Normalized for age with the mean predicted heart rate for age.
[c]Normalized with the predicted ninety-fifth percentile end-diastolic dimension for body weight.
(Adapted from Gelb BD, Garson A Jr. Noninvasive discrimination of right atrial ectopic tachycardia from sinus tachycardia in "dilated cardiomyopathy." Am Heart J 1990; 120:886–891.)

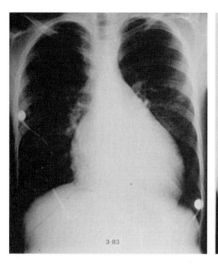
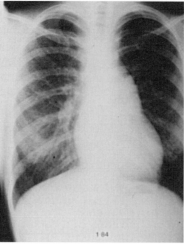

FIGURE 6.9 Secondary cardiomyopathy from automatic atrial tachycardia. Posteroanterior chest radiographs of a 12-year-old girl **(left)**. The size of the heart approached normal after cryoablative surgical treatment of the arrhythmia **(right)**. (Courtesy of Dr. Paul C. Gillette, from Kastor JA. Automatic atrial tachycardia. In Kastor JA, ed. Arrhythmias. Philadelphia: WB Saunders, 1994, with permission.)[1]

sinus tachycardia from automatic atrial tachycardia originating in the right atrium,[x] which usually has

- Faster rates.
- Longer PR intervals.
- Inverted, prolonged, or notched P waves in lead V_1.
- Echocardiographic signs of severe left ventricular dysfunction[168] (see Table 6.3).

Holter monitoring can help to identify automatic atrial tachycardia because, although the rate of the arrhythmia may decrease during sleep, sinus arrhythmia is absent.[75, 168] Exercise can increase the rate of atrial tachycardia slightly, but the changes in rate characteristic of sinus tachycardia under the influence of autonomic control do not occur.[49]

Reentrant Versus Automatic Tachycardias. Regardless of location,

- Reentrant tachycardias are more likely to be paroxysmal and automatic tachycardias incessant.[45]
- The rate of reentrant tachycardia is reached almost at once after the onset of the arrhythmia. Afterward, the rate tends to oscillate.[45] The rate of automatic atrial tachycardia gradually speeds or "warms up" after it starts[22] (Fig. 6.10).
- Vagotonic agents and beta-adrenergic–blocking drugs convert reentrant tachycardias to sinus

---

[x]Automatic atrial tachycardia from the left atrium characteristically produces inverted P waves in lead I and would not ordinarily be confused with sinus tachycardia.[70]

rhythm, but they decrease the rate of, rather than convert, automatic tachycardias.

Reentrant Versus Automatic Atrial Tachycardia

- The P wave of the first beat of reentrant atrial tachycardia is often different from those in the rest of the tachycardia, whereas in automatic atrial tachycardia, all the P waves have the same form (Fig. 6.11).
- The atrial escape beats of reentrant atrial tachycardia have the same morphology as the P waves during the tachycardia.

Reentrant Atrial Tachycardia Versus Reentrant Supraventricular Tachycardia Sustained in the Atrioventricular Node or Accessory Pathways. Each of these tachyarrhythmias is usually paroxysmal, not persistent. In addition:

- Preexcitation in the resting electrocardiogram suggests the presence of an accessory pathway that can sustain the tachycardia.
- In reentrant atrial tachycardia, the P waves, although usually abnormally formed, are easily visible and precede normal PR intervals. The PR intervals tend to be shorter in atrial tachycardia than in atrioventricular junctional or accessory pathway supraventricular tachycardia in which the P waves appear either within or just after the QRS complexes.[161]
- The P waves in reentrant supraventricular tachycardia are inverted in the inferior leads and

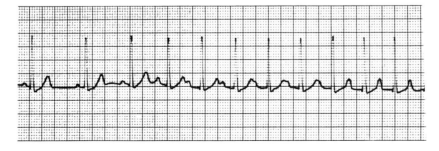

FIGURE 6.10 Typical "warming up" at the onset of automatic atrial tachycardia. After two sinus beats, the tachycardia begins, its rate increases, and the PR intervals prolong as the P waves merge with the T waves. (Adapted from Gillette PA, Garson A Jr. Electrophysiologic and pharmacologic characteristics of automatic ectopic atrial tachycardia. Circulation 1977; 56:571–575, with permission.)[1]

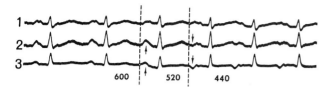

FIGURE 6.11 *Automatic atrial tachycardia.* Leads I, II, and III from one of the three adults in the first electrophysiological report of the arrhythmia. The first three P waves are sinus beats. The fourth P wave is the first of three atrial depolarizations from the abnormal focus. Note how the form of the P waves differ between sinus rhythm *(upward arrows)* and atrial tachycardia *(downward arrows)* and that each of the P waves of the abnormal tachycardia has the same form. The sinus rate is 100 beats per minute (600 milliseconds between P waves). The first abnormal P wave follows 520 milliseconds after the third sinus P wave. The tachycardia has a PP interval of 440 milliseconds or a rate of 136 beats per minute. (Adapted from Goldreyer BN, Gallagher JJ, Damato AN. The electrophysiologic demonstration of atrial ectopic tachycardia in man. Am Heart J 1973; 85:205–215, with permission. This article introduced the concept of ectopic (automatic) atrial tachycardia.)[22]

either closely precede, follow, or are buried within the QRS complexes.

• Reentrant atrial tachycardia can continue despite the development of atrioventricular block, whereas atrioventricular block disrupts supraventricular tachycardia in the atrioventricular node or accessory pathway.

Automatic Atrial Tachycardia Versus Supraventricular Tachycardia Sustained in the Atrioventricular Node or Accessory Pathways. Automatic atrial tachycardia is usually a persistent arrhythmia.[22] Reentrant arrhythmias sustained within the atrioventricular node and accessory pathways are usually, but not always, paroxysmal. In addition:

• The first P wave of automatic atrial tachycardia has the same form as the other P waves (see Fig. 6.11). In atrioventricular reentry, the first beat is a spontaneous ectopic atrial or ventricular beat that triggers the circuit. Subsequent P waves, if they are seen, have a different morphology because they do not originate from the same location as the first beat.

• The first beat of a paroxysm of automatic atrial tachycardia characteristically occurs late, just before the next sinus P wave would be expected to appear.[22] In atrioventricular reentry, the first beat must usually be sufficiently premature to block in the atrioventricular node or bypass tract and to establish the reentry.

• The P waves may be upright or inverted, depending on the site of origin, but they always precede the QRS complexes as in sinus rhythm. They are not buried within, or follow, the QRS complexes, as in atrioventricular nodal or bypass tract reentry.[45, 147]

• The PR interval of the first ectopic beat of automatic atrial tachycardia is similar to those of the other beats.[22] This finding indicates that atrioventricular nodal delay, essential to establish reentrant arrhythmias involving the atrioventricular

node, is not required for atrial automaticity to begin. Automatic, as well as reentrant, atrial tachycardia does not depend on the state of atrioventricular conduction and can thus continue in the presence of atrioventricular block.

• Ventricular premature beats often institute reentrant tachycardias in accessory pathways, but rarely do they start reentrant atrial tachycardia.[157]

• Vagotonic maneuvers and drugs convert reentrant supraventricular tachycardia, but not automatic atrial tachycardia, in which they may increase atrioventricular block or may slightly decrease the rate of the tachycardia.[45, 68, 69]

ELECTROCARDIOGRAM IN SINUS RHYTHM

The P waves are more often normal than abnormal during sinus rhythm in patients with reentrant atrial tachycardia.[47y] Sinoatrial block occasionally occurs (see Fig. 6.3).[47] The PR interval is more frequently normal than abnormal.[47z] Bundle branch and intraventricular block are uncommon.[47] Because the arrhythmia in patients with automatic atrial tachycardia is often chronic, 12-lead electrocardiograms taken during brief periods of sinus rhythm have seldom been obtained or published.[aa]

DIFFERENTIAL DIAGNOSIS

Using the surface electrocardiogram, cardiologists can often successfully differentiate atrial tachycardia from those other supraventricular tachycardias, not so far discussed.

Atrial Fibrillation

Whereas P waves are characteristically present in atrial tachycardia, organized atrial activity is absent in atrial fibrillation, and undulating, irregular F waves replace the P waves. The ventricular rhythm is irregular.

Atrial Flutter

In flutter, the P waves are replaced by the characteristic sawtooth pattern of the flutter waves. Because atrioventricular block in atrial flutter may vary, the ventricular

---

[y]In 20 patients with reentrant atrial tachycardia, P-wave morphology during sinus rhythm was normal or nearly normal in 13 (65%), whereas an intraatrial conduction disturbance was present in seven.[47] The duration of the sinus P waves was equal to, or less than, 120 milliseconds in 17 cases and more than 160 milliseconds in three cases.

[z]In the same 20 patients, the PR interval was less than 200 milliseconds in 13 and between 200 and 330 milliseconds in seven cases.[47]

[aa]In the first report of adults in which the diagnosis was made by electrophysiological study, the P waves were normal during sinus rhythm in two of the patients and notched and broad in the third.[22] Nonspecific ST- and T-wave abnormalities were present because of "post-tachycardia repolarization abnormalities." The P-wave axes during sinus rhythm in three other patients were −30, +75, and +45 degrees.[66] Each of the six patients was at least 17 years of age.[22, 66]

rhythm can be irregular, an unusual finding in atrial tachycardia.

Multifocal Atrial Tachycardia

This atrial tachyarrhythmia is recognized electrocardiographically by P waves with at least three different, abnormal forms, clearly distinguishable from atrial tachycardia with its unchanging P waves. Most of the P waves of multifocal atrial tachycardia are conducted to the ventricles, although some may be blocked when they occur sufficiently early in the cardiac cycle.

Junctional Ectopic Tachycardia

Like automatic atrial tachycardia, junctional ectopic tachycardia is much more frequent in children than in adults. It is, however, one of the rarest forms of chronic supraventricular tachycardia seen in children, most of whom also have a congenital heart defect. The characteristic electrocardiographic sign is atrioventricular dissociation in which the atria are usually controlled by the sinus node and the ventricles by the abnormal pacemaker within the junction. Rarely, retrograde capture of the atria may occur.[45]

What appears to be junctional ectopic tachycardia in adults may rarely be due to atrial tachycardia, possibly automatic, in which the atria cannot generate P waves. The diagnosis can only be made with intra-atrial recordings.[175]

Inappropriate Sinus Tachycardia

As the name implies, this arrhythmia looks like sinus tachycardia, has normal P waves, and originates, or so it is thought, in the sinus node.[176–179] Investigators using the phrases "chronic nonparoxysmal sinus tachycardia in otherwise healthy persons,"[180] "chronic sinoatrial tachycardia,"[111] and "refractory paroxysmal sinus tachycardia"[181] are probably describing what is now called inappropriate sinus tachycardia. "Paroxysmal reciprocating sinus tachycardia," however, described in eight patients with an average heart rate of 105 beats per minute, may have been slow reentrant atrial tachycardia.[182]

The heart rates of the few otherwise healthy patients with inappropriate sinus tachycardia tend to be rapid at rest and to rise more than expected during physiological stress.[176] Inappropriate sinus tachycardia develops in a few patients after ablation or modification of the atrioventricular node with radiofrequency current for treatment of supraventricular tachyarrhythmias.[179, 183–185] Abnormal autonomic responses may participate in causing this arrhythmia, but the mechanism of inappropriate sinus tachycardia has not as yet been definitively elucidated.

OTHER ELECTROCARDIOGRAPHIC STUDIES[186]

Ambulatory monitoring reveals that greater sympathetic tone, which may be present during the day, can produce more episodes and faster rates of atrial tachycardia due to reentry.[47] The technique is also useful for selecting the best drugs for treating patients with reentrant atrial tachycardia.

Holter recordings demonstrated in 47 patients that automatic atrial tachycardia was persistent[11]

- One hundred percent of the time in 76%.
- Fifty percent to 90% of the time in 13%.
- Ten percent to 49% of the time in 11%.

The P waves had the same form in each patient throughout the period of recording.[11]

The rate of persistent automatic atrial tachycardia can vary greatly in individual patients,[11, 74] and it seems likely that the autonomic nervous system significantly influences the rate of the arrhythmia. In patients with almost incessant automatic atrial tachycardia, continuous monitoring may uncover short periods of sinus rhythm[116] sometimes during sleep.[74]

Holter monitoring reveals brief arrhythmias called "benign slow paroxysmal atrial tachycardia,"[187, 188] the mechanism of which is not known. The heart rates of patients with automatic atrial tachycardia characteristically increase slightly during exercise.[49, 66, 67, 114]

ECHOCARDIOGRAPHY

Decreased left ventricular shortening fraction and ejection fraction and increased chamber size are characteristically observed in patients with cardiomyopathy due to automatic atrial tachycardia.[11, 72, 73, 75, 76, 85, 112, 114, 189bb] Echocardiographic evaluation of ventricular function may be abnormal in patients with atrial tachycardia even though cardiomegaly does not appear on the chest radiograph.[11] Echocardiograms tend to be normal when the rate of atrial tachycardia is relatively slow, thus confirming the relation of heart rate to the development of secondary cardiomyopathy.[112]

Doppler flow studies establish that retrograde flow characteristically occurs during atrial tachycardia when the right atrium contracts against the closed tricuspid valve.[190] Intracardiac[191–193] and transesophageal[194] echocardiography helps the electrophysiologist to visualize anatomic landmarks when ablating atrial tachycardia.

LABORATORY STUDIES

Hematology and Chemistry

Hematological and chemical laboratory values are usually normal in patients with atrial tachycardia. One should consider hyperthyroidism, although rare,[cc] and other causes of sinus or abnormal tachycardia such as pheochromocytoma, carcinoid syndrome, or psychiatric disturbances in patients who have symptoms consistent with these diagnoses.

[bb]Sixty-eight percent of 41 children with the arrhythmia had echocardiographic shortening fractions considered to be abnormal.[11]

[cc]Thyroid function was normal in each of 10 children with automatic atrial tachycardia.[76]

Chest Radiography

The radiograph of the chest in patients with automatic atrial tachycardia either is normal or shows cardiomegaly from secondary cardiomyopathy.[11, 72, 73, 75, 112, 116, 154] Typical findings of congestive failure in the pulmonary vasculature may also appear.

A few children with structural heart disease have abnormal chest radiographs unrelated to cardiomyopathy.[11] No findings specific for the tachycardia have been observed in adults with cardiomyopathy.[49]

Cardiac Catheterization

When performed, results of cardiac catheterization and coronary arteriography are usually normal in those patients who have not developed cardiomyopathy from atrial tachycardia.[51, 67, 69] Other abnormalities, seemingly unrelated to secondary cardiomyopathy include

- Independent origin of left anterior descending and circumflex coronary artery.[51]
- Coronary disease with reduced ejection fraction.[50]
- Left ventricular hypokinesis and mitral regurgitation.[111]

HEMODYNAMICS

Apart from the occasional child with structural congenital heart diseases associated with atrial tachycardia, the principal hemodynamic effects of the arrhythmia are due to cardiomyopathy with its associated decreased cardiac output and congestive heart failure. However, few intracardiac hemodynamic studies on patients with the arrhythmia have been reported, probably because the functional evaluation of such patients is usually conducted with echocardiography. One adult with automatic atrial tachycardia had normal findings from cardiac catheterization.[67]

PATHOLOGY

Pathological examination seldom provides consistent evidence of a process that accounts for atrial tachycardia.[195] Most of the few autopsies reported on patients in whom the arrhythmia has been established by electrophysiological study show little disease of the ventricular myocardium.[70, 196] Tissue removed at operation may have minimal increase in fibrous tissue,[51] mild hypertrophy or fibrosis,[11] and focal myocyte hypertrophy.[72] Other findings include "peculiar small cells," focal myocarditis, and chronic epicarditis.[154]

Specific findings more directly related to causing the arrhythmia include tissue at the origin of the tachycardia in one case showing abnormal amorphous cells with pale eosinophilic staining cytoplasm and absence of nuclei.[197] In another, pathological study of the tissue demonstrated "a mesenchymal tumor at the site of origin of the atrial tachycardia with tumor free borders."[67]

CLINICAL ELECTROPHYSIOLOGY[13, 42, 198–206]

Intervals and Refractory Periods

Intra-atrial conduction and sinus node recovery are often prolonged in patients with atrial tachycardia.[207–208] Split atrial electrograms may confirm the substrate for the arrhythmia.[207] The AH and HV intervals and the refractory periods of the atrioventricular node are usually normal in patients with atrial tachycardia.[22, 47, 49, 66, 69, 71, 74dd]

Defining the Mechanism of a Regular Supraventricular Tachycardia from the Electrophysiological Study[23, 45, 147, 170, 172]

Reentrant versus automatic tachycardias. These following rules apply to all reentrant and automatic tachycardias including those that start in the atria.[44, 81, 84, 146, 153, 155, 156, 198, 209]

- Reentrant tachycardias can be started or stopped by rapid pacing or premature beats. Premature beats do not start automatic tachyarrhythmias. Rapid pacing temporarily suppresses automatic tachycardias, but the arrhythmias return when the pacing stops.
- Reentry is probably the mechanism when permanent pacing prevents recurrence of the tachycardia.

Reentrant Atrial Tachycardia Versus Reentrant Supraventricular Tachycardia Sustained in the Atrioventricular Node or Accessory Pathways

- The spontaneous or paced induction of reentrant atrial tachycardia does not depend on atrioventricular nodal conduction. Thus, the onset of atrial tachycardia is unrelated to the AH, HV, or VA intervals, whereas activity in the atrioventricular node is essential to the induction and maintenance of supraventricular tachycardia sustained in the atrioventricular node or accessory pathways.
- Reentry in the atrioventricular node or accessory pathways are excluded whenever ventricular pacing at a rate slower than the rate of the tachycardia produces complete or high-grade ventriculoatrial block.[47]

Automatic Atrial Tachycardia Versus Reentrant Supraventricular Tachycardia Sustained in the Atrioventricular Node or Accessory Pathways

- Automatic atrial tachycardia cannot be instituted by pacing or programmed premature beats, as is characteristic of reentrant supraventricular tachycardia.[22, 147] This finding provides further proof that timed or "critical" conduction delays will not start an automatic arrhythmia.
- Pacing the atria faster than the tachycardia prolongs the AH interval during automatic atrial

---

[dd]These values are seldom reported during reentrant atrial tachycardia. The AH intervals should be prolonged in many cases in view of the relatively high incidence of, at least, first-degree atrioventricular nodal block during reentrant atrial tachycardia.[47]

tachycardia. Thus, "nodal conduction is a function of atrial rate"[22] in automatic atrial tachycardia. The reverse applies in atrioventricular nodal reentry in which the rate of the tachycardia is a function of the speed of conduction through the reentrant circuit.

- Atrial premature beats introduced progressively earlier during the atrial cycle reset and do not interrupt the tachycardia. Such beats often terminate reentrant supraventricular tachycardia.[22, 49] The AH interval of the first beat of automatic atrial tachycardia is identical to those in the other beats of the tachycardia.[22] This finding confirms that atrioventricular nodal delay is not required for the institution of the tachycardia, as in reentrant arrhythmias involving the atrioventricular node.
- Automatic atrial tachycardia cannot be permanently terminated by rapid pacing or premature beats, whereas reentrant arrhythmias characteristically can be stopped by this method. Pacing the atria at a rate faster than the tachycardia suppresses automatic arrhythmias temporarily. However, after the pacing has stopped, automatic atrial tachycardia usually reappears, sometimes after a few sinus beats.

Termination

Atrial reentrant supraventricular tachycardia may end with any one of at least three patterns:[47, 147, 157]

- Suddenly, without any change in the rate of the tachycardia.
- Gradually, with progressive slowing of the rate of the tachycardia.
- With alternating short and long PP intervals just before termination.

In 17 of 20 cases of atrial tachycardia, the closer the stimulating electrode to the earliest point of atrial activation, the less premature was the stimulus necessary to stop the tachycardia.[47] Careful study of the effects of overdrive pacing can help to distinguish between atrial tachycardia and supraventricular tachycardia.[210]

Location of Focus

Mapping the origin of atrial tachycardia is carried out in electrophysiology laboratories with several electrode catheters guided into particular anatomical positions under fluoroscopic control.[54] The older the patient, the more likely it is that the focus originates in the right atrium or that the patient has multiple atrial tachycardias.[62] Body-surface mapping localizes the origin of right atrial tachycardia with great precision.[211]

Reentrant Atrial Tachycardia.[147] Among 20 cases of reentrant atrial tachycardia, the atria were activated from the top to the bottom of the atria in 12 cases and in the opposite direction in 8 cases.[47] The signals conducted more rapidly from the high to the low atria

during tachycardia than in sinus rhythm in 11 of the 12 cases. Activation started in

- The mid-right atrium in nine patients.
- The low-right atrium in two.
- The left atrium in four.
- The interatrial septum in two.
- The low-right atrium in two.

The sinus node or the region immediately adjacent to it was the likely site of reentry in only one of 20 cases of reentrant atrial tachycardia.[47] In this case, intra-atrial conduction and the sequence of atrial activation were similar in both sinus rhythm and during tachycardia. Sinus node reentry, the authors of this series suggest,[47] is probably rare, and one should not use the phrase unless the intra-atrial conduction time is absolutely identical during both sinus rhythm and the tachycardia.[45] If one relies solely on finding high to low atrial activation,[64, 81, 82, 212, 213] many of the published cases and 12 of the 20 cases would erroneously be called sinus node reentry.[47] Several different circuits may participate in sustaining reentrant atrial tachycardia caused by operative repair of congenital heart disease.[90, 95]

Automatic Atrial Tachycardia. Atrial activation during tachycardia differs from that during sinus rhythm.[11] The electrocardiogram during automatic atrial tachycardia almost always reveals only one abnormal P wave, which is associated with one atrial activation sequence.[11]

Automatic atrial tachycardia originates more frequently from the right than the left atrium.[5, 51, 66, 67, 70, 72–75, 111, 112, 137, 154, 195, 214, 215] Of 50 patients in one report,[11] automatic atrial tachycardia started in the right atrium in 36 patients (72%) in the following specific locations:

- Right atrial appendage, 22 patients (mouth, 13, tip, nine).
- Midposterior right atrium, seven.
- Right side of the atrial septum, three.
- High lateral right atrium, three.
- Mouth of the coronary sinus, one.

In no patient from this series did the tachycardia originate from the superior vena cava–right atrial junction in the area of the sinus node.[11] In 28% of the 50 patients, automatic atrial tachycardia originated from the left atrium, specifically at the base of the left atrial appendage in 13 patients and in the posterior left atrium in one patient.[11] In two reports of single cases, the tachycardias were thought to come from the sinus node itself.[69, 181]

Selection of Drugs by Electrophysiological Study

Electrophysiologists occasionally use electrophysiological studies to help choose which drugs will successfully treat atrial tachycardia.[44, 206ee]

---

*ee*However, as Hein J. J. Wellens wrote (1994): "The value of the electrophysiologic study in selecting the best pharmacological long-term treatment for paroxysmal atrial tachycardia is not clear. . . ."[206]

Entrainment[216]

By capturing the reentrant circuit through the process of entrainment, investigators have revealed further information about the electrophysiology of atrial tachycardia.[217]

Basic Electrophysiology

Tissue taken from patients with right atrial automatic tachycardia reveals pacemaker activity.[67, 196, 218] In one case, the automaticity was induced by norepinephrine[67] and was probably produced by the slow inward current with spontaneous shifts in the site of the dominant pacemaker. Conduction of the tissue was slow and synchronous.[67]

TREATMENT[11, 203, 219]

Physical Maneuvers

Carotid sinus massage or the Valsalva maneuver may convert reentrant atrial tachycardia to sinus rhythm.[44, 220] In automatic atrial tachycardia, however, these techniques do not convert, but they may slow the atrial rate slightly or may increase atrioventricular block.[11, 68, 69]

Drugs

Patients with reentrant atrial tachycardia, like those with other reentrant, usually paroxysmal, tachyarrhythmias, often convert to sinus rhythm when they are given intravenously administered adenosine or beta-adrenergic or calcium-channel–blocking drugs.[221] In a series of 54 patients with automatic atrial tachycardia, a drug that successfully suppressed the arrhythmia was found in 22 (50%), and a partially successful drug was found in 13 (24%). The drugs most likely to be effective are amiodarone, flecainide, moricizine, and propranolol.[11] Automatic atrial tachycardia occasionally ceases spontaneously without treatment.[116]//

Adenosine. This drug is so effective in converting reentrant atrial tachycardia arising within or near the sinus node[43, 48, 222] that some workers believe that conversion by adenosine locates a reentrant atrial tachycardia to that region.[43, 48] Opinion is divided whether adenosine converts reentrant atrial tachycardia arising elsewhere in the atria. Some say it does,[44, 223–225] whereas others find it relatively ineffective.[43, 65, 226] When the drug does not convert the arrhythmia, it decreases the ventricular rate briefly by increasing atrioventricular block.[226, 227] As for automatic atrial tachycardia, some investigators report that adenosine converts the arrhythmia,[228] and others note that the drug only temporarily suppresses it.[43, 68, 224, 229]

Ajmalin. This drug slowed and terminated the auto-

matic atrial tachycardia for eight minutes in one patient.[68]

Amiodarone. Given intravenously, amiodarone converts most patients with reentrant atrial tachycardia to sinus rhythm, and, given orally, it suppresses recurrences of the arrhythmia in many patients.[64, 230] Amiodarone partially or fully, but not always,[66] controls automatic atrial tachycardia.[11, 52, 65, 75, 76, 113, 116, 231, 232] The response to intravenous administration of the drug can reliably predict the clinical effect when the medication is given orally.[76]

Beta-Adrenergic–Blocking Drugs. Propranolol decreases the rate of,[49, 67, 70, 71, 76, 111, 112] increases atrioventricular block in,[49, 67, 70, 71, 76, 111, 112, 233] but seldom converts[234] atrial tachycardia. The drug can sustain sinus rhythm at least temporarily in some cases[74, 76] and thereby reduce the effects of tachycardia-induced cardiomyopathy.[111] Digoxin, when given with propranolol to children with automatic atrial tachycardia, can also improve heart failure.[76]

Calcium-Channel Antagonists. These drugs convert and suppress many cases of reentrant atrial tachycardia.[64, 82, 235] Verapamil decreases the rate of,[68, 112, 115, 236] increases atrioventricular block in,[68, 112, 115, 236, 237] but is usually ineffective in converting automatic atrial tachycardia.[11, 43, 66, 72, 75, 76, 116, 236]

Digoxin.[11, 60, 234] This drug seldom exerts an antiarrhythmic effect on atrial tachycardia, whatever the mechanism,[5, 35, 45, 49, 51, 66, 67, 70–72, 74–76, 111, 112, 116]gg although occasionally the drug slightly decreases the rate.[67, 73, 112] The positive inotropic effect of digoxin, however, can reduce or relieve congestive heart failure produced by cardiomyopathy or other causes.[35, 49, 112] Patients whose paroxysmal atrial tachycardia with block has not been produced by digitalis may respond to administration of digitalis and diuretics for associated congestive heart failure or occasionally to antiarrhythmic drugs.[133–135]

Digoxin-Specific Fab Fragments. These agents slow the rate of and suppress atrial tachycardia due to digitalis intoxication, whether or not atrioventricular block is present.[238]

Disopyramide. This drug is ineffective or slightly decreases the rate of automatic atrial tachycardia.[67, 68]

Flecainide. This drug suppresses or reduces the appearance of atrial tachycardia, particularly automatic, in many of the children[239–241] and adults who receive the drug.[242–248]

Isoproterenol. This drug increases the rate of automatic atrial tachycardia.[51]

Lidocaine. This drug slightly slows the rate of automatic atrial tachycardia.[75]

//This occurred in three of nine children followed for seven years.[116] The authors suggested: "This may explain the very rare finding of automatic atrial tachycardia in adults."

ggDigoxin prevented the induction of atrial tachycardia during electrophysiological study in each of two patients.[64]

Moricizine. One of the few drugs that effectively controls automatic atrial tachycardia,[85, 249] moricizine suppressed more than 90% of episodes of automatic atrial tachycardia in 10 of 12 children (83%).[250]

Phenylephrine. This drug briefly slows the rate of automatic atrial tachycardia.[45]

Phenytoin. This drug is ineffective for automatic atrial tachycardia.[11, 67, 70, 75, 76]

Procainamide. This drug does not control automatic atrial tachycardia[11, 45, 49, 51, 66, 67, 71, 75, 76] and may produce hypotension.[76]

Propafenone. This drug partially or completely suppresses automatic atrial tachycardia in children.[251, 252]

Quinidine. This drug is ineffective[11, 45, 49, 51, 66, 67, 72, 74, 75] or deleterious[66] in the treatment of automatic atrial tachycardia.

Reserpine. This drug has occasionally been given for automatic atrial tachycardia,[70] is usually ineffective,[49, 67, 70] and may be injurious.[253]

Sotalol. This drug restored sinus rhythm in several children with automatic atrial tachycardia[116, 254] and decreased the rate of the arrhythmia in others.[51, 116]

Cardioversion

Cardioverting patients with reentrant atrial tachycardia almost certainly returns most, if not all, to sinus rhythm. The treatment is seldom required, however.[hh] Cardioverting patients with automatic atrial tachycardia, however, does not restore sinus rhythm.[45, 49, 70, 72, 75, 111]

Cardioversion may restore sinus rhythm in some patients who have "paroxysmal atrial tachycardia with block,"[255-257] but potentially dangerous ventricular arrhythmias may arise in patients with digitalis intoxication.[256, 258ii] Cardioversion should be avoided or conducted with great care in such cases.

Pacing[259-261]

Pacing the atrium interrupts reentrant atrial tachycardia and is used for this purpose during electrophysiological study. Esophageal pacing can also convert the tachycardia.[86] Long-term pacing,[262-264] however, is

rarely used alone to treat the arrhythmia, although it may be needed to prevent bradycardia in patients with paroxysmal atrial tachycardia and the sick sinus syndrome[262] or atrioventricular block.

Pacing the atria at rates faster than the arrhythmia suppresses automatic atrial tachycardia,[50, 265] but it is ineffective for long-term treatment because the arrhythmia returns when the pacing stops.[70jj] Occasionally, atrial fibrillation can be induced, the ventricular rate from which is easier to control.[266] Atrial coupled pacing, in which a paced premature beat activates the atria but is not conducted to the ventricles, decreases the ventricular rate.[71] This form of treatment has not been widely applied.

Ablation[267-275]

Atrial tachycardia can be controlled or cured by ablating the origin of the tachycardia or the bundle of His. With the arrhythmia gone, patients with tachycardia-induced cardiomyopathy usually regain normal ventricular function.[119, 120, 174, 276kk]

Source of the Arrhythmia. Ablating the site where atrial tachycardia originates with electrode catheters has become the treatment of choice for patients in whom drug therapy fails. Originally, the focus was ablated with an electric shock of 50 or more joules applied to the region where the origin of the arrhythmia has been mapped.[11, 66, 74, 75, 189, 277] Radiofrequency current, the technique now favored, cures many patients of their tachycardias whether reentrant or automatic[44, 48, 89-93, 95, 119, 120, 151, 193, 268, 278-294ll] (Fig. 6.12). Success in ablating automatic foci is most likely in relatively young

[jj]A team has used long-term overdrive pacing to suppress atrial tachycardia successfully and to reduce the amount of antiarrhythmic drugs required by the patients.[265]

[kk]In the case of a 15-year-old boy referred for cardiac transplantation because of a primary cardiomyopathy, ablation of a previously unsuspected incessant automatic atrial tachycardia led to doubling of the left ventricular ejection fraction to an almost normal value within 1 month.[174]

[ll]Including triggered activity.[44]

[hh]This is a presumption because I could find no reports of cardioverting atrial tachycardia established to be reentry by electrophysiological study.

[ii]Cardioversion restored sinus rhythm in 12 of 18 episodes of "PAT with block."[256] Digitalis toxicity was present in most of the cases when cardioversion failed, and, in these patients, the atrial rate increased and ventricular premature beats appeared after cardioversion. These data were reported in 1969 without electrophysiologic studies, so the mechanism of the arrhythmias is not known. On the basis of knowledge accumulated later, either abnormal automaticity or triggered activity was probably involved.

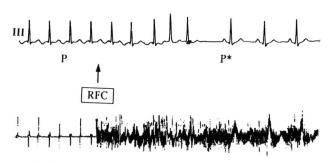

FIGURE 6.12 Catheter ablation of automatic atrial tachycardia. Radiofrequency current (**bottom**), applied at RFC, (*arrow* pointing to **top** panel of lead III) interrupts the tachycardia, and sinus rhythm (P*) resumes. (Adapted from Chiladakis JA, Vassilikos VP, Maounis TN, Cokkinos DV, Manolis AS. Successful radiofrequency catheter ablation of automatic atrial tachycardia with regression of the cardiomyopathy picture. Pacing Clin Electrophysiol 1997; 20:953–959, with permission.)[120]

patients whose tachycardias have a single morphology and in tachycardias originating in the right atrium.[62] The technique works less well in those patients with tachycardia with multiple foci,[62, 291] which may also appear after catheter ablation of a single focus.[291]

In children with congenital heart disease and reentrant atrial tachycardia, the arrhythmia not infrequently recurs after ablation, and the new tachycardia often has different forms from the original one.[95] Ablation of the atrial tachycardia caused by operative repair of congenital heart disease is more likely to be successful when the rate is slower.[90] The site of surgical repair for congenital heart disease always forms at least one aspect of the region ablated when treating atrial tachycardia caused by the operation.[92mm]

Automatic atrial tachycardia has been stopped with the injection of alcohol into a blood vessel supplying the site of origin[295nn] and "chronic nonparoxysmal sinus tachycardia" by infusion of alcohol through a catheter in the sinus nodal artery.[178] Intracardiac echocardiography[191, 192] and new mapping techniques[296] help the electrophysiologist more precisely to localize the site to be ablated.

Surgery[297-300]

Before catheter ablation with radiofrequency current was perfected, excising or isolating the ectopic focus by a surgical operation was the standard method for treating atrial tachycardia when drugs failed. Most patients so treated probably had automatic rather than reentrant atrial tachycardia.[5, 11, 51, 66-69, 72, 75, 112, 114, 116, 118, 154, 189, 195, 197, 214, 215, 218, 301-314]

First, the diagnosis and mechanism are established by electrophysiological evaluation. The origin of the arrhythmia is then mapped with catheters (Fig. 6.13) and is later confirmed during cardiac surgery unless anesthesia has suppressed the tachycardia and has prevented mapping in the operating room.[67, 154] When this happens, the arrhythmia can sometimes be reestablished by catecholamine drugs[67] or by decreasing the level of anesthesia.[154] Cardiopulmonary bypass, when required,[45, 72, 154, 302, 305] is then applied, and the site of earliest activation is resected or excluded,[11, 51, 56, 67, 69, 72, 112, 154, 195, 197, 214, 215, 218, 301-304, 307, 310, 313] isolated,[51, 112, 181, 309] or cryoablated.[5, 11, 75, 154, 189, 214, 302, 304, 305, 307, 310, 311, 313-315] Successful surgical treatment of the arrhythmia often leads to full recovery of ventricular function in patients with tachycardia-induced cardiomyopathy.[75, 116]

The rate of success is similar whether surgery or a full medical program is employed. Both forms of treatment restore sinus rhythm in 70% to 90% of

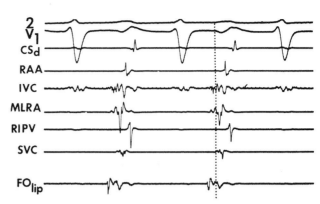

FIGURE 6.13 **Intracardiac catheter map of a patient with automatic atrial tachycardia.** Electrocardiographic leads II and V$_1$ show the abnormal P waves; the *dotted vertical line* indicates the beginning of the second one. The intracardiac electrograms (*top* to *bottom*) are taken from the distal coronary sinus (CS$_d$), the right atrial appendage (RAA), the junction of the inferior vena cava and low right atrium (IVC), the midlateral right atrium (MLRA), the atrial junction of the right inferior pulmonary vein (RIPV), the junction of the superior vena cava and right atrium (SVC), and the lip of the fossa ovalis (FO$_{lip}$), where the arrhythmia originates. The atrial electrogram is recorded earliest there, several milliseconds before any signal appears on the surface tracings. A cardiac surgeon excised the focus, and the patient was cured of the tachycardia. (Adapted from Josephson ME, Spear JF, Harken AH, Horowitz LN, Dorio RJ. Surgical excision of automatic atrial tachycardia: anatomic and electrophysiologic correlates. Am Heart J 1982; 104:1076–1085, with permission.)[67]

patients.[11, 310] The mortality from surgery is low; no deaths were reported in one of the largest series.[11, 310]

Multiple Foci. Although automatic atrial tachycardia is characteristically monofocal, other foci frequently appear after the site in the right atrium has been removed.[11, 313] Surgical techniques have been developed that can overcome the presence of multiple foci in many cases.[310] Excision of a left atrial focus of automatic atrial tachycardia is not followed by the appearance of other foci.[167, 310oo]

Bundle of His. Ablating the atrioventricular junction with shock or radiofrequency energy slows the ventricular rate, but a permanent pacemaker must be inserted. Radiofrequency catheter ablation of the origin of the tachycardia has superseded atrioventricular junctional ablation for treating most cases of resistant atrial tachycardia.[pp]

Pacing. Pacing is occasionally required after surgery for atrial tachycardia because of the sick sinus syndrome or atrioventricular block.[195, 314, 316]

[mm]This finding has led one group of investigators to suggest that atrial tachycardia caused by surgical repair of congenital heart disease should be called "incisional reentry."[92]

[nn]In this case, alcohol was injected into an atrial branch of the circumflex coronary artery that supplied the region of the sinus node. Increase in the level of creatine phosphokinase provided evidence of myocardial damage. The rate of the junctional rhythm produced by the procedure decreased from 90 beats per minute to an average of 67 beats per minute and increased to 110 beats per minute when the patient exercised.[295]

[oo]One intriguing explanation for this difference is that left atrial tachycardias may originate in remnants of denervated left sinus nodes. Once these structures have been ablated or removed, no other sites for ectopic rhythms are present. The right atrial tachycardias are presumed to arise from pathological atrial tissue, which may be broadly distributed and difficult to remove completely.[154, 167]

[pp]See Chapter 4 for references and further discussion about atrioventricular junctional ablation for atrial tachycardia.

PROGNOSIS

The younger the patient is, the more likely the arrhythmia is to resolve spontaneously; older patients tend to have recurrences.[53] Few patients die of atrial tachycardia. Most who are treated with antiarrhythmic drugs, ablation, or cardiac surgery return to sinus rhythm, and tachycardia-induced cardiomyopathy, if present, is permanently cured.[11, 45, 51, 70, 76, 317, 318] The prognosis, however, is poor for those patients who have atrial tachycardia, digitalis toxicity, and severe heart disease, whether or not they have pulmonary disease.[125] Most of these patients succumb to their underlying heart or lung disease rather than to the arrhythmia.

SUMMARY

Atrial tachycardia is a regular supraventricular tachycardia originating in the atria and the sinus node and identified by the presence of P waves before each QRS complex. Some of the clinical and electrophysiological characteristics of the arrhythmia differ when caused by reentry or automaticity.

Atrial tachycardia accounts for about 9% of all supraventricular tachycardias in adults and 23% in children. The arrhythmia occurs at all ages without predilection for males or females.

Many adults with atrial tachycardia have structural heart disease; those with reentry in the sinus node or with automatic atrial tachycardia tend to have less. Most children with atrial tachycardia have no structural heart disease, except for those who develop the tachycardia from the effects of atrial surgery for congenital abnormalities. Persistent atrial tachycardia can produce cardiomyopathy, which disappears when the arrhythmia is treated. Digitalis intoxication is a well-known cause of atrial tachycardia and is often associated with atrioventricular block.

The symptoms of atrial tachycardia are those characteristic of any tachycardia. The average heart rate in adults is about 150 beats per minute; in children, it is faster, but the rate slows as the child grows. The faster the tachycardia and the longer it persists, the more likely cardiomyopathy is to develop. When paroxysmal, the mechanism of atrial tachycardia tends to be reentrant, and when persistent, automatic.

Each of the P waves in a patient with atrial tachycardia has the same form, which is usually at least slightly different from that seen during sinus rhythm. Prolonged PR intervals and dropped QRS complexes from block in the atrioventricular node may be present. Sinus tachycardia and supraventricular tachycardia sustained in the atrioventricular node or bypass tracts are the principal arrhythmias with which atrial tachycardia may be confused. Electrophysiologic study can confirm the diagnosis of atrial tachycardia, establish its mechanism—reentry is more common among adults and automaticity among children—locate its origin, and determine which drugs are likely to be effective.

Adenosine, amiodarone, and beta- and calcium-channel–blocking drugs, given intravenously, quickly convert most patients with reentrant atrial tachycardia to sinus rhythm. Combinations of these and other antiarrhythmic drugs often suppress recurrences. Amiodarone, flecainide, moricizine, and beta-adrenergic–blocking drugs seem to be the most effective agents for suppressing automatic atrial tachycardia. Cardioversion and atrial pacing convert reentrant atrial tachycardia, but cardioversion is ineffective for reverting automatic atrial tachycardia, and pacing only temporarily suppresses the arrhythmia.

Ablating the site of origin of atrial tachycardia with radiofrequency current delivered through electrode catheters is now the preferred method for definitively treating atrial tachycardia whatever its mechanism. Antiarrhythmic surgery is seldom needed.

Few patients with atrial tachycardia die of the arrhythmia itself. The prognosis is determined by underlying cardiac or systemic disease.

REFERENCES

1. Kastor JA. Automatic atrial tachycardia. In Kastor JA (ed). Arrhythmias. Philadelphia: WB Saunders, 1994, pp. 116–132.
2. Flammang D, Coumel P. Supraventricular tachycardia with reentry in the sinus node or atria. In Kastor JA (ed). Arrhythmias. Philadelphia: WB Saunders, 1994, pp. 297–309.
3. Josephson ME, Kastor JA. Supraventricular tachycardia: mechanisms and management. Ann Intern Med 1977; 87:346–358.
4. Garson A Jr. Supraventricular tachycardia. In Gillette PC, Garson Jr A (eds). Pediatric Cardiac Dysrhythmias. New York: Grune & Stratton, 1981, pp. 177–253.
5. Gillette PC. Advances in the diagnosis and treatment of tachydysrhythmias in children. Am Heart J 1981; 102:111–120.
6. Benditt DG, Benson DW Jr, Dunnigan A, Gornick CC, Anderson RW. Atrial flutter, atrial fibrillation, and other primary atrial tachycardias. Med Clin North Am 1984; 68:895–918.
7. Fauchier JP, Cosnay P, Latour F, Rouesnel P. Atrial tachycardias: diagnosis and management. In Levy S, Scheinman MM (eds). Cardiac Arrhythmias. From Diagnosis to Therapy. Mount Kisco, NY: Futura Publishing Co., 1984, pp. 195–216.
8. Garson A Jr. Atrial tachycardia: a rare disease sheds light on common questions. J Am Coll Cardiol 1989; 14:1783–1784.
9. Porter CJ. Premature atrial contractions and atrial tachyarrhythmias. In Gillette PC, Garson A Jr (eds). Pediatric Arrhythmias. Electrophysiology and Pacing. Philadelphia: WB Saunders, 1990, pp. 328–359.
10. Ludomirsky A, Garson A Jr. Supraventricular tachycardia. In Gillette PC, Garson A Jr (eds). Pediatric Arrhythmias. Electrophysiology and Pacing. Philadelphia: WB Saunders, 1990, pp. 380–426.
11. Garson A Jr, Smith RT, Moak JP, Judd VE, Ott DA, Cooley DA. Atrial automatic ectopic tachycardia in children. In Touboul P, Waldo AL (eds). Atrial Arrhythmias. Current Concepts and Management. St. Louis: Mosby–Year Book, 1990, pp. 282–287.
12. Case CL, Gillette PC. Automatic atrial and junctional tachycardias in the pediatric patient: strategies for diagnosis and management. PACE 1993; 16:1323–1335.
13. Josephson ME. Clinical Cardiac Electrophysiology. Techniques and Interpretations. Philadelphia: Lea & Febiger, 1993, pp. 256–274.
14. Ganz LI, Friedman PL. Supraventricular tachycardia. N Engl J Med 1995; 332:162–173.
15. Goldberger JJ, Kadish AH. Atrial premature depolarizations, junctional premature depolarizations, multifocal atrial tachycardia, and atrial tachycardia. In Podrid PJ, Kowey PR (eds). Cardiac Arrhythmia. Mechanisms, Diagnosis and

Management. Baltimore: Williams & Wilkins, 1995, pp. 768–789.

16. Naccarelli GV, Shih H-T, Jalal S. Clinical arrhythmias: mechanisms, clinical features, and management. Supraventricular tachycardia. In Zipes DP, Jalife J (eds). Cardiac Electrophysiology. From Cell to Bedside. 2nd ed. Philadelphia: WB Saunders, 1995, pp. 607–619.

17. Mirowski M, Rowe RD. Atrial tachycardia with exit block around the ectopic pacemaker in an otherwise healthy infant. J Pediatr 1972; 80:457–459.

18. Schamroth L. Idioatrial tachycardia. J Electrocardiol 1971; 4:227–230.

19. Waldo AL, Cooper TB, MacLean WAH. Need for additional criteria for the diagnosis of sinus node reentrant tachycardias. J Electrocardiol 1977; 10:103–104.

20. Kirchhof CJHJ, Bonke FIM, Allessie MA. Sinus node reentry: fact or fiction? In Brugada P, Wellens HJJ (eds). Cardiac Arrhythmias. Where To Go From Here? Mount Kisco, NY: Futura Publishing Co., 1987, pp. 53–65.

21. Lesh MD, Kalman JM. To fumble flutter or tackle "tach"? Toward updated classifiers for atrial tachyarrhythmias. J Cardiovasc Electrophysiol 1996; 7:460–466.

22. Goldreyer BN, Gallagher JJ, Damato AN. The electrophysiologic demonstration of atrial ectopic tachycardia in man. Am Heart J 1973; 85:205–215.

23. Gillette PC. The mechanisms of supraventricular tachycardia in children. Circulation 1976; 54:133–139.

24. Weiss HB, McGuire J. Ectopic tachycardia, auricular in origin, of unusual duration. Am Heart J 1936; 12:585–591.

25. Miller R, Perelman JS. Chronic auricular tachycardia with unusual response to change in posture. Am Heart J 1945; 29:555–569.

26. Herson RN, Willington FL. Chronic auricular tachycardia. Br Heart J 1947; 9:19–26.

27. Hay JD, Keidan SE. Persistent ectopic auricular tachycardia in children. Br Heart J 1952; 14:345–349.

28. Nadas AS, Daeschner CW, Roth A, Blumenthal SL. Paroxysmal tachycardia in infants and children: study of 41 cases. Pediatrics 1952; 9:167–181.

29. Shachnow N, Spellman S, Rubin I. Persistent supraventricular tachycardia. Circulation 1954; 10:232–236.

30. Strom G, Zetterqvist E, Zetterqvist P. Chronic supraventricular tachycardia of continuous or repetitive type in children: a note on circulatory function and long-term prognosis. Acta Paediatr 1960; 49:827–837.

31. Morgan CL, Nadas AS. Chronic ectopic tachycardia in infancy and childhood. Am Heart J 1964; 67:617–627.

32. Dolara A, Pozzi L. Persistent supraventricular tachycardia. Am J Cardiol 1965; 16:449–451.

33. Moulopoulos SD, Anthopoulos LP, Plassaras GC, Zellos SL. Paroxysmal supraventricular tachycardia with atrio-ventricular block before and after implantation of an electrical pacemaker. Cardiology 1968; 53:51–56.

34. Walters L, Geptes LS, Noonan JA, Surawicz B. Long-term management of chronic tachycardias of childhood with orally administered propranolol. Am J Cardiol 1968; 21:119.

35. Lund-Larsen G. Permanent ectopic supraventricular tachycardia treated with an adrenergic beta-receptor antagonist: a case report. Acta Med Scand 1969; 186:183–185.

36. Simcha A, Bonham-Carter RE. Paroxysmal atrial tachycardia in infants and children. Lancet 1971; 1:832–834.

37. Keane JF, Plauth WH Jr, Nadas AS. Chronic ectopic tachycardia of infancy and childhood. Am Heart J 1972; 84:748–757.

38. Damgard Andersen E, Ramsoe Jacobsen J, Sandoe E, Videbaek J, Wennevold A. Paroxysmal tachycardia in infancy and childhood. Acta Paediatr Scand 1973; 62:341–348.

39. Hedvall G. Congenital paroxysmal tachycardia: a report of three cases. Acta Paediatr Scand 1973; 62:550–552.

40. Ramsoe Jacobsen J, Anderson ED, Sandoe E, Videbaek J, Wennevold A. Chronic supraventricular tachycardia in infancy and childhood. Acta Paediatr Scand 1975; 64:597–604.

41. Epstein ML, Benditt DG. Long-term evaluation of persistent supraventricular tachycardia in children: clinical and electrocardiographic features. Am Heart J 1981; 102:80–84.

42. Akhtar M. Mechanisms of supraventricular tachycardia originating in the atria. In Touboul P, Waldo AL (eds). Atrial Arrhythmias. Current Concepts and Management. St. Louis: Mosby–Year Book, 1990, pp. 270–281.

43. Engelstein ED, Lippman N, Stein KM, Lerman BB. Mechanism-specific effects of adenosine on atrial tachycardia. Circulation 1994; 89:2645–2654.

44. Chen SA, Chiang CE, Yang CJ, et al. Sustained atrial tachycardia in adult patients: electrophysiological characteristics, pharmacological response, possible mechanisms, and effects of radiofrequency ablation. Circulation 1994; 90:1262–1278.

45. Garson A Jr, Gillette PC. Electrophysiologic studies of supraventricular tachycardia in children. II. Prediction of specific mechanism by noninvasive features. Am Heart J 1981; 102:383–388.

46. Ko JK, Deal BJ, Strasburger JF, Benson DW Jr. Supraventricular tachycardia mechanisms and their age distribution in pediatric patients. Am J Cardiol 1992; 69:1028–1032.

47. Coumel P, Flammang D, Attuel P. Sustained intraatrial reentrant tachycardia: electrophysiologic study of 20 cases. Clin Cardiol 1979; 2:167–178.

48. Sanders WE Jr, Sorrentino RA, Greenfield RA, Shenasa H, Hamer ME, Wharton JM. Catheter ablation of sinoatrial node reentrant tachycardia. J Am Coll Cardiol 1994; 23:926–934.

49. Scheinman MM, Basu D, Hollenberg M. Electrophysiologic studies in patients with persistent atrial tachycardia. Circulation 1974; 50:266–273.

50. Friedman HS, Zaman Q. Persistent repetitive supraventricular tachycardia. Eur J Cardiol 1977; 5:405–411.

51. Anderson KP, Stinson EB, Mason JW. Surgical exclusion of focal paroxysmal atrial tachycardia. Am J Cardiol 1982; 49:869–874.

52. von Bernuth G, Engelhardt W, Kramer HH, et al. Atrial automatic tachycardia in infancy and childhood. Eur Heart J 1992; 13:1410–1415.

53. Klersy C, Chimienti M, Marangoni E, Comelli M, Salerno JA. Factors that predict spontaneous remission of ectopic atrial tachycardia. Eur Heart J 1993; 14:1654–1656.

54. Tang CW, Scheinman MM, Van Hare GF, et al. Use of P wave configuration during atrial tachycardia to predict site of origin. J Am Coll Cardiol 1995; 26:1315–1324.

55. Garson A Jr, Gillette PC, McNamara DG. Supraventricular tachycardia in children: clinical features, response to treatment, and long-term follow-up in 217 patients. J Pediatr 1981; 98:875–882.

56. Gillette PC. Supraventricular arrhythmias in children. J Am Coll Cardiol 1985; 5:122B–129B.

57. Vanagt EJ, Wellens HJJ. The electrocardiogram in digitalis intoxication. In Wellens HJJ, Kulbertus HE (eds). What's New in Electrocardiography. Boston: Martinus Nijhoff, 1981, pp. 315–343.

58. Smith TW, Haber E. Digoxin intoxication: the relationship of clinical presentation to serum digoxin concentration. J Clin Invest 1970; 49:2377–2386.

59. Moorman JR. Digitalis toxicity at Duke Hospital, 1973 to 1984. South Med J 1985; 78:561–564.

60. Aliot E. Digitalis therapy for atrial arrhythmias: rationale and controversies. In Touboul P, Waldo AL (eds). Atrial Arrhythmias. Current concepts and management. St. Louis: Mosby–Year Book, 1990, pp. 370–380.

61. Lown B, Marcus F, Levine HD. Digitalis and atrial tachycardia with block. N Engl J Med 1959; 260:301–309.

62. Chen SA, Tai CT, Chiang CE, Ding YA, Chang MS. Focal atrial tachycardia: reanalysis of the clinical and electrophysiologic characteristics and prediction of successful radiofrequency ablation. J Cardiovasc Electrophysiol 1998; 9:355–365.

63. Rodriguez LM, Oyarzun R, Smeets J, et al. Identification of patients at high risk for recurrence of sustained ventricular tachycardia after healing of acute myocardial infarction. Am J Cardiol 1992; 69:462–464.

64. Gomes JA, Hariman RJ, Kang PS, Chowdry IH. Sustained symptomatic sinus node reentrant tachycardia: incidence,

clinical significance, electrophysiologic observations and the effects of antiarrhythmic agents. J Am Coll Cardiol 1985; 5:45–57.

65. Haines DE, DiMarco JP. Sustained intraatrial reentrant tachycardia: clinical, electrocardiographic and electrophysiologic characteristics and long-term follow-up. J Am Coll Cardiol 1990; 15:1345–1354.

66. Davis J, Scheinman MM, Ruder MA, et al. Ablation of cardiac tissues by an electrode catheter technique for treatment of ectopic supraventricular tachycardia in adults. Circulation 1986; 74:1044–1053.

67. Josephson ME, Spear JF, Harken AH, Horowitz LN, Dorio RJ. Surgical excision of automatic atrial tachycardia: anatomic and electrophysiologic correlates. Am Heart J 1982; 104:1076–1085.

68. Perelman MS, Krikler DM. Termination of focal atrial tachycardia by adenosine triphosphate. Br Heart J 1987; 58:528–530.

69. Sosa E, Marcial MB, Scanavacca M, Bellotti G, Pileggi F. Incessant ectopic atrial tachycardia and sudden death. PACE 1991; 14:764–767.

70. Gillette PC, Garson A Jr. Electrophysiologic and pharmacologic characteristics of automatic ectopic atrial tachycardia. Circulation 1977; 56:571–575.

71. Arbel ER, Cohen HC, Langendorf R, Glick G. Successful treatment of drug-resistant atrial tachycardia and intractable congestive heart failure with permanent coupled atrial pacing. Am J Cardiol 1978; 41:336–340.

72. Giorgi LV, Hartzler GO, Hamaker WR. Incessant focal atrial tachycardia: a surgically remediable cause of cardiomyopathy. J Thorac Cardiovasc Surg 1984; 87:466–469.

73. Kugler JD, Baisch SD, Cheatham JP, et al. Improvement of left ventricular dysfunction after control of persistent tachycardia. J Pediatr 1984; 105:543–548.

74. Silka MJ, Gillette PC, Garson A Jr, Zinner A. Transvenous catheter ablation of a right automatic ectopic tachycardia. J Am Coll Cardiol 1985; 5:999–1001.

75. Gillette PC, Smith RT, Garson A Jr, et al. Chronic supraventricular tachycardia: a curable cause of congestive cardiomyopathy. JAMA 1985; 253:391–392.

76. Mehta AV, Sanchez GR, Sacks EJ, Casta A, Dunn JM, Donner RM. Ectopic automatic atrial tachycardia in children: clinical characteristics, management and follow-up. J Am Coll Cardiol 1988; 11:379–385.

77. Silber DL, Durnin RE. Intrauterine atrial tachycardia. Am J Dis Child 1969; 117:722–726.

78. Vaerius NH, Jacobsen JR. Intrauterine supraventricular tachycardia. Acta Obstet Gynecol Scand 1978; 57:407–410.

79. Rodriguez LM, de Chillou C, Schlapfer J, et al. Age at onset and gender of patients with different types of supraventricular tachycardias. Am J Cardiol 1992; 70:1213–1215.

80. Balaji S, Sullivan ID, Shinebourne EA. Familial neonatal atrial tachycardia. Heart 1996; 76:178–180.

81. Weisfogel GM, Batsford WP, Paulay KL. Sinus node reentrant tachycardia in man. Am Heart J 1975; 90:295–304.

82. Curry PV, Evans TR, Krikler DM. Paroxysmal reciprocating sinus tachycardia. Eur J Cardiol 1977; 6:199–228.

83. Akhtar M, Caracta AR, Lau SH. Demonstration of intraatrial conduction delay, block, gap and reentry: a report of two cases. Circulation 1978; 58:947–955.

84. Wu D, Denes P, Amat-y-Leon F, et al. Clinical, electrocardiographic and electrophysiologic observations in patients with paroxysmal supraventricular tachycardia. Am J Cardiol 1978; 41:1045–1051.

85. Evans VL, Garson A Jr, Smith RT, Moak JP, McVey P, McNamara DG. Ethmozine (moricizine hcl): a promising drug for "automatic" atrial ectopic tachycardia. Am J Cardiol 1987; 60:83F–86F.

86. Butto F, Dunnigan A, Overholt ED, Benditt DG, Benson DW Jr. Transesophageal study of recurrent atrial tachycardia after atrial baffle procedures for complete transposition of the great arteries. Am J Cardiol 1986; 57:1356–1362.

87. Muller GI, Deal BJ, Strasburger JF, Benson DW. Electrocardiographic features of atrial tachycardias after operation for congenital heart disease. Am J Cardiol 1993; 71:122–124.

88. Gelatt M, Hamilton RM, McCrindle BW, et al. Risk factors for atrial tachyarrhythmias after the Fontan operation. J Am Coll Cardiol 1994; 24:1735–1741.

89. Lesh MD, Van Hare GF, Epstein LM, et al. Radiofrequency catheter ablation of atrial arrhythmias: results and mechanisms. Circulation 1994; 89:1074–1089.

90. Triedman JK, Saul JP, Weindling SN, Walsh EP. Radiofrequency ablation of intraatrial reentrant tachycardia after surgical palliation of congenital heart disease. Circulation 1995; 91:707–714.

91. Baker BM, Lindsay BD, Bromberg BI, Frazier DW, Cain ME, Smith JM. Catheter ablation of clinical intraatrial reentrant tachycardias resulting from previous atrial surgery: localizing and transecting the critical isthmus. J Am Coll Cardiol 1996; 28:411–417.

92. Kalman JM, Van Hare GF, Olgin JE, Saxon LA, Stark SI, Lesh MD. Ablation of "incisional" reentrant atrial tachycardia complicating surgery for congenital heart disease: use of entrainment to define a critical isthmus of conduction. Circulation 1996; 93:502–512.

93. Van Hare GF, Lesh MD, Ross BA, Perry JC, Dorostkar PC. Mapping and radiofrequency ablation of intraatrial reentrant tachycardia after the Senning or Mustard procedure for transposition of the great arteries. Am J Cardiol 1996; 77:985–991.

94. Triedman JK, Jenkins KJ, Colan SD, Saul JP, Walsh EP. Intra-atrial reentrant tachycardia after palliation of congenital heart disease: characterization of multiple macroreentrant circuits using fluoroscopically based three-dimensional endocardial mapping. J Cardiovasc Electrophysiol 1997; 8:259–270.

95. Triedman JK, Bergau DM, Saul JP, Epstein MR, Walsh EP. Efficacy of radiofrequency ablation for control of intraatrial reentrant tachycardia in patients with congenital heart disease. J Am Coll Cardiol 1997; 30:1032–1038.

96. Ebels T. Can intraatrial reentry be prevented by changes in surgical technique? Pacing Clin Electrophysiol 1997; 20:2118–2120.

97. Dunnigan A, Pierpont ME, Smith SA, Breningstall G, Benditt DG, Benson DW. Cardiac and skeletal myopathy associated with cardiac dysrhythmias. Am J Cardiol 1984; 53:731–737.

98. Julian DG, Valentine PA, Miller GG. Disturbances of rate, rhythm and conduction in acute myocardial infarction: a prospective study of 100 consecutive unselected patients with the aid of electrocardiographic monitoring. Am J Med 1964; 37:915–927.

99. Kurland GS, Pressman D. The incidence of arrhythmias in acute myocardial infarction studies with a constant monitoring system. Circulation 1965; 31:834–841.

100. Langhorne WH. The coronary care unit: a year's experience in a community hospital. JAMA 1967; 201:92–95.

101. Norris RM. Acute coronary care. N Z Med J 1968; 67:470–476.

102. DeSanctis RW, Block P, Hutter AM Jr. Tachyarrhythmias in myocardial infarction. Circulation 1972; 45:681–702.

103. Scheinman MM, Abbott JA. Clinical significance of transmural versus nontransmural electrocardiographic changes in patients with acute myocardial infarction. Am J Med 1973; 55:602–607.

104. Cristal N, Szwarcberg J, Gueron M. Supraventricular arrhythmias in acute myocardial infarction: prognostic importance of clinical setting; mechanism of production. Ann Intern Med 1975; 82:35–39.

105. Liberthson RR, Salisbury KW, Hutter AM Jr, DeSanctis RW. Atrial tachyarrhythmias in acute myocardial infarction. Am J Med 1976; 60:956–960.

106. Lofmark R, Orinius E. Supraventricular tachyarrhythmias in acute myocardial infarction. Acta Med Scand 1978; 203:517–520.

107. Corazza LJ, Pastor BH. Cardiac arrhythmias in chronic cor pulmonale. N Engl J Med 1958; 259:862–865.

108. Thomas AJ, Valabhji P. Arrhythmia and tachycardia in pulmonary heart disease. Br Heart J 1969; 31:491–495.

109. Ramsdale DR, Arumugam N, Singh SS, Pearson J, Charles RG. Holter monitoring in patients with mitral stenosis and sinus rhythm. Eur Heart J 1987; 8:164–170.

110. Gallagher JJ. Tachycardia and cardiomyopathy: the chicken-egg dilemma revisited. J Am Coll Cardiol 1985; 6:1172–1173.
111. Engel TR, Bush CA, Schaal SF. Tachycardia-aggravated heart disease. Ann Intern Med 1974; 80:384–388.
112. Olsson SB, Blomstrom P, Sabel K-G, William-Olsson G. Successful surgical treatment with regression of dilated cardiomyopathy picture. Am J Cardiol 1984; 53:1127–1130.
113. Leman RB, Gillette PC, Zinner AJ. Resolution of congestive cardiomyopathy caused by supraventricular tachycardia using amiodarone. Am Heart J 1986; 112:622–624.
114. Packer DL, Bardy GH, Worley SJ, et al. Tachycardia-induced cardiomyopathy: a reversible form of left ventricular dysfunction. Am J Cardiol 1986; 57:563–570.
115. Rao PS, Najjar HN. Congestive cardiomyopathy due to chronic tachycardia: resolution of cardiomyopathy with antiarrhythmic drugs. Int J Cardiol 1987; 17:216–220.
116. Koike K, Hesslein PS, Finlay CD, Williams WG, Ikukawa T, Freedom RM. Atrial automatic tachycardia in children. Am J Cardiol 1988; 61:1127–1130.
117. Ross BA, Crawford FA, Whitman V, Gillette PC. Atrial automatic ectopic tachycardia due to an atrial tumor. Am Heart J 1988; 115:606–610.
118. Hendry PJ, Packer DL, Anstadt MP, Plunkett MD, Lowe JE. Surgical treatment of automatic atrial tachycardias. Ann Thorac Surg 1990; 49:253–259.
119. Walsh EP, Saul JP, Hulse JE, et al. Transcatheter ablation of ectopic atrial tachycardia in young patients using radiofrequency current. Circulation 1992; 86:1138–1146.
120. Chiladakis JA, Vassilikos VP, Maounis TN, Cokkinos DV, Manolis AS. Successful radiofrequency catheter ablation of automatic atrial tachycardia with regression of the cardiomyopathy picture. Pacing Clin Electrophysiol 1997; 20:953–959.
121. Fauchier JP, Cosnay P, Babuty RD. Drug-induced atrial arrhythmias. In Touboul P, Waldo AL (eds). Atrial Arrhythmias. Current Concepts and Management. St. Louis: Mosby–Year Book, 1990, pp. 288–310.
122. Heyl AF. Auricular paroxysmal tachycardia caused by digitalis. Ann Intern Med 1932; 5:858–872.
123. Decherd GM, Herrmann GR, Schwab EH. Paroxysmal supraventricular tachycardia with atrioventricular block. Am Heart J 1943; 26:444–472.
124. Lown B, Wyatt NF, Crocker AT, Goodale WT, Levine S. Interrelationship of digitalis and potassium in auricular tachycardia with block. Am Heart J 1953; 45:589–601.
125. Freiermuth LJ, Jick S. Paroxysmal atrial tachycardia with atrioventricular block. Am J Cardiol 1958; 1:584–591.
126. Hejtmancik MR, Herrmann GR, Wright JC. Paroxysmal supraventricular tachycardias complicating organic heart disease. Am Heart J 1958; 56:671–684.
127. Harris EA, Julian DG, Oliver MF. Atrial tachycardia with atrioventricular block due to digitalis poisoning. BMJ 1960; 2:1409–1413.
128. Lown B, Wyatt NF, Levine HD. Paroxysmal atrial tachycardia with block. Circulation 1960; 21:129–143.
129. Oram S, Resnekov L, Davies P. Digitalis as a cause of paroxysmal atrial tachycardia with atrioventricular block. BMJ 1960; 2:1402–1409.
130. Taguchi JT, Ryan JM. Spontaneous conversion of established atrial fibrillation: clinical significance of a change to atrial flutter or to paroxysmal atrial tachycardia with AV block. Arch Intern Med 1969; 124:468–476.
131. Goldberg LM, Bristow JD, Parker BM, Riztmann LW. Paroxysmal atrial tachycardia with atrioventricular block. Circulation 1960; 21:499–504.
132. Rose MR, Glassman E, Spencer FC. Arrhythmias following cardiac surgery: relation to serum digoxin levels. Am Heart J 1975; 89:288–294.
133. Spritz N, Frimpter GL, Braveman WS, Rubin AL. Persistent atrial tachycardia with atrioventricular block. Am J Med 1958; 25:442–448.
134. Morgan WL, Breneman GM. Atrial tachycardia with block treated with digitalis. Circulation 1962; 25:787–797.
135. Storstein O, Rasmussen K. Digitalis and atrial tachycardia with block. Br Heart J 1974; 36:171–176.
136. Marchlinski FE, Miller JM. Atrial arrhythmias exacerbated by theophylline: response to verapamil and evidence for triggered activity in man. Chest 1985; 88:931–934.
137. Borggrefe M, Breithardt G. Ectopic atrial tachycardia after transvenous catheter ablation of a posteroseptal accessory pathway. J Am Coll Cardiol 1986; 8:441–445.
138. Jacquet L, Ziady G, Stein K, et al. Cardiac rhythm disturbances early after orthotopic heart transplantation: prevalence and clinical importance of the observed abnormalities. J Am Coll Cardiol 1990; 16:832–837.
139. Randazzo DN, Schweitzer P, Stein E, Banas JS Jr, Winters SL. Flecainide induced atrial tachycardia with 1:1 ventricular conduction during exercise testing. PACE 1994; 17:1509–1514.
140. Hubbard WN, Jenkins BA, Ward DE. Persistent atrial tachycardia in pregnancy. BMJ 1983; 287:327.
141. Doig JC, McComb JM, Reid DS. Incessant atrial tachycardia accelerated by pregnancy. Br Heart J 1992; 67:266–268.
142. Lindsay AE. Tachycardia caused by swallowing: mechanisms and treatment. Am Heart J 1973; 85:679–684.
143. Engel TR, Laporte SM, Meister SG, Frankl WS. Tachycardia upon swallowing: evidence for a left atrial automatic focus. J Electrocardiol 1976; 9:69–73.
144. Terasaka R, Takemoto M, Haraoka S. Swallowing-induced paroxysmal supraventricular tachycardia. Jpn Heart J 1987; 28:555–560.
145. Saksena S, Siegel P, Rathyen W. Electrophysiologic mechanisms in postural supraventricular tachycardia. Am Heart J 1983; 106:151–154.
146. Narula OS. Sinus node re-entry: a mechanism for supraventricular tachycardia. Circulation 1974; 50:1114–1128.
147. Wu D, Amat-y-Leon F, Denes P, Dhingra RC, Pietras RJ, Rosen KM. Demonstration of sustained sinus and atrial re-entry as a mechanism of paroxysmal supraventricular tachycardia. Circulation 1975; 51:234–243.
148. Komatsu C, Ishinaga T, Tateishi O, et al. Shift of atrial reentrant tachycardia with transient entrainment to an uncommon and a common type of atrial flutter. Pacing Clin Electrophysiol 1988; 11:687–695.
149. Paulay KL, Ruskin JN, Damato AN. Sinus and atrioventricular nodal reentrant tachycardia in the same patient. Am J Cardiol 1975; 36:810–816.
150. Green M, Brugada P, Wellens HJJ. Incessant dual supraventricular tachycardia in a child. Pacing Clin Electrophysiol 1983; 6:624–630.
151. Giudici MC, Gimbel MJ. Radiofrequency catheter ablation of an intraatrial reentrant tachycardia: evidence of an area of slow conduction. PACE 1993; 16:1249–1255.
152. Wu D, Denes P, Leon FA, Chhablani RC, Rosen KM. Limitation of the surface electrocardiogram in diagnosis of atrial arrhythmias: further observations on dissimilar atrial rhythms. Am J Cardiol 1975; 36:91–97.
153. Fisher JD, Johnston DR, Kim SG, Furman S, Mercando AM. Implantable pacers for tachycardia termination: stimulation techniques and long-term efficacy. Pacing Clin Electrophysiol 1986; 9:1325–1333.
154. Iwa T, Ichihashi T, Hashizume Y, Ishida K, Okada R. Successful surgical treatment of left atrial tachycardia. Am Heart J 1985; 109:160–162.
155. Pahlajani DB, Miller RA, Serrato M. Sinus node reentry and sinus node tachycardia. Am Heart J 1975; 90:305–311.
156. Castellanos A, Aranda J, Moleiro F. Effects of the pacing site in sinus node reentrant tachycardia. J Electrocardiol 1978; 9:165–169.
157. Wellens HJJ. Unusual examples of supraventricular reentrant tachycardias. Circulation 1975; 51:997–1002.
158. Riva SI, Della Bella P, Fassini G, Maslowsky F, Tondo C. Value of analysis of ST segment changes during tachycardia in determining type of narrow QRS complex tachycardia. J Am Coll Cardiol 1996; 27:1480–1485.
159. Rosner SW. Atrial tachysystole with block. Circulation 1964; 29:614–621.
160. von Bernuth G, Belz GG, Schairer K. Repetitive paroxysmal tachycardia originating in the left atrium. Br Heart J 1973; 35:729–733.

161. Kalbfleisch SJ, el-Atassi R, Calkins H, Langberg JJ, Morady F. Differentiation of paroxysmal narrow QRS complex tachycardias using the 12-lead electrocardiogram. J Am Coll Cardiol 1993; 21:85–89.

162. Mirowski M, Neill CA, Taussig HB. Left atrial ectopic rhythm in mirror-image dextrocardia and in normally placed malformed hearts: report of twelve cases with "dome and dart" P waves. Circulation 1963; 27:864–877.

163. Beder SD, Gillette PC, Garson A Jr, McNamara DG. Clinical confirmation of ECG criteria for left atrial rhythm. Am Heart J 1982; 103:848–852.

164. MacLean WAH, Karp RB, Kouchoukos NT, James TN, Waldo AL. P waves during ectopic atrial rhythms in man: a study utilizing atrial pacing with fixed electrodes. Circulation 1975; 52:426–434.

165. Bernstein RB, Stanzler RM. Paroxysmal atrial tachycardia with latent block. Arch Intern Med 1966; 118:154–157.

166. Mehta AV. Supraventricular tachycardia in children: diagnosis and management. Ind J Pediatr 1991; 58:567–585.

167. Garson A Jr. Personal communication, 1991.

168. Gelb BD, Garson A Jr. Noninvasive discrimination of right atrial ectopic tachycardia from sinus tachycardia in "dilated cardiomyopathy." Am Heart J 1990; 120:886–891.

169. Green M, Heddle B, Dassen W, et al. Value of QRS alteration in determining the site of origin of narrow QRS supraventricular tachycardia. Circulation 1983; 68:368–373.

170. Bar FW, Brugada P, Dassen WR, Wellens HJJ. Differential diagnosis of tachycardia with narrow QRS complex (shorter than 0.12 second). Am J Cardiol 1984; 54:555–560.

171. Morady F, DiCarlo LA Jr, Baerman JM, de Buitleir M, Kou WH. Determinants of QRS alternans during narrow QRS tachycardia. J Am Coll Cardiol 1987; 9:489–499.

172. Josephson ME, Wellens HJJ. Differential diagnosis of supraventricular tachycardia. Cardiol Clin 1990; 8:411–442.

173. Wellens HJ. The value of the ECG in the diagnosis of supraventricular tachycardias. Eur Heart J 1996; 17:10–20.

174. Rabbani LE, Wang PJ, Couper GL, Friedman PL. Time course of improvement in ventricular function after ablation of incessant automatic atrial tachycardia. Am Heart J 1991; 121:816–819.

175. Zipes DP, Gaum WE, Genetos BC, Glassman RD, Noble RJ, Fisch C. Atrial tachycardia without P waves masquerading as an A-V junctional tachycardia. Circulation 1977; 55:253–260.

176. Morillo CA, Klein GJ, Thakur RK, Li H, Zardini M, Yee R. Mechanism of "inappropriate" sinus tachycardia: role of sympathovagal balance. Circulation 1994; 90:873–877.

177. Ehlert FA, Damle RS, Goldberger JJ, Kadish AH. Effect of stimulus intensity on atrial refractoriness and sinus node recovery. J Cardiovasc Electrophysiol 1994; 5:485–495.

178. de Paola AAV, Horowitz LN, Vattimo AC, et al. Sinus node artery occlusion for treatment of chronic nonparoxysmal sinus tachycardia. Am J Cardiol 1992; 70:128–130.

179. Skeberis V, Simonis F, Tsakonas K, Celiker A, Andries E, Brugada P. Inappropriate sinus tachycardia following radiofrequency ablation of AV nodal tachycardia: incidence and clinical significance. PACE 1994; 17:924–927.

180. Bauernfeind RA, Amat-y-Leon F, Dhingra RC, Kehoe R, Wyndham CRC, Rosen KM. Chronic nonparoxysmal sinus tachycardia in otherwise healthy persons. Ann Intern Med 1979; 91:702–710.

181. Yee R, Guiraudon GM, Gardner MJ, Gulamhusein SS, Klein GJ. Refractory paroxysmal sinus tachycardia: management by subtotal right atrial exclusion. J Am Coll Cardiol 1984; 3:400–404.

182. Curry PVL, Krikler DM. Paroxysmal reciprocating sinus tachycardia. In Kulbertus HE (ed). Re-entrant Arrhythmias. Mechanisms and Treatment. Baltimore: University Park Press, 1976, pp. 39–62.

183. Ehlert FA, Goldberger JJ, Brooks R, Miller S, Kadish AH. Persistent inappropriate sinus tachycardia after radiofrequency current catheter modification of the atrioventricular node. Am J Cardiol 1992; 69:1092–1095.

184. Kocovic DZ, Harada T, Shea JB, Soroff D, Friedman PL. Alterations of heart rate and of heart rate variability after radiofrequency catheter ablation of supraventricular

185. Friedman PL, Stevenson WG, Kocovic DZ. Autonomic dysfunction after catheter ablation. J Cardiovasc Electrophysiol 1996; 7:450–459.

186. Shenasa M, Nadeau R, Savard P, Lemieux R, Curtiss EI, Follansbee WP. Noninvasive evaluation of supraventricular tachycardias. Cardiol Clin 1990; 8:443–464.

187. Stemple DR, Fitzgerald JW, Winkle RA. Benign slow paroxysmal atrial tachycardia. Ann Intern Med 1977; 87:44–48.

188. Shani J, Lichstein E, Jonas S, et al. Clinical significance of slow paroxysmal atrial tachycardia. Am Heart J 1983; 106:478–483.

189. Gillette PC, Wampler DG, Garson A Jr, Zinner A, Ott DA, Cooley D. Treatment of atrial automatic tachycardia by ablation procedures. J Am Coll Cardiol 1985; 6:405–409.

190. Strasburger JF, Duffy CE, Gidding SS. Abnormal systemic venous Doppler flow patterns in atrial tachycardia in infants. Am J Cardiol 1997; 80:640–643.

191. Chu E, Anza C, Chin MC, Sudhir K, Yock PG, Lesh MD. Radiofrequency catheter ablation guided by intracardiac echocardiography. Circulation 1994; 89:1301–1305.

192. Chu E, Kalman JM, Kwasman MA, et al. Intracardiac echocardiography during radiofrequency catheter ablation of cardiac arrhythmias in humans. J Am Coll Cardiol 1994; 24:1351–1357.

193. Kalman JM, Olgin JE, Karch MR, Hamdan M, Lee RJ, Lesh MD. "Cristal tachycardias": origin of right atrial tachycardias from the crista terminalis identified by intracardiac echocardiography. J Am Coll Cardiol 1998; 31:451–459.

194. Kay GN, Holman WL, Nanda NC. Combined use of transesophageal echocardiography and endocardial mapping to localize the site of origin of ectopic atrial tachycardia. Am J Cardiol 1990; 65:1284–1286.

195. McGuire MA, Johnson DC, Nunn GR, Yung T, Uther JB, Ross DL. Surgical therapy for atrial tachycardia in adults. J Am Coll Cardiol 1989; 14:1777–1782.

196. Rossi L. Histopathologic correlates of atrial arrhythmias. In Touboul P, Waldo AL (eds). Atrial Arrhythmias. Current Concepts and Management. St. Louis: Mosby–Year Book, 1990, pp. 27–40.

197. de Bakker JMT, Hauer RNW, Bakker PFA, Becker AE, Janse MJ, Robles de Medina EO. Abnormal automaticity as mechanism of atrial tachycardia in the human heart: electrophysiologic and histologic correlation: a case report. J Cardiovasc Electrophysiol 1994; 5:335–344.

198. Wu D, Denes P. Mechanisms of paroxysmal supraventricular tachycardia. Arch Intern Med 1975; 135:437–442.

199. Waldo AL, MacLean WAH. Diagnosis and Treatment of Cardiac Arrhythmias Following Open Heart Surgery. Emphasis on the Use of Atrial and Ventricular Epicardial Wire Electrodes. Mount Kisco, NY: Futura Publishing Co., 1980.

200. Sung RJ. Incessant supraventricular tachycardia. Pacing Clin Electrophysiol 1983; 6:1306–1326.

201. Sung RJ, Shen EN, Morady F, Scheinman MM, Hess D, Botvinick EH. Electrophysiologic mechanisms of exercise-induced sustained ventricular tachycardia. Am J Cardiol 1983; 51:525–530.

202. Ross DL, Denniss AR, Uther JB. Electrophysiologic study in supraventricular arrhythmias. Cardiovasc Clin 1985; 15:187–213.

203. Manolis AS, Estes NA III. Supraventricular tachycardia: mechanisms and therapy. Arch Intern Med 1987; 147:1706–1716.

204. Leitch J, Klein GJ, Yee R, Murdock C. Invasive electrophysiologic evaluation of patients with supraventricular tachycardia. Cardiol Clin 1990; 8:465–477.

205. Shakespeare CF, Anderson M, Camm AJ. Pathophysiology of supraventricular tachycardia. Eur Heart J 1993; 14:2–8.

206. Wellens HJJ. Atrial tachycardia: how important is the mechanism? Circulation 1994; 90:1576–1577.

207. Fisher JD, Lehmann MH. Marked intra-atrial conduction delay with split atrial electrograms: substrate for reentrant supraventricular tachycardia. Am Heart J 1986; 111:781–784.

tachycardia: delineation of parasympathetic pathways in the human heart. Circulation 1993; 88:1671–1681.

208. Simpson RJ Jr, Amara I, Foster JR, Woelfel A, Gettes LS. Thresholds, refractory periods, and conduction times of the normal and diseased human atrium. Am Heart J 1988; 116:1080–1090.

209. Tenczer J, Littmann L, Molnar F, Kekes E. Atrial reentry in chronic repetitive supraventricular tachycardia. Am Heart J 1980; 99:349–353.

210. Kadish AH, Morady F. The response of paroxysmal supraventricular tachycardia to overdrive atrial and ventricular pacing: can it help determine the tachycardia mechanism? J Cardiovasc Electrophysiol 1993; 4:239–252.

211. SippensGroenewegen A, Peeters HAP, Jessurun ER, et al. Body surface mapping during pacing at multiple sites in the human atrium: P-wave morphology of ectopic right atrial activation. Circulation 1998; 97:369–380.

212. Paritzky KL, Obayashi K, Mandel WJ. Atrial tachycardia secondary to sino-atrial node reentry. Chest 1974; 66:526–529.

213. Breithardt G, Seipel L. Further evidence for the site of reentry in so-called sinus node reentrant tachycardia in man. Eur J Cardiol 1980; 11:105–113.

214. Lawrie GM, Lin HT, Wyndham CR, DeBakey ME. Surgical treatment of supraventricular arrhythmias: results in 67 patients. Ann Surg 1987; 205:700–711.

215. Johnson DC, Nunn GR, Richards DA, Uther JB, Ross DL. Surgical therapy for supraventricular tachycardia, a potentially curable disorder. J Thorac Cardiovasc Surg 1987; 93:913–918.

216. Stevenson WG, Sager PT, Friedman PL. Entrainment techniques for mapping atrial and ventricular tachycardias. J Cardiovasc Electrophysiol 1995; 6:201–216.

217. Henthorn RW, Okumura K, Olshansky B, Plumb VJ, Hess PG, Waldo AL. A fourth criterion for transient entrainment: the electrogram equivalent of progressive fusion. Circulation 1988; 77:1003–1012.

218. Moro C, Rufilanchas JJ, Tamargo J, Novo L, Martinez J. Evidence of abnormal automaticity and triggering activity in incessant ectopic atrial tachycardia. Am Heart J 1988; 116:873–877.

219. Anderson KP. Management of ectopic atrial tachycardia. J Am Coll Cardiol 1993; 22:93–94.

220. Wellens HJJ, Brugada P, Ross D, Bar FWHM, Vanagt EJ, Dassen WR. Atrial tachycardia: the paroxysmal versus the permanent form. Am J Cardiol 1981; 47:495.

221. Weindling SN, Saul JP, Walsh EP. Efficacy and risks of medical therapy for supraventricular tachycardia in neonates and infants. Am Heart J 1996; 131:66–72.

222. Griffith MJ, Garratt CJ, Ward DE, Camm AJ. The effects of adenosine on sinus node reentrant tachycardia. Clin Cardiol 1989; 12:409–411.

223. Hsieh I-C, Yeh S-J, Wen M-S, Wang C-C, Lin F-C, Wu D. Effects of adenosine on paroxysmal atrial tachycardia. Am J Cardiol 1994; 74:279–281.

224. Kall JG, Kopp D, Olshansky B, et al. Adenosine-sensitive atrial tachycardia. Pacing Clin Electrophysiol 1995; 18:300–306.

225. Iesaka Y, Takahashi A, Goya M, et al. Adenosine-sensitive atrial reentrant tachycardia originating from the atrioventricular nodal transitional area. J Cardiovasc Electrophysiol 1997; 8:854–864.

226. DiMarco JP, Sellers TD, Lerman BB, Greenberg ML, Berne RM, Belardinelli L. Diagnostic and therapeutic use of adenosine in patients with supraventricular tachyarrhythmias. J Am Coll Cardiol 1985; 6:417–425.

227. Overholt ED, Rheuban KS, Gutgesell HP, Lerman BB, DiMarco JP. Usefulness of adenosine for arrhythmias in infants and children. Am J Cardiol 1988; 61:336–340.

228. Shenasa H, Kanter RJ, Hamer ME, et al. Reappraisal of the efficacy of adenosine for termination of ectopic atrial tachycardia. J Am Coll Cardiol 1993; 21:456A.

229. Till J, Shinebourne EA, Rigby ML, Clarke B, Ward DE, Rowland E. Efficacy and safety of adenosine in the treatment of supraventricular tachycardia in infants and children. Br Heart J 1989; 62:204–211.

230. Haines DE, Lerman BB, DiMarco JP. Repetitive supraventricular tachycardia: clinical manifestations and response to therapy with amiodarone. Pacing Clin Electrophysiol 1986; 9:130–133.

231. Pongiglione G, Strasburger JF, Deal BJ, Benson DW Jr. Use of amiodarone for short-term and adjuvant therapy in young patients. Am J Cardiol 1991; 68:603–608.

232. Shuler CO, Case CL, Gillette PC. Efficacy and safety of amiodarone in infants. Am Heart J 1993; 125:1430–1432.

233. Coumel P, Escoubet B, Attuel P. Beta-blocking therapy in atrial and ventricular tachyarrhythmias: experience with nadolol. Am Heart J 1984; 108:1098–1108.

234. Dhala AA, Case CL, Gillette PC. Evolving treatment strategies for managing atrial ectopic tachycardia in children. Am J Cardiol 1994; 74:283–286.

235. Sung RJ, Elser B, McAllister RG Jr. Intravenous verapamil for termination of re-entrant supraventricular tachycardias: intracardiac studies correlated with plasma verapamil concentrations. Ann Intern Med 1980; 93:682–689.

236. Rinkenberger RL, Prystowsky EN, Heger JJ, Troup PJ, Jackman WM, Zipes DP. Effects of intravenous and chronic oral verapamil administration in patients with supraventricular tachyarrhythmias. Circulation 1980; 62:996–1010.

237. Sapire DW, Mongkolsmai C, O'Riordan AC. Control of chronic ectopic supraventricular tachycardia with verapamil. J Pediatr 1979; 94:312–314.

238. DeSantola JR, Marchlinski FE. Response of digoxin toxic atrial tachycardia to digoxin-specific Fab fragments. Am J Cardiol 1986; 58:1109–1110.

239. Till JA, Rowland E, Shinebourne EA, Ward DE. Treatment of refractory supraventricular arrhythmias with flecainide acetate. Arch Dis Child 1987; 62:247–252.

240. Zeigler V, Gillette PC, Hammill B, Ross BA, Ewing L. Flecainide for supraventricular tachycardia in children. Am J Cardiol 1988; 62:41D–43D.

241. Perry JC, McQuinn RL, Smith RT Jr, Gothing C, Fredell P, Garson A Jr. Flecainide acetate for resistant arrhythmias in the young: efficacy and pharmacokinetics. J Am Coll Cardiol 1989; 14:185–191.

242. Kunze K, Kuck K, Schluter M, Bleifeld W. Effect of encainide and flecainide on chronic ectopic atrial tachycardia. J Am Coll Cardiol 1986; 7:1121–1126.

243. Creamer JE, Nathan AW, Camm AJ. Successful treatment of atrial tachycardias with flecainide acetate. Br Heart J 1985; 53:164–166.

244. Berns E, Rinkenberger RL, Jeang MK, Dougherty AH, Jenkins M, Naccarelli GV. Efficacy and safety of flecainide acetate for atrial tachycardia or fibrillation. Am J Cardiol 1987; 59:1337–1341.

245. Goy JJ, Kappenberger L. Flecainide acetate in supraventricular arrhythmias. J Electrophysiol 1987; 1:113–119.

246. Hellestrand KJ. Intravenous flecainide acetate for supraventricular tachycardias. Am J Cardiol 1988; 62:16D–22D.

247. Kuck KH, Kunze KP, Schluter M, Duckeck W. Encainide versus flecainide for chronic atrial and junctional ectopic tachycardia. Am J Cardiol 1988; 62:37L–44L.

248. van Wijk LM, Crijns HJ, van Gilst WH, Wesseling H, Lie KI. Flecainide acetate in the treatment of supraventricular tachycardias: value of programmed electrical stimulation for long-term prognosis. Am Heart J 1989; 117:365–369.

249. Mehta AV, Subrahmanyam AB, Long JB, Kanter RJ. Experience with moricizine HCL in children with supraventricular tachycardia. Int J Cardiol 1996; 57:31–35.

250. Moak JP, Smith RT, Garson A Jr. Newer antiarrhythmic drugs in children. Am Heart J 1987; 113:179–185.

251. Beaufort-Krol GCM, Bink-Boelkens MTE. Oral propafenone as treatment for incessant supraventricular and ventricular tachycardia in children. Am J Cardiol 1993; 72:1213–1214.

252. Heusch A, Kramer HH, Krogmann ON, Rammos S, Bourgeous M. Clinical experience with propafenone for cardiac arrhythmias in the young. Eur Heart J 1994; 15:1050–1056.

253. Combs RM. Unusual response to reserpine in paroxysmal atrial tachycardia with block unassociated with digitalis. South Med J 1967; 60:839–842.

254. Colloridi V, Perri C, Ventriglia F, Critelli G. Oral sotalol in

pediatric atrial ectopic tachycardia. Am Heart J 1992; 123:254–256.

255. Corwin ND, Klein MJ, Friedberg CK. Countershock conversion of digitalis-associated paroxysmal atrial tachycardia with block. Am Heart J 1963; 66:804–808.

256. Vassaux C, Lown B. Cardioversion of supraventricular tachycardias. Circulation 1969; 39:791–802.

257. Mark H, Sham R. Non-digitalis induced paroxysmal atrial tachycardia with block. I. Management with cardioversion. J Electrocardiol 1969; 2:171–176.

258. Kleiger R, Lown B. Cardioversion and digitalis. II. Clinical studies. Circulation 1966; 33:878–887.

259. Batchelder JE, Zipes DP. Treatment of tachyarrhythmias by pacing. Arch Intern Med 1975; 135:1115–1124.

260. Cooper TB, MacLean WA, Waldo AL. Overdrive pacing for supraventricular tachycardia: a review of theoretical implications and therapeutic techniques. Pacing Clin Electrophysiol 1978; 1:196–221.

261. Gillette PC. Antitachycardia pacing. Pacing Clin Electrophysiol 1997; 20:2121–2124.

262. Leclercq JF, Rosengarten MD, Delcourt P, Attuel P, Coumel P, Slama R. Prevention of intra-atrial reentry by chronic atrial pacing. Pacing Clin Electrophysiol 1980; 3:162–170.

263. Li CK, Shandling AH, Nolasco M, Thomas LA, Messenger JC, Warren J. Atrial automatic tachycardia-reversion pacemakers: their economic viability and impact on quality-of-life. Pacing Clin Electrophysiol 1990; 13:639–645.

264. Rhodes LA, Walsh EP, Gamble WJ, Triedman JK, Saul JP. Benefits and potential risks of atrial antitachycardia pacing after repair of congenital heart disease. Pacing Clin Electrophysiol 1995; 18:1005–1016.

265. Ragonese P, Drago F, Guccione P, Santilli A, Silvetti MS, Agostino DA. Permanent overdrive atrial pacing in the chronic management of recurrent postoperative atrial reentrant tachycardia in patients with complex congenital heart disease. PACE 1997; 20:2917–2923.

266. Moreira DA, Shepard RB, Waldo AL. Chronic rapid atrial pacing to maintain atrial fibrillation: use to permit control of ventricular rate in order to treat tachycardia induced cardiomyopathy. Pacing Clin Electrophysiol 1989; 12:761–775.

267. Gillette PC. Successful transcatheter ablation of ectopic atrial tachycardia in young patients using radiofrequency current. Circulation 1992; 86:1339–1340.

268. Lesh MD, Van Hare GF. Status of ablation in patients with atrial tachycardia and flutter. Pacing Clin Electrophysiol 1994; 17:1026–1033.

269. Manolis AS, Wang PJ, Estes NA III. Radiofrequency catheter ablation for cardiac tachyarrhythmias. Ann Intern Med 1994; 121:452–461.

270. Scheinman MM. Catheter ablation for atrial tachycardia. In Touboul P, Waldo AL (eds). Atrial Arrhythmias. Current Concepts and Management. St. Louis: Mosby–Year Book, 1990, pp. 458–461.

271. Klein LS. Radiofrequency catheter ablation: safety and practicality. Circulation 1991; 84:2594–2597.

272. American College of Cardiology Cardiovascular Technology Assessment Committee. Catheter ablation for cardiac arrhythmias: clinical applications, personnel and facilities: American College of Cardiology cardiovascular technology assessment committee. J Am Coll Cardiol 1994; 24:828–833.

273. Scheinman MM. Patterns of catheter ablation practice in the United States: results of the 1992 NASPE survey. PACE 1994; 17:873–875.

274. Saul JP, Triedman JK. Radiofrequency ablation of intraatrial reentrant tachycardia after surgery for congenital heart disease. Pacing Clin Electrophysiol 1997; 20:2112–2117.

275. Stevenson WG, Ellison KE, Lefroy DC, Friedman PL. Ablation therapy for cardiac arrhythmias. Am J Cardiol 1997; 80:56G–66G.

276. Scheinman MM, Laks MM, DiMarco J, Plumb V. Current role of catheter ablative procedures in patients with cardiac arrhythmias. Circulation 1991; 83:2146–2153.

277. Young M-L, Dai Z-K, Chang J-S, Chen M-R. Catheter fulguration ablation of left atrial ectopic tachycardia in a child. Am Heart J 1992; 123:253–254.

278. Case CL, Gillette PC, Oslizlok PC, Knick BJ, Blair HL. Radiofrequency catheter ablation of incessant, medically resistant supraventricular tachycardia in infants and small children. J Am Coll Cardiol 1992; 20:1405–1410.

279. Kall JG, Wilber DJ. Radiofrequency catheter ablation of an automatic atrial tachycardia in an adult. Pacing Clin Electrophysiol 1992; 15:281–287.

280. Lau YR, Gillette PC, Wienecke MM, Case CL. Successful radiofrequency catheter ablation of an atrial ectopic tachycardia in an adolescent. Am Heart J 1992; 123:1384–1386.

281. Chen SA, Chiang CE, Yang CJ, et al. Radiofrequency catheter ablation of sustained intra-atrial reentrant tachycardia in adult patients: identification of electrophysiological characteristics and endocardial mapping techniques. Circulation 1993; 88:578–587.

282. Goldberger J, Kall J, Ehlert F, et al. Effectiveness of radiofrequency catheter ablation for treatment of atrial tachycardia. Am J Cardiol 1993; 72:787–793.

283. Kay GN, Epstein AE, Dailey SM, Plumb VJ. Role of radiofrequency ablation in the management of supraventricular arrhythmias: experience in 760 consecutive patients. J Cardiovasc Electrophysiol 1993; 4:371–389.

284. Kay GN, Chong F, Epstein AE, Dailey SM, Plumb VJ. Radiofrequency ablation for treatment of primary atrial tachycardias. J Am Coll Cardiol 1993; 21:901–909.

285. Van Hare GF, Lesh MD, Stanger P. Radiofrequency catheter ablation of supraventricular arrhythmias in patients with congenital heart disease: results and technical considerations. J Am Coll Cardiol 1993; 22:883–890.

286. Tracy CM, Swartz JF, Fletcher RD, et al. Radiofrequency catheter ablation of ectopic atrial tachycardia using paced activation sequence mapping. J Am Coll Cardiol 1993; 21:910–917.

287. Kugler JD, Danford DA, Deal BJ, et al. Radiofrequency catheter ablation for tachyarrhythmias in children and adolescents: the Pediatric Electrophysiology Society. N Engl J Med 1994; 330:1481–1487.

288. Van Hare GF, Witherell CL, Lesh MD. Follow-up of radiofrequency catheter ablation in children: results in 100 consecutive patients. J Am Coll Cardiol 1994; 23:1651–1659.

289. Waspe LE, Chien WW, Merillat JC, Stark SI. Sinus node modification using radiofrequency current in a patient with persistent inappropriate sinus tachycardia. PACE 1994; 17:1569–1576.

290. Wu T-J, Chen S-A, Chiang C-E, et al. Radiofrequency catheter ablation of sustained intraatrial reentrant tachycardia in a patient with mirror-image dextrocardia. J Cardiovasc Electrophysiol 1994; 5:790–794.

291. Poty H, Saoudi N, Haissaguerre M, Daou A, Clementy J, Letac B. Radiofrequency catheter ablation of atrial tachycardias. Am Heart J 1996; 131:481–489.

292. Ivanov MY, Evdokimov VP, Vlasenco VV. Predictors of successful radiofrequency catheter ablation of sinoatrial tachycardia. PACE 1998; 21:311–315.

293. Lai W, Kao A, Silka MJ, et al. Recipient to donor conduction of atrial tachycardia following orthotopic heart transplantation. PACE 1998; 21:1331–1335.

294. Lin JL, Huang SKS, Lai LP, Ko WC, Tseng YZ, Lien WP. Clinical and electrophysiological characteristics and long-term efficacy of slow-pathway catheter ablation in patients with spontaneous supraventricular tachycardia and dual atrioventricular node pathways without inducible tachycardia. J Am Coll Cardiol 1998; 31:855–860.

295. Sosa EM, Arie S, Scanavacca MI, Vanzini P, Bellotti G, Pileggi F. Transcoronary chemical ablation of incessant atrial tachycardia. J Cardiovasc Electrophysiol 1990; 1:116–120.

296. Kottkamp H, Hindricks G, Breithardt G, Borggrefe M. Three-dimensional electromagnetic catheter technology: electroanatomical mapping of the right atrium and ablation of ectopic atrial tachycardia. J Cardiovasc Electrophysiol 1997; 8:1332–1337.

297. Klein GJ, Guiraudon GM. Surgical therapy of cardiac arrhythmias. Cardiol Clin 1983; 1:323–340.

298. Garson A Jr, Moak JP, Friedman RA, Perry JC, Ott DA.

Surgical treatment of arrhythmias in children. Cardiol Clin 1989; 7:319–329.

299. Guiraudon GM, Klein GJ, Sharma AD, Yee R. Surgical alternatives for supraventricular tachycardias. In Touboul P, Waldo AL (eds). Atrial Arrhythmias. Current Concepts and Management. St. Louis: Mosby–Year Book, 1990, pp. 488–497.

300. Guiraudon GM, Klein GJ, Yee R. Supraventricular tachycardias: the role of surgery. Pacing Clin Electrophysiol 1993; 16:658–670.

301. Wyndham CRC, Arnsdorf MF, Levitsky S, et al. Successful surgical excision of focal paroxysmal atrial tachycardia. Circulation 1980; 62:1365–1372.

302. Ott DA, Garson A, Cooley DA, McNamara DG. Definitive operation for refractory cardiac tachyarrhythmias in children. J Thorac Cardiovasc Surg 1985; 90:681–689.

303. Ott DA, Gillette PC, Garson A Jr, Cooley DA, Reul GJ, McNamara DG. Surgical management of refractory supraventricular tachycardia in infants and children. J Am Coll Cardiol 1985; 5:124–129.

304. Frank G, Baumgart D, Klein H, Luhmer I, Kallfelz HC, Borst HG. Successful surgical treatment of focal atrial tachycardia: a case report and review of the literature. Thorac Cardiovasc Surg 1986; 34:398–402.

305. Ott DA, Garson A Jr, Cooley DA, Smith RT, Moak J. Cryoablative techniques in the treatment of cardiac tachyarrhythmias. Ann Thorac Surg 1987; 43:138–143.

306. Kerr CR, Klein GG, Guiraudon GM, Webb JG. Surgical therapy for sinoatrial reentrant tachycardia. Pacing Clin Electrophysiol 1988; 11:776–783.

307. Seals AA, Lawrie GM, Magro S, et al. Surgical treatment of right atrial focal tachycardia in adults. J Am Coll Cardiol 1988; 11:1111–1117.

308. Case CL, Crawford FA, Gillette PC, Ross BA, Lee A, Zeigler V. Management strategies for surgical treatment of dysrhythmias in infants and children. Am J Cardiol 1989; 63:1069–1073.

309. Chang JP, Chang CH, Yeh SJ, Yamamoto T, Wu D. Surgical cure of automatic atrial tachycardia by partial left atrial isolation. Ann Thorac Surg 1990; 49:466–468.

310. Garson A Jr, Gillette PC, Moak JP, Perry JC, Ott DA, Cooley DA. Supraventricular tachycardia due to multiple atrial ectopic foci: a relatively common problem. J Cardiovasc Electrophysiol 1990; 1:132–138.

311. Bredikis J, Lekas R, Benetis R, et al. Diagnosis and surgical treatment of ectopic atrial tachycardia. Eur J Cardiothorac Surg 1991; 5:199–204.

312. Graffigna A, Vigano M, Pagani F, Salerno G. Surgical treatment for ectopic atrial tachycardia. Ann Thorac Surg 1992; 54:338–343.

313. Ott DA, Cooley DA, Moak J, Friedman RA, Perry J, Garson A Jr. Computer-guided surgery for tachyarrhythmias in children: current results and expectations. J Am Coll Cardiol 1993; 21:1205–1210.

314. Prager NA, Cox JL, Lindsay BD, Ferguson TB, Osborn JL, Cain ME. Long-term effectiveness of surgical treatment of ectopic atrial tachycardia. J Am Coll Cardiol 1993; 22:85–92.

315. Klein GJ, Hackel DB, Gallagher JJ. Anatomic substrate of impaired antegrade conduction over an accessory atrioventricular pathway in the Wolff-Parkinson-White syndrome. Circulation 1980; 61:1249–1256.

316. Giannelli Jr. S, Ayres SM, Gomprecht RF, Conklin EF, Kennedy RJ. Therapeutic surgical division of the human conduction system. JAMA 1967; 199:155–160.

317. Gillette PC, Garson A Jr, Hesslein PS, et al. Successful surgical treatment of atrial, junctional, and ventricular tachycardia unassociated with accessory connections in infants and children. Am Heart J 1981; 102:984–991.

318. Garson A Jr, Gillette PC. Electrophysiologic studies of supraventricular tachycardia in children. I. Clinical-electrophysiologic correlations. Am Heart J 1981; 102:233–250.

Multifocal Atrial Tachycardia[1-8a]

The electrocardiographic and clinical features of multifocal atrial tachycardia were first described systematically in 1968[9] and confirmed in papers published in the late 1960s and early 1970s.[10-14] Before then, examples of the arrhythmia had been reported, but they were not recognized as part of a clinical syndrome.[15-21] Several different names have been applied to what we now call multifocal atrial tachycardia[10, 12, 14-18, 20, 22-31] (Table 7.1).[b]

Few electrocardiographers before 1968 commented on specific characteristics of the patients whose electrocardiograms showed this arrhythmia. However, 10 years earlier, Corazza and Pastor published an example (Fig. 7.1) of what we would now call multifocal atrial tachycardia, which they described as follows:[18]

> In several cases very irregular bizarre atrial arrhythmias were observed, with beats arising in multiple atrial foci, occasionally with partial atrio-ventricular block.

Corazza and Pastor suggested that an association could exist between arrhythmias originating in the right atrium and patients with severe pulmonary disease:[18]

> Distention of the right atrium in cor pulmonale presents a situation analogous to the distention of the left atrium in mitral stenosis that is considered an important factor in the production of atrial arrhythmias.

Also in 1958, Scherf and Boyd printed another characteristic example of multifocal atrial tachycardia, which they described as follows:[19]

> A typical disturbance, appearing in any age but found especially often in elderly patients. . . . Atrial extrasystoles originating in many foci and shifting of the pacemaker with varying forms of T waves are seen. This arrhythmia often precedes atrial fibrillation.

In the 1968 report of 32 patients,[9] the phrase "multifocal atrial tachycardia" was first used for tachycardias characterized by multiform P waves. Most of the afflicted patients were elderly and severely ill, often from acute or chronic pulmonary disease. Their hospital mortality was high. They frequently had underlying cardiac disease, hypokalemia, and occasionally recent major surgery. The arrhythmia seemed rarely, if ever, due to digitalis, but injudicious use of the drug could hasten death.

The relatively high incidence of diabetes in patients with multifocal atrial tachycardia was first suggested in 1969[10] and was confirmed in subsequent series.[12, 14, 32] Little, however, was then understood about the pathogenesis of multifocal atrial tachycardia, except for the importance of extracardiac diseases and the likelihood that the arrhythmia was due to forces affecting the right rather than the left atrium.

Physicians treating multifocal atrial tachycardia concentrated on improving the nonarrhythmic conditions and reducing, if possible, the amount of chronotropic agents and bronchodilators often prescribed for the associated pulmonary disease. Reports provided little favorable information about the use of antiarrhythmic drugs. Effective acute treatment for multifocal atrial tachycardia with a beta-blocking drug, metoprolol, was established in 1984,[33] and treatment with a calcium-

---

[a]Revised from Chapter 5 in the first edition of this book.
[b]Most writers on the subject, including myself, favor the word "multifocal" over "chaotic" (from *chaos,* "a state of utter confusion"),[28] a word more suited to describing the electrocardiographic appearance of atrial fibrillation.

Table 7.1	OTHER NAMES FOR MULTIFOCAL ATRIAL TACHYCARDIA

Auricular paroxysmal tachycardia showing polymorphic auricular complexes[15]
Auricular paroxysmal tachycardia with irregular rhythm of the ventricles[17]
Chaotic atrial rhythm[12, 22, 24, 26, 27, 29]
Chaotic atrial mechanism[10, 14]
Chaotic atrial tachycardia[23, 25, 26, 30, 31]
Multifocal auricular extrasystoles[16]
Rapid or irregular atrial tachycardia[18]
Repetitive multifocal paroxysmal atrial (or auricular) tachycardia[17, 20]

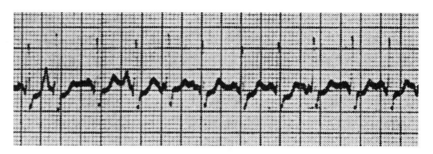

FIGURE 7.1 Multifocal atrial tachycardia. Electrocardiogram from a 1958 publication showing what we now call multifocal atrial tachycardia. (From Corazza LJ, Pastor BH. Cardiac arrhythmias in chronic cor pulmonale. N Engl J Med 1958; 259:862. Reprinted by permission of the New England Journal of Medicine.)[18]

channel–blocking drug, verapamil, was established a year later.[34]

PREVALENCE

Multifocal atrial tachycardia occurs infrequently when compared with the incidence of other arrhythmias. Investigators have reported finding multifocal atrial tachycardia in 0.05% to 0.32% of electrocardiograms interpreted in general hospitals[9, 11, 14] and in 0.36% of patients admitted to a hospital.[32] The incidence in children is lower.[30c]

AGE AND GENDER

Multifocal atrial tachycardia most commonly develops in elderly patients.[1, 9–12, 14, 32, 35d] Men and women are afflicted almost equally.[9, 11, 12, 35e] Multifocal atrial tachycardia, or a similar rhythm that pediatricians often call "chaotic atrial tachycardia," occurs occasionally in children.[36] More are boys than girls.[22, 24, 26, 29, 30, 32, 37–40f] Young adults occasionally have multifocal atrial tachycardia.[20, 41, 42] The arrhythmia often has little adverse clinical effect in this group.[42]

CLINICAL SETTING

Patients with multifocal atrial tachycardia are often acutely ill and, consequently, are frequently treated in units specializing in the critical care of patients with respiratory and heart failure, burns, and sepsis.

Pulmonary Disease

At least 60% of patients with multifocal atrial tachycardia have clinically important pulmonary disease.[1, 9–12, 14, 32, 35, 43, 44] The arrhythmia was observed in 17% of

patients with chronic airway obstruction who were admitted to the hospital for acute respiratory failure.[45] Chronic obstructive lung disease is the most common pulmonary diagnosis; pulmonary infections and, less frequently, pulmonary embolism are also found.

Drugs such as isoproterenol[14] and aminophylline,[9, 32, 46–48] administered to treat pulmonary disease, can exacerbate multifocal atrial tachycardia when therapeutic and especially when toxic blood levels are present. Aminophylline increases the atrial rate and the number of ectopic atrial beats as the concentration in the blood rises.[32]

Heart Disease

Patients with multifocal atrial tachycardia frequently have cardiac disease, which is hardly surprising in view of their advanced age. Coronary artery disease is the usual cause,[1, 9–12, 14, 32] and, although infrequent, multifocal atrial tachycardia occasionally complicates the course of myocardial infarction.[49] Valvular heart disease is rarely present,[9] although ambulatory monitoring has documented paroxysms of multifocal atrial tachycardia in patients with mitral stenosis.[50]

The severity of the cardiac problems can be difficult to evaluate clinically because pulmonary findings often dominate the physical examination of the chest. Congestive heart failure, however, frequently accompanies multifocal atrial tachycardia when the diagnosis is first made.[9, 11, 12, 14, 32, 35]

Metabolic Disorders

Patients with multifocal atrial tachycardia not infrequently have diabetes,[12, 14, 32g] hypokalemia,[9, 11, 12, 14] or azotemia.[10, 12, 14h]

Recent Operations

Multifocal atrial tachycardia tends to develop in patients after major surgery,[9, 32, 51] particularly when com-

---

cOf 1,500 children admitted to a pediatric cardiology service known for its expertise in arrhythmias, 0.2% had multifocal atrial tachycardia, called by the authors "chaotic atrial tachycardia." The incidence of the arrhythmia in all pediatric electrocardiograms must be much lower.

dThe average age of 315 patients reported in eight series was 70.1 years.[1, 9–12, 14, 32, 35]

eIn reports from community and university hospitals, 50% of 105 patients were male.[9, 11, 12, 35] Several groups of patients with multifocal atrial tachycardia, all males, have been reported from Department of Veterans Affairs Hospitals.[32, 35]

fThe ages of 42 children collected from eight reports[22, 24, 26, 29, 30, 37–39] ranged from *in utero* in one, from birth to one week of age in 13, from one week to one month in nine, from one month to one year in 11, to more than one year in eight. Sixty-seven percent of the children were male.

gAmong 118 patients in three series, 24% had diabetes. Specific testing of 31 patients with multifocal atrial tachycardia showed 74% with abnormalities of glucose tolerance.[10]

hHypokalemia was observed in 14% of 131 patients,[9, 11, 12, 14] and azotemia was found in 14% of 99 patients with multifocal atrial tachycardia.[10, 12, 14]

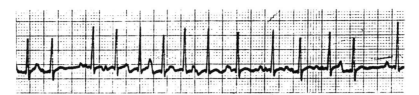

FIGURE 7.2 Multiple waves. Characteristic electrocardiogram of multifocal atrial tachycardia from a patient with chronic obstructive pulmonary disease and congestive heart failure. All the P waves except the last probably originate from abnormal atrial foci. Notice the irregularity of the rhythm, which can lead to confusion with atrial fibrillation when examining a patient at the bedside.

plicated by pneumonia, infections, or congestive heart failure.[9][i]

Associated Diseases in Children and Young Adults

Children have the serious illnesses that accompany multifocal atrial tachycardia less frequently than adults.[22, 24, 26, 37, 38, 52][j] Young adults with multifocal atrial tachycardia are often otherwise well or have asymptomatic abnormalities such as mitral valve prolapse.[23]

OTHER ARRHYTHMIAS

Patients often have a history of other atrial arrhythmias before, and may develop such disturbances after, multifocal atrial tachycardia develops. Because multifocal atrial tachycardia can be seen as constituting bursts of multiform atrial premature beats, it is not surprising that single atrial beats are frequently found in such patients.

---

[i]In a series of 32 patients, 28% developed multifocal atrial tachycardia after major surgery.[9] However, multifocal atrial tachycardia was the least common of five different supraventricular tachyarrhythmias that developed after major noncardiac surgery in 35 patients from another series:[51] atrial fibrillation in 17; regular supraventricular in six; atrial flutter in five; paroxysmal atrial tachycardia in four; and multifocal atrial tachycardia in three.

[j]Fifty-two percent of 29 children had no sickness other than multifocal atrial tachycardia, 20% had congenital heart disease, and 28% had a variety of other diagnoses.[22, 24, 26, 37, 38, 52]

Sinus tachycardia and arrest,[53] atrial fibrillation, and, less frequently atrial flutter or atrial tachycardia, including paroxysmal atrial tachycardia with block resulting from digitalis toxicity, have been observed in patients before or after they demonstrate multifocal atrial tachycardia.[2, 10–12, 14, 32, 35] The same diseases and metabolic abnormalities that are associated with multifocal atrial tachycardia and some of the drugs that such patients take can increase the sinus rate and produce other atrial arrhythmias.

HISTORY

Physicians usually discover that patients have multifocal atrial tachycardia from routine electrocardiograms or from monitors used in the intensive care units where such patients are often treated. Many patients with multifocal atrial tachycardia are unaware of the arrhythmia's presence, in my experience.[k] Decreased mental functioning during their acute illnesses probably contributes to this lack of awareness.

Symptoms not specific for arrhythmias such as dyspnea, which is usually the most common complaint, may increase during the tachycardia.[10] Weakness, chest pain, and operative pain are often present. Fainting during multifocal atrial tachycardia has been reported.[11] Some patients, however, volunteer that their hearts are beating rapidly or that they have palpitations.

PHYSICAL EXAMINATION

The physical examination of patients with multifocal atrial tachycardia reveals a rapid, irregular pulse, the discovery of which may make the unwary suspect atrial fibrillation. Specific, characteristic waveforms in the

---

[k]Symptoms are rarely mentioned in the series of patients with multifocal atrial tachycardia reported since 1968.

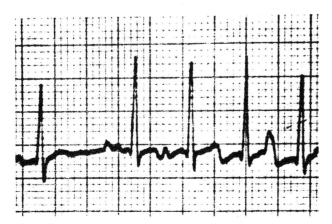

FIGURE 7.3 Form of P waves. Enlargement of beats 2 to 6 from Figure 7.2. The abnormally shaped P waves are easily seen.

Table 7.2 **GENERALLY ACCEPTED ELECTROCARDIOGRAPHIC CRITERIA FOR MULTIFOCAL ATRIAL TACHYCARDIA**
Rate more than 100 beats/min
Organized, discrete nonsinus P waves with at least three different forms in the same electrocardiographic lead
Isoelectric baseline between P waves
Irregular PP, PR, and RR intervals

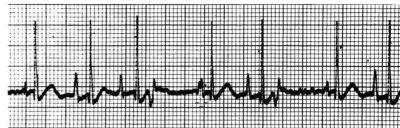

FIGURE 7.4 Chaotic atrial rhythm in an infant. Because the rate is relatively slow, "chaotic atrial rhythm" is the name the authors assigned to the arrhythmia of this 3-month-old girl who also had ectopic atrial tachycardia. (Adapted from Yeager SB, Hougen TJ, Levy AM. Sudden death in infants with chaotic atrial rhythm. Am J Dis Child 1984; 138:689–692, with permission.)

neck veins have not been reported in the literature, and I have not observed them. Findings typical of chronic obstructive pulmonary disease, congestive heart failure, and hypoperfusion of vital organs are frequent observations and may relate as much to the severity of underlying cardiopulmonary diseases as to the arrhythmia itself.[l] Almost all adults with multifocal atrial tachycardia report a history of underlying, usually severe cardiopulmonary or other systemic diseases.

ELECTROCARDIOGRAPHY

Rate

Because the word "tachycardia" appears in the name, most writers consider 100 beats per minute to be the slowest rate for multifocal atrial tachycardia[m] (Table 7.2). In adults, the fastest ventricular rate seldom exceeds 180 beats per minute;[9, 12] it ranged from 104 to 166 with an average of 127 beats per minute in one of the few studies[2] in which the rate of each patient was given. The atrial rate, up to 250 beats per minute,[9] but averaging about 142[2], is usually faster because

some P waves may be blocked from conducting to the ventricles.

P Waves

Frequent multiform P waves are the most characteristic feature of the electrocardiogram of multifocal atrial tachycardia (Figs. 7.2 to 7.5). They have the appearance of atrial premature beats with a form different from the patient's P waves in sinus rhythm and may be upright, inverted, biphasic, peaked, or bifid. Their form is due to their ectopic origin and to abnormal conduction through fibrosed, hypertrophied, or dilated atrial myocardium. Because the abnormal P waves have several forms, the range of their axes has never been reported.

Three Different P Waves. The requirement of at least three differently shaped P waves for the diagnosis of multifocal atrial tachycardia has been applied since the condition was first described. Does this mean two ectopic P waves plus the sinus P wave[1] or a minimum of three ectopic P waves? Although investigators do not always specify this point, the general consensus—with which I agree—favors a minimum of three abnormal P waves in addition to those from the sinus node. Whatever their number, the P waves with their different forms in multifocal atrial tachycardia tend to be most easily recognized in leads II, III, and V[1].[27]

PR Interval

The PR interval varies in patients with multifocal atrial tachycardia because the premature, ectopic atrial activity frequently reaches the atrioventricular node when it is partially refractory.[1, 9–12, 27, 35] The PR intervals of the ectopic P waves may be shorter, longer, or the same length as the PR intervals of the sinus beats. Atrioventricular block, usually of the first degree, has

[l] Writers seldom discuss the physical examination of patients with multifocal atrial tachycardia. This omission probably reflects the particular interest of many of the authors in arrhythmias and the retrospective nature of most series, which have often been collected from electrocardiography laboratories.

[m] Some authors suggest that requiring a rate of more than 100 beats per minute is too restrictive because a few patients with slower rates are encountered whose electrocardiograms fulfill all the other criteria and who have the clinical features characteristic of patients with multifocal atrial tachycardia.[10] Multifocal atrial *rhythm*, multifocal atrial *bradycardia* if the heart rate is less than 60 beats per minute, and *slow multifocal atrial tachycardia* have been used to describe the arrhythmia in such cases. Controversy arises when to consider such an arrhythmia wandering atrial pacemaker or a slow variant of multifocal atrial tachycardia. In such cases, correlating the clinical setting with the arrhythmia helps to provide a definitive diagnosis. Wandering atrial pacemaker almost always occurs in patients who are asymptomatic or much less severely ill than those with multifocal atrial tachycardia.

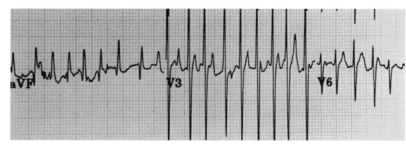

FIGURE 7.5 Multifocal atrial tachycardia in a child. Electrocardiographic leads aVF, V₃, and V₆ from the electrocardiogram of a child with chaotic atrial rhythm (multifocal atrial tachycardia). The rate is very rapid, as can be found in young children, and the P waves have several different forms. (Adapted from Dodo H, Gow RM, Hamilton RM, Freedom RM. Chaotic atrial rhythm in children. Am Heart J 1995; 129:990–995, with permission.)[29]

been reported in up to 20% of cases. The prematurity of some of the atrial beats may produce greater degrees of block.

QRS Complex

The QRS complexes are seldom normal in patients with multifocal atrial tachycardia.[12] Intraventricular conduction disturbances occur in up to 32% of patients,[10] right bundle branch block in about 16%,[10, 12, 32] and left bundle branch block occasionally.[10, 12] Right bundle branch block may appear intermittently because of the rapid rate.[1]

The electrocardiogram of left ventricular hypertrophy appears in 3% to 29% of patients with multifocal atrial tachycardia.[10, 12n] Electrocardiographic findings of right ventricular hypertrophy or of abnormal right axis deviation have seldom been noted despite the frequency of chronic lung disease in patients with multifocal atrial tachycardia.[12] Signs of myocardial infarction appear in the QRS complexes of one-third of patients with multifocal atrial tachycardia.[12]

ST and T Waves

The ST and T waves are abnormal in 39% to 58% of patients with multifocal atrial tachycardia.[10, 12, 32] Intrinsic myocardial disease, hypokalemia, hypoxia, and the effects of antiarrhythmic drugs and digitalis contribute to these findings.

OTHER ELECTROCARDIOGRAPHIC STUDIES

Holter monitoring reveals that multifocal atrial tachycardia is one of the arrhythmias that occur in patients with mitral stenosis.[50]

DIFFERENTIAL DIAGNOSIS

A supraventricular tachycardia with an irregular ventricular rate, multifocal atrial tachycardia must be distinguished from other arrhythmias with these fundamental characteristics.[1, 9]

Wandering Atrial Pacemaker

In this arrhythmia, the form of the P waves changes as the pacemaker varies its location.[10–12] Patients with wandering atrial pacemaker are usually well.

Sinus Arrhythmia

The duration of the PP intervals vary during sinus arrhythmia, but the form of the P waves does not change. Sinus arrhythmia, which occurs in healthy people related to respiration, may also develop in a more exaggerated form in elderly people with heart disease.

Atrial Fibrillation

The electrocardiogram of atrial fibrillation and multifocal atrial tachycardia can appear quite similar both to physicians and to the diagnostic computers that are routinely now employed in electrocardiography.[9, 11, 12, 32, 49] To make the correct diagnosis, particular attention should be given to the morphology of the atrial activity. The P waves in multifocal atrial tachycardia are well formed and discrete, whereas atrial activity in fibrillation is continuous, undulating, and changing. This is particularly noticeable in the baseline between the T waves and the QRS complexes.

When the ventricular rate is especially fast and P waves are particularly difficult to discern, the administration of a small amount of a beta-adrenergic or calcium-blocking drug usually decreases the ventricular rate sufficiently to allow the physician to recognize the P waves of multifocal atrial tachycardia or the characteristic forms of atrial fibrillation.

Atrial Flutter

During flutter, the atrial electrical activity, with its characteristic sawtooth appearance at a rate of about 250 to 400 beats per minute, is regular, as may be the ventricular rhythm. However, the speed of atrioventricular conduction can vary producing an irregular ventricular pattern.

Atrial Tachycardia

P waves with the same but usually abnormal form that occurs at regular intervals characterize automatic and reentrant atrial tachycardia. Partial atrioventricular block, if present, can produce an irregular ventricular rhythm.

Junctional Ectopic Tachycardia

Atrioventricular dissociation is the salient feature of this supraventricular tachycardia, most frequently found in children. When the dissociation is incomplete, some of the atrial activity captures the ventricles and thus produces an irregular rhythm.

LABORATORY STUDIES
Hematology and Chemistry

The blood urea nitrogen and creatinine of patients with multifocal atrial tachycardia are frequently elevated, reflecting at least some impairment of renal function during the arrhythmia.[10, 12, 14] Normal values often return after the acute illness has passed. However, because of the advanced age and chronic diseases of many patients with multifocal atrial tachycardia, evidence of abnormal renal function may persist.

Hypokalemia frequently accompanies multifocal atrial tachycardia.[9, 11, 12, 14] The cause usually is treatment with diuretics for concurrent congestive heart failure or hypertension. Hypomagnesemia has been

---

nThe wide range suggests that investigators may have applied different criteria in diagnosing hypertrophy.

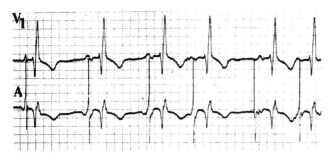

FIGURE 7.6 Several origins of P waves during multifocal atrial tachycardia. Notice how the different sources of the P waves cause the electrical activity in the right atrium to occur at different times during atrial activation. Electrocardiographic lead V₁ and the electrograms from within the right atrium (A) were recorded simultaneously in this patient with multifocal atrial tachycardia. Vertical lines connect the P waves on the surface tracing with the intracardic electrograms.

reported in a few patients with multifocal atrial tachycardia.[54, 55]

Radiology

The chest radiographs of patients with multifocal atrial tachycardia show no findings specific for the arrhythmia. Signs of chronic and acute pulmonary disease, congestive heart failure, or cardiomegaly are frequently found.[32]

Echocardiography

Slight biatrial enlargement, less than in atrial fibrillation, characterizes the echocardiograms of many patients with multifocal atrial tachycardia.[56] Moderate to severe left ventricular dysfunction occurs in a few patients.[56] Left or right atrial size are similar in patients with chronic obstructive pulmonary disease whether or not they have multifocal atrial tachycardia.[2] Echocardiograms were normal in nine children with multifocal atrial tachycardia.[22, 26]

Hemodynamics

The cardiac function of only a few patients with multifocal atrial tachycardia has been evaluated systematically with invasive or noninvasive studies during the acute illness or later after recovery. In a report of 13 patients, pulmonary capillary wedge and pulmonary artery mean pressures were elevated, and the average cardiac index was low normal.[57, 58o]

PATHOLOGY

Autopsies on 22 patients with multifocal atrial tachycardia revealed the following:[10, 32]

• Coronary artery disease in 68%.

---

*The wedge pressure was 15.5 ± 2.1 mm Hg, the pulmonary artery mean pressure 27.5 ± 3.2 mm Hg, and the cardiac index 2.85 ± 0.34 L/min/m².[58]

• Chronic pulmonary disease in 59%.
• Pulmonary edema in 59%.
• Bronchitis in 59%.
• Pneumonia in 50%.
• Myocardial infarction in 36%.
• Pulmonary emboli in 23%.

CLINICAL ELECTROPHYSIOLOGY

The word "multifocal" implies that the arrhythmia originates from several different places in the atria, a thesis favored by the different forms of the P waves and the irregular PP and PR intervals. A few intracardiac studies recorded in such patients support this thesis (Figs. 7.6 and 7.7). In one report, intra-atrial conduction was abnormal in most patients, and atrioventricular nodal conduction was prolonged in some.[22] Atrionodal conduction varied from beat to beat in half the patients.[22]

Standard electrophysiological and pharmacological testing have not defined the mechanisms causing multifocal atrial tachycardia in most cases. Programmed electrical stimulation, which characteristically elicits and terminates reentrant arrhythmias, does not substantially affect multifocal atrial tachycardia. Some workers favor triggered activity as the mechanism because verapamil, which blocks the calcium channels fundamental to this type of abnormality, can suppress some of the extra beats.[47, 48]

Why lung disease, present in many patients with multifocal atrial tachycardia, should produce the arrhythmia has not been established. However, certain effects of severe pulmonary disease such as right atrial enlargement, hypercarbia, hypoxia, acidosis, and adrenergic stimulation can arouse ectopic foci.

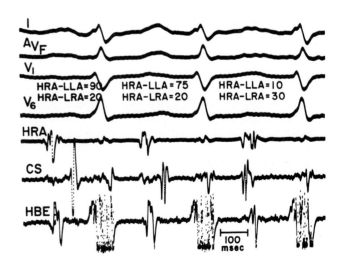

FIGURE 7.7 Atrial activation during multifocal atrial tachycardia. Notice the change in the sequence of atrial activation among the three sites in this electrophysiological recording of three beats from a patient with multifocal atrial tachycardia. Electrocardiographic leads I, aVF, V₁, and V₆ plus intracardiac electrograms recorded from the high right atrium (HRA), the low left atrium (LLA) in the coronary sinus (CS), and the low right atrium (LRA) at the His bundle electrogram position (HBE). The numbers indicate milliseconds.

| Table 7.3 | **EFFECTS OF MAGNESIUM- AND OF CALCIUM-CHANNEL- AND BETA-ADRENERGIC–BLOCKING DRUGS ON PATIENTS WITH MULTIFOCAL ATRIAL TACHYCARDIA** | | | |

Drug	Average Decrease of Ventricular Rate (beats/min)	Patients Converted to Sinus Rhythm	Reference	Dose
Acebutolol	44 (1 patient not converted)	1 of 4 (25%)	74	See reference 74, p. 150
			76	0.3 + 1.0 mg/kg intravenously (2 patients)
Esmolol	45	0 of 2	77	See reference 77, p. 395
Magnesium	—	7 of 8 (88%)	54	See reference 54, p. 790
Metoprolol	51	30 of 38 (79%)	73	25 or 50 mg orally
			72	25 mg q6h orally or 2–3 mg intravenously every 2 min, maximum 15 mg
Verapamil	31	18 of 42 (43%)	34	1 mg intravenous test dose, then 4 mg in 5 min
			68	2.5 mg intravenously, every 2–4 min, maximum 15 mg
			65	80 mg orally q8h
			67	1 mg/min intravenously

TREATMENT

General Therapy

Treating multifocal atrial tachycardia should begin by improving the cardiac, pulmonary, metabolic, and infectious conditions that have given rise to the arrhythmia.[59] Frequently, multifocal atrial tachycardia resolves after such measures without specific antiarrhythmic therapy. Multifocal atrial tachycardia, however, frequently recurs during exacerbations of the underlying diseases.

Physical Maneuvers

Carotid sinus massage transiently reduces the atrial rate and decreases the number of ectopic atrial beats.[54] The maneuver is seldom needed to make the diagnosis.

Magnesium and Potassium

Magnesium, administered intravenously[60, 61] and intramuscularly[60] to patients with multifocal atrial tachycardia and hypomagnesemia, can decrease the ventricular rate[61] and can suppress the ectopic atrial activity. This treatment has occasionally helped even when magnesium levels are within the normal range[54] (Table 7.3). Potassium may also be useful when given to patients with hypokalemia before or after administration of magnesium.[55]

Amiodarone

Intravenously and orally administered amiodarone restored and maintained sinus rhythm in a few patients with multifocal atrial tachycardia to whom it was given.[39, 62p]

Calcium-Channel–Blocking Drugs

Verapamil. The calcium-channel–blocking drug verapamil,[63] when given in sufficient amounts, decreases the ventricular rate[64] by reducing the number of atrial beats, not by increasing atrioventricular nodal blocking of them[34, 58, 65–68] (see Table 7.3). The drug also decreases the number of abnormally formed atrial beats.[34]

Despite its salutary effect on rate, verapamil does not convert all patients with multifocal atrial tachycardia to sinus rhythm (see Table 7.3), and some of those resuming sinus rhythm still have atrial premature beats.[34, 48, 58, 66, 67] Multifocal atrial tachycardia recurs in some patients if verapamil is not given on a long-term basis.[34, 65–67]

Transient hypotension is the most common side effect produced by intravenous verapamil in patients with multifocal atrial tachycardia, but clinically injurious decreases are unusual.[58, 67] Calcium gluconate, when given before the verapamil, reduces the drop in blood pressure.[67q]

Verapamil decreases arterial oxygen tension and increases the alveolar-arterial oxygen gradient in patients with multifocal atrial tachycardia.[58r] Calcium-channel–blocking drugs may lower arterial oxygen tension by relieving hypoxic pulmonary vasoconstriction, which leads to perfusion of poorly ventilated lung units,[58, 69] or by reducing right ventricular function in patients with severe lung disease.[70] Although this effect may not cause significant clinical deterioration, physicians should be aware of the potential danger of the finding.[71]

Beta-Adrenergic–Blocking Drugs

In the 1968 report, my colleagues and I wrote:[9]

---

pSinus rhythm returned in four patients given amiodarone intravenously and in five given the drug orally.[62] The authors suggested: "Amiodarone may be the drug of choice for treatment of MAT, for which up to now no effective therapy has been established."[62] Amiodarone also successfully converted multifocal atrial tachycardia in a 3-year old boy with congenital heart disease and congestive heart failure in whom verapamil and digoxin had failed.[39]

---

qFrom 27% without the calcium to 11% with calcium.[67]
rIn 13 patients with multifocal atrial tachycardia, arterial oxygen tension dropped from 105.2 ± 16.8 mm Hg before verapamil to 78.3 ± 7.3 mm Hg after verapamil ($P < 0.025$).[57, 58] Alveolar-arterial oxygen gradient increased from 139.9 ± 23.3 mm Hg before verapamil to 167.7 ± 29.2 mm Hg after verapamil.[58]

Propranolol had no effect in one moribund patient, but completely abolished multifocal atrial tachycardia, which had been recurrent, in a man with coronary-artery disease.

Despite this and other[12, 14, 35] references to the possible value of beta-blocking drugs, clinicians hesitated to administer them to patients with multifocal atrial tachycardia because of concern that the drugs would exacerbate the spastic component of the patients' lung disease or would dangerously decrease cardiac function producing hypotension or congestive heart failure. Theoretically, this class of drugs should be useful by slowing or suppressing ectopic foci, increasing atrioventricular block, or calming the effects of sympathetic stimulation on the heart.[32]

By 1979, reports began appearing that showed that beta-blocking drugs could favorably affect multifocal atrial tachycardia relatively quickly with few side effects. Metoprolol, the cardioselective beta blocker, decreases the ventricular rates of most patients with multifocal atrial tachycardia[33, 72, 73] as do acebutolol[74–76] and esmolol,[77] the ultrashort-acting intravenously administered beta-adrenergic–blocking agent, which, in one case, suppressed the arrhythmia entirely[78] (see Table 7.3). Long-term oral treatment of the arrhythmia is sometimes required for continued suppression.[72s]

Beta-Adrenergic–Blocking Versus Calcium-Channel–Blocking Drugs

A randomized, blinded evaluation of 13 subjects with multifocal atrial tachycardia showed that more patients responded favorably to metoprolol than to verapamil or placebo.[68] As for verapamil,[72]

> Our own impression with verapamil for multifocal atrial tachycardia left us unimpressed with its value. Indeed, 6 study patients had received verapamil without any conversion or an unacceptable reduction in rate before metoprolol was used.

In view of these results, I advise choosing a beta blocker before verapamil unless specific conditions strongly contraindicate its use. A trial with esmolol is unlikely to cause serious problems. Beta- or calcium-channel–blocking agents should be given whenever the rapid rate of multifocal atrial tachycardia produces ischemia, dangerous ventricular arrhythmias, hypoxia, pulmonary congestion, or systemic hypoperfusion.[79] Despite the rate-lowering and converting effects of verapamil and metoprolol on multifocal atrial tachycardia, these drugs have not been shown to reduce mortality in patients with multifocal atrial tachycardia.

Digitalis

Digitalis, all but one reporter[1] has agreed, seldom, if ever, produces multifocal atrial tachycardia.[9–12, 35] Neither, however, is the drug particularly effective in suppressing the arrhythmia.[9, 14, 35] General improvement of cardiopulmonary function, rather than any specific antiarrhythmic action, probably accounts for suppression of the arrhythmia when digitalis is given.[9, 32]

Digitalis intoxication can easily develop in patients with multifocal atrial tachycardia because they frequently have severe myocardial disease and may be hypokalemic, hypomagnesemic, hypoxic, or uremic. Atrioventricular block, ventricular arrhythmias, and death have been reported when too much digitalis has been administered in a misguided effort to slow the ventricular rate when atrial fibrillation has been incorrectly diagnosed.[9, 26, 35, 79] However, in the absence of toxicity, digitalis need not be withheld if the drug is otherwise indicated.[1, 32]

Flecainide

Flecainide, given intravenously and by mouth, has suppressed a few cases of multifocal atrial tachycardia in adults[80, 81] and children.[40, 82]

Other Antiarrhythmic Drugs

Until the use of beta-adrenergic and calcium-channel–blocking drugs was described, no pharmacological treatment seemed to suppress multifocal atrial tachycardia reliably. Investigators have been continuously frustrated by the ineffectiveness of lidocaine, quinidine, procainamide, phenytoin, and other antiarrhythmic agents.[1, 9, 10, 14, 22, 24, 26, 32, 35, 38] Intravenous propafenone controlled multifocal atrial tachycardia completely in one of four and partially in two of four infants.[83]

Cardioversion

In the few reports of cardioversion of multifocal atrial tachycardia, the arrhythmia has usually persisted after the shock.[13, 14, 35] Consequently, cardioversion should not be used in the treatment of multifocal atrial tachycardia.

PROGNOSIS

Adults

Forty-four percent of 280 adult patients with multifocal atrial tachycardia in nine series published from 1968 to 1988 died during the hospitalization in which the arrhythmia was first documented.[2, 9–12, 14, 35, 68, 84t] Death usually results from the severe diseases that afflict most patients with multifocal atrial tachycardia, rather than from the arrhythmia itself, which is often no longer present near the time of death.[32]

Few data are available about the survival of patients with multifocal atrial tachycardia who leave the initial hospitalization alive. Shorter survival, however, seems to coincide with faster heart rates and the use of aminophylline and digitalis.[32] These factors tend to occur in the presence of advanced pulmonary and cardiac disease, the severity of which is more likely the underlying cause of a poor prognosis.

'Twenty-seven percent in one series.[72]

'The range of mortality was 29% to 56%.[2, 9–12, 14, 35, 68, 84]

Children

Most children have a favorable course. Only 4 of 28 (14%) died, none directly from multifocal atrial tachycardia.[22, 24, 26, 37–39] However, the outlook for infants with the arrhythmia may be more ominous.[26]

SUMMARY

Multifocal atrial tachycardia is an abnormal, rapid supraventricular tachyarrhythmia characterized by irregular P waves with several different forms. Patients usually are elderly and have severe pulmonary and cardiovascular diseases. Treating the underlying disease is the basic form of therapy. Beta-adrenergic and calcium-channel–blocking drugs usually decrease the heart rate and improve patients' cardiovascular function. The prognosis in adults depends more on the severity of the underlying disease than on the arrhythmia.

REFERENCES

1. Chung EK. Appraisal of multifocal atrial tachycardia. Br Heart J 1971; 33:500–504.
2. Scher DL, Arsura EL. Multifocal atrial tachycardia: mechanisms, clinical correlates, and treatment. Am Heart J 1989; 118:574–580.
3. Kastor JA. Multifocal atrial tachycardia. N Engl J Med 1990; 322:1713–1717.
4. Porter CJ. Premature atrial contractions and atrial tachyarrhythmias. In Gillette PC, Garson A Jr (eds). Pediatric Arrhythmias. Electrophysiology and Pacing. Philadelphia: WB Saunders, 1990; pp. 328–359.
5. Schwartz M, Rodman D, Lowenstein SR. Recognition and treatment of multifocal atrial tachycardia: a critical review. J Emerg Med 1994; 12:353–360.
6. Ganz LI, Friedman PL. Supraventricular tachycardia. N Engl J Med 1995; 332:162–173.
7. Goldberger JJ, Kadish AH. Atrial premature depolarizations, junctional premature depolarizations, multifocal atrial tachycardia, and atrial tachycardia. In Podrid PJ, Kowey PR (eds). Cardiac Arrhythmia. Mechanisms, Diagnosis and Management. Baltimore: Williams & Wilkins, 1995, pp. 768–789.
8. Naccarelli GV, Shih H-T, Jalal S. Clinical arrhythmias: mechanisms, clinical features, and management. Supraventricular tachycardia. In Zipes DP, Jalife J (eds). Cardiac Electrophysiology. From Cell to Bedside. 2nd ed. Philadelphia: WB Saunders, 1995, pp. 607–619.
9. Shine KI, Kastor JA, Yurchak PM. Multifocal atrial tachycardia: clinical and electrocardiographic features in 32 patients. N Engl J Med 1968; 279:344–349.
10. Phillips J, Spano J, Burch G. Chaotic atrial mechanism. Am Heart J 1969; 78:171–179.
11. Lipson MJ, Naimi S. Multifocal atrial tachycardia (chaotic atrial tachycardia): clinical associations and significance. Circulation 1970; 42:397–407.
12. Berlinerblau R, Feder W. Chaotic atrial rhythm. J Electro-cardiol 1972; 5:135–144.
13. Ticzon AR, Andres R, Whalen R. Refractory supraventricular tachycardias. Circulation 1973; 47:642–653.
14. Kones RJ, Phillips J, Hersh J. Mechanism and management of chaotic atrial mechanism. Cardiology 1974; 59:92–101.
15. Mackinnon AU. The rhythm of paroxysmal tachycardia: an electrocardiographic study. Q J Med 1934; 3:1–14.
16. Parkinson J, Papp C. Repetitive paroxysmal tachycardia. Br Heart J 1947; 9:241–262.
17. Katz LN, Pick A. Clinical Electrocardiography. Part I. The Arrhythmias. Philadelphia: Lea & Febiger, 1956, pp. 327, 594–595.
18. Corazza LJ, Pastor BH. Cardiac arrhythmias in chronic cor pulmonale. N Engl J Med 1958; 259:862–865.
19. Scherf D, Boyd LJ. Cardiovascular Diseases. 3rd ed. New York: Grune & Stratton, 1958, p. 641.
20. Abrams DL, Eaddy JA. Repetitive multifocal paroxysmal atrial tachycardia. Am J Cardiol 1965; 15:871–873.
21. Thomas AJ, Valabhji P. Arrhythmia and tachycardia in pulmonary heart disease. Br Heart J 1969; 31:491–495.
22. Gavrilescu S, Luca C. Chaotic atrial rhythm. Eur Heart J 1974; 2:153–159.
23. Bisset GS III, Seigel SF, Gaum WE, Kaplan S. Chaotic atrial tachycardia in childhood. Am Heart J 1981; 101:268–272.
24. Liberthson RR, Colan SD. Multifocal or chaotic atrial rhythm: report of nine infants, delineation of clinical course and management, and review of the literature. Pediatr Cardiol 1982; 2:179–184.
25. Abinader EG, Cooper M. Chaotic atrial tachycardia in the mitral valve prolapse syndrome. Am Heart J 1983; 106:1161–1162.
26. Yeager SB, Hougen TJ, Levy AM. Sudden death in infants with chaotic atrial rhythm. Am J Dis Child 1984; 138:689–692.
27. Strasburger JF, Smith RT Jr, Moak JP, Gothing C, Garson A Jr. Encainide for resistant supraventricular tachycardia in children: follow-up report. Am J Cardiol 1988; 62:50L–54L.
28. Anonymous. Merriam Webster's Collegiate Dictionary. 10th ed. Springfield, MA: Merriam-Webster, 1993, p. 191.
29. Dodo H, Gow RM, Hamilton RM, Freedom RM. Chaotic atrial rhythm in children. Am Heart J 1995; 129:990–995.
30. Salim MA, Case CL, Gillette PC. Chaotic atrial tachycardia in children. Am Heart J 1995; 129:831–833.
31. Zipes DP. Specific arrhythmias: diagnosis and treatment. In Braunwald E (ed). Heart Disease. A Textbook of Cardiovascular Medicine. 5th ed. Philadelphia: WB Saunders, 1997:675–677.
32. Habibzadeh MA. Multifocal atrial tachycardia: a 66 month follow-up of 50 patients. Heart Lung 1980; 9:328–335.
33. Hanau SP, Solar M, Arsura EL. Metoprolol in the treatment of multifocal atrial tachycardia. Cardiovasc Rev Rep 1984; 5:1182, 1191–1194.
34. Levine JH, Michael JR, Guarnieri T. Treatment of multifocal atrial tachycardia with verapamil. N Engl J Med 1985; 312:21–25.
35. Wang K, Goldfarb BL, Gobel FL, Richman HG. Multifocal atrial tachycardia. Arch Intern Med 1977; 137:161–164.
36. Zuckerman GB, Conway EE Jr, Singh J, Walsh C. Multifocal atrial tachycardia in a child presenting with chest pain. Pediatr Emerg Care 1993; 9:348–350.
37. Farooki ZQ, Green EW. Multifocal atrial tachycardia in two neonates. Br Heart J 1977; 39:872–874.
38. Southall DP, Johnson AM, Shinebourne EA, Johnston PG, Vulliamy DG. Frequency and outcome of disorders of cardiac rhythm and conduction in a population of newborn infants. Pediatrics 1981; 68:58–66.
39. Zeevi B, Berant M, Sclarovsky S, Blieden LC. Treatment of multifocal atrial tachycardia with amiodarone in a child with congenital heart disease. Am J Cardiol 1986; 57:344–345.
40. Perry JC, McQuinn RL, Smith RT Jr, Gothing C, Fredell P, Garson A Jr. Flecainide acetate for resistant arrhythmias in the young: efficacy and pharmacokinetics. J Am Coll Cardiol 1989; 14:185–191.
41. Omori Y. Repetitive multifocal paroxysmal atrial tachycardia: with cyclic Wenckebach phenomenon under observation for thirteen years. Am Heart J 1971; 82:527–530.
42. D'Cruz IA, Mehta AB, Kelkar PN, Pahlajani DB. Benign repetitive multifocal ectopic atrial tachycardia: response to intracardiac atrial stimulation. Am Heart J 1974; 88:671–672.
43. Levine PA, Klein MD. Mechanisms of arrhythmias in chronic obstructive lung disease. Geriatrics 1976; 31:47–56.
44. Biggs FD, Lefrak SS, Kleiger RE, Senior RM, Oliver GC. Disturbances of rhythm in chronic lung disease. Heart Lung 1977; 6:256–261.
45. Hudson LD, Kurt TL, Petty TL, Genton E. Arrhythmias associated with acute respiratory failure in patients with chronic airway obstruction. Chest 1973; 63:661–665.

46. Greenberg A, Piraino BH, Kroboth PD, Weiss J. Severe theophylline toxicity: role of conservative measures, antiarrhythmic agents, and charcoal hemoperfusion. Am J Med 1984; 76:854–860.

47. Levine JH, Michael JR, Guarnieri T. Multifocal atrial tachycardia: a toxic effect of theophylline. Lancet 1985; 1:12–14.

48. Marchlinski FE, Buxton AE, Doherty JU, et al. Use of programmed electrical stimulation to predict sudden death after myocardial infarction. Cardiovasc Clin 1985; 15:163–169.

49. White RD. Prehospital recognition of multifocal atrial tachycardia: association with acute myocardial infarction. Ann Emerg Med 1992; 21:753–756.

50. Ramsdale DR, Arumugam N, Singh SS, Pearson J, Charles RG. Holter monitoring in patients with mitral stenosis and sinus rhythm. Eur Heart J 1987; 8:164–170.

51. Goldman L. Supraventricular tachyarrhythmias in hospitalized adults after surgery: clinical correlates in patients over 40 years of age after major noncardiac surgery. Chest 1978; 73:450–454.

52. Singsen B, Goldreyer B, Stanton R, Hanson V. Childhood polymyositis with cardiac conduction defects. Am J Dis Child 1976; 130:72–74.

53. Nakazato Y, Nakata Y, Hisaoka T, Sumiyoshi M, Ogura S, Yamaguchi H. Clinical and electrophysiological characteristics of atrial standstill. Pacing Clin Electrophysiol 1995; 18:1244–1254.

54. Iseri LT, Fairshter RD, Hardemann JL, Brodsky MA. Magnesium and potassium therapy in multifocal atrial tachycardia. Am Heart J 1985; 110:789–794.

55. Strickberger SA, Miller CB, Levine JH. Multifocal atrial tachycardia from electrolyte imbalance. Am Heart J 1988; 115:680–682.

56. Santos-Ocampo CD, Sadaniantz A, Elion JL, Garber CE, Malone LL, Parisi AF. Echocardiographic assessment of the cardiac anatomy in patients with multifocal atrial tachycardia: a comparison with atrial fibrillation. Am J Med Sci 1994; 307:264–268.

57. Arsura EL, Scher DL. Verapamil and multifocal atrial tachycardia. Ann Intern Med 1988; 108:486.

58. Arsura E, Lefkin AS, Scher DL, Solar M, Tessler S. A randomized, double-blind, placebo-controlled study of verapamil and metoprolol in treatment of multifocal atrial tachycardia. Am J Med 1988; 85:519–524.

59. Payne RM. Management of arrhythmias in patients with severe lung disease. Clin Pulm Med 1994; 1:232–236.

60. Cohen L, Kitzes R, Shnaider H. Multifocal atrial tachycardia responsive to parenteral magnesium. Magnes Res 1988; 1:239–242.

61. McCord JK, Borzak S, Davis T, Gheorghiade M. Usefulness of intravenous magnesium for multifocal atrial tachycardia in patients with chronic obstructive pulmonary disease. Am J Cardiol 1998; 81:91–93.

62. Kouvaras G, Cokkinos DV, Halal G, Chronopoulos G, Ioannou N. The effective treatment of multifocal atrial tachycardia with amiodarone. Jpn Heart J 1989; 30:301–312.

63. Graboys TB. The treatment of supraventricular tachycardias. N Engl J Med 1985; 312:43–44.

64. Aronow WS, Plasencia G, Wong R, Landa D, Karlsberg R, Ferlinz J. Effect of verapamil versus placebo on PAT and MAT (paroxysmal atrial tachycardia and multifocal atrial tachycardia). Curr Ther Res 1980; 27:823–829.

65. Schettini B, Katz S, Zeldis SM. Verapamil in tachycardia therapy. Chest 1986; 89:616.

66. Mukerji V, Alpert MA, Diaz-Arias M, Sanfelippo JF. Termination and suppression of multifocal atrial tachycardia with verapamil. South Med J 1987; 80:269–270.

67. Salerno DM, Anderson B, Sharkey PJ, Iber C. Intravenous verapamil for treatment of multifocal atrial tachycardia with and without calcium pretreatment. Ann Intern Med 1987; 107:623–628.

68. Hazard PB, Burnett CR. Verapamil in multifocal atrial tachycardia: hemodynamic and respiratory changes. Chest 1987; 91:68–70.

69. Melto C, Hallemans R, Naeije R, Mols P, Lejeune P. Deleterious effect of nifedipine on pulmonary gas exchange in chronic obstructive pulmonary disease. Am Rev Respir Dis 1984; 130:612–616.

70. Packer M, Medina N, Yushak M. Adverse hemodynamic and clinical effects of calcium channel blockade in pulmonary hypertension secondary to obliterative pulmonary vascular disease. J Am Coll Cardiol 1984; 4:890–901.

71. Rotkin LG. Verapamil for multifocal atrial tachycardia. N Engl J Med 1985; 312:1126.

72. Hazard PB, Burnett CR. Treatment of multifocal atrial tachycardia with metoprolol. Crit Care Med 1987; 15:20–25.

73. Arsura EL, Solar M, Lefkin AS, Scher DL, Tessler S. Metoprolol in the treatment of multifocal atrial tachycardia. Crit Care Med 1987; 15:591–594.

74. Aronow WS, Van Camp S, Turbow M, Whittaker K, Lurie M. Acebutolol in supraventricular arrhythmias. Clin Pharmacol Ther 1979; 25:149–153.

75. Aronow WS, Landa D, Plasencia G, Wong R, Karlsberg RP, Ferlinz J. Verapamil in atrial fibrillation and atrial flutter. Clin Pharmacol Ther 1979; 26:578–583.

76. Williams DO, Tatelbaum R, Most AS. Effective treatment of supraventricular arrhythmias with acebutolol. Am J Cardiol 1979; 44:521–525.

77. Byrd RC, Sung RJ, Marks J, Parmley WW. Safety and efficacy of esmolol (ASL-8052: an ultrashort-acting beta-adrenergic blocking agent) for control of ventricular rate in supraventricular tachycardias. J Am Coll Cardiol 1984; 3:394–399.

78. Hill GA, Owens SD. Esmolol in the treatment of multifocal atrial tachycardia. Chest 1992; 101:1726–1728.

79. Parrillo JE. Treating multifocal atrial tachycardia (MAT) in a critical care unit: new data regarding verapamil and metoprolol. Update Crit Care Med 1987; 2:3–5.

80. Creamer JE, Nathan AW, Camm AJ. Successful treatment of atrial tachycardias with flecainide acetate. Br Heart J 1985; 53:164–166.

81. Barranco F, Sanchez M, Rodriguez J, Guerrero M. Efficacy of flecainide in patients with supraventricular arrhythmias and respiratory insufficiency. Intensive Care Med 1994; 20:42–44.

82. Houyel L, Fournier A, Davignon A. Successful treatment of chaotic atrial tachycardia with oral flecainide. Int J Cardiol 1990; 27:27–29.

83. Reimer A, Paul T, Kallfelz HC. Efficacy and safety of intravenous and oral propafenone in pediatric cardiac dysrhythmias. Am J Cardiol 1991; 68:741–744.

84. Clark ANG. Multifocal atrial tachycardia (MAT): the misdiagnosed atrial arrhythmia of old age. Gerontology 1977; 23:445–451.

8

Paroxysmal Supraventricular Tachycardia, Including Wolff-Parkinson-White Syndrome[a, 1–24]

Paroxysmal supraventricular tachycardia a common, relatively benign affliction, has many names (Table 8.1), and even today, knowledgeable practitioners and investigators use different titles for the arrhythmia.[25] This variation gives me the opportunity to select the nomenclature I prefer.

For decades, the regular tachyarrhythmias have been differentiated by their site of origin: (1) ventricular tachycardia, with its wide QRS complexes, originating in the ventricles; and (2) atrial tachycardia, with "normal" QRS complexes, coming from the atria. Two problems with this distinction are immediately apparent. Electrocardiographically, not all atrial tachycardias have normal QRS complexes, and electrophysiologically, most supraventricular tachycardias do not originate in the atria.

Even today, the terms atrial and supraventricular tachycardia are often used interchangeably, confusing our efforts to understand which arrhythmia authors are describing. For example, the phrase "supraventricular tachycardia" is employed in at least two ways: (1) for all arrhythmias arising "above" the ventricles; and (2) for those regular tachyarrhythmias, usually with narrow QRS complexes, that are sustained within the atrioventricular node or in accessory pathways. I use the second definition in this chapter and add the work

"paroxysmal" because paroxysms are such a fundamental clinical feature of most cases of the arrhythmia. Thus, when we call an arrhythmia "paroxysmal supraventricular tachycardia" or PSVT,[b] we are implying that it is due to a particular electrophysiological mechanism, *reentry* that courses through specific structures. PSVT in this context is an electrophysiological as well as an electrocardiographic definition, and, as we shall see, the recognition and management of the arrhythmia derive from our understanding of what sustains it.[26c]

Our contemporary knowledge of PSVT started with the development of the clinical electrophysiology laboratory and the tools of His bundle electrocardiography[27] and programmed stimulation, both products of the late 1960s. That appropriately timed atrial or ventricular beats could start or stop a paroxysm of supraventricular tachycardia[28–30] strongly suggested that reentry was the mechanism,[28, 30, 31] and further study revealed that the structures sustaining the reentry were the atrioventricular node[32, 33] and accessory pathways.[28] Dual pathways within the atrioventricular node sustain

---

[a]This chapter includes material from Chapter 10, "Supraventricular Tachycardia with Reentry in the Atrioventricular Node," by Hein J. J. Wellens,[1] and Chapter 11, "Supraventricular Tachycardia with Reentry in Accessory Pathways," by John J. Gallagher[2] in the first edition of this book.

[b]I have avoided using abbreviations throughout this book, but "paroxysmal supraventricular tachycardia" is such a mouthful and PSVT is so frequently employed that I will make an exception in this case. (I thank Dr. Hugh Calkins of Johns Hopkins for convincing me of the wisdom of this approach.)

[c]The principal objection to using the letters "PSVT" for all cases of reentrant tachycardia sustained in the atrioventricular node or accessory pathways is that a few cases of this arrhythmia are persistent and not paroxysmal. I suggest we try to live with this linguistic complication.

| Table 8.1 | **OTHER NAMES FOR PAROXYSMAL SUPRAVENTRICULAR TACHYCARDIA** |

General names
    Supraventricular tachycardia
    Paroxysmal atrial tachycardia
PSVT sustained in the atrioventricular node
    Atrioventricular junctional reentrant tachycardia
    Atrioventricular nodal reciprocating tachycardia
PSVT sustained in accessory pathways
    Atrioventricular reentrant tachycardia
    Atrioventricular reciprocating tachycardia
        Atrioventricular nodal (reciprocating) rhythm
        Atrioventricular junctional reciprocating tachycardia
    Circus movement tachycardia
    Permanent junctional reciprocating tachycardia

PSVT, paroxysmal supraventricular tachycardia.

| Table 8.2 | **PREVALENCE OF THE ELECTROCARDIOGRAM OF WOLFF-PARKINSON-WHITE SYNDROME** |

Year of Report	Authors	Prevalence (%)
1944	Ohnell[3a]	0.06
1954	Manning[45]	0.12
1954	Packard et al.[43]	0.2
1956	Katz and Pick[44]	0.61
1957	Hejtmancik and Herrmann[46]	0.15
1960	Averill et al.[47]	0.16
1985	Guize et al.[49b]	0.15 in men; 0.08 in women
1993	Munger et al.[50]	4/100,000 detected/year

[a]As quoted by Chung, Walsh, and Massie.[3]
[b]As quoted in Marriott, page 294, 8th edition.[200]

atrioventricular nodal reentrant PSVT, and accessory pathways provide one of the pathways for the PSVT that bothers many patients with the Wolff-Parkinson-White syndrome.

The importance of accessory pathways was not immediately evident to Louis Wolff, John Parkinson, and Paul Dudley White when they described, in 1930, 11 otherwise healthy, young people with recurrent tachycardia and a peculiar electrocardiogram in sinus rhythm that had short PR intervals and QRS complexes that looked to them like bundle branch block.[34–36d] We learned that rapid conduction through an accessory pathway skirting the atrioventricular node accounts for the short PR interval and that abnormal, early ventricular activation via the accessory pathway produces the unusual QRS complexes with their "delta waves." For those who eschew eponyms, the term "ventricular preexcitation" or, simply, "preexcitation" was invented to describe the characteristic electrocardiographic features of the syndrome during sinus rhythm.

SOME ADVANCES SINCE THE FIRST EDITION OF THIS BOOK

- Proof that paroxysms of PSVT appear with a circadian pattern in many patients.
- Further knowledge of the clinical electrophysiology of the arrhythmia.
- Refinement of techniques of catheter ablation with radiofrequency current of accessory pathways and intranodal pathways in patients with PSVT.
- Improvement in locating circuits sustaining PSVT

[d]In 1917, Dr. White recorded an electrocardiogram with short PR interval and an abnormal QRS complex from a 24-year-old man who had been rejected for military service during World War I because of a heart murmur. According to his colleague, Dr. Gordon S. Myers, "Dr. White told the patient that the heart murmur was functional and the electrocardiogram *unusual* [my italics] but there was no evidence of heart disease."[36] The patient, who was not included in the original 11 patients with the syndrome, served in the army in both world wars and never had tachyarrhythmias. He was well without symptoms of heart disease at the age of 68 years when last examined by Dr. Myers. According to Dr. Louis Wolff, the first patient in the original report of what came to be called the Wolff-Parkinson-White syndrome was initially seen in Dr. White's laboratory at the Massachusetts General Hospital in Boston on April 2, 1928.

with such techniques as intracardiac echocardiography and body-surface mapping.

PREVALENCE

Based on the prevalence of PSVT in the region surrounding Marshfield, Wisconsin, 570,000 persons in the United States have PSVT, and about 89,000 new cases are diagnosed each year.[37, 38e] PSVT is the arrhythmia in about 85% of adults with regular supraventricular tachyarrhythmias.[39] Atrioventricular nodal reentry is the most frequent mechanism.[f] In children, atrioventricular nodal and accessory pathway reentry account for a smaller fraction[40] of those with regular tachycardias.[41g] Arrhythmias are rare in newborns, but PSVT does occur in them.[42h]

Few patients, with or without arrhythmias, have the electrocardiogram of Wolff-Parkinson-White syndrome despite the impression one might receive from the immense amount of work which clinical electrophysiologists have devoted to the subject during the past 25 years.[43, 44] The incidence ranges from 0.06% to 0.61% of patients, the latter figure reported in 1956 from the electrocardiograms taken in a large Chicago general hospital[3, 43–50] (Table 8.2).

AGE

The first episode of PSVT appears in more than half of patients with accessory pathway reentry before the

[e]The prevalence of paroxysmal supraventricular tachycardia is 2.25 in 1,000 persons and the incidence is 35 in 100,000 person-years in the 50,000 patients of the Marshfield, Wisconsin Epidemiological Study Area.[38]
[f]In 561 patients evaluated electrophysiologically in Philadelphia and in Maastricht, the Netherlands, reentrant supraventricular tachycardia was sustained in the atrioventricular node in 60% and in accessory pathways in 40%.[39]
[g]Seventy-one (69%) of 103 children, each studied electrophysiologically.[41]
[h]Of 3,383 apparently healthy newborns in two British maternity hospitals, two (0.06%) had supraventricular tachycardia and two had the electrocardiogram of Wolff-Parkinson-White syndrome without arrhythmias.[42]

age of 20 years, seldom after middle age,[34, 51–53] and only occasionally after the age of 50 years.[54i] On average, patients are older when their first paroxysm of supraventricular tachycardia develops if the arrhythmia is sustained within the atrioventricular node.[52, 53, 55] The first episodes of intranodal tachycardia cluster between 15 and 35 years and at about the age of 55 years.[56]

Compared with patients with PSVT who have structural heart disease, those without cardiac abnormalities other than the arrhythmia are younger.[38] Among women, PSVT develops more frequently in the childbearing years in those without other cardiac lesions and more often later in life in women with structural heart disease.[38] The intervals between paroxysms of supraventricular tachycardia shorten in older patients,[57] and the frequency of paroxysms increases with age in patients with Wolff-Parkinson-White syndrome.[49]

Among children, the first episode occurs most often from birth to two months of age,[58, 59] and next most frequently from ages five to 10 years.[59] Fetuses,[60–71] premature newborns,[72] and infants[42, 73–75] may develop PSVT.[j] Among children with the arrhythmia, reentry in accessory pathways is the more common mechanism.[76, 77k]

As with adults, PSVT from accessory pathway reentry usually appears at a younger age than atrioventricular nodal reentrant PSVT,[76] which is rare before the age of two years.[77] As infants, children, and adults grow older, the electrocardiogram of Wolff-Parkinson-White syndrome may disappear, and paroxysms of supraventricular tachycardia,[78] including that due to accessory pathway reentry, may decrease or cease.[73, 74, 78–83l]

GENDER

Probably as many men as women develop PSVT.[51, 84, 85m] Men predominate when the mechanism is reentry through accessory pathways, and women predominate with reentry in the atrioventricular node.[52, 53n] Cardiac disease other than the arrhythmia is more likely to be present in men than in women with PSVT.[38]

Wolff-Parkinson-White syndrome appears more often in males than females.[49, 50, 59, 86, 87o] This difference decreases with age because of loss of preexcitation and not because of the earlier mortality of men.[49]

GENETICS

The electrocardiogram characteristic of Wolff-Parkinson-White syndrome in patients with or without PSVT usually occurs sporadically. However, preexcitation may be familial.[88–92] The characteristic electrocardiogram appears in a greater number of the first-degree relatives of those with preexcitation than would be expected in the general population.[93p]

CLINICAL SETTING
Precipitating Events

Patients can frequently recall events in their lives that seem to precipitate, or at least be associated with, the onset of paroxysms[94–96] (Table 8.3). As observed by Louis N. Katz and Alfred Pick in their classic 1956 text on arrhythmias:[97]

> Sometimes, a particular event, e.g., a certain body movement, an emotional upset, or a dream . . . may be the trigger mechanism. At least the patient may be convinced of this relationship. . . . When associated with the menstrual cycle attacks may recur each lunar month.

Pregnancy. Patients infrequently sustain their first episode of PSVT during pregnancy, but when this does occur, reentry in accessory pathways is more likely.[55q] Some women report that pregnancy seems to increase the number of paroxysms.[55, 67, 98] The arrhythmia does not, however, usually interfere with the normal course of pregnancy.[55]

---

[p]Electrocardiographic preexcitation was documented in one or more first-degree relatives of 13 (3.4%) of 383 index patients with electrophysiologically proven accessory pathways.[93]

[q]First episode of supraventricular tachycardia during pregnancy: seven (6.5%) of 107 women with accessory pathways; one (1%) of 100 women with atrioventricular nodal reentry.[55]

Table 8.3   EVENTS PRECIPITATING PAROXYSMAL TACHYARRHYTHMIAS[a]

Precipitating Event	Examples
Chemicals and drugs[94]	Epinephrine, amyl nitrate, alcohol
Gastrointestinal events[94]	Bloating and belching after a large meal
Infection[94]	Upper respiratory, urinary, pneumonia, prostatitis
Menstruation[97]	
Psychic events[94]	Anger, fright, intense excitement
Sudden movement[94]	Bending over, turning around quickly, standing up suddenly, rapidly taking a deep breath
Sustained exercise[94, 96]	Marching, dancing, running, swimming, climbing stairs
Swallowing[95]	—

[a]Most of the patients in one of the reports[94] had PSVT, but some had atrial fibrillation, atrial flutter, or ventricular tachycardia. Drinking coffee and smoking cigarettes, popularly thought to cause arrhythmias, were seldom documented to be precipitating factors.[94]

---

[i]In their original report, Wolff, Parkinson, and White found that the disorder principally affects young adults.[34]

[j]In several of the references cited about children, the mechanism of the supraventricular tachycardia was not defined electrophysiologically, and some of these children almost certainly had atrial tachycardia (see Chapter 6).

[k]The mechanism of supraventricular tachycardia in 240 children from two series was reentry in accessory pathways in 151 (63%) and in the atrioventricular node in 43 (18%).[76, 77] Atrial or junctional tachycardia accounted for the arrhythmia in 46 (19%) patients.[76, 77]

[l]Probably in part because of decreasing ability of accessory pathways to conduct as patients age.[83]

[m]At least such was the observation of Maurice Campbell in a 1947 report of 165 cases of "paroxysmal supraventricular tachycardia."[85]

[n]According to a study of 623 consecutive patients evaluated by electrophysiological study, the male-to-female gender ratio was 2.00 (273 male, 136 female) for reentry through accessory pathways and 0.46 (52 male, 113 female) within the atrioventricular node.[52]

[o]Of 140 children with Wolff-Parkinson-White syndrome referred to a children's hospital with particular interest in arrhythmias, 62% were male.[59] Eight of the 11 patients described by Wolff, Parkinson, and White were men.[34]

Duration and Frequency of Paroxysms of Supraventricular Tachycardia

Paroxysms of supraventricular tachycardia usually are of shorter duration than attacks of atrial fibrillation.[85] Their duration varies greatly. Maurice Campbell observed in 1947:[85]

> Paroxysms last hours much more commonly than days. Though variable, they tend to have a more or less customary length in any one person, who can generally report that the attacks last between, say, two and eight hours, or less than half an hour . . . and is surprised if his past experience does not prove a useful guide to what to expect.

In addition, Katz and Pick noted:[97]

> The frequency of recurrence and the duration of a single attack vary from patient to patient, from many attacks per day to only an occasional one per year, but tend to maintain a certain pattern in the individual case. The more often paroxysms have occurred in the past the more apt they are to recur.

Predicting when a paroxysm will appear, however, is almost impossible. Thus, in general, the time of a previous episode does not predict when the next episode will occur,[99] and, among children with Wolff-Parkinson-White syndrome, the presence or disappearance of preexcitation does not affect when the arrhythmia will occur.[59]

However, a circadian pattern does apply in some cases.[100–103] PSVT recurs most often during the daytime,[101, 103, 104] peaking at about 4 to 6 p.m., three to five times as often as from 4 to 6 a.m., when the arrhythmia is least likely to be seen.[57, 101] Persistence of the electrocardiogram of Wolff-Parkinson-White syndrome predicts which infants with PSVT will more likely have recurrences.[105]

Paroxysmal versus incessant. PSVT whether sustained in the atrioventricular node or accessory pathways is most often paroxysmal, and afflicted patients are usually in normal rhythm and only occasionally in tachycardia. In a few patients, however, the arrhythmia may persist for hours, days, weeks, or longer without spontaneously reverting to sinus rhythm.[106–136r]

> Even among these longer attacks, relatively few lasted more than two or three days . . . . These long attacks . . . are more serious but they may occur without there being any disease of the heart. . . . Attacks lasting more than a month are extremely rare.[85]

Incessant or permanent tachycardia occurs more of-

ten, among those with PSVT, in children than in adults.[108, 110s]

Structural Heart Disease

Compared with patients who also have structural heart disease, those with PSVT and no other cardiac lesions are more likely to[38]

- Be female.
- Be younger.
- Have a faster heart rate during a paroxysm of tachycardia.
- Have had their arrhythmia first documented in an emergency department.

Organic heart disease occurs more often in patients whose PSVT is sustained in the atrioventricular node than in accessory pathways.[137] This coincidence is particularly notable, as one would expect, in patients whose first episode of intranodal tachycardia occurs at an older age.[56]

Congenital Heart Disease

In children with Wolff-Parkinson-White syndrome, congenital heart disease is frequently present,[58, 59, 87] most often Ebstein's anomaly (Table 8.4). However, children with Wolff-Parkinson-White syndrome and no other congenital lesions are as apt to have PSVT as children with anatomical defects.[59t] Dual atrioventricular nodal pathways, the electrophysiological substrate for PSVT, are equally prevalent in children with corrected and uncorrected congenital heart disease.[138]

---

sPermanent supraventricular tachycardia was observed in 20 patients, whereas the paroxysmal form appeared in about 250, according to one group.[108] The incessant variety was seen in half of the children with supraventricular tachycardia.[110]

tIn one series, 52 (32%) of 140 children had anatomical lesions in addition to the accessory pathways.[59] In referring to "other congenital lesions," I am assuming that an accessory pathway is also a congenital cardiac abnormality.

Table 8.4	CONGENITAL HEART DISEASE IN 52 PATIENTS WITH WOLFF-PARKINSON-WHITE SYNDROME	
Lesion		No. of Patients
Ebstein's anomaly		12
Ventricular septal defect		7
Cardiomyopathy/endocardial fibroelastosis		5
Aortic stenosis		4
Primum atrial septal defect		4
Corrected transposition of the great arteries		3
Aortic coarctation		2
Secundum atrial septal defect		2
Tetralogy of Fallot		2
Tricuspid atresia		2
Other		9

(From Perry JC, Garson A Jr. Supraventricular tachycardia due to Wolff-Parkinson-White syndrome in children: early disappearance and late recurrence. J Am Coll Cardiol 1990; 16:1215–1220. Reprinted with permission from the American College of Cardiology.)[59]

---

rOne patient lived quite comfortably for 50 years with persistent and, in her case, permanent supraventricular tachycardia at a rate of 140 to 160 beats per minute.[133] A fairly large literature exists about "chronic atrial tachycardia," as the permanent or persistent form of supraventricular tachycardia was formerly called, particularly in children, before electrophysiological studies were available to define the mechanisms. Some of these cases were almost certainly due to reentrant supraventricular tachycardia, and others were caused by atrial automaticity (see Chapter 6).

Congestive Heart Failure

Congestive heart failure frequently accompanies the first episode of PSVT in young children.[139u] Heart failure occurs with greater frequency among children with accessory pathway PSVT than when the mechanism is atrioventricular nodal reentry,[76] probably because many patients with Wolff-Parkinson-White syndrome are young when they develop tachycardia, and their heart rates can be extremely fast.[76]

Cardiac Surgery

PSVT develops in a few patients after surgical repair of atrial septal defect.[140v]

Coronary Heart Disease

PSVT rarely, if ever, develops for the first time during myocardial infarction.[141–143]

Miscellaneous Factors

Alcohol. Alcohol consumption seems to precipitate atrioventricular nodal PSVT in some patients,[144] although no significant association has been established between the time alcohol is ingested and when a paroxysm of PSVT begins.[102]

Hypertrophic cardiomyopathy. The electrocardiogram of preexcitation is said to occur with a frequency greater than expected in patients with hypertrophic cardiomyopathy.[92] Both conditions may appear in an inherited pattern.[92]

Mitral valve prolapse. Patients with mitral valve prolapse and PSVT seem to have a relatively high incidence of left-sided accessory pathways that participate in sustaining the arrhythmia.[145] Whether PSVT occurs with greater than expected frequency in patients with mitral valve prolapse is not known.

Neoplasms. Rhabdomyoma, a benign cardiac tumor and the most common cardiac tumor in children, is associated with Wolff-Parkinson-White syndrome to a greater degree than expected.[146]

Position. Lying on his right side prompted short bursts of PSVT in a medical intern, particularly noticeable during periods of stress.[147]

Swallowing. Swallowing and balloon distention of the esophagus produced paroxysms of PSVT of unknown mechanism.[148]

Thyrotoxicosis. Unlike atrial fibrillation, PSVT is rarely related to thyrotoxicosis.[94, 142]

OTHER ARRHYTHMIAS IN PATIENTS WITH PAROXYSMAL SUPRAVENTRICULAR TACHYCARDIA

Atrial Fibrillation[w]

Atrial Flutter

One report suggests that there may be a high incidence of accessory pathways in fetuses and young infants with atrial flutter.[149] Sonography has demonstrated the presence of both atrial flutter and PSVT in a fetus.[70]

Atrial Tachycardia

PSVT due to atrioventricular nodal reentry and atrial reentry can coexist in the same patient.[150]

Ventricular Tachycardia

Other arrhythmias, such as ventricular tachycardia, with no particular relation to PSVT occur in patients with preexcitation.[151]

SYMPTOMS[x]

PSVT lasting for at least 30 seconds produces symptoms that few patients ignore.[152y] Most decrease their activity during an attack, and many find it necessary to sit or lie down.[94] A few are unaware that they are having a paroxysm.[85] The symptoms of PSVT are often misdiagnosed as due to panic, anxiety, or stress.[153z]

About one-third of asymptomatic patients less than 40 years of age when their preexcited electrocardiograms are discovered will eventually develop symptoms.[50] Few patients who are more than 40 years old when preexcitation is discovered develop symptoms.[50] The symptoms that patients 50 years of age or older with Wolff-Parkinson-White syndrome experience are similar to those of younger patients.[154]

Palpitations

Although palpitations are a frequent,[155, 156] although not universal,[94] complaint of patients with PSVT, they do not always indicate a clinical arrhythmia. For example, more than two-thirds of patients whose PSVT has been cured with ablation and in whom no arrhythmia

---

[u]Thirty-eight percent of children four months of age or younger presented in heart failure with their first episode of supraventricular tachycardia.[139]

[v]The electrophysiological mechanism of most postoperative supraventricular tachycardias has not been established, and many may be due to intra-atrial reentry or automaticity, rather than atrioventricular nodal reentry.

[w]See Chapter 4 for the principal discussion of atrial fibrillation in patients with Wolff-Parkinson-White syndrome.

[x]Much of the recent literature omits clinical descriptions of symptoms and findings of patients with supraventricular tachycardia. For this information, I have returned to the writings of leading clinical cardiologists of previous generations for descriptions, many of which are difficult to match for clarity and style.

[y]Each of 14 patients detected each episode of supraventricular tachycardia recorded by Holter recordings.[152] In contrast, patients are often unaware of paroxysms of atrial fibrillation lasting at least 30 seconds.[152]

[z]In 32 (54%) of 59 patients in one series.[153]

can be reinduced at electrophysiological study report the persistence of symptoms similar to those before the arrhythmia was treated.[157]

Other clinicians may detect the tachycardia in patients unaware of their own rapid heart action, as reported by M. H. Luria in 1971:[94]

> Cigarettes in a shirt pocket moving in time to the heart beat, or, as noted by the wife of a patient, movement of the bed in time to the rate of the heart.

Pounding in the Neck

Many patients with PSVT sustained in the atrioventricular node report the sensation of rapid, regular pounding in the neck.[158aa]

Chest Pain

Chest pain or pressure often suggesting ischemia frequently accompanies PSVT,[85, 94, 159] even in young patients who are unlikely to have coronary heart disease. The cause of this common symptom in those having PSVT has never been satisfactorily explained.

Dizziness, Lightheadedness, and Syncope

Few patients with PSVT faint from the arrhythmia,[85] although many become lightheaded or dizzy. Among those who do faint, older patients predominate.[160] Dizziness and syncope occur more frequently in patients with accessory pathway reentry who have antidromic than those who have orthodromic tachycardia.[156bb]

Contrary to conventional wisdom, heart rate during tachycardia is often not the primary factor producing symptoms.[161, 162] Vasomotor factors may play a more important role.[162] For example, *slower* resting heart rates during paroxysms of PSVT sustained in accessory pathways determine which children will feel that they may faint while exercising during the arrhythmia.[163]

Among young patients with Wolff-Parkinson-White syndrome, syncope more likely occurs in those with atrial fibrillation and a rapid ventricular rate.[164] However, whether a patient with Wolff-Parkinson-White syndrome faints does *not* usually relate to the following:[165]

- Age.
- Clinical history.
- Frequency of arrhythmic events.
- Gender.
- Incidence or characteristics of the arrhythmia.
- Presence of associated cardiac disease.

PSVT is not the only arrhythmia that can cause syncope in patients with Wolff-Parkinson-White syndrome electrocardiogram. Some patients may also have ventricular tachycardia unrelated to their preexcitation.[151]

---

aaOf 244 patients with palpitations, rapid, regular pounding in the neck was felt by 50 (94%) of 54 patients with atrioventricular nodal supraventricular tachycardia but by none of 190 patients with other arrhythmias.[158]

bbSee later for an explanation of orthodromic and antidromic tachycardia.

Cardiac Arrest

When PSVT is incriminated in producing cardiac arrest, the usual arrhythmia is atrial fibrillation or atrial flutter in patients with accessory pathways.[cc] However, cardiac arrest does occur in an occasional patient during atrioventricular nodal PSVT.[166dd]

Beginning and End of Paroxysms

Paroxysms of PSVT characteristically begin and end suddenly. However, confirming these features is often quite difficult. As Paul Wood reported in his excellent 1968 text:[167]

> Experience shows that most careful cross-examination is required to establish the true sequence of events. It is not enough to determine that the onset is sudden, it is necessary to be sure that it is abrupt: that the full velocity of the attack is reached immediately in the space of one beat; that from no sensation whatsoever, maximum palpitation develops within one second. To assess the rate and rhythm it is helpful to ask the patient to represent them by tapping with his finger. . . . The manner in which the attack ends may be more difficult to establish; some patients become accustomed to the palpitations and gradually fail to perceive them; others pass from a true paroxysm to sinus tachycardia without appreciating the change, and their description of the end refers to the gradual slowing down of the sinus rhythm.

PHYSICAL EXAMINATION

Although most physicians make the diagnosis of PSVT from the electrocardiogram, clues in the physical examination can lead one to the same result.[168]

Rhythm

The rhythm of PSVT is regular.

First Heart Sound

The atria contract with each ventricular beat, or, put another way, atrioventricular dissociation is absent. Consequently, the level of the blood pressure, the height of neck vein pulsations, and the loudness of the first heart sound and systolic murmurs do not vary from beat to beat.

Pulsations in the Neck

When the atria contract at or about the same time as the ventricles, large waves with each beat appear in the veins of the neck from the right atrium contracting against the closed tricuspid valve (Fig. 8.1). This sequence of atrioventricular contraction produces the rapid pulsations in the neck ("frog sign") that may be

---

ccThis topic is discussed in Chapter 4.

ddSupraventricular tachycardia sustained in the atrioventricular node was the apparent cause of "aborted sudden death" in three (1%) of 290 patients in one series.[166]

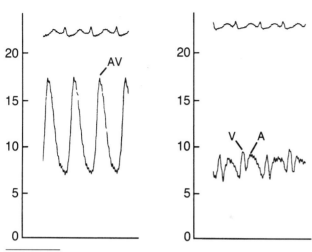

FIGURE 8.1 **Large venous waves depend on the mechanism of PSVT.** The waves of right atrial pressure (millimeters of mercury) are greater when the arrhythmia is sustained in the atrioventricular node **(left)** than in an accessory pathway **(right)** because the right atrium contracts against the closed tricuspid valve during atrioventricular nodal reentry. (Adapted from Gursoy S, Steurer G, Brugada J, Andries E, Brugada P. Brief report: the hemodynamic mechanism of pounding in the neck in atrioventricular nodal reentrant tachycardia. N Engl J Med 1992; 327:772–774. Reprinted by permission of the New England Journal of Medicine.)[158]

Table 8.5	**HEMODYNAMIC CONSEQUENCES OF PAROXYSMAL SUPRAVENTRICULAR TACHYCARDIA IN EIGHT PATIENTS**[a]	
Characteristics	During Sinus Rhythm	During Paroxysmal Supraventricular Tachycardia
Heart rate (beats/min)	79 (58–103)	183 (130–210)
PR interval (msec)	154 (130–180)	256 (180–390)
Mean systolic pressure (brachial artery)	141	99
Cardiac output (L/min/m²)	3.6	2.2
Pulmonary artery systolic pressure	18 (10–25)	26 (13–46)
Right atrial maximum pressure	5 (4–7)	17 (7–25)

[a]After measurements during sinus rhythm were taken, the arrhythmia was induced with programmed stimulation. The right atrial pressures were recorded in five of the patients. Mean values, with ranges in parentheses. Pressures in millimeters of mercury. Values recorded 60 to 90 seconds after the onset of arrhythmia.

(From Goldreyer BN, Kastor JA, Kershbaum KL. The hemodynamic effects of induced supraventricular tachycardia in man. Circulation 1976; 54:783–789, with permission of the American Heart Association, Inc.)[169]

seen when the arrhythmia is sustained in the atrioventricular node but less often in accessory pathways.[158]

On examination, the physician may misinterpret the pulsations as originating in the carotid arteries rather than the veins. However, the low blood pressure and stroke volume characteristic of PSVT would be unlikely to produce strong arterial pulsations.[169]

HEMODYNAMICS

When PSVT begins, the arterial pressure rapidly falls,[169–176] explaining why patients with PSVT, most of whom have no structural heart disease, become weak, lightheaded, or faint (Table 8.5) (Fig. 8.2). Soon the blood pressure rises, although not quite to the levels achieved during sinus rhythm.[169, 174, 175] Partial restoration of the blood pressure reflects, at least in part, compensation by the autonomic nervous system. The blood pressure falls to lower levels and the autonomic response is greater if the tachycardia begins when the patient is upright rather than prone.[175]

PSVT also

- Decreases cardiac output and index,[169, 176, 177] particularly when the rate of the tachycardia is fast.[178]
- Decreases stroke volume.[169, 176–178]
- Decreases ejection fraction when the rate is very fast or organic heart disease is present.[178]
- Raises pulmonary artery mean,[176] systolic,[177] and diastolic[169, 177] pressures.

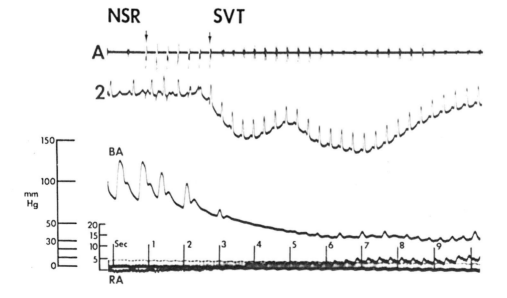

FIGURE 8.2 Hemodynamic changes produced by the induction of PSVT (SVT) in a patient in sinus rhythm (NSR). Notice how low the blood pressure falls during the first seconds after the arrhythmia begins. It is a small wonder that patients feel so ill. (A, intra–right atrial electrogram; 2, electrocardiographic lead II; BA, brachial pressure; RA, right atrial pressure. (From Goldreyer BN, Kastor JA, Kershbaum KL. The hemodynamic effects of induced supraventricular tachycardia in man. Circulation 1976; 54:783–789, by permission of the American Heart Association, Inc.)[169]

- Raises right[158, 169, 177, 179, 180] and left atrial pressures.[177]
- Produces pulsus alternans, in some cases, which is most notable just as the tachycardia begins and disappears as the arrhythmia continues.[174]

Timing of Atrial Contraction

Given that the heart rates during PSVT often approximate those achieved during vigorous exercise, why are the hemodynamic and clinical consequences of the arrhythmia so severe? The answer lies in the timing of atrial contraction, which occurs when the mitral and tricuspid valves are closed in most patients with PSVT,[169, 177] whether it is sustained in the atrioventricular node or accessory pathways[177] (Fig. 8.3). The ventricles are deprived of the blood normally contributed by atrial contraction, a hemodynamic event of particular importance during tachycardia. Furthermore, the retrograde emptying of the atria during simultaneous atrioventricular contraction[181] decreases the amount of blood entering the ventricles during early diastole and mid-diastole.

The location of reentry affects the atrial and ventricular hemodynamics. In atrioventricular nodal PSVT, reversal of flow from the right atrium to the great veins is greater than during accessory pathway PSVT.[158] The atria and ventricles often contract simultaneously during atrioventricular nodal reentry and produce large, fused venous A and V waves. Because atrial contraction occurs slightly later than ventricular contrac-

tion in most cases of accessory pathway reentry, distinct, separate A and V waves can be seen[158] (see Fig. 8.1). These differences help to explain why rapid, regular pounding in the neck from the venous pulse is reported and is detected more often when the tachycardia is sustained in the atrioventricular node.[158]

Furthermore, the deleterious hemodynamic effects of PSVT are greater in patients with "slow-fast" intranodal tachycardia, in which atrial contraction occurs when the atrioventricular valves are closed, than during the infrequently encountered "fast-slow" variety with its more normal PR intervals that preserve the atrial contribution to ventricular filling.[182ee]

Rapid atrial pacing does not produce the severe hemodynamic changes associated with spontaneous PSVT,[172] presumably because atrial filling of the ventricles is preserved. However, simultaneous atrial and ventricular activation produced by pacing at rates comparable to those achieved during PSVT markedly reduces ventricular end-diastolic and stroke volumes.[183] These findings further support the significance of losing the atrial contribution to ventricular filling during PSVT.

Vasomotor Effects

Fainting during PSVT appears to depend more on vasomotor reactions to the tachycardia than on the heart rate.[162]

Effects of Drugs

Propranolol decreases heart rate, systolic aortic pressure, and cardiac index and raises arteriovenous oxygen difference when the drug is given intravenously during persistence of PSVT.[177] The drug can therefore worsen the symptoms of PSVT if it does not convert the arrhythmia promptly.[177]

Polyuria During Tachycardia

As many as half the patients with paroxysmal tachyarrhythmias report polyuria during or after the episode.[184] PSVT joins paroxysmal atrial fibrillation, the arrhythmia most frequently involved, in producing polyuria.[94, 185–189ff] Atrial natriuretic factor (protein) rises[190] and vasopressin concentrations fall[189] during PSVT induced by electrophysiological stimulation and may contribute to the polyuria associated with the arrhythmia.

Secondary Cardiomyopathy

PSVT[191–194] sustained in the atrioventricular node[130, 195] or accessory pathways[196–199] occasionally produces reversible cardiomyopathy, although less frequently than does atrial tachycardia.[gg] The condition can develop in fetuses with PSVT.[71]

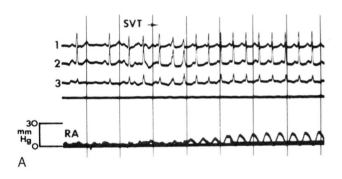

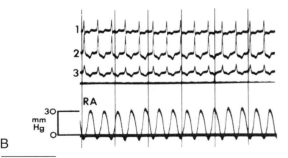

FIGURE 8.3 **Large A waves during PSVT** (SVT) (30 mm Hg) produced by atrial contraction when the atrioventricular valves are closed during the arrhythmia. Thirty seconds elapsed between the end of **A** and the beginning of **B**. 1, 2, 3, electrocardiographic leads; RA, right atrial pressure. (From Goldreyer BN, Kastor JA, Kershbaum KL. The hemodynamic effects of induced supraventricular tachycardia in man. Circulation 1976; 54:783–789, by permission of the American Heart Association, Inc.)[169]

---

*ee*See the paragraphs on electrophysiology later for an explanation of "slow-fast" and "fast-slow" tachycardia.

*ff*See Chapter 4 for further information and references.

*gg*See Chapter 6.

ELECTROCARDIOGRAM DURING SINUS RHYTHM

Rate

Most patients with PSVT sustained either in the atrioventricular node or accessory pathways have normal heart rates during sinus rhythm.[200]

P Waves

The form and axis of the P waves are usually normal during sinus rhythm in patients with PSVT. Abnormalities reflect the effects of intrinsic heart disease, rather than the tendency to have the arrhythmia.

PR Interval

The PR interval during sinus rhythm is usually normal in patients with atrioventricular nodal reentrant PSVT. Patients may occasionally indicate that they have dual atrioventricular nodal pathways with abrupt, persistent prolongations and other variations of the PR intervals,[201, 202] often instituted by spontaneous ventricular[203] and other premature beats.[204]

The short PR intervals so characteristic of the electrocardiogram of Wolff-Parkinson-White syndrome reflect transmission of the signal from atria to ventricles over accessory pathways that conduct more rapidly than does the atrioventricular node. The PR intervals may be normal during sinus rhythm, however, in those patients with concealed accessory pathway reentrant PSVT whose accessory pathways do not conduct from atria to ventricles.

QRS Complex

The QRS complex of patients with atrioventricular nodal reentrant PSVT during sinus rhythm is usually the same as during tachycardia. Both may be similarly abnormal from intrinsic heart disease. Ventricular *preexcitation*, the characteristic electrocardiographic feature of the QRS complex during Wolff-Parkinson-White syndrome, is produced by the rapidly conducting accessory pathway inserting directly into ventricular myocardium. The ventricles are then activated from the abnormal site of union with the accessory pathway, rather than via the bundle of His, bundle branches, and Purkinje network. This process produces the *delta wave*, a slow, abnormal deflection that begins in, and extends to a variable degree through, the QRS complex.

Fusion. The QRS complex during sinus rhythm of a patient with Wolff-Parkinson-White syndrome is a fusion beat, incorporating contributions from both accessory pathway and atrioventricular nodal conduction. The early part of the QRS complex is most notably distorted because ventricular activation from the accessory pathway precedes activation via the normal conduction system. Conduction through the atrioventricular node contributes to the later appearance of the QRS complex. The extent of contribution from

these two sources depends upon the relative speed of conduction in each.

Concealed accessory pathways. Not all accessory pathways announce their presence with the electrocardiogram of Wolff-Parkinson-White syndrome during sinus rhythm.[205, 206] Thus, we have *manifest* accessory pathways identified by short PR intervals and delta waves during sinus rhythm and *concealed* accessory pathways that participate in the arrhythmia but show no evidence of their presence during sinus rhythm even when they are studied with electrophysiological techniques designed to maximize conduction in accessory pathways from atria to ventricles.

Electrocardiographic prediction of location of accessory pathways. Characteristics of the delta wave and of the remainder of the QRS complex can point to the location of accessory pathways in patients with Wolff-Parkinson-White syndrome.[207–210] The basis for such evaluation depends on where the accessory pathway inserts into the ventricle. Historically,[211hh] the first attempt at locating the course of the accessory pathway followed the description of the electrocardiograms of preexcitation as *type A* and *type B*, depending on the major deflection in right-sided chest leads.

In type A preexcitation, the QRS complexes are upright in the precordial lead simulating right bundle branch block. In type B, most of the precordial deflection is negative, as in left bundle branch block. Accessory pathways inserting into the left ventricle were assumed to produce type A, and type B was taken to indicate insertion of the accessory pathway into the right ventricle. PSVT is more likely in those with type A preexcitation.[49] In infants and children, structural heart disease is more frequently present with the type B electrocardiogram (right ventricular connection)[59] than with the type A electrocardiogram.[87] However, the location of the accessory pathway does not affect the clinical course of tachycardia in children with Wolff-Parkinson-White syndrome.[59]

With contemporary methods, the routes of accessory pathways can be much more precisely defined than was possible with the A versus B descriptions. Many formulas have been developed to predict accurately where the operator will find the pathway to ablate.[207, 209, 212–238] Describing these criteria is beyond the scope of this book.

Lown-Ganong-Levine syndrome defines patients, without definable structural heart disease, who have repetitive supraventricular tachyarrhythmias and whose electrocardiograms show short PR intervals but no delta waves in the QRS complexes.[239] When the arrhythmias are PSVT—patients with Lown-Ganong-Levine syndrome have other supraventricular arrhythmias as well, according to the original description[239]—they are sustained in either dual intranodal or in accessory pathways, just as in reentrant PSVT with normal PR inter-

---

hh In 1945, when this much-referenced work from the laboratory of Frank N. Wilson was published.[211]

vals or with preexcitation.[240][ii] Patients with structural heart disease may, of course, sustain ventricular tachyarrhythmias that have no relation to the incidental presence of short PR intervals and no delta waves.[241]

ST Segments and T Waves

Ventricular repolarization during sinus rhythm in patients with PSVT sustained in the atrioventricular node or in concealed accessory pathways shows no specific abnormalities, except those expected from the effects of intrinsic heart disease. The ST segments and T waves, however, are characteristically abnormal during sinus rhythm in patients with Wolff-Parkinson-White syndrome corresponding to the abnormal ventricular activation produced by conduction through the accessory pathway.

Post-paroxysm tachycardia syndrome. T waves may be inverted for days or even weeks in patients with no structural heart disease after PSVT converts to sinus rhythm.[242]

Evaluation of Patients with the Electrocardiogram of Wolff-Parkinson-White Syndrome and No Symptoms

What evaluation is indicated when the electrocardiogram of Wolff-Parkinson-White syndrome is unexpectedly discovered in an asymptomatic patient?[24] This question is important because the first manifestation of Wolff-Parkinson-White syndrome in a few patients may be cardiac arrest resulting from ventricular fibrillation. This calamity is caused by the ability of accessory pathways, which lack the blocking properties of the atrioventricular node, to conduct too many signals from atrial fibrillation or atrial flutter to the ventricles. Ventricular fibrillation may develop when the ventricles are driven by extremely rapid rates and are influenced by the catecholamine response that such a condition may produce.

Intermittent preexcitation in the electrocardiogram. Inconstant preexcitation, the intermittent presence and absence of the characteristic short PR intervals and delta waves, suggests that the accessory pathway will not readily conduct all atrial impulses, and the risk of cardiac arrest in such patients is low (Fig. 8.4). The electrophysiological properties of accessory pathways deteriorate in many infants with Wolff-Parkinson-White syndrome and accessory pathway PSVT as they grow older, a finding accounting for the disappearance of preexcitation and relief from PSVT.[81]

Disappearance of preexcitation during exercise implies that the electrophysiological characteristics of the accessory pathway are such that production of rapid ventricular rates during atrial fibrillation or atrial flutter is unlikely.[243–245] Several leads should be recorded simultaneously to prevent overlooking preservation of preexcitation not seen in all leads.

Effects of drugs. Procainamide, and other drugs that lengthen the refractory period of accessory pathways,[246] will prevent preexcitation in patients whose accessory pathways are unlikely to be able to transmit dangerously rapid impulses. This test, however, does not appear to screen out all patients with the potential to develop ventricular fibrillation.[247]

Electrophysiological study. If preexcitation persists despite these studies, electrophysiological study should be considered to prevent the unlikely but real possibility of sudden death.[ii]

ELECTROCARDIOGRAM DURING PAROXYSMAL SUPRAVENTRICULAR TACHYCARDIA

Rate

Several factors affect the rate of PSVT[38, 57, 163, 248–252] (Table 8.6). One that does not is gender.[57] The rate of PSVT slows slightly (the duration of the RR intervals slightly increases) in the last beats before converting to sinus rhythm.[253–255] This slowing may last somewhat longer before conversion if a catecholamine agonist has been given.[254] The ventricular rate of PSVT is usually faster than during untreated atrial fibrillation.[57]

[ii]The short PR intervals characteristic of Lown-Ganong-Levine syndrome may be produced by other causes, such as, in one case, a pheochromocytoma.[240]

[ii]See the section on electrophysiology of atrial fibrillation and Wolff-Parkinson-White syndrome in Chapter 4.

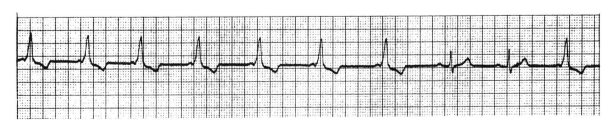

FIGURE 8.4 Intermittent conduction in an accessory pathway produces some preexcited (1–7 and 10) and some normally conducted (8 and 9) beats (lead I). The accessory pathway in this case has a long refractory period and is unlikely to conduct rapidly and to produce dangerous ventricular tachyarrhythmias. (Adapted from Gallagher JJ: Supraventricular tachycardia with reentry in accessory pathways. In Kastor JA, ed. Arrhythmias. Philadelphia: WB Saunders, 1994, with permission.)

Table 8.6	FACTORS AFFECTING HEART RATE DURING PAROXYSMAL SUPRAVENTRICULAR TACHYCARDIA		
Factor	**Faster**	**Slower**	
Activity[120, 163]	Exercise	Rest	
Age[57, 251, 437]	Younger	Older	
Structural heart disease[38]	None	Present	
Setting[252]	Spontaneous	Induced in electrophysiology laboratory[a]	
Time since last paroxysm of tachycardia in untreated patients[250]	Longer	Shorter	

[a] The average rate of spontaneous supraventricular tachycardia in 38 patients was 16 beats per minute faster than when induced by electrophysiological techniques.[252] These differences are probably due to variation in the hemodynamic and autonomic states in the two settings.

P Wave and PR Interval

P waves are usually hidden within the QRS complexes during PSVT sustained in the atrioventricular node[120, 256, 257] (Table 8.7). However, part of them may appear at the end of or rarely just before the QRS complexes (Fig. 8.5). The P'R intervals are characteristically longer than the RP' intervals.[kk]

During paroxysmal supraventricular tachycardia sustained in accessory pathways, the P waves usually appear just after the QRS complex, but the P'R intervals are still longer than the RP' intervals. When the arrhythmia is incessant, the P waves usually appear later between the QRS complexes. In these cases, the P'R intervals are shorter than the RP' intervals (Fig. 8.6).[120]

When the P'R interval is shorter than the RP' interval during tachycardia, a positive P wave in lead I favors atypical atrioventricular nodal reentry, an unusual type in which the course of reentry is the opposite to the route in most cases.[257]

Axis. The axis of the P waves in the frontal plane during PSVT, when these waves can be seen, is usually negative in inferior leads II, III, and aVF, in accordance with the abnormal activation of the atria upward from the atrioventricular node or the base of the atria.[256, 257]

[kk] The apostrophe in P'R and RP' indicates that atrial activation arises from the tachycardia and not from the sinus node.

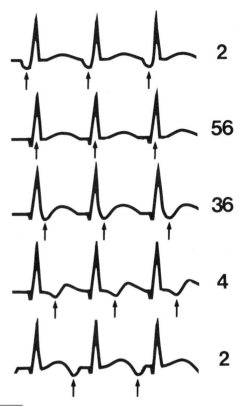

FIGURE 8.5 Where the P waves occur during PSVT sustained in dual atrioventricular nodal pathways in 100 patients each studied electrophysiologically. The most frequent locations (*arrows*) are within or just after the QRS complexes. (Adapted from Wellens HJJ. Supraventricular tachycardia with reentry in the atrioventricular node. In Kastor JA, ed. Arrhythmias. Philadelphia: WB Saunders, 1994, with permission.)

QRS Complex During Atrioventricular Nodal Reentry

The QRS complexes of patients whose tachycardia is sustained within the atrioventricular node usually have the same form as during sinus rhythm because the ventricles are activated through the atrioventricular node and bundle of His (Table 8.8). When one of the bundle branches blocks because of the rapid rate, one must differentiate the arrhythmia from ventricular tachycardia.[ll]

[ll] See Chapter 12 for diagnosing the mechanism of wide complex tachycardias from symptoms, electrocardiogram, and electrophysiological study.

Table 8.7	RELATION OF P WAVES TO QRS COMPLEXES DURING PAROXYSMAL SUPRAVENTRICULAR TACHYCARDIA[256]			
Location of Reentry	**Character**	**P Wave Within QRS**	**P Wave Before QRS (PR > RP)**	**P Wave After QRS (PR < RP)**
Atrioventricular node	Paroxysmal	Almost always	Never	Seldom
	Incessant	No[a]	Yes	Not usually
Accessory pathways	Paroxysmal	Seldom	Occasionally	Usually
	Incessant	No	Yes	Not usually

[a] The P waves in lead I during atrioventricular nodal are usually upright or isoelectric.[257]
(From Bar FW, Brugada P, Dassen WR, Wellens HJJ. Differential diagnosis of tachycardia with narrow QRS complex (shorter than 0.12 sec). Am J Cardiol 1984; 54:555–560, with permission.)

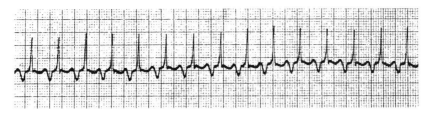

FIGURE 8.6 Incessant PSVT. The electrocardiogram (lead II) shows a PSVT at a rate of about 140 beats per minute. Notice the inverted P waves that precede each QRS complex and mimic atrial tachycardia. (Adapted from Gallagher JJ: Supraventricular tachycardia with reentry in accessory pathways. In Kastor JA, ed. Arrhythmias. Philadelphia: WB Saunders, 1994, with permission.)

QRS Complex During Accessory Pathway Reentry

During PSVT sustained in accessory pathways, the QRS complexes usually look like non-preexcited supraventricular beats because, in most cases, the ventricles are activated through the normal conduction system (see Table 8.8). This route of reentry "down" the atrioventricular node and "up" the accessory pathway is known as "orthodromic."[mm] The pathway is reversed in "antidromic" PSVT. Then the ventricles are activated through the accessory pathway, and the QRS complexes are preexcited.

ST Segments and T Waves

Inverted T waves may appear on conversion of PSVT to sinus rhythm in the absence of any evidence of

[mm]"Orthodromic" (from the Greek words *ortho*, "straight" or "upright," and *dromic*, "running"). "Antidromic" (from *anti*, "against" or "opposite to," and *dromic*).

Table 8.8 **ELECTROCARDIOGRAPHIC CLUES THAT HELP TO PREDICT THE MECHANISM OF PAROXYSMAL SUPRAVENTRICULAR TACHYCARDIA IN A GROUP OF PATIENTS WHOSE DIAGNOSIS WAS ESTABLISHED BY ELECTROPHYSIOLOGICAL STUDY**[272a]

Criteria	Atrioventricular Nodal Reentry (%)	Accessory Pathway Reentry (%)
During Sinus Rhythm		
Preexcitation	2	45
During Paroxysmal Supraventricular Tachycardia		
P waves visible	35	68[b]
Pseudo r' in lead V_1	12	58
Pseudo S waves in leads II, III, or aVF	14	0
Alternans of QRS complexes	13	27

[a]Each comparison is statistically significant.
[b]P waves are detected during supraventricular tachycardia sustained in accessory pathways with equal frequency whether or not preexcitation is present during sinus rhythm.

(From Kalbfleisch SJ, el-Atassi R, Calkins H, Langberg JJ, Morady F. Differentiation of paroxysmal narrow QRS complex tachycardias using the 12-lead electrocardiogram. J Am Coll Cardiol 1993; 21:85–89. Reprinted with permission from the American College of Cardiology.)

structural heart disease.[258] T-wave abnormalities present during Wolff-Parkinson-White syndrome may persist for as long as 5 weeks[259] after ablation of accessory pathways in patients with preexcitation,[259–263] although not in patients with concealed accessory pathways.[261] These changes may reflect "cardiac memory" in which repolarization abnormalities brought about by pacing,[264] preexcitation, or other influences may persist after the force producing the abnormality has been removed[260] (Fig. 8.7).

Diagnosis of Mechanism of Regular Supraventricular Tachyarrhythmia with Narrow QRS Complexes

Several criteria assist physicians in determining which mechanism accounts for regular tachyarrhythmias with QRS complexes of less than 0.12 second in duration[220, 256, 265–272] (see Table 8.8). However, despite carefully applying the "rules," experts cannot determine in advance of the electrophysiological study what mechanism will be found in every case.[256, 269]

Rate of the tachycardia. Although some series suggest that, on average, PSVT sustained in accessory pathways tends to be faster than atrioventricular nodal reentry,[76, 137, 267, 269] other reports show that no consistent difference exists.[256, 267, 272] In an individual case, diagnosis on the basis of rate is unreliable.

P waves. These waves usually occur within the QRS complexes during atrioventricular nodal reentry (Table 8.9). Part of the P waves can frequently be seen, however, protruding from the end of the QRS complex and distorting the terminal portion of the QRS complex. This helpful clue is often called *pseudo-incomplete bundle branch block pattern* because, in lead V_1, the end of the P wave may produce a small positive deflection. The diagnosis is best made by carefully comparing the morphology of the QRS complexes in lead V_1 during PSVT and sinus rhythm[256] (Fig. 8.8).

When P waves occur midway or later in the RR interval, as they occasionally do in this form of arrhythmia, the tachycardia is usually incessant, rather than paroxysmal.[107–110, 112, 115, 117, 120–123, 125, 126, 134, 135] Finally, P waves, when seen during PSVT sustained in the atrioventricular node, are almost invariably inverted in the inferior leads.[256]

The P waves of most patients with accessory pathway reentry occur after the QRS complexes. They are usually inverted in lead II, but in some patients, the P waves may be positive or biphasic in that lead.[256] Moreover, although the P waves reflect retrograde activation of the atria in both atrioventricular nodal and accessory pathway reentrant tachycardia and should therefore be negative in the inferior electrocardiogram leads, using differences in P-wave axis adds relatively little to making a mechanistic diagnosis.[272]

Occasionally, the retrograde P waves of PSVT sustained in dual pathways may *precede* the QRS complexes and may produce what has been called "pseudo Q waves," small, negative deflections in the inferior leads (see Fig. 8.8).

PR intervals. Atrioventricular block rarely occurs during PSVT sustained in either the atrioventricular

	Table 8.9 ELECTROCARDIOGRAPHIC CLUES THAT HELP TO DIAGNOSE WHEN PAROXYSMAL SUPRAVENTRICULAR TACHYCARDIA DEPENDS ON ATRIOVENTRICULAR NODAL REENTRY OR A CONCEALED ACCESSORY PATHWAY		
Criteria	**Atrioventricular Node**	**Concealed Accessory Pathways**
Location of P wave	Within QRS complex	Follows QRS complex
P wave in lead I	Positive	Negative[a]
Bundle branch block during tachycardia	No	Yes

[a]In the presence of left-sided accessory pathways.[267]

node[273-278] or an accessory pathway.[275, 279] When it does appear, the arrhythmia usually stops. When block develops in what seems to be PSVT, one should consider whether the patient really has atrial tachycardia or atrial flutter.

QRS complexes

Bundle branch block. Functional bundle branch block develops more often at the onset of PSVT when the tachycardia is sustained in concealed accessory pathways than in the atrioventricular node[20, 267, 280-286] (see Tables 8.8 and 8.9) (Fig. 8.9).[nn] The block occurs in the ventricle into which the accessory pathway inserts (the ipsilateral ventricle).[20, 267]

The rate of PSVT decreases when bundle branch block develops in the ipsilateral ventricle connected to the accessory pathway but not if the bundle branch block involves the contralateral ventricle unattached to the accessory pathway.[280, 282, 285, 287] The rate does not change when bundle branch block appears during PSVT sustained within the atrioventricular node.

Pseudo-S waves. Again best seen by comparing tracings during the arrhythmia and during sinus rhythm, these waves appear in a few cases of PSVT because of atrioventricular nodal reentry but not during accessory pathway reentry[272] (Fig. 8.10).

Alternation of the QRS complexes. This phenomenon, seen during PSVT, in which the amplitude of every other QRS complex varies,[288] favors accessory pathway reentry, although it appears in atrioventricular nodal reentry,[256, 268, 272] and it is more frequently seen at faster rates regardless of the mechanism[269-272] (see Table 8.8).[oo]

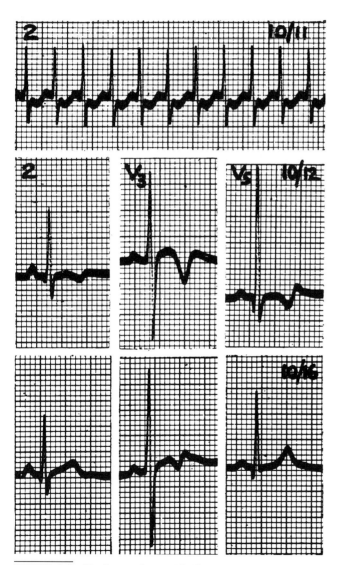

FIGURE 8.7 Electrocardiographic "memory" of abnormal T waves. The T waves remain abnormally inverted one day **(middle)** after termination of PSVT on 10/11 **(top)**, but they return toward normal 4 days later **(bottom)**. (Adapted from Marriott HJL. Practical Electrocardiography. 8th ed. Baltimore: Williams & Wilkins, 1988, with permission.)[1388]

[nn]Bundle branch block at the onset of supraventricular tachycardia occurred in 75% of patients with concealed accessory pathways and in 13% of those with atrioventricular nodal reentrant tachycardia, according to one series.[20]

[oo]What investigators think that alternans during supraventricular tachycardia predicts has changed from accessory pathway reentry only (in 1983 and 1984)[256, 268] to faster rate only (in 1987 and 1990)[269-271] to, more recently, accessory pathway reentry *and* faster rate (in 1993).[272] In one case, electrical (and mechanical) alternans developed during supraventricular tachycardia in a patient with a concealed accessory pathway when the rate *decreased* after propranolol was given.[288]

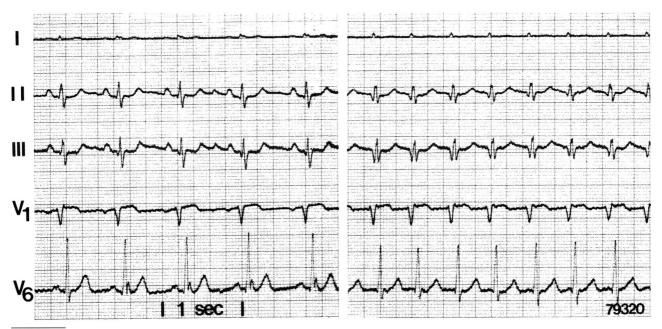

FIGURE 8.8 **"Pseudo-Q waves"** identifying atrioventricular nodal reentry as the mechanism of PSVT. Inverted P waves just before the beginning of ventricular activation produce what look like small Q waves during PSVT sustained in dual pathways **(right)**. Compare with the QRS complexes during sinus rhythm **(left)**. Pseudo-Q waves are an unusual finding even among patients whose PSVT depends on dual pathways, and they rarely, if ever, appear when the arrhythmia is sustained in accessory pathways. (From Wellens HJJ. Supraventricular tachycardia with reentry in the atrioventricular node. In Kastor JA, ed. Arrhythmias. Philadelphia: WB Saunders, 1994, with permission.)

ST segments and T waves. ST segments are frequently depressed during PSVT. Exercise testing[289] and measurement of myocardial lactate production[159] show that the ST depressions are not due to myocardial ischemia in most of these patients even if they have coronary disease.[159] ST segments are depressed by at least 2 mm and T waves are inverted during narrow complex PSVT more frequently when the arrhythmia is sustained through accessory pathways than within the atrioventricular node.[290][pp]

[pp] These findings were present in 57% of supraventricular tachycardias sustained in accessory pathways and in 25% of supraventricular tachycardias sustained in the atrioventricular node.[290]

Diagnosis of Electrophysiological Mechanism of Regular Tachycardias with Wide QRS Complexes in Patients with Accessory Pathways[qq]

Atrial flutter with antegrade conduction down accessory pathways is the most frequent cause of regular tachycardias with QRS complexes greater than or equal to 0.12 second in patients with accessory pathways[291] (Table 8.10). Next in frequency comes antidromic PSVT.[291] The ventricular rate is usually faster in patients

---

[qq] See Chapter 12 for a general discussion of the diagnosis of a tachycardia with wide QRS complex.

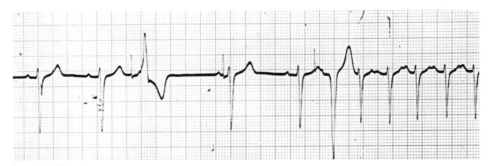

FIGURE 8.9 **Incomplete left bundle branch block during the onset of PSVT** in a patient without spontaneous preexcitation. The third pacing stimulus *(right side)* captures the atria sufficiently early to cause antegrade block in the accessory pathway and establish orthodromic PSVT. The left bundle branch transmitting the first beat is partially refractory. This finding strongly suggests that the arrhythmia is sustained in an accessory pathway and not within the atrioventricular node. The first atrial pacing stimulus (beat 3 to the *left*) proves the presence of an accessory pathway by producing marked preexcitation with a very short PR interval, a large delta wave, and deep inversion of the T wave. (This beat looks like, but is not, a ventricular premature beat.) The second atrial pacing stimulus occurs during the refractory period of the atria.

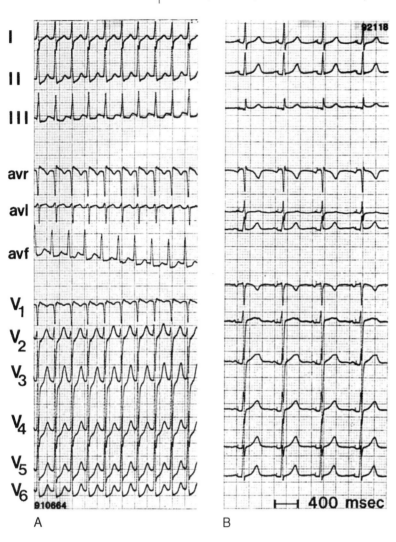

FIGURE 8.10 "Pseudo-S waves" and "pseudo-incomplete right bundle branch block" identifying atrioventricular nodal reentry as the mechanism of PSVT. Retrograde P waves and not terminal activation of the ventricles produce the small S waves in leads II, III, and aVF and the small r' in lead V$_1$ **(A)**. Compare with the end of the QRS complexes in the electrocardiogram of the same patient during sinus rhythm in which these findings are absent **(B)**. Inverted P waves hugging the end of the QRS complexes in this fashion are typical of PSVT sustained in dual pathways. (From Wellens HJJ. Supraventricular tachycardia with reentry in the atrioventricular node. In Kastor JA, ed. Arrhythmias. Philadelphia: WB Saunders, 1994, with permission.)

with flutter than in those with antidromic tachycardia.[291]

Onset of PSVT

Atrial premature beats are the most frequent event which institute PSVT. *Ventricular premature beats* can occasionally, but much less frequently than atrial premature beats, start PSVT sustained in the atrioventricular node.

Sinus captures during junctional rhythm[292] or after a junctional escape[293] can produce the electrophysiological conditions necessary to start PSVT. This mechanism seems more common in children than adults.[293]

OTHER ELECTROCARDIOGRAPHIC TESTS

Exercise Testing

Exercise during sinus rhythm in patients with preexcitation only occasionally[96, 124, 243, 294–298] induces PSVT,[rr] even in patients who have spontaneous paroxysms of the arrhythmia.[299] However, exercising brings out the tachycardia in some of those patients, including young athletes, whose arrhythmias are associated with high levels of activity.[96] Esophageal pacing during exercise occasionally induces PSVT in athletes with palpitations and no arrhythmia on standard electrocardiographic evaluation.[300] As a general rule, however, exercising is a relatively unreliable method of predicting which

Table 8.10 **MECHANISMS OF REGULAR TACHYCARDIAS WITH WIDE QRS COMPLEXES FOUND IN 26 (15%) OF 163 PATIENTS WITH ACCESSORY PATHWAYS**[291]

Arrhythmia	Number (%)	Ventricular Rate
Atrial flutter with 1:1 antegrade conduction in the accessory pathway	15 (58%)	262 ± 42
Antidromic paroxysmal supraventricular tachycardia	7 (27%)	217 ± 22
Ventricular tachycardia	1 (4%)	—
Other	2 (8%)	—

(From Benditt DG, Pritchett EL, Gallagher JJ. Spectrum of regular tachycardias with wide QRS complexes in patients with accessory atrioventricular pathways. Am J Cardiol 1978; 42:828–838, with permission.)

[rr]Some of the "supraventricular tachycardias" recorded during exercise may have been atrial tachycardias.

patients with Wolff-Parkinson-White syndrome electrocardiogram will develop PSVT.[299]

Exercise reveals information about the refractoriness of accessory pathways. If preexcitation disappears during exercise, the accessory pathway is unlikely to be able to conduct rapidly enough to produce ventricular fibrillation during atrial fibrillation or atrial flutter.[243–245] Exercising during reentrant PSVT usually increases the rate of the tachycardia.[120] Exercise testing reveals that ST segment depressions during PSVT are not due to coronary heart disease in most patients.[289]

Ambulatory Monitoring

Ambulatory monitoring documents PSVT,[296, 298, 301] reveals its temporal characteristics in symptomatic and asymptomatic patients, and defines the circadian appearance of the arrhythmia.[57, 152] Ambulatory monitoring reveals when PSVT is the cause of syncope better than does exercise testing.[302] However, event monitors help to make the diagnosis of PSVT more successfully than does Holter monitoring.[153ss]

ECHOCARDIOGRAPHY

Echocardiography reveals, in patients with PSVT, that, compared with sinus rhythm, the size of the left atrium increases during atrioventricular nodal and accessory pathway PSVT.[180] Echocardiographic studies also

* Help to identify the location of accessory pathways.[303]
* Show that ventricular function improves, to a variable degree,[196, 304] after successful treatment of incessant PSVT causing cardiomyopathy.[198]

VALUES BEFORE AND AFTER TREATMENT[198ff]

Left Ventricular Measurements	During Tachycardia	After Conversion to Sinus Rhythm
Ejection fraction	36%	59%
End-diastolic diameter	56 mm	49 mm
End-systolic diameter	44 mm	32 mm

Doppler flow studies establish that retrograde flow characteristically occurs during PSVT when the right atrium contracts against the closed tricuspid valve.[181] Intracardiac echocardiography assists in performing ablation to cure the patient of PSVT and other arrhythmias.[305–309] Transesophageal echocardiography shows that catheter ablation with radiofrequency current rarely produces thrombi.[310]

Fetal echocardiography and electrocardiographic monitoring confirm the presence of PSVT in utero.[68–71, 311, 312] Sonography has shown that a fetus had, at different times, atrial flutter and PSVT, proven after birth to be due to accessory pathway reentry.[70] When compared with normal atrioventricular conduction and activa-

tion, Doppler studies show that preexcitation diminishes atrial transport function and decreases stroke volume.[313]

NUCLEAR CARDIOLOGY

Nuclear studies show the following during PSVT:

* Left ventricular end-diastolic and stroke volumes markedly decrease without change in ejection fraction.[178]
* In paced patients cured of PSVT by surgical division of accessory pathways, the hemodynamic consequences of PSVT are due primarily to decreased ventricular volume, rather than to reduced ventricular function.[183] These changes are ascribed principally to loss of the atrial contribution to ventricular filling.[183]

PATHOLOGY

Autopsy examinations of the hearts of patients known to have Wolff-Parkinson-White syndrome often reveal accessory pathways in the locations predicted from the electrocardiogram.[314, 315] However, pathological studies do not, with one published exception,[316] reveal separate tracts that correspond to dual pathways within the atrioventricular node of patients with intranodal PSVT.[317]

An infant with hypertrophic cardiomyopathy and recurrent PSVT who died suddenly had myofiber disarray around an abnormally formed central fibrous body, numerous nodoventricular fibers, and fibrosis of the left bundle branch. These findings suggest that the arrhythmias were due to reentry in a concealed accessory pathway or malformed atrioventricular junction.[318]

Fibrosis of the accessory pathways may account for the inability of some tracts to conduct in both directions.[319] Endomyocardial biopsy in patients with cardiomyopathy secondary to PSVT shows focal degenerative changes, mild to moderate interstitial edema, or myocardial fibrosis without inflammation.[196]

ELECTROPHYSIOLOGY OF PAROXYSMAL SUPRAVENTRICULAR TACHYCARDIA SUSTAINED IN THE ATRIOVENTRICULAR NODE

PSVT in patients without accessory pathways is a reentrant arrhythmia[20, 30, 31, 320–348] sustained within the atrioventricular node.[32, 33] In most cases, the arrhythmia depends on the presence of two (dual) pathways,[349, 350] each with different rates of conduction and duration of refractoriness and located in, or closely adjacent to,[351, 352] the atrioventricular node. The more slowly conducting pathway is known as the "slow" or "alpha" pathway and is located posterior to the more anteriorly located "fast" or "beta" pathway. The retrograde fast pathway has electrophysiological properties of atrioventricular nodal tissue,[353] and it may not be an anatomically discrete structure.[354, 355] The dual pathway

---

ss Event monitors revealed the diagnosis in 8 (47%) of 17 patients, and Holter monitoring showed it in 6 (9%) of 64 patients.[153]

ff These values were recorded before and after successful treatment of six patients with cardiomyopathy due to incessant supraventricular tachycardia.[198]

concept, although relatively easy to comprehend in understanding the genesis of the arrhythmia, probably simplifies the nature of the atrioventricular junction, a three-dimensional structure with complex electrophysiological properties.[355]

Few adults have dual pathways[356, 357uu] and not everyone with dual pathways has PSVT.[357–362vv] Furthermore, dual pathways cannot be demonstrated in everyone who has PSVT sustained in the atrioventricular node.[356, 363] In children and young adults, dual atrioventricular nodal pathways occur with greater frequency in those with, than in those without, PSVT.[138]

Patients with PSVT sustained within the atrioventricular node can have preexcited electrocardiograms indicating the presence of accessory pathways that may not participate in the arrhythmia.[284, 364–371] Conversely, patients with PSVT sustained in accessory pathways may have dual atrioventricular nodal pathways that play no role in their arrhythmias.[372, 373] A few patients have more than two pathways within the atrioventricular node[374–382ww] or, in addition, accessory pathways[374, 377, 383, 384] that may participate in tachycardia. Furthermore, some intranodal pathways can mimic features of accessory pathways on electrophysiological study.[385]

Fast and Slow Pathways

During sinus rhythm, in patients with dual atrioventricular nodal pathways, the signal that activates the atria enters both the fast and slow pathways[347] (Fig. 8.11). The impulse in the fast pathway reaches and activates the bundle of His first for further transmission to the ventricles. The signal traveling through the slow pathway finds the bundle of His refractory from the signal previously reaching it through the fast pathway.

During PSVT, a reentrant circuit within the fast and slow pathway must be established. The signal that sustains PSVT can take several courses:

- In antegrade fashion through the slow pathway from atria to ventricles and in retrograde fashion through the fast pathway. This course, known as "slow-fast," accounts for most cases of PSVT sustained in the atrioventricular node.
- The reverse—the "fast-slow" course—with antegrade conduction in the fast pathway and retrograde transmission in the slow pathway, the route for most cases of *incessant* or permanent atrioventricular nodal PSVT.[111, 114]
- An uncommon mechanism of "slow-slow" transmission in which both the antegrade and retrograde pathways conduct slowly.[131]

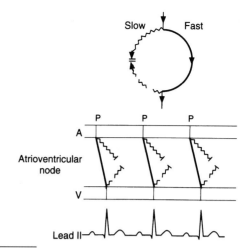

FIGURE 8.11 Conduction in dual atrioventricular nodal pathways during sinus rhythm. The signal from the atria enters the fast (*solid diagonal line,* **top** and **middle**) and slow (*wavy lines*) pathways. The signal in the fast pathway activates the bundle of His and the ventricles. Meanwhile, the signal in the slow pathway arrives too late to activate the now refractory bundle of His or is blocked from completing its antegrade course by retrograde conduction of the signal transmitted previously in the fast pathway (*upward arrow,* **top**). A, atria; P, P waves; V, ventricles; VPD, ventricular premature depolarization. (Adapted from Ganz LI, Friedman PL. Supraventricular tachycardia. N Engl J Med 1995; 332:162–173. Reprinted by permission of the New England Journal of Medicine.)[22]

A few patients with atrioventricular nodal PSVT have more than two intranodal pathways[386, 387] or more than one type of tachycardia.[388xx] Not each of the antegrade slow pathways may participate in the arrhythmia.[387] Whether atrial tissue does,[127, 389–394] or does not,[316, 395–401] form part of the reentrant circuit remains a subject of continuing controversy.

Slow-Fast Conduction

The most common form of PSVT sustained in dual pathways starts and is sustained by the following events, in sequence (Fig. 8.12):

1. An atrial premature beat occurs sufficiently early to block in the fast pathway but to enter the slow pathway.
2. The signal traverses the slow pathway antegrade (forward).
3. The signal meets the fast pathway in the distal (caudal) part of the node and proceeds retrograde (backward) to the proximal (cephalic) junction with the slow pathway.
4. The signal *reenters* the slow pathway.
5. The tachycardia begins.

The ventricles are activated after the reentrant signal, arriving at its distal site, prompts transmission through the bundle of His and bundle branches producing the characteristic narrow QRS complexes (in

---

[uu]The prevalence of dual pathways, documented by electrophysiological techniques, ranges from 4.2% (17 of 405 patients)[357] to 10.3% (41 of 397 patients).[356] Among 78 children evaluated before or after surgery for congenital or acquired heart disease, electrophysiological studies demonstrated dual pathways in one-third.[360] Thus, the incidence of dual pathways is almost certainly greater in children than in adults.

[vv]None of the 78 children with dual pathways had a history of arrhythmia or could be induced into supraventricular tachycardia.[360]

[ww]In a series of 550 patients with atrioventricular nodal reentrant supraventricular tachycardia, 36 (6.5%) had more than one form of supraventricular tachycardia.[982]

[xx]Of 550 patients with atrioventricular nodal supraventricular tachycardia, 26 (5.2%) had three or more intranodal pathways,[387] and 36 (6.5%) had multiple types of the arrhythmia.[388]

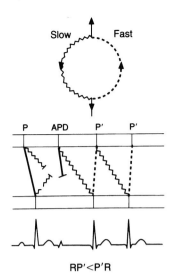

FIGURE 8.12 Mechanism of slow-fast atrioventricular nodal reentrant PSVT. An atrial premature beat (APD, atrial premature depolarization or beat, **middle**) occurs sufficiently early to block in the fast pathway, with its longer refractory period, but to transmit slowly in the slow pathway, (very long PR interval, **bottom**), which has a shorter refractory period. The signal in retrograde fashion enters the fast pathway (*dashed lines*, **top** and **middle**), which has recovered from its partial penetration previously, and on reaching the proximal part of the node, it *reenters* the slow pathway, thereby establishing the arrhythmia. The atria are activated retrograde from the node (P', **middle**, and small negative P wave just after the QRS complex, **bottom**), a process that makes the RP' interval less than the P'R interval (or the P'R interval longer than the RP' interval). (Adapted from Ganz LI, Friedman PL. Supraventricular tachycardia. N Engl J Med 1995; 332:162–173. Reprinted by permission of the New England Journal of Medicine.)[22]

the absence of bundle branch block). The atria are activated from the proximal reentrant site retrograde from the atrioventricular node to the superior parts of the chambers producing in most cases inverted P waves in the inferior electrocardiographic leads.

Refractoriness and the onset of PSVT. The beginning of a paroxysm of PSVT depends on different refractoriness in the two pathways. In the most frequent example, an atrial premature beat occurs sufficiently early to find refractory the fast conducting pathway through which sinus beats ordinarily reach the ventricles. However, the signal from the atrial premature beat finds the slowly conducting pathway excitable and enters it. When this signal reaches the distal connection with the fast pathway, retrograde transmission can occur if the fast pathway is excitable. If the slow pathway has recovered when the retrograde signal in the fast pathway reaches its proximal junction, another cycle can begin, and the tachycardia is established.

One can easily see that different refractoriness of the two pathways is essential to the onset of PSVT and determines the route of the reentry. As a general rule, fast pathways have longer refractory periods, and slow pathways have shorter refractory periods.

Chamber contraction and rate. The atria and ventricles contract at about the same time during atrioven-

tricular nodal PSVT, a feature that accounts for the absence of visible P waves in many patients with the arrhythmia and the characteristic hemodynamic events that follow. This coincidence occurs because of the relation between retrograde and antegrade conduction from the distal junction of the two pathways. The amount of time taken for the signal to travel through the bundle of His and bundle branches into the ventricles is similar to the time taken for the signal to traverse the fast pathway in retrograde fashion and to begin activating of the atria.

Most of the interval between the QRS complexes, which corresponds to the rate of the arrhythmia, is established by the time the reentrant signal takes to traverse the slow pathway in antegrade fashion.[402, 403] The minimal role played by the retrograde fast pathway is supported by the observation that when isoproterenol increases or verapamil and adenosine decrease the rate of the arrhythmia, retrograde conduction over the fast pathway does not change.[75]

Fast-Slow Conduction

PSVT can also be sustained, in both adults and children,[114] by antegrade conduction through a fast conducting pathway and retrograde conduction via a slowly conducting pathway, both within the atrioventricular node (Fig. 8.13).[126, 130, 277, 278, 389, 404–406] This course is much less frequently the mechanism of PSVT than is the slow-fast course.[y] Most cases of incessant or

---

[y]Three (7%) of 42 cases of supraventricular tachycardias sustained in the atrioventricular node.[404]

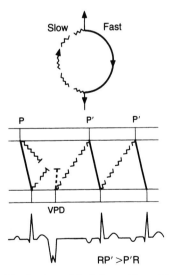

FIGURE 8.13 Mechanism of fast-slow atrioventricular nodal reentrant PSVT. The signal from a ventricular premature beat **(middle)** blocks in retrograde fashion in the fast pathway but conducts in the slow pathway. In the proximal portion of the node, it activates the atria (P', **middle**, inverted P wave, **bottom**) and enters the fast pathway in antegrade fashion. The arrhythmia is established by the signal's reentering the slow pathway retrograde. (Adapted from Ganz LI, Friedman PL. Supraventricular tachycardia. N Engl J Med 1995; 332:162–173. Reprinted by permission of the New England Journal of Medicine.)[22]

persistent atrioventricular nodal PSVT are sustained in the fast-slow mode.

Ventricular pacing or spontaneous ventricular premature beats can institute fast-slow PSVT more easily that atrial premature beats. The ventricular beat blocks in the fast pathway, which must have a longer retrograde refractory period than the slow pathway, and proceeds toward the atria through the slow pathway. Where the two pathways meet proximally, the signal enters the excitable fast pathway and is transmitted in antegrade fashion to the distal union with the slow pathway. If the slow pathway has recovered, PSVT ensues.

Atrial activation occurs later than during slow-fast PSVT because the signal travels more slowly up the slow pathway than down the bundle of His and bundle branches to the ventricles. This process produces the characteristic electrocardiographic appearance of inverted P waves (in the inferior leads) often well seen between the QRS complexes. Put another way, in fast-slow PSVT, the P′R interval is often shorter than RP′ interval, whereas in slow-fast tachycardia in which the P wave is within or peeking out from the end of the QRS complex, the P′R interval is longer than the RP′ interval.

Another electrocardiographic clue favoring slow-fast atrioventricular nodal reentry is the appearance of the P waves in lead I. They tend to be upright or isoelectric in slow-fast atrioventricular nodal reentry, whereas they are usually inverted during low atrial tachycardia or PSVT sustained in accessory pathways.[257]

Slow-Slow Conduction

Occasionally, PSVT, usually incessant, is sustained in pathways that conduct slowly in both directions.[131] It appears that the tracts sustaining this form of tachycardia are located posterior to the usually more anteriorly positioned atrioventricular nodal limbs that support PSVT.[127, 131]

Institution of Paroxysmal Supraventricular Tachycardia

PSVT begins in patients with atrioventricular nodal reentry when the conditions are established whereby one of the two pathways is rendered refractory.

Atrial premature stimuli. These stimuli induce the arrhythmia in most patients with spontaneous PSVT sustained in the atrioventricular node. The site of stimulation does not significantly affect the ease of demonstrating dual pathways or inducing the tachycardia.[407]

Atrial pacing. Atrial pacing at sufficiently rapid rates can cause block in the fast pathway and can lead to PSVT.[352, 363, 408, 409] Esophageal pacing of the left atrium during exercise induces atrioventricular nodal PSVT in some athletes with palpitations and no arrhythmia on standard electrocardiographic evaluation.[300]

Ventricular premature stimuli. These stimuli[404, 408] or, more frequently, ventricular pacing,[409] will occasion-

ally start a paroxysm in patients with atrioventricular nodal PSVT but less often than will atrial premature stimulation[39, 404] (Fig. 8.14).[zz] Incessant PSVT is more easily started with ventricular than with atrial stimulation.

Sinus captures during junctional rhythm. In this relatively unusual circumstance, a sinus beat occurs sufficiently early to enter one, usually the fast, pathway alone because the slow pathway has been rendered refractory by retrograde penetration from the previous junctional beat.[292] The same mechanism explains the onset of a paroxysm when a sinus capture follows a junctional escape.[293] Because this mechanism is seen more frequently in children than adults, it may depend on the greater tendency in children for sudden sinus slowing and junctional escapes.[293]

Position. Atrioventricular nodal PSVT can be induced more readily in some patients when they are standing than when lying flat, presumably because of increased sympathetic tone.[410]

Termination of Paroxysmal Supraventricular Tachycardia

Paroxysms of PSVT in the atrioventricular node terminate when the electrophysiological substrate, usually

---

[zz]Ventricular stimulation starts atrioventricular nodal reentrant supraventricular tachycardia in 10%,[409] 19%,[404] or 40%[20] of patients with the arrhythmia, according to different series.

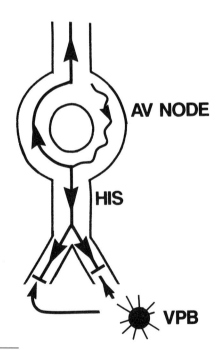

FIGURE 8.14 *Ventricular premature beats seldom start PSVT sustained in the dual pathways* because refractoriness of the His-Purkinje system prevents the ventricular beat (VPB) from reaching the atrioventricular (AV) node to dissociate the pathways. (Adapted from Wellens HJJ. Supraventricular tachycardia with reentry in the atrioventricular node. In Kastor JA, ed. Arrhythmias. Philadelphia: WB Saunders, 1994, with permission.)

the refractoriness of one of the pathways, changes sufficiently so that reentry can no longer be sustained. Spontaneous beats or programmed stimuli from atria or ventricles can accomplish this.

Atrial premature beats. Introduction of atrial stimuli that interrupt the reentrant circuit terminates PSVT.[411] In typical (slow-fast) PSVT, an atrial premature beat terminates the tachycardia, in most cases, by blocking in the slow pathway and entering the fast pathway, where it collides with the retrograde signal sustaining the tachycardia.[20] In atypical (fast-slow) PSVT, the atrial premature beat again enters the fast pathway, but it blocks in the slow pathway, which is refractory from its recent use by the reentrant signal; the tachycardia then stops.[20]

Ventricular premature beats. These beats can terminate typical (slow-fast) PSVT by blocking either in the fast pathway retrograde or in the slow pathway after traversing the fast pathway,[20] particularly when the rate of tachycardia is slow. On many occasions, however, single ventricular premature beats do not terminate because refractoriness of the bundle branches or bundle of His prevent the signal's reaching the dual pathways in the atrioventricular node. In atypical (fast-slow) PSVT, ventricular premature beats terminate the arrhythmia by blocking in the retrograde slow pathway.[20]

Another pathway. Rarely, conduction over a third reentrant pathway may terminate PSVT.[412]

Atrioventricular block. Characteristic of termination is the production of block in at least one of the pathways sustaining PSVT whether sustained in dual atrioventricular nodal or accessory pathways. Consequently, clinical atrioventricular block is inconsistent with perpetuation of the reentry.

Occasionally, however, atrioventricular block does appear and not stop the arrhythmia. In such cases, the block is due to inhibited conduction below the region of reentry,[276] for example, within the His-Purkinje system during intranodal PSVT.[273]

Requirements for Atrioventricular Nodal Paroxysmal Supraventricular Tachycardia

In summary, PSVT within dual pathways depends on three electrophysiological events:

- Sustaining the tachycardia's "engine," reentry within the closed circuit of fast conducting and slowly conducting pathways in the atrioventricular nodal region.
- Ventricular activation beginning each time the reentrant signal reaches the distal union of the two pathways.
- Retrograde atrial activation beginning each time the reentrant signal reached the proximal union of the two pathways.

Lown-Ganong-Levine Syndrome

The short PR interval in patients with Lown-Ganong-Levine syndrome[239, 413–415] usually reflects conduction through an intranodal fast pathway that is either anatomically short or, more frequently, has a shorter refractory period and conducts faster than normal in the antegrade[403, 416–431] and retrograde[432] directions. Short PR intervals in the absence of preexcitation may be considered to be one end of the range of conduction in the normal atrioventricular node and not necessarily a pathological condition.[433] Occasionally, a rapidly conducting extranodal tract that connects the atria to the bundle of His accounts for the short PR interval.[425, 429, 434aaa]

Reentrant tachycardia is favored in patients with Lown-Ganong-Levine syndrome who also have slow pathways[420, 425, 428bbb] because of the large differences in conduction and refractoriness between the two pathways. The rate of reentrant PSVT is usually faster in patients with Lown-Ganong-Levine syndrome than in patients with normal PR intervals because conduction in the slow pathway, which is the most important determinant of rate during the arrhythmia, is quicker.[402, 425, 429]

Drugs[ccc]

Miscellaneous Factors

Antegrade conduction over two pathways. This rare condition can produce a nonreentrant PSVT from two QRS complexes from each sinus beat.[435]

Coronary sinus. The ostium and the first 10 mm of the coronary sinus are larger in patients with PSVT sustained in the atrioventricular node than in other subjects.[436] The significance of this finding is unknown.

Retrograde dual pathways. In a few patients, dual retrograde pathways elicited by ventricular stimulation can participate in PSVT.[376ddd]

Differences in rate. The slowing of the rate of PSVT as patients age appears to be due to prolongation of conduction in the retrograde pathway.[437]

Posture. Upright posture enhances conduction in patients with dual atrioventricular nodal pathways and facilitates atrioventricular nodal reentry.[438] The rate of the tachycardia is faster in the upright position because of faster conduction in the antegrade slow pathway.[438]

[aaa]Because these extranodal connections insert into the bundle of His and not into ventricular myocardium, no delta wave of abnormal ventricular activation is seen.

[bbb]As many as half the patients with the Lown-Ganong-Levine syndrome also have slow pathways, according to one series.[429]

[ccc]The electropharmacologic effects of drugs used to treat supraventricular tachycardia sustained in dual atrioventricular nodal pathways are discussed with accessory pathways later.

[ddd]Retrograde dual pathways were demonstrated in only 31 (3.5%) of 887 patients.[376]

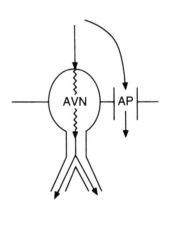

Fiber Crossing
Electrical Insulation

FIGURE 8.15   Ventricular activation during preexcitation. In addition to signals conducted down the normal atrioventricular nodal–His-Purkinje system *(thick black arrows)*, the ventricles also receive impulses through an accessory pathway (Fiber) coursing from the left atrium to the left ventricle *(thin black arrows)*. (From Gallagher JJ: Supraventricular tachycardia with reentry in accessory pathways. In Kastor JA, ed. Arrhythmias. Philadelphia: WB Saunders, 1994, with permission.)

Other advances. In addition to the references cited, other publications report advances in our knowledge of the electrophysiology of patients with PSVT sustained in the atrioventricular node.[274, 342, 349, 350, 439–481]

ELECTROPHYSIOLOGY OF PAROXYSMAL SUPRAVENTRICULAR TACHYCARDIA SUSTAINED IN ACCESSORY PATHWAYS

Two Pathways

PSVT in patients with accessory pathways, whether or not they have Wolff-Parkinson-White syndrome, is, like PSVT, sustained in dual pathways in the atrioventricular node, also a reentrant arrhythmia, but this time the two basic parts of the circuit are the normal conducting system (atrioventricular node, bundle of His, bundle branches and Purkinje network) and the accessory pathway.[20, 24, 320, 324–327, 330, 332, 335, 337–339, 345, 482–495eee]

Sinus rhythm. During sinus rhythm, the atrial signal conducts through both the atrioventricular node and the accessory pathway (Figs. 8.15 and 8.16). The PR interval is short and the delta wave is large when conduction in the accessory pathway dominates, whereas the PR interval is normal and the delta wave is small or absent when nodal conduction is favored or if the accessory pathway does not conduct in antegrade fashion.

---

eeeThe European Study Group for Preexcitation prefers that the term "connection" be used for accessory pathways that insert into myocardium and "tract" for those unusual pathways that insert into specialized conduction tissue.[495]

Orthodromic conduction. In most cases of PSVT, the signal courses from atria to ventricles down the normal conducting system—the antegrade route—and up the accessory pathway from ventricles to atria—the retrograde pathway (Figs. 8.17 and 8.18). Part of the

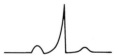

FIGURE 8.16   Conduction during sinus rhythm in patients with accessory pathways. A signal from the atria conducts to the ventricles through both the atrioventricular node (AVN) and accessory pathway (AP) **(top)**. The PR interval will be short and the delta wave large if conduction in the accessory pathway is favored **(bottom)**. The PR interval will be normal and the delta wave small or absent if little or no conduction occurs over the accessory pathway. (Adapted from Ganz LI, Friedman PL. Supraventricular tachycardia. N Engl J Med 1995; 332:162–173. Reprinted by permission of the New England Journal of Medicine.)[22]

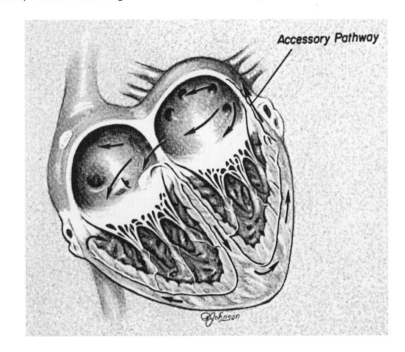

FIGURE 8.17 Cardiac activation during orthodromic tachycardia. The ventricles are activated through the normal conducting system (*arrows* traveling in the interventricular septum and to left and right through the ventricular myocardium). The signal also traverses an accessory pathway between the lateral wall of the left ventricle and the left atrium. The circuit is completed by the signal's reentering the atrioventricular node. Atrial activation, which is, accordingly, abnormal, produces the characteristic negative P waves in the electrocardiogram. (From Gallagher JJ: Supraventricular tachycardia with reentry in accessory pathways. In Kastor JA, ed. Arrhythmias. Philadelphia: WB Saunders, 1994, with permission.)

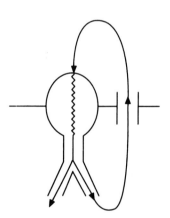

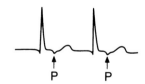

FIGURE 8.18 Course of orthodromic reentrant PSVT sustained in an accessory pathway. The route of the signal that sustains the tachycardia during the more common type of this arrhythmia is down the slowly conducting atrioventricular node and up the accessory pathway. Retrograde atrial activation produces the inverted P waves in the inferior leads **(bottom)**, which are characteristically further from the end of the QRS complexes than during nodal reentrant tachycardia. (Adapted from Ganz LI, Friedman PL. Supraventricular tachycardia. N Engl J Med 1995; 332:162–173. Reprinted by permission of the New England Journal of Medicine.)[22]

antegrade limb lies within the node in what we call the fast pathway during atrioventricular nodal reentry and through which conduction occurs during normal sinus rhythm. However, all tracts in the atrioventricular nodes conduct more slowly than do most accessory pathways. Consequently, what functions as the "fast pathway" during atrioventricular nodal PSVT becomes the "slow pathway" during accessory pathway reentry. The more rapidly the atrioventricular nodal pathway conducts, the faster the tachycardia.[496]

Another important difference from atrioventricular nodal reentrant PSVT is that in accessory pathway tachycardia, the atria and ventricles participate in sustaining the reentry. The accessory pathways insert into these chambers, and transmission through atrial and ventricular tissue is essential to maintain the circuit. Patients with accessory pathways with or without Wolff-Parkinson-White syndrome may also have dual atrioventricular nodal pathways that sustain,[284, 364–371, 373, 377, 497] or do not sustain,[373, 498] PSVT.[fff]

Not all patients with preexcitation develop PSVT. Characteristics of the accessory pathways of asymptomatic patients with Wolff-Parkinson-White syndrome, when compared with patients with Wolff-Parkinson-White syndrome who have PSVT, include the following:

- Longer anterograde refractory periods,[499] which prolong in some patients as they age.[83]
- Less rapid conduction of atrial fibrillation.[499]
- Inability to conduct in retrograde fashion, which is required to support the arrhythmia.[368]

The electrophysiological substrate for PSVT, however, can be demonstrated in many asymptomatic patients with preexcitation.[500]

Antidromic conduction. As in atrioventricular nodal reentry, an infrequently encountered antidromic course exists in which antegrade conduction flows through the accessory pathway and retrograde conduc-

---

[fff] Thirty-two (8%) of 402 patients with accessory pathways requiring surgical ablation had dual atrioventricular nodal physiology or intranodal supraventricular tachycardia.[373]

tion flows through the standard conducting system (Fig. 8.19).[368, 501–505ggg] The prevalence of males is greater among those with antidromic than with orthodromic tachycardia.[156hhh]

Concealed Accessory Pathways

Electrophysiological studies reveal when PSVT can be sustained in concealed accessory pathways that produce no preexcitation during sinus rhythm.[136, 205, 206, 267, 273, 281–283, 285, 319, 366, 496, 506–519] Although able to conduct in retrograde fashion during PSVT and thereby to sustain the tachycardia, these pathways are refractory to antegrade conduction (Fig. 8.20). Most concealed accessory pathways insert into the left ventricle.[267] The antegrade block appears to be located near the interface of the accessory pathway and the ventricle into which it inserts.[520] Concealed accessory pathways form part of the circuit sustaining PSVT in many patients.[iii]

[gggAntidromic tachycardia was induced in 52 (7.6%) of 685 patients with Wolff-Parkinson-White syndrome studied in two electrophysiology laboratories.[504, 505] Of the 52, *spontaneous* antidromic tachycardia was observed in 21 (40%) and in only 3.1% of those with Wolff-Parkinson-White syndrome.[504, 505]]

[hhhSeventy percent of patients with antidromic tachycardia are male, whereas 60% with orthodromic tachycardia are male.[156]]

[iiiConcealed accessory pathways formed the retrograde limb of supraventricular tachycardia in 106 (38%) of 280 patients with supraventricular tachycardia and no preexcitation during sinus rhythm.[20]]

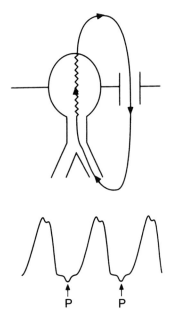

FIGURE 8.19 Course of antidromic reentrant PSVT sustained in an accessory pathway. The route of the signal in antidromic PSVT is the opposite of orthodromic tachycardia—up the slowly conducting atrioventricular node and down the rapidly conducting accessory pathway. Accordingly, the QRS complexes are fully preexcited, wide, and abnormal **(bottom)**. Retrograde atrial activation (inverted P waves in the inferior electrocardiographic leads, **bottom**) can usually be seen between the QRS complexes. (Adapted from Ganz LI, Friedman PL. Supraventricular tachycardia. N Engl J Med 1995; 332:162–173. Reprinted by permission of the New England Journal of Medicine.)[22]

Induction

Starting PSVT sustained in accessory pathways depends on differences in refractoriness and speed of conduction in the two limbs of the circuit, just as in atrioventricular nodal reentrant tachycardia.[521, 522] In most cases, the antegrade electrophysiological properties of the normal conducting system and the retrograde electrophysiological properties of the accessory pathways determine whether PSVT will develop.[523] Antegrade electrophysiological properties of the accessory pathways have little importance.[523]

Atrial pacing and atrial premature beats. These beats institute the arrhythmia in most patients with spontaneous PSVT due to reentry in accessory pathways, whether manifest or concealed (Fig. 8.21).[20, 28, 492, 524, 525] The early atrial beat

1. Finds the accessory pathway refractory and courses through the atrioventricular node slowly because the beat, being premature, traverses the node when it is partially refractory.
2. Travels rapidly through the bundle of His, bundle branches, and Purkinje network.
3. Activates the ventricles.
4. Reaches and then courses up the accessory pathway in retrograde fashion.
5. Activates and traverses the atria.
6. Reenters the atrioventricular node if it is no longer refractory, thereby establishing the tachycardia. Atrial premature beats can also induce one or more intra-atrial reentrant beats that may facilitate the beginning of PSVT in accessory pathways.[526]

Ventricular premature beats and ventricular pacing. These features start the arrhythmia in about 80% of patients with PSVT sustained in accessory pathways[492] (Fig. 8.22). When the accessory pathways are concealed and do not conduct in antegrade fashion, ventricular stimulation starts the arrhythmia in about 50% of cases.[20] Ventricular stimulation starts PSVT sustained in accessory pathways more than twice as frequently than when the arrhythmia is sustained solely within the atrioventricular node.

The signal generated by ventricular pacing or by a ventricular premature beat, in sequence

1. Blocks retrograde in the His-bundle branch-Purkinje system.[527, 528jjj]
2. Proceeds in retrograde fashion to the atria through the accessory pathway.
3. Activates and traverses the atria.
4. Engages the atrioventricular node, which is not refractory because no signal has recently proceeded through it.
5. Travels in antegrade fashion through the atrioventricular node–bundle of His–bundle branch–Purkinje network to the ventricles.

[jjjBefore reproducible demonstration of retrogradely activated bundle of His deflections, the site of retrograde block in the normal conduction system was uncertain[1389] or was thought to be located, incorrectly as later studies showed, in the atrioventricular node.]

MANIFEST

CONCEALED

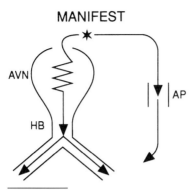 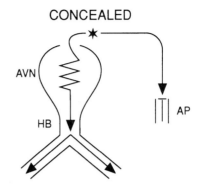

FIGURE 8.20   Manifest and concealed preexcitation. In patients with Wolff-Parkinson-White syndrome, the ventricles are activated from both the standard pathway through the atrioventricular node (AVN) and bundle of His (HB) and via an accessory pathway (AP) **(left)**, a process that produces the familiar electrocardiogram (*manifest* preexcitation). If the accessory pathway cannot conduct in antegrade fashion, preexcitation is said to be *concealed* **(right)**, and signs of Wolff-Parkinson-White syndrome are absent during sinus rhythm. Some concealed accessory pathways, however, can conduct in retrograde fashion and, thereby, sustain PSVT. (From Gallagher JJ: Supraventricular tachycardia with reentry in accessory pathways. In Kastor JA, ed. Arrhythmias. Philadelphia: WB Saunders, 1994, with permission.)

6. While activating the ventricles, reenters the accessory pathway, thereby establishing the tachycardia.

Whereas ventricular beating can establish PSVT in accessory pathways by other mechanisms, this is by far the most common method in orthodromic tachycardia.[492] Because the accessory pathways insert in different locations in the ventricles, the site of stimulation can affect whether or not tachycardia is induced.[529]

Increasing the sinus rate. This occasionally induces PSVT, usually incessant,[113, 116, 530] and more frequently in younger patients.[530]

Junctional escape beats. These beats can establish the conditions for reentry to occur in patients with PSVT sustained in an accessory pathway.[531]

Transient ventricular tachycardia. Transient ventricular tachycardia of no clinical significance can occasionally be induced in patients with Wolff-Parkinson-White syndrome.[532,kkk] This finding does not relate to the electrophysiological properties of accessory pathways.[532]

Position. As with PSVT sustained in the atrioventricular node, accessory pathway PSVT can also be in-

---

[kkk]Nonclinical transient ventricular tachycardia was induced in 15 (10%) of 148 patients with Wolff-Parkinson-White syndrome.[532]

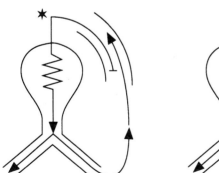 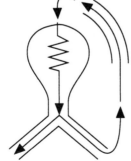

FIGURE 8.21   Induction of orthodromic PSVT sustained in an accessory pathway. An atrial premature beat (*asterisk*, **left**) conducts slowly (*jagged arrow*) through the atrioventricular node but is blocked in the accessory pathway (*curved line terminated with horizontal dash*). The signal in the ventricles travels in retrograde fashion up the accessory pathway that is no longer refractory, courses through the atria and reenters the node, establishing the tachycardia **(right)**. (Adapted from Gallagher JJ: Supraventricular tachycardia with reentry in accessory pathways. In Kastor JA, ed. Arrhythmias. Philadelphia: WB Saunders, 1994, with permission.)

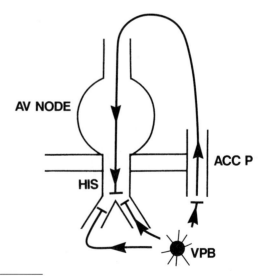

FIGURE 8.22   Ventricular premature beats often start PSVT sustained in accessory pathways. In such patients, the ventricular beat (VPB) can enter the accessory pathway (ACC P), but it is blocked from activating the atrioventricular (AV) node–His-bundle branch system, which is refractory to retrograde penetration. The dissociation produced between the two pathways allows the arrhythmia to start. (Adapted from Wellens HJJ. Supraventricular tachycardia with reentry in the atrioventricular node. In Kastor JA, ed. Arrhythmias. Philadelphia: WB Saunders, 1994, with permission.)

duced more readily in some patients when they are standing rather than when lying flat, presumably because of increased sympathetic tone.[410]

Termination

PSVT sustained in accessory pathways stops spontaneously when block occurs in the atrioventricular node, His-Purkinje system, or accessory pathway.[533] Programmed stimulation terminates PSVT most frequently through block in the atrioventricular node.[492, 534] Single atrial or ventricular stimuli can usually terminate an episode of tachycardia when its rate is less than 200 beats per minute;[492] more beats may be required when the rate is faster.[492lll]

Effects of Bundle Branch Block

In addition to the decreasing heart rate,[20, 267, 280–286, 535] the duration of ventriculoatrial conduction increases when bundle branch block develops in the ventricle into which an accessory pathway inserts (Fig. 8.23).[535] Because this does not occur when the bundle branch block involves the other ventricle or during intranodal tachycardia, the finding indicates that an accessory pathway participates in the arrhythmia[280, 535] and helps to localize the route of the accessory pathway.[535] These changes occur because the bundle branch block enlarges the reentry circuit, and the signal must traverse more ventricular myocardium.

Electrophysiological Recognition of Patients with Wolff-Parkinson-White Syndrome Who Are at Risk of Cardiac Arrest[mmm]

Most electrophysiologists advise that each patient with arrhythmia and Wolff-Parkinson-White syndrome

---

[lll]Although one group reported that single atrial stimuli terminated supraventricular tachycardia in none of 11 patients.[525]

[mmm]See Chapter 4 for additional information about electrophysiological testing of patients with Wolff-Parkinson-White syndrome who develop atrial fibrillation.

---

should have an electrophysiological study to make certain that no patient at risk of ventricular fibrillation and cardiac arrest goes untreated.[24, 536] Asymptomatic patients, however, do not require electrophysiological evaluation because the incidence of sudden cardiac death in this group is virtually nil.[50, 500]

Two tests measuring conducting ability and refractoriness reveal which accessory pathways may transmit signals from atria to ventricles too rapidly if atrial fibrillation or atrial flutter should develop:

- Premature beats. One measures the refractory periods of accessory pathways by introducing atrial premature beats and observing which conduct to the ventricles through the abnormal tracts. Most electrophysiologists consider an effective refractory period of less than 270 milliseconds to indicate that the pathway has the ability, under suitable circumstances, to conduct so rapidly that, in the presence of atrial fibrillation or atrial flutter, ventricular fibrillation could develop.

- RR interval during induced atrial fibrillation. Induction of atrial fibrillation by rapid atrial pacing in the electrophysiology laboratory also tests the conducting ability of accessory pathways under controlled conditions. One measures the shortest interval in milliseconds between preexcited ventricular beats as an indication of the maximum ventricular rate that antegrade conduction within the accessory pathway can produce. If this interval is less than 260 milliseconds, the patient may be at risk of ventricular fibrillation.

Incessant Paroxysmal Supraventricular Tachycardia

The accessory pathway that constitutes the retrograde limb of the reentrant circuit during incessant (also called "permanent," "persistent," or "almost continuously present") PSVT usually conducts abnormally

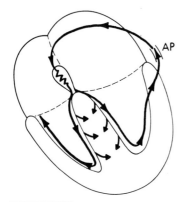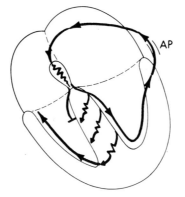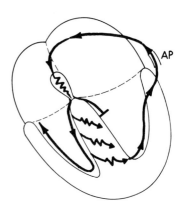

FIGURE 8.23   Effects of bundle branch block during orthodromic PSVT sustained in accessory pathways. The diagrams illustrate activation during PSVT sustained in a left lateral accessory pathway (AP) when the QRS complexes are normal **(left)** and during right bundle branch block **(middle)**. With normal conduction preserved in the ventricle with the accessory pathway, the rate of the arrhythmia does not change when the bundle branch block appears. When left bundle branch block develops, however **(right)**, the impulse must course into the right ventricle and cross the intraventricular septum to reach the left ventricle and enter the accessory pathway. Transseptal conduction lengthens the circuit sustaining the tachycardia, increases the intervals between the QRS complexes, and slows the rate. (Adapted from Gallagher JJ: Supraventricular tachycardia with reentry in accessory pathways. In Kastor JA, ed. Arrhythmias. Philadelphia: WB Saunders, 1994, with permission.)

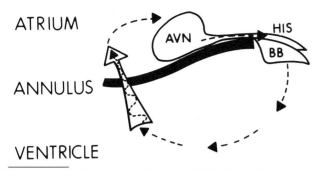

FIGURE 8.24 Mechanism of incessant PSVT. The unique electrophysiological feature of this arrhythmia is the slowly conducting accessory pathway (large arrow, left), which transmits the signal from the ventricles to the atria. The atrioventricular nodal (AVN)–bundle of His–bundle branch (BB) pathway constitutes the antegrade limb. (Adapted from Gallagher JJ: Supraventricular tachycardia with reentry in accessory pathways. In Kastor JA, ed. Arrhythmias. Philadelphia: WB Saunders, 1994, with permission.)

slowly (Fig. 8.24).[108–110, 112, 113, 115–117, 119–126, 128, 132, 134, 135, 197, 537, 538] These pathways, also present in some patients without incessant tachycardia,[539] are often "rate-dependent." They demonstrate decremental conduction, which means that as ventricular premature beats are introduced sooner after the previous ventricular beat, conduction in these pathways slows further. This behavior is more typical of the atrioventricular node than of accessory pathways, which tend to conduct or not conduct ("all or nothing" phenomenon) as coupling intervals are varied, a property they share with normal bundles of His and bundle branches.[112, 126, 134, 540, 541][nnn] Because of the slow retrograde conduction, atrial activation is delayed, and the P waves appear between the QRS complexes, with the P′R intervals usually shorter than the RP′ intervals.[109, 112, 115, 117, 120–123, 126, 134]

These slowly conducting accessory pathways are usually located in the posterior septum.[121, 132, 542] This position accounts for the positive P waves in lead I usually seen in this form of tachycardia.[257] Rarely, the slowly conducting pathway may be located elsewhere, for example, in the lateral wall of the left ventricle.[123] Incessant PSVT sustained in accessory pathways may occur in patients without preexcitation.[123]

[nnn] Decremental accessory pathways were demonstrated in 74 (10%) of 759 patients with accessory pathway-mediated tachyarrhythmia.[134]

Unusual Pathways

Most accessory pathways connect atrial to ventricular myocardium (Kent bundles). A few, however, take different routes and, accordingly, may or may not sustain PSVT or produce short PR intervals or ventricular preexcitation during sinus rhythm[543, 544] (Table 8.11).

Atriofascicular tracts. These tracts, which have decremental properties like the atrioventricular node,[545–548] seldom conduct in retrograde fashion.[549] Consequently, the PSVT they sustain are antidromic—down the atriofascicular pathway and up the bundle of His and atrioventricular node—and the QRS complexes are preexcited during the tachycardia (Fig. 8.25).[549]

Nodofascicular and nodoventricular tracts (Mahaim fibers).[ooo] The tachycardias these tracts support are antidromic, with antegrade conduction down the abnormal pathway and retrograde conduction up the bundle of His and atrioventricular node, producing a retrograde His potential.[361, 550–562] Because the atria do not participate in the reentrant circuit of the arrhythmia sustained in Mahaim fibers, atrioventricular dissociation can occur as in ventricular tachycardia.[552, 563, 564] The characteristic electrocardiogram of left bundle branch block during the tachycardia corresponds to the insertion of Mahaim fibers into the right side of the heart. The accessory pathways that occur with greater than expected frequency in patients with Ebstein's anomaly are often nodofascicular/ventricular tracts.[565][ppp]

Fasciculoventricular tracts. These fibers do not sustain tachycardia.[552]

Bystander tracts. Occasionally, accessory pathways influence the form of the QRS complex during tachycardia through antegrade conduction to the ventricles without participating in sustaining the tachycardia. These connections, often one of the unusual pathways

[ooo] Writers have broadened the eponym "Mahaim fibers," once applied only to connections between the atrioventricular node and the myocardium or fascicles of the ventricles, to include atriofascicular fibers that possess similar electrophysiological properties.[559]
[ppp] Four (13%) of 30 accessory pathways in 22 patients with Ebstein's anomaly were Mahaim fibers.[218]

Table 8.11 **CHARACTERISTICS OF UNUSUAL ACCESSORY PATHWAYS**[544]				
Pathways	Course	PR Interval	Form of Delta Wave	Paroxysmal Supraventricular Tachycardia
Atriofascicular	Atrium to right ventricle	Normal	Left bundle branch block	Occasionally, antidromic
Nodoventricular and nodofascicular	Atrioventricular node to right ventricle	Normal	Left bundle branch block	Yes, antidromic
Fasciculoventricular	Fascicles to ventricles	Normal	Varies	No, bystanders

(From Kottkamp H, Hindricks G, Shenasa H, et al. Variants of preexcitation—specialized atriofascicular pathways, nodofascicular pathways, and fasciculoventricular pathways: electrophysiologic findings and target sites for radiofrequency catheter ablation. J Cardiovasc Electrophysiol 1996; 7:916–930, with permission.)

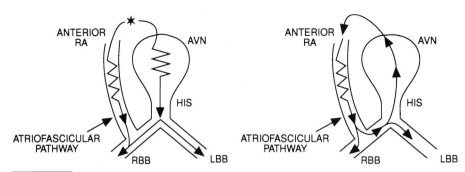

FIGURE 8.25 Conduction in the atriofascicular pathway. During sinus rhythm **(left)**, the signal conducts in antegrade fashion, down the atrioventricular node (AVN) and the atriofascicular pathway, a slowly conducting fiber connecting, in this case, the anterior right atrium (RA) with the right bundle branch (RBB). The QRS complexes are fusion beats combining information transmitted through the normal and abnormal pathways. During PSVT **(right)**, the reentry is sustained in antegrade fashion down the accessory pathway and in retrograde fashion up the atrioventricular node. The route is antidromic, and the QRS complexes are maximally preexcited. LBB, left bundle branch. (Adapted from Gallagher JJ: Supraventricular tachycardia with reentry in accessory pathways. In Kastor JA, ed. Arrhythmias. Philadelphia: WB Saunders, 1994, with permission.)

discussed in the previous section, are known as by-stander tracts.[371, 545, 553, 566*qqq*]

Multiple Accessory Pathways

Some patients with Wolff-Parkinson-White syndrome have more than one accessory pathway, each of which may participate in sustaining PSVT.[124, 377, 498, 504, 550, 555, 565, 567–579*rrr*] Multiple accessory pathways occur with greater than expected frequency in patients with

- Antidromic, preexcited tachycardia.[504, 573]
- Ebstein's anomaly[59, 218, 504, 573*sss*] and other forms of structural congenital heart disease.[59]
- Familial preexcitation.[93]

Mapping

The course that accessory pathways take within the heart can be located with several techniques:[209, 210, 491, 580–586*ttt*]

- Electrophysiological study with catheter electrodes.[146, 219, 230, 232–234, 236, 237, 587–594]
- Epicardial mapping at surgery.[207, 212, 213, 215, 218, 224, 225, 230, 232, 573, 595–602]

- Isopotential body-surface maps.[214, 217, 603–608]
- Scintigraphic phase mapping.[609]
- Magnetocardiography.[610–613]
- Gated single-photon emission computed tomography (SPECT).[614]
- A non-fluoroscopic (CARTO) mapping system.[615–617]

Esophageal Pacing and Recordings

Pacing and recording from the esophagus, techniques found particularly useful when evaluating arrhythmias in children, provide useful information about the electrophysiology of PSVT, especially, but not exclusively, when sustained in accessory pathways.[77, 81, 163, 300, 471, 618–644]

Electrophysiological Diagnosis of Paroxysmal Supraventricular Tachycardia Sustained in Accessory Pathways Versus the Atrioventricular Node

In summary, here are the principal criteria electrophysiologists use in deciding which mechanism sustains the arrhythmia:[26, 39, 645–648*uuu*]

- Atrial activation. In both atrioventricular nodal and accessory pathway reentrant PSVT, the atria are activated in retrograde fashion. During dual pathway reentry, activation begins at the atrioventricular node, whereas in accessory pathway reentry, atrial activation starts where the accessory pathway inserts, which is often somewhere else, except, of course, in the case of septal tracts, in which case the activation pattern may simulate that due to nodal reentry.

---

*qqq*Bystander tracts are uncommon. Of 190 patients with Wolff-Parkinson-White syndrome, only three (1.6%) demonstrated wide QRS complexes because of antegrade accessory pathway bystander conduction during supraventricular tachycardia sustained in the atrioventricular node.[371]

*rrr*Multiple accessory pathways were present in 52 (13%) of 388 patients studied electrophysiologically for accessory pathways.[573]

*sss*Eight (36%) of 22 patients with Ebstein's anomaly had multiple pathways.[218]

*ttt*In one series of 218 accessory pathways located by catheter and open-heart surgical mapping, the pathways were located in the
- Left ventricular free wall in 46%.[210]
- Posterior septal region in 26%.[210]
- Right ventricular free wall in 18%.[210] (The pathways in patients with Ebstein's anomaly invariably insert into the atrialized right ventricle.)[218]
- Anterior septal region in 10%.[210]

---

*uuu*Electrophysiologists recognize that other findings help to distinguish between atrioventricular nodal and accessory pathway reentry, to define antidromic tachycardia, and to characterize atrial tachycardia and ventricular tachycardia. Here are some relevant references,[647, 648] but further discussion of each of these criteria is beyond the scope of this book.

- Atrial preexcitation. The atria can only be preexcited by ventricular premature stimuli during PSVT if an accessory pathway, conducting in retrograde fashion, participates in the circuit.
- Bundle branch block developing during PSVT sustained by an accessory pathway in the same ventricle prolongs the duration of ventriculoatrial conduction. This measurement does not change when bundle branch block appears during atrioventricular nodal PSVT or PSVT sustained in accessory pathways distant from the ventricle with the bundle branch block.
- Ventriculoatrial intervals of less than 60 milliseconds exclude reentry in accessory pathways.[649, 650]

Other Advances

In addition to the references cited, other publications have reported advances in our knowledge of the electrophysiology of patients with PSVT sustained in accessory pathways.[154, 608, 635, 651–694]

DRUGS IN THE ELECTROPHYSIOLOGICAL EVALUATION OF PATIENTS WITH PAROXYSMAL SUPRAVENTRICULAR TACHYCARDIA SUSTAINED IN DUAL ATRIOVENTRICULAR NODAL AND ACCESSORY PATHWAYS[vvv]

Electrophysiological studies reveal the sites of action of the various antiarrhythmic drugs employed to treat PSVT, whether sustained in dual atrioventricular nodal or accessory pathways[339, 695, 696] (Table 8.12).

- Type IA drugs (disopyramide, procainamide, quinidine) and type IC drugs (flecainide, propafenone, moricizine) usually delay conduction

---

[vvv]See Chapter 4 for further discussion of the electrophysiological effects of drugs in patients with Wolff-Parkinson-White syndrome and that arrhythmia.

and prolong refractoriness in accessory pathways and in retrograde fast conducting intranodal pathways. Type IB drugs (lidocaine, mexiletine, tocainide) have little useful electrophysiological effect on these structures.
- Type II drugs (beta-adrenergic–blocking drugs) act only on intranodal slow pathways.
- Type III drugs (amiodarone, *d,l* sotalol) prolong refractoriness or slow conduction in both intranodal and accessory pathways.
- Type IV drugs (calcium-channel–blocking drugs with electrophysiological properties such as diltiazem and verapamil) act principally on nodal and not on accessory pathways.

The action of drugs on PSVT induced in the electrophysiology laboratory can predict their success or failure in suppressing future spontaneous paroxysms of PSVT.[623, 637, 697–711]

Adenosine. Adenosine[712–714] interrupts PSVT by depressing anterograde atrioventricular nodal conduction[715–719] in the slow pathways of patients with intranodal reentry.[715, 718] In addition, adenosine slows conduction in the intranodal fast pathway in adults,[720] although not in infants.[75] During atrial pacing in patients with dual intranodal pathways, adenosine first blocks the fast pathway, producing abrupt prolongation of the AH and PR interval.[721]

Most,[715, 716, 718, 722] but not all,[717] reports show that adenosine has limited and inconstant effect on the electrophysiology of the retrograde fast pathway[723] in atrioventricular nodal reentry or on accessory pathways. However, it shortens antegrade refractoriness in some accessory pathways, an effect partly mediated by beta-adrenergic stimulation,[724] and it can slow conduction in those accessory pathways with decremental properties that support incessant PSVT.[126, 725, 726] Furthermore, by suppressing atrioventricular nodal conduction, adenosine can reveal the presence of accessory pathways[229, 727–731] and may unmask conduction remaining after ablation.[726, 732] Adenosine can help to indicate whether a patient with PSVT has dual path-

---

Table 8.12 LOCATION OF ACTION OF DRUGS AND MANEUVERS ON THE PATHWAYS THAT SUSTAIN PAROXYSMAL SUPRAVENTRICULAR TACHYCARDIA

Drug	Vaughan Williams Classification	Atrioventricular Node		Accessory Pathway
		Slow Pathway	*Fast Pathway*	
Adenosine	—	X	—	—
Amiodarone	III	X	X	X
Beta-adrenergic blockers	II	X	—	—
Digitalis	—	X	—	—
Diltiazem	IV	X	—	—
Disopyramide	IA	—	X	X
Flecainide	IC	—	X	X
Lidocaine	IB	—	—	?
Propafenone	IC	X	X	X
Procainamide	IA	—	X	X
Quinidine	IA	—	X	X
Sotalol	III	X	X	X
Vagal stimulation	—	X	—	—
Verapamil	IV	X	—	—

ways during sinus rhythm by producing a sudden increase in the PR interval resulting from the shifting of antegrade conduction from the fast to the slow pathway.[733]

Ajmaline. This drug, studied in Europe and Asia but not employed in the United States, depresses conduction in accessory pathways like type IA agents and, by this mechanism, converts PSVT sustained in accessory pathways.[734, 735]

Amiodarone. This drug prolongs refractoriness within the atrioventricular node,[736] in both fast and slow intranodal pathways,[737, 738] as well as in accessory pathways,[624, 739, 740] both manifest and concealed.[737, 741] The drug also makes the induction of PSVT more difficult.[739, 742]

Aprindine. Not prescribed clinically, aprindine depresses conduction in accessory pathways and makes more difficult the induction of PSVT in some patients.[743]

Atropine. This drug facilitates conduction in the slow antegrade[744, 745] and fast retrograde[744] pathways and shortens the refractoriness of both pathways[746] supporting orthodromic intranodal PSVT. Atropine thereby enhances induction and maintenance of atrioventricular nodal reentrant PSVT.[298, 744, 747] Autonomic blockade with atropine and propranolol prolongs the refractoriness of concealed atrioventricular and atrio-His accessory pathways and decreases the rate of PSVT sustained in these structures.[748]

Beta-adrenergic–blocking drugs. These drugs[699] slow conduction in the atrioventricular node[702, 749-751] and thereby decrease the rate of the arrhythmia[632, 702, 749] and the ability for the tachycardia to be induced or sustained.[702, 749, 752] These drugs convert PSVT to sinus rhythm by their effects on the electrophysiological properties of either or both of the intranodal pathways.[699] The drugs do not, however, similarly influence accessory pathways[702, 750] although, when they are given with digoxin, conduction in the accessory pathway may be affected.[753] The electrophysiological effects of beta-adrenergic–blocking drugs on PSVT have been demonstrated with esmolol,[754, 755] metoprolol,[750, 756] nadolol,[702, 752] propranolol,[632, 699, 702, 749, 751, 753, 757] and timolol.[758]

Calcium-channel–blocking drugs. These drugs[759, 760] stop PSVT usually by blocking the antegrade slowly conducting pathway.[704, 761-765] Verapamil seems to have a similar effect on the retrograde fast[766, 767] pathway in atrioventricular nodal PSVT.[751, 761, 768] Slowing of the heart rate[769] and alternation of the length of the intervals between QRS complexes ("cycle length alternation")[769-772] herald termination of the arrhythmia in many cases. This class of drugs also prevents induction of PSVT in some patients,[703, 705, 711, 751, 764, 765, 773-777] and it decreases the rate of PSVT in most patients,[75, 632, 704, 773-775, 778] thanks to the ability of these drugs to slow

conduction and to prolong refractoriness in atrioventricular nodal pathways.[632, 703, 711, 765, 771, 773, 774, 776, 779-785]

Calcium-channel–blocking drugs have little[711, 786] or no[126, 281, 763-765, 768, 771, 773, 779, 780, 784, 785, 787] effect on the electrophysiological properties of accessory pathways, whether manifest or concealed. Verapamil can, however, precipitate rapid ventricular arrhythmias, including, rarely, ventricular fibrillation and cardiac arrest in patients with atrial fibrillation or atrial flutter[775, 788] resulting from facilitation of antegrade conduction in accessory pathways.[775, 789] This action may be due to less concealed conduction of signals transmitted through the atrioventricular node and, consequently, less depression of antegrade conduction in the accessory pathways.[768] Verapamil can block conduction in catecholamine-sensitive accessory pathways.[790] The electrophysiological effects of calcium-channel–blocking drugs on PSVT and Wolff-Parkinson-White syndrome have been demonstrated most often with verapamil[126, 281, 703, 711, 751, 766-768, 770, 771, 773-776, 778, 780-783, 786-788, 790] but also with diltiazem.[704, 762-764, 776, 778, 784, 785]

Digitalis. Digitalis prolongs the refractoriness of the atrioventricular node and reduces its ability to sustain PSVT in some patients.[791, 792] Digitalis has no consistent effect on the refractoriness of accessory pathways, sometimes shortening, sometimes prolonging, and sometimes not affecting it.[368, 793www] In those patients in whom digitalis does shorten the refractory period of the accessory pathway, the drug may encourage rapid and more frequent transmission of atrial impulses to the ventricles.[368, 793-796] Digitalis does not decrease the inducibility of accessory pathway–mediated PSVT.[793]

Disopyramide. This drug decreases the heart rate during PSVT,[797] depresses retrograde conduction in accessory pathways[798-801] and, thereby, according to some workers,[797, 799, 801] but not others,[798] decreases the ability to induce PSVT.

Flecainide. By depressing conduction in accessory pathways,[802-808] flecainide reduces the ability to induce accessory pathway–mediated PSVT[706, 803, 806, 807] and leads to conversion of the arrhythmia sustained in them.[805] Its effectiveness in patients with intranodal reentrant tachycardia is due to a similar effect on the retrograde fast pathway.[706, 802-804, 806]

Isoproterenol. This drug facilitates induction of PSVT[298, 809] in patients with accessory pathways mainly by improving antegrade conduction in the atrioventricular node.[810] The drug also shortens refractoriness in retrograde accessory pathways.[726] Isoproterenol facilitates induction of atrioventricular nodal PSVT in some patients by enhancing antegrade[811, 812] and retrograde[144, 811, 812] intranodal conduction.[144] The drug does not, at least in infants,[75] speed conduction in the retrograde fast pathway.

[www] In one study of patients with Wolff-Parkinson-White syndrome, the combination of digoxin and propranolol reduced the ability to induce or sustain supraventricular tachycardia.[753]

Lidocaine. Lidocaine's action on accessory pathway varies. It may slow,[813, 814] speed,[815] or not affect[816] conduction.

Magnesium. Magnesium decreases the rate of PSVT in normomagnesemic patients by slowing conduction in the antegrade limb of the reentrant circuit in the atrioventricular node for both nodal and accessory pathway reentrant PSVT.[719, 817]

Procainamide. This drug prolongs refractoriness and slows conduction in the fast pathway conducting in retrograde fashion during atrioventricular nodal PSVT,[699, 818–820] and thereby usually, but not always,[821] it inhibits induction of the arrhythmia.[818] Procainamide has a similar effect on accessory pathways,[247, 740, 777] more so for antegrade than for retrograde conduction.[822] The drug produced incessant PSVT in a patient with Wolff-Parkinson-White syndrome.[823]

Propafenone. This drug slows conduction and prolongs antegrade and retrograde refractoriness in accessory pathways and often inhibits induction of PSVT in patients with PSVT mediated through accessory pathways.[824] In patients with atrioventricular nodal reentry, propafenone depresses conduction in the retrograde fast pathway and reduces the ability to induce the arrhythmia.[825]

Quinidine. Quinidine depresses conduction on the retrograde fast pathway during intranodal PSVT[826] and, by this affect, converts the arrhythmia.[699]

Sotalol. Sotalol (d,l)[827] prevents induction of PSVT in many patients[707, 828] by affecting either the antegrade or the retrograde limb supporting the tachycardia.[756] Its beta-adrenergic–blocking properties are also helpful.

Autonomic drugs and physical maneuvers. Administration of parasympathetic and adrenergic agonists and the physical maneuvers, such as carotid sinus pressure, long used to convert PSVT work by activating the parasympathetic nervous system either directly or by a reflex stimulated by the production of catecholamines from the hypotension produced by the arrhythmia. This output so prolongs conduction and refractoriness within the circuit maintaining the tachycardia that the

reentry can no longer be sustained. In atrioventricular nodal reentry, parasympathetic stimulation converts the arrhythmia most often by its effect on the slow pathway and less often by its effect on the retrograde conducting fast pathway.[829]

TREATMENT

Patients with recurrent PSVT should be instructed how to convert the arrhythmia themselves because many episodes do not require visiting a doctor's office or a hospital emergency department.[26, 337, 830–832] When self-treatment fails, the staff of appropriately trained mobile coronary care units can often convert the arrhythmia in the patient's home.[833]

Physical Maneuvers

Most patients with PSVT discover or are instructed to perform various physical actions that may convert PSVT.[834] The maneuvers are more effective in younger patients and in those whose PSVT is sustained within the atrioventricular node than in accessory pathways.[835] Decreasing the autonomic response by administering drugs that block the parasympathetic or beta-adrenergic system prevents these maneuvers from converting the arrhythmia.[836]

Among the maneuvers in general use are the following:[94, 835]xxx

- Assuming the dependent position with the head below the rest of the body[836, 837] or leaning over with the head down, especially from the squatting or sitting position.[94] Some patients know this maneuver while squatting as "hunkering down."[94]
- Carotid sinus massage[253, 254, 838–840] (Fig. 8.26).
- Eyeball pressure.[94]
- Gagging.[94]
- Insertion of a nasogastric tube.[841]
- Sighing[94] or deep respirations.[94, 837]
- Valsalva maneuver,[94, 253, 255] which is more effective when the patient is supine than when standing[835] (Fig. 8.27).

---

xxxIn 35 patients, physical maneuvers converted supraventricular tachycardia, as follows:[835]
- Valsalva maneuver, supine in 19 (54%), standing in nine (20%).
- Right carotid sinus pressure in six (17%).
- Left carotid sinus pressure in two (5%).
- Diving reflex in six (17%).

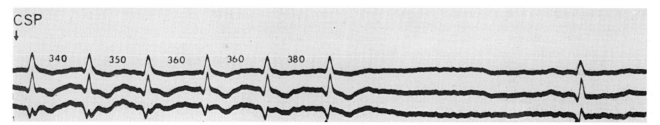

FIGURE 8.26 Carotid sinus pressure converting PSVT. When carotid sinus pressure (CSP) is applied (*arrow*), the rate slows (increasing RR intervals) and the PR intervals are prolonged because of decreasing conduction in the slow pathway just before termination of the tachycardia (leads I, II, and III). (Adapted from Josephson ME, Seides SE, Batsford WB, Caracta AR, Damato AN, Kastor JA. The effects of carotid sinus pressure in re-entrant paroxysmal supraventricular tachycardia. Am Heart J 1974; 88:694–697, with permission.)[253]

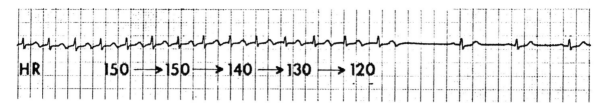

FIGURE 8.27   Valsalva maneuver converts PSVT. The patient performed the maneuver as the electrocardiographic tracing begins. The heart rate (HR) gradually decreases (numbers are beats per minute) as rising vagal tone slows conduction in the atrioventricular node. The electrophysiological properties of the reentrant circuit change so that eventually reentry can no longer be maintained, and the arrhythmia stops. (Adapted from Josephson ME, Seides SE, Batsford WB, Caracta AR, Damato AN, Kastor JA. The effects of carotid sinus pressure in re-entrant paroxysmal supraventricular tachycardia. Am Heart J 1974; 88:694–697, with permission.)

- Diving reflex.[842] The parasympathetic autonomic nervous system can also be aroused to convert PSVT through activating the diving reflex by immersing the patient's face in cold water.[843–847] Energetic patients can perform this maneuver themselves to convert their arrhythmia. The maneuver seems to be particularly effective in infants.[844–847]

Drugs

The primary treatment of PSVT, whether sustained in the atrioventricular node or accessory pathways, is pharmacological.[848–856] A drug given intravenously usually converts a paroxysm, and, in oral form, prevents or reduces the number of recurrences in many patients. Admitting a patient to the hospital for up to 72 hours to develop an antiarrhythmic drug program is cost-effective for most patients with PSVT.[857]

Most patients with sustained paroxysms come to a doctor's office or the hospital for the intravenous administration of a drug. Favorite choices are adenosine, diltiazem, and verapamil. Some patients become accustomed to taking a drug or combination of drugs to convert paroxysms at home.[858] A computer program has been developed to help choose treatment of paroxysms of PSVT in the elderly.[859]

For long-term suppression, most physicians first choose beta-adrenergic or calcium-channel–blocking drugs. Amiodarone and flecainide, among others, are also effective. Digoxin and beta-adrenergic–blocking drugs are often prescribed for infants and children, and they seem effectively to prevent recurrences in most of these patients.[644, 860] Perpetual treatment is often not required, and patients may reasonably try stopping drugs when paroxysms cease. When and how best to treat fetal PSVT are specialized topics beyond the scope of this book or my experience.[69]

Adenosine. Probably the most popular drug for acute treatment, adenosine[713, 714] converts most paroxysms of PSVT[716, 718, 719, 861–867] in adults and children,[868–870] faster[871] and with similar[839] or slightly better success than does verapamil.[718, 864, 872] After doses of 3, 6, 9, and 12 mg given sequentially, as required, PSVT usually terminates, at least temporarily.[871] Adenosine converts the arrhythmia more quickly than verapamil, but it produces more side effects, albeit of short duration.[718]

Adenosine converts antidromic, wide QRS complex tachycardia,[865, 873] as well as the more common orthodromic tachycardia, and it converts the arrhythmia whether or not dependent on catecholamine stimulation.[874] The drug may also be used to help make the diagnosis of a regular tachycardia because adenosine converts most arrhythmias that incorporate the atrioventricular node in the reentrant circuit, but adenosine only rarely converts such arrhythmias as ventricular tachycardia.[865, 875]

The most commonly encountered side effects, which are brief and seldom prevent using the drug, are facial flushing, dyspnea, and chest pain or pressure. In some patients, adenosine provokes other supraventricular arrhythmias.[876yyy] Induction of atrial fibrillation in patients with accessory pathways may produce so rapid a ventricular rhythm that ventricular fibrillation results.[877] Accordingly, adenosine should be used with caution and with a defibrillator standing by in patients with manifest or suspected accessory pathways. Sinus slowing and some degree of atrioventricular block may briefly appear after conversion, and attention should be paid to these bradyarrhythmias in patients in whom sick sinus syndrome is suspected.

Amiodarone. Amiodarone[878–880] prevents or reduces the frequency of paroxysms of PSVT in many patients[738, 741, 742, 881–886] including children.[887] Given intravenously, this drug often converts the arrhythmia.[888] However, because of its side effects and the availability of other effective drugs and ablation, amiodarone is seldom the first choice for suppressing paroxysms of PSVT.

Beta-adrenergic–blocking drugs. These drugs,[889, 890] given intravenously, convert one-half to three-fourths of patients with PSVT into sinus rhythm.[781, 891] Propranolol, however, converted none of 24 infants in one study.[632] Uncontrolled studies and case reports indicate that beta-adrenergic–blocking drugs prevent or decrease the incidence of paroxysms of PSVT.[62, 100, 710, 750, 892–897] One study found propranolol equal to verapamil and digoxin in suppressing recurrences of PSVT unassociated with Wolff-Parkinson-White syndrome.[898] No other comparative study has shown that beta-adren-

---

yyyAdenosine-induced atrial fibrillation or flutter in 24 (12%) of 200 patients with supraventricular tachycardia.[876]

ergic–blocking drugs are superior to, or equal to, calcium-channel–blocking drugs in suppressing paroxysms of PSVT.

The peripheral effects of propranolol account for most of the decrease in systemic blood pressure and cardiac index seen after giving these drugs to patients with PSVT.[177] These actions may have important hemodynamic consequences if the arrhythmia does not convert promptly.[177] The hypotension usually resolves within 30 minutes after receiving esmolol, the ultrashort-acting beta blocker, sooner than after propranolol.[891] Beta-blocking drugs studied for the treatment of PSVT include atenolol,[894, 896, 897] esmolol,[891, 899, 900] metoprolol,[750, 901] nadolol,[100, 702, 710, 890] and propranolol.[62, 632, 702, 710, 891–893, 895, 902]

Calcium-channel–blocking drugs. These drugs,[760, 903] specifically diltiazem and verapamil,[904, 905] are frequently chosen both to convert and prevent paroxysms of PSVT. Intravenous administration of diltiazem[778, 785, 906, 907] or verapamil[632, 763, 768, 771, 777, 779, 839, 872, 908–916] converts most patients to sinus rhythm.[zzz] Given intravenously, these drugs briefly decrease the blood pressure in some patients, but seldom to clinically significant levels,[176, 764, 778, 906, 915] and they may produce sinus slowing[771] and a few ventricular premature beats.[771, 910]

Diltiazem[704, 776] and verapamil[700, 711, 774, 779, 783, 784, 917–919] in adequate oral doses abolish or reduce the frequency and duration of episodes of spontaneous PSVT whether sustained in the atrioventricular node or accessory pathways. Large *oral* doses of verapamil, however, seldom convert PSVT to sinus rhythm.[920]

Potentially serious complications that may develop when calcium-channel–blocking drugs are given to patients with PSVT include the following:

* Atrial and ventricular fibrillation.[921] If the atrial fibrillation produces a sufficiently rapid ventricular response in patients with accessory pathways, ventricular fibrillation can follow. This unlikely but possible complication dictates that a defibrillator be available when the drug is given intravenously to such patients.[775, 788, 789, 922]
* Hemodynamic decompensation, particularly in infants and children.[923, 924]

Catecholamine agonists. Catecholamine agonists that elevate the blood pressure, such as phenylephrine[254, 255, 837] or metaraminol,[254] often convert PSVT by stimulating the parasympathetic system in reflex fashion. Except in hypotensive patients, this approach is seldom now used.

Digitalis. This was the principal drug given in the past to convert PSVT[58, 87] and to prevent recurrences.[58, 65, 87, 106, 623aaaa] I know of no properly controlled study in adults, however, showing that digoxin suppresses paroxysms of PSVT. Comparative studies in infants

show this drug to be less effective than verapamil for conversion[915] and less effective than flecainide in preventing paroxysms.[925] One group of pediatricians concluded in 1995:[925]

> Comparison with previous natural history studies suggests that digoxin is ineffective in the prophylaxis of PSVT.

Because digitalis facilitates antegrade conduction of signals within accessory pathways in some patients and decreases passage within the atrioventricular node in all, the drug may occasionally produce ventricular tachycardia or ventricular fibrillation and cardiac arrest during atrial fibrillation or atrial flutter.[926bbbb] This albeit uncommon calamity, combined with its unproved efficacy in preventing PSVT and the availability of more effective drugs and ablation, leads me to advise choosing drugs other than digitalis to treat recurrent PSVT.

Disopyramide. This drug converts PSVT to sinus rhythm in some patients,[777, 916, 927] and it may reduce the frequency of paroxysms of PSVT sustained in accessory pathways.[798] However, the drug is seldom used now for treating PSVT.

Edrophonium. This strongly vagotonic agent[928] usually terminates PSVT when it is administered intravenously.[929] The drug is seldom employed for this purpose now, having been superseded by more effective agents with fewer side effects.

Flecainide. Given intravenously, flecainide terminates PSVT[930] sustained in the atrioventricular node or accessory pathways.[804, 931] The drug reduces recurrences of PSVT[460, 706, 806, 925, 931–933] in children,[930, 934] as well as in adults, and as effectively as verapamil.[935]

Parasympathometic agonists. Drugs like edrophonium were in vogue for converting PSVT before drugs of greater effectiveness and fewer side effects were available.[254, 255]

Procainamide. This drug suppresses and converts PSVT,[777, 936cccc] including patients with orthodromic accessory pathway PSVT when taken orally.[937dddd] The drug induced incessant PSVT in a patient with Wolff-Parkinson-White syndrome. Procainamide is seldom used now to convert or suppress PSVT.

Propafenone. This drug stops and reduces the frequency of paroxysms of PSVT in adults[824, 938–940] and in children.[941–944]

Quinidine. Quinidine suppresses or reduces the frequency of recurrences of atrioventricular nodal PSVT.[826]

[zzz]Diltiazem converted 13 (87%) of 15 with supraventricular tachycardia to sinus rhythm.[906]

[aaaa]In one case, administering digoxin to a mother seemed to convert her fetus's supraventricular tachycardia to sinus rhythm.[65]

[bbbb]See Chapter 4 for a discussion of treating this arrhythmia in patients with Wolff-Parkinson-White syndrome.

[cccc]Even in a fetus when delivered transplacentally.[936]

[dddd]In a regimen called "periodic procainamide" by its developers.[937]

Sotalol. Sotalol (d,l),[827, 945, 946] which combines beta-adrenergic–blocking and type III antiarrhythmic properties, terminates, when given intravenously, many episodes of PSVT.[947–949] Given orally, the drug also reduces the likelihood that PSVT will recur,[950] and it can suppress paroxysms in newborns.[945]

Combinations of drugs. Beta-adrenergic and calcium-channel–blocking drugs, given together, may suppress spontaneous episodes of PSVT better than one drug alone.[751] However, the amount of data supporting this conclusion is limited.

Recurrences. Infants who require more than one drug to maintain sinus rhythm during hospitalization for Wolff-Parkinson-White syndrome have more recurrences of PSVT than those needing fewer drugs.[87] Recurrences in infants occur more often in those with type B than type A preexcitation.[87]

Ineffective drugs. *Bidisomide*, a class I antiarrhythmic drug, does not reduce the frequency of paroxysms of PSVT.[951] *Lidocaine* has little value in treating PSVT although it has been reported to convert a few paroxysms of PSVT.[952, 953] In patients with Wolff-Parkinson-White syndrome and atrial fibrillation, lidocaine may decrease,[813, 814] or increase,[815] the ventricular rate. Although intravenous *magnesium* slows the rate of PSVT and converts some patients to sinus rhythm, the electrolyte seems to have little value in treating PSVT.[719, 817]

Catheter Ablation

PSVT can be cured by ablating the function of one, preferably the slow, pathway in patients with atrioventricular nodal reentry or the accessory pathway (Fig. 8.28) in patients with manifest or concealed PSVT sustained in accessory pathways.[493, 954–976] Ablation treatment is effective in patients of all ages, including children[977–986] and the elderly.[251, 987] Catheter ablation of accessory pathways provides a superior equality of life[988] and better exercise tolerance than does treatment with drugs.[988] As the operator's experience with ablation grows, the rate of success rises,[989, 990] the number of complications falls,[981] and patients with more complex or difficult-to-ablate lesions can be treated.[983, 991]

Risks. Risks to patients having ablation are small compared with those associated with other forms of definitive treatment for arrhythmias.[992] Exposure to radiation of patients and operators during ablation is well within established guidelines,[993] and with additional experience, the amount of exposure decreases[994] as the time required for the procedure falls.[983, 995] Mural thrombi are rarely, if ever, produced by the current.[310]

Costs. Successful catheter ablation of PSVT costs less than surgical[978, 996, 997] or pharmacological treatment of symptomatic, drug-refractory patients with atrioventricular nodal reentry.[998] In children 5 years of age or older with Wolff-Parkinson-White syndrome, catheter ablation is less expensive and has lower mortality and morbidity than either medical management or surgery.[999] Ablation to cure PSVT sustained in the atrioventricular node[1000] or accessory pathways[1001] can be safely performed on an outpatient basis and at less expense than with admission to the hospital.

Indications. Most electrophysiolgists reserve ablation in patients with atrioventricular nodal reentrant PSVT to those in whom treatment with antiarrhythmic drugs, in particular, beta-adrenergic or calcium-channel–blocking drugs,[1002] fails. Some suggest, however, that each patient, when first evaluated, should be given the option of choosing an electrophysiological study.[536]

Opinion is divided about whether ablation should be undertaken as primary treatment for *all* patients with PSVT sustained in accessory pathways.[989, 1002] However, many electrophysiologists advise evaluating and then using ablation, if suitable, in all patients with arrhythmias and Wolff-Parkinson-White syndrome, and few would debate the wisdom of evaluating in the electrophysiology laboratory all patients who present with syncope or severe compromise of hemodynamic function.[536] Asymptomatic patients with preexcitation, however, do not require electrophysiological study and ablation because the prognosis for them is so favorable.[50]

In neonates and infants, drugs prevent recurrences so often that observers advise withholding ablation except in patients with the following:[644]

• Severe symptoms.
• Complications such as ventricular dysfunction.
• Complex congenital heart disease.
• Failure of aggressive drug therapy.

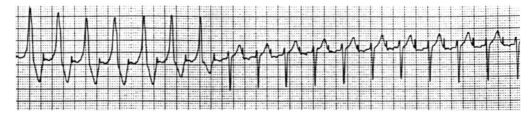

FIGURE 8.28   Radiofrequency ablation of an accessory pathway. Current, applied in the beginning of the tracing, ablates conduction in the accessory pathway, so that from the eighth complex onward, preexcitation ceases (lead V_1). (Preexcitation is maximized by atrial pacing.) (Adapted from Gallagher JJ: Supraventricular tachycardia with reentry in accessory pathways. In Kastor JA, ed. Arrhythmias. Philadelphia: WB Saunders, 1994, with permission.)

However, catheter ablation is the treatment of choice for children 5 years of age or older with Wolff-Parkinson-White syndrome and frequent episodes of PSVT.[999]

Techniques. Radiofrequency current delivered through electrode catheters in the electrophysiology laboratory is the preferred technique. Formerly, direct current shocks were used to ablate accessory pathways[504, 1003–1030] or, occasionally, to modify atrioventricular nodal function in intranodal reentry,[1031, 1032] but this method requires general anesthesia,[1033] has more complications,[1034, 1035] and gives less precise ablation. Similarly, ablating the atrioventricular junction with insertion of a ventricular pacemaker[eeee] and modifying atrioventricular nodal conduction with radiofrequency current[1036] are seldom used for treating intranodal PSVT. There is a troublingly high incidence of complete atrioventricular block following modification.[1037, 1038] Laser coagulation with catheters to treat PSVT is under investigation.[1039, 1040]

Slow versus fast pathway ablation. In atrioventricular nodal reentry, ablation of the slow pathway is preferred, thereby preserving the fast pathway through which normal rhythm is transmitted. Furthermore, slow pathway ablation eliminates PSVT more successfully[1038, 1041–1045] and less often produces atrioventricular block than does fast pathway ablation.[991, 1044–1049] The success of the procedure in eliminating spontaneous or induced tachycardia is not limited by the retention of residual function in some slow pathways[466, 1042, 1043, 1050–1057] or the ability to induce new, nonclinical PSVT.[1058] Successful slow pathway ablation does not affect the electrophysiological properties of the fast pathway.[1051, 1059] Fast pathway ablation, as one would expect, leaves patients with longer PR intervals and sometimes first or greater degrees of atrioventricular block because conduction during sinus rhythm must now proceed in the slow pathway.[1044, 1060–1062]

Accessory pathways. Ablation of accessory pathways in patients with manifest or concealed Wolff-Parkinson-White syndrome cures patients of PSVT and prevents excessively rapid ventricular rates during atrial fibrillation and atrial flutter resulting from antegrade conduction in accessory pathways.

Results

Atrioventricular nodal PSVT. Experienced teams report few failures in ablating the slow pathway to prevent induction of atrioventricular nodal PSVT.[579, 979, 995, 1042–1044, 1046, 1047, 1050, 1051, 1055–1057, 1059, 1061, 1063–1079ffff] Most patients no longer have spontaneous PSVT after this treatment.

Those few in whom the arrhythmia returns can usually be cured with another treatment.[1054, 1080] Other atrial arrhythmias, which can be mistaken for atrioventricular nodal reentry, sometimes appear for the first time after successful ablation of atrioventricular nodal reentrant PSVT and may raise concern that the ablation was not successful.[1054] Ablating retrograde slowly conducting pathways rids patients of fast-slow,[130, 195, 385, 406, 1047, 1066, 1081] incessant PSVT and relieves secondary cardiomyopathy caused by the arrhythmia.[130] Ablation with radiofrequency current can eliminate PSVT in those relatively few patients who have more than two intranodal pathways[387] or more than one type of intranodal tachycardia.[388]

Accessory pathway reentrant PSVT. Ablation of accessory pathways with radiofrequency current to cure patients of PSVT[135, 1082] is similarly successful both electrophysiologically and clinically[978, 989, 990, 1035, 1046, 1083–1097gggg] in children,[978, 995, 1098–1102] as well as adults, including patients with congenital heart disease.[1103–1106]

Ablation is particularly helpful in relieving patients of permanent or incessant PSVT sustained in slowly conducting accessory pathways,[128, 132, 135] in children[1107] as well as in adults. Ablation can also be applied successfully to eliminate multiple tracts[576, 578, 1107] or those in unusual locations or settings:

- Atrio-His,[544, 549, 1108] atriofascicular,[559, 1066, 1109, 1110] and intermediate septal tracts that insert into the bundle of His and the atrioventricular node.[1111] Success with ablation is lower than for the standard atrioventricular tracts, and the production of atrioventricular and right bundle branch block is relatively high.[1111]
- Nodofascicular/nodoventricular (Mahaim) fibers.[544, 559, 1066, 1112–1114]
- Right ventricular tracts in Ebstein's anomaly.[1115, 1116]
- Accessory pathways in patients with intracardiac tumors.[146]

In a few patients, antegrade and retrograde conduction must be ablated in the same accessory pathway at different sites.[1117] Occasionally, conduction in accessory pathways remaining immediately after the ablation disappears later.[1118–1120] Ablation of accessory pathways may reveal signs of old myocardial infarction hidden by the preexcitation.[1121]

[eeee]See Chapter 4 for further information and references on atrioventricular junctional ablation.

[ffff]The North American Society of Pacing and Electrophysiology (NASPE) reported, in 1995, that catheter ablation of the slow pathway with radiofrequency current in United States hospitals cured 97% of patients of supraventricular tachycardia sustained in the atrioventricular node.[1082]

[gggg]The North American Society of Pacing and Electrophysiology reported, in 1995, successful ablation by experienced groups[1038] in tracts located in the
- Left ventricular free wall, 93%.
- Septal region, 94%.
- Right ventricular free wall, 8%.

In a survey started in 1991, The Pediatric Radiofrequency Catheter Ablation (RCA) Registry reported (in 1997) successful ablation in 90% of 4,136 children and adolescents.[995] Three years after the procedure, 75% of the children had no recurrences. The rates of successful ablation were
- Left lateral accessory pathways, 95%.
- Septal accessory pathways, 87%.
- Right free wall accessory pathways, 87%.
- Atrioventricular nodal reentry, 96%.

Recurrence. Conduction, with or without tachycardia, returns in the ablated pathway in a few patients after electrophysiological treatment of atrioventricular nodal or accessory tracts.[1122–1125][hhhh] A second treatment is usually successful.[1122] In patients with atrioventricular nodal reentry, recurrences are more likely if slow pathway conduction or atrioventricular nodal beats persist after ablation.[1052]

Event monitoring and electrophysiological study show that the cause of postablation palpitations is seldom due to a recurrence of the arrhythmia for which ablation was performed.[157, 1126] Clinical follow-up and event monitoring answer most of the questions about arrhythmias occurring after ablation, and electrophysiological study is infrequently necessary.[1127]

Nevertheless, PSVT and preexcitation may reappear in patients with concealed or "dormant"[1128] accessory pathways *after* radiofrequency current ablation of the manifest pathway.[1128, 1129] Further ablation obliterates the preexcitation and the tachycardia.[1129]

Complications. Complications[1037, 1038, 1130] occur more frequently during an electrophysiological study that includes radiofrequency current ablation than during a diagnostic electrophysiological study,[1131] and in the elderly compared with the young.[1131] Arrhythmias seldom develop after recovery from the procedure,[1132] and fatalities are rare.[995]

Electrophysiological complications include the following:

- Transient accelerated junctional rhythm,[1133] which successful atrioventricular nodal ablation almost uniformly produces; its absence often indicates unsuccessful ablation.[1069, 1072, 1075, 1134] Accordingly, some clinicians suggest that this arrhythmia should not be considered a "complication" of ablation.[536]
- Temporary atrioventricular block,[982, 1049, 1065, 1069, 1076, 1135, 1136][iiii] which is almost always preceded by accelerated junctional rhythm.[1049, 1135, 1137] The junctional rate tends to be faster and may be associated with ventriculoatrial block in those patients more likely to develop atrioventricular block.[1137]
- Permanent atrioventricular block,[983, 991, 1048, 1072, 1076, 1082, 1086, 1093, 1135] an infrequent complication now that the fast pathway is seldom ablated, usually appears during or soon after the procedure, but occasionally it develops after the patient leaves the hospital.[1049, 1138] This complication, in particular, convinces some physicians not to offer ablation as primary treatment for all, and particularly young, patients with PSVT.

- Autonomic dysfunction,[1139, 1140] manifested as sudden sinus slowing,[1139, 1141] reversible cardiac arrest,[1142] inappropriate sinus tachycardia,[1139, 1143–1147] or change in the variability of the heart rate.[1144, 1148] The dysfunction may last for months but is seldom permanent.[1139, 1146]
- Inadvertent fast pathway ablation while attempting to ablate the slow pathway.[1076]
- Failure of sensing of pacemakers in patients being treated with ablation.[1149]

Nonelectrophysiological complications may also develop (Table 8.13):[983, 1038, 1150–1156]

Miscellaneous. The slow pathway in atrioventricular nodal PSVT can be successfully ablated in those few patients whose PSVT is complicated by atrioventricular block.[279] A patient with tachycardia sustained by a ventricular pacemaker and an extremely slowly conducting retrograde pathway was successfully treated by ablating the pathway.[1157] Most parameters of pacemaker function are not affected by ablation with radiofrequency current.[1158]

Since the technique of ablating pathways supporting PSVT with radiofrequency current was introduced in the late 1980s and applied widely in the 1990s, several developments have increased its success, reduced the complications, simplified the procedure, and revealed further information about the electrophysiology of ablation.[129, 306, 307, 309, 355, 577, 607, 969, 1053, 1086, 1092, 1096, 1105, 1119, 1145, 1159–1218] Detailed discussion of these important advances is beyond the scope of this chapter.

Pacing

Pacing the atria or ventricles temporarily or with implanted pacemakers can convert patients with PSVT to sinus rhythm just as does programmed stimulation in

Table 8.13	NONELECTROPHYSIOLOGICAL COMPLICATIONS OF CATHETER ABLATION IN PATIENTS WITH PAROXYSMAL SUPRAVENTRICULAR TACHYCARDIA

Aortic regurgitation[1151]
Catheter entrapment requiring surgical removal from the femoral vein[983] and mitral valve[1155]
Coronary artery spasm[1150]
Dissection of a coronary artery[1154]
Damage to peripheral arteries[1038]
Emboli[1152, 1153a]
Perforation of an aortic leaflet[1387]
Pericardial effusion[983]
Pericarditis[1038]
Pneumothorax[1038]
Postcardiac injury syndrome following production of bloody pericardial effusion[1156]
Puncture of the left atrium[983]
Tamponade[1038]
Thrombosis of the coronary sinus[983]
Venous thrombosis[1038]

a Transcranial Doppler frequently detects signals of intracranial microemboli after left-sided ablation.[1153] Neurological symptoms or signs, however, seldom appear.[1153]

[hhhh]Conduction recurred in 35 (6.5%) of 538 patients in atrioventricular nodal or accessory pathways ablated for treatment of supraventricular tachycardia.[1125] The frequency of recurrence was greater after ablation of accessory pathways compared with atrioventricular nodal pathways.[1125]

[iiii]Temporary second- or third-degree atrioventricular block developed in 12 (2.1%) of 580 patients undergoing radiofrequency current ablation for intranodal supraventricular tachycardia.[1135] The block in these patients lasted from five seconds to 10 minutes (mean, 72 sec).[1135]

the electrophysiology laboratory.[627, 848, 1127, 1219–1289] The development of effective drugs and ablation with radiofrequency current has, for the most part, eliminated the need for permanent pacemakers to convert or suppress PSVT.

Surgery

Before catheter ablation was developed, the only definitive treatment for patients with PSVT was surgical interruption,[16, 584, 1290–1296] sometimes with cryoablation[113, 215, 1297–1305] or lasers[1306] of conduction in accessory pathways[113, 197, 198, 215, 373, 402, 501, 506, 509, 558, 568, 598, 601, 602, 978, 1297–1299, 1301, 1302, 1305–1364] and occasionally in atrioventricular nodal tracts.[127, 1300, 1303, 1304, 1342, 1361, 1365–1374] The surgeon was guided to the pathways by mapping the structures to be treated, first with catheters in the electrophysiology laboratory and then under direct vision during the operation.

Occasionally, surgical interruption of the bundle of His was employed in patients with PSVT.[iiii] Catheter ablation with radiofrequency current has replaced surgical treatment for most patients.

Cardioversion

Although almost universally effective[1375–1380kkkk] and with relatively small amounts of power, cardioversion for reentrant PSVT is rarely needed now because intravenous drugs suppress the arrhythmia in most patients.

Implantable Cardioverter-Defibrillator

Few patients with PSVT require implantable cardioverter-defibrillators to treat that arrhythmia because cardiac arrest produced by PSVT is rare, and ablation can prevent ventricular fibrillation produced by rapid conduction of atrial fibrillation or flutter through accessory pathways.[166] Some patients with PSVT, of course, may need defibrillators for other indications.

Electrical Stimulation of the Carotid Sinus

Activation of an implantable stimulator producing radiofrequency current to the carotid sinus nerves can reliably convert PSVT to sinus rhythm.[1381–1383] An intriguing approach, the device enjoyed only transient popularity.

PROGNOSIS

The prognosis of patients with PSVT is excellent.[58, 186, 1384] Although the untreated condition can annoy and frustrate affected patients, they seldom die or sustain serious damage from a paroxysm.

The incidence of sudden cardiac death among adults and children with the electrocardiogram of Wolff-Parkinson-White syndrome is extremely low, and this calamity seldom, if ever, occurs in those who are asymptomatic.[50, 500, 1385llll] The loss of preexcitation in some patients as they age contributes to the excellent prognosis of asymptomatic patients with Wolff-Parkinson-White syndrome.[82] Even the prognosis for patients with syncope is no worse than for those who do not faint.[165] The most notable exceptions are those few patients with accessory pathways who develop atrial fibrillation or flutter, a rapid ventricular response, and cardiac arrest.[1386mmmm]

SUMMARY

Paroxysmal supraventricular tachycardia or PSVT, a common arrhythmia, arises from reentry within dual pathways in the atrioventricular node or accessory pathways in Wolff-Parkinson-White syndrome. It is the most frequent regular tachyarrhythmia in adults, and atrioventricular nodal reentry is the more common mechanism. PSVT first appears in relatively young subjects, and the reentry in them is more often sustained in accessory pathways. Reentry in accessory pathways is more common in men, and intranodal reentry is more common in women.

The tachycardia is usually paroxysmal and is occasionally persistent or permanent, a pattern that occurs less often in adults than in children, in whom the persistent arrhythmia may produce reversible cardiomyopathy. Most patients with PSVT have no structural heart disease. Palpitations are the most frequent symptoms, and many patients can recognize that the paroxysms characteristically start and stop suddenly. Pounding in the neck is due to large venous waves produced by contraction of the right atrium against a closed tricuspid valve, a phenomenon more pronounced in patients with atrioventricular nodal reentry.

PSVT decreases the systemic blood pressure, cardiac output, stroke volume, and ejection fraction and raises pulmonary artery, right atrial, and left atrial pressure. Fainting seems to depend more on vasomotor instability than on the hemodynamic effects of the tachycardia alone.

During sinus rhythm, the Wolff-Parkinson-White electrocardiogram of short PR intervals and delta waves identifies the presence of accessory pathways and the electrophysiological substrate for PSVT. The electrocardiogram during the arrhythmia shows a rapid, regular rhythm, usually with normal QRS complexes. Rate-related bundle branch aberrancy or antegrade conduction through accessory pathways can produce abnormal QRS complexes. The P waves are

---

iiii See Chapter 4 for references and further discussion of this topic.

kkkk Early reports, in the 1960s particularly, on cardioversion of supraventricular tachyarrhythmias, discussed arrhythmias with different mechanisms, not all of which were reentrant supraventricular sustained in the atrioventricular node or accessory pathways. By only including those that *appear* to be the subject of this chapter, the efficacy of cardioversion for supraventricular tachycardia stands.

llll Two (1.7%) patients of 113 who had the electrocardiogram of Wolff-Parkinson-White syndrome died suddenly when followed for 1,338 patient-years. The sudden cardiac death rate in this study, conducted in Olmsted County, Minnesota, which includes the Mayo Clinic, was 0.0015% per patient-year. Both of those who died had symptoms from arrhythmias.[50]

mmmm Only one of 100 cases personally followed by Paul Dudley White (the White of Wolff-Parkinson-White) died. "This was a physician of middle age, who at the time of her last paroxysm of tachycardia showed an excessive heart rate and was about to be examined by electrocardiograph when she died."[1386]

inverted in the inferior leads when they can be found. In most cases of dual pathway reentry, these waves are invisible, hidden within the QRS complexes. Parts of the P waves may produce what appears to be small Q waves, small S waves, or incomplete right bundle branch block.

Few adults have dual pathways, and not all who do, have PSVT. Most tachycardias in these patients are sustained by antegrade conduction through the atrioventricular node over the slower conducting pathway, which has a longer refractory period, and retrograde conduction over the faster conducting pathway with shorter refractory period ("slow-fast" sequence). In a few cases, the reverse course is followed ("fast-slow" sequence), and many of these patients have persistent tachycardia. A rare "slow-slow" sequence also occurs. The arrhythmia usually starts after an atrial premature beat that dissociates the pathways and allows reentry to begin. In the Lown-Ganong-Levine syndrome, the PR intervals are short, but no delta waves are present. Some of these patients have PSVT sustained in dual pathways.

In patients with Wolff-Parkinson-White syndrome, the atrioventricular node is usually the antegrade limb supporting the tachycardia and the accessory pathway is the retrograde pathway. The circuit sustaining the tachycardia includes the ventricles and the atria. Incessant or persistent PSVT in these patients courses in the opposite direction. Concealed accessory pathways cannot conduct in the antegrade direction and do not produce ventricular preexcitation, the electrocardiographic hallmark of Wolff-Parkinson-White syndrome. Ventricular premature beats more easily start PSVT sustained within accessory pathways than within dual atrioventricular nodal pathways. Arrhythmias are also sustained through pathways that connect structures other than the atria and ventricles, and some patients have multiple pathways. Electrophysiological study can predict which drugs are most likely to convert or suppress reentrant PSVT.

Conversion is usually produced by slowing conduction in the atrioventricular node. This is the effect of carotid sinus pressure or the Valsalva maneuver, which patients can administer to produce sinus rhythm. Drugs that slow conduction include adenosine and calcium-channel blockers, which, given intravenously, convert most paroxysms. Beta-adrenergic–blocking drugs are also, but somewhat less often, effective. The same drugs are frequently prescribed to prevent recurrences, but long-term suppression is usually less successful than acute conversion. Consequently, many patients are now treated by catheter ablation with radiofrequency current, which permanently cures most patients of the arrhythmia, whether it occurs sustained in dual atrioventricular nodal or in accessory pathways.

PSVT rarely affects prognosis. A few patients with accessory pathways are at risk of potentially fatal ventricular arrhythmias, but they can usually be identified and cured with catheter ablation.

REFERENCES

1. Wellens HJJ. Supraventricular tachycardia with reentry in the atrioventricular node. In Kastor JA (ed). Arrhythmias. Philadelphia: WB Saunders, 1994, pp. 250–261.
2. Gallagher JJ. Supraventricular tachycardia with reentry in accessory pathways. In Kastor JA (ed). Arrhythmias. Philadelphia: WB Saunders, 1994, pp. 262–296.
3. Chung K-Y, Walsh TJ, Massie E. Wolff-Parkinson-White syndrome. Am Heart J 1965; 69:116–133.
4. Newman BJ, Donoso E, Friedberg CK. Arrhythmias in the Wolff-Parkinson-White syndrome. Prog Cardiovas Dis 1966; 9:147–165.
5. Orinius E. Pre-excitation: studies on criteria, prognosis and heredity. Acta Med Scand Suppl 1966; 465:1–55.
6. Ferrer MI. New concepts relating to the preexcitation syndrome. JAMA 1967; 201:1038–1039.
7. James TN. The Wolff-Parkinson-White syndrome. Ann Intern Med 1969; 71:399–405.
8. James TN. The Wolff-Parkinson-White syndrome: evolving concepts of its pathogenesis. Prog Cardiovasc Dis 1970; 13:159–189.
9. Durrer D, Schuilenburg RM, Wellens HJJ. Pre-excitation revisited. Am J Cardiol 1970; 25:690–697.
10. Wallace AG, Boineau JP, Davidson RM, Sealy WC. Wolff-Parkinson-White syndrome: a new look. Am J Cardiol 1971; 28:509–515.
11. Narula OS. Wolff-Parkinson-White syndrome: a review. Circulation 1973; 47:872–887.
12. Durrer D, Wellens HJJ. The Wolff-Parkinson-White syndrome anno 1973. Eur J Cardiol 1974; 1:347–367.
13. Gallagher JJ, Gilbert M, Svenson RH, Sealy WC, Kasell J, Wallace AG. Wolff-Parkinson-White syndrome: the problem, evaluation, and surgical correction. Circulation 1975; 51:767–785.
14. Josephson ME, Kastor JA. Supraventricular tachycardia: mechanisms and management. Ann Intern Med 1977; 87:346–358.
15. Wellens HJJ, Lubbers WJ, Losekoot TG. Preexcitation. In Roberts NK, Gelband H (eds). Arrhythmias. Infant, and Child. New York: Appleton-Century-Crofts, 1977, pp. 231–263.
16. Gallagher JJ, Pritchett EL, Sealy WC, Kasell J, Wallace AG. The preexcitation syndromes. Prog Cardiovasc Dis 1978; 20:285–327.
17. Sung RJ, Castellanos A. Supraventricular tachycardia: mechanisms and treatment. Cardiovasc Clin 1980; 11:27–34.
18. Sung RJ, Castellanos A. Preexcitation syndrome. Cardiovasc Clin 1980; 11:103–112.
19. Till JA, Shinebourne EA. Supraventricular tachycardia: diagnosis and current acute management. Arch Dis Child 1991; 66:647–652.
20. Josephson ME. Clinical Cardiac Electrophysiology. Techniques and Interpretations. 2nd ed. Philadelphia: Lea & Febiger, 1993, pp. 140–143.
21. Oren JW IV, Beckman KJ, McClelland JH, Wang X, Lazzara R, Jackman WM. A functional approach to the preexcitation syndromes. Cardiol Clin 1993; 11:121–149.
22. Ganz LI, Friedman PL. Supraventricular tachycardia. N Engl J Med 1995; 332:162–173.
23. Morillo CA, Klein GJ, Yee R, Guiraudon GM. The Wolff-Parkinson-White syndrome. In Camm AJ (ed). Clinical Approaches to Tachycardias. Vol. 6. Armonk, NY: Futura Publishing Co., 1997, p. 1143.
24. Wellens HJJ, Rodriguez LM, Timmermans C, Smeets JP. The asymptomatic patient with the Wolff-Parkinson-White electrocardiogram. Pacing Clin Electrophysiol 1997; 20:2082–2086.
25. Campbell RW. Supraventricular tachycardia: doing the right things. Eur Heart J 1997; 18:C50–C53.
26. Kastor JA. Supraventricular tachyarrhythmias: classification and general principles of therapy. In Horowitz LN (ed). Current Management of Arrhythmias. Philadelphia: B.C. Decker, 1991, pp. 44–47.
27. Scherlag BJ, Lau SH, Helfant RH, Berkowitz WD, Stein E,

Damato AN. Catheter technique for recording His bundle activity in man. Circulation 1969; 39:13–18.

28. Durrer D, Schoo L, Schuilenburg RM, Wellens HJJ. The role of premature beats in the initiation and the termination of supraventricular tachycardia in the Wolff-Parkinson-White syndrome. Circulation 1967; 36:644–662.

29. Barold SS, Linhart JW, Samet P, Lister JW. Supraventricular tachycardia initiated and terminated by a single electrical stimulus. Am J Cardiol 1969; 24:37–41.

30. Goldreyer BN, Bigger JT Jr. Spontaneous and induced reentrant tachycardia. Ann Intern Med 1969; 70:87–98.

31. Bigger JT Jr, Goldreyer BN. The mechanism of supraventricular tachycardia. Circulation 1970; 42:673–688.

32. Goldreyer BN, Damato AN. The essential role of atrioventricular conduction delay in the initiation of paroxysmal supraventricular tachycardia. Circulation 1971; 43:679–687.

33. Goldreyer BN, Bigger JT Jr. Site of reentry in paroxysmal supraventricular tachycardia in man. Circulation 1971; 43:15–26.

34. Wolff L, Parkinson J, White PD. Bundle-branch block with short P-R interval in healthy young people prone to paroxysmal tachycardia. Am Heart J 1930; 5:685–704.

35. Wolff L. Wolff-Parkinson-White syndrome: historical and clinical features. Prog Cardiovasc Dis 1960; 2:677–690.

36. Myers GS. A forty-four year follow-up. Am J Cardiol 1965; 15:513.

37. Campbell RW. Supraventricular tachycardia: occasional nuisance or frequent threat? Eur Heart J 1996; 17:C21–C25.

38. Orejarena LA, Vidaillet H, De Stefano F, et al. Paroxysmal supraventricular tachycardia in the general population. J Am Coll Cardiol 1998; 31:150–157.

39. Josephson ME. Clinical Cardiac Electrophysiology. Techniques and Interpretations. 2nd ed. Philadelphia: Lea & Febiger, 1993, pp. 181–274.

40. Gillett PC. The mechanisms of supraventricular tachycardia in children. Circulation 1976; 54:133–139.

41. Garson A Jr, Gillette PC. Electrophysiologic studies of supraventricular tachycardia in children. II. Prediction of specific mechanism by noninvasive features. Am Heart J 1981; 102:383–388.

42. Southall DP, Johnson AM, Shinebourne EA, Johnston PG, Vulliamy DG. Frequency and outcome of disorders of cardiac rhythm and conduction in a population of newborn infants. Pediatrics 1981; 68:58–66.

43. Packard JM, Graettinger JS, Graybiel A. Analysis of the electrocardiograms obtained from 1,000 young healthy aviators: ten year follow-up. Circulation 1954; 10:384–400.

44. Katz LN, Pick A. Clinical Electrocardiography. Part I. The Arrhythmias. Philadelphia: Lea & Febiger, 1956, p. 43.

45. Manning GW. Electrocardiography in the selection of Royal Canadian Air Force aircrew. Circulation 1954; 10:401–412.

46. Hejtmancik MR, Herrmann GR. The electrocardiographic syndrome of short P-R interval and broad QRS complexes. Am Heart J 1957; 54:708–721.

47. Averill KH, Fosmoe RJ, Lamb LE. Electrocardiographic findings in 67,375 asymptomatic subjects. IV. Wolff-Parkinson-White syndrome. Am J Cardiol 1960; 6:108–129.

48. Manning GW. An electrocardiographic study of 17,000 fit, young Royal Canadian Air Force aircrew applicants. Am J Cardiol 1960; 6:70–74.

49. Guize L, Soria R, Chaouat JC, Chretien JM, Houe D, Le Heuzey JY. Prevalence and course of Wolff-Parkinson-White syndrome in a population of 138,048 subjects. Ann Med Interne 1985; 136:474–478.

50. Munger TM, Packer DL, Hammill SC, et al. A population study of the natural history of Wolff-Parkinson-White syndrome in Olmsted County, Minnesota, 1953–1989. Circulation 1993; 87:866–873.

51. Larsen JA, Kadish AH. Effects of gender on cardiac arrhythmias. J Cardiovasc Electrophysiol 1998; 9:655–664.

52. Rodriguez LM, de Chillou C, Schlapfer J, et al. Age at onset and gender of patients with different types of supraventricular tachycardias. Am J Cardiol 1992; 70:1213–1215.

53. Rodriguez LM. Age at onset and gender of patients with different types of supraventricular tachycardias. In Rodriguez LM (ed). New Observations on Cardiac Arrhythmias. Maastricht: Universitaire Pers Maastricht, 1994, pp. 19–25.

54. Rosenfeld LE, Van Zetta AM, Batsford WP. Comparison of clinical and electrophysiologic features of preexcitation syndromes in patients presenting initially after age 50 years with those presenting at younger ages. Am J Cardiol 1991; 67:709–712.

55. Lee SH, Chen SA, Wu TJ, et al. Effects of pregnancy on first onset and symptoms of paroxysmal supraventricular tachycardia. Am J Cardiol 1995; 76:675–678.

56. Pentinga ML, Meeder JG, Crijns HJ, de Muinck ED, Wiesfeld AC, Lie KI. Late onset atrioventricular nodal tachycardia. Int J Cardiol 1993; 38:293–298.

57. Clair WK, Wilkinson WE, McCarthy EA, Page RL, Pritchett EL. Spontaneous occurrence of symptomatic paroxysmal atrial fibrillation and paroxysmal supraventricular tachycardia in untreated patients. Circulation 1993; 87:1114–1122.

58. Giardina AC, Ehlers KH, Engle MA. Wolff-Parkinson-White syndrome in infants and children: a long-term follow-up study. Br Heart J 1972; 34:839–846.

59. Perry JC, Garson A Jr. Supraventricular tachycardia due to Wolff-Parkinson-White syndrome in children: early disappearance and late recurrence. J Am Coll Cardiol 1990; 16:1215–1220.

60. Levkoff AH. Perinatal outcome of paroxysmal tachycardia of the newborn with onset in utero. Report of 2 cases: review of the literature and a discussion of a clinical approach to fetal tachycardia. Am J Obstet Gynecol 1969; 104:73–79.

61. Klapholz H, Schifrin BS, Rivo E. Paroxysmal supraventricular tachycardia in the fetus. Obstet Gynecol 1974; 43:718–721.

62. Teuscher A, Bossi E, Imhof P, Erb E, Stocker FP, Weber JW. Effect of propranolol on fetal tachycardia in diabetic pregnancy. Am J Cardiol 1978; 42:304–307.

63. Newburger JW, Keane JF. Intrauterine supraventricular tachycardia. J Pediatr 1979; 95:780–786.

64. Kerenyi TD, Gleicher N, Meller J, et al. Transplacental cardioversion of intrauterine supraventricular tachycardia with digitalis. Lancet 1980; 2:393–394.

65. Lingman G, Ohrlander S, Ohlin P. Intrauterine digoxin treatment of fetal paroxysmal tachycardia: case report. Br J Obstet Gynaecol 1980; 87:340–342.

66. Harrigan JT, Kangos JJ, Sikka A, et al. Successful treatment of fetal congestive heart failure secondary to tachycardia. N Engl J Med 1981; 304:1527–1529.

67. Gleicher N, Meller J, Sandler RZ, Sullum S. Wolff-Parkinson-White syndrome in pregnancy. Obstet Gynecol 1981; 58:748–752.

68. Kleinman CS, Copel JA, Weinstein EM, Santulli TV Jr, Hobbins JC. Treatment of fetal supraventricular tachyarrhythmias. J Clin Ultrasound 1985; 13:265–273.

69. Kleinman CS, Copel JA, Weinstein EM, Santulli TV Jr, Hobbins JC. In utero diagnosis and treatment of fetal supraventricular tachycardia. Semin Perinatol 1985; 9:113–129.

70. Johnson WH Jr, Dunnigan A, Fehr P, Benson DW. Association of atrial flutter with orthodromic reciprocating fetal tachycardia. Am J Cardiol 1987; 59:374–375.

71. Gembruch U, Redel DA, Bald R, Hansmann M. Longitudinal study in 18 cases of fetal supraventricular tachycardia: Doppler echocardiographic findings and pathophysiologic implications. Am Heart J 1993; 125:1290–1301.

72. Moene RJ, Roos JP. Transient Wolff-Parkinson-White syndrome and neonatal reciprocating tachycardia. Circulation 1973; 48:443–447.

73. Wolff GS, Han J, Curran J. Wolff-Parkinson-White syndrome in the neonate. Am J Cardiol 1978; 41:559–563.

74. Lundberg A. Paroxysmal atrial tachycardia in infancy: long-term follow-up study of 49 subjects. Pediatrics 1982; 70:638–642.

75. Crosson JE, Hesslein PS, Thilenius OG, Dunnigan A. AV node reentry tachycardia in infants. Pacing Clin Electrophysiol 1995; 18:2144–2149.

76. Garson A Jr, Gillette PC. Electrophysiologic studies of supraventricular tachycardia in children. I. Clinical-electrophysiologic correlations. Am Heart J 1981; 102:233–250.

77. Ko JK, Deal BJ, Strasburger JF, Benson DW Jr. Supraventricular tachycardia mechanisms and their age distribution in pediatric patients. Am J Cardiol 1992; 69:1028–1032.

78. Lundberg A. Paroxysmal tachycardia in infancy: follow-up study of 47 subjects ranging in age from 10 to 26 years. Pediatrics 1973; 51:26–35.

79. Roelandt J, Roos JP. On the mechanism of paroxysmal tachycardias in neonates. Am Heart J 1971; 81:842–843.

80. Mantakas ME, McCue CM, Miller WW. Natural history of Wolff-Parkinson-White syndrome discovered in infancy. Am J Cardiol 1978; 41:1097–1103.

81. Benson DW Jr, Dunnigan A, Benditt DG. Follow-up evaluation of infant paroxysmal atrial tachycardia: transesophageal study. Circulation 1987; 75:542–549.

82. Klein GJ, Yee R, Sharma AD. Longitudinal electrophysiologic assessment of asymptomatic patients with the Wolff-Parkinson-White electrocardiographic pattern. N Engl J Med 1989; 320:1229–1233.

83. Michelucci A, Padeletti L, Mezzani A, et al. Relationship between age and anterograde refractoriness of the accessory pathway in Wolff-Parkinson-White patients. Cardiology 1989; 76:270–273.

84. Rubart M, von der Lohe E. Sex steroids and cardiac arrhythmias: more questions than answers. J Cardiovasc Electrophysiol 1998; 9:665–667.

85. Campbell M. The paroxysmal tachycardias. Lancet 1947; 1:641–647.

86. Lubbers WJ, Losekoot TG, Anderson RH, Wellens HJJ. Paroxysmal supraventricular tachycardia in infancy and childhood. Eur J Cardiol 1974; 2:91–99.

87. Deal BJ, Keane JF, Gillette PC, Garson A Jr. Wolff-Parkinson-White syndrome and supraventricular tachycardia during infancy: management and follow-up. J Am Coll Cardiol 1985; 5:130–135.

88. Harnischfeger WW. Hereditary occurrence of the pre-excitation (Wolff-Parkinson-White) syndrome with re-entry mechanism and concealed conduction. Circulation 1959; 19:28–40.

89. Schneider RG. Familial occurrence of Wolff-Parkinson-White syndrome. Am Heart J 1969; 78:34–36.

90. Krikler DM, Davies MJ, Rowland E, Goodwin JF, Evans RC, Shaw DB. Sudden death in hypertrophic cardiomyopathy: associated accessory atrioventricular pathways. Br Heart J 1980; 43:245–251.

91. Vidaillet HJ Jr, Burton CS III, Ramirez NM, et al. An unusual variant of familial preexcitation. Am J Cardiol 1987; 59:371–373.

92. Shibata M, Yamakado T, Hendricks FH, Isaka N, Nakano T. Familial hypertrophic cardiomyopathy with Wolff-Parkinson-White syndrome progressing to ventricular dilation. Am Heart J 1996; 131:1223–1225.

93. Vidaillet HJ Jr, Pressley JC, Henke E, Harrell FE Jr, German LD. Familial occurrence of accessory atrioventricular pathways (preexcitation syndrome). N Engl J Med 1987; 317:65–69.

94. Luria MH. Selected clinical features of paroxysmal tachycardia: a prospective study in 120 patients. Br Heart J 1971; 33:351–357.

95. Goldberger AL, Johnson AD. Swallowing-induced paroxysmal supraventricular tachycardia. J Electrocardiol 1980; 13:83–84.

96. Coelho A, Palileo E, Ashley W, et al. Tachyarrhythmias in young athletes. J Am Coll Cardiol 1986; 7:237–243.

97. Katz LN, Pick A. Clinical Electrocardiography. Part I. The Arrhythmias. Philadelphia: Lea & Febiger, 1956, pp. 275–276.

98. Widerhorn J, Widerhorn AL, Rahimtoola SH, Elkayam U. WPW syndrome during pregnancy: increased incidence of supraventricular arrhythmias. Am Heart J 1992; 123:796–798.

99. Pritchett EL, Smith MS, McCarthy EA, Lee KL. The spontaneous occurrence of paroxysmal supraventricular tachycardia. Circulation 1984; 70:1–6.

100. Mir MA. Effect of a long acting beta-adrenoceptor blocker on diurnal variation of cardiac dysrhythmias. Postgrad Med J 1986; 62:175–178.

101. Irwin JM, McCarthy EA, Wilkinson WE, Pritchett EL. Circadian occurrence of symptomatic paroxysmal supraventricular tachycardia in untreated patients. Circulation 1988; 77:298–300.

102. Kupari M, Koskinen P, Leinonen H. Double-peaking circadian variation in the occurrence of sustained supraventricular tachyarrhythmias. Am Heart J 1990; 120:1364–1369.

103. Rostagno C, Taddei T, Paladini B, Modesti PA, Utari P, Bertini G. The onset of symptomatic atrial fibrillation and paroxysmal supraventricular tachycardia is characterized by different circadian rhythms. Am J Cardiol 1993; 71:453–455.

104. Porterfield JG, Porterfield LM, Nestor JR. Daily variations in the occurrence of symptomatic supraventricular tachycardia as determined by ambulatory event monitoring. Am J Cardiol 1997; 80:889–891.

105. Lemler MS, Schaffer MS. Neonatal supraventricular tachycardia: predictors of successful treatment withdrawal. Am Heart J 1997; 133:130–131.

106. Keane JF, Plauth WH Jr, Nadas AS. Chronic ectopic tachycardia of infancy and childhood. Am Heart J 1972; 84:748–757.

107. Coumel P. Junctional reciprocating tachycardias. The permanent and paroxysmal forms of A-V nodal reciprocating tachycardias. J Electrocardiol 1975; 8:79–90.

108. Coumel P, Attuel P, Mugica J. Junctional reciprocating tachycardia: the permanent form. In Kulbertus HE (ed). Re-entrant Arrhythmias. Mechanisms and Treatment. Baltimore: University Park Press, 1976, pp. 170–183.

109. Gallagher JJ, Sealy WC. The permanent form of junctional reciprocating tachycardia: further elucidation of the underlying mechanism. Eur J Cardiol 1978; 8:413–430.

110. Coumel P, Attuel P, Leclercq JF. Permanent form of junctional reciprocating tachycardia: Mechanism, clinical and therapeutic implications. In Narula OS (ed). Cardiac Arrhythmias. Electrophysiology, Diagnosis and Management. Baltimore: Williams & Wilkins, 1979, pp. 347–363.

111. Denes P, Kehoe R, Rosen KM. Multiple reentrant tachycardias due to retrograde conduction of dual atrioventricular bundles with atrioventricular nodal-like properties. Am J Cardiol 1979; 44:162–170.

112. Epstein ML, Stone FM, Benditt DG. Incessant atrial tachycardia in childhood: association with rate-dependent conduction in an accessory atrioventricular pathway. Am J Cardiol 1979; 44:498–504.

113. Ward DE, Camm AJ, Pearce RC, Spurrell RAJ, Rees GM. Incessant atrioventricular tachycardia involving an accessory pathway: preoperative and intraoperative electrophysiologic studies and surgical correction. Am J Cardiol 1979; 44:428–434.

114. Wolff GS, Sung RJ, Pickoff A, et al. The fast-slow form of atrioventricular nodal reentrant tachycardia in children. Am J Cardiol 1979; 43:1181–1188.

115. Brugada P, Vanagt EJ, Bar FW, Wellens HJJ. Incessant reciprocating atrioventricular tachycardia: factors playing a role in the mechanism of the arrhythmia. Pacing Clin Electrophysiol 1980; 3:670–677.

116. Brugada P, Bar FW, Vanagt EJ, Friedman PL, Wellens HJJ. Observations in patients showing A-V junctional echoes with a shorter P-R than R-P interval. Am J Cardiol 1981; 48:611–622.

117. Klein GJ, Kostuk WJ, Ko P, Gulamhusein S. Permanent junctional reciprocating tachycardia in an asymptomatic adult: further evidence for an accessory ventriculoatrial nodal structure. Am Heart J 1981; 102:282–286.

118. Prystowsky EN, Heger JJ, Jackman WM, Naccarelli GV, Zipes DP. Post-myocardial infarction incessant supraventricular tachycardia due to concealed accessory pathway. Am Heart J 1982; 103:426–430.

119. Sung RJ. Incessant supraventricular tachycardia. Pacing Clin Electrophysiol 1983; 6:1306–1326.

120. Brugada P, Farre J, Green M, Heddle B, Roy D, Wellens HJJ.

Observations in patients with supraventricular tachycardia having a P-R interval shorter than the R-P interval: differentiation between atrial tachycardia and reciprocating atrioventricular tachycardia using an accessory pathway with long conduction times. Am Heart J 1984; 107:556–570.

121. Critelli G, Gallagher JJ, Monda V, Coltorti F, Scherillo M, Rossi L. Anatomic and electrophysiologic substrate of the permanent form of junctional reciprocating tachycardia. J Am Coll Cardiol 1984; 4:601–610.

122. Guarnieri T, Sealy WC, German LD, Gallagher JJ. Utilization of an accessory pathway as the anterograde limb during the permanent form of junctional reciprocating tachycardia. Am J Cardiol 1984; 53:365–368.

123. Okumura K, Henthorn RW, Epstein AE, Plumb VJ, Waldo AL. "Incessant" atrioventricular (AV) reciprocating tachycardia utilizing left lateral AV bypass pathway with a long retrograde conduction time. Pacing Clin Electrophysiol 1986; 9:332–342.

124. Yeh SJ, Lin FC, Wu D. Exercise provocation of multiple reentrant tachycardias in a patient with permanent form of junctional tachycardia and intermittent ventricular preexcitation. Am Heart J 1986; 112:1109–1114.

125. Guarnieri T, German LD, Gallagher JJ. The long R-P' tachycardias. Pacing Clin Electrophysiol 1987; 10:103–117.

126. Lerman BB, Greenberg M, Overholt ED, et al. Differential electrophysiologic properties of decremental retrograde pathways in long RP' tachycardia. Circulation 1987; 76:21–31.

127. McGuire MA, Lau KC, Johnson DC, Richards DA, Uther JB, Ross DL. Patients with two types of atrioventricular junctional (AV nodal) reentrant tachycardia: evidence that a common pathway of nodal tissue is not present above the reentrant circuit. Circulation 1991; 83:1232–1246.

128. Chien WW, Cohen TJ, Lee MA, et al. Electrophysiological findings and long-term follow-up of patients with the permanent form of junctional reciprocating tachycardia treated by catheter ablation. Circulation 1992; 85:1329–1336.

129. Ticho BS, Saul JP, Hulse JE, De W, Lulu J, Walsh EP. Variable location of accessory pathways associated with the permanent form of junctional reciprocating tachycardia and confirmation with radiofrequency ablation. Am J Cardiol 1992; 70:1559–1564.

130. Corey WA, Markel ML, Hoit BD, Walsh RA. Regression of a dilated cardiomyopathy after radiofrequency ablation of incessant supraventricular tachycardia. Am Heart J 1993; 126:1469–1473.

131. McGuire MA, Yip AS, Lau KC, et al. Posterior ("atypical") atrioventricular junctional reentrant tachycardia. Am J Cardiol 1994; 73:469–477.

132. Gaita F, Haissaguerre M, Giustetto C, et al. Catheter ablation of permanent junctional reciprocating tachycardia with radiofrequency current. J Am Coll Cardiol 1995; 25:648–654.

133. Lindsay DC, Garratt CJ, Rowland E. Fifty years of tachycardia. Br Heart J 1995; 74:334.

134. Chen SA, Tai CT, Chiang CE, et al. Electrophysiologic characteristics, electropharmacologic responses and radiofrequency ablation in patients with decremental accessory pathway. J Am Coll Cardiol 1996; 28:732–737.

135. Critelli G. Recognizing and managing permanent junctional reciprocating tachycardia in the catheter ablation era. J Cardiovasc Electrophysiol 1997; 8:226–236.

136. Zivin A, Morady F. Incessant tachycardia using a concealed atrionodal bypass tract. J Cardiovasc Electrophysiol 1998; 9:191–195.

137. Wu D, Denes P, Amat-y-Leon F, et al. Clinical, electrocardiographic and electrophysiologic observations in patients with paroxysmal supraventricular tachycardia. Am J Cardiol 1978; 41:1045–1051.

138. Thapar MK, Gillette PC. Dual atrioventricular nodal pathways: a common electrophysiologic response in children. Circulation 1979; 60:1369–1374.

139. Garson A Jr, Gillette PC, McNamara DG. Supraventricular tachycardia in children: clinical features, response to treatment, and long-term follow-up in 217 patients. J Pediatr 1981; 98:875–882.

140. Brandenburg RO Jr, Holmes DR Jr, Brandenburg RO, McGoon DC. Clinical follow-up study of paroxysmal supraventricular tachyarrhythmias after operative repair of a secundum type atrial septal defect in adults. Am J Cardiol 1983; 51:273–276.

141. Josephson ME, Horowitz LN, Kastor JA. Supraventricular tachyarrhythmias in acute myocardial infarction. In Donoso E, Lipski J (eds). Acute Myocardial Infarction. New York: Stratton Intercontinental Medical Book Corp, 1977, pp. 99–111.

142. Vazifdar JP, Levine SA. Rarity of atrial tachycardia in acute myocardial infarction and in thyrotoxicosis. Arch Intern Med 1966; 118:41–42.

143. Sung RJ, Catellanos A. A-V nodal reentrant tachycardia vs accelerated A-V junctional rhythm in acute inferior myocardial infarction. Chest 1978; 74:570–571.

144. Hariman RJ, Gomes JA, el-Sherif N. Catecholamine-dependent atrioventricular nodal reentrant tachycardia. Circulation 1983; 67:681–686.

145. Josephson ME, Horowitz LN, Kastor JA. Paroxysmal supraventricular tachycardia in patients with mitral valve prolapse. Circulation 1978; 57:111–115.

146. Van Hare GF, Phoon CK, Munkenbeck F, Patel CR, Fink DL, Silverman NH. Electrophysiologic study and radiofrequency ablation in patients with intracardiac tumors and accessory pathways: is the tumor the pathway? J Cardiovasc Electrophysiol 1996; 7:1204–1210.

147. Falk RH, Tarko HB, Levine PA. Positional supraventricular tachycardia. N Engl J Med 1981; 304:1364.

148. Bajaj SC, Ragaza EP, Silva H, Goyal RK. Deglutition tachycardia. Gastroenterology 1972; 62:632–635.

149. Till J, Wren C. Atrial flutter in the fetus and young infant: an association with accessory connections. Br Heart J 1992; 67:80–83.

150. Paulay KL, Ruskin JN, Damato AN. Sinus and atrioventricular nodal reentrant tachycardia in the same patient. Am J Cardiol 1975; 36:810–816.

151. Lloyd EA, Hauer RN, Zipes DP, Heger JJ, Prystowsky EN. Syncope and ventricular tachycardia in patients with ventricular preexcitation. Am J Cardiol 1983; 52:79–82.

152. Page RL, Wilkinson WE, Clair WK, McCarthy EA, Pritchett EL. Asymptomatic arrhythmias in patients with symptomatic paroxysmal atrial fibrillation and paroxysmal supraventricular tachycardia. Circulation 1994; 89:224–227.

153. Lessmeier TJ, Gamperling D, Johnson-Liddon V, et al. Unrecognized paroxysmal supraventricular tachycardia: potential for misdiagnosis as panic disorder. Arch Intern Med 1997; 157:537–543.

154. Fan W, Peter CT, Gang ES, Mandel W. Age-related changes in the clinical and electrophysiologic characteristics of patients with Wolff-Parkinson-White syndrome: comparative study between young and elderly patients. Am Heart J 1991; 122:741–747.

155. Zimetbaum P, Josephson ME. Evaluation of patients with palpitations. N Engl J Med 1998; 338:1369–1373.

156. Atie J, Brugada P, Brugada J, et al. Clinical and electrophysiologic characteristics of patients with antidromic circus movement tachycardia in the Wolff-Parkinson-White syndrome. Am J Cardiol 1990; 66:1082–1091.

157. Mann DE, Kelly PA, Adler SW, Fuenzalida CE, Reiter MJ. Palpitations occur frequently following radiofrequency catheter ablation for supraventricular tachycardia, but do not predict pathway recurrence. Pacing Clin Electrophysiol 1993; 16:1645–1649.

158. Gursoy S, Steurer G, Brugada J, Andries E, Brugada P. Brief report: the hemodynamic mechanism of pounding in the neck in atrioventricular nodal reentrant tachycardia. N Engl J Med 1992; 327:772–774.

159. Nelson SD, Kou WH, Annesley T, de Buitleir M, Morady F. Significance of ST segment depression during paroxysmal supraventricular tachycardia. J Am Coll Cardiol 1988; 12:383–387.

160. Wu TJ, Chen SA, Chiang CE, et al. Clinical features and electrophysiologic characteristics of accessory atrioventricular pathways and atrioventricular nodal

reentrant tachycardia: comparative study between young and elderly patients. Am Heart J 1993; 126:1341–1348.

161. Yee R, Klein GJ. Syncope in the Wolff-Parkinson-White syndrome: incidence and electrophysiologic correlates. Pacing Clin Electrophysiol 1984; 7:381–388.

162. Leitch JW, Klein GJ, Yee R, Leather RA, Kim YH. Syncope associated with supraventricular tachycardia: an expression of tachycardia rate or vasomotor response? Circulation 1992; 85:1064–1071.

163. Drago F, Turchetta A, Calzolari A, et al. Reciprocating supraventricular tachycardia in children: low rate at rest as a major factor related to propensity to syncope during exercise. Am Heart J 1996; 132:280–285.

164. Paul T, Guccione P, Garson A Jr. Relation of syncope in young patients with Wolff-Parkinson-White syndrome to rapid ventricular response during atrial fibrillation. Am J Cardiol 1990; 65:318–321.

165. Auricchio A, Klein H, Trappe HJ, Wenzlaff P. Lack of prognostic value of syncope in patients with Wolff-Parkinson-White syndrome. J Am Coll Cardiol 1991; 17:152–158.

166. Wang YS, Scheinman MM, Chien WW, Cohen TJ, Lesh MD, Griffin JC. Patients with supraventricular tachycardia presenting with aborted sudden death: incidence, mechanism and long-term follow-up. J Am Coll Cardiol 1991; 18:1711–1719.

167. Anonymous. Paul Wood's Diseases of the Heart and Circulation. 3rd ed. Philadelphia: JB Lippincott, 1968, pp. 272–275.

168. Marriott HJL. Bedside Cardiac Diagnosis. Philadelphia: JB Lippincott, 1993, pp. 265–279.

169. Goldreyer BN, Kastor JA, Kershbaum KL. The hemodynamic effects of induced supraventricular tachycardia in man. Circulation 1976; 54:783–789.

170. Samet P. Hemodynamic sequelae of cardiac arrhythmias. Circulation 1973; 47:399–407.

171. McIntosh HD, Kong Y, Morris JJ Jr. Hemodynamic effects of supraventricular tachycardia. Am J Med 1964; 37:712–727.

172. Benchimol A, Ellis JG, Dimond EG, Wu T-L. Hemodynamic consequences of atrial and ventricular arrhythmias in man. Am Heart J 1965; 70:775–788.

173. McIntosh HD, Morris J Jr. The hemodynamic consequences of arrhythmias. Prog Cardiovasc Dis 1966; 8:330–363.

174. Saunders DE Jr, Ord JW. The hemodynamic effects of paroxysmal supraventricular tachycardia in patients with the Wolff-Parkinson-White syndrome. Am J Cardiol 1962; 9:223–236.

175. Curry PV, Rowland E, Fox KM, Krikler DM. The relationship between posture, blood pressure and electrophysiological properties in patients with paroxysmal supraventricular tachycardia. Arch Mal Coeur Vaiss 1978; 71:293–299.

176. Schlepper M, Weppner HG, Merle H. Haemodynamic effects of supraventricular tachycardias and their alterations by electrically and verapamil induced termination. Cardiovasc Res 1978; 12:28–33.

177. Alboni P, Fuca G, Paparella N, Scarfo S, Pirani R. Effects of intravenous propranolol on cardiovascular hemodynamics during supraventricular tachycardia. Am J Cardiol 1996; 78:347–350.

178. Swiryn S, Pavel D, Byrom E, et al. Assessment of left ventricular function by radionuclide angiography during induced supraventricular tachycardia. Am J Cardiol 1981; 47:555–561.

179. Ferrer MI, Harvey RM, Weiner HM, Cathgart RT, Cournand A. Hemodynamic studies in two cases of Wolff-Parkinson-White syndrome with paroxysmal AV nodal tachycardia. Am J Med 1949; 6:725–733.

180. Klein LS, Miles WM, Zipes DP. Effect of atrioventricular interval during pacing or reciprocating tachycardia on atrial size, pressure, and refractory period: contraction-excitation feedback in human atrium. Circulation 1990; 82:60–68.

181. Strasburger JF, Duffy CE, Gidding SS. Abnormal systemic venous Doppler flow patterns in atrial tachycardia in infants. Am J Cardiol 1997; 80:640–643.

182. Sganzerla P, Fabbiocchi F, Grazi S, Cipolla C, Moruzzi P, Guazzi MD. Electrophysiologic and haemodynamic

correlates in supraventricular tachycardia. Eur Heart J 1989; 10:32–39.

183. Hung J, Kelly DT, Hutton BF, Uther JB, Baird DK. Influence of heart rate and atrial transport on left ventricular volume and function: relation to hemodynamic changes produced by supraventricular arrhythmia. Am J Cardiol 1981; 48:632–638.

184. Kaye GC, Nathan AW, Camm AJ. Polyuria associated with paroxysmal tachycardia. Clin Prog Pacing Electrophysiol 1984; 2:349–359.

185. Wood P. Polyuria in paroxysmal tachycardia and paroxysmal atrial flutter and fibrillation. Br Heart J 1963; 25:273–282.

186. Flensted-Jensen E. Wolff-Parkinson-White syndrome: a long-term follow-up of 47 cases. Acta Med Scand 1969; 186:65–74.

187. Luria MH, Adelson EI, Lochaya S. Paroxysmal tachycardia with polyuria. Ann Intern Med 1966; 65:461–470.

188. Kinney MJ, Stein RM, DiScala VA. The polyuria of paroxysmal atrial tachycardia. Circulation 1974; 50:429–435.

189. Canepa-Anson R, Williams M, Marshall J, Mitsuoka T, Lightman S, Sutton R. Mechanism of polyuria and natriuresis in atrioventricular nodal tachycardia. BMJ 1984; 289:861–868.

190. Roy D, Paillard F, Cassidy D, et al. Atrial natriuretic factor during atrial fibrillation and supraventricular tachycardia. J Am Coll Cardiol 1987; 9:509–514.

191. Gallagher JJ. Tachycardia and cardiomyopathy: the chicken-egg dilemma revisited. J Am Coll Cardiol 1985; 6:1172–1173.

192. Shinbane JS, Wood MA, Jensen DN, Ellenbogen KA, Anza C, Scheinman MM. Tachycardia-induced cardiomyopathy: a review of animal models and clinical studies. J Am Coll Cardiol 1997; 29:709–715.

193. Ferrer MI. Hemodynamic effects of prolonged supraventricular tachycardia in normal heart. N Y State J Med 1970; 70:2120–2124.

194. Epstein ML, Benditt DG. Long-term evaluation of persistent supraventricular tachycardia in children: clinical and electrocardiographic features. Am Heart J 1981; 102:80–84.

195. Anselme F, Frederiks J, Boyle NG, Papageorgiou P, Josephson ME. An unusual cause of tachycardia-induced myopathy. Pacing Clin Electrophysiol 1996; 19:115–119.

196. McLaran CJ, Gersh BJ, Sugrue DD, Hammill SC, Seward JB, Holmes DR Jr. Tachycardia induced myocardial dysfunction: a reversible phenomenon? Br Heart J 1985; 53:323–327.

197. O'Neill BJ, Klein GJ, Guiraudon GM, et al. Results of operative therapy in the permanent form of junctional reciprocating tachycardia. Am J Cardiol 1989; 63:1074–1079.

198. Cruz FE, Cheriex EC, Smeets JL, et al. Reversibility of tachycardia-induced cardiomyopathy after cure of incessant supraventricular tachycardia. J Am Coll Cardiol 1990; 16:739–744.

199. Sanchez C, Benito F, Moreno F. Reversibility of tachycardia-induced cardiomyopathy after radiofrequency ablation of incessant supraventricular tachycardia in infants. Br Heart J 1995; 74:332–333.

200. Marriott HJL. Practical Electrocardiography. 8th ed. Baltimore: Williams & Wilkins, 1988, pp. 285–309.

201. Schamroth L, Perlman MM. Periodic variation in A-V conduction time: the "supernormal" phase of A-V conduction: a study in differential dual A-V pathway conductivity and refractoriness. J Electrocardiol 1973; 6:81–84.

202. Ezri MD, Huang SK, Chhablani R, Denes P. Dual AV nodal pathways: vagal influences on AV nodal conduction. Pacing Clin Electrophysiol 1983; 6:697–701.

203. Wu D, Hull J, Rosen KM. Unmasking of dual atrioventricular nodal pathways with spontaneous premature ventricular contractions. Chest 1976; 69:414–415.

204. Fisch C, Mandrola JM, Rardon DP. Electrocardiographic manifestations of dual atrioventricular node conduction during sinus rhythm. J Am Coll Cardiol 1997; 29:1015–1022.

205. Krikler D, Rowland E. Concealed pre-excitation. J Electrocardiol 1978; 11:209–211.

206. Ross DL, Uther JB. Diagnosis of concealed accessory pathways in supraventricular tachycardia. Pacing Clin Electrophysiol 1984; 7:1069–1085.

207. Boineau JP, Moore EN, Spear JF, Sealy WC. Basis of static and dynamic electrocardiographic variations in Wolff-Parkinson-White syndrome: anatomic and electrophysiologic observations in right and left ventricular preexcitation. Am J Cardiol 1973; 32:32–45.

208. Puech P, Grolleau R, Cinca J. Reciprocating tachycardia using a latent left-sided accessory pathway: diagnostic approach by conventional ECG. In Kulbertus HE (ed). Re-entrant Arrhythmias. Mechanisms and Treatment. Baltimore: University Park Press, 1976, pp. 117–131.

209. Reddy GV, Schamroth L. The localization of bypass tracts in the Wolff-Parkinson-White syndrome from the surface electrocardiogram. Am Heart J 1987; 113:984–993.

210. Gallagher JJ. Supraventricular tachycardia with reentry in accessory pathways. In Kastor JA (ed). Arrhythmias. Philadelphia: WB Saunders, 1994, p. 270.

211. Rosenbaum FF, Hecht HH, Wilson FN, Johnston FD. The potential variations of the thorax and the esophagus in anomalous atrioventricular excitation (Wolff-Parkinson-White syndrome). Am Heart J 1945; 29:281.

212. Neutze JM, Kerr AR, Whitlock RM. Epicardial mapping in a variant of type a Wolff-Parkinson-White syndrome. Circulation 1973; 48:662–666.

213. Tonkin AM, Wagner GS, Gallagher JJ, Cope GD, Kasell J, Wallace AG. Initial forces of ventricular depolarization in the Wolff-Parkinson-White syndrome: analysis based upon localization of the accessory pathway by epicardial mapping. Circulation 1975; 52:1030–1036.

214. Yamada K, Toyama J, Wada M, Sugiyama S, Sugenoya J. Body surface isopotential mapping in Wolff-Parkinson-White syndrome: noninvasive method to determine the localization of the accessory atrioventricular pathway. Am Heart J 1975; 90:721–734.

215. Benson DW Jr, Gallagher JJ, Spach MS, et al. Accessory atrioventricular pathway in an infant: prediction of location with body surface maps and ablation with cryosurgery. J Pediatr 1980; 96:41–46.

216. Okumura M, Okajima S, Sotobata I. Non-invasive localization of the pre-excitation site in patients with the Wolff-Parkinson-White syndrome: vectorcardiographic and echocardiographic correlations. Jpn Heart J 1980; 21:157–169.

217. Benson DW Jr, Sterba R, Gallagher JJ, Walston A II, Spach MS. Localization of the site of ventricular preexcitation with body surface maps in patients with Wolff-Parkinson-White syndrome. Circulation 1982; 65:1259–1268.

218. Smith WM, Gallagher JJ, Kerr CR, et al. The electrophysiologic basis and management of symptomatic recurrent tachycardia in patients with Ebstein's anomaly of the tricuspid valve. Am J Cardiol 1982; 49:1223–1234.

219. Bardy GH, Fedor JM, German LD, Packer DL, Gallagher JJ. Surface electrocardiographic clues suggesting presence of a nodofascicular Mahaim fiber. J Am Coll Cardiol 1984; 3:1161–1168.

220. Wellens HJJ, Brugada P, Heddle WF. Value of the 12 lead electrocardiogram in diagnosing type and mechanism of a tachycardia: a survey among 22 cardiologists. J Am Coll Cardiol 1984; 4:176–179.

221. Giorgi C, Ackaoui A, Nadeau R, Savard P, Primeau R, Page P. Wolff-Parkinson-White VCG patterns that mimic other cardiac pathologies: a correlative study with the preexcitation pathway localization. Am Heart J 1986; 111:891–902.

222. Kamakura S, Shimomura K, Ohe T, Matsuhisa M, Toyoshima H. The role of initial minimum potentials on body surface maps in predicting the site of accessory pathways in patients with Wolff-Parkinson-White syndrome. Circulation 1986; 74:89–96.

223. Lemery R, Hammill SC, Wood DL, et al. Value of the resting 12 lead electrocardiogram and vectorcardiogram for locating the accessory pathway in patients with the Wolff-Parkinson-White syndrome. Br Heart J 1987; 58:324–332.

224. Lindsay BD, Crossen KJ, Cain ME. Concordance of distinguishing electrocardiographic features during sinus rhythm with the location of accessory pathways in the Wolff-Parkinson-White syndrome. Am J Cardiol 1987; 59:1093–1102.

225. Milstein S, Sharma AD, Guiraudon GM, Klein GJ. An algorithm for the electrocardiographic localization of accessory pathways in the Wolff-Parkinson-White syndrome. Pacing Clin Electrophysiol 1987; 10:555–563.

226. Giorgi C, Nadeau R, Primeau R, et al. Comparative accuracy of the vectorcardiogram and electrocardiogram in the localization of the accessory pathway in patients with Wolff-Parkinson-White syndrome: validation of a new vectorcardiographic algorithm by intraoperative epicardial mapping and electrophysiologic studies. Am Heart J 1990; 119:592–598.

227. Teo WS, Klein GJ, Yee R, Leitch JW, Murdock CJ. Significance of minimal preexcitation in Wolff-Parkinson-White syndrome. Am J Cardiol 1991; 67:205–207.

228. Yuan SW, Iwa T, Misaki T, et al. Comparative study of five preoperative methods for the localization of accessory pathways in the Wolff-Parkinson-White syndrome. Jpn Circ J 1991; 55:685–691.

229. Cohen TJ, Tucker KJ, Abbott JA, et al. Usefulness of adenosine in augmenting ventricular preexcitation for noninvasive localization of accessory pathways. Am J Cardiol 1992; 69:1178–1185.

230. Scheinman MM, Wang YS, Van Hare GF, Lesh MD. Electrocardiographic and electrophysiologic characteristics of anterior, midseptal and right anterior free wall accessory pathways. J Am Coll Cardiol 1992; 20:1220–1229.

231. Yuan S, Iwa T, Tsubota M, Bando H. Comparative study of eight sets of ECG criteria for the localization of the accessory pathway in Wolff-Parkinson-White syndrome. J Electrocardiol 1992; 25:203–214.

232. Rodriguez LM, Smeets JL, de Chillou C, et al. The 12-lead electrocardiogram in midseptal, anteroseptal, posteroseptal and right free wall accessory pathways. Am J Cardiol 1993; 72:1274–1280.

233. Anza C, Gonzales RP, Lesh MD, Modin GW, Lee RJ, Scheinman MM. New algorithm for the localization of accessory atrioventricular connections using a baseline electrocardiogram. J Am Coll Cardiol 1994; 23:107–116.

234. Haissaguerre M, Marcus F, Poquet F, Gencel L, Le Metayer P, Clementy J. Electrocardiographic characteristics and catheter ablation of parahissian accessory pathways. Circulation 1994; 90:1124–1128.

235. Rodriguez LM. The 12-lead electrocardiogram in mid-septal, anteroseptal, posteroseptal and right free wall accessory pathways. In Rodriguez LM (ed). New Observations on Cardiac Arrhythmias. Maastricht: Universitaire Pers Maastricht, 1994, pp. 27–42.

236. Xie B, Heald SC, Bashir Y, et al. Localization of accessory pathways from the 12-lead electrocardiogram using a new algorithm. Am J Cardiol 1994; 74:161–165.

237. Chiang CE, Chen SA, Teo WS, et al. An accurate stepwise electrocardiographic algorithm for localization of accessory pathways in patients with Wolff-Parkinson-White syndrome from a comprehensive analysis of delta waves and R/S ratio during sinus rhythm. Am J Cardiol 1995; 76:40–46.

238. Arruda MS, McClelland JH, Wang X, et al. Development and validation of an ECG algorithm for identifying accessory pathway ablation site in Wolff-Parkinson-White syndrome. J Cardiovasc Electrophysiol 1998; 9:2–12.

239. Lown B, Ganong WF, Levine SA. The syndrome of short P-R interval, normal QRS complex and paroxysmal heart action. Circulation 1952; 5:693–706.

240. Huang SK, Rosenberg MJ, Denes P. Short PR interval and narrow QRS complex associated with pheochromocytoma: electrophysiologic observations. J Am Coll Cardiol 1984; 3:872–875.

241. Myerburg RJ, Sung RJ, Castellanos A. Ventricular tachycardia and ventricular fibrillation in patients with short P-R intervals and narrow QRS complexes. Pacing Clin Electrophysiol 1979; 2:568–578.

242. Kernohan RJ. Post-paroxysmal tachycardia syndrome. Br Heart J 1969; 31:803–806.

243. Bricker JT, Porter CJ, Garson A Jr, et al. Exercise testing in

children with Wolff-Parkinson-White syndrome. Am J Cardiol 1985; 55:1001–1004.

244. Eshchar Y, Belhassen B, Laniado S. Comparison of exercise and ajmaline tests with electrophysiologic study in the Wolff-Parkinson-White syndrome. Am J Cardiol 1986; 57:782–786.

245. Sharma AD, Yee R, Guiraudon G, Klein GJ. Sensitivity and specificity of invasive and noninvasive testing for risk of sudden death in Wolff-Parkinson-White syndrome. J Am Coll Cardiol 1987; 10:373–381.

246. Wellens HJJ, Bar FW, Gorgels AP, Vanagt EJ. Use of ajmaline in patients with the Wolff-Parkinson-White syndrome to disclose short refractory period of the accessory pathway. Am J Cardiol 1980; 45:130–133.

247. Fananapazir L, Packer DL, German LD, et al. Procainamide infusion test: inability to identify patients with Wolff-Parkinson-White syndrome who are potentially at risk of sudden death. Circulation 1988; 77:1291–1296.

248. Rinne C, Klein GJ, Sharma AD, Yee R. Clinical usefulness of the 12-lead electrocardiogram in the Wolff-Parkinson-White syndrome. Cardiol Clin 1987; 5:499–509.

249. Garratt CJ, Griffith MJ. Electrocardiographic Diagnosis of Tachycardias. Armonk, NY: Futura Publishing Co., 1994.

250. Sintetos AL, Roark SF, Smith MS, McCarthy EA, Lee KL, Pritchett EL. Incidence of symptomatic tachycardia in untreated patients with paroxysmal supraventricular tachycardia. Arch Intern Med 1986; 146:2205–2209.

251. Chen S-A, Chiang C-E, Yang C-J, et al. Accessory pathway and atrioventricular node reentrant tachycardia in elderly patients: clinical features, electrophysiologic characteristics and results of radiofrequency ablation. J Am Coll Cardiol 1994; 23:702–708.

252. Hamer ME, Wilkinson WE, McCarthy EA, Page RL, Pritchett EL. Heart rate during spontaneous and induced paroxysmal supraventricular tachycardia. Pacing Clin Electrophysiol 1995; 18:2155–2157.

253. Josephson ME, Seides SE, Batsford WB, Caracta AR, Damato AN, Kastor JA. The effects of carotid sinus pressure in re-entrant paroxysmal supraventricular tachycardia. Am Heart J 1974; 88:694–697.

254. Klein HO, Hoffman BF. Cessation of paroxysmal supraventricular tachycardias by parasympathomimetic interventions. Ann Intern Med 1974; 81:48–50.

255. Waxman MB, Wald RW, Sharma AD, Huerta F, Cameron DA. Vagal techniques for termination of paroxysmal supraventricular tachycardia. Am J Cardiol 1980; 46:655–664.

256. Bar FW, Brugada P, Dassen WR, Wellens HJJ. Differential diagnosis of tachycardia with narrow QRS complex (shorter than 0.12 second). Am J Cardiol 1984; 54:555–560.

257. Ng KS, Lauer MR, Young C, Liem LB, Sung RJ. Correlation of P-wave polarity with underlying electrophysiologic mechanisms of long RP′ tachycardia. Am J Cardiol 1996; 77:1129–1132.

258. Sargin O, Demirkol C. Deeply inverted T-waves after supraventricular paroxysmal tachycardia. Dis Chest 1965; 48:321–323.

259. Wood MA, DiMarco JP, Haines DE. Electrocardiographic abnormalities after radiofrequency catheter ablation of accessory bypass tracts in the Wolff-Parkinson-White syndrome. Am J Cardiol 1992; 70:200–204.

260. Rosenbaum MB, Blanco HH, Elizari MV, Lazzari JO, Davidenko JM. Electrotonic modulation of the T wave and cardiac memory. Am J Cardiol 1982; 50:213–222.

261. Kalbfleisch SJ, Sousa J, el-Atassi R, Calkins H, Langberg J, Morady F. Repolarization abnormalities after catheter ablation of accessory atrioventricular connections with radiofrequency current. J Am Coll Cardiol 1991; 18:1761–1766.

262. Poole JE, Bardy GH. Further evidence supporting the concept of T-wave memory: observation in patients having undergone high-energy direct current catheter ablation of the Wolff-Parkinson-White syndrome. Eur Heart J 1992; 13:801–807.

263. Yanagawa T, Hirai M, Hayashi H, et al. QRST time integral values in 12-lead electrocardiograms before and after radiofrequency catheter ablation in patients with Wolff-

Parkinson-White syndrome. J Am Coll Cardiol 1995; 25:1584–1590.

264. Goyal R, Syed ZA, Mukhopadhyay PS, et al. Changes in cardiac repolarization following short periods of ventricular pacing. J Cardiovasc Electrophysiol 1998; 9:269–280.

265. Josephson ME, Wellens HJJ. Differential diagnosis of supraventricular tachycardia. Cardiol Clin 1990; 8:411–442.

266. Wellens HJ. The value of the ECG in the diagnosis of supraventricular tachycardias. Eur Heart J 1996; 17:10–20.

267. Farshidi A, Josephson ME, Horowitz LN. Electrophysiologic characteristics of concealed bypass tracts: clinical and electrocardiographic correlates. Am J Cardiol 1978; 41:1052–1060.

268. Green M, Heddle B, Dassen W, et al. Value of QRS alteration in determining the site of origin of narrow QRS supraventricular tachycardia. Circulation 1983; 68:368–373.

269. Kay GN, Pressley JC, Packer DL, Pritchett EL, German LD, Gilbert MR. Value of the 12-lead electrocardiogram in discriminating atrioventricular nodal reciprocating tachycardia from circus movement atrioventricular tachycardia utilizing a retrograde accessory pathway. Am J Cardiol 1987; 59:296–300.

270. Morady F, DiCarlo LA Jr, Baerman JM, de Buitleir M, Kou WH. Determinants of QRS alternans during narrow QRS tachycardia. J Am Coll Cardiol 1987; 9:489–499.

271. Pulignano G, Patruno N, Urbani P, Greco C, Critelli G. Electrophysiological significance of QRS alternans in narrow QRS tachycardia. Pacing Clin Electrophysiol 1990; 13:144–150.

272. Kalbfleisch SJ, el-Atassi R, Calkins H, Langberg JJ, Morady F. Differentiation of paroxysmal narrow QRS complex tachycardias using the 12-lead electrocardiogram. J Am Coll Cardiol 1993; 21:85–89.

273. Wellens HJJ, Wesdorp JC, Duren DR, Lie KI. Second degree block during reciprocal atrioventricular nodal tachycardia. Circulation 1976; 53:595–599.

274. Bauernfeind RA, Wu D, Denes PO, Rosen KM. Retrograde block during dual pathway atrioventricular nodal reentrant paroxysmal tachycardia. Am J Cardiol 1978; 42:499–505.

275. Ko PT, Naccarelli GV, Gulamhusein S, Prystowsky EN, Zipes DP, Klein GJ. Atrioventricular dissociation during paroxysmal junctional tachycardia. Pacing Clin Electrophysiol 1981; 4:670–678.

276. DiMarco JP, Sellers TD, Belardinelli L. Paroxysmal supraventricular tachycardia with Wenckebach block: evidence for reentry within the upper portion of the atrioventricular node. J Am Coll Cardiol 1984; 3:1551–1555.

277. Vassallo JA, Cassidy DM, Josephson ME. Atrioventricular nodal supraventricular tachycardia. Am J Cardiol 1985; 56:193–195.

278. Yeh SJ, Yamamoto T, Lin FC, Wu D. Atrioventricular block in the atypical form of junctional reciprocating tachycardia: evidence supporting the atrioventricular node as the site of reentry. J Am Coll Cardiol 1990; 15:385–392.

279. Lee SH, Chen SA, Tai CT, et al. Electrophysiologic characteristics and radiofrequency catheter ablation in atrioventricular node reentrant tachycardia with second-degree atrioventricular block. J Cardiovasc Electrophysiol 1997; 8:502–511.

280. Coumel P, Attuel P. Reciprocating tachycardia in overt and latent preexcitation: influence of functional bundle branch block on the rate of the tachycardia. Eur J Cardiol 1974; 1:423–436.

281. Spurrell RA, Krikler DM, Sowton E. Concealed bypasses of the atrioventricular node in patients with paroxysmal supraventricular tachycardia revealed by intracardiac electrical stimulation and verapamil. Am J Cardiol 1974; 33:590–595.

282. Neuss H, Schlepper M, Thormann J. Analysis of re-entry mechanisms in the three patients with concealed Wolff-Parkinson-White syndrome. Circulation 1975; 51:75–81.

283. Tonkin AM, Gallagher JJ, Svenson RH, Wallace AG, Sealy WC. Anterograde block in accessory pathways with retrograde conduction in reciprocating tachycardia. Eur J Cardiol 1975; 3:143–152.

284. Wellens HJJ, Durrer D. The role of an accessory atrioventricular pathway in reciprocal tachycardia: observations in patients with and without the Wolff-Parkinson-White syndrome. Circulation 1975; 52:58–72.

285. Sung RJ, Castellanos A, Gelband H, Myerburg RJ. Mechanism of reciprocating tachycardia initiated during sinus rhythm in concealed Wolff-Parkinson-White syndrome: report of a case. Circulation 1976; 54:338–344.

286. Lehmann MH, Denker S, Mahmud R, Tchou P, Dongas J, Akhtar M. Electrophysiologic mechanisms of functional bundle branch block at onset of induced orthodromic tachycardia in the Wolff-Parkinson-White syndrome: role of stimulation method. J Clin Invest 1985; 76:1566–1574.

287. Spurrell RA, Krikler DM, Sowton E. Retrograde invasion of the bundle branches producing aberration of the QRS complex during supraventricular tachycardia studied by programmed electrical stimulation. Circulation 1974; 50:487–495.

288. Crosson JE, Dunnigan A. Propranolol induced electrical and mechanical alternans in orthodromic reciprocating tachycardia. Pacing Clin Electrophysiol 1993; 16:496–500.

289. Petsas AA, Anastassiades LC, Antonopoulos AG. Exercise testing for assessment of the significance of ST segment depression observed during episodes of paroxysmal supraventricular tachycardia. Eur Heart J 1990; 11:974–979.

290. Riva SI, Della Bella P, Fassini G, Maslowsky F, Tondo C. Value of analysis of ST segment changes during tachycardia in determining type of narrow QRS complex tachycardia. J Am Coll Cardiol 1996; 27:1480–1485.

291. Benditt DG, Pritchett EL, Gallagher JJ. Spectrum of regular tachycardias with wide QRS complexes in patients with accessory atrioventricular pathways. Am J Cardiol 1978; 42:828–838.

292. Goldreyer BN, Weiss MB, Damato AN. Supraventricular tachycardia initiated by sinus beats. Circulation 1971; 44:820–825.

293. Levy AM, Bonazinga BJ. Sudden sinus slowing with junctional escape: a common mode of initiation of juvenile supraventricular tachycardia. Circulation 1983; 67:84–87.

294. Podrid PJ, Graboys TB, Lampert S, Blatt C. Exercise stress testing for exposure of arrhythmias. Circulation 1987; 75:(Suppl III):III-60–III-68.

295. Podrid PJ, Venditti FJ, Levine PA, Klein MD. The role of exercise testing in evaluation of arrhythmias. Am J Cardiol 1988; 62:24H–33H.

296. Force T, Graboys TB. Exercise testing and ambulatory monitoring in patients with preexcitation syndrome. Arch Intern Med 1981; 141:88–90.

297. Pantano JA, Oriel RJ. Prevalence and nature of cardiac arrhythmias in apparently normal well-trained runners. Am Heart J 1982; 104:762–768.

298. Toda I, Kawahara T, Murakawa Y, et al. Electrophysiological study of young patients with exercise related paroxysms of palpitation: role of atropine and isoprenaline for initiation of supraventricular tachycardia. Br Heart J 1989; 61:268–273.

299. Strasberg B, Ashley WW, Wyndham CR, et al. Treadmill exercise testing in the Wolff-Parkinson-White syndrome. Am J Cardiol 1980; 45:742–748.

300. Biffi A, Ammirati F, Caselli G, et al. Usefulness of transesophageal pacing during exercise for evaluating palpitations in top-level athletes. Am J Cardiol 1993; 72:922–926.

301. Gazes PC, Sovell BF, Dellastatious JW. Continuous radioelectrocardiographic monitoring of football and basketball coaches during games. Am Heart J 1969; 78:509–512.

302. Boudoulas H, Schaal SF, Lewis RP, Robinson JL. Superiority of 24-hour outpatient monitoring over multi-stage exercise testing for the evaluation of syncope. J Electrocardiol 1979; 12:103–108.

303. Okumura M, Sotobata I, Isomura S, et al. Echocardiographic evaluation of right ventricular anterior wall motion in the Wolff-Parkinson-White syndrome. Jpn Heart J 1979; 20:577–585.

304. Warnowicz MA, Santucci BA, Bucheleres HG, Denes P.

305. Goldman AP, Irwin JM, Glover MU, Mick W. Transesophageal echocardiography to improve positioning of radiofrequency ablation catheters in left-sided Wolff-Parkinson-White syndrome. Pacing Clin Electrophysiol 1991; 14:1245–1250.

306. Chu E, Anza C, Chin MC, Sudhir K, Yock PG, Lesh MD. Radiofrequency catheter ablation guided by intracardiac echocardiography. Circulation 1994; 89:1301–1305.

307. Chu E, Kalman JM, Kwasman MA, et al. Intracardiac echocardiography during radiofrequency catheter ablation of cardiac arrhythmias in humans. J Am Coll Cardiol 1994; 24:1351–1357.

308. Fisher WG, Pelini MA, Bacon ME. Adjunctive intracardiac echocardiography to guide slow pathway ablation in human atrioventricular nodal reentrant tachycardia: anatomic insights. Circulation 1997; 96:3021–3029.

309. Kalman JM, Olgin JE, Karch MR, Lesh MD. Use of intracardiac echocardiography in interventional electrophysiology. Pacing Clin Electrophysiol 1997; 20:2248–2262.

310. Goli VD, Prasad R, Hamilton K, et al. Transesophageal echocardiographic evaluation for mural thrombus following radiofrequency catheter ablation of accessory pathways. Pacing Clin Electrophysiol 1991; 14:1992–1997.

311. Hochberg HM, Poppers PJ, George ME. Fetal paroxysmal supraventricular tachycardia recorded by intrauterine scalp electrocardiography. J Perinat Med 1976; 4:51–54.

312. Valerius NH, Jacobsen JR. Intrauterine supraventricular tachycardia. Acta Obstet Gynecol Scand 1978; 57:407–410.

313. Jue J, Winslow T, Ossipov M, Lesh MD, Schiller NB. Effect of preexcitation on Doppler indexes of left ventricular filling. Am J Cardiol 1993; 71:1462–1464.

314. Becker AE, Anderson RH. The Wolff-Parkinson-White syndrome and its anatomical substrates. Anat Rec 1981; 201:169–177.

315. Becker AE, Anderson RH, Durrer D, Wellens HJJ. The anatomical substrates of Wolff-Parkinson-White syndrome: a clinicopathologic correlation in seven patients. Circulation 1978; 57:870–879.

316. Scheinman MM, Gonzalez R, Thomas A, Ullyot D, Bharati S, Lev M. Reentry confined to the atrioventricular node: electrophysiologic and anatomic findings. Am J Cardiol 1982; 49:1814–1818.

317. Ho SY, McComb JM, Scott CD, Anderson RH. Morphology of the cardiac conduction system in patients with electrophysiologically proven dual atrioventricular nodal pathways. J Cardiovasc Electrophysiol 1993; 4:504–512.

318. Kanter RJ, Gravatt A, Bharati S. Pathologic findings following sudden death in an infant with hypertrophic cardiomyopathy and supraventricular tachycardia. J Cardiovasc Electrophysiol 1997; 8:222–225.

319. Klein GJ, Hackel DB, Gallagher JJ. Anatomic substrate of impaired antegrade conduction over an accessory atrioventricular pathway in the Wolff-Parkinson-White syndrome. Circulation 1980; 61:1249–1256.

320. Goldreyer BN. Intracardiac electrocardiography in the analysis and understanding of cardiac arrhythmias. Ann Intern Med 1972; 77:117–136.

321. Kastor JA, Goldreyer BN. Reciprocal rhythms. In Dreifus LS, Likoff W (eds). Cardiac Arrhythmias. New York: Grune & Stratton, 1973, pp. 391–403.

322. Kastor JA, Goldreyer BN, Moore EN, Spear JF. Re-entry: an important mechanism of cardiac arrhythmias. Cardiovasc Clin 1974; 6:111–135.

323. Goldreyer BN. Mechanisms of supraventricular tachycardias. Annu Rev Med 1975; 26:219–228.

324. Wu D, Denes P. Mechanisms of paroxysmal supraventricular tachycardia. Arch Intern Med 1975; 135:437–442.

325. Barold SS, Fracp MB, Coumel P. Mechanisms of atrioventricular junctional tachycardia: role of reentry and concealed accessory bypass tracts. Am J Cardiol 1977; 39:97–106.

326. Josephson ME. Paroxysmal supraventricular tachycardia: an

electrophysiologic approach. Am J Cardiol 1978; 41:1123–1126.

327. Wellens HJJ. Value and limitations of programmed electrical stimulation of the heart in the study and treatment of tachycardias. Circulation 1978; 57:845–853.

328. Akhtar M. Paroxysmal atrioventricular nodal reentrant tachycardia. In Narula OS (ed). Cardiac Arrhythmias. Electrophysiology, Diagnosis and Management. Baltimore: Williams & Wilkins, 1979, pp. 294–317.

329. Rosen KM, Bauernfeind RA, Wyndham CR, Dhingra RC. Retrograde properties of the fast pathway in patients with paroxysmal atrioventricular nodal reentrant tachycardia. Am J Cardiol 1979; 43:863–865.

330. Rosen KM, Bauernfeind RA, Swiryn S, Dhingra RC, Wyndham CR. The significance of normal and anomalous atrioventricular conducting pathways in cardiac arrhythmias. Adv Intern Med 1980; 25:277–302.

331. Rosen KM, Bauernfeind RA, Swiryn S, Strasberg B, Palileo EV. Dual AV nodal pathways and AV nodal reentrant paroxysmal tachycardia. Am Heart J 1981; 101:691–695.

332. Wiener I. Current applications of clinical electrophysiologic study in the diagnosis and treatment of cardiac arrhythmias. Am J Cardiol 1982; 49:1287–1292.

333. Wu D. Dual atrioventricular nodal pathways: a reappraisal. Pacing Clin Electrophysiol 1982; 5:72–89.

334. Wu D. A-V nodal re-entry. Pacing Clin Electrophysiol 1983; 6:1190–1200.

335. Ross DL, Denniss AR, Uther JB. Electrophysiologic study in supraventricular arrhythmias. Cardiovasc Clin 1985; 15:187–213.

336. Scheinman MM. Atrioventricular nodal or atriojunctional reentrant tachycardia? J Am Coll Cardiol 1985; 6:1393–1394.

337. Manolis AS, Estes NA III. Supraventricular tachycardia: mechanisms and therapy. Arch Intern Med 1987; 147:1706–1716.

338. Wellens HJJ, Brugada P. Mechanisms of supraventricular tachycardia. Am J Cardiol 1988; 62:10D–15D.

339. Leitch J, Klein GJ, Yee R, Murdock C. Invasive electrophysiologic evaluation of patients with supraventricular tachycardia. Cardiol Clin 1990; 8:465–477.

340. Akhtar M, Jazayeri MR, Sra J, Blanck Z, Deshpande S, Dhala A. Atrioventricular nodal reentry: clinical, electrophysiological, and therapeutic considerations. Circulation 1993; 88:282–295.

341. Janse MJ, Anderson RH, McGuire MA, Ho SY. "AV nodal" reentry. I. "AV nodal" reentry revisited. J Cardiovasc Electrophysiol 1993; 4:561–572.

342. Jazayeri MR, Sra JS, Akhtar M. Atrioventricular nodal reentrant tachycardia: electrophysiologic characteristics, therapeutic interventions, and specific reference to anatomic boundary of the reentrant circuit. Cardiol Clin 1993; 11:151–181.

343. McGuire MA, Janse MJ, Ross DL. "AV nodal" reentry. II. AV nodal, AV junctional, or atrionodal reentry? J Cardiovasc Electrophysiol 1993; 4:573–586.

344. Perry JC, Garson A Jr. Complexities of junctional tachycardias. J Cardiovasc Electrophysiol 1993; 4:224–238.

345. Shakespeare CF, Anderson M, Camm AJ. Pathophysiology of supraventricular tachycardia. Eur Heart J 1993; 14:2–8.

346. Ward DE, Garratt CJ. The substrate for atrioventricular "nodal" reentrant tachycardia: is there a "third pathway"? J Cardiovasc Electrophysiol 1993; 4:62–67.

347. Lerman BB. Redefining dual AV nodal physiology. J Cardiovasc Electrophysiol 1997; 8:1145–1147.

348. Strickberger SA, Morady F. Evaluation of fast pathway function: the importance of autonomic tone. J Cardiovasc Electrophysiol 1997; 8:639–641.

349. Denes P, Wu D, Dhingra RC, Chuquimia R, Rosen KM. Demonstration of dual A-V nodal pathways in patients with paroxysmal supraventricular tachycardia. Circulation 1973; 48:549–555.

350. Rosen KM, Mehta A, Miller RA. Demonstration of dual atrioventricular nodal pathways in man. Am J Cardiol 1974; 33:291–294.

351. Gomes JA, Dhatt MS, Damato AN, Akhtar M, Holder CA.

352. Gomes JA, Dhatt MS, Rubenson DS, Damato AN. Electrophysiologic evidence for selective retrograde utilization of a specialized conducting system in atrioventricular nodal reentrant tachycardia. Am J Cardiol 1979; 43:687–698.

353. Lee CS, Lai WT, Wu JC, Sheu SH, Wu SN, Belardinelli L. Differential effects of adenosine on antegrade and retrograde fast pathway conduction in atrioventricular nodal reentry. Am Heart J 1997; 134:799–806.

354. Anselme F, Hook B, Monahan K, et al. Heterogeneity of retrograde fast-pathway conduction pattern in patients with atrioventricular nodal reentry tachycardia: observations by simultaneous multisite catheter mapping of Koch's triangle. Circulation 1996; 93:960–968.

355. Chen SA, Tai CT, Lee SH, Chang MS. AV nodal reentrant tachycardia with unusual characteristics: lessons from radiofrequency catheter ablation. J Cardiovasc Electrophysiol 1998; 9:321–333.

356. Denes P, Wu D, Dhingra R, Amat-y-Leon F, Wyndham C, Rosen KM. Dual atrioventricular nodal pathways: a common electrophysiological response. Br Heart J 1975; 37:1069–1076.

357. Csapo G. Paroxysmal nonreentrant tachycardias due to simultaneous conduction in dual atrioventricular nodal pathways. Am J Cardiol 1979; 43:1033–1045.

358. Levites R, Haft JI. Evidence suggesting dual A-V nodal pathways in patients without supraventricular tachycardias. Chest 1975; 67:36–42.

359. Mirvis DM, Bandura JP. Atrioventricular nodal gap conduction as a manifestation of dual nodal pathways. Am J Cardiol 1978; 41:1115–1118.

360. Casta A, Wolff GS, Mehta AV, et al. Dual atrioventricular nodal pathways: a benign finding in arrhythmia-free children with heart disease. Am J Cardiol 1980; 46:1013–1018.

361. Weiss J, Cabeen WR Jr, Roberts NK. Nodoventricular accessory atrioventricular connection associated with dual atrioventricular pathways: a case report and review of the literature. J Electrocardiol 1981; 14:185–190.

362. Kinoshita S, Kawasaki T, Fujiwara S, Okimori K. Periodic variation in atrioventricular conduction time: mechanisms of initiation, maintenance and termination of periods of long PR intervals. Am J Cardiol 1984; 53:1288–1291.

363. Tai CT, Chen SA, Chiang CE, et al. Complex electrophysiological characteristics in atrioventricular nodal reentrant tachycardia with continuous atrioventricular node function curves. Circulation 1997; 95:2541–2547.

364. Rosen KM. A-V nodal reentrance: an unexpected mechanism of paroxysmal tachycardia in a patient with preexcitation. Circulation 1973; 47:1267–1273.

365. Neuss H, Schlepper M. Unusual re-entry mechanisms in patients with Wolff-Parkinson-White syndrome. Br Heart J 1974; 36:880–887.

366. Zipes DP, DeJoseph RL, Rothbaum DA. Unusual properties of accessory pathways. Circulation 1974; 49:1200–1211.

367. Mandel WJ, Laks MM, Obayashi K. Atrioventricular nodal reentry in the Wolff-Parkinson-White syndrome. Chest 1975; 68:321–325.

368. Gillette PC, Garson A Jr, Kugler JD. Wolff-Parkinson-White syndrome in children: electrophysiologic and pharmacologic characteristics. Circulation 1979; 60:1487–1495.

369. Rubenson DS, Akhtar M, Lau SH, Caracta AR, Damato AN. Multiple mechanisms of tachycardias in a patient with the Wolff-Parkinson-White syndrome. J Electrocardiol 1979; 12:221–226.

370. Adams JR, Hess D, Scheinman MM. Mechanisms of spontaneous tachycardia termination in a patient with the Wolff-Parkinson-White syndrome and dual atrioventricular nodal pathways. Pacing Clin Electrophysiol 1981; 4:367–375.

371. Smith WM, Broughton A, Reiter MJ, Benson DW, Grant AO, Gallagher JJ. Bystander accessory pathway during AV node re-entrant tachycardia. Pacing Clin Electrophysiol 1983; 6:537–547.

Incidence, determinants and significance of fixed retrograde conduction in the region of the atrioventricular node: evidence for retrograde atrioventricular nodal bypass tracts. Am J Cardiol 1979; 44:1089–1098.

372. Sung RJ, Styperek JL. Electrophysiologic identification of dual atrioventricular nodal pathway conduction in patients with reciprocating tachycardia using anomalous bypass tracts. Circulation 1979; 60:1464–1476.

373. Zardini M, Leitch JW, Guiraudon GM, Klein GJ, Yee R. Atrioventricular nodal reentry and dual atrioventricular node physiology in patients undergoing accessory pathway ablation. Am J Cardiol 1990; 66:1388–1389.

374. Spurrell RA, Krikler D, Sowton E. Two or more intra AV nodal pathways in association with either a James or Kent extranodal bypass in 3 patients with paroxysmal supraventricular tachycardia. Br Heart J 1973; 35:113–122.

375. Dopirak MR, Schaal SF, Leier CV. Triple AV nodal pathways in man? J Electrocardiol 1980; 13:185–188.

376. Strasberg B, Swiryn S, Bauernfeind RU, et al. Retrograde dual atrioventricular nodal pathways. Am J Cardiol 1981; 48:639–646.

377. Portillo B, Portillo-Leon N, Zaman L, Castellanos A. Quintuple pathways participating in three distinct types of atrioventricular reciprocating tachycardia in a patient with Wolff-Parkinson-White syndrome. Am J Cardiol 1982; 50:347–352.

378. Swiryn S, Bauernfeind RA, Palileo EA, Strasberg B, Duffy CE, Rosen KM. Electrophysiologic study demonstrating triple antegrade AV nodal pathways in patients with spontaneous and/or induced supraventricular tachycardia. Am Heart J 1982; 103:168–176.

379. Kuck KH, Kuch B, Bleifeld W. Multiple anterograde and retrograde AV nodal pathways: demonstration by multiple discontinuities in the AV nodal conduction curves and echo time intervals. Pacing Clin Electrophysiol 1984; 7:656–662.

380. Kuhlkamp V, Haasis R, Seipel L. AV nodal reentrant tachycardia using three different AV nodal pathways. Eur Heart J 1990; 11:857–862.

381. Sublett KL, Fujimura O. Atrioventricular node reentry that utilizes triple nodal pathways. Am Heart J 1992; 124:777–779.

382. Yamashita T, Murakawa Y, Ajiki K, Omata M. Triple atrioventricular nodal pathways can be masked. Am J Cardiol 1996; 77:1365–1367.

383. Amat-y-Leon F, Wyndham C, Wu D, Denes P, Dhingra RC, Rosen KM. Participation of fast and slow A-V nodal pathways in tachycardias complicating the Wolff-Parkinson-White syndrome: report of a case. Circulation 1977; 55:663–668.

384. Pimenta J, Miranda M, Silva LA. Double ventricular response to an extrastimulus in a patient with triple atrioventricular pathways. Chest 1978; 74:593–596.

385. Hwang C, Martin DJ, Goodman JS, et al. Atypical atrioventricular node reciprocating tachycardia masquerading as tachycardia using a left-sided accessory pathway. J Am Coll Cardiol 1997; 30:218–225.

386. Sebag C, Chevalier P, Davy JM, Laine JF, Motte G. Triple antegrade nodal pathway in a patient with supraventricular paroxysmal tachycardia. J Electrocardiol 1986; 19:85–90.

387. Tai CT, Chen SA, Chiang CE, et al. Multiple anterograde atrioventricular node pathways in patients with atrioventricular node reentrant tachycardia. J Am Coll Cardiol 1996; 28:725–731.

388. Tai C-T, Chen S-A, Chiang C-E, et al. Electrophysiologic characteristics and radiofrequency catheter ablation in patients with multiple atrioventricular nodal reentry tachycardias. Am J Cardiol 1996; 77:52–58.

389. Suzuki F, Kawara T, Sato T, et al. Fast-slow form of "atrioventricular nodal" reentrant tachycardia suggesting atrial participation in the reentrant circuit. Am J Cardiol 1989; 63:1413–1416.

390. Chang BC, Schuessler RB, Stone CM, et al. Computerized activation sequence mapping of the human atrial septum. Ann Thorac Surg 1990; 49:231–241.

391. Keim S, Werner P, Jazayeri M, Akhtar M, Tchou P. Localization of the fast and slow pathways in atrioventricular nodal reentrant tachycardia by intraoperative ice mapping. Circulation 1992; 86:919–925.

392. Satoh M, Miyajima S, Koyama S, Ishiguro J, Okabe M. Orthodromic capture of the atrial electrogram during transient entrainment of atrioventricular nodal reentrant tachycardia. Circulation 1993; 88:2329–2336.

393. Gamache MC, Bharati S, Lev M, Lindsay BD. Histopathological study following catheter guided radiofrequency current ablation of the slow pathway in a patient with atrioventricular nodal reentrant tachycardia. Pacing Clin Electrophysiol 1994; 17:247–251.

394. Olgin JE, Ursell P, Kao AK, Lesh MD. Pathological findings following slow pathway ablation for AV nodal reentrant tachycardia. J Cardiovasc Electrophysiol 1996; 7:625–631.

395. Wu D, Denes P, Dhingra R, Pietras RJ, Rosen KM. New manifestations of dual A-V nodal pathways. Eur J Cardiol 1975; 2:459–466.

396. Josephson ME, Kastor JA. Paroxysmal supraventricular tachycardia: is the atrium a necessary link? Circulation 1976; 54:430–435.

397. Hariman RJ, Chen CM, Caracta AR, Damato AN. Evidence that AV nodal re-entrant tachycardia does not require participation of the entire AV node. Pacing Clin Electrophysiol 1983; 6:1252–1257.

398. Kerr CR, Benson DW, Gallagher JJ. Role of specialized conducting fibers in the genesis of "AV nodal" re-entry tachycardia. Pacing Clin Electrophysiol 1983; 6:171–184.

399. Portillo B, Mejias J, Leon-Portillo N, Zaman L, Myerburg RJ, Castellanos A. Entrainment of atrioventricular nodal reentrant tachycardias during overdrive pacing from high right atrium and coronary sinus. With special reference to atrioventricular dissociation and 2:1 retrograde block during tachycardias. Am J Cardiol 1984; 53:1570–1576.

400. Josephson ME, Miller JM. Atrioventricular nodal reentry: evidence supporting an intranodal location. Pacing Clin Electrophysiol 1993; 16:599–614.

401. McGuire MA, Bourke JP, Robotin MC, et al. High resolution mapping of Koch's triangle using sixty electrodes in humans with atrioventricular junctional (AV nodal) reentrant tachycardia. Circulation 1993; 88:2315–2328.

402. Prystowsky EN, Pritchett LC, Smith WM, Wallace AG, Sealy WC, Gallagher JJ. Electrophysiologic assessment of the atrioventricular conduction system after surgical correction of ventricular preexcitation. Circulation 1979; 59:789–796.

403. Bauernfeind RA, Ayres BF, Wyndham CC, et al. Cycle length in atrioventricular nodal reentrant paroxysmal tachycardia with observations on the Lown-Ganong-Levine syndrome. Am J Cardiol 1980; 45:1148–1153.

404. Sung RJ, Styperek JL, Myerburg RJ, Castellanos A. Initiation of two distinct forms of atrioventricular nodal reentrant tachycardia during programmed ventricular stimulation in man. Am J Cardiol 1978; 42:404–415.

405. Matsuhisa M, Shimomura K, Ohe T, Kamakura S, Aihara N. Double atrial and double ventricular responses during slow-fast fast-slow atrioventricular nodal reentrant tachycardia. Pacing Clin Electrophysiol 1989; 12:1381–1386.

406. Goldberger J, Brooks R, Kadish A. Physiology of "atypical" atrioventricular junctional reentrant tachycardia occurring following radiofrequency catheter modification of the atrioventricular node. Pacing Clin Electrophysiol 1992; 15:2270–2282.

407. Ross DL, Brugada P, Bar FW, et al. Comparison of right and left atrial stimulation in demonstration of dual atrioventricular nodal pathways and induction of intranodal reentry. Circulation 1981; 64:1051–1058.

408. Walter P, Lesser L. Refractory paroxysmal supraventricular tachycardia incited by multiple mechanisms. J Electrocardiol 1975; 8:343–349.

409. Wu D, Hung JS, Kuo CT. Determinants of sustained slow pathway conduction and relation to reentrant tachycardia in patients with dual atrioventricular nodal transmission. Am Heart J 1981; 101:521–528.

410. Hashimoto T, Fukatani M, Mori M, Hashiba K. Effects of standing on the induction of paroxysmal supraventricular tachycardia. J Am Coll Cardiol 1991; 17:690–695.

411. Ross DL, Brugada P, Vanagt EJ, Bar FW, Wellens HJJ. Delayed termination of re-entrant atrioventricular nodal tachycardia. Pacing Clin Electrophysiol 1983; 6:104–112.

412. Brugada P, Ross D, Bar FW, Vanagt EJ, Dassen WR, Wellens

HJJ. Observations on spontaneous termination of atrioventricular nodal reentrant tachycardia. Am J Cardiol 1981; 47:703–707.

413. Castellanos A, Zaman L, Moleiro F, Aranda JM, Myerburg RJ. The Lown-Ganong-Levine syndrome. Pacing Clin Electrophysiol 1982; 5:715–740.

414. Wiener I. Syndromes of Lown-Ganong-Levine and enhanced atrioventricular nodal conduction. Am J Cardiol 1983; 52:637–639.

415. Ward DE, Camm J. Mechanisms of junctional tachycardias in the Lown-Ganong-Levine syndrome. Am Heart J 1983; 105:169–175.

416. Castellanos A Jr, Castillo CA, Agha AS, Tessler M. His bundle electrograms in patients with short P-R intervals, narrow QRS complexes, and paroxysmal tachycardias. Circulation 1971; 43:667–678.

417. Mandel WJ, Danzig R, Hayakawa H. Lown-Ganong-Levine syndrome: a study using His bundle electrograms. Circulation 1971; 44:696–708.

418. Bissett JK, Thompson AJ, deSoyza N, Murphy ML. Atrioventricular conduction in patients with short PR intervals and normal QRS complexes. Br Heart J 1973; 35:123–127.

419. Caracta AR, Damato AN, Gallagher JJ, et al. Electrophysiologic studies in the syndrome of short P-R interval, normal QRS complex. Am J Cardiol 1973; 31:245–253.

420. Denes P, Wu D, Rosen KM. Demonstration of dual A-V pathways in a patient with Lown-Ganong-Levine syndrome. Chest 1974; 65:343–346.

421. Bissett JK, de Soyza N, Kane JJ, Murphy ML. Altered refractory periods in patients with short P-R intervals and normal QRS complex. Am J Cardiol 1975; 35:487–491.

422. Iannone LA. Electrophysiology of atrial pacing in patients with short PR interval, normal QRS complex. Am Heart J 1975; 89:74–78.

423. Befeler B, Castellanos A, Aranda J, Gutierrez R, Lazzara R. Intermittent bundle-branch block in patients with accessory atrio-His or atrio-AV nodal pathways: variants of the Lown-Ganong-Levine syndrome. Br Heart J 1976; 38:173–179.

424. Josephson ME, Kastor JA. Supraventricular tachycardia in Lown-Ganong-Levine syndrome: atrionodal versus intranodal reentry. Am J Cardiol 1977; 40:521–527.

425. Benditt DG, Pritchett LC, Smith WM, Wallace AG, Gallagher JJ. Characteristics of atrioventricular conduction and the spectrum of arrhythmias in Lown-Ganong-Levine syndrome. Circulation 1978; 57:454–465.

426. Moro C, Cosio FG. Electrophysiologic study of patients with short P-R interval and normal QRS complex. Eur J Cardiol 1980; 11:81–90.

427. Moleiro F, Mendoza IJ, Medina-Ravell V, Castellanos A, Myerburg RJ. One to one atrioventricular conduction during atrial pacing at rates of 300/minute in absence of Wolff-Parkinson-White syndrome. Am J Cardiol 1981; 48:789–796.

428. Holmes DR Jr, Hartzler GO, Merideth J. The clinical and electrophysiologic characteristics of patients with accelerated atrioventricular nodal conduction. Mayo Clin Proc 1982; 57:339–344.

429. Ward DE, Bexton R, Camm AJ. Characteristics of atrio-His conduction in the short PR interval, normal QRS complex syndrome: evidence for enhanced slow-pathway conduction. Eur Heart J 1983; 4:882–888.

430. Benditt DG, Klein GJ, Kriett JM, Dunnigan A, Benson DW. Enhanced atrioventricular nodal conduction in man: electrophysiologic effects of pharmacologic autonomic blockade. Circulation 1984; 69:1088–1095.

431. Ometto R, Thiene G, Corrado D, Vincenzi M, Rossi L. Enhanced A-V nodal conduction (Lown-Ganong-Levine syndrome) by congenitally hypoplastic A-V node. Eur Heart J 1992; 13:1579–1584.

432. Bauernfeind RA, Swiryn S, Strasberg B, et al. Analysis of anterograde and retrograde fast pathway properties in patients with dual atrioventricular nodal pathways: observations regarding the pathophysiology of the Lown-Ganong-Levine syndrome. Am J Cardiol 1982; 49:283–290.

433. Jackman WM, Prystowsky EN, Naccarelli GV, et al. Reevaluation of enhanced atrioventricular nodal conduction: evidence to suggest a continuum of normal atrioventricular nodal physiology. Circulation 1983; 67:441–448.

434. Brechenmacher C. Atrio-His bundle tracts. Br Heart J 1975; 37:853–855.

435. Vora AM, Green MS, Tang AS. An unusual mechanism of incessant supraventricular tachycardia. Pacing Clin Electrophysiol 1997; 20:982–984.

436. Doig JC, Saito J, Harris L, Downar E. Coronary sinus morphology in patients with atrioventricular junctional reentry tachycardia and other supraventricular tachyarrhythmias. Circulation 1995; 92:436–441.

437. Anselme F, Frederiks J, Papageorgiou P, et al. Nonuniform anisotropy is responsible for age-related slowing of atrioventricular nodal reentrant tachycardia. J Cardiovasc Electrophysiol 1996; 7:1145–1153.

438. Mann DE, Reiter MJ. Effects of upright posture on atrioventricular nodal reentry and dual atrioventricular nodal pathways. Am J Cardiol 1988; 62:408–412.

439. Mazgalev TN. The dual AV nodal pathways: are they dual and where are they? J Cardiovasc Electrophysiol 1997; 8:1408–1412.

440. Sung RJ. Can alteration of dual atrioventricular nodal pathway physiology be related to sinus node dysfunction? J Cardiovasc Electrophysiol 1998; 9:479–480.

441. Denes P, Wyndham CR, Wu D, Rosen KM. "Supernormal conduction" of a premature impulse utilizing the fast pathway in a patient with dual atrioventricular nodal pathways. Circulation 1975; 51:811–814.

442. Wu D, Denes P, Dhingra R, Wyndham C, Rosen KM. Determinants of fast- and slow-pathway conduction in patients with dual atrioventricular nodal pathways. Circ Res 1975; 36:782–790.

443. Amat-y-Leon F, Dhingra RC, Wu D, Denes P, Wyndham C, Rosen KM. Catheter mapping of retrograde atrial activation: observations during ventricular pacing and AV nodal re-entrant paroxysmal tachycardia. Br Heart J 1976; 38:355–362.

444. Schlepper M. Mechanisms underlying sudden changes in heart rate during paroxysmal supraventricular tachycardia. In Kulbertus HE (ed). Reentrant Arrhythmias. Mechanisms and Treatment. Baltimore: University Park Press, 1976, pp. 184–192.

445. Touboul P, Huerta F, Porte J, Delahaye JP. Reciprocal rhythm in patients with normal electrocardiogram: evidence for dual conduction pathways. Am Heart J 1976; 91:3–10.

446. Denes P, Wu D, Amat-y-Leon F, Dhingra R, Wyndham CR, Rosen KM. The determinants of atrioventricular nodal re-entrance with premature atrial stimulation in patients with dual A-V nodal pathways. Circulation 1977; 56:253–259.

447. Satake S, Heijima K, Sakamoto Y, Suzuki F, Sano T. Demonstration of bidirectional dual A-V nodal pathways in the same patient. J Electrocardiol 1977; 10:71–76.

448. Wu D, Denes P, Amat-y-Leon F, Wyndham CR, Dhingra R, Rosen KM. An unusual variety of atrioventricular nodal re-entry due to retrograde dual atrioventricular nodal pathways. Circulation 1977; 56:50–59.

449. Akhtar M, Damato A, Ruskin JN, et al. Antegrade and retrograde conduction characteristics in three patterns of paroxysmal atrioventricular junctional reentrant tachycardia. Am Heart J 1978; 95:22–42.

450. Akhtar M, Gilbert CJ, Al-Nouri M, Schmidt DH. Electrophysiologic mechanisms for modification and abolition of atrioventricular junctional tachycardia with simultaneous and sequential atrial and ventricular pacing. Circulation 1979; 60:1443–1454.

451. Sung RJ, Waxman HL, Saksena S, Juma Z. Sequence of retrograde atrial activation in patients with dual atrioventricular nodal pathways. Circulation 1981; 64:1059–1067.

452. Neuss H, Buss J, Schlepper M, Mitrovic V. Double ventricular response in dual AV nodal pathways mimicking supraventricular as well as ventricular tachycardia. Eur Heart J 1982; 3:146–154.

453. Brodine WN, Lyons C, Han J. Dual atrioventricular nodal pathways associated with a gap phenomenon in atrioventricular nodal conduction. J Am Coll Cardiol 1983; 2:582–584.

454. Sutton FJ, Lee Y. Supraventricular nonreentrant tachycardia due to simultaneous conduction through dual atrioventricular nodal pathways. Am J Cardiol 1983; 51:897–900.

455. Brugada P, Heddle B, Green M, Wellens HJJ. Initiation of atrioventricular nodal reentrant tachycardia in patients with discontinuous anterograde atrioventricular nodal conduction curves with and without documented supraventricular tachycardia: observations on the role of a discontinuous retrograde conduction curve. Am Heart J 1984; 107:685–697.

456. Lin FC, Yeh SJ, Wu D. Determinants of simultaneous fast and slow pathway conduction in patients with dual atrioventricular nodal pathways. Am Heart J 1985; 109:963–970.

457. Brugada P, Waldo AL, Wellens HJJ. Transient entrainment and interruption of atrioventricular node tachycardia. J Am Coll Cardiol 1987; 9:769–775.

458. Miller JM, Rosenthal ME, Vassallo JA, Josephson ME. Atrioventricular nodal reentrant tachycardia: studies on upper and lower "common pathways." Circulation 1987; 75:930–940.

459. Schuger CD, Steinman RT, Lehmann MH. The excitable gap in atrioventricular nodal reentrant tachycardia: characterization with ventricular extrastimuli and pharmacologic intervention. Circulation 1989; 80:324–334.

460. Henthorn RW, Waldo AL, Anderson JL, et al. Flecainide acetate prevents recurrence of symptomatic paroxysmal supraventricular tachycardia: the Flecainide Supraventricular Tachycardia Study Group. Circulation 1991; 83:119–125.

461. Wang PJ, Sosa-Suarez G, Friedman PL. Modification of human atrioventricular nodal function by selective atrioventricular nodal artery catheterization. Circulation 1990; 82:817–829.

462. Miller JM, Rosenthal ME, Gottlieb CD, Vassallo JA, Josephson ME. Usefulness of the delta HA interval to accurately distinguish atrioventricular nodal reentry from orthodromic septal bypass tract tachycardias. Am J Cardiol 1991; 68:1037–1044.

463. Schuger CD, Steinman RT, Lehmann MH. Recovery of retrograde fast pathway excitability in the atrioventricular node reentrant circuit after concealed anterograde impulse penetration. J Am Coll Cardiol 1991; 17:1129–1137.

464. Sakurada H, Sakamoto M, Hiyoshi Y, et al. Double ventricular responses to a single atrial depolarization in a patient with dual AV nodal pathways. Pacing Clin Electrophysiol 1992; 15:28–33.

465. Chien WW, Wang YS, Epstein LM, et al. Ventricular septal summit stimulation in atrioventricular nodal reentrant tachycardia. Am J Cardiol 1993; 72:1268–1273.

466. Jazayeri MR, Sra JS, Deshpande SS, et al. Electrophysiologic spectrum of atrioventricular nodal behavior in patients with atrioventricular nodal reentrant tachycardia undergoing selective fast or slow pathway ablation. J Cardiovasc Electrophysiol 1993; 4:99–111.

467. Shimizu A, Fukatani M, Centurion OA, et al. Double response of the ventricle during transient entrainment in a common atrioventricular nodal reentrant tachycardia. Pacing Clin Electrophysiol 1993; 16:39–45.

468. de Bakker JM, Coronel R, McGuire MA, et al. Slow potentials in the atrioventricular junctional area of patients operated on for atrioventricular node tachycardias and in isolated porcine hearts. J Am Coll Cardiol 1994; 23:709–715.

469. Glotzer T, Evans S, Bernstein N, Chinitz L. Specificity of retrograde conduction in screening for atrioventricular nodal reentrant tachycardia. Pacing Clin Electrophysiol 1994; 17:2134–2136.

470. Natale A, Klein G, Yee R, Thakur R. Shortening of fast pathway refractoriness after slow pathway ablation: effects of autonomic blockade. Circulation 1994; 89:1103–1108.

471. Rhodes LA, Walsh EP, Saul JP. Programmed atrial stimulation via the esophagus for management of supraventricular arrhythmias in infants and children. Am J Cardiol 1994; 74:353–356.

472. Lai WT, Lee CS, Sheu SH, Hwang YS, Sung RJ. Electrophysiological manifestations of the excitable gap of slow-fast AV nodal reentrant tachycardia demonstrated by single extrastimulation. Circulation 1995; 92:66–76.

473. Niebauer MJ, Daoud E, Williamson B, et al. Atrial electrogram characteristics in patients with and without atrioventricular nodal reentrant tachycardia. Circulation 1995; 92:77–81.

474. Wagshal AB, Huang SK, Pires LA, Mittleman RS, Greene TO, Schuger CD. Use of double ventricular extrastimulation to determine the preexcitation index in atrioventricular nodal reentrant tachycardia. Pacing Clin Electrophysiol 1995; 18:2041–2052.

475. Sheahan RG, Klein GJ, Yee R, Le Feuvre CA, Krahn AD. Atrioventricular node reentry with "smooth" AV node function curves: a different arrhythmia substrate? Circulation 1996; 93:969–972.

476. Akiyama J, Aonuma K, Ogahara S, et al. Longitudinal dissociation in the His bundle: a possible mechanism of two distinct cycle lengths in atrioventricular reentrant tachycardia. Pacing Clin Electrophysiol 1997; 20:2016–2018.

477. Haines DE, Nath S, DiMarco JP, Lobban JH. Entrainment mapping in patients with sustained atrioventricular nodal reentrant tachycardia: insights into the sites of conduction slowing in the slow atrioventricular nodal pathway. Am J Cardiol 1997; 80:883–888.

478. Lee SH, Chen SA, Tai CT, et al. Atrioventricular node reentrant tachycardia in patients with a long fast pathway effective refractory period: clinical features, electrophysiologic characteristics, and results of radiofrequency ablation. Am Heart J 1997; 134:387–394.

479. Kreiner G, Frey B, Gossinger HD. Atrioventricular nodal reentry tachycardia in patients with sinus node dysfunction: electrophysiologic characteristics, clinical presentation, and results of slow pathway ablation. J Cardiovasc Electrophysiol 1998; 9:470–478.

480. Lin LJ, Lin JL, Lai LP, Chen JH, Tseng YZ, Lien WP. Effects of pharmacological autonomic blockade on dual atrioventricular nodal pathways: physiology in patients with slow-fast atrioventricular nodal reentrant tachycardia. PACE 1998; 21:1375–1379.

481. Young C, Lauer MR, Liem B, Chun H, Sung RJ. Demonstration of a posterior atrial input to the atrioventricular node during sustained anterograde slow pathway conduction. J Am Coll Cardiol 1998; 31:1615–1621.

482. Castellanos A Jr, Castillo C, Cunha D, Myerburg RJ. Value of His bundle recordings in the evaluation of the pre-excitation (Wolff-Parkinson-White) syndrome. Proc Koninklijke Ned Akad Wetenschappen 1972; 75:402–421.

483. Castellanos A Jr, Castillo CA, Martinez A, Agha AS. Mechanisms of AV conduction in ventricular pre-excitation. In Schlandt RC, Hurst JW (eds). Advances in Electrocardiography. Orlando, Florida, Grune & Stratton, 1972, pp. 249–258.

484. Moore EN, Spear JF, Boineau JP. Recent electrophysiologic studies on the Wolff-Parkinson-White syndrome. N Engl J Med 1973; 289:956–963.

485. Wellens HJJ. Contribution of cardiac pacing to our understanding of the Wolff-Parkinson-White syndrome. Br Heart J 1975; 37:231–241.

486. Touboul P, Gressard A, Vexler RM, Chatelain MT. Unusual re-entrant tachycardias associated with accessory pathways. In Kulbertus HE (ed). Reentrant Arrhythmias. Mechanisms and Treatment. Baltimore: University Park Press, 1976, pp. 132–143.

487. Wallace AG, Sealy WC, Gallagher JJ, Kasell J. Ventricular excitation in the Wolff-Parkinson-White syndrome. In Wellens HJJ, Lie KI, Janse MJ (eds). The Conduction System of the Heart. Structure, Function and Clinical Implications. Philadelphia: Lea & Febiger, 1976, pp. 613–630.

488. Wellens HJJ, Farre J, Bar FW. Wolff Parkinson-White syndrome: value and limitations of programmed electrical

stimulation. In Narula OS (ed). Cardiac Arrhythmias. Electrophysiology, Diagnosis and Management. Baltimore: Williams & Wilkins, 1979, pp. 589–617.

489. German LD, Gallagher JJ. Functional properties of accessory atrioventricular pathways in Wolff-Parkinson-White syndrome: clinical implications. Am J Med 1984; 76:1079–1086.

490. Waldo AL, Akhtar M, Benditt DG, et al. Appropriate electrophysiologic study and treatment of patients with the Wolff-Parkinson-White syndrome. J Am Coll Cardiol 1988; 11:1124–1129.

491. Cain ME, Luke RA, Lindsay BD. Diagnosis and localization of accessory pathways. Pacing Clin Electrophysiol 1992; 15:801–824.

492. Josephson ME. Clinical Cardiac Electrophysiology. Techniques and Interpretations. 2nd ed. Philadelphia: Lea & Febiger, 1993, pp. 71–95.

493. Callans DJ, Schwartzman D, Gottlieb CD, Marchlinski FE. Insights into the electrophysiology of accessory pathway-mediated arrhythmias provided by the catheter ablation experience: "learning while burning, part III." J Cardiovasc Electrophysiol 1996; 7:877–904.

494. Li H, Easley A, Windle J. Problematic palpitations and exercise induced preexcitation. Pacing Clin Electrophysiol 1997; 20:122–124.

495. Anderson RH, Becker AE, Brechenmacher C, Davies MJ, Rossi L. Ventricular preexcitation: a proposed nomenclature for its substrates. Eur J Cardiol 1975; 3:27–36.

496. Benditt DG, Epstein ML, Arentzen CE, Kriett JM, Klein GJ. Enhanced atrioventricular conduction in patients without preexcitation syndrome: relation to heart rate in paroxysmal reciprocating tachycardia. Circulation 1982; 65:1474–1479.

497. Rosen KM, Bauernfeind RA, Strasberg B, Duffy E. Electrocardiographic diagnosis of dual AV nodal pathways complicating the Wolff-Parkinson-White syndrome. Chest 1982; 81:639–642.

498. Rosenfeld LE, Batsford WP. Two accessory pathways, dual AV nodal conduction, and 1:2 ventriculoatrial conduction in a patient with multiple supraventricular tachycardias. Pacing Clin Electrophysiol 1990; 13:171–178.

499. Milstein S, Sharma AD, Klein GJ. Electrophysiologic profile of asymptomatic Wolff-Parkinson-White pattern. Am J Cardiol 1986; 57:1097–1100.

500. Leitch JW, Klein GJ, Yee R, Murdock C. Prognostic value of electrophysiology testing in asymptomatic patients with Wolff-Parkinson-White pattern. Circulation 1990; 82:1718–1723.

501. Gillette PC, Garson A Jr, Cooley DA, McNamara DG. Prolonged and decremental antegrade conduction properties in right anterior accessory connections: wide QRS antidromic tachycardia of left bundle branch block pattern without Wolff-Parkinson-White configuration in sinus rhythm. Am Heart J 1982; 103:66–74.

502. Inoue H, Matsuo H, Takayanagi K, Ishimitsu T, Murao S. Antidromic reciprocating tachycardia via a slow Kent bundle in Ebstein's anomaly. Am Heart J 1983; 106:147–149.

503. Kuck KH, Brugada P, Wellens HJJ. Observations on the antidromic type of circus movement tachycardia in the Wolff-Parkinson-White syndrome. J Am Coll Cardiol 1983; 2:1003–1010.

504. Bardy GH, Packer DL, German LD, Gallagher JJ. Preexcited reciprocating tachycardia in patients with Wolff-Parkinson-White syndrome: incidence and mechanisms. Circulation 1984; 70:377–391.

505. Wellens HJJ. Personal communication, 1984.

506. Denes P, Wyndham CR, Rosen KM. Intractable paroxysmal tachycardia caused by a concealed retrogradely conducting Kent bundle: demonstration by epicardial mapping and cure of tachycardias by surgical interruption of the His bundle. Br Heart J 1976; 38:758–763.

507. Gould L, Ramana Reddy CV, Del Nunzio R. Recurrent tachycardias due to an accessory pathway. J Electrocardiol 1976; 9:259–264.

508. Pritchett EL, Tonkin AM, Dugan FA, Wallace AG, Gallagher JJ. Ventriculo-atrial conduction time during reciprocating tachycardia with intermittent bundle-branch block in Wolff-Parkinson-White syndrome. Br Heart J 1976; 38:1058–1064.

509. Gillette PC. Concealed anomalous cardiac conduction pathways: a frequent cause of supraventricular tachycardia. Am J Cardiol 1977; 40:848–852.

510. Orzan F, Gillette PC. Reciprocating tachycardia due to a right-sided unidirectional retrograde anomalous pathway (URAP). Pacing Clin Electrophysiol 1978; 1:306–312.

511. Salerno JA, Tavazzi L, Chimienti M, Ray M, Bobba P. Paroxysmal atrioventricular tachycardia involving an anomalous pathway with antegrade unidirectional block. Eur J Cardiol 1979; 9:285–305.

512. Holmes DR Jr, Hartzler GO, Maloney JD. Concealed retrograde bypass tracts and enhanced atrioventricular nodal conduction: an unusual subset of patients with refractory paroxysmal supraventricular tachycardia. Am J Cardiol 1980; 45:1053–1060.

513. Ito M, Shinoda S, Nagashima M, Chimori K, Kinoshita Y, Suzuki H. Electrophysiological diagnosis of participation of accessory pathway in patients with paroxysmal supraventricular tachycardia. Jpn Circ J 1981; 45:472–482.

514. Ohe T, Kamakura S, Matsuhisa M, Hirata Y, Sato I, Shimomura K. Limiting factor for the initiation of reentrant tachycardia in concealed Wolff-Parkinson-White syndrome. Int J Cardiol 1983; 3:207–213.

515. Hariman RJ, Kvaternik D, Chen CM, Caracta AR, Damato AN. Paroxysmal supraventricular tachycardia utilizing concealed bypass tract induced by ventricular pacemaker. Am J Cardiol 1983; 52:1149–1151.

516. Henglein D, Gillette PC, Garson A Jr, Porter CJ. Antegrade conduction and AV node function in patients with unidirectional retrograde accessory pathways. Am Heart J 1984; 107:411–417.

517. Steinbeck G, Bach P, Haberl R, Markewitz A. Ventricular preexcitation following catheter ablation of the His bundle in concealed WPW syndrome. Eur Heart J 1986; 7:444–448.

518. Suzuki F, Kawara T, Tanaka K, et al. Electrophysiological demonstration of anterograde concealed conduction in accessory atrioventricular pathways capable only of retrograde conduction. Pacing Clin Electrophysiol 1989; 12:591–603.

519. Martinez-Alday JD, Almendral J, Arenal A, et al. Identification of concealed posteroseptal Kent pathways by comparison of ventriculoatrial intervals from apical and posterobasal right ventricular sites. Circulation 1994; 89:1060–1067.

520. Kuck KH, Friday KJ, Kunze KP, Schluter M, Lazzara R, Jackman WM. Sites of conduction block in accessory atrioventricular pathways: basis for concealed accessory pathways. Circulation 1990; 82:407–417.

521. Krikler D, Curry P. Atypical initiation of reciprocating tachycardia in the Wolff-Parkinson-White syndrome. In Kulbertus HE (ed). Re-entrant Arrhythmias. Mechanisms and Treatment. Baltimore: University Park Press, 1976, pp. 144–152.

522. Wellens HJJ. Modes of initiation of circus movement tachycardia in 139 patients with the Wolff-Parkinson-White syndrome studied by programmed electrical stimulation. In Kulbertus HE (ed). Re-entrant arrhythmias. Mechanisms and Treatment. Baltimore: University Park Press, 1976, pp. 153–169.

523. Denes P, Wu D, Amat-y-Leon F, et al. Determinants of atrioventricular reentrant paroxysmal tachycardia in patients with Wolff-Parkinson-White syndrome. Circulation 1978; 58:415–425.

524. Kuck KH, Kunze KP, Schluter M, Bleifeld W. Tachycardia prevention by programmed stimulation. Am J Cardiol 1984; 54:550–554.

525. Kuck KH, Kunze KP, Schluter M, Bleifeld W. Prevention of reentrant tachycardia by single beat or repetitive stimulation. Eur Heart J 1985; 6:67–74.

526. Odakura H, Ito M, Namekawa A, et al. Effect of intraatrial reentry on initiation of atrioventricular reentrant tachycardia. Pacing Clin Electrophysiol 1996; 19:1070–1074.

527. Akhtar M, Shenasa M, Schmidt DH. Role of retrograde His

Purkinje block in the initiation of supraventricular tachycardia by ventricular premature stimulation in the Wolff-Parkinson-White syndrome. J Clin Invest 1981; 67:1047–1055.

528. Akhtar M, Lehmann MH, Denker ST, Mahmud R, Tchou P, Jazayeri M. Electrophysiologic mechanisms of orthodromic tachycardia initiation during ventricular pacing in the Wolff-Parkinson-White syndrome. J Am Coll Cardiol 1987; 9:89–100.

529. Wellens HJJ, Schuilenberg RM, Durrer D. Electrical stimulation of the heart in patients with Wolff-Parkinson-White syndrome, type A. Circulation 1971; 43:99–114.

530. Krikler D, Curry P, Attuel P, Coumel P. "Incessant" tachycardias in Wolff-Parkinson-White syndrome. I. Initiation without antecedent extrasystoles or PR lengthening, with reference to reciprocation after shortening of cycle length. Br Heart J 1976; 38:885–896.

531. Coumel P, Attuel P, Slama R, Curry P, Krikler D. "Incessant" tachycardias in Wolff-Parkinson-White syndrome. II. Role of atypical cycle length dependency and nodal-His escape beats in initiating reciprocating tachycardias. Br Heart J 1976; 38:897–905.

532. Milstein S, Sharma AD, Klein GJ. Nonclinical ventricular tachycardia in the Wolff-Parkinson-White syndrome. PACE 1985; 8:678–683.

533. Ross DL, Farre J, Bar FW, et al. Spontaneous termination of circus movement tachycardia using an atrioventricular accessory pathway: incidence, site of block and mechanisms. Circulation 1981; 63:1129–1139.

534. Lai WT, Huycke EC, Keung EC, Nguyen NX, Tseng CD, Sung RJ. Electrophysiologic manifestations of the excitable gap of orthodromic atrioventricular reciprocating tachycardia demonstrated by single extrastimulation. Am J Cardiol 1989; 63:545–555.

535. Kerr CR, Gallagher JJ, German LD. Changes in ventriculoatrial intervals with bundle branch block aberration during reciprocating tachycardia in patients with accessory atrioventricular pathways. Circulation 1982; 66:196–201.

536. Calkins H. Personal communication, 1998.

537. Levine HD, Smith C Jr. Repetitive paroxysmal tachycardia in adults. Cardiology 1970; 55:2–21.

538. Klein GJ, Yee R, Guiraudon G. Accessory pathways with decremental properties. In Josephson ME, Wellens HJJ (eds). Tachycardias. Mechanisms and Management. Mount Kisco, NY: Futura Publishing Co., 1993, pp. 297–312.

539. Deng Z, Rosenthal ME, Oseran DS, Gang ES, Mandel WJ, Peter T. Retrograde Wenckebach conduction in atrioventricular bypass tracts: further evidence for AV nodal-like conduction in accessory pathways. Am Heart J 1985; 110:1074–1077.

540. Klein GJ, Prystowsky EN, Pritchett EL, Davis D, Gallagher JJ. Atypical patterns of retrograde conduction over accessory atrioventricular pathways in the Wolff-Parkinson-White syndrome. Circulation 1979; 60:1477–1486.

541. Murdock CJ, Leitch JW, Teo WS, Sharma AD, Yee R, Klein GJ. Characteristics of accessory pathways exhibiting decremental conduction. Am J Cardiol 1991; 67:506–510.

542. Farre J, Ross D, Weiner I, Bar FW, Vanagt EJ, Wellens HJJ. Reciprocal tachycardias using accessory pathways with long conduction times. Am J Cardiol 1979; 44:1099–1109.

543. Anderson RH, Ho SY. Anatomy of the atrioventricular junctions with regard to ventricular preexcitation. Pacing Clin Electrophysiol 1997; 20:2072–2076.

544. Kottkamp H, Hindricks G, Shenasa H, et al. Variants of preexcitation—specialized atriofascicular pathways, nodofascicular pathways, and fasciculoventricular pathways: electrophysiologic findings and target sites for radiofrequency catheter ablation. J Cardiovasc Electrophysiol 1996; 7:916–930.

545. Kou WH, Morady F, de Buitleir M, Nelson SD. Electrophysiologic demonstration of an atriofascicular accessory pathway. Pacing Clin Electrophysiol 1988; 11:166–173.

546. Tchou P, Lehmann MH, Jazayeri M, Akhtar M.

Atriofascicular connection or a nodoventricular Mahaim fiber? Electrophysiologic elucidation of the pathway and associated reentrant circuit. Circulation 1988; 77:837–848.

547. Okishige K, Friedman PL. New observations on decremental atriofascicular and nodofascicular fibers: implications for catheter ablation. Pacing Clin Electrophysiol 1995; 18:986–998.

548. Mecca A, Telfer A, Lanzarotti C, Olshansky B. Symptomatic atrioventricular block in an atriofascicular pathway inserting into the left bundle branch without apparent atrioventricular node function. J Cardiovasc Electrophysiol 1997; 8:922–926.

549. Kreiner G, Heinz G, Frey B, Gossinger HD. Demonstration of retrograde conduction over an atriofascicular accessory pathway. J Cardiovasc Electrophysiol 1997; 8:74–79.

550. Castellanos A, Agha AS, Befeler B, Myerburg RJ. Double accessory pathways in Wolff-Parkinson-White syndrome. Circulation 1975; 51:1020–1025.

551. Ward DE, Camm AJ, Spurrell RA. Ventricular preexcitation due to anomalous nodo-ventricular pathways: report of 3 patients. Eur J Cardiol 1979; 9:111–127.

552. Gallagher JJ, Smith WM, Kasell JH, Benson DW, Sterba R, Grant AO. Role of Mahaim fibers in cardiac arrhythmias in man. Circulation 1981; 64:176–189.

553. Morady F, Scheinman MM, Gonzalez R, Hess D. His-ventricular dissociation in a patient with reciprocating tachycardia and a nodoventricular bypass tract. Circulation 1981; 64:839–844.

554. Zaman L, Garcia N, Luceri RM, Castellanos A, Myerburg RJ. Ectopic left atrial rhythm that produces QRS changes in absence of Wolff-Parkinson-White syndrome. Circulation 1983; 68:701–706.

555. Benditt DG, Epstein ML, Benson DW Jr. Dual accessory nodoventricular pathways: role in paroxysmal wide QRS reciprocating tachycardia. Pacing Clin Electrophysiol 1983; 6:577–586.

556. Gmeiner R, Ng CK, Hammer I, Becker AE. Tachycardia caused by an accessory nodoventricular tract: a clinco-pathologic correlation. Eur Heart J 1984; 5:233–242.

557. Ellenbogen KA, Ramirez NM, Packer DL, et al. Accessory nodoventricular (Mahaim) fibers: a clinical review. Pacing Clin Electrophysiol 1986; 9:868–884.

558. Klein GJ, Guiraudon GM, Kerr CR, et al. "Nodoventricular" accessory pathway: evidence for a distinct accessory atrioventricular pathway with atrioventricular node-like properties. J Am Coll Cardiol 1988; 11:1035–1040.

559. Grogin HR, Lee RJ, Kwasman M, et al. Radiofrequency catheter ablation of atriofascicular and nodoventricular Mahaim tracts. Circulation 1994; 90:272–281.

560. Andersen HR, Nielsen JC. Pacing in sick sinus syndrome: need for a prospective, randomized trial comparing atrial with dual chamber pacing. PACE 1998; 21:1175–1179.

561. Touboul P, Vexler RM, Chatelain MT. Re-entry via Mahaim fibres as a possible basis for tachycardia. Br Heart J 1978; 40:806–811.

562. Lerman BB, Waxman HL, Proclemer A, Josephson ME. Supraventricular tachycardia associated with nodoventricular and concealed atrioventricular bypass tracts. Am Heart J 1982; 104:1097–1102.

563. Hamdan MH, Page RL, Scheinman MM. Diagnostic approach to narrow complex tachycardia with VA block. PACE 1997; 20:2984–2988.

564. Hamdan MH, Kalman JM, Lesh MD, et al. Narrow complex tachycardia with VA block: diagnostic and therapeutic implications. PACE 1998; 21:1196–1206.

565. Tonkin AM, Dugan FA, Svenson RH, Sealy WC, Wallace AG, Gallagher JJ. Coexistence of functional Kent and Mahaim-type tracts in the pre-excitation syndrome: demonstration by catheter techniques and epicardial mapping. Circulation 1975; 52:193–200.

566. Kuo CT, Lauer MR, Young C, et al. Role of atrial extrastimulation in the diagnosis of atrioventricular node reentrant tachycardia with antegrade atrioventricular conduction via bystander accessory connection. Am Heart J 1996; 131:839–842.

567. Coumel P, Waynberger M, Fabiato A, Slama R, Aigueperse J, Bouvrain Y. Wolff-Parkinson-White syndrome: problems in evaluation of multiple accessory pathways and surgical therapy. Circulation 1972; 45:1216–1230.
568. Denes P, Amat-y-Leon F, Wyndham C, Wu D, Levitsky S, Rosen KM. Electrophysiologic demonstration of bilateral anomalous pathways in a patient with Wolff-Parkinson-White syndrome (type B preexcitation). Am J Cardiol 1976; 37:93–101.
569. Cinca J, Valle V, Gutierrez L, Figueras J, Rius J. Reciprocating tachycardia using bilateral anomalous pathways: electrophysiologic and clinical implications. Circulation 1980; 62:657–661.
570. Kaku T, Fukatani M, Kiya F, Hashiba K. Wolff-Parkinson-White syndrome with bilateral accessory pathways both exhibiting antegrade and retrograde conduction. Am Heart J 1981; 102:296–299.
571. Heddle WF, Brugada P, Wellens HJJ. Multiple circus movement tachycardias with multiple accessory pathways. J Am Coll Cardiol 1984; 4:168–175.
572. Murabit I, Sosa E, Pileggi F, Denes P. Multiple reentry tachycardia in patients with ventricular preexcitation: report of three cases. Am Heart J 1986; 111:69–80.
573. Colavita PG, Packer DL, Pressley JC, et al. Frequency, diagnosis and clinical characteristics of patients with multiple accessory atrioventricular pathways. Am J Cardiol 1987; 59:601–606.
574. Fananapazir L, German LD, Gallagher JJ, Lowe JE, Prystowsky EN. Importance of preexcited QRS morphology during induced atrial fibrillation to the diagnosis and localization of multiple accessory pathways. Circulation 1990; 81:578–585.
575. Wellens HJJ, Atie J, Smeets JL, Cruz FE, Gorgels AP, Brugada P. The electrocardiogram in patients with multiple accessory atrioventricular pathways. J Am Coll Cardiol 1990; 16:745–751.
576. Chen SA, Hsia CP, Chiang CE, et al. Reappraisal of radiofrequency ablation of multiple accessory pathways. Am Heart J 1993; 125:760–771.
577. Levine JC, Walsh EP, Saul JP. Radiofrequency ablation of accessory pathways associated with congenital heart disease including heterotaxy syndrome. Am J Cardiol 1993; 72:689–693.
578. Yeh SJ, Wang CC, Wen MS, Lin FC, Wu D. Radiofrequency ablation in multiple accessory pathways and the physiologic implications. Am J Cardiol 1993; 71:1174–1180.
579. Iesaka Y, Yamane T, Takahashi A, et al. Retrograde multiple and multifiber accessory pathway conduction in the Wolff-Parkinson-White syndrome: potential precipitating factor of atrial fibrillation. J Cardiovasc Electrophysiol 1998; 9:141–151.
580. Boineau JP, Moore EN, Sealy WC, Kasell JH. Epicardial mapping in Wolff-Parkinson-White syndrome. Arch Intern Med 1975; 135:422–431.
581. Gallagher JJ, Sealy WC, Wallace AG, Kasell J. Correlation between catheter electrophysiological studies and findings on mapping of ventricular excitation in the W.P.W. syndrome. In Wellens HJJ, Lie KI, Janse MJ (eds). The Conduction System of the Heart. Structure, Function and Clinical Implications. Philadelphia: Lea & Febiger, 1976, pp. 588–612.
582. Gallagher JJ, Kasell J, Sealy WC, Pritchett EL, Wallace AG. Epicardial mapping in the Wolff-Parkinson-White syndrome. Circulation 1978; 57:854–866.
583. Gallagher JJ, Sealy WC, Kasell J. Intraoperative mapping studies in the Wolff-Parkinson-White syndrome. Pacing Clin Electrophysiol 1979; 2:523–537.
584. Klein GJ, Guiraudon GM. Surgical therapy of cardiac arrhythmias. Cardiol Clin 1983; 1:323–340.
585. Gallagher JJ. Localization of accessory atrioventricular pathways: what's the "gold standard"? Pacing Clin Electrophysiol 1987; 10:583–584.
586. Szabo TS, Klein GJ, Guiraudon GM, Yee R, Sharma AD. Localization of accessory pathways in the Wolff-Parkinson-White syndrome. Pacing Clin Electrophysiol 1989; 12:1691–1705.
587. Denes P, Wyndham CR, Amat-y-Leon F, et al. Atrial pacing at multiple sites in the Wolff-Parkinson-White syndrome. Br Heart J 1977; 39:506–514.
588. Gallagher JJ, Pritchett EL, Benditt DG, et al. New catheter techniques for analysis of the sequence of retrograde atrial activation in man. Eur J Cardiol 1977; 6:1–14.
589. Ward DE, Camm AJ, Spurrell RA. Patterns of atrial activation during right ventricular pacing in patients with concealed left-sided Kent pathways. Br Heart J 1979; 42:192–200.
590. Mitchell LB, Mason JW, Scheinman MM, Winkle RA, Burchell HB. Recordings of basal ventricular preexcitation from electrode catheters in patients with accessory atrioventricular connections. Circulation 1984; 69:233–241.
591. Lacombe P, Sadr-Ameli MA, Page P, Cardinal R, Nadeau RA, Shenasa M. Catheter recording of left atrial activation from left pulmonary artery in the Wolff-Parkinson-White syndrome: validation of the technique with intraoperative mapping results. Pacing Clin Electrophysiol 1988; 11:2168–2179.
592. Jackman WM, Friday KJ, Fitzgerald DM, Bowman AJ, Yeung-Lai-Wai JA, Lazzara R. Localization of left free-wall and posteroseptal accessory atrioventricular pathways by direct recording of accessory pathway activation. Pacing Clin Electrophysiol 1989; 12:204–214.
593. Packer DL, Ellenbogen KA, Colavita PG, O'Callaghan WG, German LD, Prystowsky EN. Utility of introducing ventricular premature complexes during reciprocating tachycardia in specifying the location of left free wall accessory pathways. Am J Cardiol 1989; 63:49–57.
594. Cappato R, Schluter M, Weiss C, Willems S, Meinertz T, Kuck KH. Mapping of the coronary sinus and great cardiac vein using a 2-French electrode catheter and a right femoral approach. J Cardiovasc Electrophysiol 1997; 8:371–376.
595. Durrer D, Roos JP. Epicardial excitation of the ventricles in a patient with Wolff-Parkinson-White syndrome (type B). Circulation 1967; 35:15–21.
596. Boineau JP, Moore EN. Evidence for propagation of activation across an accessory atrioventricular connection in types A and B pre-excitation. Circulation 1970; 41:375–397.
597. Lister JW, Worthington FX Jr, Gentsch TO, Swenson JA, Nathan DA, Gosselin AJ. Preexcitation and tachycardias in Wolff-Parkinson-White syndrome, type B: a case report. Circulation 1972; 45:1081–1090.
598. Sealy WC, Gallagher JJ, Pritchett EL. The surgical anatomy of Kent bundles based on electrophysiological mapping and surgical exploration. J Thorac Cardiovasc Surg 1978; 76:804–815.
599. Kramer JB, Corr PB, Cox JL, Witkowski FX, Cain ME. Simultaneous computer mapping to facilitate intraoperative localization of accessory pathways in patients with Wolff-Parkinson-White syndrome. Am J Cardiol 1985; 56:571–576.
600. Vidaillet HJ Jr, Lowe JE, German LD, et al. Computer-assisted intraoperative mapping of the entire ventricular epicardium in the Wolff-Parkinson-White syndrome. Am J Cardiol 1986; 58:940–948.
601. Guiraudon GM, Klein GJ, Sharma AD, Yee R, Pineda EA. "Atypical" posteroseptal accessory pathway in Wolff-Parkinson-White syndrome. J Am Coll Cardiol 1988; 12:1605–1608.
602. Murdock CJ, Leitch JW, Klein GJ, Guiraudon GM, Yee R, Teo WS. Epicardial mapping in patients with "nodoventricular" accessory pathways. Am J Cardiol 1991; 68:208–214.
603. De Ambroggi L, Taccardi B, Macchi E. Body-surface maps of heart potentials: tentative localization of pre-excited areas in forty-two Wolff-Parkinson-White patients. Circulation 1976; 54:251–263.
604. Oguri H. Experimental and clinical study of WPW syndrome: detection of preexcitation site through the use of body surface maps. Jpn Circ J 1978; 42:65–75.
605. Giorgi C, Nadeau R, Savard P, Shenasa M, Page PL, Cardinal R. Body surface isopotential mapping of the entire QRST complex in the Wolff-Parkinson-White syndrome: correlation with the location of the accessory pathway. Am Heart J 1991; 121:1445–1453.

606. Liebman J, Zeno JA, Olshansky B, et al. Electrocardiographic body surface potential mapping in the Wolff-Parkinson-White syndrome. Noninvasive determination of the ventricular insertion sites of accessory atrioventricular connections. Circulation 1991; 83:886–901.
607. Dubuc M, Nadeau R, Tremblay G, Kus T, Molin F, Savard P. Pace mapping using body surface potential maps to guide catheter ablation of accessory pathways in patients with Wolff-Parkinson-White syndrome. Circulation 1993; 87:135–143.
608. Akahoshi M, Hirai M, Inden Y, et al. Body-surface distribution of changes in activation-recovery intervals before and after catheter ablation in patients with Wolff-Parkinson-White syndrome: clinical evidence for ventricular "electrical remodeling" with prolongation of action-potential duration over a preexcited area. Circulation 1997; 96:1566–1574.
609. Chan WW, Kalff V, Dick M II, et al. Topography of preemptying ventricular segments in patients with Wolff-Parkinson-White syndrome using scintigraphic phase mapping and esophageal pacing. Circulation 1983; 67:1139–1146.
610. Weismuller P, Abraham-Fuchs K, Schneider S, et al. Biomagnetic noninvasive localization of accessory pathways in Wolff-Parkinson-White syndrome. Pacing Clin Electrophysiol 1991; 14:1961–1965.
611. Weismuller P, Abraham-Fuchs K, Schneider S, Richter P, Kochs M, Hombach V. Magnetocardiographic non-invasive localization of accessory pathways in the Wolff-Parkinson-White syndrome by a multichannel system. Eur Heart J 1992; 13:616–622.
612. Makijarvi M, Nenonen J, Toivonen L, Montonen J, Katila T, Siltanen P. Magnetocardiography: supraventricular arrhythmias and preexcitation syndromes. Eur Heart J 1993; 14:46–52.
613. Nenonen J, Makijarvi M, Toivonen L, et al. Non-invasive magnetocardiographic localization of ventricular pre-excitation in the Wolff-Parkinson-White syndrome using a realistic torso model. Eur Heart J 1993; 14:168–174.
614. Weismuller P, Clausen M, Weller R, et al. Non-invasive three-dimensional localization of arrhythmogenic foci in Wolff-Parkinson-White syndrome and in ventricular tachycardia by radionuclide ventriculography: phase analysis of double-angulated integrated single photon emission computed tomography (SPECT). Br Heart J 1993; 69:201–210.
615. Gepstein L, Evans SJ. Electroanatomical mapping of the heart: basic concepts and implications for the treatment of cardiac arrhythmias. PACE 1998; 21:1268–1278.
616. Nakagawa H, Jackman WM. Use of a three-dimensional, nonfluoroscopic mapping system for catheter ablation of typical atrial flutter. PACE 1998; 21:1279–1286.
617. Smeets JLRM, Ben-Haim SA, Rodriguez LM, Timmermans C, Wellens HJJ. New method for nonfluoroscopic endocardial mapping in humans: accuracy assessment and first clinical results. Circulation 1998; 97:2426–2432.
618. Gallagher JJ, Smith WM, Kasell J, Grant AO, Benson DW Jr. Use of the esophageal lead in the diagnosis of mechanisms of reciprocating supraventricular tachycardia. Pacing Clin Electrophysiol 1980; 3:440–451.
619. Gallagher JJ, Smith WM, Kerr CR, et al. Esophageal pacing: a diagnostic and therapeutic tool. Circulation 1982; 65:336–341.
620. Ward DE, Camm AJ. Ventriculo-atrial conduction over accessory pathways exhibiting decremental properties. Eur Heart J 1982; 3:267–275.
621. Benson DW Jr, Dunnigan A, Benditt DG, Pritzker MR, Thompson TR. Transesophageal study of infant supraventricular tachycardia: electrophysiologic characteristics. Am J Cardiol 1983; 52:1002–1006.
622. Critelli G, Grassi G, Perticone F, Coltorti F, Monda V, Condorelli M. Transesophageal pacing for prognostic evaluation of preexcitation syndrome and assessment of protective therapy. Am J Cardiol 1983; 51:513–518.
623. Benson DW Jr, Dunnigan A, Benditt DG, Thompson TR, Narayan A, Boros S. Prediction of digoxin treatment failure in infants with supraventricular tachycardia: role of transesophageal pacing. Pediatrics 1985; 75:288–293.
624. Gonzalez MD, Guillen RH, Pellizzon OA, Raimondi EC. Study of Wolff-Parkinson-White syndrome by transesophageal pacing and assessment of long-term amiodarone therapy. Am J Cardiol 1985; 55:852–856.
625. Butto F, Dunnigan A, Overholt ED, Benditt DG, Benson DW Jr. Transesophageal study of recurrent atrial tachycardia after atrial baffle procedures for complete transposition of the great arteries. Am J Cardiol 1986; 57:1356–1362.
626. Schnittger I, Rodriguez IM, Winkle RA. Esophageal electrocardiography: a new technology revives an old technique. Am J Cardiol 1986; 57:604–607.
627. Dick M II, Scott WA, Serwer GS, et al. Acute termination of supraventricular tachyarrhythmias in children by transesophageal atrial pacing. Am J Cardiol 1988; 61:925–927.
628. Pongiglione G, Saul JP, Dunnigan A, Strasburger JF, Benson DW. Role of transesophageal pacing in evaluation of palpitations in children and adolescents. Am J Cardiol 1988; 62:566–570.
629. Vergara G, Furlanello F, Disertori M, et al. Induction of supraventricular tachyarrhythmia at rest and during exercise with transesophageal atrial pacing in the electrophysiological evaluation of asymptomatic athletes with Wolff-Parkinson-White syndrome. Eur Heart J 1988; 9:1119–1125.
630. Zales VR, Dunnigan A, Benson DW. Clinical and electrophysiologic features of fetal and neonatal paroxysmal atrial tachycardia resulting in congestive heart failure. Am J Cardiol 1988; 62:225–228.
631. Goldstein M, Dunnigan A, Milstein S, Benson DW. Bundle branch block during orthodromic reciprocating tachycardia onset in infants. Am J Cardiol 1989; 63:301–306.
632. Silberbach M, Dunnigan A, Benson DW. Effect of intravenous propranolol or verapamil on infant orthodromic reciprocating tachycardia. Am J Cardiol 1989; 63:438–442.
633. Colloridi V, Boscioni M, Patruno N, Pulignano G, Critelli G. Transesophageal electropharmacologic test in a newborn with familial Wolff-Parkinson-White syndrome. Pediatr Cardiol 1990; 11:213–215.
634. Brembilla-Perrot B, Spatz F, Khaldi E, Terrier de la Chaise A, Le Van D, Pernot C. Value of esophageal pacing in evaluation of supraventricular tachycardia. Am J Cardiol 1990; 65:322–330.
635. Brembilla-Perrot B. Study of P wave morphology in lead V_1 during supraventricular tachycardia for localizing the reentrant circuit. Am Heart J 1991; 121:1714–1720.
636. Drago F, Turchetta A, Calzolari A, et al. Detection of atrial tachyarrhythmias by transesophageal pacing and recording at rest and during exercise in children with ventricular preexcitation. Am J Cardiol 1992; 69:1098–1099.
637. Guarnerio M, Furlanello F, Vergara G, et al. Electropharmacological testing by transesophageal atrial pacing in inducible supraventricular tachyarrhythmias: a good approach for selection of long-term anti-arrhythmic therapy. Eur Heart J 1992; 13:763–769.
638. Vignati G, Mauri L, Lunati M, Gasparini M, Figini A. Transesophageal electrophysiological evaluation of paediatric patients with Wolff-Parkinson-White syndrome. Eur Heart J 1992; 13:220–222.
639. Brembilla-Perrot B, Ghawi R. Electrophysiological characteristics of asymptomatic Wolff-Parkinson-White syndrome. Eur Heart J 1993; 14:511–515.
640. Drago F, Turchetta A, Calzolari A, et al. Detection of atrial vulnerability by transesophageal atrial pacing and the relation of symptoms in children with Wolff-Parkinson-White syndrome and in a symptomatic control group. Am J Cardiol 1994; 74:400–401.
641. D'Este D, Pasqual A, Bertaglia M, et al. Evaluation of atrial vulnerability with transesophageal stimulation in patients with atrioventricular junctional reentrant tachycardia: comparison with patients with ventricular pre-excitation and with normal subjects. Eur Heart J 1995; 16:1632–1636.
642. Samson RA, Deal BJ, Strasburger JF, Benson DW Jr. Comparison of transesophageal and intracardiac

electrophysiologic studies in characterization of supraventricular tachycardia in pediatric patients. J Am Coll Cardiol 1995; 26:159–163.

643. Fenici R, Ruggieri MP, di Lillo M, Fenici P. Reproducibility of transesophageal pacing in patients with Wolff-Parkinson-White syndrome. Pacing Clin Electrophysiol 1996; 19:1951–1957.

644. Weindling SN, Saul JP, Walsh EP. Efficacy and risks of medical therapy for supraventricular tachycardia in neonates and infants. Am Heart J 1996; 131:66–72.

645. Josephson ME. Clinical Cardiac Electrophysiology. Techniques and Interpretations. 2nd ed. Philadelphia: Lea & Febiger, 1993, pp. 311–416.

646. Miles WM, Klein LS, Rardon DP, Mitrani RD, Zipes DP. Atrioventricular reentry and variants: mechanisms, clinical features, and management. In Zipes DP, Jalife J (eds). Cardiac Electrophysiology. From Cell to Bedside. 2nd ed. Philadelphia: WB Saunders, 1995, pp. 638–655.

647. Crozier I, Wafa S, Ward D, Camm J. Diagnostic value of comparison of ventriculoatrial interval during junctional tachycardia and right ventricular apical pacing. Pacing Clin Electrophysiol 1989; 12:942–953.

648. Yamashita T, Inoue H, Nozaki A, et al. A new method for estimating preexcitation index without extrastimulus technique and its usefulness in determining the mechanism of supraventricular tachycardia. Am J Cardiol 1991; 67:830–834.

649. Benditt DG, Pritchett EL, Smith WM, Gallagher JJ. Ventriculoatrial intervals: diagnostic use in paroxysmal supraventricular tachycardia. Ann Intern Med 1979; 91:161–166.

650. Schaffer MS, Gillette PC. Ventriculoatrial intervals during narrow complex reentrant tachycardia in children. Am Heart J 1991; 121:1699–1702.

651. Roelandt J, Van der Hauwaert LG. Atrial reciprocal rhythm and reciprocating tachycardia in Wolff-Parkinson-White syndrome. Circulation 1968; 38:64–72.

652. Wellens HJJ, Durrer D. Supraventricular tachycardia with left aberrant conduction due to retrograde invasion into the left bundle branch. Circulation 1968; 38:474–479.

653. Wellens HJJ, Durrer D. Combined conduction disturbances in two AV pathways in patients with Wolff-Parkinson-White syndrome. Eur J Cardiology 1973; 1:23–28.

654. Miles WM, Yee R, Klein GJ, Zipes DP, Prystowsky EN. The preexcitation index: an aid in determining the mechanism of supraventricular tachycardia and localizing accessory pathways. Circulation 1986; 74:493–500.

655. Wellens HJJ, Durrer D. Patterns of ventriculo-atrial conduction in the Wolff-Parkinson-White syndrome. Circulation 1974; 49:22–31.

656. Svenson RH, Miller HC, Gallagher JJ, Wallace AG. Electrophysiological evaluation of the Wolff-Parkinson-White syndrome: problems in assessing antegrade and retrograde conduction over the accessory pathway. Circulation 1975; 52:552–562.

657. Sellers TD Jr, Gallagher JJ, Cope GD, Tonkin AM, Wallace AG. Retrograde atrial preexcitation following premature ventricular beats during reciprocating tachycardia in the Wolff-Parkinson-White syndrome. Eur J Cardiol 1976; 4:283–294.

658. Castellanos A, Agha AS, Mendoza IJ, Sung RJ. Evaluation of intracardiac recordings in diagnosis of impulse formation and concealed conduction in atrioventricular nodal bypass tracts. Br Heart J 1977; 39:726–732.

659. Przybylski J, Chiale PA, Halpern MS, Lazzari JO, Elizari MV, Rosenbaum MB. Existence of automaticity in anomalous bundle of Wolff-Parkinson-White syndrome. Br Heart J 1978; 40:672–680.

660. Ward DE, Camm AJ, Spurrell RA. The response of regular re-entrant supraventricular tachycardia to right heart stimulation. Pacing Clin Electrophysiol 1979; 2:586–595.

661. Hammill SC, Pritchett EL, Klein GJ, Smith WM, Gallagher JJ. Accessory atrioventricular pathways that conduct only in the antegrade direction. Circulation 1980; 62:1335–1340.

662. Wellens HJJ, Bar FW, Dassen WR, Brugada P, Vanagt EJ,

Farre J. Effect of drugs in the Wolff-Parkinson-White syndrome: importance of initial length of effective refractory period of the accessory pathway. Am J Cardiol 1980; 46:665–669.

663. Broughton A, Gallagher JJ, German LD, Guarnieri T, Trantham JL. Differentiation of septal from free wall accessory pathway location: observations during bundle branch block in reciprocating tachycardia in the presence of type I antiarrhythmic drugs. Am J Cardiol 1983; 52:751–754.

664. Belhassen B, Misrahi D, Shapira I, Laniado S. Longitudinal dissociation in an anomalous accessory atrioventricular pathway. Am Heart J 1983; 106:1441–1443.

665. Jackman WM, Friday KJ, Scherlag BJ, et al. Direct endocardial recording from an accessory atrioventricular pathway: localization of the site of block, effect of antiarrhythmic drugs, and attempt at nonsurgical ablation. Circulation 1983; 68:906–916.

666. Morady F, Wang YS, Scheinman MM, Sung RJ, Shen E, Shapiro WA. Extent of atrial participation in atrioventricular-reciprocating tachycardia. Circulation 1983; 67:646–650.

667. Prystowsky EN, Browne KF, Zipes DP. Intracardiac recording by catheter electrode of accessory pathway depolarization. J Am Coll Cardiol 1983; 1:468–470.

668. Waldo AL, Plumb VJ, Arciniegas JG, et al. Transient entrainment and interruption of the atrioventricular bypass pathway type of paroxysmal atrial tachycardia: a model for understanding and identifying reentrant arrhythmias. Circulation 1983; 67:73–83.

669. Cinca J, Valle V, Figueras J, Gutierrez L, Montoyo J, Rius J. Shortening of ventriculoatrial conduction in patients with left-sided Kent bundles. Am Heart J 1984; 107:912–918.

670. Portillo B, Castellanos A, Mejias J, Zaman L, Leon-Portillo N, Myerburg RJ. Right atrial-ventricular dissociation and entrainment while pacing from high right atrium and coronary sinus during circus movement tachycardias. Pacing Clin Electrophysiol 1984; 7:710–719.

671. Klein GJ, Yee R, Sharma AD. Concealed conduction in accessory atrioventricular pathways: an important determinant of the expression of arrhythmias in patients with Wolff-Parkinson-White syndrome. Circulation 1984; 70:402–411.

672. Bardy GH, Packer DL, German LD, Coltorti F, Gallagher JJ. Paradoxical delay in accessory pathway conduction during long R-P' tachycardia after interpolated ventricular premature complexes. Am J Cardiol 1985; 55:1223–1225.

673. Lin FC, Yeh SJ, Wu D. Double atrial responses to a single ventricular impulse due to simultaneous conduction via two retrograde pathways. J Am Coll Cardiol 1985; 5:168–175.

674. Okumura K, Henthorn RW, Epstein AE, Plumb VJ, Waldo AL. Further observations on transient entrainment: importance of pacing site and properties of the components of the reentry circuit. Circulation 1985; 72:1293–1307.

675. Morady F, Scheinman MM, DiCarlo LA Jr, et al. Coexistent posteroseptal and right-sided atrioventricular bypass tracts. J Am Coll Cardiol 1985; 5:640–646.

676. Svinarich JT, Tai DY, Mickelson J, Keung EC, Sung RJ. Electrophysiologic demonstration of concealed conduction in anomalous atrioventricular bypass tracts. J Am Coll Cardiol 1985; 5:898–903.

677. O'Callaghan WG, Colavita PG, Kay GN, Ellenbogen KA, Gilbert MR, German LD. Characterization of retrograde conduction by direct endocardial recording from an accessory atrioventricular pathway. J Am Coll Cardiol 1986; 7:167–171.

678. Winters SL, Gomes JA. Intracardiac electrode catheter recordings of atrioventricular bypass tracts in Wolff-Parkinson-White syndrome: techniques, electrophysiologic characteristics and demonstration of concealed and decremental propagation. J Am Coll Cardiol 1986; 7:1392–1403.

679. Benditt DG, Benson DW, Dunnigan A, et al. Role of extrastimulus site and tachycardia cycle length in inducibility of atrial preexcitation by premature ventricular stimulation during reciprocating tachycardia. Am J Cardiol 1987; 60:811–819.

680. Crossen KJ, Lindsay BD, Cain ME. Reliability of retrograde atrial activation patterns during ventricular pacing for localizing accessory pathways. J Am Coll Cardiol 1987; 9:1279–1287.

681. Zaman L, Castellanos A, Saoudi NC, et al. Significance of pacing cycle lengths in manifest entrainment of orthodromic circus movement tachycardia by ventricular pacing. Am J Cardiol 1987; 59:1325–1331.

682. Jackman WM, Friday KJ, Yeung-Lai-Wah JA, et al. New catheter technique for recording left free-wall accessory atrioventricular pathway activation: identification of pathway fiber orientation. Circulation 1988; 78:598–611.

683. Henthorn RW, Okumura K, Olshansky B, Plumb VJ, Hess PG, Waldo AL. A fourth criterion for transient entrainment: the electrogram equivalent of progressive fusion. Circulation 1988; 77:1003–1012.

684. Baerman JM, Bauernfeind RA, Swiryn S. Shortening of ventriculoatrial intervals with left bundle branch block during orthodromic reciprocating tachycardia in three patients with a right-sided accessory atrioventricular pathway. J Am Coll Cardiol 1989; 13:215–219.

685. Blomstrom P, Jonsson R. The relationship between intraoperatively assessed atrial and ventricular insertions of accessory pathways. Clin Cardiol 1989; 12:701–708.

686. Kou WH, Morady F, Dick M, Nelson SD, Baerman JM. Concealed anterograde accessory pathway conduction during the induction of orthodromic reciprocating tachycardia. J Am Coll Cardiol 1989; 13:391–398.

687. Goldberger J, Wang Y, Scheinman M. Stimulation of the summit of the right ventricular aspect of the ventricular septum during orthodromic atrioventricular reentrant tachycardia. Am J Cardiol 1992; 70:78–85.

688. Gonzalez MD, Greenspon AJ, Kidwell GA. Linking in accessory pathways: functional loss of antegrade preexcitation. Circulation 1991; 83:1221–1231.

689. Calkins H, Kim YN, Schmaltz S, et al. Electrogram criteria for identification of appropriate target sites for radiofrequency catheter ablation of accessory atrioventricular connections. Circulation 1992; 85:565–573.

690. Langberg JJ, Calkins H, el-Atassi R, et al. Temperature monitoring during radiofrequency catheter ablation of accessory pathways. Circulation 1992; 86:1469–1474.

691. Centurion OA, Fukatani M, Shimizu A, et al. Anterograde and retrograde decremental conduction over left-sided accessory atrioventricular pathways in the Wolff-Parkinson-White syndrome. Am Heart J 1993; 125:1038–1047.

692. Chang HJ, Wang CC, Yeh SJ, Wu D. Double atrial responses to a single ventricular premature impulse resulting from simultaneous ventriculoatrial conductions through the normal pathway and a slow paraseptal accessory pathway. Am Heart J 1993; 125:1434–1436.

693. Ormaetxe JM, Almendral J, Arenal A, et al. Ventricular fusion during resetting and entrainment of orthodromic supraventricular tachycardia involving septal accessory pathways: implications for the differential diagnosis with atrioventricular nodal reentry. Circulation 1993; 88:2623–2631.

694. Tanaka K, Suzuki F, Hiejima K, Fujimura O. Quantitative analysis of concealed conduction into accessory atrioventricular pathways in Wolff-Parkinson-White syndrome. Pacing Clin Electrophysiol 1997; 20:1342–1353.

695. Wu D, Wyndham CR, Denes P, Amat-y-Leon F, Miller RH, Dhingra RC. Chronic electrophysiological study in patients with recurrent paroxysmal tachycardia: a new method for developing successful oral antiarrhythmic therapy. In Kulbertus HE (ed). Re-entrant Arrhythmias. Mechanisms and Treatment. Baltimore: University Park Press, 1976, pp. 294–311.

696. Jackman WM, Friday KJ, Fitzgerald DM, Yeung-Lai-Wah JA, Lazzara R. Use of intracardiac recordings to determine the site of drug action in paroxysmal supraventricular tachycardia. Am J Cardiol 1988; 62:8L–19L.

697. Wellens HJJ, Duren DR, Liem DL, Lie KI. Effect of digitalis in patients with paroxysmal atrioventricular nodal tachycardia. Circulation 1975; 52:779–788.

698. Wu D, Amat-y-Leon F, Simpson RJ Jr, et al. Electrophysiological studies with multiple drugs in patients with atrioventricular re-entrant tachycardias utilizing an extranodal pathway. Circulation 1977; 56:727–736.

699. Bauernfeind RA, Wyndham CR, Dhingra RC, et al. Serial electrophysiologic testing of multiple drugs in patients with atrioventricular nodal reentrant paroxysmal tachycardia. Circulation 1980; 62:1341–1349.

700. Porter CJ, Gillette PC, Garson A Jr, et al. Effects of verapamil on supraventricular tachycardia in children. Am J Cardiol 1981; 48:487–491.

701. Wiener I, Rubin D, Pitchon R, Boccardo D. Rapid AV nodal re-entrant tachycardias presenting with syncope or pre-syncope: use of electrophysiological studies to select therapy. Pacing Clin Electrophysiol 1982; 5:173–179.

702. Chang MS, Sung RJ, Tai TY, Lin SL, Liu PH, Chiang BN. Nadolol and supraventricular tachycardia: an electrophysiologic study. J Am Coll Cardiol 1983; 2:894–903.

703. Wu D, Kou HC, Yeh SJ, Lin FC, Hung JS. Effects of oral verapamil in patients with atrioventricular reentrant tachycardia incorporating an accessory pathway. Circulation 1983; 67:426–433.

704. Hung JS, Yeh SJ, Lin FC, Fu M, Lee YS, Wu D. Usefulness of intravenous diltiazem in predicting subsequent electrophysiologic and clinical responses to oral diltiazem. Am J Cardiol 1984; 54:1259–1262.

705. Yeh SJ, Fu M, Lin FC, Lee YS, Hung JS, Wu D. Serial electrophysiologic studies of the effects of oral diltiazem on paroxysmal supraventricular tachycardia. Chest 1985; 87:639–643.

706. Kim SS, Lal R, Ruffy R. Treatment of paroxysmal reentrant supraventricular tachycardia with flecainide acetate. Am J Cardiol 1986; 58:80–85.

707. Kunze KP, Schluter M, Kuck KH. Sotalol in patients with Wolff-Parkinson-White syndrome. Circulation 1987; 75:1050–1057.

708. Niazi I, Naccarelli G, Dougherty A, Rinkenberger R, Tchou P, Akhtar M. Treatment of atrioventricular node reentrant tachycardia with encainide: reversal of drug effect with isoproterenol. J Am Coll Cardiol 1989; 13:904–910.

709. Nagi HM, Pinski SL, Mokhtar S, Saad Y, Maloney JD. Serial electrophysiologic testing of drug therapy in supraventricular tachycardia related to accessory pathways. Clev Clin J Med 1990; 57:622–626.

710. Mehta AV, Chidambaram B. Efficacy and safety of intravenous and oral nadolol for supraventricular tachycardia in children. J Am Coll Cardiol 1992; 19:630–635.

711. Lai WT, Voon WC, Yen HW, et al. Comparison of the electrophysiologic effects of oral sustained-release and intravenous verapamil in patients with paroxysmal supraventricular tachycardia. Am J Cardiol 1993; 71:405–408.

712. DiMarco JP. Electrophysiology of adenosine. J Cardiovasc Electrophysiol 1990; 1:340–348.

713. Camm AJ, Garratt CJ. Adenosine and supraventricular tachycardia. N Engl J Med 1991; 325:1621–1629.

714. DiMarco JP. Adenosine. In Podrid PJ, Kowey PR (eds). Cardiac Arrhythmia. Mechanisms, Diagnosis, and Management. Baltimore: Williams & Wilkins, 1995, pp. 488–498.

715. Belhassen B, Pelleg A, Shoshani D. Electrophysiologic effects of adenosine-5′-triphosphate on atrioventricular reentrant tachycardia. Circulation 1983; 68:827–833.

716. DiMarco JP, Sellers TD, Berne RM, West GA, Belardinelli L. Adenosine: electrophysiologic effects and therapeutic use for terminating paroxysmal supraventricular tachycardia. Circulation 1983; 68:1254–1263.

717. Perrot B, Clozel JP, Faivre G. Effect of adenosine triphosphate on the accessory pathways. Eur Heart J 1984; 5:382–393.

718. Belhassen B, Glick A, Laniado S. Comparative clinical and electrophysiologic effects of adenosine triphosphate and verapamil on paroxysmal reciprocating junctional tachycardia. Circulation 1988; 77:795–805.

719. Viskin S, Belhassen B, Sheps D, Laniado S. Clinical and electrophysiologic effects of magnesium sulfate on

paroxysmal supraventricular tachycardia and comparison with adenosine triphosphate. Am J Cardiol 1992; 70:879–885.

720. Lee CS, Lai WT, Wu JC, Sheu SH, Wu SN, Belardinelli L. Differential effects of adenosine on antegrade and retrograde fast pathway conduction in atrioventricular nodal reentry. Am Heart J 1997; 134:799–806.

721. Curtis AB, Belardinelli L, Woodard DA, Brown CS, Conti JB. Induction of atrioventricular node reentrant tachycardia with adenosine: differential effect of adenosine on fast and slow atrioventricular node pathways. J Am Coll Cardiol 1997; 30:1778–1784.

722. Rinne C, Sharma AD, Klein GJ, Yee R, Szabo T. Comparative effects of adenosine triphosphate on accessory pathway and atrioventricular nodal conduction. Am Heart J 1988; 115:1042–1047.

723. Fishberger SB, Mehta D, Rossi AF, Langan MN, Marx SO, Gomes JA. Variable effects of adenosine on retrograde conduction in patients with atrioventricular nodal reentry tachycardia. PACE 1998; 21:1254–1257.

724. Garratt CJ, Griffith MJ, O'Nunain S, Ward DE, Camm AJ. Effects of intravenous adenosine on antegrade refractoriness of accessory atrioventricular connections. Circulation 1991; 84:1962–1968.

725. Wienecke MM, Case CL, Gillette PC. Adenosine's effectiveness in long RP' re-entrant tachycardia: additional evidence of the decremental qualities of the retrograde limb. Clin Cardiol 1992; 15:114–116.

726. Engelstein ED, Wilber D, Wadas M, Stein KM, Lippman N, Lerman BB. Limitations of adenosine in assessing the efficacy of radiofrequency catheter ablation of accessory pathways. Am J Cardiol 1994; 73:774–779.

727. Belhassen B, Shoshani D, Laniado S. Unmasking of ventricular preexcitation by adenosine triphosphate: its usefulness in the assessment of ajmaline test. Am Heart J 1989; 118:634–636.

728. Garratt CJ, Antoniou A, Griffith MJ, Ward DE, Camm AJ. Use of intravenous adenosine in sinus rhythm as a diagnostic test for latent preexcitation. Am J Cardiol 1990; 65:868–873.

729. Morgan-Hughes NJ, Griffith MJ, McComb JM. Intravenous adenosine can reveal accessory pathways not revealed by routine electrophysiological testing. Pacing Clin Electrophysiol 1993; 16:2059–2063.

730. Morgan-Hughes NJ, Griffith MJ, McComb JM. Intravenous adenosine reveals intermittent preexcitation by direct and indirect effects on accessory pathway conduction. Pacing Clin Electrophysiol 1993; 16:2098–2103.

731. Canby RC, Horton RP, Kessler DJ, Roman CA, Page RL. Use of transesophageal atrial pacing with adenosine infusion to evaluate ventricular preexcitation. Am J Cardiol 1995; 75:548–550.

732. Walker KW, Silka MJ, Haupt D, Kron J, McAnulty JH, Halperin BD. Use of adenosine to identify patients at risk for recurrence of accessory pathway conduction after initially successful radiofrequency catheter ablation. Pacing Clin Electrophysiol 1995; 18:441–446.

733. Belhassen B, Fish R, Glikson M, et al. Noninvasive diagnosis of dual AV node physiology in patients with AV nodal reentrant tachycardia by administration of adenosine-5'-triphosphate during sinus rhythm. Circulation 1998; 98:47–53.

734. Khalilullah M, Sathyamurthy I, Singhal NK. Ajmaline in WPW syndrome: an electrophysiologic study. Am Heart J 1980; 99:766–771.

735. Sethi KK, Jaishankar S, Gupta MP. Salutary effects of intravenous ajmaline in patients with paroxysmal supraventricular tachycardia mediated by dual atrioventricular nodal pathways: blockade of the retrograde fast pathway. Circulation 1984; 70:876–883.

736. Waleffe A, Bruninx P, Kulbertus HE. Effects of amiodarone studied by programmed electrical stimulation of the heart in patients with paroxysmal re-entrant supraventricular tachycardia. J Electrocardiol 1978; 11:253–260.

737. Gomes JA, Kang PS, Hariman RJ, el-Sherif N, Lyons, J. Electrophysiologic effects and mechanisms of termination of supraventricular tachycardia by intravenous amiodarone. Am Heart J 1984; 107:214–221.

738. Maggioni AP, Volpi A, Cavalli A, Giani P. Incessant atrioventricular nodal reciprocating tachycardia successfully treated with intravenous amiodarone. Am Heart J 1985; 110:159–161.

739. Wellens HJJ, Lie KI, Bar FW, et al. Effect of amiodarone in the Wolff-Parkinson-White syndrome. Am J Cardiol 1976; 38:189–194.

740. Brugada P, Dassen WR, Braat S, Gorgels AP, Wellens HJJ. Value of the ajmaline-procainamide test to predict the effect of long-term oral amiodarone on the anterograde effective refractory period of the accessory pathway in the Wolff-Parkinson-White syndrome. Am J Cardiol 1983; 52:70–72.

741. Alboni P, Shantha N, Pirani R, et al. Effects of amiodarone on supraventricular tachycardia involving bypass tracts. Am J Cardiol 1984; 53:93–98.

742. Rasmussen V, Berning J. Effect of amiodarone in the Wolff-Parkinson-White syndrome: a clinical and electrophysiological study. Acta Med Scand 1979; 205:31–37.

743. Zipes DP, Gaum WE, Foster PR, et al. Aprindine for treatment of supraventricular tachycardias: with particular application to Wolff-Parkinson-White syndrome. Am J Cardiol 1977; 40:586–596.

744. Wu D, Denes P, Bauernfeind R, Dhingra RC, Wyndham C, Rosen KM. Effects of atropine on induction and maintenance of atrioventricular nodal reentrant tachycardia. Circulation 1979; 59:779–788.

745. Senges J, Rizos I, Hennig E, Jauernig R, Lengfelder W, Kubler W. Atrioventricular nodal reentrant tachycardia with second-degree AV nodal block. Am Heart J 1983; 106:766–770.

746. Neuss H, Schlepper M, Spies HF. Effects of heart rate and atropine on "dual AV conduction." Br Heart J 1975; 37:1216–1227.

747. Akhtar M, Damato AN, Batsford WP, et al. Induction of atrioventricular nodal reentrant tachycardia after atropine: report of five cases. Am J Cardiol 1975; 36:286–291.

748. Alboni P, Paparella N, Cappato R, et al. Intrinsic electrophysiologic properties of reentrant supraventricular tachycardia involving bypass tracts. Am J Cardiol 1986; 58:266–272.

749. Wu D, Denes P, Dhingra R, Khan A, Rosen KM. The effects of propranolol on induction of A-V nodal reentrant paroxysmal tachycardia. Circulation 1974; 50:665–677.

750. Gmeiner R, Ng CK. Metoprolol in the treatment and prophylaxis of paroxysmal reentrant supraventricular tachycardia. J Cardiovasc Pharmacol 1982; 4:5–13.

751. Yee R, Gulamhusein SS, Klein GJ. Combined verapamil and propranolol for supraventricular tachycardia. Am J Cardiol 1984; 53:757–763.

752. Saksena S, Klein GJ, Kowey PR, et al. Electrophysiologic effects, clinical efficacy and safety of intravenous and oral nadolol in refractory supraventricular tachyarrhythmias. Am J Cardiol 1987; 59:307–312.

753. Hung JS, Kou HC, Wu D. Digoxin, propranolol, and atrioventricular reentrant tachycardia in the Wolff-Parkinson-White syndrome. Ann Intern Med 1982; 97:175–182.

754. Greenspan AM, Spielman SR, Horowitz LN, Senior S, Steck J, Laddu A. Electrophysiology of esmolol. Am J Cardiol 1985; 56:19F–26F.

755. Philippon F, Plumb VJ, Kay GN. Differential effect of esmolol on the fast and slow AV nodal pathways in patients with AV nodal reentrant tachycardia. J Cardiovasc Electrophysiol 1994; 5:810–817.

756. Rizos I, Senges J, Jauernig R, et al. Differential effects of sotalol and metoprolol on induction of paroxysmal supraventricular tachycardia. Am J Cardiol 1984; 53:1022–1027.

757. Barrett PA, Jordan JL, Mandel WJ, Yamaguchi I, Laks MM. The electrophysiologic effects of intravenous propranolol in the Wolff-Parkinson-White syndrome. Am Heart J 1979; 98:213–224.

758. White HD, Antman EM, Glynn MA, et al. Efficacy and safety of timolol for prevention of supraventricular tachyarrhythmias after coronary artery bypass surgery. Circulation 1984; 70:479–484.

759. Mitchell LB, Schroeder JS, Mason JW. Comparative clinical electrophysiologic effects of diltiazem, verapamil and nifedipine: a review. Am J Cardiol 1982; 49:629–635.

760. Akhtar M, Tchou P, Jazayeri M. Use of calcium channel entry blockers in the treatment of cardiac arrhythmias. Circulation 1989; 80(Suppl IV):IV-31–IV-39.

761. Hamer A, Peter T, Mandel W. Atrioventricular node reentry: intravenous verapamil as a method of defining multiple electrophysiologic types. Am Heart J 1983; 105:629–642.

762. Roy D, Marchand E, Chabot M, Gagne P, Waters DD, Bourassa MG. Electrophysiologic effects of intravenous diltiazem in patients with recurrent supraventricular tachycardias. Can J Cardiol 1985; 1:302–305.

763. Waleffe A, Hastir F, Kulbertus HE. Effects of intravenous diltiazem administration in patients with inducible tachycardia. Eur Heart J 1985; 6:882–890.

764. Frabetti L, Capucci A, Gerometta PS, Cavallini C, Leto di Priolo S, Magnani B. Intravenous diltiazem in patients with paroxysmal re-entrant supraventricular tachycardia. Int J Cardiol 1989; 23:215–221.

765. Rizos I, Seidl KH, Aidonidis I, Stamou S, Senges J, Toutouzas P. Intraindividual comparison of diltiazem and verapamil on induction of paroxysmal supraventricular tachycardia. Cardiology 1994; 85:388–396.

766. Shenasa M, Denker S, Mahmud R, Lehmann M, Murthy VS, Akhtar M. Effect of verapamil on retrograde atrioventricular nodal conduction in the human heart. J Am Coll Cardiol 1983; 2:545–550.

767. Reddy CP, McAllister RG Jr. Effect of verapamil on retrograde conduction in atrioventricular nodal reentrant tachycardia. Am J Cardiol 1984; 54:535–543.

768. Sung RJ, Elser B, McAllister RG. Intravenous verapamil for termination of re-entrant supraventricular tachycardias: intracardiac studies correlated with plasma verapamil concentrations. Ann Intern Med 1980; 93:682–689.

769. Feigl D, Ravid M. Electrocardiographic observations on the termination of supraventricular tachycardia by verapamil. J Electrocardiol 1979; 12:129–136.

770. Vohra J, Hunt D, Stuckey J, Sloman G. Cycle length alternation in supraventricular tachycardia after administration of verapamil. Br Heart J 1974; 36:570–576.

771. Hamer A, Peter T, Platt M, Mandel WJ. Effects of verapamil on supraventricular tachycardia in patients with overt and concealed Wolff-Parkinson-White syndrome. Am Heart J 1981; 101:600–612.

772. Ross DL, Dassen WR, Vanagt EJ, Brugada P, Bar FW, Wellens HJJ. Cycle length alternation in circus movement tachycardia using an atrioventricular accessory pathway: a study of the role of the atrioventricular node using a computer model of tachycardia. Circulation 1982; 65:862–868.

773. Wellens HJJ, Tan SL, Bar FW, Duren DR, Lie KI, Dohmen HM. Effect of verapamil studied by programmed electrical stimulation of the heart in patients with paroxysmal re-entrant supraventricular tachycardia. Br Heart J 1977; 39:1058–1066.

774. Tonkin AM, Aylward PE, Joel SE, Heddle WF. Verapamil in prophylaxis of paroxysmal atrioventricular nodal reentrant tachycardia. J Cardiovasc Pharmacol 1980; 2:473–486.

775. Harper RW, Whitford E, Middlebrook K, Federman J, Anderson S, Pitt A. Effects of verapamil on the electrophysiologic properties of the accessory pathway in patients with the Wolff-Parkinson-White syndrome. Am J Cardiol 1982; 50:1323–1330.

776. Yeh SJ, Kou HC, Lin FC, Hung JS, Wu D. Effects of oral diltiazem in paroxysmal supraventricular tachycardia. Am J Cardiol 1983; 52:271–278.

777. Komatsu C, Ishinaga T, Tateishi O, Tokuhisa Y, Yoshimura S. Effects of four antiarrhythmic drugs on the induction and termination of paroxysmal supraventricular tachycardia. Jpn Circ J 1986; 50:961–972.

778. Dougherty AH, Jackman WM, Naccarelli GV, Friday KJ, Dias VC. Acute conversion of paroxysmal supraventricular tachycardia with intravenous diltiazem. IV. Diltiazem study group. Am J Cardiol 1992; 70:587–592.

779. Rinkenberger RL, Prystowsky EN, Heger JJ, Troup PJ, Jackman WM, Zipes DP. Effects of intravenous and chronic oral verapamil administration in patients with supraventricular tachyarrhythmias. Circulation 1980; 62:996–1010.

780. Matsuyama E, Konishi T, Okazaki H, Matsuda H, Kawai C. Effects of verapamil on accessory pathway properties and induction of circus movement tachycardia in patients with the Wolff-Parkinson-White syndrome. J Cardiovasc Pharmacol 1981; 3:11–24.

781. Klein GJ, Gulamhusein S, Prystowsky EN, Carruthers SG, Donner AP, Ko PT. Comparison of the electrophysiologic effects of intravenous and oral verapamil in patients with paroxysmal supraventricular tachycardia. Am J Cardiol 1982; 49:117–124.

782. Rozanski JJ, Zaman L, Castellanos A. Electrophysiologic effects of diltiazem hydrochloride on supraventricular tachycardia. Am J Cardiol 1982; 49:621–628.

783. Sakurai M, Yasuda H, Kato N, et al. Acute and chronic effects of verapamil in patients with paroxysmal supraventricular tachycardia. Am Heart J 1983; 105:619–628.

784. Shenasa M, Fromer M, Faugere G, et al. Efficacy and safety of intravenous and oral diltiazem for Wolff-Parkinson-White syndrome. Am J Cardiol 1987; 59:301–306.

785. Huycke EC, Sung RJ, Dias VC, Milstein S, Hariman RJ, Platia EV. Intravenous diltiazem for termination of reentrant supraventricular tachycardia: a placebo-controlled, randomized, double-blind, multicenter study. J Am Coll Cardiol 1989; 13:538–544.

786. Rosenthal M, Oseran DS, Gang E, Deng Z, Mandel WJ, Peter T. Verapamil-induced retrograde conduction block in a concealed atrioventricular bypass tract. Am J Cardiol 1985; 55:1222–1223.

787. Spurrell RA, Krikler DM, Sowton E. Effects of verapamil on electrophysiological properties of anomalous atrioventricular connection in Wolff-Parkinson-White syndrome. Br Heart J 1974; 36:256–264.

788. McGovern B, Garan H, Ruskin JN. Precipitation of cardiac arrest by verapamil in patients with Wolff-Parkinson-White syndrome. Ann Intern Med 1986; 104:791–794.

789. Gulamhusein S, Ko P, Carruthers SG, Klein GJ. Acceleration of the ventricular response during atrial fibrillation in the Wolff-Parkinson-White syndrome after verapamil. Circulation 1982; 65:348–354.

790. Horio Y, Matsuyama K, Morikami Y, et al. Blocking effect of verapamil on conduction over a catecholamine-sensitive bypass tract in exercise-induced Wolff-Parkinson-White syndrome. J Am Coll Cardiol 1984; 4:186–191.

791. Wellens HJJ, Cats VM, Duren DR. Symptomatic sinus node abnormalities following lithium carbonate therapy. Am J Med 1975; 59:285–287.

792. Wu D, Denes P, Wyndham C, Amat-y-Leon F, Dhingra RC, Rosen KM. Demonstration of dual atrioventricular nodal pathways utilizing a ventricular extrastimulus in patients with atrioventricular nodal re-entrant paroxysmal supraventricular tachycardia. Circulation 1975; 52:789–798.

793. Dhingra RC, Palileo EV, Strasberg B, et al. Electrophysiologic effects of ouabain in patients with preexcitation and circus movement tachycardia. Am J Cardiol 1981; 47:139–144.

794. Wellens HJJ, Durrer D. Effects of digitalis on atrioventricular conduction and circus-movement tachycardias in patients with Wolff-Parkinson-White syndrome. Circulation 1973; 47:1229–1233.

795. Sellers TD Jr, Bashore TM, Gallagher JJ. Digitalis in the pre-excitation syndrome: analysis during atrial fibrillation. Circulation 1977; 56:260–267.

796. Jedeikin R, Gillette PC, Garson A Jr, et al. Effect of ouabain on the anterograde effective refractory period of accessory atrioventricular connections in children. J Am Coll Cardiol 1983; 1:869–872.

797. Swiryn S, Bauernfeind RA, Wyndham CR, et al. Effects of oral disopyramide phosphate on induction of paroxysmal supraventricular tachycardia. Circulation 1981; 64:169–175.

798. Kerr CR, Prystowsky EN, Smith WM, Cook L, Gallagher JJ. Electrophysiologic effects of disopyramide phosphate in

patients with Wolff-Parkinson-White syndrome. Circulation 1982; 65:869–878.

799. Kou HC, Hung JS, Lee YS, Wu D. Effects of oral disopyramide phosphate on induction and sustenance of atrioventricular reentrant tachycardia incorporating retrograde accessory pathway conduction. Circulation 1982; 66:454–462.

800. Tajima T, Dohi Y. Electrophysiological effects of intravenous disopyramide phosphate on the Wolff-Parkinson-White syndrome. Pacing Clin Electrophysiol 1982; 5:741–747.

801. Sethi KK, Jaishankar S, Khalilullah M, Gupta MP. Selective blockade of retrograde fast pathway by intravenous disopyramide in paroxysmal supraventricular tachycardia mediated by dual atrioventricular nodal pathways. Br Heart J 1983; 49:532–543.

802. Hellestrand KJ, Bexton RS, Nathan AW, Spurrell RA, Camm AJ. Acute electrophysiological effects of flecainide acetate on cardiac conduction and refractoriness in man. Br Heart J 1982; 48:140–148.

803. Bexton RS, Hellestrand KJ, Nathan AW, Spurrell RA, Camm AJ. A comparison of the antiarrhythmic effects on AV junctional re-entrant tachycardia of oral and intravenous flecainide acetate. Eur Heart J 1983; 4:92–102.

804. Hellestrand KJ, Nathan AW, Bexton RS, Spurrell RA, Camm AJ. Cardiac electrophysiologic effects of flecainide acetate for paroxysmal reentrant junctional tachycardias. Am J Cardiol 1983; 51:770–776.

805. Neuss H, Buss J, Schlepper M, et al. Effects of flecainide on electrophysiological properties of accessory pathways in the Wolff-Parkinson-White syndrome. Eur Heart J 1983; 4:347–353.

806. Hoff PI, Tronstad A, Oie B, Ohm OJ. Electrophysiologic and clinical effects of flecainide for recurrent paroxysmal supraventricular tachycardia. Am J Cardiol 1988; 62:585–589.

807. Manolis AS, Salem DN, Estes NA III. Electrophysiologic effects, efficacy and tolerance of class Ic antiarrhythmic agents in Wolff-Parkinson-White syndrome. Am J Cardiol 1989; 63:746–750.

808. Goldberger J, Helmy I, Katzung B, Scheinman M. Use-dependent properties of flecainide acetate in accessory atrioventricular pathways. Am J Cardiol 1994; 73:43–49.

809. Brembilla-Perrot B, Terrier de la Chaise A, Pichene M, Aliot E, Cherrier F, Pernot C. Isoprenaline as an aid to the induction of catecholamine dependent supraventricular tachycardias during programmed stimulation. Br Heart J 1989; 61:348–355.

810. Brugada P, Facchini M, Wellens HJJ. Effects of isoproterenol and amiodarone and the role of exercise in initiation of circus movement tachycardia in the accessory atrioventricular pathway. Am J Cardiol 1986; 57:146–149.

811. Brownstein SL, Hopson RC, Martins JB, et al. Usefulness of isoproterenol in facilitating atrioventricular nodal reentry tachycardia during electrophysiologic testing. Am J Cardiol 1988; 61:1037–1041.

812. Huycke EC, Lai WT, Nguyen NX, Keung EC, Sung RJ. Role of intravenous isoproterenol in the electrophysiologic induction of atrioventricular node reentrant tachycardia in patients with dual atrioventricular node pathways. Am J Cardiol 1989; 64:1131–1137.

813. Rosen KM, Barwolf C, Ehsani A, Rahimtoola SH. Effects of lidocaine and propranolol on the normal and anomalous pathways in patients with preexcitation. Am J Cardiol 1972; 30:801–809.

814. Josephson ME, Kastor JA, Kitchen JG III. Lidocaine in Wolff-Parkinson-White syndrome with atrial fibrillation. Ann Intern Med 1976; 84:44–45.

815. Akhtar M, Gilbert CJ, Shenasa M. Effect of lidocaine on atrioventricular response via the accessory pathway in patients with Wolff-Parkinson-White syndrome. Circulation 1981; 63:435–441.

816. Barrett PA, Laks MM, Mandel WJ, Yamaguchi I. The electrophysiologic effects of intravenous lidocaine in the Wolff-Parkinson-White syndrome. Am Heart J 1980; 100:23–33.

817. Sager PT, Widerhorn J, Petersen R, et al. Prospective evaluation of parenteral magnesium sulfate in the treatment of patients with reentrant AV supraventricular tachycardia. Am Heart J 1990; 119:308–316.

818. Wu D, Denes P, Bauernfeind R, Kehoe R, Amat-y-Leon F, Rosen KM. Effects of procainamide on atrioventricular nodal re-entrant paroxysmal tachycardia. Circulation 1978; 57:1171–1179.

819. Gomes JA, Kang PS, Kelen G, Khan R, el-Sherif N. Simultaneous anterograde fast-slow atrioventricular nodal pathway conduction after procainamide. Am J Cardiol 1980; 46:677–684.

820. Shenasa M, Gilbert CJ, Schmidt DH, Akhtar M. Procainamide and retrograde atrioventricular nodal conduction in man. Circulation 1982; 65:355–362.

821. Fukatani M, Kiya F, Yano K, Hashiba K. Paradoxical effects of procainamide-facilitation of the induction of sustained reciprocating tachycardia after procainamide administration in Wolff-Parkinson-White syndrome. Jpn Circ J 1983; 47:124–131.

822. Leitch JW, Klein GJ, Yee R, Feldman RD, Brown J. Differential effect of intravenous procainamide on anterograde and retrograde accessory pathway refractoriness. J Am Coll Cardiol 1992; 19:118–124.

823. Eldar M, Ruder MA, Davis JC, et al. Procainamide-induced incessant supraventricular tachycardia in the Wolff-Parkinson-White syndrome. Pacing Clin Electrophysiol 1986; 9:652–659.

824. Breithardt G, Borggrefe M, Wiebringhaus E, Seipel L. Effect of propafenone in the Wolff-Parkinson-White syndrome: electrophysiologic findings and long-term follow-up. Am J Cardiol 1984; 54:29D–39D.

825. Garcia-Civera R, Sanjuan R, Morell S, et al. Effects of propafenone on induction and maintenance of atrioventricular nodal reentrant tachycardia. Pacing Clin Electrophysiol 1984; 7:649–655.

826. Wu D, Hung JS, Kuo CT, Hsu KS, Shieh WB. Effects of quinidine on atrioventricular nodal reentrant paroxysmal tachycardia. Circulation 1981; 64:823–831.

827. Hohnloser SH, Woosley RL. Sotalol. N Engl J Med 1994; 331:31–38.

828. Mitchell LB, Wyse DG, Duff HJ. Electropharmacology of sotalol in patients with Wolff-Parkinson-White syndrome. Circulation 1987; 76:810–818.

829. Belz MK, Stambler BS, Wood MA, Pherson C, Ellenbogen KA. Effects of enhanced parasympathetic tone on atrioventricular nodal conduction during atrioventricular nodal reentrant tachycardia. Am J Cardiol 1997; 80:878–882.

830. Gallagher JJ, Svenson RH, Sealy WC, Wallace AG. The Wolff-Parkinson-White syndrome and the preexcitation dysrhythmias: medical and surgical management. Med Clin North Am 1976; 60:101–123.

831. Wilkinson JL. Management of paroxysmal tachycardia. Arch Dis Child 1983; 58:945–946.

832. Ornato JP. Management of paroxysmal supraventricular tachycardia. Circulation 1986; 74(Suppl IV):IV-108–IV-110.

833. Rostagno C, Paladini B, Pini C, et al. Feasibility of out-of-hospital treatment of supraventricular tachycardias. Am J Cardiol 1991; 68:119–122.

834. Waxman MB, Wald RW, Cameron D. Interactions between the autonomic nervous system and tachycardias in man. Cardiol Clin 1983; 1:143–185.

835. Mehta D, Wafa S, Ward DE, Camm AJ. Relative efficacy of various physical manoeuvres in the termination of junctional tachycardia. Lancet 1988; 1:1181–1185.

836. Waxman MB, Sharma AD, Cameron DA, Huerta F, Wald RW. Reflex mechanisms responsible for early spontaneous termination of paroxysmal supraventricular tachycardia. Am J Cardiol 1982; 49:259–272.

837. Waxman MB, Bonet JF, Finley JP, Wald RW. Effects of respiration and posture on paroxysmal supraventricular tachycardia. Circulation 1980; 62:1011–1020.

838. Anonymous. Hazard of carotid-sinus stimulation. N Engl J Med 1966; 275:165–166.

839. Hood MA, Smith WM. Adenosine versus verapamil in the treatment of supraventricular tachycardia: a randomized double-crossover trial. Am Heart J 1992; 123:1543–1549.

840. Davies AJ, Kenny RA. Frequency of neurologic complications following carotid sinus massage. Am J Cardiol 1998; 81:1256–1257.
841. Gupta A, Lennmarken C, Lemming D, Lindqvist J. Termination of paroxysmal supraventricular tachycardia with a nasogastric tube: a case report. Acta Anaesthesiol Scand 1991; 35:786–787.
842. Wildenthal K, Atkins JM. Use of the "diving reflex" for the treatment of paroxysmal supraventricular tachycardia. Am Heart J 1979; 98:536–537.
843. Wildenthal K, Leshin SJ, Atkins JM, Skelton CL. The diving reflex used to treat paroxysmal atrial tachycardia. Lancet 1975; 1:12–14.
844. Whitman V, Sakeosian GM. The diving reflex in termination of supraventricular tachycardia in childhood. J Pediatr 1976; 89:1032–1033.
845. Whitman V, Friedman Z, Berman W Jr, Maisels MJ. Supraventricular tachycardia in newborn infants: an approach to therapy. J Pediatr 1977; 91:304–305.
846. Hamilton J, Moodie D, Levy J. The use of the diving reflex to terminate supraventricular tachycardia in a 2-week-old infant. Am Heart J 1979; 97:371–374.
847. Sperandeo V, Pieri D, Palazzolo P, Donzelli M, Spataro G. Supraventricular tachycardia in infants: use of the "diving reflex." Am J Cardiol 1983; 51:286–287.
848. Krikler D, Rowland E. Management of supraventricular tachycardia with drugs and artificial pacing. In Narula OS (ed). Cardiac Arrhythmias. Electrophysiology, Diagnosis and Management. Baltimore: Williams & Wilkins, 1979, pp. 382–396.
849. Belhassen B, Pelleg A. Acute management of paroxysmal supraventricular tachycardia: verapamil, adenosine triphosphate or adenosine? Am J Cardiol 1984; 54:225–227.
850. Moak JP, Smith RT, Garson A Jr. Newer antiarrhythmic drugs in children. Am Heart J 1987; 113:179–185.
851. Schoenfeld MH. Pediatric pre-excitation: say "no" to drugs? J Am Coll Cardiol 1990; 16:1221–1223.
852. Viskin S, Belhassen B. Acute management of paroxysmal atrioventricular junctional reentrant supraventricular tachycardia: pharmacologic strategies. Am Heart J 1990; 120:180–188.
853. Belhassen B, Viskin S. What is the drug of choice for the acute termination of paroxysmal supraventricular tachycardia: verapamil, adenosine triphosphate, or adenosine? Pacing Clin Electrophysiol 1993; 16:1735–1741.
854. Luderitz B, Manz M. Pharmacologic treatment of supraventricular tachycardia: the German experience. Am J Cardiol 1992; 70:66A–73A.
855. Manz M, Luderitz B. Supraventricular tachycardia and pre-excitation syndromes: pharmacological therapy. Eur Heart J 1993; 14:E91–E98.
856. Levy S, Ricard P. Using the right drug: a treatment algorithm for regular supraventricular tachycardias. Eur Heart J 1997; 18:C27–C32.
857. Simons GR, Eisenstein EL, Shaw LJ, Mark DB, Pritchett ELC. Cost effectiveness of inpatient initiation of antiarrhythmic therapy for supraventricular tachycardias. Am J Cardiol 1997; 80:1551–1557.
858. Margolis B, DeSilva RA, Lown B. Episodic drug treatment in the management of paroxysmal arrhythmias. Am J Cardiol 1980; 45:621–626.
859. Wang S, Xie J, Sada M, Doherty TM, French WJ. TACHY: an expert system for the management of supraventricular tachycardia in the elderly. Am Heart J 1998; 135:82–87.
860. Pfammatter JP, Stocker FP. Results of a restrictive use of antiarrhythmic drugs in the chronic treatment of atrioventricular reentrant tachycardias in infancy and childhood. Am J Cardiol 1998; 82:72–75.
861. Munoz A, Leenhardt A, Sassine A. Therapeutic use of adenosine for terminating spontaneous paroxysmal supraventricular tachycardia. Eur Heart J 1984; 5:735–738.
862. DiMarco JP, Sellers TD, Lerman BB, Greenberg ML, Berne RM, Belardinelli L. Diagnostic and therapeutic use of adenosine in patients with supraventricular tachyarrhythmias. J Am Coll Cardiol 1985; 6:417–425.
863. Saito D, Ueeda M, Abe Y, et al. Treatment of paroxysmal supraventricular tachycardia with intravenous injection of adenosine triphosphate. Br Heart J 1986; 55:291–294.
864. Garratt C, Linker N, Griffith M, Ward D, Camm AJ. Comparison of adenosine and verapamil for termination of paroxysmal junctional tachycardia. Am J Cardiol 1989; 64:1310–1316.
865. Rankin AC, Oldroyd KG, Chong E, Rae AP, Cobbe SM. Value and limitations of adenosine in the diagnosis and treatment of narrow and broad complex tachycardias. Br Heart J 1989; 62:195–203.
866. Sharma AD, Klein GJ, Yee R. Intravenous adenosine triphosphate during wide QRS complex tachycardia: safety, therapeutic efficacy, and diagnostic utility. Am J Med 1990; 88:337–343.
867. Domanovits H, Laske H, Stark G, et al. Adenosine for the management of patients with tachycardias: a new protocol. Eur Heart J 1994; 15:589–593.
868. Clarke B, Till J, Rowland E, Ward DE, Barnes PJ, Shinebourne EA. Rapid and safe termination of supraventricular tachycardia in children by adenosine. Lancet 1987; 1:299–301.
869. Overholt ED, Rheuban KS, Gutgesell HP, Lerman BB, DiMarco JP. Usefulness of adenosine for arrhythmias in infants and children. Am J Cardiol 1988; 61:336–340.
870. Till J, Shinebourne EA, Rigby ML, Clarke B, Ward DE, Rowland E. Efficacy and safety of adenosine in the treatment of supraventricular tachycardia in infants and children. Br Heart J 1989; 62:204–211.
871. DiMarco JP, Miles W, Akhtar M, et al. Adenosine for paroxysmal supraventricular tachycardia: dose ranging and comparison with verapamil: assessment in placebo-controlled, multicenter trials. The adenosine for PSVT study group. Ann Intern Med 1990; 113:104–110.
872. Rankin AC, Rae AP, Oldroyd KG, Cobbe SM. Verapamil or adenosine for the immediate treatment of supraventricular tachycardia. Q J Med 1990; 74:203–208.
873. Garratt CJ, O'Nunain S, Griffith MJ, et al. Effects of intravenous adenosine in patients with preexcited junctional tachycardias: therapeutic efficacy and incidence of proarrhythmic events. Am J Cardiol 1994; 74:401–404.
874. Lauer MR, Young C, Liem LB, Sung RJ. Efficacy of adenosine in terminating catecholamine-dependent supraventricular tachycardia. Am J Cardiol 1994; 73:38–42.
875. Conti JB, Belardinelli L, Curtis AB. Usefulness of adenosine in diagnosis of tachyarrhythmias. Am J Cardiol 1995; 75:952–955.
876. Strickberger SA, Man KC, Daoud EG, et al. Adenosine-induced atrial arrhythmia: a prospective analysis. Ann Intern Med 1997; 127:417–422.
877. Exner DV, Muzyka T, Gillis AM. Proarrhythmia in patients with the Wolff-Parkinson-White syndrome after standard doses of intravenous adenosine. Ann Intern Med 1995; 122:351–352.
878. Marcus FI, Fontaine GH, Frank R, Grosgogeat Y. Clinical pharmacology and therapeutic applications of the antiarrhythmic agent amiodarone. Am Heart J 1981; 101:480–493.
879. Coumel P, Lucet V, Do Ngoc D. The use of amiodarone in children. Pacing Clin Electrophysiol 1983; 6:930–939.
880. Desai AD, Chun S, Sung RJ. The role of intravenous amiodarone in the management of cardiac arrhythmias. Ann Intern Med 1997; 127:294–303.
881. Rosenbaum MB, Chiale PA, Ryba D, Elizari MV. Control of tachyarrhythmias associated with Wolff-Parkinson-White syndrome by amiodarone hydrochloride. Am J Cardiol 1974; 34:215–223.
882. Wheeler PJ, Puritz R, Ingram DV, Chamberlain DA. Amiodarone in the treatment of refractory supraventricular and ventricular arrhythmias. Postgrad Med J 1979; 55:1–9.
883. Coumel P, Fidelle J, Loges-en-Josas L. Amiodarone in the treatment of cardiac arrhythmias in children: one hundred thirty-five cases. Am Heart J 1980; 100:1063–1069.
884. Rowland E, Krikler DM. Electrophysiological assessment of amiodarone in treatment of resistant supraventricular arrhythmias. Br Heart J 1980; 44:82–90.

885. Ward DE, Camm AJ, Spurrell RA. Clinical antiarrhythmic effects of amiodarone in patients with resistant paroxysmal tachycardias. Br Heart J 1980; 44:91–95.
886. Shuler CO, Case CL, Gillette PC. Efficacy and safety of amiodarone in infants. Am Heart J 1993; 125:1430–1432.
887. Garson A Jr, Gillette PC, McVey P, et al. Amiodarone treatment of critical arrhythmias in children and young adults. J Am Coll Cardiol 1984; 4:749–755.
888. Cybulski J, Kulakowski P, Makowska E, Czepiel A, Sikora-Frac M, Ceremuzynski L. Intravenous amiodarone is safe and seems to be effective in termination of paroxysmal supraventricular tachyarrhythmias. Clin Cardiol 1996; 19:563–566.
889. Gibson D, Sowton E. The use of beta-adrenergic receptor blocking drugs in dysrhythmias. Prog Cardiovasc Dis 1969; 12:16–39.
890. Coumel P, Escoubet B, Attuel P. Beta-blocking therapy in atrial and ventricular tachyarrhythmias: experience with nadolol. Am Heart J 1984; 108:1098–1108.
891. Abrams J, Allen J, Allin D, et al. Efficacy and safety of esmolol vs propranolol in the treatment of supraventricular tachyarrhythmias: a multicenter double-blind clinical trial. Am Heart J 1985; 110:913–922.
892. Frieden J, Rosenblum R, Enselberg CD, Rosenberg A. Propranolol treatment of chronic intractable supraventricular arrhythmias. Am J Cardiol 1968; 22:711–717.
893. Pickoff AS, Zies L, Ferrer PL, et al. High-dose propranolol therapy in the management of supraventricular tachycardia. J Pediatr 1979; 94:144–146.
894. Pimenta J, Pereira CB. Effects of atenolol in patients with reciprocating supraventricular tachycardia. Clin Cardiol 1986; 9:191–195.
895. McBride JW, McCoy HG, Goldenberg IF. Supraventricular tachycardia treated with continuous infusions of propranolol. Clin Pharmacol Ther 1988; 44:93–99.
896. Trippel DL, Gillette PC. Atenolol in children with supraventricular tachycardia. Am J Cardiol 1989; 64:233–236.
897. Mehta AV, Subrahmanyam AB, Anand R. Long-term efficacy and safety of atenolol for supraventricular tachycardia in children. Pediatr Cardiol 1996; 17:231–236.
898. Winniford MD, Fulton KL, Hillis LD. Long-term therapy of paroxysmal supraventricular tachycardia: a randomized, double-blind comparison of digoxin, propranolol and verapamil. Am J Cardiol 1984; 54:1138–1139.
899. Morganroth J, Horowitz LN, Anderson J, Turlapaty P. Comparative efficacy and tolerance of esmolol to propranolol for control of supraventricular tachyarrhythmia. Am J Cardiol 1985; 56:33F–39F.
900. Anderson S, Blanski L, Byrd RC, et al. Comparison of the efficacy and safety of esmolol, a short-acting beta blocker, with placebo in the treatment of supraventricular tachyarrhythmias: the esmolol vs placebo multicenter study group. Am Heart J 1986; 111:42–48.
901. Hepner SI, Davoli E. Successful treatment of supraventricular tachycardia with metoprolol, a cardioselective beta blocker. Clin Pediatr 1983; 22:522–523.
902. Gettes LS, Yoshonis KF. Rapidly recurring supraventricular tachycardia: a manifestation of reciprocating tachycardia and an indication for propranolol therapy. Circulation 1970; 41:689–700.
903. Krikler D. Verapamil in cardiology. Eur J Cardiol 1974; 2:3–10.
904. McGoon MD, Vlietstra RE, Holmes DR Jr, Osborn JE. The clinical use of verapamil. Mayo Clin Proc 1982; 57:495–510.
905. Roy D. Efficacy of diltiazem in recurrent supraventricular tachyarrhythmias. Can J Cardiol 1995; 11:538–540.
906. Betriu A, Chaitman BR, Bourassa MG, et al. Beneficial effect of intravenous diltiazem in the acute management of paroxysmal supraventricular tachyarrhythmias. Circulation 1983; 67:88–94.
907. Sternbach GL, Schroeder JS, Eliastam M, Beier-Scott L. Intravenous diltiazem for the treatment of supraventricular tachycardia. Clin Cardiol 1986; 9:145–149.
908. Schamroth L, Krikler DM, Garrett C. Immediate effects of intravenous verapamil in cardiac arrhythmias. Br Med J 1972; 1:660–662.
909. Krikler DM, Spurrell RA. Verapamil in the treatment of paroxysmal supraventricular tachycardia. Postgrad Med J 1974; 50:447–453.
910. Vohra J, Peter T, Hunt D, Sloman G. Verapamil induced premature ventricular beats before reversion of supraventricular tachycardia. Br Heart J 1974; 36:1186–1193.
911. Heng MK, Singh BN, Roche AH, Norris RM, Mercer CJ. Effects of intravenous verapamil on cardiac arrhythmias and on the electrocardiogram. Am Heart J 1975; 90:487–498.
912. Hartel G, Hartikainen M. Comparison of verapamil and practolol in paroxysmal supraventricular tachycardia. Eur J Cardiol 1976; 4:87–90.
913. Soler-Soler J, Sagrista-Sauleda J, Cabrera A, et al. Effect of verapamil in infants with paroxysmal supraventricular tachycardia. Circulation 1979; 59:876–879.
914. Gonzalez R, Scheinman MM. Treatment of supraventricular arrhythmias with intravenous and oral verapamil. Chest 1981; 80:465–470.
915. Greco R, Musto B, Arienzo V, Alborino A, Garofalo S, Marsico F. Treatment of paroxysmal supraventricular tachycardia in infancy with digitalis, adenosine-5'-triphosphate, and verapamil: a comparative study. Circulation 1982; 66:504–508.
916. Boudonas G, Lefkos N, Efthymiadis AP, Styliadis IG, Tsapas G. Intravenous administration of diltiazem in the treatment of supraventricular tachyarrhythmias. Acta Cardiol 1995; 50:125–134.
917. Mauritson DR, Winniford MD, Walker WS, Rude RE, Cary JR, Hillis LD. Oral verapamil for paroxysmal supraventricular tachycardia: a long-term, double-blind randomized trial. Ann Intern Med 1982; 96:409–412.
918. Lie KI, Duren DR, Cats VM, David GK, Durrer D. Long-term efficacy of verapamil in the treatment of paroxysmal supraventricular tachycardias. Am Heart J 1983; 105:688.
919. Satake S, Hiejima K, Moroi Y, Hirao K, Kubo I, Suzuki F. Usefulness of invasive and non-invasive electrophysiologic studies in the selection of antiarrhythmic drugs for the patients with paroxysmal supraventricular tachyarrhythmia. Jpn Circ J 1985; 49:345–350.
920. Hamer AW, Tanasescu DE, Marks JW, Peter T, Waxman AD, Mandel WJ. Failure of episodic high-dose oral verapamil therapy to convert supraventricular tachycardia: a study of plasma verapamil levels and gastric motility. Am Heart J 1987; 114:334–342.
921. Belhassen B, Viskin S, Laniado S. Sustained atrial fibrillation after conversion of paroxysmal reciprocating junctional tachycardia by intravenous verapamil. Am J Cardiol 1988; 62:835–837.
922. Jacob AS, Nielsen DH, Gianelly RE. Fatal ventricular fibrillation following verapamil in Wolff-Parkinson-White syndrome with atrial fibrillation. Ann Emerg Med 1985; 14:159–160.
923. Epstein ML, Kiel EA, Victorica BE. Cardiac decompensation following verapamil therapy in infants with supraventricular tachycardia. Pediatrics 1985; 75:737–740.
924. Kirk CR, Gibbs JL, Thomas R, Radley-Smith R, Qureshi SA. Cardiovascular collapse after verapamil in supraventricular tachycardia. Arch Dis Child 1987; 62:1265–1266.
925. O'Sullivan JJ, Gardiner HM, Wren C. Digoxin or flecainide for prophylaxis of supraventricular tachycardia in infants? J Am Coll Cardiol 1995; 26:991–994.
926. Byrum CJ, Wahl RA, Behrendt DM, Dick M. Ventricular fibrillation associated with use of digitalis in a newborn infant with Wolff-Parkinson-White syndrome. J Pediatr 1982; 101:400–403.
927. Luoma PV, Kujala PA, Juustila HJ, Takkunen JT. Efficacy of intravenous disopyramide in the termination of supraventricular arrhythmias. J Clin Pharmacol 1978; 18:293–301.
928. Moss AJ, Aledort LM. Use of edrophonium (Tensilon) in the evaluation of supraventricular tachycardias. Am J Cardiol 1966; 17:58–62.
929. Cantwell JD, Dawson JE, Fletcher GF. Supraventricular

tachyarrhythmias: treatment with edrophonium. Arch Intern Med 1972; 130:221–224.

930. Till JA, Shinebourne EA, Rowland E, et al. Paediatric use of flecainide in supraventricular tachycardia: clinical efficacy and pharmacokinetics. Br Heart J 1989; 62:133–139.

931. Ward DE, Jones S, Shinebourne EA. Use of flecainide acetate for refractory junctional tachycardias in children with the Wolff-Parkinson-White syndrome. Am J Cardiol 1986; 57:787–790.

932. Neuss H. Long term use of flecainide in patients with supraventricular tachycardia. Drugs 1985; 29:21–25.

933. van Wijk LM, Crijns HJ, van Gilst WH, Wesseling H, Lie KI. Flecainide acetate in the treatment of supraventricular tachycardias: value of programmed electrical stimulation for long-term prognosis. Am Heart J 1989; 117:365–369.

934. Perry JC, McQuinn RL, Smith RT Jr, Gothing C, Fredell P, Garson A Jr. Flecainide acetate for resistant arrhythmias in the young: efficacy and pharmacokinetics. J Am Coll Cardiol 1989; 14:185–191.

935. Dorian P, Naccarelli GV, Coumel P, Hohnloser SH, Maser MJ. A randomized comparison of flecainide versus verapamil in paroxysmal supraventricular tachycardia: the Flecainide Multicenter Investigators Group. Am J Cardiol 1996; 77:89A–95A.

936. Dumesic DA, Silverman NH, Tobias S, Golbus MS. Transplacental cardioversion of fetal supraventricular tachycardia with procainamide. N Engl J Med 1982; 307:1128–1131.

937. Benson DW Jr, Dunnigan A, Green TP, Benditt DG, Schneider SP. Periodic procainamide for paroxysmal tachycardia. Circulation 1985; 72:147–152.

938. Ludmer PL, McGowan NE, Antman EM, Friedman PL. Efficacy of propafenone in Wolff-Parkinson-White syndrome: electrophysiologic findings and long-term follow-up. J Am Coll Cardiol 1987; 9:1357–1363.

939. Pritchett EL, McCarthy EA, Wilkinson WE. Propafenone treatment of symptomatic paroxysmal supraventricular arrhythmias: a randomized, placebo-controlled, crossover trial in patients tolerating oral therapy. Ann Intern Med 1991; 114:539–544.

940. UK Propafenone PSVT Study Group. A randomized, placebo-controlled trial of propafenone in the prophylaxis of paroxysmal supraventricular tachycardia and paroxysmal atrial fibrillation. Circulation 1995; 92:2550–2557.

941. Guccione P, Drago F, Di Donato RM, et al. Oral propafenone therapy for children with arrhythmias: efficacy and adverse effects in midterm follow-up. Am Heart J 1991; 122:1022–1027.

942. Beaufort-Krol GCM, Bink-Boelkens MTE. Oral propafenone as treatment for incessant supraventricular and ventricular tachycardia in children. Am J Cardiol 1993; 72:1213–1214.

943. Vignati G, Mauri L, Figini A. The use of propafenone in the treatment of tachyarrhythmias in children. Eur Heart J 1993; 14:546–550.

944. Heusch A, Kramer HH, Krogmann ON, Rammos S, Bourgeous M. Clinical experience with propafenone for cardiac arrhythmias in the young. Eur Heart J 1994; 15:1050–1056.

945. Bowman E, Paes BA, Way RC. Oral sotalol in neonatal supraventricular tachycardia. Acta Paediatr Scand 1988; 77:171.

946. Camm AJ, Paul V. Sotalol for paroxysmal supraventricular tachycardias. Am J Cardiol 1990; 65:67A–73A.

947. Prakash R, Parmley WW, Allen HN, Matloff JM. Effect of sotalol on clinical arrhythmias. Am J Cardiol 1972; 29:397–400.

948. Jordaens L, Gorgels A, Stroobandt R, Temmerman J. Efficacy and safety of intravenous sotalol for termination of paroxysmal supraventricular tachycardia: the sotalol versus placebo multicenter study group. Am J Cardiol 1991; 68:35–40.

949. Sung RJ, Tan HL, Karagounis L, et al. Intravenous sotalol for the termination of supraventricular tachycardia and atrial fibrillation and flutter: a multicenter, randomized, double-blind, placebo-controlled study. Sotalol Multicenter Study Group. Am Heart J 1995; 129:739–748.

950. Wanless RS, Anderson K, Joy M, Joseph SP. Multicenter comparative sutdy of the efficacy and safety of sotalol in the prophylactic treatment of patients with paroxysmal supraventricular tachyarrhythmias. Am Heart J 1997; 133:441–446.

951. Atrial Fibrillation Investigation with Bidisomide (AFIB) Investigators. Treatment of atrial fibrillation and paroxysmal supraventricular tachycardia with bidisomide. Circulation 1997; 96:2625–2632.

952. Dye CL. Atrial tachycardia in Wolff-Parkinson-White syndrome: conversion to normal sinus rhythm with lidocaine. Am J Cardiol 1969; 24:265–268.

953. Rosen KM, Denes P, Wu D, Cummings J. Conversion of paroxysmal supraventricular tachycardia due to a concealed extranodal pathway with intravenous bolus of lidocaine. Chest 1977; 71:78–80.

954. Buxton AE. Catheter ablation of atrioventricular bypass tracts: still an investigational procedure. Circulation 1989; 79:1388–1390.

955. Huang SK. Radiofrequency catheter ablation of cardiac arrhythmias: appraisal of an evolving therapeutic modality. Am Heart J 1989; 118:1317–1323.

956. Borggrefe M, Hindricks G, Haverkamp W, Breithardt G. Catheter ablation using radiofrequency energy. Clin Cardiol 1990; 13:127–131.

957. Huang SK. Advances in applications of radiofrequency current to catheter ablation therapy. Pacing Clin Electrophysiol 1991; 14:28–42.

958. Klein LS. Radiofrequency catheter ablation: safety and practicality. Circulation 1991; 84:2594–2597.

959. Ruskin JN. Catheter ablation for supraventricular tachycardia. N Engl J Med 1991; 324:1660–1662.

960. Kalbfleisch SJ, Langberg JJ. Catheter ablation with radiofrequency energy: biophysical aspects and clinical applications. J Cardiovasc Electrophysiol 1992; 3:173–186.

961. Scheinman MM. North American Society of Pacing and Electrophysiology (NASPE) survey on radiofrequency catheter ablation: implications for clinicians, third party insurers, and government regulatory agencies. Pacing Clin Electrophysiol 1992; 15:2228–2231.

962. Duckeck W, Engelstein ED, Kuck KH. Radiofrequency current therapy in atrial tachyarrhythmias: modulation versus ablation of atrioventricular nodal conduction. Pacing Clin Electrophysiol 1993; 16:629–636.

963. Fisher JD. Direct current and radiofrequency catheter ablation: so far and yet so near. J Am Coll Cardiol 1993; 21:565–566.

964. Gursoy S, Schluter M, Kuck KH. Radiofrequency current catheter ablation for control of supraventricular arrhythmias. J Cardiovasc Electrophysiol 1993; 4:194–205.

965. Plumb VJ. What price success? J Am Coll Cardiol 1993; 21:1622–1623.

966. Smith JM, Cain ME. Radiofrequency catheter ablation for supraventricular tachycardias: blazing paths or burning bridges? J Cardiovasc Electrophysiol 1993; 4:390–392.

967. Wood M, Ellenbogen K, Stambler B. Radiofrequency catheter ablation for the management of cardiac tachyarrhythmias. Am J Med Sci 1993; 306:241–247.

968. American College of Cardiology Cardiovascular Technology Assessment Committee. Catheter ablation for cardiac arrhythmias: clinical applications, personnel and facilities: American College of Cardiology Cardiovascular Technology Assessment Committee. J Am Coll Cardiol 1994; 24:828–833.

969. Bashir Y, Ward DE. Radiofrequency catheter ablation: a new frontier in interventional cardiology. Br Heart J 1994; 71:119–124.

970. Haissaguerre M, Gaita F, Marcus FI, Clementy J. Radiofrequency catheter ablation of accessory pathways: a contemporary review. J Cardiovasc Electrophysiol 1994; 5:532–552.

971. Kugler JD. Radiofrequency catheter ablation for supraventricular tachycardia: should it be used in infants and small children? Circulation 1994; 90:639–641.

972. Manolis AS, Wang PJ, Estes NA III. Radiofrequency catheter ablation for cardiac tachyarrhythmias. Ann Intern Med 1994; 121:452–461.

973. Trohman RG, Pinski SL, Sterba R, Schutzman JJ, Kleman JM, Kidwell GA. Evolving concepts in radiofrequency catheter ablation of atrioventricular nodal reentry tachycardia. Am Heart J 1994; 128:586–595.

974. Zipes DP, DiMarco JP, Gillette PC, et al. Guidelines for clinical intracardiac electrophysiological and catheter ablation procedures: a report of the American College of Cardiology/American Heart Association Task Force on Practice Guidelines (Committee on Clinical Intracardiac Electrophysiologic and Catheter Ablation Procedures), developed in collaboration with the North American Society of Pacing and Electrophysiology. J Am Coll Cardiol 1995; 26:555–573.

975. Kottkamp H, Hindricks G, Borggrefe M, Breithardt G. Radiofrequency catheter ablation of the anterosuperior and posteroinferior atrial approaches to the AV node for treatment of AV nodal reentrant tachycardia: techniques for selective ablation of "fast" and "slow" AV node pathways. J Cardiovasc Electrophysiol 1997; 8:451–468.

976. Stevenson WG, Ellison KE, Lefroy DC, Friedman PL. Ablation therapy for cardiac arrhythmias. Am J Cardiol 1997; 80:56G–66G.

977. Van Hare GF, Lesh MD, Scheinman M, Langberg JJ. Percutaneous radiofrequency catheter ablation for supraventricular arrhythmias in children. J Am Coll Cardiol 1991; 17:1613 1620.

978. Sreeram N, Smeets JL, Pulles-Heintzberger CF, Wellens HJJ. Radiofrequency catheter ablation of accessory atrioventricular pathways in children and young adults. Br Heart J 1993; 70:160–165.

979. Dhala A, Bremner S, Deshpande S, et al. Efficacy and safety of atrioventricular nodal modification for atrioventricular nodal reentrant tachycardia in the pediatric population. Am Heart J 1994; 128:903–907.

980. Erickson CC, Walsh EP, Triedman JK, Saul JP. Efficacy and safety of radiofrequency ablation in infants and young children < 18 months of age. Am J Cardiol 1994; 74:944–947.

981. Kugler JD, Danford DA, Deal BJ, et al. Radiofrequency catheter ablation for tachyarrhythmias in children and adolescents: the Pediatric Electrophysiology Society. N Engl J Med 1994; 330:1481–1487.

982. Teixeira OH, Balaji S, Case CL, Gillette PC. Radiofrequency catheter ablation of atrioventricular nodal reentrant tachycardia in children. Pacing Clin Electrophysiol 1994; 17:1621–1626.

983. Bubolz B, Case CL, McKay CA, O'Connor BK, Knick BJ, Gillette PC. Learning curve for radiofrequency catheter ablation in pediatrics at a single institution. Am Heart J 1996; 131:956–960.

984. Epstein MR, Saul JP, Fishberger SB, Triedman JK, Walsh EP. Spontaneous accelerated junctional rhythm: an unusual but useful observation prior to radiofrequency catheter ablation for atrioventricular node reentrant tachycardia in young patients. Pacing Clin Electrophysiol 1997; 20:1654–1661.

985. Van Hare GF. Radiofrequency ablation of accessory pathways associated with congenital heart disease. Pacing Clin Electrophysiol 1997; 20:2077–2081.

986. Van Hare GF. Indications for radiofrequency ablation in the pediatric population. J Cardiovasc Electrophysiol 1997; 8:952–962.

987. Epstein LM, Chiesa N, Wong MN, et al. Radiofrequency catheter ablation in the treatment of supraventricular tachycardia in the elderly. J Am Coll Cardiol 1994; 23:1356–1362.

988. Lau CP, Tai YT, Lee PW. The effects of radiofrequency ablation versus medical therapy on the quality-of-life and exercise capacity in patients with accessory pathway-mediated supraventricular tachycardia: a treatment comparison study. Pacing Clin Electrophysiol 1995; 18:424–432.

989. Leather RA, Leitch JW, Klein GJ, Guiraudon GM, Yee R, Kim YH. Radiofrequency catheter ablation of accessory pathways: a learning experience. Am J Cardiol 1991; 68:1651–1655.

990. Schluter M, Geiger M, Siebels J, Duckeck W, Kuck KH. Catheter ablation using radiofrequency current to cure symptomatic patients with tachyarrhythmias related to an accessory atrioventricular pathway. Circulation 1991; 84:1644–1661.

991. Hindricks G. Incidence of complete atrioventricular block following attempted radiofrequency catheter modification of the atrioventricular node in 880 patients: results of the Multicenter European Radiofrequency Survey (MERFS) of the Working Group on Arrhythmias of the European Society of Cardiology. Eur Heart J 1996; 17:82–88.

992. Calkins H, Niklason L, Sousa J, el-Atassi R, Langberg J, Morady F. Radiation exposure during radiofrequency catheter ablation of accessory atrioventricular connections. Circulation 1991; 84:2376–2382.

993. Lindsay BD, Eichling JO, Ambos HD, Cain ME. Radiation exposure to patients and medical personnel during radiofrequency catheter ablation for supraventricular tachycardia. Am J Cardiol 1992; 70:218–223.

994. Katritsis D, Bashir Y, Heald S, Poloniecki J, Ward DE. Radiofrequency ablation of accessory pathways: implications of accumulated experience and time dedicated to procedures. Eur Heart J 1994; 15:339–344.

995. Kugler JD, Danford DA, Houston K, Felix G. Radiofrequency catheter ablation for paroxysmal supraventricular tachycardia in children and adolescents without structural heart disease: Pediatric EP Society, Radiofrequency Catheter Ablation Registry. Am J Cardiol 1997; 80:1438–1443.

996. de Buitleir M, Bove EL, Schmaltz S, Kadish AH, Morady F. Cost of catheter versus surgical ablation in the Wolff-Parkinson-White syndrome. Am J Cardiol 1990; 66:189–192.

997. Case CL, Gillette PC, Crawford FA, Knick BJ. Comparison of medical care costs between successful radiofrequency catheter ablation and surgical ablation of accessory pathways in the pediatric age group. Am J Cardiol 1994; 73:600–601.

998. Kalbfleisch SJ, Calkins H, Langberg JJ, et al. Comparison of the cost of radiofrequency catheter modification of the atrioventricular node and medical therapy for drug-refractory atrioventricular node reentrant tachycardia. J Am Coll Cardiol 1992; 19:1583–1587.

999. Garson A Jr, Kanter RJ. Management of the child with Wolff-Parkinson-White syndrome and supraventricular tachycardia: model for cost effectiveness. J Cardiovasc Electrophysiol 1997; 8:1320–1326.

1000. Man KC, Kalbfleisch SJ, Hummel JD, et al. Safety and cost of outpatient radiofrequency ablation of the slow pathway in patients with atrioventricular nodal reentrant tachycardia. Am J Cardiol 1993; 72:1323–1324.

1001. Kalbfleisch SJ, el-Atassi R, Calkins H, Langberg JJ, Morady F. Safety, feasibility and cost of outpatient radiofrequency catheter ablation of accessory atrioventricular connections. J Am Coll Cardiol 1993; 21:567–570.

1002. Andresen D, Behrens S, Bruggemann T, Schroder R. Should radiofrequency therapy be performed in every symptomatic patient with supraventricular tachycardia? (pro drug position). Pacing Clin Electrophysiol 1993; 16:653–657.

1003. Critelli G, Perticone F, Coltorti F, Monda V, Gallagher J. Closed chest modification of atrioventricular conduction system in man for treatment of refractory supraventricular tachycardia. Br Heart J 1983; 49:544–549.

1004. Critelli G, Perticone F, Coltorti F, Monda V, Gallagher JJ. Antegrade slow bypass conduction after closed-chest ablation of the His bundle in permanent junctional reciprocating tachycardia. Circulation 1983; 67:687–692.

1005. Bardy GH, Poole JE, Coltorti F, et al. Catheter ablation of a concealed accessory pathway. Am J Cardiol 1984; 54:1366–1368.

1006. Bhandari A, Morady F, Shen EN, Schwartz AB, Botvinick E, Scheinman MM. Catheter-induced His bundle ablation in a patient with reentrant tachycardia associated with a nodoventricular tract. J Am Coll Cardiol 1984; 4:611–616.

1007. Fisher JD, Brodman R, Kim SG, et al. Attempted nonsurgical electrical ablation of accessory pathways via the coronary sinus in the Wolff-Parkinson-White syndrome. J Am Coll Cardiol 1984; 4:685–694.

1008. Josephson ME. Catheter ablation of arrhythmias. Ann Intern Med 1984; 101:234–237.

1009. Morady F, Scheinman MM. Transvenous catheter ablation of a posteroseptal accessory pathway in a patient with the Wolff-Parkinson-White syndrome. N Engl J Med 1984; 310:705–707.

1010. Gang ES, Oseran D, Rosenthal M, et al. Closed chest catheter ablation of an accessory pathway in a patient with permanent junctional reciprocating tachycardia. J Am Coll Cardiol 1985; 6:1167–1171.

1011. Morady F, Scheinman MM, Winston SA, et al. Efficacy and safety of transcatheter ablation of posteroseptal accessory pathways. Circulation 1985; 72:170–177.

1012. Ward DE, Camm AJ. Treatment of tachycardias associated with the Wolff-Parkinson-White syndrome by transvenous electrical ablation of accessory pathways. Br Heart J 1985; 53:64–68.

1013. Scheinman MM, Davis JC. Catheter ablation for treatment of tachyarrhythmias: present role and potential promise. Circulation 1986; 73:10–13.

1014. Smith RT Jr, Gillette PC, Massumi A, McVey P, Garson A Jr. Transcatheter ablative techniques for treatment of the permanent form of junctional reciprocating tachycardia in young patients. J Am Coll Cardiol 1986; 8:385–390.

1015. Bardy GH, Ivey TD, Coltorti F, Stewart RB, Johnson G, Greene HL. Developments, complications and limitations of catheter-mediated electrical ablation of posterior accessory atrioventricular pathways. Am J Cardiol 1988; 61:309–316.

1016. Evans GT Jr, Scheinman MM, Zipes DP, et al. The percutaneous cardiac mapping and ablation registry: final summary of results. Pacing Clin Electrophysiol 1988; 11:1621–1626.

1017. Warin JF, Haissaguerre M, Lemetayer P, Guillem JP, Blanchot P. Catheter ablation of accessory pathways with a direct approach: results in 35 patients. Circulation 1988; 78:800–815.

1018. Webb JG, Downar E, Harris L, Rossall RE. Direct endocardial recording and catheter ablation of an accessory pathway in a patient with incessant supraventricular tachycardia. Pacing Clin Electrophysiol 1988; 11:1533–1539.

1019. Borggrefe M, Breithardt G, Podczeck A, Rohner D, Budde T, Martinez-Rubio A. Catheter ablation of ventricular tachycardia using defibrillator pulses: electrophysiological findings and long-term results. Eur Heart J 1989; 10:591–601.

1020. Bromberg BI, Dick M II, Scott WA, Morady F. Transcatheter electrical ablation of accessory pathways in children. Pacing Clin Electrophysiol 1989; 12:1787–1796.

1021. Haissaguerre M, Warin JF, Lemetayer P, Saoudi N, Guillem JP, Blanchot P. Closed-chest ablation of retrograde conduction in patients with atrioventricular nodal reentrant tachycardia. N Engl J Med 1989; 320:426–433.

1022. Sanjuan R, Morell S, Garcia Civera R, et al. Transvenous ablation with high frequency energy for atrioventricular junctional (AV nodal) reentrant tachycardia. Pacing Clin Electrophysiol 1989; 12:1631–1639.

1023. Scheinman MM. Catheter techniques for ablation of supraventricular tachycardia. N Engl J Med 1989; 320:460–461.

1024. Haissaguerre M, Warin JF, Le Metayer P, et al. Catheter ablation of Mahaim fibers with preservation of atrioventricular nodal conduction. Circulation 1990; 82:418–427.

1025. Haissaguerre M, Warin JF, d'Ivernois C, Le Metayer PH, Montserrat P. Fulguration for AV nodal tachycardia: results in 42 patients with a mean follow-up of 23 months. Pacing Clin Electrophysiol 1990; 13:2000–2007.

1026. Oslizlok P, Case CL, Gillette PC. Successful transcatheter ablation of an accessory connection in a child following failed surgery: an ideal case? Am Heart J 1990; 119:1424–1426.

1027. Warin JF, Haissaguerre M, d'Ivernois C, Le Metayer P, Montserrat P. Catheter ablation of accessory pathways: technique and results in 248 patients. Pacing Clin Electrophysiol 1990; 13:1609–1614.

1028. Haissaguerre M, Dartigues JF, Warin JF, Le Metayer P, Montserrat P, Salamon R. Electrogram patterns predictive of successful catheter ablation of accessory pathways: value of unipolar recording mode. Circulation 1991; 84:188–202.

1029. Lemery R, Talajic M, Roy D, et al. Success, safety, and late electrophysiological outcome of low-energy direct-current ablation in patients with the Wolff-Parkinson-White syndrome. Circulation 1992; 85:957–962.

1030. Haissaguerre M, Puel V, Bekheit S, et al. Catheter ablation of accessory pathways in children. Eur Heart J 1994; 15:200–205.

1031. Epstein LM, Scheinman MM, Langberg JJ, Chilson D, Goldberg HR, Griffin JC. Percutaneous catheter modification of the atrioventricular node: a potential cure for atrioventricular nodal reentrant tachycardia. Circulation 1989; 80:757–768.

1032. Moro C, Madrid AH, Rayo I, et al. Cardiac fulguration, a new alternative therapy for atrioventricular nodal reentrant tachycardia. Eur Heart J 1992; 13:61–66.

1033. Lemery R, Talajic M, Roy D, et al. Results of a comparative study of low energy direct current with radiofrequency ablation in patients with the Wolff-Parkinson-White syndrome. Br Heart J 1993; 70:580–584.

1034. Sebag C, Lavergne T, Millat B, et al. Rupture of the stomach and the esophagus after attempted transcatheter ablation of an accessory pathway by direct current shock. Am J Cardiol 1989; 63:890–891.

1035. Chen SA, Tsang WP, Hsia CP, et al. Catheter ablation of accessory atrioventricular pathways in 114 symptomatic patients with Wolff-Parkinson-White syndrome: a comparative study of direct-current and radiofrequency ablation. Am Heart J 1992; 124:356–365.

1036. Lee MA, Morady F, Kadish A, et al. Catheter modification of the atrioventricular junction with radiofrequency energy for control of atrioventricular nodal reentry tachycardia. Circulation 1991; 83:827–835.

1037. Hindricks G. The Multicentre European Radiofrequency Survey (MERFS): complications of radiofrequency catheter ablation of arrhythmias. The Multicentre European Radiofrequency Survey (MERFS) investigators of the Working Group on Arrhythmias of the European Society of Cardiology. Eur Heart J 1993; 14:1644–1653.

1038. Scheinman MM. NASPE survey on catheter ablation. Pacing Clin Electrophysiol 1995; 18:1474–1478.

1039. Weber HP, Heinze A. Laser catheter ablation of atrial flutter and of atrioventricular nodal reentrant tachycardia in a single session. Eur Heart J 1994; 15:1147–1149.

1040. Weber HP, Kaltenbrunner W, Heinze A, Steinbach K. Laser catheter coagulation of atrial myocardium for ablation of atrioventricular nodal reentrant tachycardia: first clinical experience. Eur Heart J 1997; 18:487–495.

1041. Garratt CJ. Fast or slow pathway ablation (or neither) for AV nodal tachycardia? Heart 1997; 78:3–4.

1042. Jazayeri MR, Hempe SL, Sra JS, et al. Selective transcatheter ablation of the fast and slow pathways using radiofrequency energy in patients with atrioventricular nodal reentrant tachycardia. Circulation 1992; 85:1318–1328.

1043. Chen SA, Chiang CE, Tsang WP, et al. Selective radiofrequency catheter ablation of fast and slow pathways in 100 patients with atrioventricular nodal reentrant tachycardia. Am Heart J 1993; 125:1–10.

1044. Mitrani RD, Klein LS, Hackett FK, Zipes DP, Miles WM. Radiofrequency ablation for atrioventricular node reentrant tachycardia: comparison between fast (anterior) and slow (posterior) pathway ablation. J Am Coll Cardiol 1993; 21:432–441.

1045. Simmers TA, Wever EF, Wittkampf FH, Hauer RN. Change in delay of atrioventricular conduction after radiofrequency catheter ablation for atrioventricular nodal re-entry tachycardia. Br Heart J 1995; 73:442–444.

1046. Calkins H, Sousa J, el-Atassi R, et al. Diagnosis and cure of the Wolff-Parkinson-White syndrome or paroxysmal supraventricular tachycardias during a single electrophysiologic test. N Engl J Med 1991; 324:1612–1618.

1047. Jazayeri MR, Akhtar M. Electrophysiological behavior of atrioventricular node after selective fast or slow pathway ablation in patients with atrioventricular nodal reentrant tachycardia. Pacing Clin Electrophysiol 1993; 16:623–628.

1048. Greene TO, Huang SK, Wagshal AB, et al. Cardiovascular complications after radiofrequency catheter ablation of supraventricular tachyarrhythmias. Am J Cardiol 1994; 74:615–617.

1049. Fenelon G, d'Avila A, Malacky T, Brugada P. Prognostic significance of transient complete atrioventricular block during radiofrequency ablation of atrioventricular node reentrant tachycardia. Am J Cardiol 1995; 75:698–702.

1050. Kay GN, Epstein AE, Dailey SM, Plumb VJ. Selective radiofrequency ablation of the slow pathway for the treatment of atrioventricular nodal reentrant tachycardia: evidence for involvement of perinodal myocardium within the reentrant circuit. Circulation 1992; 85:1675–1688.

1051. Moulton K, Miller B, Scott J, Woods WT Jr. Radiofrequency catheter ablation for AV nodal reentry: a technique for rapid transection of the slow AV nodal pathway. Pacing Clin Electrophysiol 1993; 16:760–768.

1052. Baker JH II, Plumb VJ, Epstein AE, Kay GN. Predictors of recurrent atrioventricular nodal reentry after selective slow pathway ablation. Am J Cardiol 1994; 73:765–769.

1053. Manolis AS, Wang PJ, Estes NA III. Radiofrequency ablation of slow pathway in patients with atrioventricular nodal reentrant tachycardia: do arrhythmia recurrences correlate with persistent slow pathway conduction or site of successful ablation? Circulation 1994; 90:2815–2819.

1054. Chen SA, Wu TJ, Chiang CE, et al. Recurrent tachycardia after selective ablation of slow pathway in patients with atrioventricular nodal reentrant tachycardia. Am J Cardiol 1995; 76:131–137.

1055. Kreiner G, Heinz G, Siostrzonek P, Gossinger HD. Effect of slow pathway ablation on ventricular rate during atrial fibrillation: dependence on electrophysiological properties of the fast pathway. Circulation 1996; 93:277–283.

1056. Markowitz SM, Stein KM, Lerman BB. Mechanism of ventricular rate control after radiofrequency modification of atrioventricular conduction in patients with atrial fibrillation. Circulation 1996; 94:2856–2864.

1057. Tondo C, Bella PD, Maslowsky F, Riva S. Persistence of single echo beat inducibility after selective ablation of the slow pathway in patients with atrioventricular nodal reentrant tachycardia: relationship to the functional properties of the atrioventricular node and clinical implications. J Cardiovasc Electrophysiol 1996; 7:689–696.

1058. Langberg JJ, Kim YN, Goyal R, et al. Conversion of typical to "atypical" atrioventricular nodal reentrant tachycardia after radiofrequency catheter modification of the atrioventricular junction. Am J Cardiol 1992; 69:503–508.

1059. Shen WK, Munger TM, Stanton MS, Osborn MJ, Hammill SC, Packer DL. Effects of slow pathway ablation on fast pathway function in patients with atrioventricular nodal reentrant tachycardia. J Cardiovasc Electrophysiol 1997; 8:627–638.

1060. Kim YH, O'Nunain S, Trouton T, et al. Pseudo-pacemaker syndrome following inadvertent fast pathway ablation for atrioventricular nodal reentrant tachycardia. J Cardiovasc Electrophysiol 1993; 4:178–182.

1061. Kottkamp H, Hindricks G, Willems S, et al. An anatomically and electrogram-guided stepwise approach for effective and safe catheter ablation of the fast pathway for elimination of atrioventricular node reentrant tachycardia. J Am Coll Cardiol 1995; 25:974–981.

1062. Mehta D, Gomes JA. Long term results of fast pathway ablation in atrioventricular nodal reentry tachycardia using a modified technique. Br Heart J 1995; 74:671–675.

1063. Goy JJ, Fromer M, Schlaepfer J, Kappenberger L. Clinical efficacy of radiofrequency current in the treatment of patients with atrioventricular node reentrant tachycardia. J Am Coll Cardiol 1990; 16:418–423.

1064. Jackman WM, Beckman KJ, McClelland JH, et al. Treatment of supraventricular tachycardia due to atrioventricular nodal reentry, by radiofrequency catheter ablation of slow-pathway conduction. N Engl J Med 1992; 327:313–318.

1065. Wathen M, Natale A, Wolfe K, Yee R, Newman D, Klein G. An anatomically guided approach to atrioventricular node slow pathway ablation. Am J Cardiol 1992; 70:886–889.

1066. Kay GN, Epstein AE, Dailey SM, Plumb VJ. Role of radiofrequency ablation in the management of supraventricular arrhythmias: experience in 760 consecutive patients. J Cardiovasc Electrophysiol 1993; 4:371–389.

1067. Li HG, Klein GJ, Stites HW, et al. Elimination of slow pathway conduction: an accurate indicator of clinical success after radiofrequency atrioventricular node modification. J Am Coll Cardiol 1993; 22:1849–1853.

1068. Lindsay BD, Chung MK, Gamache MC, et al. Therapeutic end points for the treatment of atrioventricular node reentrant tachycardia by catheter-guided radiofrequency current. J Am Coll Cardiol 1993; 22:733–740.

1069. Jentzer JH, Goyal R, Williamson BD, et al. Analysis of junctional ectopy during radiofrequency ablation of the slow pathway in patients with atrioventricular nodal reentrant tachycardia. Circulation 1994; 90:2820–2826.

1070. Miles WM, Hubbard JE, Zipes DP, Klein LS. Elimination of AV nodal reentrant tachycardia with 2:1 VA block by posteroseptal ablation. J Cardiovasc Electrophysiol 1994; 5:510–516.

1071. Blanck Z, Dhala AA, Sra J, et al. Characterization of atrioventricular nodal behavior and ventricular response during atrial fibrillation before and after a selective slow-pathway ablation. Circulation 1995; 91:1086–1094.

1072. Epstein LM, Lesh MD, Griffin JC, Lee RJ, Scheinman MM. A direct midseptal approach to slow atrioventricular nodal pathway ablation. Pacing Clin Electrophysiol 1995; 18:57–64.

1073. Kuo C, Lauer MR, Young C, et al. Electrophysiologic significance of discrete slow potentials in dual atrioventricular node physiology: implications for selective radiofrequency ablation of slow pathway conduction. Am Heart J 1996; 131:490–498.

1074. Ueng KC, Chen SA, Chiang CE, et al. Dimension and related anatomical distance of Koch's triangle in patients with atrioventricular nodal reentrant tachycardia. J Cardiovasc Electrophysiol 1996; 7:1017–1023.

1075. Yu JC, Lauer MR, Young C, Liem LB, Hou C, Sung RJ. Localization of the origin of the atrioventricular junctional rhythm induced during selective ablation of slow-pathway conduction in patients with atrioventricular node reentrant tachycardia. Am Heart J 1996; 131:937–946.

1076. Basta MN, Krahn AD, Klein GJ, Rosenbaum M, Le Feuvre C, Yee R. Safety of slow pathway ablation in patients with atrioventricular node reentrant tachycardia and a long fast pathway effective refractory period. Am J Cardiol 1997; 80:155–159.

1077. Lai LP, Lin JL, Chen TF, Ko WC, Lien WP. Clinical, electrophysiological characteristics, and radiofrequency catheter ablation of atrial tachycardia near the apex of Koch's triangle. PACE 1998; 21:367–374.

1078. De Lima GG, Roy D, Talajic M, Dubuc M. One-to-two atrioventricular conduction causing nonreentrant tachycardia: successful treatment with radiofrequency ablation. PACE 1998; 21:1152–1154.

1079. Tada H, Nogami A, Naito S, et al. Selected slow pathway ablation in a patient with corrected transposition of the great arteries and atrioventricular nodal reentrant tachycardia. J Cardiovasc Electrophysiol 1998; 9:436–440.

1080. Langberg JJ, Calkins H, Kim YN, et al. Recurrence of conduction in accessory atrioventricular connections after initially successful radiofrequency catheter ablation. J Am Coll Cardiol 1992; 19:1588–1592.

1081. Boyce K, Henjum S, Helmer G, Chen PS. Radiofrequency catheter ablation of the accessory pathway in the permanent form of junctional reciprocating tachycardia. Am Heart J 1993; 126:716–719.

1082. Scheinman MM. Patterns of catheter ablation practice in the United States: results of the 1992 NASPE survey: North American Society of Pacing and Electrophysiology. Pacing Clin Electrophysiol 1994; 17:873–875.

1083. Borggrefe M, Budde T, Podczeck A, Breithardt G. High frequency alternating current ablation of an accessory pathway in humans. J Am Coll Cardiol 1987; 10:576–582.

1084. Kuck KH, Kunze KP, Schluter M, Geiger M, Jackman WM, Naccarelli GV. Modification of a left-sided accessory atrioventricular pathway by radiofrequency current using a bipolar epicardial-endocardial electrode configuration. Eur Heart J 1988; 9:927–932.

1085. Kuck KH, Kunze KP, Schluter M, Geiger M, Jackman WM. Ablation of a left-sided free-wall accessory pathway by percutaneous catheter application of a radiofrequency current in a patient with the Wolff-Parkinson-White syndrome. Pacing Clin Electrophysiol 1989; 12:1681–1690.

1086. Jackman WM, Wang XZ, Friday KJ, et al. Catheter ablation of accessory atrioventricular pathways (Wolff-Parkinson-White syndrome) by radiofrequency current. N Engl J Med 1991; 324:1605–1611.

1087. Kuck KH, Schluter M, Geiger M, Siebels J, Duckeck W. Radiofrequency current catheter ablation of accessory atrioventricular pathways. Lancet 1991; 337:1557–1561.

1088. Okishige K, Strickberger SA, Walsh EP, Saul JP, Friedman PL. Catheter ablation of the atrial origin of a decrementally conducting atriofascicular accessory pathway by radiofrequency current. J Cardiovasc Electrophysiol 1991; 2:465–475.

1089. Calkins H, Langberg J, Sousa J, et al. Radiofrequency catheter ablation of accessory atrioventricular connections in 250 patients: abbreviated therapeutic approach to Wolff-Parkinson-White syndrome. Circulation 1992; 85:1337–1346.

1090. Chen SA, Tsang WP, Hsia CP, et al. Catheter ablation of free wall accessory atrioventricular pathways in 89 patients with Wolff-Parkinson-White syndrome: comparison of direct current and radiofrequency ablation. Eur Heart J 1992; 13:1329–1338.

1091. Lesh MD, Van Hare GF, Schamp DJ, et al. Curative percutaneous catheter ablation using radiofrequency energy for accessory pathways in all locations: results in 100 consecutive patients. J Am Coll Cardiol 1992; 19:1303–1309.

1092. Lesh MD, Van Hare GF, Scheinman MM, Ports TA, Epstein LA. Comparison of the retrograde and transseptal methods for ablation of left free wall accessory pathways. J Am Coll Cardiol 1993; 22:542–549.

1093. Swartz JF, Tracy CM, Fletcher RD. Radiofrequency endocardial catheter ablation of accessory atrioventricular pathway atrial insertion sites. Circulation 1993; 87:487–499.

1094. Timmermans C, Smeets JL, Rodriguez LM, et al. Recurrence rate after accessory pathway ablation. Br Heart J 1994; 72:571–574.

1095. Wen ZC, Chen SA, Tai CT, et al. Temperature monitoring in radiofrequency catheter ablation of atrial flutter using the linear ablation technique. J Cardiovasc Electrophysiol 1996; 7:1050–1057.

1096. Brugada J, Garcia-Bolao I, Figueiredo M, Puigfel M, Matas M, Navarro-Lopez F. Radiofrequency ablation of concealed left free-wall accessory pathways without coronary sinus catheterization: results in 100 consecutive patients. J Cardiovasc Electrophysiol 1997; 8:249–253.

1097. Soejima K, Mitamura H, Miyazaki T, et al. Catheter ablation of accessory atrioventricular connection between right atrial appendage to right ventricle: a case report. J Cardiovasc Electrophysiol 1998; 9:523–528.

1098. Dick M II, O'Connor BK, Serwer GA, LeRoy S, Armstrong B. Use of radiofrequency current to ablate accessory connections in children. Circulation 1991; 84:2318–2324.

1099. Schluter M, Kuck KH. Radiofrequency current for catheter ablation of accessory atrioventricular connections in children and adolescents: emphasis on the single-catheter technique. Pediatrics 1992; 89:930–935.

1100. Case CL, Schaffer MS, Dhala AA, Gillette PC, Fletcher SE. Radiofrequency catheter ablation of an accessory atrioventricular connection in a Fontan patient. Pacing Clin Electrophysiol 1993; 16:1434–1436.

1101. Lemery R, Talajic M, Roy D, et al. Catheter ablation using radiofrequency or low-energy direct current in pediatric patients with the Wolff-Parkinson-White syndrome. Am J Cardiol 1994; 73:191–194.

1102. Benito F, Sanchez C. Radiofrequency catheter ablation of accessory pathways in infants. Heart 1997; 78:160–162.

1103. Van Hare GF, Lesh MD, Stanger P. Radiofrequency catheter ablation of supraventricular arrhythmias in patients with

congenital heart disease: results and technical considerations. J Am Coll Cardiol 1993; 22:883–890.

1104. Abe H, Araki M, Nagatomo T, Miura Y, Nakashima Y. Radiofrequency catheter ablation of an accessory pathway in dextrocardia. Pacing Clin Electrophysiol 1997; 20:2284–2285.

1105. Fischbach P, Campbell RM, Hulse E, et al. Transhepatic access to the atrioventricular ring for delivery of radiofrequency energy. J Cardiovasc Electrophysiol 1997; 8:512–516.

1106. Okishige K, Azegami K, Goseki Y, et al. Radiofrequency ablation of tachyarrhythmias in patients with Ebstein's anomaly. Int J Cardiol 1997; 60:171–180.

1107. Case CL, Gillette PC, Oslizlok PC, Knick BJ, Blair HL. Radiofrequency catheter ablation of incessant, medically resistant supraventricular tachycardia in infants and small children. J Am Coll Cardiol 1992; 20:1405–1410.

1108. Okumura K, Yamabe H, Yasue H. Radiofrequency catheter ablation of concealed atrio-His bypass tract involved in paroxysmal supraventricular tachycardia. Pacing Clin Electrophysiol 1994; 17:1686–1690.

1109. McClelland JH, Wang X, Beckman KJ, et al. Radiofrequency catheter ablation of right atriofascicular (Mahaim) accessory pathways guided by accessory pathway activation potentials. Circulation 1994; 89:2655–2666.

1110. Okishige K, Friedman PL. New observations on decremental atriofascicular and nodofascicular fibers: implications for catheter ablation. PACE 1995; 18:986–998.

1111. Yeh SJ, Wang CC, Wen MS, et al. Characteristics and radiofrequency ablation therapy of intermediate septal accessory pathway. Am J Cardiol 1994; 73:50–56.

1112. Klein LS, Hackett FK, Zipes DP, Miles WM. Radiofrequency catheter ablation of Mahaim fibers at the tricuspid annulus. Circulation 1993; 87:738–747.

1113. Cappato R, Schluter M, Weib C, et al. Catheter-induced mechanical conduction block of right-sided accessory fibers with Mahaim-type preexcitation to guide radiofrequency ablation. Circulation 1994; 90:282–290.

1114. Wen MS, Yeh SJ, Wang CC, Lin FC, Wu D. Successful radiofrequency ablation in reentrant tachycardia incorporating a nodoventricular tract. Am Heart J 1994; 127:1413–1419.

1115. Kocheril AG, Rosenfeld LE. Radiofrequency ablation of an accessory pathway in a patient with corrected Ebstein's anomaly. Pacing Clin Electrophysiol 1994; 17:986–990.

1116. Cappato R, Schluter M, Weib C, et al. Radiofrequency current catheter ablation of accessory atrioventricular pathways in Ebstein's anomaly. Circulation 1996; 94:376–383.

1117. Chen SA, Tai CT, Lee SH, et al. Electrophysiologic characteristics and anatomical complexities of accessory atrioventricular pathways with successful ablation of anterograde and retrograde conduction at different sites. J Cardiovasc Electrophysiol 1996; 7:907–915.

1118. Dick M II, Dorostkar PC, Serwer G, LeRoy S, Armstrong B. Delayed response to radiofrequency ablation of accessory connections. Pacing Clin Electrophysiol 1993; 16:2143–2145.

1119. Lanberg JJ, Harvey M, Calkins H, el-Atassi R, Kalbfleisch SJ, Morady F. Titration of power output during radiofrequency catheter ablation of atrioventricular nodal reentrant tachycardia. Pacing Clin Electrophysiol 1993; 16:465–470.

1120. Stein KM, Lerman BB. Delayed success following radiofrequency catheter ablation. PACE 1993; 16:698–701.

1121. Preminger MW, Callans DJ, Gottlieb CD, Marchlinski FE. Radiofrequency catheter ablation used to unmask infarction Q waves in Wolff-Parkinson-White syndrome. Am Heart J 1994; 128:1040–1042.

1122. Twidale N, Wang XZ, Beckman KJ, et al. Factors associated with recurrence of accessory pathway conduction after radiofrequency catheter ablation. Pacing Clin Electrophysiol 1991; 14:2042–2048.

1123. Leitch JW, Klein GJ, Yee R, Leather RA, Kim YH. Does delayed loss of preexcitation after unsuccessful radiofrequency catheter ablation of accessory pathways result in permanent cure? Am J Cardiol 1992; 70:830–832.

1124. Chen SA, Chiang CE, Tsang WP, et al. Recurrent conduction in accessory pathway and possible new arrhythmias after

radiofrequency catheter ablation. Am Heart J 1993;
125:381–387.

1125. Calkins H, Prystowsky E, Berger RD, et al. Recurrence of
conduction following radiofrequency catheter ablation
procedures: relationship to ablation target and electrode
temperature: the ATAKR Multicenter Investigators Group. J
Cardiovasc Electrophysiol 1996; 7:704–712.

1126. Grossman DS, Cohen TJ, Goldner B, Jadonath R.
Pseudorecurrence of paroxysmal supraventricular
tachycardia after radiofrequency catheter ablation. Am Heart
J 1994; 128:516–519.

1127. Griffin JC, Mason JW, Calfee RV. Clinical use of an
implantable automatic tachycardia-terminating pacemaker.
Am Heart J 1980; 100:1093–1096.

1128. Schluter M, Cappato R, Ouyang F, Antz M, Schluter CA,
Kuck KH. Clinical recurrences after successful accessory
pathway ablation: the role of "dormant" accessory pathways.
J Cardiovasc Electrophysiol 1997; 8:1366–1372.

1129. Willems S, Shenasa M, Borggrefe M, et al. Unexpected
emergence of manifest preexcitation following transcatheter
ablation of concealed accessory pathways. J Cardiovasc
Electrophysiol 1993; 4:467–472.

1130. Chiang CE, Chen SA, Wang DC, et al. Arrhythmogenicity of
catheter ablation in supraventricular tachycardia. Am Heart J
1993; 125:388–395.

1131. Chen SA, Chiang CE, Tai CT, et al. Complications of
diagnostic electrophysiologic studies and radiofrequency
catheter ablation in patients with tachyarrhythmias: an eight-
year survey of 3,966 consecutive procedures in a tertiary
referral center. Am J Cardiol 1996; 77:41–46.

1132. Johnson TB, Varney FL Jr, Gillette PC, et al. Lack of
proarrhythmia as assessed by Holter monitor after atrial
radiofrequency ablation of supraventricular tachycardia in
children. Am Heart J 1996; 132:120–124.

1133. Alison JF, Yeung-Lai-Wah JA, Schulzer M, Kerr CR.
Characterization of junctional rhythm after atrioventricular
node ablation. Circulation 1995; 91:84–90.

1134. Boyle NG, Anselme F, Monahan K, et al. Origin of
junctional rhythm during radiofrequency ablation of
atrioventricular nodal reentrant tachycardia in patients
without structural heart disease. Am J Cardiol 1997;
80:575–580.

1135. Chen SA, Chiang CE, Tai CT, et al. Transient complete
atrioventricular block during radiofrequency ablation of slow
pathway for atrioventricular nodal reentrant tachycardia. Am
J Cardiol 1996; 77:1367–1370.

1136. Stamato NJ, Eddy SL, Whiting DJ. Transient complete heart
block during radiofrequency ablation of a left lateral bypass
tract. Pacing Clin Electrophysiol 1996; 19:1351–1354.

1137. Thakur RK, Klein GJ, Yee R, Stites HW. Junctional
tachycardia: a useful marker during radiofrequency ablation
for atrioventricular node reentrant tachycardia. J Am Coll
Cardiol 1993; 22:1706–1710.

1138. Fujimura O, Schoen WJ, Kuo CS, Leonelli FM. Delayed
recurrence of atrioventricular block after radiofrequency
ablation of atrioventricular node reentry: a word of caution.
Am Heart J 1993; 125:901–904.

1139. Friedman PL, Stevenson WG, Kocovic DZ. Autonomic
dysfunction after catheter ablation. J Cardiovasc
Electrophysiol 1996; 7:450–459.

1140. Kowallik P, Escher S, Peters W, Braun C, Meesmann M.
Preserved autonomic modulation of the sinus and
atrioventricular nodes following posteroseptal ablation for
treatment of atrioventricular nodal reentrant tachycardia. J
Cardiovasc Electrophysiol 1998; 9:567–573.

1141. Schlapfer J, Kappenberger L, Fromer M. Bezold-Jarisch–like
phenomenon induced by radiofrequency ablation of a left
posteroseptal accessory pathway via the coronary sinus. J
Cardiovasc Electrophysiol 1996; 7:445–449.

1142. Tsai CF, Chen SA, Chiang CE, et al. Radiofrequency
ablation-induced asystole during transaortic approach for a
left anterolateral accessory pathway: a Bezold-Jarisch–like
phenomenon. J Cardiovasc Electrophysiol 1997; 8:694–699.

1143. Ehlert FA, Goldberger JJ, Brooks R, Miller S, Kadish AH.
Persistent inappropriate sinus tachycardia after

radiofrequency current catheter modification of the
atrioventricular node. Am J Cardiol 1992; 69:1092–1095.

1144. Kocovic DZ, Harada T, Shea JB, Soroff D, Friedman PL.
Alterations of heart rate and of heart rate variability after
radiofrequency catheter ablation of supraventricular
tachycardia: delineation of parasympathetic pathways in the
human heart. Circulation 1993; 88:1671–1681.

1145. Simmers TA, Hauer RN, Wever EF, Wittkampf FH, Robles de
Medina EO. Unipolar electrogram models for prediction of
outcome in radiofrequency ablation of accessory pathways.
Pacing Clin Electrophysiol 1994; 17:186–198.

1146. Madrid AH, Mestre JL, Moro C, et al. Heart rate variability
and inappropriate sinus tachycardia after catheter ablation
of supraventricular tachycardia. Eur Heart J 1995;
16:1637–1640.

1147. Pappone C, Stabile G, Oreto G, et al. Inappropriate sinus
tachycardia after radiofrequency ablation of para-Hisian
accessory pathways. J Cardiovasc Electrophysiol 1997;
8:1357–1365.

1148. Frey B, Heinz G, Kreiner G, Schmidinger H, Weber H,
Gossinger H. Increased heart rate variability after
radiofrequency ablation. Am J Cardiol 1993; 71:1460–1461.

1149. Pfeiffer D, Tebbenjohanns J, Schumacher B, Jung W,
Luderitz B. Pacemaker function during radiofrequency
ablation. Pacing Clin Electrophysiol 1995; 18:1037–1044.

1150. Hartzler GO, Giorgi LV, Diehl AM, Hamaker WR. Right
coronary spasm complicating electrode catheter ablation of
a right lateral accessory pathway. J Am Coll Cardiol 1985;
6:250–253.

1151. Minich LL, Snider AR, Dick M II. Doppler detection of
valvular regurgitation after radiofrequency ablation of
accessory connections. Am J Cardiol 1992; 70:116–117.

1152. Thakur RK, Klein GJ, Yee R, Zardini M. Embolic
complications after radiofrequency catheter ablation. Am J
Cardiol 1994; 74:278–279.

1153. Georgiadis D, Lindner A, Manz M, et al. Intracranial
microembolic signals in 500 patients with potential cardiac
or carotid embolic source and in normal controls. Stroke
1997; 28:1203–1207.

1154. Janeira LF. Coronary artery dissection complicating
radiofrequency catheter ablation via the retrograde
approach. PACE 1998; 21:1327–1328.

1155. Mandawat MK, Turitto G, el-Sherif N. Catheter entrapment
in the mitral valve apparatus requiring surgical removal: an
unusual complication of radiofrequency ablation. PACE
1998; 21:772–773.

1156. Turitto G, Abordo MG, Mandawat MK, Togay VS, el-Sherif
N. Radiofrequency ablation for cardiac arrhythmias causing
postcardiac injury syndrome. Am J Cardiol 1998; 81:369–370.

1157. Timmermans C, Rodriguez LM, Den Dulk K, Dijkman B,
Smeets JL, Wellens HJJ. Cure of incessant pacemaker circus
movement tachycardia by radiofrequency catheter ablation. J
Cardiovasc Electrophysiol 1996; 7:862–866.

1158. Ellenbogen KA, Wood MA, Stambler BS. Acute effects of
radiofrequency ablation of atrial arrhythmias on implanted
permanent pacing systems. Pacing Clin Electrophysiol 1996;
19:1287–1295.

1159. Haissaguerre M, Jais P, Shah DC, et al. Analysis of
electrophysiological activity in Koch's triangle relevant to
ablation of the slow AV nodal pathway. PACE 1997;
20:2470–2481.

1160. Kuck KH, Schluter M. Single-catheter approach to
radiofrequency current ablation of left-sided accessory
pathways in patients with Wolff-Parkinson-White syndrome.
Circulation 1991; 84:2366–2375.

1161. Lesh MD, Van Hare G, Kao AK, Scheinman MM.
Radiofrequency catheter ablation for Wolff-Parkinson-White
syndrome associated with a coronary sinus diverticulum.
Pacing Clin Electrophysiol 1991; 14:1479–1484.

1162. Borganelli M, el-Atassi R, Leon A, et al. Determinants of
impedance during radiofrequency catheter ablation in
humans. Am J Cardiol 1992; 69:1095–1097.

1163. Chen X, Borggrefe M, Shenasa M, Haverkamp W, Hindricks
G, Breithardt G. Characteristics of local electrogram
predicting successful transcatheter radiofrequency ablation

of left-sided accessory pathways. J Am Coll Cardiol 1992; 20:656–665.

1164. Harvey M, Kim YN, Sousa J, et al. Impedance monitoring during radiofrequency catheter ablation in humans. Pacing Clin Electrophysiol 1992; 15:22–27.

1165. Fisher WG, Swartz JF. Three-dimensional electrogram mapping improves ablation of left-sided accessory pathways. Pacing Clin Electrophysiol 1992; 15:2344–2356.

1166. Haissaguerre M, Gaita F, Fischer B, Egloff P, Lemetayer P, Warin JF. Radiofrequency catheter ablation of left lateral accessory pathways via the coronary sinus. Circulation 1992; 86:1464–1468.

1167. Haissaguerre M, Gaita F, Fischer B, et al. Elimination of atrioventricular nodal reentrant tachycardia using discrete slow potentials to guide application of radiofrequency energy. Circulation 1992; 85:2162–2175.

1168. Hood MA, Cox JL, Lindsay BD, Ferguson TB Jr, Schechtman KB, Cain ME. Improved detection of accessory pathways that bridge posterior septal and left posterior regions in the Wolff-Parkinson-White syndrome. Am J Cardiol 1992; 70:205–210.

1169. Kuck KH, Schluter M, Gursoy S. Preservation of atrioventricular nodal conduction during radiofrequency current catheter ablation of midseptal accessory pathways. Circulation 1992; 86:1743–1752.

1170. Schluter M, Kuck KH. Catheter ablation from right atrium of anteroseptal accessory pathways using radiofrequency current. J Am Coll Cardiol 1992; 19:663–670.

1171. Silka MJ, Kron J, Halperin BD, et al. Analysis of local electrogram characteristics correlated with successful radiofrequency catheter ablation of accessory atrioventricular pathways. Pacing Clin Electrophysiol 1992; 15:1000–1007.

1172. Tai YT, Lau CP, Li JP. Successful sequential radiofrequency catheter ablation of anatomically discrete antegrade and retrograde accessory pathway conduction in the Wolff-Parkinson-White syndrome. Clin Cardiol 1992; 15:211–216.

1173. Bashir Y, Heald SC, Katritsis D, Hammouda M, Camm AJ, Ward DE. Radiofrequency ablation of accessory atrioventricular pathways: predictive value of local electrogram characteristics for the identification of successful target sites. Br Heart J 1993; 69:315–321.

1174. Chen SA, Chiang CE, Chiou CW, et al. Serial electrophysiological studies in the late outcome of radiofrequency ablation for accessory atrioventricular pathway-mediated tachyarrhythmias. Eur Heart J 1993; 14:734–743.

1175. Chiang CE, Chen SA, Yang CR, et al. Radiofrequency ablation of posteroseptal accessory pathways in patients with abnormal coronary sinus. Am Heart J 1993; 126:1213–1216.

1176. Interian A Jr, Cox MM, Jimenez RA, et al. A shared pathway in atrioventricular nodal reentrant tachycardia and atrial flutter: implications for pathophysiology and therapy. Am J Cardiol 1993; 71:297–303.

1177. Saul JP, Hulse JE, De W, et al. Catheter ablation of accessory atrioventricular pathways in young patients: use of long vascular sheaths, the transseptal approach and a retrograde left posterior parallel approach. J Am Coll Cardiol 1993; 21:571–583.

1178. Solomon AJ, Tracy CM, Swartz JF, Reagan KM, Karasik PE, Fletcher RD. Effect on coronary artery anatomy of radiofrequency catheter ablation of atrial insertion sites of accessory pathways. J Am Coll Cardiol 1993; 21:1440–1444.

1179. Walker KW, McAnulty JH, Kron J, Silka MJ, Halperin BD. Unmasking accessory pathway conduction with adenosine-induced atrioventricular nodal block after radiofrequency catheter ablation. Chest 1993; 104:1614–1616.

1180. Wu D, Yeh SJ, Wang CC, Wen MS, Lin FC. A simple technique for selective radiofrequency ablation of the slow pathway in atrioventricular node reentrant tachycardia. J Am Coll Cardiol 1993; 21:1612–1621.

1181. Calkins H, Mann C, Kalbfleisch S, Langberg JJ, Morady F. Site of accessory pathway block after radiofrequency catheter ablation in patients with the Wolff-Parkinson-White syndrome. J Cardiovasc Electrophysiol 1994; 5:20–27.

1182. Calkins H, Prystowsky E, Carlson M, Klein LS, Saul JP, Gillette P. Temperature monitoring during radiofrequency catheter ablation procedures using closed loop control: ATAKR Multicenter Investigators Group. Circulation 1994; 90:1279–1286.

1183. Cappato R, Schluter M, Kuck K-H. Anatomic, electrical, and mechanical factors affecting bipolar endocardial electrograms: impact on catheter ablation of manifest left free-wall accessory pathways. Circulation 1994; 90:884–894.

1184. Dhala AA, Deshpande SS, Bremner S, et al. Transcatheter ablation of posteroseptal accessory pathways using a venous approach and radiofrequency energy. Circulation 1994; 90:1799–1810.

1185. Grimm W, Miller J, Josephson ME. Successful and unsuccessful sites of radiofrequency catheter ablation of accessory atrioventricular connections. Am Heart J 1994; 128:77–87.

1186. Holman WL, Anderson PG, Spruell RD, Pacifico AD. Anatomic definition of a vulnerable extranodal site in AV node reentry. Ann Thorac Surg 1994; 57:1273–1280.

1187. Hummel J, Strickberger SA, Kalbfleisch S, et al. Effect of pacing site on the atrial electrogram at target sites for slow pathway ablation in patients with atrioventricular nodal reentrant tachycardia. Pacing Clin Electrophysiol 1994; 17:585–589.

1188. Li HG, Klein GJ, Natale A, Thakur RK, Yee R. Nonreentrant supraventricular tachycardia due to simultaneous conduction over fast and slow AV node pathways: successful treatment with radiofrequency ablation. Pacing Clin Electrophysiol 1994; 17:1186–1193.

1189. Rodriguez LM. Radiofrequency catheter ablation of three accessory pathways in a single session. In Rodriguez LM (ed). New Observations on Cardiac Arrhythmias. Maastricht: Universitaire Pers Maastricht, 1994, pp. 43–54.

1190. Strickberger SA, Vorperian VR, Man KC, et al. Relation between impedance and endocardial contact during radiofrequency catheter ablation. Am Heart J 1994; 128:226–229.

1191. Vijgen JM, Carlson MD. Independent ablation of retrograde and anterograde accessory connection conduction at the atrial and ventricular insertion sites: evidence supporting the impedance mismatch hypothesis for unidirectional block. J Cardiovasc Electrophysiol 1994; 5:782–789.

1192. Xie B, Heald SC, Bashir Y, Camm AJ, Ward DE. Radiofrequency catheter ablation of septal accessory atrioventricular pathways. Br Heart J 1994; 72:281–284.

1193. Davis LM, Richards DA, Uther JB, Ross DL. Simultaneous mapping of the tricuspid and mitral valve annuli at electrophysiological study. Br Heart J 1995; 73:377–382.

1194. Heald SC, Davies DW, Ward DE, Garratt CJ, Rowland E. Radiofrequency catheter ablation of Mahaim tachycardia by targeting Mahaim potentials at the tricuspid annulus. Br Heart J 1995; 73:250–257.

1195. Nath S, DiMarco JP, Mounsey JP, Lobban JH, Haines DE. Correlation of temperature and pathophysiological effect during radiofrequency catheter ablation of the AV junction. Circulation 1995; 92:1188–1192.

1196. Giorgberidze I, Saksena S, Krol RB, Mathew P. Efficacy and safety of radiofrequency catheter ablation of left-sided accessory pathways through the coronary sinus. Am J Cardiol 1995; 76:359–365.

1197. Hindricks G, Kottkamp H, Chen X, Willems S, Breithardt G, Borggrefe M. Successful radiofrequency catheter ablation of right sided accessory pathways during sustained atrial fibrillation. Eur Heart J 1995; 16:967–970.

1198. Hintringer F, Hartikainen J, Davies DW, et al. Prediction of atrioventricular block during radiofrequency ablation of the slow pathway of the atrioventricular node. Circulation 1995; 92:3490–3496.

1199. Lin JL, Schie JT, Tseng CD, et al. Value of local electrogram characteristics predicting successful catheter ablation of left-versus right-sided accessory atrioventricular pathways by radiofrequency current. Cardiology 1995; 86:135–142.

1200. Lin JL, Lin FY, Lo HM, et al. Perinodal slow potential as a local guide for transcatheter radiofrequency ablation of atrioventricular nodal reentrant tachycardia: therapeutic efficacy and electrophysiological mechanisms of success. Br Heart J 1995; 74:268–276.

1201. Strickberger SA, Hummel J, Gallagher M, et al. Effect of accessory pathway location on the efficiency of heating during radiofrequency catheter ablation. Am Heart J 1995; 129:54–58.

1202. Chiang CE, Chen SA, Tai CT, et al. Prediction of successful ablation site of concealed posteroseptal accessory pathways by a novel algorithm using baseline electrophysiological parameters: implication for an abbreviated ablation procedure. Circulation 1996; 93:982–991.

1203. Strickberger SA, Zivin A, Daoud EG, et al. Temperature and impedance monitoring during slow pathway ablation in patients with AV nodal reentrant tachycardia. J Cardiovasc Electrophysiol 1996; 7:295–300.

1204. Willems S, Shenasa H, Kottkamp H, et al. Temperature-controlled slow pathway ablation for treatment of atrioventricular nodal reentrant tachycardia using a combined anatomical and electrogram guided strategy. Eur Heart J 1996; 17:1092–1102.

1205. Xie B, Heald SC, Camm AJ, Rowland E, Ward DE. Successful radiofrequency ablation of accessory pathways with the first energy delivery: the anatomic and electrical characteristics. Eur Heart J 1996; 17:1072–1079.

1206. Berger RD, Nsah E, Calkins H. Signal-averaged intracardiac electrograms: a new method to detect Kent potentials. J Cardiovasc Electrophysiol 1997; 8:155–160.

1207. Brignole M, Delise P, Menozzi C, et al. Multiple mechanisms of successful slow-pathway catheter ablation of common atrioventricular nodal re-entrant tachycardia. Eur Heart J 1997; 18:985–993.

1208. Kavesh NG, Gosnell MR, Shorofsky SR, Gold MR, Polaris Investigator Group. Comparison of power- and temperature-guided radiofrequency modification of the atrioventricular node. Am J Cardiol 1997; 80:1444–1447.

1209. Laohaprasitiporn D, Walsh EP, Saul JP, Triedman JK. Predictors of permanence of successful radiofrequency lesions created with controlled catheter tip temperature. Pacing Clin Electrophysiol 1997; 20:1283–1291.

1210. Stellbrink C, Ziegert K, Schauerte P, Hanrath P. A prospective, randomized comparison of temperature-controlled vs manually delivered radiofrequency catheter ablation in patients undergoing atrioventricular nodal modification or accessory pathway ablation. Eur Heart J 1997; 18:1780–1786.

1211. Suguta M, Nogami A, Naito S, et al. Retrograde supernormal conduction in concealed accessory atrioventricular pathway following catheter ablation. J Cardiovasc Electrophysiol 1997; 8:1291–1295.

1212. Vorperian VR, Langberg JJ, Strickberger SA, Morady F. Effect of electrophysiologic properties and location of manifest accessory pathways on local electrogram intervals at effective radiofrequency ablation sites. Am Heart J 1997; 134:173–180.

1213. Brugada J, Puigfel M, Mont L, et al. Radiofrequency ablation of anteroseptal, para-Hisian, and mid-septal accessory pathways using a simplified femoral approach. PACE 1998; 21:735–741.

1214. Chinushi M, Aizawa Y, Ogawa Y, et al. Successful slow pathway ablation in a patient with atrioventricular nodal reentrant tachycardia having a proximal common pathway. PACE 1998; 21:1316–1318.

1215. Hii JTY, Wuttke RD, Kalaburnis M, Velisarris G. Feasibility and safety of a minimally invasive approach to catheter ablation for atrioventricular nodal reentrant tachycardia. PACE 1998; 21:308–310.

1216. Okishige K, Goseki Y, Itoh A, et al. New electrophysiologic features and catheter ablation of atrioventricular and atriofascicular accessory pathways: evidence of decremental conduction and the anatomic structure of the Mahaim pathway. J Cardiovasc Electrophysiol 1998; 9:22–33.

1217. Psychari SN, Theodorakis GN, Koutelou M, Livanis EG, Kremastinos DT. Cardiac denervation after radiofrequency ablation of supraventricular tachycardias. Am J Cardiol 1998; 81:725–731.

1218. Shinbane JS, Lesh MD, Stevenson WG, et al. Anatomic and electrophysiologic relation between the coronary sinus and mitral annulus: implications for ablation of left-sided accessory pathways. Am Heart J 1998; 135:93–98.

1219. Mowry FM. Cardiac pacing in the prevention and treatment of tachyarrhythmias. Med Clin North Am 1969; 53:1287–1295.

1220. Barold SS, Linhart JW. Recent advances in the treatment of ectopic tachycardias by electrical pacing. Am J Cardiol 1970; 25:698–706.

1221. Cheng TO. Atrial pacing: its diagnostic and therapeutic applications. Prog Cardiovasc Dis 1971; 14:230–247.

1222. DeSanctis RW. Diagnostic and therapeutic uses of atrial pacing. Circulation 1971; 43:748–761.

1223. Zipes DP. The contribution of artificial pacemaking to understanding the pathogenesis of arrhythmias. Am J Cardiol 1971; 28:211–222.

1224. Barold SS. Therapeutic uses of cardiac pacing in tachyarrhythmias. In Narula OS (ed). His Bundle. Electrocardiography and Clinical Electrophysiology. Philadelphia: FA Davis, 1975, pp. 407–435.

1225. Batchelder JE, Zipes DP. Treatment of tachyarrhythmias by pacing. Arch Intern Med 1975; 135:1115–1124.

1226. Dreifus LS, Berkovits BV, Kimibiris D, et al. Use of atrial and bifocal cardiac pacemakers for treating resistant dysrhythmias. Eur J Cardiol 1975; 3:257–266.

1227. Spurrell RAJ, Sowton E. Pacing techniques in the management of supraventricular tachycardias. I. J Electrocardiol 1975; 8:287–295.

1228. Cohen HC, Arbel ER. Tachycardias and electrical pacing. Med Clin North Am 1976; 60:343–367.

1229. Spurrell RAJ. The use of programmed pacing techniques in the management of re-entrant tachycardias. In Kulbertus HE (ed). Re-entrant Arrhythmias. Mechanisms and Treatment. Baltimore: University Park Press, 1976, pp. 327–333.

1230. Fisher JD, Cohen HL, Mehra R, Altschuler H, Escher DJW, Furman S. Cardiac pacing and pacemakers. II. Serial electrophysiologic-pharmacologic testing for control of recurrent tachyarrhythmias. Am Heart J 1977; 93:658–668.

1231. Cooper TB, MacLean WA, Waldo AL. Overdrive pacing for supraventricular tachycardia: a review of theoretical implications and therapeutic techniques. Pacing Clin Electrophysiol 1978; 1:196–221.

1232. Wellens HJJ, Bar FW, Gorgels AP, Muncharaz JF. Electrical management of arrhythmias with emphasis on the tachycardias. Am J Cardiol 1978; 41:1025–1034.

1233. Castellanos A, Waxman HL, Berkovits BV, Sung RJ. Implantable pacemakers for cardiac tachyarrhythmias. In Castellanos A (ed). Cardiac Arrhythmias. Mechanisms and Management. Philadelphia: FA Davis, 1980, pp. 159–173.

1234. Wiener I. Pacing techniques in the treatment of tachycardias. Ann Intern Med 1980; 93:326–329.

1235. Wirtzfeld A, Schmidt G, Klein G, Worzewski W. External electrical stimulation in the management of acute tachyarrhythmias. Pacing Clin Electrophysiol 1981; 4:679–691.

1236. Luderitz B, d'Alnoncourt CN, Steinbeck G, Beyer J. Therapeutic pacing in tachyarrhythmias by implanted pacemakers. Pacing Clin Electrophysiol 1982; 5:366–371.

1237. Cohen HE, Kahn M, Donoso E. Treatment of supraventricular tachycardias with catheter and permanent pacemakers. Am J Cardiol 1967; 20:735–738.

1238. Cheng TO. Transvenous ventricular pacing in the treatment of paroxysmal atrial tachyarrhythmias alternating with sinus bradycardia and standstill. Am J Cardiol 1968; 22:874–879.

1239. Lister JW, Cohen LS, Bernstein WH, Samet P. Treatment of supraventricular tachycardias by rapid atrial stimulation. Circulation 1968; 38:1044–1059.

1240. Ryan GF, Easley RM Jr, Zaroff LI, Goldstein S. Paradoxical use of a demand pacemaker in treatment of supraventricular tachycardia due to the Wolff-Parkinson-White syndrome: observation on termination of reciprocal rhythm. Circulation 1968; 38:1037–1043.

1241. Sowton E, Balcon R, Preston T, Leaver D, Yacoub M. Long-term control of intractable supraventricular tachycardia by ventricular pacing. Br Heart J 1969; 31:700–706.

1242. Zeft HJ, McGowan RL. Termination of paroxysmal junctional tachycardia by right ventricular stimulation. Circulation 1969; 40:919–926.

1243. Castellanos A Jr, Chapunoff E, Castillo C, Maytin O, Lemberg L. His bundle electrograms in two cases of Wolff-Parkinson-White (pre-excitation) syndrome. Circulation 1970; 41:399–411.

1244. Preston TA, Kirsh MM. Permanent pacing of the left atrium for treatment of WPW tachycardia. Circulation 1970; 42:1073–1077.

1245. Dreifus LS, Arriaga J, Watanabe Y, Downing D, Haiat R, Morse D. Recurrent Wolff-Parkinson-White tachycardia in an infant: successful treatment by a radiofrequency pacemaker. Am J Cardiol 1971; 28:586–591.

1246. Kitchen JG III, Goldreyer BN. Demand pacemaker for refractory paroxysmal supraventricular tachycardia. N Engl J Med 1972; 287:596–599.

1247. Lister JW, Gulotta SJ, Keller JW Jr, et al. Treatment of supraventricular tachycardias by right atrial alternating current stimulation. Am J Cardiol 1972; 29:208–212.

1248. Vergara GS, Hildner FJ, Schoenfeld CB, Javier RP, Cohen LS, Samet P. Conversion of supraventricular tachycardias with rapid atrial stimulation. Circulation 1972; 46:788–793.

1249. Arthur A, Basta LL. Termination of recurrent supraventricular tachycardia by right ventricular endocardial pacing but not by left ventricular epicardial pacing. J Electrocardiol 1973; 6:345–351.

1250. Montoyo JV, Angel J, Valle V, Gausi C. Cardioversion of tachycardias by transesophageal atrial pacing. Am J Cardiol 1973; 32:85–90.

1251. Pittman DE, Makar JS, Kooros KS, Joyner CR. Rapid atrial stimulation: successful method of conversion of atrial flutter and atrial tachycardia. Am J Cardiol 1973; 32:700–706.

1252. Fruehan CT, Meyer JA, Klie JH, et al. Refractory paroxysmal supraventricular tachycardia: treatment with patient controlled permanent radiofrequency atrial pacemaker. Am Heart J 1974; 87:229–237.

1253. Moss AJ, Rivers RJ Jr. Termination and inhibition of recurrent tachycardias by implanted pervenous pacemakers. Circulation 1974; 50:942–947.

1254. Iwa T, Wada J. Treatment of tachycardia by atrial pacing. Jpn Circ J 1974; 38:82–86.

1255. Williams DO, Davison PH. Long-term treatment of refractory supraventricular tachycardia by patient-controlled inductive atrial pacing. Br Heart J 1974; 36:336–340.

1256. Wise JR Jr. Patient-activated atrial pacing in the treatment of recurrent supraventricular tachycardia. Chest 1974; 65:212–215.

1257. Goyal SL, Lichstein E, Gupta PK, Chadda KD. Refractory reentrant atrial tachycardia: successful treatment with a permanent radiofrequency triggered atrial pacemaker. Am J Med 1975; 58:586–590.

1258. Moss AJ. Therapeutic uses of permanent pervenous atrial pacemakers: a review. J Electrocardiol 1975; 8:373–380.

1259. Kahn A, Morris JJ, Citron P. Patient-initiated rapid atrial pacing to manage supraventricular tachycardia. Am J Cardiol 1976; 38:200–204.

1260. Krikler D, Curry P, Buffet J. Dual-demand pacing for reciprocating atrioventricular tachycardia. Br Med J 1976; 1:1114–1116.

1261. Spurrell RA, Sowton E. Pacing techniques in the management of supraventricular tachycardias. II. An implanted atrial synchronous pacemaker with a short atrioventricular delay for the prevention of paroxysmal supraventricular tachycardias. J Electrocardiol 1976; 9:89–96.

1262. Peters RW, Shafton E, Frank S, Thomas AN, Scheinman MM. Radiofrequency-triggered pacemakers: uses and limitations: a long-term study. Ann Intern Med 1978; 88:17–22.

1263. Waxman MB, Wald RW, Bonet JF, MacGregor DC, Goldman BS. Self-conversion of supraventricular tachycardia by rapid atrial pacing. Pacing Clin Electrophysiol 1978; 1:35–48.

1264. Curry PV, Rowland E, Krikler DM. Dual-demand pacing for refractory atrioventricular re-entry tachycardia. Pacing Clin Electrophysiol 1979; 2:137–151.

1265. Hyman AL. Permanent programmable pacemakers in the management of recurrent tachycardias. Pacing Clin Electrophysiol 1979; 2:28–39.

1266. Sung RJ, Styperek JL, Castellanos A. Complete abolition of the reentrant supraventricular tachycardia zone using a new modality of cardiac pacing with simultaneous atrioventricular stimulation. Am J Cardiol 1980; 45:72–78.

1267. Critelli G, Grassi G, Adinolfi L, Perticone F, Condorelli M. Arrhythmia control by cardiac stimulation. Eur J Cardiol 1981; 12:297–307.

1268. Critelli G, Adinolfi L, Perticone F, Condorelli M. Programmed electrical stimulation and amiodarone therapy for the control of persistent junctional tachycardia. Bull Texas Heart Inst 1981; 2:232–236.

1269. Hartzler GO, Holmes DR Jr, Osborn MJ. Patient-activated transvenous cardiac stimulation for the treatment of supraventricular and ventricular tachycardia. Am J Cardiol 1981; 47:903–909.

1270. Kappenberger L, Sowton E. Programmed stimulation for long-term treatment and non-invasive investigation of recurrent tachycardia. Lancet 1981; 1:909–914.

1271. Nathan A, Hellestrand K, Ward D, Spurrell R, Camm J. Rate-related accelerating (autodecremental) atrial pacing for reversion of paroxysmal supraventricular tachycardia. J Electrocardiol 1982; 15:77–84.

1272. Nathan A, Hellestrand K, Bexton R, Nappholz T, Spurrel R, Camm J. Clinical evaluation of an adaptive tachycardia intervention pacemaker with automatic cycle length adjustment. Pacing Clin Electrophysiol 1982; 5:201–207.

1273. Portillo B, Medina-Ravell V, Portillo-Leon N, et al. Treatment of drug resistant A-V reciprocating tachycardias with multiprogrammable dual demand A-V sequential (DVI,MN) pacemakers. Pacing Clin Electrophysiol 1982; 5:814–825.

1274. Solti F, Szabo Z, Czako E, Bodor A, Renyi-Vamos F Jr. Refractory supraventricular reentry tachycardia treated by radiofrequency atrial pacemaker. Pacing Clin Electrophysiol 1982; 5:275–277.

1275. Spurrell RA, Nathan AW, Bexton RS, Hellestrand KJ, Nappholz T, Camm AJ. Implantable automatic scanning pacemaker for termination of supraventricular tachycardia. Am J Cardiol 1982; 49:753–760.

1276. Den Dulk K, Bertholet M, Brugada P, et al. A versatile pacemaker system for termination of tachycardias. Am J Cardiol 1983; 52:731–738.

1277. Lerman BB, Waxman HL, Buxton AE, Sweeney M, Josephson ME. Tachyarrhythmias associated with programmable automatic atrial antitachycardia pacemakers. Am Heart J 1983; 106:1029–1035.

1278. Medina-Ravell V, Castellanos A, Portillo-Acosta B, et al. Management of tachyarrhythmias with dual-chamber pacemakers. Pacing Clin Electrophysiol 1983; 6:333–345.

1279. Den Dulk K, Bertholet M, Brugada P, et al. Clinical experience with implantable devices for control of tachyarrhythmias. Pacing Clin Electrophysiol 1984; 7:548–556.

1280. German LD, Strauss HC. Electrical termination of tachyarrhythmias by discrete pulses. Pacing Clin Electrophysiol 1984; 7:514–521.

1281. Lyons C, Schroeder P, Shankar K, Brodine W. Transtelephonic monitoring of a tachycardia-terminating pacemaker. Pacing Clin Electrophysiol 1984; 7:34–36.

1282. Waldecker B, Brugada P, Den Dulk K, Zehender M, Wellens HJJ. Arrhythmias induced during termination of supraventricular tachycardia. Am J Cardiol 1985; 55:412–417.

1283. Schluter M, Kunze KP, Kuck KH. Train stimulation at the atria for prevention of atrioventricular tachycardia: dependence on accessory pathway location. J Am Coll Cardiol 1987; 9:1288–1293.

1284. Gang ES, Peter T, Nalos PC, et al. Subthreshold atrial pacing in patients with a left-sided accessory pathway: an effective new method for terminating reciprocating tachycardia. J Am Coll Cardiol 1988; 11:515–521.

1285. Fromer M, Gloor H, Kus T, Shenasa M. Clinical experience with a new software-based antitachycardia pacemaker for recurrent supraventricular and ventricular tachycardias. Pacing Clin Electrophysiol 1990; 13:890–899.

1286. Fromer M, Gloor H, Kus T, Kappenberger L, Shenasa M. Clinical experience with the Intertach 262–12 pulse generator in patients with recurrent supraventricular and ventricular tachycardia. Pacing Clin Electrophysiol 1990; 13:1955–1959.

1287. Li CK, Shandling AH, Nolasco M, Thomas LA, Messenger JC, Warren J. Atrial automatic tachycardia-reversion pacemakers: their economic viability and impact on quality-of-life. Pacing Clin Electrophysiol 1990; 13:639–645.

1288. Connelly DT, de Belder MA, Cunningham D, Lopes AN, Rickards AF, Rowland E. Long-term follow up of patients treated with a software based antitachycardia pacemaker. Br Heart J 1993; 69:250–254.

1289. Griffith MJ, Bexton RS, McComb JM. Financial audit of antitachycardia pacing for the control of recurrent supraventricular tachycardia. Br Heart J 1993; 69:272–275.

1290. Gallagher JJ. Surgical treatment of arrhythmias: current status and future directions. Am J Cardiol 1978; 41:1035–1044.

1291. Sealy WC, Pritchett ELC, Gallagher JJ, Kasell J. The surgical problems with the identification and interruption of the bundle of Kent. In Narula OS (ed). Cardiac Arrhythmias. Electrophysiology, Diagnosis and Management. Baltimore: Williams & Wilkins, 1979, pp. 636–651.

1292. Burchell HB. The surgical treatment of reentrant atrioventricular tachycardia (Wolff-Parkinson-White syndrome). Mayo Clin Proc 1982; 57:387–389.

1293. Campbell RM, Hammon JW Jr, Echt DS, Graham TP Jr. Surgical treatment of pediatric cardiac arrhythmia. J Pediatr 1987; 110:501–508.

1294. Gallagher JJ, Selle JG, Svenson RH, et al. Surgical treatment of arrhythmias. Am J Cardiol 1988; 61:27A–44A.

1295. Garson A Jr, Moak JP, Friedman RA, Perry JC, Ott DA. Surgical treatment of arrhythmias in children. Cardiol Clin 1989; 7:319–329.

1296. Guiraudon GM, Klein GJ, Yee R. Surgery for the Wolff-Parkinson-White syndrome and supraventricular tachycardias. In Josephson ME, Wellens HJJ (eds). Tachycardias. Mechanisms and Management. Mount Kisco, NY: Futura Publishing Co., 1993, pp. 479–504.

1297. Gallagher JJ, Sealy WC, Anderson RW, et al. Cryosurgical ablation of accessory atrioventricular connections: a method for correction of the pre-excitation syndrome. Circulation 1977; 55:471–479.

1298. Klein GJ, Guiraudon GM, Perkins DG, Jones DL, Yee R, Jarvis E. Surgical correction of the Wolff-Parkinson-White syndrome in the closed heart using cryosurgery: a simplified approach. J Am Coll Cardiol 1984; 3:405–409.

1299. Guiraudon GM, Klein GJ, Sharma AD, Jones DL, McLellan DG. Surgery for Wolff-Parkinson-White syndrome: further experience with an epicardial approach. Circulation 1986; 74:525–529.

1300. Cox JL, Holman WL, Cain ME. Cryosurgical treatment of atrioventricular node reentrant tachycardia. Circulation 1987; 76:1329–1336.

1301. Lawrie GM, Lin HT, Wyndham CR, DeBakey ME. Surgical treatment of supraventricular arrhythmias: results in 67 patients. Ann Surg 1987; 205:700–711.

1302. Ott DA, Garson A Jr, Cooley DA, Smith RT, Moak J. Cryoablative techniques in the treatment of cardiac tachyarrhythmias. Ann Thorac Surg 1987; 43:138–143.

1303. Wood DL, Hammill SC, Porter CB, et al. Cryosurgical modification of atrioventricular conduction for treatment of atrioventricular node reentrant tachycardia. Mayo Clin Proc 1988; 63:988–992.

1304. Cox JL, Ferguson TB Jr, Lindsay BD, Cain ME. Perinodal cryosurgery for atrioventricular node reentry tachycardia in 23 patients. J Thorac Cardiovasc Surg 1990; 99:440–449.

1305. Ott DA, Cooley DA, Moak J, Friedman RA, Perry J, Garson A Jr. Computer-guided surgery for tachyarrhythmias in children: current results and expectations. J Am Coll Cardiol 1993; 21:1205–1210.

1306. Selle JG, Svenson RH, Gallagher JJ, Littmann L, Sealy WC, Robicsek F. Surgical treatment of ventricular tachycardia with ND:YAG laser photocoagulation. Pacing Clin Electrophysiol 1992; 15:1357–1361.

1307. Burchell HB, Frye RL, Anderson MW, McGoon DC. Atrioventricular and ventriculoatrial excitation in Wolff-Parkinson-White syndrome (type B): temporary ablation at surgery. Circulation 1967; 36:663–672.

1308. Cobb FR, Blumenschein SD, Sealy WC, Boineau JP, Wagner GS, Wallace AG. Successful surgical interruption of the bundle of Kent in a patient with Wolff-Parkinson-White syndrome. Circulation 1968; 38:1018–1029.

1309. Sealy WC, Hattler BG Jr, Blumenschein SD, Cobb FR. Surgical treatment of Wolff-Parkinson-White syndrome. Ann Thorac Surg 1969; 8:1–11.

1310. Cole JS, Wills RE, Winterscheid LC, Reichenbach DD, Blackmon JR. The Wolff-Parkinson-White syndrome: problems in evaluation and surgical therapy. Circulation 1970; 42:111–121.

1311. Sealy WC, Boineau JP, Wallace AG. The identification and division of the bundle of Kent for premature ventricular excitation and supraventricular tachycardia. Surgery 1970; 68:1009–1017.

1312. Lindsay AE, Nelson RM, Abildskov JA, Wyatt R. Attempted surgical division of the preexcitation pathway in the Wolff-Parkinson-White syndrome. Am J Cardiol 1971; 28:581–585.

1313. Svenson RH, Gallagher JJ, Sealy WC, Wallace AG. An electrophysiologic approach to the surgical treatment of the Wolff-Parkinson-White syndrome: report of two cases utilizing catheter recording and epicardial mapping techniques. Circulation 1974; 49:799–804.

1314. Wallace AG, Sealy WC, Gallagher J, Svenson RH, Strauss HC, Kasell J. Surgical correction of anomalous left ventricular pre-excitation: Wolff-Parkinson-White (type A). Circulation 1974; 49:206–213.

1315. Gallagher JJ, Sealy WC, Kasell J, Wallace AG. Multiple accessory pathways in patients with the pre-excitation syndrome. Circulation 1976; 54:571–591.

1316. Sealy WC, Gallagher JJ, Wallace AG. The surgical treatment of Wolff-Parkinson-White syndrome: evolution of improved methods for identification and interruption of the Kent bundle. Ann Thorac Surg 1976; 22:443–457.

1317. Sealy WC, Anderson RW, Gallagher JJ. Surgical treatment of supraventricular tachyarrhythmias. J Thorac Cardiovasc Surg 1977; 73:511–522.

1318. Kugler JD, Gillette PC, Duff DF, Cooley DA, McNamara DG. Elective mapping and surgical division of the bundle of Kent in a patient with Ebstein's anomaly who required tricuspid valve replacement. Am J Cardiol 1978; 41:602–605.

1319. Pritchett EL, Gallagher JJ, Sealy WC, et al. Supraventricular tachycardia dependent upon accessory pathways in the absence of ventricular preexcitation. Am J Med 1978; 64:214–220.

1320. Sealy WC, Gallagher JJ, Pritchett EL, Wallace AG. Surgical treatment of tachyarrhythmias in patients with both an Ebstein anomaly and a Kent bundle. J Thorac Cardiovasc Surg 1978; 75:847–853.

1321. Benson DW Jr, Gallagher JJ. Electrophysiologic evaluation and surgical correction of Wolff-Parkinson-White syndrome in children. Clin Pediatr 1980; 19:575–583.

1322. Benson DW Jr, Gallagher JJ, Oldham HN, Sealy WC, Sterba R, Spach MS. Corrected transposition with severe intracardiac deformities with Wolff-Parkinson-White syndrome in a child: electrophysiologic investigation and surgical correction. Circulation 1980; 61:1256–1261.

1323. Gillette PC, Garson A Jr, Kugler JD, Cooley DA, Zinner A, McNamara DG. Surgical treatment of supraventricular tachycardia in infants and children. Am J Cardiol 1980; 46:281–284.

1324. Iwa T, Magara T, Watanabe Y, Kawasuji M, Misaki T. Interruption of multiple accessory conduction pathways in the Wolff-Parkinson-White syndrome. Ann Thorac Surg 1980; 30:313–325.

1325. Iwa T, Teranaka M, Tsuchiya K, Misaki T, Watanabe Y. Simultaneous surgery for Wolff-Parkinson-White syndrome combined with Ebstein's anomaly: interruption of multiple accessory conduction pathways. Thorac Cardiovasc Surg 1980; 28:42–47.

1326. Untereker WJ, Litwak RS, Mindich BP, et al. Superficial accessory pathway in the Wolff-Parkinson-White syndrome: electrophysiological, surgical and histologic demonstration. J Electrocardiol 1980; 13:393–400.

1327. Dick M II, Behrendt DM, Byrum CJ, et al. Tricuspid atresia and the Wolff-Parkinson-White syndrome: evaluation methodology and successful surgical treatment of the combined disorders. Am Heart J 1981; 101:496–500.

1328. Iwa T, Kawasuji M, Misaki T, Magara T, Mukai K, Kobayashi H. Surgical treatment of the Wolff-Parkinson-White syndrome in infants and children. Jpn J Surg 1981; 11:297–304.

1329. Holmes DR Jr, Osborn MJ, Gersh B, Maloney JD, Danielson GK. The Wolff-Parkinson-White syndrome: a surgical approach. Mayo Clin Proc 1982; 57:345–350.

1330. Smith WM, Gallagher JJ, Kerr CR, et al. The electrophysiologic basis and management of symptomatic recurrent tachycardia in patients with Ebstein's anomaly of the tricuspid valve. Am J Cardiol 1982; 49:1223–1233.

1331. Guiraudon GM, Klein GJ, Jones D, Kerr CR. Surgical treatment of Wolff-Parkinson-White syndrome. Can J Surg 1983; 26:147–149.

1332. Sealy WC, Mikat EM. Anatomical problems with identification and interruption of posterior septal Kent bundles. Ann Thorac Surg 1983; 36:584–595.

1333. Guarnieri T, Sealy WC, Kasell JH, German LD, Gallagher JJ. The nonpharmacologic management of the permanent form of junctional reciprocating tachycardia. Circulation 1984; 69:269–277.

1334. Guiraudon GM, Klein GJ, Gulamhusein S, et al. Surgical repair of Wolff-Parkinson-White syndrome: a new closed-heart technique. Ann Thorac Surg 1984; 37:67–71.

1335. Bredikis J, Bukauskas F, Zebrauskas R, et al. Cryosurgical ablation of right parietal and septal accessory atrioventricular connections without the use of extracorporeal circulation: a new surgical technique. J Thorac Cardiovasc Surg 1985; 90:206–211.

1336. Cox JL, Gallagher JJ, Cain ME. Experience with 118 consecutive patients undergoing operation for the Wolff-Parkinson-White syndrome. J Thorac Cardiovasc Surg 1985; 90:490–501.

1337. Gallagher JD, Del Rossi AJ, Fernandez J, et al. Cryothermal mapping of recurrent ventricular tachycardia in man. Circulation 1985; 71:732–739.

1338. Holmes DR Jr, Danielson GK, Gersh BJ, et al. Surgical treatment of accessory atrioventricular pathways and symptomatic tachycardia in children and young adults. Am J Cardiol 1985; 55:1509–1512.

1339. Ott DA, Gillette PC, Garson A Jr, Cooley DA, Reul GJ, McNamara DG. Surgical management of refractory supraventricular tachycardia in infants and children. J Am Coll Cardiol 1985; 5:124–129.

1340. Sharma AD, Klein GJ, Guiraudon GM, Milstein S. Atrial fibrillation in patients with Wolff-Parkinson-White syndrome: incidence after surgical ablation of the accessory pathway. Circulation 1985; 72:161–169.

1341. Guiraudon GM, Klein GJ, Sharma AD, Jones DL, McLellan DG. Surgical ablation of posterior septal accessory pathways in the Wolff-Parkinson-White syndrome by a closed heart technique. J Thorac Cardiovasc Surg 1986; 92:406–413.

1342. Guiraudon GM, Klein GJ, Sharma AD, Yee R, McLellan DG. Surgical treatment of supraventricular tachycardia: a five-year experience. Pacing Clin Electrophysiol 1986; 9:1376–1380.

1343. Guiraudon GM, Klein GJ, Sharma AD, Milstein S, McLellan DG. Closed-heart technique for Wolff-Parkinson-White syndrome: further experience and potential limitations. Ann Thorac Surg 1986; 42:651–657.

1344. Iwa T, Mitsui T, Misaki T, Mukai K, Magara T, Kamata E. Radical surgical cure of Wolff-Parkinson-White syndrome: the Kanazawa experience. J Thorac Cardiovasc Surg 1986; 91:225–233.

1345. Lowe JE. Surgical treatment of the Wolff-Parkinson-White syndrome and other supraventricular tachyarrhythmias. J Cardiac Surg 1986; 1:117–134.

1346. Packer DL, Bardy GH, Worley SJ, et al. Tachycardia-induced cardiomyopathy: a reversible form of left ventricular dysfunction. Am J Cardiol 1986; 57:563–570.

1347. Fischell TA, Stinson EB, Derby GC, Swerdlow CD. Long-term follow-up after surgical correction of Wolff-Parkinson-White syndrome. J Am Coll Cardiol 1987; 9:283–287.

1348. Johnson DC, Nunn GR, Richards DA, Uther JB, Ross DL. Surgical therapy for supraventricular tachycardia, a potentially curable disorder. J Thorac Cardiovasc Surg 1987; 93:913–918.

1349. Selle JG, Sealy WC, Gallagher JJ, Fedor JM, Svenson RH, Zimmern SH. Technical considerations in the surgical approach to multiple accessory pathways in the Wolff-Parkinson-White syndrome. Ann Thorac Surg 1987; 43:579–584.

1350. Guiraudon GM, Guiraudon CM, Klein GJ, Sharma AD, Yee R. The coronary sinus diverticulum: a pathologic entity associated with the Wolff-Parkinson-White syndrome. Am J Cardiol 1988; 62:733–735.

1351. Guiraudon GM, Klein GJ, Sharma AD, Yee R, Pineda EA, McLellan DG. Surgical approach to anterior septal accessory pathways in 20 patients with the Wolff-Parkinson-White syndrome. Eur J Cardiothorac Surg 1988; 2:201–206.

1352. Mahomed Y, King RD, Zipes DP, et al. Surgical division of Wolff-Parkinson-White pathways utilizing the closed-heart technique: a 2-year experience in 47 patients. Ann Thorac Surg 1988; 45:495–504.

1353. Case CL, Crawford FA, Gillette PC, Ross BA, Lee A, Zeigler V. Management strategies for surgical treatment of dysrhythmias in infants and children. Am J Cardiol 1989; 63:1069–1073.

1354. Lezaun R, Brugada P, Smeets J, et al. Cost-benefit analysis of medical vs surgical treatment of symptomatic patients with accessory atrioventricular pathways. Eur Heart J 1989; 10:1105–1109.

1355. Menasche P, Leclercq JF, Cauchemez B, et al. Surgery for the Wolff-Parkinson-White syndrome in 73 consecutive patients: what have we learnt from intraoperative mapping? Eur J Cardiothorac Surg 1989; 3:387–390.

1356. Selle JG, Sealy WC, Gallagher JJ, et al. The complex posterior septal space in the Wolff-Parkinson-White syndrome: surgical experience with 47 patients. Thorac Cardiovasc Surg 1989; 37:299–304.

1357. Crawford FA Jr, Gillette PC, Zeigler V, Case C, Stroud M. Surgical management of Wolff-Parkinson-White syndrome in infants and small children. J Thorac Cardiovasc Surg 1990; 99:234–239.

1358. McGiffin DC, Masterson ML, Stafford WJ. Wolff-Parkinson-White syndrome associated with a coronary sinus diverticulum: ablative surgical approach. Pacing Clin Electrophysiol 1990; 13:966–969.

1359. Page PL, Pelletier LC, Kaltenbrunner W, Vitali E, Roy D, Nadeaua R. Surgical treatment of the Wolff-Parkinson-White syndrome: endocardial versus epicardial approach. J Thorac Cardiovasc Surg 1990; 100:83–87.

1360. Bolling SF, Morady F, Calkins H, et al. Current treatment for Wolff-Parkinson-White syndrome: results and surgical implications. Ann Thorac Surg 1991; 52:461–468.

1361. Davis LM, Johnson DC, Uther JB, et al. What is the best method for assessing the long-term outcome of surgery for accessory pathways and atrioventricular junctional reentrant tachycardias? Circulation 1991; 83:528–535.

1362. Epstein AE, Kirklin JK, Holman WL, Plumb VJ, Kay GN. Intermediate septal accessory pathways: electrocardiographic characteristics, electrophysiologic observations and their surgical implications. J Am Coll Cardiol 1991; 17:1570–1578.

1363. Lowes D, Frank G, Klein J, Manz M. Surgical treatment of the Wolff-Parkinson-White syndrome: experiences in 120 patients. Eur Heart J 1993; 14:E99–E102.

1364. Milstein S, Dunnigan A, Tang C, Pineda E. Right atrial appendage to right ventricle accessory atrioventricular connection: a case report. Pacing Clin Electrophysiol 1997; 20:1877–1880.

1365. Pritchett EL, Anderson RW, Benditt DG, et al. Reentry within the atrioventricular node: surgical cure with preservation of atrioventricular conduction. Circulation 1979; 60:440–446.

1366. Marquez-Montes J, Rufilanchas JJ, Esteve JJ, et al. Paroxysmal nodal reentrant tachycardia: surgical cure with preservation of atrioventricular conduction. Chest 1983; 83:690–694.

1367. Ross DL, Johnson DC, Denniss AR, Cooper MJ, Richards DA, Uther JB. Curative surgery for atrioventricular junctional ("AV nodal") reentrant tachycardia. J Am Coll Cardiol 1985; 6:1383–1392.

1368. Gartman DM, Bardy GH, Williams AB, Ivey TD. Direct surgical treatment of atrioventricular node reentrant tachycardia. J Thorac Cardiovasc Surg 1989; 98:63–71.

1369. Fujimura O, Guiraudon GM, Yee R, Sharma AD, Klein GJ. Operative therapy of atrioventricular node reentry and results of an anatomically guided procedure. Am J Cardiol 1989; 64:1327–1332.

1370. Guiraudon GM, Klein GJ, Sharma AD, Yee R, Kaushik RR, Fujimura O. Skeletonization of the atrioventricular node for AV node reentrant tachycardia: experience with 32 patients. Ann Thorac Surg 1990; 49:565–572.

1371. Guiraudon GM, Klein GJ, van Hemel N, Guiraudon CM, Yee R, Vermeulen FE. Anatomically guided surgery to the AV node: AV nodal skeletonization: experience in 46 patients with AV nodal reentrant tachycardia. Eur J Cardiothorac Surg 1990; 4:461–464.

1372. Lo HM, Lin FY, Jong YS, Tseng CD, Tseng YZ, Hung CR. Reappraisals of atrioventricular node reentrant tachycardia: lessons learned from surgical treatment. Int J Cardiol 1990; 29:173–178.

1373. Ruder MA, Mead RH, Smith NA, Gaudiani VA, Winkle RA. Comparison of pre- and postoperative conduction patterns in patients surgically cured of atrioventricular node reentrant tachycardia. J Am Coll Cardiol 1991; 17:397–402.

1374. Lo H-M, Lin F-Y, Tseng C-D, Jong Y-S, Chern T-H, Tseng Y-Z. Selective surgical ablation of the slow atrioventricular nodal pathway by posterior perinodal dissection. Am J Cardiol 1993; 71:1457–1459.

1375. Knoebel SB, King H, Fisch C. Termination of supraventricular tachycardia complicating the Wolff-Parkinson-White syndrome with external countershock. Circulation 1963; 28:111–113.

1376. Castellanos A Jr, Johnson D, Mas I, Lemberg L. Electrical conversion of paroxysmal atrial fibrillation in the Wolff-Parkinson-White (pre-excitation) syndrome. Am J Cardiol 1966; 17:91–93.

1377. Castellanos A Jr, Lemberg L, Scheib RJ, Budkin A. Cardioversion of A-V nodal tachycardias. Am J Cardiol 1966; 18:884–887.

1378. Meyer AD, Greenberg HB. Cardioversion of recurrent postoperative supraventricular tachycardia in Wolff-Parkinson-White syndrome. Am J Cardiol 1966; 18:904–906.

1379. Vassaux C, Lown B. Cardioversion of supraventricular tachycardias. Circulation 1969; 39:791–802.

1380. Schroeder JS, Harrison DC. Repeated cardioversion during pregnancy: treatment of refractory paroxysmal atrial tachycardia during 3 successive pregnancies. Am J Cardiol 1971; 27:445–446.

1381. Braunwald E, Sobel BE, Braunwald NS. Treatment of paroxysmal supraventricular tachycardia by electrical stimulation of the carotid-sinus nerves. N Engl J Med 1969; 281:885–887.

1382. Braunwald E, Vatner SF, Braunwald NS, Sobel BE. Carotid sinus nerve stimulation in the treatment of angina pectoris and supraventricular tachycardia. Calif Med 1970; 112:41–50.

1383. Waxman MB, Felderhof CH, Downar E, Goldman BS, Morch JE. Self-conversion of drug-resistant paroxysmal atrial tachycardia. Can Med Assoc J 1975; 112:600–603.

1384. Krikler DM. Wolff-Parkinson-White syndrome: long follow-up and an Anglo-American historical note. J Am Coll Cardiol 1983; 2:1216–1218.

1385. Beckman KJ, Gallastegui JL, Bauman JL, Hariman RJ. The predictive value of electrophysiologic studies in untreated patients with Wolff-Parkinson-White syndrome. J Am Coll Cardiol 1990; 15:640–647.

1386. White PD, Donovan H. Hearts. Their Long Follow-up. Philadelphia: WB Saunders, 1967, pp. 289–299.

1387. Seifert MJ, Morady F, Calkins HG, Langberg JJ. Aortic leaflet perforation during radiofrequency ablation. Pacing Clin Electrophysiol 1991; 14:1582–1585.

1388. Marriott HJL. Practical Electrocardiography. 8th ed. Baltimore: Williams & Wilkins, 1988.

1389. Sung RJ, Castellanos A, Mallon SM, Gelband H, Mendoza I, Myerburg RJ. Mode of initiation of reciprocating tachycardia during programmed ventricular stimulation in the Wolff-Parkinson-White syndrome: with reference to various patterns of ventriculoatrial conduction. Am J Cardiol 1977; 40:24–31.

Junctional Ectopic Tachycardia[1-3a]

Junctional ectopic tachycardia is an uncommon, rapid, irregular supraventricular tachyarrhythmia. Coumel and associates first defined it in 1975 as "tachycardias focales hissienes congénitales."[4] The mechanism and the English name were established 4 years later.[5]

Electrophysiologically, junctional ectopic tachycardia is similar to automatic atrial tachycardia, but it differs electrocardiographically in that atrioventricular dissociation is present in the junctional arrhythmia and absent in the atrial tachycardia. Junctional ectopic tachycardia occurs predominantly in children.

PREVALENCE

Congenital junctional ectopic tachycardia is the rarest of the supraventricular tachycardias,[2] which are the most common sustained symptomatic tachyarrhythmias in children.[6b] The arrhythmia also develops occasionally as a complication of open-heart surgery.[c] Adults rarely have junctional ectopic tachycardia.[7-11]

AGE

Among children, junctional ectopic tachycardia frequently presents in infancy, including in premature infants,[12] and it has been detected in fetuses. Junctional ectopic tachycardia usually appears in the youngest children who develop supraventricular tachycardia.[2]

The arrhythmia occurs occasionally in adults.[8, 10, 13] In two reports of seven adults, the average age when the arrhythmia developed was 20 years, with a range of 13 to 23 years.[8, 10]

GENETICS

Fifty percent of children with congenital junctional ectopic tachycardia have a family history of the arrhythmia.[5, 14, 15d]

CLINICAL SETTING

Congenital Heart Disease

Most infants with congenital junctional ectopic tachycardia have no structural cardiac defects.[5, 14-17] Of seven adults with junctional ectopic tachycardia, one had an atrial septal defect,[10] another had a ventricular septal defect,[10] and a third had the combination of atrial septal defect, ventricular septal defect, and congenital aortic regurgitation.[8]

After Cardiac Surgery

Surgical repair of congenital cardiac defects can produce junctional ectopic tachycardia.[5, 18-26] Because suturing near the atrioventricular node and bundle of His appears to arouse the arrhythmia, junctional ectopic tachycardia develops most frequently after the Fontan and Senning procedures and after repair of tetralogy of Fallot, ventricular septal defect, transposition of the great arteries, and atrioventricular canal.[22e] In adults, the arrhythmia may arise, but rarely, after surgical treatment for ventricular tachycardia.[7, 27]

---

[a]This chapter is based on Chapter 8, "Junctional Ectopic Tachycardia," by Paul C. Gillette, Christopher L. Case, and myself[1] in the first edition of this book.

[b]Of 178 children with supraventricular tachycardia studied in the electrophysiology laboratory at the Texas Children's Hospital, junctional ectopic tachycardia was the diagnosis in only seven (4%).[2]

[c]Twelve (7.8%) patients developed symptomatic junctional ectopic tachycardia during 154 pediatric open-heart procedures.[21]

[d]In a cooperative study of 26 infants with the arrhythmia admitted to several institutions from 1970 to 1987, 10 were siblings, four were pairs of nonidentical twins, and two infants were cousins, and the father of one patient had an accelerated junctional rhythm.[15]

[e]In 12 patients, the following congenital defects were present: transposition of the great arteries in four; tetralogy of Fallot in two; total anomalous pulmonary venous return in two; and one case each of atrioventricular canal, mitral regurgitation, tricuspid atresia, and double outlet right ventricle.[21]

No Structural Heart Disease

An occasional case of junctional ectopic tachycardia has been reported in patients without any documented heart disease.[28]

PATIENT HISTORY

Congenital junctional ectopic tachycardia is usually recognized within the first 6 months of life, and most infants present before 4 weeks of age.[15] Occasionally, the tachycardia is diagnosed during fetal life.[15] Junctional ectopic tachycardia after cardiac surgery appears most often in younger children who have had severe congenital cardiac defects repaired and are consequently sicker and require inotropic support after operation.[21, 22]

In the few adults reported with junctional ectopic tachycardia, the arrhythmia occurred infrequently or several times a day and lasted from seconds to hours.[10] In some cases, exercise and stress precipitated episodes[10] or accelerated the rate.[8] Syncope occurred in two of five patients.

ELECTROCARDIOGRAPHY

Ventricular Rate

The average ventricular rate of 26 infants with congenital junctional ectopic tachycardia was 230 beats per minute (range, 140–370 beats/min), and in most the rate exceeded 200 beats per minute.[15] The ventricular rate was 210 beats per minute (range, 165–250 beats/min) in 12 symptomatic patients with junctional ectopic tachycardia after cardiac surgery.[21] The ventricular rate in patients with congestive heart failure is faster than in those without heart failure.[15f]

Among children, the rate of junctional ectopic tachycardia often determines the symptoms. When the rate is relatively slow—less than about 130 beats per minute—patients may be asymptomatic. Slower tachycardias often resolve spontaneously. Newborns and infants whose heart rates exceed 170 beats per minute usually develop symptoms and signs of congestive heart failure. In the five reported adults, heart rates ranged from 130 to 250 beats per minute.[10]

---

fTwo hundred forty-eight ±26 beats per minute with heart failure versus 220 ±18 beats per minute without heart failure.[15] Age does not predict the presence or absence of congestive heart failure.[15]

P Waves

The atria are usually controlled by a sinus mechanism, and P waves are visible in almost all patients with congenital junctional ectopic tachycardia.[15, 29] Occasionally, retrograde conduction modifies the form of the P waves,[15, 20] which will then be negative in the inferior leads and will follow the QRS complexes.[20] The P waves can be more difficult to detect in junctional ectopic tachycardia after cardiac surgery.[30]

PR Intervals

Atrioventricular dissociation is characteristically present in junctional ectopic tachycardia because the ventricles are driven by the ectopic junctional pacemaker faster than the sinus tachycardia present in the atria[15] (Figs. 9.1 and 9.2). Consequently, PR intervals change throughout the electrocardiogram. Determining the degree of atrioventricular block may be difficult because relatively few P waves conduct to the ventricles when the ventricular rate is especially rapid. However, atrioventricular block is not a characteristic feature of the arrhythmia.

QRS Complexes

Because junctional ectopic tachycardia originates above the bifurcation of the bundle of His, the QRS complexes are usually normal, with the same appearance as during sinus rhythm.[5]

DIFFERENTIAL DIAGNOSIS

Atrial Rhythm

Atrioventricular dissociation is the most characteristic feature of junctional ectopic tachycardia when compared with other supraventricular tachyarrhythmias. In sinus and atrial tachycardia, P waves are usually visible, but they precede the QRS complexes with fixed PR intervals. P waves are absent or follow the QRS complexes in most supraventricular tachycardias that are sustained by reentry in the atrioventricular node or accessory pathways. In atrial fibrillation, no P waves are present, and in multifocal atrial tachycardia, the morphology of the P waves changes.

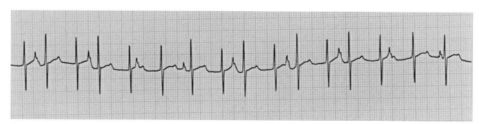

FIGURE 9.1 **Congenital junctional ectopic tachycardia** in a 6-month-old infant (lead II). When the rate of the sinus rhythm is less than that of the junctional tachycardia, the atrial rhythm sometimes, but not always, captures the ventricles and produces the irregularity of the ventricular rhythm. (From Gillette PC, Case CL, Kastor JA. Junctional ectopic tachycardia. In Kastor JA (ed). Arrhythmias. Philadelphia: WB Saunders, 1994, with permission.)[1]

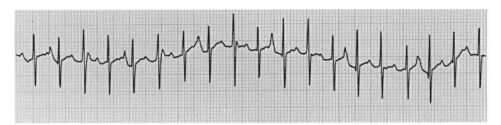

FIGURE 9.2 **Atrioventricular dissociation during junctional ectopic tachycardia** (lead II) in the same patient as in Figure 9.1. The junctional ectopic tachycardia is now faster, and sinus rhythm rarely captures the ventricles. It is typical of congenital junctional ectopic tachycardia that few sinus captures occur when the junctional rate is fast. (From Gillette PC, Case CL, Kastor JA. Junctional ectopic tachycardia. In Kastor JA (ed). Arrhythmias. Philadelphia: WB Saunders, 1994, with permission.)[1]

Ventricular Rhythm

The ventricular rhythm in junctional ectopic tachycardia is characteristically irregular, whereas the ventricular rhythm in sinus tachycardia, atrial tachycardia, and most reentrant supraventricular tachycardias is regular. The ventricular rhythm is irregular in atrial fibrillation and multifocal atrial tachycardia, but these arrhythmias can be differentiated from junctional ectopic tachycardia by the absence of, or characteristic appearance of, the P waves. Accelerated junctional rhythm, which occurs in adults with digitalis intoxication and myocardial infarction and in children and adults with myocarditis and after cardiac surgery, is slower than junctional ectopic tachycardia.

LABORATORY STUDIES

Echocardiography

Consistent with the frequency of congestive heart failure in patients with junctional ectopic tachycardia, echocardiography typically shows a reduced shortening fraction.[15] Even in asymptomatic children, echocardiography reveals dilatation and a decreased shortening fraction of the left ventricle.[15g]

HEMODYNAMICS

Congenital junctional ectopic tachycardia often produces congestive heart failure from left ventricular dysfunction.[31] Hypotension is frequent in postoperative infants with the arrhythmia.[30, 31h]

PATHOLOGY

In addition to the usual signs of congestive heart failure with ventricular hypertrophy and dilatation,[32] pathological examination of a few children with junctional ectopic tachycardia has revealed the following:

- Splitting of the His bundle into several thin and irregular longitudinally oriented strands, with many areas of focal degeneration.[14]
- Partial displacement of the atrioventricular node within the central fibrous body and a left-sided atrioventricular bundle with acute necrosis at the summit of the ventricular septum, adjacent to the atrioventricular node and bundle in a 6-month-old girl.[32]
- Cranial displacement of the coronary sinus, producing entrapment, distortion, and division of the atrioventricular node and bundle into two distinct components within the central fibrous body in a 5-month-old boy.[32]
- Purkinje cell tumors of the bifurcation of the bundle of His and throughout the conduction system in a 13-month-old boy.[33]
- Fibroelastosis in two patients.[15]

ELECTROPHYSIOLOGY

Abnormally enhanced automaticity causes junctional ectopic tachycardia. The following characteristics distinguish junctional ectopic tachycardia from the reentrant tachyarrhythmias:[5, 21, 22, 34, 35]

- The ventricular rate of junctional ectopic tachycardia gradually increases ("warms up") and decreases.
- The atria are not integral to sustaining junctional ectopic tachycardia.
- Drugs such as adenosine or verapamil, which characteristically convert reentrant supraventricular arrhythmias, seldom, if ever, produce sinus rhythm in patients with junctional ectopic tachycardia.
- Rapid atrial and ventricular pacing may capture the ventricles in junctional ectopic tachycardia, but when the pacing is stopped, the arrhythmia returns. Atrial pacing does not change the RR intervals.
- Rapid or programmed stimulation and electrical cardioversion do not convert junctional ectopic tachycardia to sinus rhythm.

The His bundle electrocardiogram of patients with junctional ectopic tachycardia shows that the arrhythmia is supraventricular (Fig. 9.3). The A waves, which reflect atrial activation, are dissociated from the ventricular complexes. The V waves, which correspond to

---

[g]This was seen in five of eight asymptomatic patients whose mean shortening fraction of the left ventricle was 23% (range, 20% to 26%).[15]

[h]Intracardiac hemodynamic measurements have not been reported in patients with junctional ectopic tachycardia, but the effects of the arrhythmia on patients after open-heart surgery "make JET [junctional ectopic tachycardia] perhaps the most hemodynamically malignant of all supraventricular arrhythmias."[31]

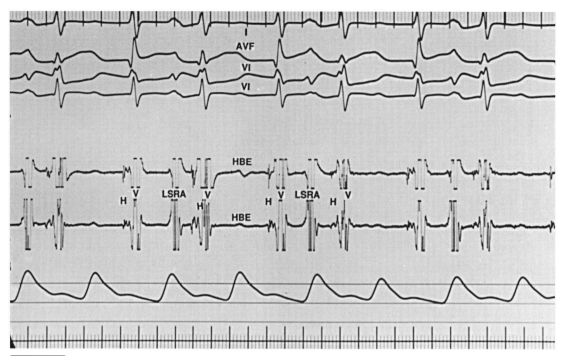

FIGURE 9.3 **Electrophysiological record of junctional ectopic tachycardia.** Each ventricular activation (V in the lines labeled HBE) is preceded by depolarization from the bundle of His (H). QRS complexes 3, 5, and 7 have been captured by the atria. These intracardiac recordings are from the patient in Figures 9.1 and 9.2. From **top** to **bottom**, electrocardiographic are leads I, aVF, V₁, and V₆ (labeled V₁); two His bundle electrocardiograms (HBE); and arterial pressure. The atrial deflection is recorded from the low septal right atrial (LSRA) area. (From Gillette PC, Case CL, Kastor JA. Junctional ectopic tachycardia. In Kastor JA (ed). Arrhythmias. Philadelphia: WB Saunders, 1994, with permission.)[1]

ventricular activation, are preceded by H deflections from activation of the bundle of His. The HV intervals, which indicate the time of conduction from the bundle of His to the ventricles, are normal.

TREATMENT

General Principles

Because many patients with junctional ectopic tachycardia are severely ill with congestive heart failure and hypotension, primary treatment consists of increasing cardiac output, sustaining blood pressure, maintaining adequate oxygenation, and preventing cardiac arrest. Specific antiarrhythmic treatment should be undertaken in all patients with congenital junctional ectopic tachycardia.[15] Catheter or surgical ablation is reserved for patients with severe congestive heart failure that is unresponsive to medical management.

In children who develop junctional ectopic tachycardia after repair of congenital cardiac defects, treatment should be instituted as soon as minimal acceleration of junctional ectopic tachycardia is detected and before cardiogenic shock has developed:[22]

• Levels of potassium, calcium, and magnesium should be frequently measured and maintained in the upper range of normal.
• Sympathetic and catecholamine stimulation should be minimized, and agents such as amrinone should be avoided whenever possible.

• Vagotonia should be enhanced. Consequently, morphine is the drug of choice for sedation, and vagolytic agents such as meperidine and barbiturates should be avoided. Curare or metacurare should be used for paralysis rather than pancuronium bromide, which may increase sympathetic tone and decrease vagal tone.
• Digitalis should be given to all patients with postsurgical junctional ectopic tachycardia to improve myocardial function without increasing automaticity.
• Central venous and atrial pressures should be maintained at appropriate levels.
• The atria should be paced at a rate slightly faster than that of the junctional ectopic tachycardia to increase cardiac output by reestablishing atrioventricular synchrony.

Drugs

Drugs seldom convert junctional ectopic tachycardia to sinus rhythm, but several of them decrease the heart rate so that the deleterious effects of the arrhythmia can be reduced.[36]

Adenosine. This drug briefly decreases the rate of,[27, 37] but seldom converts, junctional ectopic tachycardia.[37, 38] By decreasing ventriculoatrial conduction, the drug may help to reveal the diagnosis[37] (Fig. 9.4).

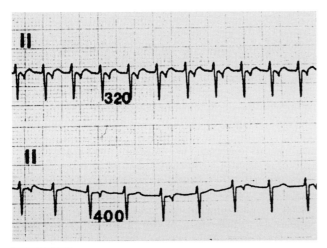

FIGURE 9.4   Adenosine and junctional ectopic tachycardia. Adenosine was administered intravenously to a 3-week-old male infant with postoperative supraventricular tachycardia that was unlikely to be junctional ectopic tachycardia because of the absence of atrioventricular dissociation (**top**). Intravenously administered adenosine, however, established the diagnosis by producing 2:1 ventriculoatrial block; every other QRS complex is followed by a retrograde P wave (**bottom**). The drug also briefly decreased the ventricular rate; the RR intervals increased from 320 to 400 milliseconds. (Adapted from Rossi AF, Kipel G, Golinko RJ, Griepp RB. Use of adenosine in postoperative junctional ectopic tachycardia with 1:1 retrograde atrial conduction. Am Heart J 1991; 121:1237–1239, with permission.)[37]

Amiodarone. Amiodarone decreases the ventricular rate, but it seldom converts the arrhythmia.[2, 15, 16, 39, 40] The authors of the largest series of patients with congenital junctional ectopic tachycardia suggest that amiodarone be given when the combination of digoxin and propranolol does not decrease the heart rate to less than 150 beats per minute.[15] The combination of amiodarone and flecainide controlled the arrhythmia in each of three infants in whom treatment with one of the drugs was ineffective.[41]

Beta-adrenergic–blocking drugs. Beta blockers do not convert patients with junctional ectopic tachycardia to sinus rhythm, but they usually—although not always—reduce the ventricular rate of the arrhythmia.[8, 10, 15, 17] The combination of beta-blocking drugs and digoxin may be particularly useful.[2]

Digitalis. Digitalis improves myocardial function and reduces congestive heart failure in patients with junctional ectopic tachycardia, but it has little, if any, effect on the rate of the arrhythmia.[5, 15] Digoxin was incriminated in producing ventricular fibrillation in a 4-week-old child with severe heart failure, and atrial tachycardia and then atrial flutter may have been produced in a 10-day-old infant.[15]

Edrophonium. Edrophonium slowed the tachycardia in one patient[7] and was ineffective in another.[17]

Flecainide. In a few patients who received the drug, flecainide suppressed junctional ectopic tachycardia acutely, when given intravenously, and on a long-term

basis, when given orally.[11, 42] Given with amiodarone, flecainide controlled the arrhythmia in each of three infants.[41]

Moricizine. This drug suppressed junctional ectopic tachycardia in a few children to whom it was given.[43]

Phenytoin. Phenytoin may have helped in two cases.[7, 17]

Procainamide. This drug helped to suppress junctional ectopic tachycardia in an adult with the arrhythmia.[13]

Propafenone. Propafenone decreased the heart rate in all patients with junctional ectopic tachycardia,[20, 44i] and it suppressed the arrhythmia in some.[44, 45]

Quinidine. Quinidine suppressed the arrhythmia in a few cases.[12, 17]

Sotalol. This drug decreased the rate of junctional ectopic tachycardia and may have led to the suppression of the arrhythmia months later in one infant.[46]

Other drugs. Lidocaine,[5] phenylephrine,[17] and verapamil[17, 28] are seldom effective for treating junctional ectopic tachycardia.

Pacing

Pacing at a rate faster than the tachycardia can temporarily capture the atria and the ventricles and may increase the cardiac output by reestablishing atrioventricular synchrony.[40, 47] However, as is characteristic of automatic rhythms, the arrhythmia returns after the pacing is stopped.[7, 17, 30]

The deaths of several patients with bradycardia and the destructive lesions found in the bundle of His[14, 32] have led some workers to suggest that permanent ventricular pacing should be applied more frequently.[48] This recommendation is controversial.[15]

Cardioversion

Junctional ectopic tachycardia cannot be converted with electric shock.[5, 7, 11, 17]

Ablation

Catheter ablation with radiofrequency current can eliminate junctional ectopic tachycardia.[49–58] In most, but not all,[51, 52] cases, the technique produces atrioventricular block, and a pacemaker, preferably a synchronous unit, must be inserted. Radiofrequency current has supplanted direct current shock of the atrioventricular junction, previously the preferred method.[8, 10, 16, 59]

---

iPropafenone decreased the ventricular rate an average of 109 beats per minute (range, 60–180 beats/min) in seven patients.[20]

Surgery

Surgical ligation or cryoablation can obliterate the focus of junctional ectopic tachycardia.[5, 18, 23, 60] Pacing is required afterward.

Hypothermia

Lowering the body temperature of infants who have developed junctional ectopic tachycardia after cardiac surgery can temporarily decrease the rate of the arrhythmia and can improve myocardial function while awaiting spontaneous reversion or other treatment.[25, 30, 61, 62]*j*

PROGNOSIS

It is fortunate that junctional ectopic tachycardia is rare, because its mortality is high, although some children have a benign course.[12] In the 1990 report of 26 infants with congenital junctional ectopic tachycardia, the overall mortality was 35%.[15] Among survivors, treatment may sometimes be stopped without complications, but frequently drugs must be continued to keep the rate of the arrhythmia sufficiently slow when it persists.[15] Long-term follow-up of patients with junctional ectopic tachycardia is not yet available. Junctional ectopic tachycardia resolves spontaneously in most infants who develop the arrhythmia after cardiac surgery if they survive the first 48 to 72 hours after operation.[22]

SUMMARY

Junctional ectopic tachycardia is an abnormal automatic tachyarrhythmia that arises in the atrioventricular conduction system above the bifurcation of the bundle of His. Children develop junctional ectopic tachycardia as a congenital disease without associated structural defects and from cardiac surgery. The arrhythmia is rare in adults.

Many children with congenital junctional ectopic tachycardia have a family history of the arrhythmia. Associated congenital cardiac defects are uncommon. Congenital junctional ectopic tachycardia usually presents early in life. When the arrhythmia follows cardiac surgery, the children have often had operations involving the atrioventricular junction. Congestive heart failure and hypotension accompany rapid heart rates.

The characteristic electrocardiographic finding is atrioventricular dissociation. The arrhythmia has the electrophysiological features of an automatic, not a reentrant, mechanism.

Congenital junctional ectopic tachycardia is usually treated with beta-adrenergic–blocking drugs and amiodarone, which will decrease the ventricular rate.

Digitalis is administered to improve cardiac function. Atrial pacing can temporarily reestablish atrioventricular synchrony and can increase cardiac output. Ablation of the atrioventricular junction often obliterates the arrhythmia, but a pacemaker is then required.

Because junctional ectopic tachycardia can severely compromise cardiac function when it develops after cardiac surgery, usually in children with congenital heart disease, acute treatment is essential. Digitalis should be given to raise cardiac output. Drugs that increase catecholamine stimulation and may accelerate automatic foci should be avoided, and agents with vagotonic effects should be administered. Amiodarone, beta-adrenergic–blocking drugs, and propafenone decrease the rate of the tachycardia, but other antiarrhythmic drugs are usually ineffective. Ablation of the atrioventricular junction and ventricular pacing may occasionally be needed. The arrhythmia can be expected to resolve spontaneously in most cases if the patient survives the early postoperative period.

REFERENCES

1. Gillette PC, Case CL, Kastor JA. Junctional ectopic tachycardia. In Kastor JA (ed). Arrhythmias. Philadelphia: WB Saunders, 1994, pp. 218–224.
2. Ludomirsky A, Garson A Jr. Supraventricular tachycardia. In Gillette PC, Garson A Jr (eds). Pediatric Arrhythmias. Electrophysiology and Pacing. Philadelphia: WB Saunders, 1990, pp. 380–426.
3. Case CL, Gillette PC. Automatic atrial and junctional tachycardias in the pediatric patient: strategies for diagnosis and management. PACE 1993; 16:1323–1335.
4. Coumel P, Fidelle JE, Attuel P, et al. Tachycardias focales hissiennes congénitales. Arch Mal Coeur 1975; 69:899.
5. Garson A, Gillette PC. Junctional ectopic tachycardia in children: electrocardiography, electrophysiology and pharmacology response. Am J Cardiol 1979; 44:298–302.
6. Garson A Jr, Gillette PC, McNamara DG. Supraventricular tachycardia in children: clinical features, response to treatment, and long-term follow-up in 217 patients. J Pediatr 1981; 98:875–882.
7. Kerr CR, Gallagher JJ, Cox JL, Smith WM, Sterba R. Accelerated junctional tachycardia at a rate of 190 beats/minute following cryosurgery and aneurysmectomy for ventricular tachycardia: a case report. Pacing Clin Electrophysiol 1982; 5:442–454.
8. Davis J, Scheinman MM, Ruder MA, et al. Ablation of cardiac tissues by an electrode catheter technique for treatment of ectopic supraventricular tachycardia in adults. Circulation 1986; 74:1044–1053.
9. Laurent M, Almange C, Biron Y, et al. Junctional ectopic tachycardia in a young woman with chronic complete heart block. Am Heart J 1986; 111:597–599.
10. Ruder MA, Davis JC, Eldar M, et al. Clinical and electrophysiologic characterization of automatic junctional tachycardia in adults. Circulation 1986; 73:930–937.
11. Cook JR, Steinberg JS. An incessant form of junctional ectopic tachycardia in an adult responsive to a class Ic agent. Am Heart J 1991; 122:1487–1489.
12. Bolens M, Friedli B. Junctional ectopic tachycardia with a benign course in a premature infant. Pediatr Cardiol 1990; 11:216–218.
13. Kumagai K, Yamato H, Yamanouchi Y, et al. Automatic junctional tachycardia in an adult. Clin Cardiol 1990, 13:813–816.
14. Brechenmacher C, Coumel P, James TN. De subitaneis mortibus. XVI. Intractable tachycardia in infancy. Circulation 1976; 53:377–381.

---

*j*In each of three patients, the body temperature was reduced to 31.1° to 34.4°C, which decreased the heart rate sufficiently to sustain more normal cardiac function. The value of hypothermia for converting the arrhythmia is not known.[30]

CHAPTER 9 | Junctional Ectopic Tachycardia 275

15. Villain E, Vetter VL, Garcia JM, Herre J, Cifarelli A, Garson A Jr. Evolving concepts in the management of congenital junctional ectopic tachycardia: a multicenter study. Circulation 1990; 81:1544–1549.
16. Gillette PC, Garson A Jr, Porter CJ, et al. Junctional automatic ectopic tachycardia: new proposed treatment by transcatheter His bundle ablation. Am Heart J 1983; 106:619–623.
17. Karpawich PP. Junctional automatic ectopic tachycardia: new proposed treatment by transcatheter His bundle ablation. Am Heart J 1988; 109:159–160.
18. Gillette PC, Garson A Jr, Hesslein PS, et al. Successful surgical treatment of atrial, junctional, and ventricular tachycardia unassociated with accessory connections in infants and children. Am Heart J 1981; 102:984–991.
19. Krongrad E. Postoperative arrhythmias in patients with congenital heart disease. Chest 1984; 85:107–113.
20. Garson A, Moak JP, Smith RT, Norton JB. Usefulness of intravenous propafenone for control of postoperative junctional ectopic tachycardia. Am J Cardiol 1987; 59:1422–1424.
21. Grant JW, Serwer GA, Armstrong BE, Oldham HN, Anderson PA. Junctional tachycardia in infants and children after open heart surgery for congenital heart disease. Am J Cardiol 1987; 59:1216–1218.
22. Gillette PC. Diagnosis and management of postoperative junctional ectopic tachycardia. Am Heart J 1989; 118:192–194.
23. Braunstein PW Jr, Sade RM, Gillette PC. Life-threatening postoperative junctional ectopic tachycardia. Ann Thora Surg 1992; 53:726–728.
24. Gewillig M, Wyse RK, de Leval MR, Deanfield JE. Early and late arrhythmias after the Fontan operation: predisposing factors and clinical consequences. Br Heart J 1992; 67:72–79.
25. Matthys D, Verhaaren H, Deryck Y. Fatal pneumonia complicating hypothermia for the treatment of postoperative junctional ectopic tachycardia. Pediatr Cardiol 1995; 16:294–296.
26. Seghaye MC, Duchateau J, Grabitz RG, et al. Histamine liberation related to cardiopulmonary bypass in children: possible relation to transient postoperative arrhythmias. J Thorac Cardiovasc Surg 1996; 111:971–981.
27. Platt SB, Fisher JD, Zilo P, Kim SG, Ferrick KJ, Roth JA. Mutually independent atrial, junctional, and ventricular rhythms following radiofrequency ablation in a patient with postoperative junctional ectopic tachycardia. Pacing Clin Electrophysiol 1994; 17:1306–1310.
28. Santinelli V, Chiariello M, Condorelli M. Junctional ectopic tachycardia and verapamil. Chest 1984; 85:121–122.
29. Hamdan MH, Page RL, Scheinman MM. Diagnostic approach to narrow complex tachycardia with VA block. PACE 1997; 20:2984–2988.
30. Bash SE, Shah JJ, Albers WH, Geiss DM. Hypothermia for the treatment of postsurgical greatly accelerated junctional ectopic tachycardia. J Am Coll Cardiol 1987; 10:1095–1099.
31. Fyfe DA, Lowe JE, Damiano RJ, Christopher TD. Hemodynamic function in arrhythmias. In Gillette PC, Garson A (eds). Pediatric Arrhythmias: Electrophysiology and Pacing. Philadelphia: WB Saunders, 1990, p. 510.
32. Bharati S, Moskowitz WB, Scheinman M, Estes NAM, Lev M. Junctional tachycardias: anatomic substrate and its significance in ablative procedures. J Am Coll Cardiol 1991; 18:179–186.
33. Rossi L, Piffer R, Turolla E, Frigerio B, Coumel P, James TN. Multifocal Purkinje-like tumor of the heart: occurrence with other anatomic abnormalities in the atrioventricular junction of an infant with junctional tachycardia, Lown-Ganong-Levine syndrome, and sudden death. Chest 1985; 87:340–345.
34. Garson A Jr, Gillette PC. Electrophysiologic studies of supraventricular tachycardia in children. I. Clinical-electrophysiologic correlations. Am Heart J 1981; 102:233–250.
35. Goren C, Santucci BA, Bucheleres HG, Denes P. Chronic recurrent ectopic junctional tachycardia resembling triggered automaticity in mitral valve prolapse syndrome. Am Heart J 1981; 101:504–507.
36. Moak JP, Smith RT, Garson A Jr. Newer antiarrhythmic drugs in children. Am Heart J 1987; 113:179–185.
37. Rossi AF, Kipel G, Golinko RJ, Griepp RB. Use of adenosine in postoperative junctional ectopic tachycardia with 1:1 retrograde atrial conduction. Am Heart J 1991; 121:1237–1239.
38. Till J, Shinebourne EA, Rigby ML, Clarke B, Ward DE, Rowland E. Efficacy and safety of adenosine in the treatment of supraventricular tachycardia in infants and children. Br Heart J 1989; 62:204–211.
39. Perry JC, Knilans TK, Marlow D, Denfield SW, Fenrich AL, Friedman RA. Intravenous amiodarone for life-threatening tachyarrhythmias in children and young adults. J Am Coll Cardiol 1993; 22:95–98.
40. Raja P, Hawker RE, Chaikitpinyo A, et al. Amiodarone management of junctional ectopic tachycardia after cardiac surgery in children. Br Heart J 1994; 72:261–265.
41. Fenrich AL Jr, Perry JC, Friedman RA. Flecainide and amiodarone: combined therapy for refractory tachyarrhythmias in infancy. J Am Coll Cardiol 1995; 25:1195–1198.
42. Kuck KH, Kunze KP, Schluter M, Duckeck W. Encainide versus flecainide for chronic atrial and junctional ectopic tachycardia. Am J Cardiol 1988; 62:37L–44L.
43. Mehta AV, Subrahmanyam AB, Long JB, Kanter RJ. Experience with moricizine HCl in children with supraventricular tachycardia. Int J Cardiol 1996; 57:31–35.
44. Paul T, Reimer A, Janousek J, Kallfelz HC. Efficacy and safety of propafenone in congenital junctional ectopic tachycardia. J Am Coll Cardiol 1992; 20:911–914.
45. Heusch A, Kramer HH, Krogmann ON, Rammos S, Bourgeous M. Clinical experience with propafenone for cardiac arrhythmias in the young. Eur Heart J 1994; 15:1050–1056.
46. Maragnes P, Fournier A, Davignon A. Usefulness of oral sotalol for the treatment of junctional ectopic tachycardia. Int J Cardiol 1992; 35:165–167.
47. Till JA, Rowland E. Atrial pacing as an adjunct to the management of post-surgical His bundle tachycardia. Br Heart J 1991; 66:225–229.
48. Gillette PC. Evolving concepts in the management of congenital junctional ectopic tachycardia. Circulation 1990; 81:1713–1714.
49. Van Hare GF, Velvis H, Langberg JJ. Successful transcatheter ablation of congenital junctional ectopic tachycardia in a ten-month-old infant using radiofrequency energy. Pacing Clin Electrophysiol 1990; 13:730–735.
50. Van Hare GF, Lesh MD, Scheinman M, Langberg JJ. Percutaneous radiofrequency catheter ablation for supraventricular arrhythmias in children. J Am Coll Cardiol 1991; 17:1613–1620.
51. Ehlert FA, Goldberger JJ, Deal BJ, Benson DW, Kadish AH. Successful radiofrequency energy ablation of automatic junctional tachycardia preserving normal atrioventricular nodal conduction. Pacing Clin Electrophysiol 1993; 16:54–61.
52. Young ML, Mehta MB, Martinez RM, Wolff GS, Gelband H. Combined alpha-adrenergic blockade and radiofrequency ablation to treat junctional ectopic tachycardia successfully without atrioventricular block. Am J Cardiol 1993; 71:883–885.
53. Van Hare GF, Witherell CL, Lesh MD. Follow-up of radiofrequency catheter ablation in children: results in 100 consecutive patients. J Am Coll Cardiol 1994; 23:1651–1659.
54. Sanchez C, Benito F, Moreno F. Reversibility of tachycardia-induced cardiomyopathy after radiofrequency ablation of incessant supraventricular tachycardia in infants. Br Heart J 1995; 74:332–333.
55. Wu MH, Lin JL, Chang YC. Catheter ablation of junctional ectopic tachycardia by guarded low dose radiofrequency energy application. Pacing Clin Electrophysiol 1996; 19:1655–1658.
56. Cilliers AM, du Plessis JP, Clur SA, Dateling F, Levin SE. Junctional ectopic tachycardia in six paediatric patients. Heart 1997; 78:413–415.
57. Rychik J, Marchlinski FE, Sweeten TL, et al. Transcatheter radiofrequency ablation for congenital junctional ectopic tachycardia in infancy. Pediatr Cardiol 1997; 18:447–450.
58. Andersen HR, Nielsen JC. Pacing in sick sinus syndrome: need for a prospective, randomized trial comparing atrial with dual chamber pacing. PACE 1998; 21:1175–1179.

59. Perry JC, Kearney DL, Friedman RA, Moak JP, Garson A Jr. Late ventricular arrhythmia and sudden death following direct-current catheter ablation of the atrioventricular junction. Am J Cardiol 1992; 70:765–768.

60. Garson A Jr, Moak JP, Friedman RA, Perry JC, Ott DA. Surgical treatment of arrhythmias in children. Cardiol Clin 1989; 7:319–329.

61. Balaji S, Sullivan I, Deanfield J, James I. Moderate hypothermia in the management of resistant automatic tachycardias in children. Br Heart J 1991; 66:221–224.

62. Pfammatter JP, Paul T, Ziemer G, Kallfelz HC. Successful management of junctional tachycardia by hypothermia after cardiac operations in infants Ann Thorac Surg 1995; 60:556–560.

CHAPTER

10

Accelerated Junctional and Idioventricular Rhythms[1-5a]

Junctional and idioventricular rhythms arise in tissues with automatic properties located in the atrioventricular junction and ventricles. These arrhythmias are normally suppressed and only appear to protect the heart from asystole when the primary pacemaker, usually the sinus node, or atrioventricular conduction fails. These arrhythmias may also develop when inflammation or drugs accelerate the automatic pacemakers at their origins.

ACCELERATED JUNCTIONAL RHYTHM

Junctional rhythms were born as atrioventricular nodal rhythms, the name used during the first half of the twentieth century. By the 1960s, when studies suggested that these arrhythmias more likely arose in tissues adjacent to the node itself, writers began to use the word "junctional" rather than "nodal."[6, 8, 10, 16–22b] The atrioventricular junction includes the approaches to the atrioventricular node, the node itself, and the nonbranching portion of the atrioventricular bundle including the bundle of His.[23]

The atrioventricular junction, the only normal electrophysiological connection between atria and ventricles, transmits impulses in both directions and has pacemaker capacity that protects the ventricles from asystole during sinus node dysfunction or atrioventricular block.[24] However, drugs and disease may acceler-

ate junctional pacemakers to rates that are faster than normal and compete with sinus or other atrial rhythms. Accelerated junctional rhythm often produces atrioventricular dissociation, a phrase currently used to describe this electrocardiographic finding but in the past employed as the name of a specific arrhythmia.

In 1957, Pick and Dominguez described 30 patients with "nonparoxysmal atrioventricular nodal tachycardia" who, in all important respects, had accelerated junctional rhythm.[25] Use of the word "tachycardia" in the title has distressed some writers, who assert that an arrhythmia with a heart rate lower than 100 beats per minute cannot be called a tachycardia.[26] Similarly, accelerated junctional "rhythm" can be faulted as the best name when the rate exceeds 100 beats per minute.[26] I am not equipped to settle these semantic conflicts. For convenience, I avoid using the term tachycardia for the arrhythmia described in this chapter regardless of its rate, to distinguish accelerated junctional rhythm from the rapid tachyarrhythmias due to reentry or enhanced automaticity that arise or are sustained within the atrioventricular junction. The phrase "junctional rhythm," rather than "junctional bradycardia," is used even when the rate is slow.

ACCELERATED IDIOVENTRICULAR RHYTHM

Accelerated idioventricular rhythms arise in ventricular tissues with automatic function such as the bundle branches and Purkinje network. Abnormally wide QRS complexes identify these arrhythmias. They prevent

---

[a]Revised from Chapter 7, "Accelerated Junctional Rhythm," by myself and Michael R. Gold in the first edition of this book.[1]

[b]Not all workers favor the change in the name.[22]

asystole when infranodal atrioventricular block prevents transmission of supraventricular signals from activating the ventricles and junctional pacemakers are prevented from performing their normal function. Accelerated idioventricular rhythm also appears when diseases such as acute myocardial infarction activate these pacemaking tissues.

PREVALENCE

Accelerated junctional rhythm, formerly often called atrioventricular dissociation, is an uncommon but not a rare disorder:

- Atrioventricular dissociation was found in 0.68% of 100,000 electrocardiograms taken in 50,000 patients at a teaching hospital in a 25-year period ending in 1956.[27]
- A frequency of 0.48% was observed in 10,000 consecutive tracings at a Baltimore hospital at about the same time.[3c]

Atrioventricular junctional escape beats were found by 24-hour electrocardiography in 22% of normal men, but junctional rhythms were not observed.[28]

AGE

The average age of 102 patients with accelerated junctional rhythm was 62.9 years.[25, 29–31d] Most of these patients had either myocardial infarction or digitalis intoxication, and their age probably reflects the characteristics of the causes more than any particular feature of the arrhythmia.

The average age of 54 children collected from a pediatric service was 10.7 years.[32] Most of the children had acute rheumatic fever, digitalis intoxication, or recent cardiac surgery.[e]

GENDER

Fifty-nine percent of 59 patients with accelerated junctional rhythm due to myocardial infarction were male.[30, 31] This figure probably indicates the incidence of coronary disease among the patients reviewed.

CLINICAL SETTING
Digitalis Intoxication

Patients intoxicated from digitalis overdosage given for treatment of severe cardiac disease often develop accelerated junctional rhythm.[4, 8, 25, 29, 32–45f] The combination seems to be required because accelerated junctional rhythm rarely[46] develops when people with normally functioning hearts take large overdoses of digoxin by accident or for suicide.[47, 48] Digitalis intoxication may produce accelerated junctional rhythm as many as three times more frequently than paroxysmal atrial tachycardia with block.[38] Digitalis toxicity also produces accelerated idioventricular rhythm,[49–51] and in these cases, multiform QRS complexes may appear.[52]

Myocardial Infarction

Acute myocardial infarction causes accelerated junctional rhythm to develop in about 10% of such patients.[30, 31, 53–55g] Over half the patients have inferior infarctions, and about one-third have anterior infarctions.[30, 31, 56–59h] The arrhythmia is present on admission to the coronary care unit in the majority of patients,[30] and it develops in more than 80% within 36 to 72 hours after symptoms begin.[30, 31]

Accelerated idioventricular rhythm occurs during acute myocardial infarction:[60–70]

- With an incidence of about 12.5%.[64, 65, 68i]
- Probably more frequently during inferior than anterior myocardial infarction,[53, 61, 64, 65] although not all observers have found this difference.[68, 71]
- When the sinus rhythm is slow during sleeping and after administration of vagotonic agents such as morphine and digitalis.[53, 65]
- Usually within the first 24 hours after admission[61, 64–66, 68] but occasionally days or weeks afterwards.[72]
- Rarely with QRS complexes having several forms, possibly from origin in more than one ventricular site.[73, 74]

Accelerated idioventricular rhythm also develops occasionally in patients after they have recovered from myocardial infarction.[75]

---

[c]The incidence of accelerated junctional rhythm may be different now. Both these reports were published several decades ago, when rheumatic fever and digitalis intoxication were more frequently encountered. The reporters were cardiologists with special interest in arrhythmias, and most of the tracings, it appears, were taken in hospitalized patients.

[d]The ages ranged from 25 to 92 years.[25, 29–31]

[e]The average age and range of ages for the diagnoses were as follows: acute rheumatic fever, 11 years, range 5 to 13 years; digitalis intoxication, 13 years, range 8 days to 15 years; cardiac surgery, 9 years, range 16 months to 15 years; other conditions, 6 years, range 3 weeks to 13 years.[32]

[f]Digitalis was thought to be the primary factor producing junctional rhythm in 57% of 274 patients with the arrhythmia in 4 series,[4, 25, 32, 38] as well as in several patients in small group[29] and individual case reports.[34–37, 39–41] The availability of serum digoxin concentrations to guide treatment with the drug seems to have reduced the incidence of arrhythmias resulting from digitalis toxicity.

[g]Sixty-nine (10%) of 672 patients in two relatively large series[30, 31] developed accelerated junctional rhythm during myocardial infarction. Computerized review of monitoring shows the incidence to be even greater. This technique revealed that 12 (40%) of 30 patients had accelerated junctional rhythm during the first 24 hours after admission for myocardial infarction.[55] The arrhythmia was not recognized by conventional monitoring in five of the 12 patients.

[h]Although several authors have commented that junctional rhythms more frequently complicate inferior than anterior infarctions,[25, 57, 59] no data definitively support this assumption. According to two relatively large studies of myocardial infarction, electrocardiographic signs of inferior infarction occur with the same or slightly greater frequency than signs of anterior infarction.[56, 58] By comparing the data from the arrhythmia series[30, 31] with the infarction studies,[56, 58] one could infer that accelerated junctional rhythm may occur slightly more often with inferior than with anterior infarctions.

[i]One hundred sixty-six of 1,328 patients with acute myocardial infarction developed accelerated idioventricular rhythm, as reported in three relatively large series from 1970 to 1975.[64, 65, 68]

Thrombolysis. Accelerated idioventricular rhythm that appears after reperfusion of an occluded coronary artery during myocardial infarction:[76–88]

- Usually develops during the first 8 to 12 hours after reperfusion.[81]
- Occurs more often when thrombolysis normalizes the ST segments quickly.[89]
- Rarely compromises the clinical course even when not treated.[81]
- Is seldom present when patients are discharged from the hospital.[81]

Although accelerated idioventricular rhythm develops more frequently when thrombolysis successfully restores patency of coronary arteries during myocardial infarction,[78, 80, 85–87] the arrhythmia may still appear if the vessels remain occluded.[80, 82, 86] Persistent ischemic pain in the presence of the arrhythmia should suggest both myocardial necrosis and reperfusion of the vessel producing the infarction.[90]

Cardiomyopathy

Accelerated idioventricular rhythm occurs occasionally in patients with cardiomyopathy.[50] The arrhythmia appears in apparently healthy people who may have early arrhythmogenic right ventricular dysplasia established by echocardiographic documentation of right ventricular wall motion abnormalities.[91]

Cardiac Surgery

Accelerated junctional rhythm occurs after valvular, more often aortic than mitral, surgery,[92–94] but less often after coronary artery bypass grafting.[94j] The only factor, other than the type of operation, that appears to predispose to the arrhythmia is a slower sinus rate.[94] Age, potassium concentration, cross-clamp and bypass time, left ventricular ejection fraction, and diastolic pressure do not influence whether the arrhythmia will develop.[94] Accelerated junctional rhythm also appears in children after repair of congenital heart disease,[95–98] particularly atrial and ventricular septal defects present either alone or in association with more complex anomalies.[32]

Acute Rheumatic Fever

Accelerated junctional rhythm is also caused by acute rheumatic fever.[25, 32, 99k] Patients who develop the arrhythmia almost always have it when they arrive at the hospital. The duration is relatively brief and averaged only 4 days (range, 1–8 days) in one series.[32] Acceler-

ated junctional rhythm predicts the presence but not the severity of carditis and often precedes other evidence of cardiac involvement.[32]

Supraventricular Tachycardia

Accelerated junctional rhythm occasionally coexists in patients with supraventricular tachycardia sustained within the atrioventricular node but not in accessory pathways.[100]

Catheter Ablation

Successful ablation of atrioventricular nodal structures to prevent conduction or to suppress supraventricular tachycardia sustained within the node usually produces temporary accelerated junctional rhythm.[101–108]

No Structural Heart Disease

A few patients with accelerated junctional[19, 25, 32, 109, 110] or idioventricular rhythm[50, 111–117] have no discernible cardiac disease. Children rarely develop accelerated idioventricular rhythm, and those who do may have no heart disease or symptoms.[97, 118]

Miscellaneous Causes

Other factors that are thought to produce, or are associated with, occasional cases of accelerated junctional rhythm include:

- Cardiac catheterization.[32]
- Cocaine.[119, 120]
- Chronic obstructive pulmonary disease.[121]
- Direct current cardioversion.[32]
- Flexible fiberoptic bronchoscopy.[122]
- Long QT interval syndrome with syncope.[123]
- Myocarditis.[124]
- Severe infection.[32]
- Systemic amyloidosis.[125]
- Uremia with hyperkalemia.[126]
- Verapamil use.[127]

OTHER ARRHYTHMIAS IN PATIENTS WITH ACCELERATED IDIOVENTRICULAR RHYTHM

Rapid ventricular tachycardia and accelerated idioventricular rhythm may coexist,[66, 128, 129] and during myocardial infarction, accelerated idioventricular rhythm occasionally transforms into rapid ventricular tachycardia or fibrillation.[66, 71, 128, 129] Moreover, paroxysmal rapid ventricular tachycardia occurs during myocardial infarction more frequently in patients with, than in patients without, accelerated idioventricular rhythm.[71]

HISTORY

Accelerated junctional rhythm seldom produces symptoms.[l] However, many patients with the arrhythmia are

---

[j]The arrhythmia appeared during the postoperative period in one-third of 30 patients having valve replacement (18 aortic, 11 mitral, and one aortic and mitral) and in 13% with coronary surgery.[94]

[k]Twenty-eight percent of the cases of accelerated junctional rhythm were due to acute rheumatic fever in a report from a Chicago pediatric service in the late 1960s.[32] However, earlier in the same decade, only one (0.6%) of 160 cases of junctional rhythm was thought to be due to acute rheumatic fever in a study from an adult medical service in a Philadelphia teaching hospital.[38]

[l]Or at least they have rarely been reported in the literature.

quite ill with severe heart disease, digitalis intoxication, myocardial infarction, or the effects of recent cardiac surgery. The symptoms from these conditions predominate.

Accelerated junctional rhythm is not paroxysmal; it appears and recedes gradually. This characteristic distinguishes accelerated junctional rhythm from paroxysmal supraventricular tachycardia, some cases of which were formerly called "junctional tachycardia." Rarely, accelerated junctional rhythm is chronic.[121] Accelerated idioventricular rhythm is usually present intermittently for short periods of time, but occasionally may be chronic.[111, 115]

PHYSICAL EXAMINATION

One expects that when an accelerated junctional rhythm exceeds the rate of the sinus mechanism, the characteristic physical signs of atrioventricular dissociation will appear.[6, 11] These include variation in the pulse pressure, intermittent cannon A waves in the neck veins, independent atrial sounds, and varying intensity of the first heart sound and of systolic murmurs.[m] Because the usual ventricular rate of accelerated junctional rhythm is in the range of sinus rhythm or slow sinus tachycardia, medical personnel easily overlook the arrhythmia's presence during examination of the arterial pulse.[11]

A mid-to-late "nonejection systolic sound" was reported in a 35-year-old woman without cardiovascular disease during intervals of accelerated junctional rhythm at a rate of about 70 beats per minute. The sound disappeared when sinus rhythm was present. An echocardiogram showed no signs of mitral valve prolapse.[110]

ELECTROCARDIOGRAPHY
Rhythm

Accelerated junctional and idioventricular rhythms are regular unless the atrial rhythm successfully competes for control of the ventricles.[7, 10, 130]

Rate

The ventricular rate of accelerated junctional rhythm exceeds the normal escape rate of junctional pacemakers, which is said to be about 30 to 60 beats per minute in adults.[57, 131] The range of rates of nonparoxysmal atrioventricular nodal tachycardia was defined as 70 to 130 beats per minute when the arrhythmia was first described.[25]

In children with congenital complete atrioventricular block, the average rate of the junctional pacemaker is 49 beats per minute, with a range of 31 to 73 beats per minute.[132] Because the rate in a crying infant may be 70 to 75 beats per minute, the authors of the largest series of accelerated junctional rhythm in children use

80 beats per minute as the minimum rate for the arrhythmia.[32]

For accelerated junctional rhythm to be detected, the sinus rate must be less than that of the ectopic pacemaker unless atrioventricular block is also present. This feature helps to explain why the sinus rate tends to be slower in patients whose accelerated junctional rhythm can be recorded after cardiac surgery than in patients without the arrhythmia.[94] The ventricular rate of the arrhythmia tends to be faster during anterior than during inferior myocardial infarction.[31]

The rate of accelerated idioventricular rhythm in adults is usually 60 to 110 beats per minute. In children, it can be faster.[15n]

P Waves

Sinus rhythm is the usual atrial mechanism in patients with accelerated junctional or idioventricular rhythm. Accordingly, the P waves have the normal appearance for this mechanism, but they may be distorted by anatomic or electrophysiological abnormalities of the atria.

Accelerated junctional or idioventricular rhythm can also develop during atrial arrhythmias such as fibrillation, flutter, and ectopic automatic or reentrant atrial tachycardias. If the atrial arrhythmia is faster than the accelerated rhythm, then some degree of atrioventricular block must be present for the junctional or idioventricular rhythm to be detected.

Isorhythmic dissociation. In isorhythmic[o] dissociation, the rates of the atria and ventricles are almost the same even though dissociation is present.[133] The P waves of sinus rhythm hug the QRS complexes appearing just before, within, and after the QRS complex before gradually reversing the sequence (Fig. 10.1). As Henry J. L. Marriott observed: "When there is reason to conclude some influence, rather than chance, is holding the pacemakers in phase,"[6] the relationship may be called "synchronization"[3, 4, 6, 36, 134, 135] or "accrochage,"[134, 135p] the word used when the synchrony is short-lived (see Fig. 10.1).

PR Intervals

Changing PR intervals are characteristic of atrioventricular dissociation, which is usually present, either constantly or intermittently, during accelerated junctional and idioventricular rhythms. This occurs because the rate of the abnormally functioning pacemaker exceeds that of the sinus node (Fig. 10.2). The atria may intermittently capture the ventricles, except when atrioventricular block of sufficient degree is concurrently present. P waves that are inverted in the inferior electrocardiographic leads may follow each QRS complex producing RP' intervals in those cases

---

[m]However, few reports of the arrhythmia include observations on physical findings.

[n]One authority suggests "an arbitrary cut off of 120 to 150 beats per minute."[15]
[o]From *isos* (Greek) meaning "equal."
[p]From the French for "a hooking together."[134]

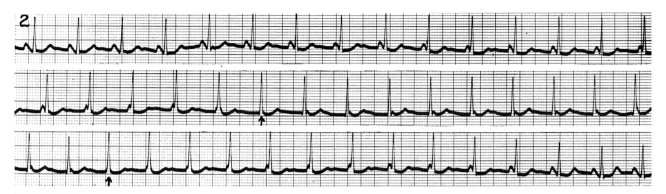

FIGURE 10.1 Isorhythmic dissociation. An accelerated junctional rhythm is present at the rate of about 95 beats per minute. The sinus rate is slightly slower, and the P waves approach and disappear within the QRS complexes (end of **top** and first part of **middle**). At the first arrow, the P waves begin to appear at the end of the QRS complexes. At the second arrow (**bottom**), this sinus rate has increased slightly, and the P waves can be seen just before the QRS complexes. (Adapted from Marriott HJ, Menendez MM. A-V dissociation revisited. Prog Cardiovasc Dis 1966; 8:522–538, with permission.)[6]

when the accelerated rhythm captures the atria in retrograde fashion (Fig. 10.3, *lower panel*).

QRS Complexes

The QRS complexes during accelerated junctional rhythm have normal width unless concurrent bundle branch block is present. Of course, cardiac abnormalities that affect the QRS complex during sinus rhythm, such as myocardial infarction and ventricular hypertrophy, are also present during the arrhythmia.

The morphology of the QRS complexes during arrhythmias thought to be junctional or nodal rhythms may be slightly different than during sinus rhythm. Formerly, the mechanism was thought to be aberrant conduction to the ventricles from junctional pacemakers.[136-140] Cardiologists now know that these rhythms usually arise within the fascicles of the bundle branches and consequently should be called fascicular rhythms[141-143] (Fig. 10.4).

The QRS complexes in accelerated idioventricular rhythm are always abnormally wide, as befits an arrhythmia originating in the ventricles (Fig. 10.5). The morphology can suggest where in the ventricle the arrhythmia arises[144] and, during thrombolysis, which vessel produces the arrhythmia:[90]

- Left anterior descending—the duration is shortest.
- Circumflex—does not have the form of left bundle branch block.
- Right—does not have an inferior axis.

Among children, the QRS complexes usually look like left bundle branch block.[15] When atrial beats capture the ventricles during this arrhythmia, fusion beats appear in which the QRS complexes are narrower than during the idioventricular beat and display characteristics of both conducted beats and ventricular beats (Fig. 10.6).

ST and T Waves

The ST and T waves are normal in most junctional rhythms, except when abnormalities of depolarization have been produced in the same patient during sinus rhythm as well. Occasionally, the P waves that may appear during the ST and T waves can distort their appearance.

DIFFERENTIAL DIAGNOSIS
Atrioventricular Dissociation

The authors of many texts, reviews, and articles have long employed the phrase "atrioventricular dissocia-

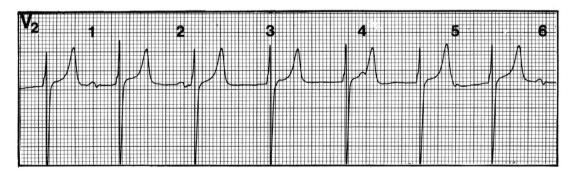

FIGURE 10.2 Accelerated junctional rhythm with atrioventricular dissociation. The ventricular rhythm is regular, a finding indicating that the dissociation is complete and that the atria do not capture the ventricles. The ventricular rate is 70 beats per minute; the sinus rate is 60 beats per minute. The P waves are numbered. P wave 3, which occurs during ventricular activation, slightly distorts the terminal portion of the QRS complex. (From Kastor JA, Gold MR. Accelerated junctional rhythm. In Kastor JA (ed). Arrhythmias. Philadelphia: WB Saunders, 1994, with permission.)[1]

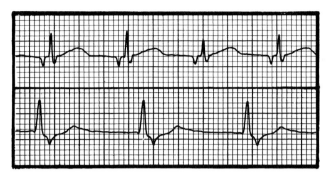

FIGURE 10.3 Low atrial and His bundle rhythms. Top (lead II): a supraventricular rhythm at a rate of 100 beats per minute; negative P waves precede each QRS complex with a short PR interval. The arrhythmia probably originates in the lower portions of the atria near the entrance to the atrioventricular node. Formerly, this finding was called a high-nodal rhythm. **Bottom** (also lead II): an accelerated His bundle rhythm at a rate of 70 beats per minute; retrograde conduction to the atria produces the negative P waves after the QRS complexes. Formerly, this was called a low-nodal rhythm. (From Kastor JA, Gold MR. Accelerated junctional rhythm. In Kastor JA (ed). Arrhythmias. Philadelphia: WB Saunders, 1994, with permission.)[1]

tion" to describe an arrhythmia characterized by narrow QRS complexes at a rate that slightly exceeds the sinus rhythm and includes, in many cases, some beats conducted from atria to ventricles.[3, 4, 6, 16, 35, 126, 135, 145–147] Many of the examples of this abnormality appear to be accelerated junctional rhythm. Atrioventricular dissociation, I suggest, is better seen as an electrocardiographic finding that is the result of other arrhythmias rather than as an arrhythmia itself.[5, 148, 149q]

---

[q]Atrioventricular dissociation "is never a primary disturbance," wrote Alfred Pick,[5] "arises secondary to some other more fundamental disorder," according to Samuel Bellet,[148] and "like jaundice is not in itself a diagnosis," suggests Henry J. L. Marriott and Robert J. Myerburg.[149]

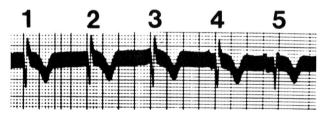

FIGURE 10.4 Accelerated fascicular rhythm in a patient with a recent inferior myocardial infarction (lead III). The ventricular rate is 75 beats per minute. In ventricular beats 1 and 2, the P waves cannot be seen because they are hidden within the QRS complexes. A P wave originating in the sinus node can be seen at the beginning of beat 3. In beat 4, the wave precedes, but does not capture, the QRS complex. Beat 5 is a sinus beat. The QRS complexes during atrioventricular dissociation (beats 1–4) have a slightly different form from that of the final conducted beat. This finding indicates that the origin of the accelerated rhythm is below the atrioventricular junction in one of the fascicles of the ventricles. In this record, from the paper that first described nonparoxysmal atrioventricular nodal tachycardia, the form of QRS complexes 1 to 4 was thought to be due to "the use of preferential AV pathway by the nodal impulses." (Adapted from Pick A, Dominguez P. Nonparoxysmal A-V nodal tachycardia. Circulation 1957; 16:1022–1032, with permission.)[25]

Lead 2

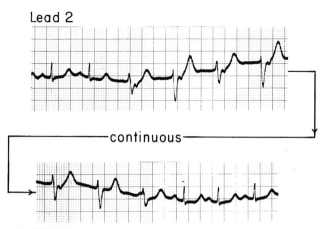

—continuous—

FIGURE 10.5 Accelerated idioventricular rhythm in a 61-year-old woman with an anterior myocardial infarction. The sinus rate slows after the first two sinus beats, and an idioventricular focus captures the ventricles and the atria by retrograde conduction. The sinus rate then increases (**lower panel**) and gains partial control of the ventricles in the third fusion beat. Sinus rhythm is then reestablished. The wide QRS complexes and the fusion beats differentiate this arrhythmia from accelerated junctional rhythm. (From Kastor JA, Goldreyer BN, Moore EN, Spear JF. Re-entry: an important mechanism of cardiac arrhymias. Cardiovasc Clin 1974; 6:111–135, with permission.)[220]

The rhythms in the atria and ventricles dissociate from each other when[5, 8]

- The sinus node malfunctions or defaults[6] in its role of primary cardiac pacemaker, as in sinus arrest, sinoatrial block, or marked sinus bradycardia, and lower pacemakers escape to sustain an adequately rapid ventricular rhythm.
- Atrioventricular block prevents the normal atrial pacemaker signal from reaching the ventricles.
- Junctional, fascicular, or ventricular foci discharge faster than normal and usurp[6] the role of ventricular pacemaker.

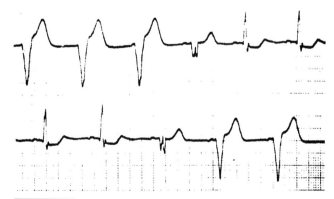

FIGURE 10.6 Fusion beats during accelerated junctional rhythm. The first three beats (**top**) arise from the accelerated junctional rhythm, and the fifth and sixth beats are conducted normally. **Bottom:** beats one and two are supraventricular and the last two beats from the arrhythmia. Beat four (**top**) and beat three (**bottom**) are fusion beats. These beats arise partly from atrioventricular conduction and partly from the idioventricular site. The PR intervals of fusion beats are shorter than normal because part of the ventricles are activated from the abnormal site before the signal starting in the sinus node reaches them.

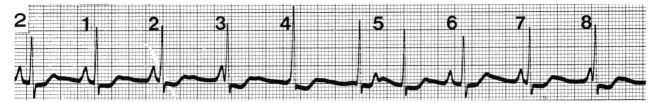

FIGURE 10.7 Accelerated junctional rhythm with atrial captures (lead II). P wave 1 conducts to the ventricles. Then an accelerated junctional rhythm at a rate of about 78 beats per minute appears that is slightly faster than the sinus rhythm at 75 beats per minute. P waves 2 and 3 are not conducted, and P wave 4 is buried within the QRS complex. P waves 5 and 6 capture the ventricles, and the RR intervals preceding them are shorter than those during the junctional rhythm. The cycle then repeats. (Adapted from Marriott HJ, Menendez MM. A-V dissociation revisited. Prog Cardiovasc Dis 1966; 8:522–538, with permission.)[6]

- Any of the three previously described abnormalities occur together.

The degree of dissociation is established by the amount of atrial capture of the ventricles. In the absence of atrioventricular block, some of the atrial signals conduct to the ventricles and disrupt their regularity[149, 150] (Fig. 10.7).[r]

Atrioventricular Block

The ventricular rate characteristically exceeds the sinus rate during accelerated junctional rhythm, whereas the atrial rate is faster than the ventricular rate during atrioventricular block. The diseases that produce accelerated junctional rhythm may also cause atrioventricular block.[25, 38, 43] When the two arrhythmias occur together, the atria and ventricles are likely to be completely dissociated.

Atrial Ectopic Rhythms

Abnormal atrial pacemakers may usurp the rhythm of the atria from the sinus node and may produce atrial rhythms with rates similar to accelerated junctional rhythm. These are recognized by P waves of abnormal morphology that precede each QRS complex; atrioventricular dissociation is not present.

The site of the ectopic atrial pacemakers may be estimated from the form of the P waves.[151–162s] For example, when the P waves are inverted in leads II, III, and aVF, the origin is likely to be in the floor of the atria[2, 16, 19, 39, 163–167] (see Fig. 10.3, *upper panel*).[t] The left

atrium is probably the focus when the P waves are inverted in lead I and are either inverted or biphasic in lead V_6[168] or have the *dome and dart* form[169–172] (Fig. 10.8).[u]

Atrioventricular Nodal Tachycardia with Block

This rapid, irregular supraventricular arrhythmia, the nature of which has not been established by electro-

---

[u]This is the phrase devised by Mirowski[169, 170] to describe the atrial activity in lead V_1 that he found "inherently related to a particularly posterior location of the pacemaker in the left atria."[171] Dome and dart P waves in lead V_1 are "bifid with an initial smooth, low voltage component, related to the initial left atrial activation followed by a high, sharply peaked component, related mainly to right atrial activation."[169, 172] They help us recognize the presence of left atrial rhythm but are not present in every case.[168]

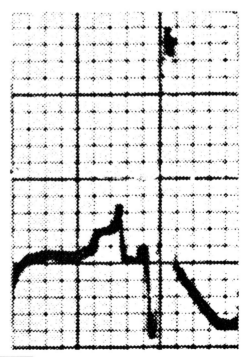

FIGURE 10.8 Dome and dart P wave. One beat from lead V_1 shows the characteristic initial smooth component and the sharply peaked termination often found in left atrial rhythms. (Adapted from Mirowski M, Neill CA, Taussig HB. Left atrial ectopic rhythm in mirror-image dextrocardia and in normally placed malformed hearts: report of twelve cases with "dome and dart" P waves. Circulation 1963; 27:864–877, with permission.)[169]

---

[r]Since the 1920s, the arrhythmia that is produced has been called "interference dissociation" or "atrioventricular dissociation with interference." (See the biographical sketch on Woldemar Mobitz in Chapter 3.) I join others[149, 150] in preferring not to use this phrase. The somewhat cumbersome but more descriptive "accelerated junctional rhythm with intermittent atrial capture" describes the arrhythmia more precisely.

[s]However, atrial pacing studies have shown the limitations of locating the focus by this method.[151–162]

[t]Ectopic atrial arrhythmias originating from this region have been called "high nodal rhythm" or "coronary sinus rhythm" when the PR interval is normal.[39, 163, 166, 167] The name "coronary nodal rhythm" was once assigned to the finding of normal P waves, short PR intervals, and QRS complexes without the delta waves of the Wolff-Parkinson-White syndrome.[2, 16, 165] Workers thought that this rhythm originated near the tail of the sinus node and that the PR interval was short from accelerated conduction or because the atrial signal had less tissue to traverse before reaching the atrioventricular junction. The name should not be used because the electrocardiographic finding represents sinus rhythm or an ectopic atrial rhythm with accelerated conduction within or around the atrioventricular node.[19] When tachyarrhythmias coexist, the Lown-Ganong-Levine syndrome is said to be present.[164]

physiological study, has been described in patients with severe myocardial disease and digitalis intoxication.[173, 174] The ventricular rate is usually faster than during accelerated junctional rhythm. The atria may be fibrillating. Exit block from the origin of the tachycardia within the atrioventricular junction is presumed to cause the characteristic irregularity.[v]

Atrial Fibrillation and Atrial Flutter

Accelerated junctional rhythm may develop when the atria are in fibrillation or flutter for the same reasons that the arrhythmia appears during sinus rhythm. Digitalis intoxication is an important cause and can be easily overlooked.

During fibrillation, regularization of the ventricular response, first at a relatively slow rate (Fig. 10.9) and then at a rate that is faster than the normal junctional escape rate, indicates the presence of an accelerated ectopic pacemaker and sufficient atrioventricular nodal block to prevent capture of the ventricles by the fibrillating atria. In flutter, the diagnosis of complete atrioventricular dissociation due to accelerated junctional rhythm may be even more difficult to establish. One must prove that the regular ventricular beats occur at a frequency that bears no numerical relationship to the rate of the flutter waves.

Double Tachycardia

Occasionally, tachyarrhythmias develop in which the atria are driven by an atrial arrhythmia (or, as formerly thought, by the atrioventricular node) and the ventricles are controlled simultaneously by an arrhythmia within the atrioventricular junction or ventricles.[7, 41, 175–185] These arrhythmias are known as double or simultaneous tachycardias, and, in some cases, the ventricular disturbance is an accelerated junctional rhythm. The phrase "double tachycardia" is not usually employed when the atria are in fibrillation or flutter.

The RR intervals are usually regular, and atrial capture of the ventricles is unusual. The ventricular rates in a series of 11 cases ranged from 88 to 177 beats per minute but were less than 150 beats per minute in nine patients.[180] The atrial rates were 118 to 250 beats per minute and greater than 150 beats per minute in nine patients. Patients with double tachycardia tend to be very ill, and they often have digitalis intoxication, poor circulatory function, hypoxia, and high mortality.[180, 186][w]

Junctional Rhythm

The rate of (nonaccelerated) junctional, formerly called atrioventricular nodal, rhythm equals the escape rate of the junctional pacemaker of about 30 to 60 beats per minute and consequently is slower than accelerated junctional rhythm.[7, 10, 21, 187] Junctional rhythm develops whenever the sinus pacemaker is excessively slow, as in the sick sinus syndrome, from damage during cardiac surgery,[188] or from hypervagotonia or the administration of beta-adrenergic–blocking and calcium-channel–blocking drugs.[189] Junctional rhythm protects the ventricles from asystole during high-grade atrioventricular block.[x]

The junctional pacemaker may capture the atria in addition to the ventricles when ventriculoatrial conduction is intact. The P waves in such cases follow the QRS complexes and are inverted in the inferior electrocardiographic leads from caudad-to-cephalic activation of the atria.[16, 21, 190–192][y] In these cases, atrioventricular dissociation, characteristic of many cases of accelerated junctional rhythm, is absent.

When sinus rhythm spontaneously returns in patients with a long history of atrial fibrillation, a rare phenomenon, the regular rhythm may be misinterpreted as junctional because the P waves are so small that they cannot be seen on the surface electrocardiogram. Intracardiac recordings are needed to make the correct diagnosis.[193]

Junctional Ectopic Tachycardia

Both accelerated junctional rhythm and junctional ectopic tachycardia are automatic arrhythmias that probably originate from the same tissue, and each is often characterized by atrioventricular dissociation. Junctional ectopic tachycardia is faster and occurs most often in infants and children either spontaneously or after cardiac surgery.

Paroxysmal Junctional Tachycardia

Some rapid, regular tachycardias with narrow QRS complexes that start and stop suddenly have been

---

[v]Until the characteristics of this arrhythmia have been further described by electrophysiological study, the diagnosis of atrioventricular nodal (junctional) tachycardia with block should not be used.

[w]Eleven patients with double tachycardia, eight of whom died, were reported during 1972 at a large teaching hospital. Each was thought to be intoxicated from digitalis.[180] The incidence of double tachycardia has almost certainly decreased with the availability of digoxin assays.[186]

[x]One can logically consider (nonaccelerated) junctional and accelerated junctional rhythms as elements of a single phenomenon, an arrhythmia arising in the atrioventricular junction with rates from about 30 beats per minute to more than 100 beats per minute. The slower examples reflect the protective properties of the junction and are manifested as escape rhythms, whereas faster, accelerated rhythms are produced by specific pathological influences on the junctional pacemakers.

[y]According to earlier nomenclature,[21] low nodal rhythm was characterized by inverted P waves after each QRS complex in the inferior electrocardiographic leads. The P waves in mid-nodal rhythm occurred at the same time as the QRS complexes and were not visible. Inverted P waves preceded the QRS complexes in high nodal rhythm.[16] Although experimental evidence has yet to establish the point, we suspect that most high-nodal rhythms originate in the atria close to the atrioventricular node and that low-nodal rhythms begin in the bundle of His. The origin of mid-nodal rhythms remains unknown. Data suggest that patients with junctional rhythm and inverted P waves preceding the QRS complexes, which may originate low in the atria, often have no significant heart disease, but they may be receiving beta-blocking– or calcium-channel–blocking drugs.[192] Earlier studies suggested that patients with atrial ectopic rhythms often have heart disease.[171, 191] Patients with junctional rhythms and P waves after the QRS complexes frequently have cardiac disease, are taking digitalis, and have a higher mortality.[192]

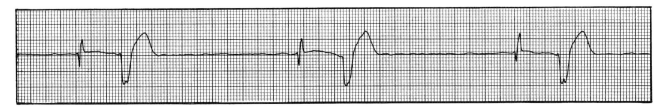

FIGURE 10.9 Slow junctional rhythm with ventricular bigeminy caused by digitalis intoxication. This electrocardiogram of a 74-year-old woman shows atrial fibrillation, a high degree of block within the atrioventricular node, and a depressed junctional escape rhythm with each beat followed by a ventricular ectopic beat. The digoxin level was 7.9 µg/mL. When the digoxin was discontinued, the ventricular beats ceased, and the ventricular rate gradually increased as atrioventricular block disappeared. The QRS complexes in lead V_1 were identical during digitalis intoxication and normal conduction. Digitalis may also increase the rate of the subsidiary pacemaker and may produce an accelerated junctional rhythm. (From Kastor JA, Gold MR. Accelerated junctional rhythm. In Kastor JA (ed). Arrhythmias. Philadelphia: WB Saunders, 1994, with permission.)[1]

called junctional for many decades. Electrophysiologists seldom use this name now, because these arrhythmias are paroxysmal supraventricular tachycardias sustained by reentry within the atrioventricular node or through atrioventricular accessory pathways. In many cases, P waves cannot be seen—they are usually buried in the QRS complexes—and this finding, more than any other, probably gave rise to the name paroxysmal junctional tachycardia.

Sinus Rhythm

Because the rate of accelerated junctional rhythm is the same as that of sinus rhythm and slow sinus tachycardia, one may mistake the arrhythmia for sinus rhythm during brief periods of isorhythmic dissociation when the PR intervals are normal or are slightly shorter than normal. Examination of an extended electrocardiographic record reveals the presence of atrioventricular dissociation.

Sinoventricular Conduction

Hyperkalemia produces this uncommon arrhythmia in which the atria are quiescent, P waves are absent, and the QRS complexes suggest idioventricular rhythm or an accelerated junctional rhythm with an intraventricular conduction disturbance.[194, 195] In sinoventricular conduction, the sinus node remains the cardiac pacemaker, but the atria do not respond electrically or mechanically because of the electrolyte disturbance that also produces the wide QRS complexes. The diagnosis should be entertained in patients whose potassium is severely elevated.

ELECTROCARDIOGRAM DURING SINUS RHYTHM

The electrocardiograms of patients who have accelerated junctional rhythm can indicate the presence of severe cardiac disease with signs of myocardial infarction, ventricular hypertrophy, or conduction disturbances. Digitalis effect in the ST and T waves may also be seen as a precursor to toxicity. Accelerated junctional rhythm can develop in patients with concurrent atrial fibrillation and flutter. These arrhythmias may be present before and after the junctional rhythm.

OTHER ELECTROCARDIOGRAPHIC STUDIES

Continuous Recordings

Holter monitoring has occasionally revealed the presence of intermittent junctional rhythm in some patients,[196] but not in healthy men.[28]

Late Potentials

The retrograde P waves that followed the QRS complexes of a slightly accelerated junctional rhythm in a man with a subendocardial myocardial infarction and transient ventricular tachycardia produced a signal-averaged electrocardiogram that simulated the presence of late potentials. The absence of these potentials during sinus rhythm confirmed that the retrograde P waves rather than slow ventricular conduction had produced the potentials.[197]

ECHOCARDIOGRAPHY

Echocardiograms show abnormalities in the wall motion of the right ventricle in some patients with accelerated idioventricular rhythm and no apparent structural heart disease.[91]

LABORATORY STUDIES

Hypokalemia is the principal abnormal laboratory finding reported in patients with accelerated junctional rhythm, particularly when digitalis intoxication produces the arrhythmia.

HEMODYNAMICS

Decreased blood pressure and cardiac output frequently follow the development of junctional rhythm after cardiac surgery.[94‡]

Isorhythmic Dissociation

The apparent relationship between the QRS complexes and the P waves in the presence of complete

---

‡These findings developed in 9 of 14 patients with the arrhythmia after cardiac surgery.[94] The cause is probably loss of synchronized atrial contraction.

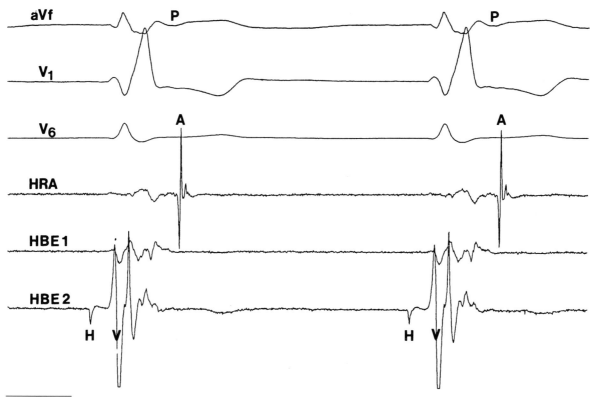

FIGURE 10.10   His bundle rhythm. This intracardiac recording shows (from **top** to **bottom**) electrocardiographic leads aVF, V_1, and V_6 and electrograms from the high right atria (HRA) and the region of the bundle of His (HBE 1 and HBE 2). Complete right bundle branch block is present. The deflection from the bundle of His (H) precedes the ventricular activation (V) with a normal HV interval. Retrograde atrial activation (A) follows the QRS complexes, producing inverted P waves (P) in lead aVF. (From Kastor JA, Gold MR. Accelerated junctional rhythm. In Kastor JA (ed). Arrhythmias. Philadelphia: WB Saunders, 1994, with permission.)[1]

atrioventricular dissociation due to accelerated junctional rhythm (or heart block) is produced by retrograde capture of the atria from the accelerated junctional pacemaker[198] or slight variations in the autonomic control of the sinus rate.[133] When the stroke volume is greater because of a relatively normal PR relationship, the sinus node discharges slightly less often, and the P wave disappears within and then emerges behind the QRS complex. The stroke volume then drops slightly, and autonomic stimulation raises the sinus rate so that the P wave passes back through and then precedes the QRS complex again.[199][aa]

ELECTROPHYSIOLOGY

Mechanism

Accelerated junctional and idioventricular rhythms have the electrophysiological characteristics of automatic rather than reentrant arrhythmias:[200]

- They appear, increase in rate, slow, and disappear gradually or nonparoxysmally and not suddenly.

- Pacing at rates faster than the arrhythmias can suppress them, but the arrhythmias return after the pacing is stopped if its causes are still present.
- Electric shock does not convert accelerated junctional or idioventricular rhythm.
- The arrhythmias cannot be started or stopped by programmed stimulation.

An occasional case of atrioventricular junctional rhythm may be due to triggered activity[201] or delayed afterdepolarizations.[200]

Intracardiac Electrocardiography

In accelerated junctional rhythm, the His bundle electrogram shows a V deflection with every QRS complex preceded by an H deflection from the bundle of His that indicates that the arrhythmia rises within or near the bundle of His[13, 19, 20, 39, 202, 203] (Fig. 10.10).[bb] A similar pattern but at a slower rate characterizes junctional escape rhythm.

In the electrophysiology laboratory, accelerated idioventricular rhythm can be differentiated from accelerated junctional rhythm because the ventricular foci pro-

---

[aa]Levy and Edelstein explain: "The mechanism responsible for . . . A-V synchronization represents a typical biologic feedback control system. The P-R interval is a determinant of stroke volume, which in turn influences the arterial pressure. The blood pressure has an inverse effect on the discharge frequency of the S-A node through the baro-receptor reflex. The S-A nodal reflex then affects the P-R interval, to close the feedback loop."[199]

[bb]No electrophysiological studies that I know about have shown accelerated junctional rhythms to originate elsewhere than in the bundle of His. However, workers have suggested that different sites within the atrioventricular junction may have pacemaker potential in humans.[20]

duce signals in the His bundle electrogram that consist only of V waves, not preceded by H deflections.[115, 204]

The atrial rhythm is identified from the atrial and bundle of His electrodes. If the atrial rhythm, such as atrial fibrillation, atrial flutter, automatic atrial tachycardia, or sinus tachycardia, is faster than the accelerated rhythm, then atrioventricular block will probably be concurrently present so that the accelerated junctional or idioventricular rhythm will not be suppressed and can be recognized. If block is absent, then some of the atrial beats will conduct through the atrioventricular node and capture the bundle of His and the ventricles.[205cc]

Autonomic Influence

The autonomic nervous system influences the rate of junctional rhythms. This is best demonstrated by the administration of atropine, the vagolytic agent, which increases the rate of junctional rhythms.

Concealed Conduction

Concealed conduction refers to the ability of beats to change conduction or impulse formation, the signs of which are delayed and are not immediately evident on the electrocardiogram.[206] In accelerated junctional rhythm, concealed conduction can be observed when a nonconducted sinus beat delays the appearance of the next accelerated junctional beat through partial penetration of the junctional pacemaker.[207] Concealed conduction of the impulses from the fibrillating atria may also reach and discharge a junctional pacemaker and may thereby delay the expected appearance of a junctional escape beat.[208]

Retrograde Conduction

Junctional rhythms, whether or not they are accelerated, may capture the atria by retrograde conduction when the atria are not controlled by their own pacemakers as during the sick sinus syndrome. The signal from the His bundle region travels slowly through the atrioventricular node before activating the atria in a caudad-to-cephalic pattern. The His bundle and atrial electrograms show early activation in the floor of the right atrium where the atrioventricular node joins the atrium and later activation in the superior region of the right atrium near the sinus node and in the left atrium.

Because of the delay within the atrioventricular node, the atria are activated after the ventricles in junctional rhythms that originate in the bundle of His. Accordingly, the P waves and the atrial signals in the electrograms usually follow the QRS complexes and the V waves. The duration of the interval from the QRS complex to the retrograde P wave reflects the difference between the time of conduction from the bundle of His pacemaker to the atria and the ventricles.

TREATMENT

General Principles

Most patients with accelerated junctional or idioventricular rhythm do not require specific antiarrhythmic treatment unless the arrhythmia produces hemodynamic deterioration. Therapy is primarily directed toward the causes of the arrhythmia.

Drugs

Atropine. Atropine can restore sinus rhythm in patients with accelerated rhythms by decreasing atrioventricular block and increasing the rate of the sinus pacemaker.[19] However, atropine can also accelerate the rate of junctional pacemakers.[9, 121, 209]

Beta-adrenergic–blocking drugs. These drugs can suppress accelerated idioventricular rhythm.[210]

Captopril. Given to patients during thrombolytic treatment for first myocardial infarctions, captopril decreases the incidence of accelerated idioventricular rhythm.[211]

Catecholamines. Catecholamine support of the circulation may be required when accelerated junctional rhythm develops after cardiac surgery.[94]

Digitalis. Digitalis must be discontinued as soon as it is recognized as a possible cause of the arrhythmia. Digitalis is not administered to treat accelerated junctional rhythm.

Digoxin-specific Fab antibody fragments. These agents specifically reverse digoxin intoxication and should be administered when digitalis-induced arrhythmias endanger the patient. This rarely occurs when accelerated junctional rhythm is present without associated ventricular tachyarrhythmias or hyperkalemia.[48]

Isoproterenol. This drug increases the rate of accelerated junctional rhythm.[121, 212]

Lidocaine. This drug decreases the rate in some cases of accelerated junctional rhythm.[213]

Procainamide. Procainamide suppresses accelerated idioventricular rhythm,[72] but antiarrhythmic drugs are seldom needed.[115dd]

[cc]A rare and complicated case has been reported of a patient with digitalis intoxication in whom accelerated junctional rhythm at a rate of 65 to 85 beats per minute was demonstrated by intracardiac electrocardiography but could not be seen in the electrocardiogram in the presence of an idioventricular escape rhythm at 45 beats per minute and complete trifascicular atrioventricular block.[205]

[dd]Idioventricular rhythms may respond to manipulation of parasympathetic and sympathetic stimulation. One patient, a 28-year-old man without cardiac disease, had chronic accelerated idioventricular rhythm at 85 beats per minute.[115] Carotid sinus massage, Valsalva maneuver, phenylephrine, edrophonium, and propranolol decreased the rate of the rhythm, and hyoscine, passive upright tilt, exercise, and isoproterenol increased its rate.[115]

Potassium. Potassium should be administered to patients with accelerated junctional rhythm who are hypokalemic, but the potassium concentration should not be allowed to rise above the normal range.

Theophylline. In a few reported cases,[214] theophylline suppressed accelerated idioventricular rhythm appearing after successful reperfusion by streptokinase during myocardial infarction. Relief of the arrhythmia by theophylline, a competitive antagonist of adenosine receptors, suggests that endogenous adenosine released by the ischemic tissue produced the arrhythmia.[214]

Tocainide. This drug reduces the likelihood of accelerated idioventricular rhythm appearing during myocardial infarction as well as, and possibly better than, lidocaine.[215]

Pacing

When loss of atrial synchrony compromises the circulation in patients with accelerated junctional or idioventricular rhythm, pacing,[94, 216] preferably atrial or atrioventricular sequential pacing, may be instituted to establish the normal atrioventricular relationship and to overdrive the accelerated focus.[213, 217] Of course, this method of treatment is inapplicable when atrial fibrillation or atrial flutter is present.[218]

Cardioversion

Electric shock does not convert automatic arrhythmias such as accelerated junctional or idioventricular rhythm.

PROGNOSIS

The prognosis of patients who develop accelerated junctional rhythm depends primarily on the severity of underlying cardiac or other diseases.[4, 16] Thus, accelerated idioventricular rhythm developing during[53, 61, 64, 65, 68] or after[219] myocardial infarction does not worsen the prognosis. The mortality is lower in outpatients with accelerated idioventricular rhythm if the rate of the arrhythmia is less than 100 beats per minute compared with patients whose arrhythmia is faster.[219ee] Patients whose arrhythmia is due to digitalis intoxication seem to have a particularly poor prognosis, probably because of the severity of the cardiac disease for which the drug has been administered.[43]

SUMMARY

Adults develop accelerated junctional and idioventricular rhythms from digitalis intoxication usually in the presence of severe myocardial disease and during acute myocardial infarction. Cardiac surgery and ablation of the atrial fibrillation node can produce transient accelerated junctional rhythm. Successful coronary thrombolysis often induces transient accelerated idioventricular rhythm. Children with acute rheumatic fever also can develop both accelerated arrhythmias, which may also occur in patients without heart disease.

Accelerated junctional and idioventricular rhythms are not paroxysmal, and patients are often unaware of their presence. The physical examination may reveal the signs of atrioventricular dissociation.

The rate of accelerated junctional rhythm is about 70 to 130 beats per minute, and the rate of accelerated idioventricular rhythm is between 60 and 100 beats per minute, both faster than the normal escape rate of junctional or ventricular pacemakers. The ventricular rate is characteristically greater than the sinus rate, and partial atrioventricular dissociation with intermittent atrial capture of the ventricles frequently occurs. The phrase "atrioventricular dissociation," formerly used to describe accelerated junctional rhythm, should be employed only to identify a lack of relationship between atrial and ventricular activation. During isorhythmic dissociation in patients with accelerated junctional rhythm, the discharge of atria and ventricles may appear to relate to one another. In accelerated junctional rhythm, the QRS complexes are usually of normal width unless concurrent bundle branch block is present. Prolonged, abnormal QRS complexes characterize accelerated idioventricular rhythm.

Accelerated junctional rhythm is recognized at electrophysiological study by the presence of H deflections before every V deflection and often by complete or intermittent dissociation from atrial activation. During accelerated idioventricular rhythm, H deflections do not appear before the QRS complexes. Both arrhythmias have the characteristics of an automatic rather than a reentrant abnormality.

Specific treatment of accelerated junctional or idioventricular rhythms is seldom required. Increasing the atrial rate with atropine, catecholamines, or atrial pacing can suppress both arrhythmias. When digitalis causes the arrhythmias, the drug must be discontinued. Cardioversion does not restore normal rhythm.

The prognosis depends primarily on the severity of the underlying cardiac disease.

---

*ee*From the Cardiac Arrhythmia Suppression Trial (CASS).[219]

REFERENCES

1. Kastor JA, Gold MR. Accelerated junctional rhythm. In Kastor JA (ed). Arrhythmias. Philadelphia: WB Saunders, 1994:201–217.
2. Katz LN, Pick A. Clinical Electrocardiograph. Part I. The Arrhythmias. Philadelphia: Lea & Febiger, 1956, pp. 100–108.
3. Marriott HJL, Schubart AF, Bradley SM. A-V dissociation: a reappraisal. Am J Cardiol 1958; 2:586–605.
4. Jacobs DR, Donoso E, Friedberg CK. A-V dissociation: a relatively frequent arrhythmia: analysis of thirty cases with detailed discussion of the etiologic differential diagnosis. Medicine 1961; 40:101–117.
5. Pick A. A-V dissociation: a proposal for a comprehensive

classification and consistent terminology. Am Heart J 1963; 66:147–150.

6. Marriott HJL, Menendez MM. A-V dissociation revisited. Prog Cardiovas Dis 1966; 8:522–538.

7. Scherf D, Cohen J. Atrioventricular rhythms. Prog Cardiovas Dis 1966; 8:499–521.

8. Pick A, Langendorf R. Recent advances in the differential diagnosis of A-V junctional rhythms. Am Heart J 1968; 76:553–575.

9. Schamroth L. Idioventricular tachycardia. Dis Chest 1969; 56:466–468.

10. Fisch C, Knoebel SB. Junctional rhythms. Prog Cardiovasc Dis 1970; 13:141–158.

11. Bellet S. Clinical Disorders of the Heart Beat. Philadelphia: Lea & Febiger, 1971, p. 479.

12. Zipes DP, Fisch C. Accelerated ventricular rhythm. Arch Intern Med 1972; 129:650–652.

13. Josephson ME. Clinical Cardiac Electrophysiology. Techniques and Interpretations. 2nd ed. Philadelphia: Lea & Febiger, 1993, pp. 169–173.

14. Grimm W, Marchlinski FE. Accelerated idioventricular rhythm, bidirectional ventricular tachycardia. In Zipes DP, Jalife J (eds). Cardiac Electrophysiology. From Cell to Bedside. 2nd ed. Philadelphia: W B Saunders, 1995:920–926.

15. Perry JC. Ventricular tachycardia in neonates. Pacing Clin Electrophysiol 1997; 20:2061–2064.

16. Friedberg CK. Diseases of the Heart. 3rd ed. Philadelphia: W B Saunders, 1966. pp. 488–496.

17. Marriott HJL. Nodal mechanisms with dependent activation of atria and ventricles In Dreifus LS, Likoff W(eds). Mechanisms and Therapy of Cardiac Arrhythmias. New York: Grune & Stratton, 1966, pp. 412–418.

18. Scherf D. Problems of nomenclature in cardiac arrhythmias. Am J Cardiol 1967; 19:327–330.

19. Rosen KM. Junctional tachycardia: mechanisms, diagnosis, differential diagnosis, and management. Circulation 1973; 47:654–664.

20. Scherlag BJ, Lazzara R, Helfant RH. Differentiation of "A-V junctional rhythms." Circulation 1973; 48:304–312.

21. Waldo AL, James TN. A retrospective look at A-V nodal rhythms. Circulation 1973; 47:222–224.

22. Guntheroth WB, Selzer A, Spodick DH. Atrioventricular nodal rhythm reconsidered. Am J Cardiol 1983; 52:416–417.

23. Hecht HH, Kossmann CE, Childers RW, et al. Atrioventricular and intraventricular conduction: revised nomenclature and concepts. Am J Cardiol 1973; 31:232–244.

24. Pick A, Langendorf R. The dual functional of the A-V junction. Am Heart J 1974; 88:790–797.

25. Pick A, Dominguez P. Nonparoxysmal A-V nodal tachycardia. Circulation 1957; 16:1022–1032.

26. Marriott HJL, Myerburg RJ. Recognition of cardiac arrhythmias. In Hurst JW (ed). The Heart, Arteries and Veins. 7th ed. New York: McGraw-Hill, 1990, p. 529.

27. Katz LN, Pick A. Clinical Electrocardiography. Part I. The Arrhythmias. Philadelphia: Lea & Febiger, 1956, p. 43.

28. Brodsky M, Wu D, Denes P, Kanakis C, Rosen KM. Arrhythmias documented by 24-hour continuous electrocardiographic monitoring in 50 male medical students without apparent heart disease. Am J Cardiol 1977; 39:390–395.

29. Soffer A. The importance of atrio-ventricular dissociation in the diagnosis of digitalis intoxication. Dis Chest 1962; 41:422–424.

30. Konecke LL, Knoebel SB. Nonparoxysmal junctional tachycardia complicating acute myocardial infarction. Circulation 1972; 45:367–374.

31. Fishenfeld J, Desser KB, Benchimol A. Non-paroxysmal A-V junctional tachycardia associated with acute myocardial infarction. Am Heart J 1973; 86:754–758.

32. Rodriguez-Coronel A, Miller RA. Accelerated nodal pacemaker. Pediatrics 1969; 43:430–441.

33. Vanagt EJ, Wellens HJJ. The electrocardiogram in digitalis intoxication. In Wellens HJJ, Kulbertus HE (eds). What's New in Electrocardiography. Boston: Martinus Nijhoff, 1981, pp. 315–343.

34. Bradley SM, Marriott HJL. Escape-capture bigeminy. Am J Cardiol 1958; 1:640–643.

35. Castellanos A, Azan L, Calvino JM. Dissociation with interference between pacemakers located within the A-V conducting system. Am Heart J 1958; 56:562–569.

36. Schubart AF, Marriott HJL, Gorten RJ. Isorhythmic dissociation. Am J Med 1958; 24:209–214.

37. Chevalier RB, Bowers JA. An unusual form of atrioventricular nodal rhythm due to digitalis. J Indiana State Med Assoc 1963; 56:178–182.

38. Dreifus LS, Katz M, Watanabe Y, Likoff W. Clinical significance of disorders of impulse formation and conduction in the atrioventricular junction. Am J Cardiol 1963; 11:384–391.

39. Damato AN, Lau SH. His bundle rhythm. Circulation 1969; 40:527–534.

40. Schamroth L. Principles governing 2:1 A-V block with interference dissociation. Br Heart J 1969; 31:780–786.

41. Chung EK. Unusual form of digitalis-induced triple A-V nodal rhythm. Am Heart J 1970; 79:250–253.

42. Chung EK. Unusual form of atrioventricular nodal bigeminy. Jpn Heart J 1970; 11:104–112.

43. De Azevedo IM, Watanabe Y, Dreifus LS. Atrioventricular junctional rhythm: classification and clinical significance. Chest 1973; 64:732–740.

44. Rose MR, Glassman E, Spencer FC. Arrhythmias following cardiac surgery: relation to serum digoxin levels. Am Heart J 1975; 89:288–294.

45. Moorman JR. Digitalis toxicity at Duke Hospital, 1973 to 1984. South Med J 1985; 78:561–564.

46. Hancock EW. AV block versus AV dissociation. Hosp Prac (Off Ed) 1985; 20:33–37.

47. Smith TW, Willerson JT. Suicidal and accidental digoxin ingestion: report of five cases with serum digoxin level correlations. Circulation 1971; 44:29–36.

48. Smith TW, Butler VP Jr. Haber E, et al. Treatment of life-threatening digitalis intoxication with digoxin-specific Fab antibody fragments. N Engl J Med 1982; 307:1357–1400.

49. Schott A. Idioventricular rhythm due to digitalis intoxication. Dis Chest 1965; 47:557–559.

50. Massumi RA, Ali N. Accelerated isorhythmic ventricular rhythms. Am J Cardiol 1970; 26:170–185.

51. Castellanos A, Azan L, Bierfield J, Myerburg RJ. Digitalis-induced accelerated idioventricular rhythms: revisited. Heart Lung 1975; 4:104–110.

52. Rothfeld EL, Zucker IR. Multiform accelerated idioventricular rhythm. Angiology 1974; 25:457–461.

53. Norris RM, Mercer CJ. Significance of idioventricular rhythms in acute myocardial infarction. Prog Cardiovasc Dis 1974; 16:455–468.

54. Julian DG, Valentine PA, Miller GG. Disturbances of rate, rhythm and conduction in acute myocardial infarction: a prospective study of 100 consecutive unselected patients with the aid of electrocardiographic monitoring. Am J Med 1964; 37:915–927.

55. Knoebel SB, Rasmussen S, Lovelace DE, Anderson GJ. Nonparoxysmal junctional tachycardia in acute myocardial infarction: computer-assisted detection. Am J Cardiol 1975; 35:825–830.

56. Multicenter Diltiazem Postinfarction Trial Research Group. The effect of diltiazem on mortality and reinfarction after myocardial infarction. N Engl J Med 1988; 319:385–392.

57. Marriott HJL, Myerburg RJ. Recognition of cardiac arrhythmias. In Hurst JW (ed). The Heart, Arteries and Veins. 7th ed. New York: McGraw-Hill, 1990, p. 526.

58. Third International Study of Infarct Survival Collaborative Group. ISIS-3: a randomised comparison of streptokinase vs. tissue plasminogen activator vs. anistreplase and of aspirin plus heparin vs. aspirin alone among 41,299 cases of suspected acute myocardial infarction. Lancet 1992; 339:753–770.

59. Zipes DP. Specific arrhythmias: diagnosis and treatment. In Braunwald E (ed). Heart Disease. A Textbook of Cardiovascular Medicine. 4th ed. Philadelphia: WB Saunders, 1992, pp. 685–688.

60. Bashour FA, Jones E, Edmonson R. Cardiac arrhythmias in acute myocardial infarction. II. Incidence of the common arrhythmias with special reference to ventricular tachycardia. Dis Chest 1967; 51:520–529.

61. Rothfeld EL, Zucker IR, Parsonnet V, Alinsonorin CA. Idioventricular rhythm in acute myocardial infarction. Circulation 1968; 37:203–209.

62. Castellanos A, Lemberg L, Arcebal AG. Mechanisms of slow ventricular tachycardias in acute myocardial infarction. Chest 1969; 56:470–476.

63. Mogensen L. Ventricular tachyarrhythmias and lignocaine prophylaxis in acute myocardial infarction. Acta Med Scand 1970; 513:1–89.

64. Norris RM, Mercer CJ, Yeates SE. Idioventricular rhythm complicating acute myocardial infarction. Br Heart J 1970; 32:617–621.

65. Rothfeld EL, Zucker IR, Leff WA, Parsonnet V. Idioventricular rhythm (IVR) in acute myocardial infarction (AMI): a reappraisal. Circulation 1970; 193:41–42.

66. Vohra JK, Dowling JT, Sloman G. Idioventricular tachycardia in acute myocardial infarction. Med J Aus 1971; 2:196–198.

67. Castellanos A, Sung RJ, Mayorga-Cortes A, Myerburg RJ. Double ectopic accelerated ventricular and nonaccelerated ventricular or supraventricular rhythms. Eur J Cardiol 1975; 3:153–156.

68. Lichstein E, Ribas-Meneclier C, Gupta PK, Chadda KD. Incidence and description of accelerated ventricular rhythm complicating acute myocardial infarction. Am J Med 1975; 58:192–198.

69. Hasin Y, Rogel S. Ventricular rhythms in acute myocardial infarction. Cardiology 1976; 61:195–207.

70. Yusuf S, Lopez R, Sleight P. Heart rate and ectopic prematurity in relation to sustained ventricular arrhythmias. Br Heart J 1980; 44:233–239.

71. de Soyza N, Bissett JK, Kane JJ, Murphy ML, Doherty JE. Association of accelerated idioventricular rhythm and paroxysmal ventricular tachycardia in acute myocardial infarction. Am J Cardiol 1974; 34:667–670.

72. Basu D, Scheinman M. Sustained accelerated idioventricular rhythm. Am Heart J 1975; 89:227–231.

73. Sclarovsky S, Strasberg G, Agmon J. Multiform accelerated idioventricular rhythm in acute myocardial infarction. J Electrocardiol 1978; 11:197–200.

74. Sclarovsky S, Strasberg B, Fuchs J, et al. Multiform accelerated idioventricular rhythm in acute myocardial infarction: electrocardiographic characteristics and response to verapamil. Am J Cardiol 1983; 52:43–47.

75. Hutchinson RG. Accelerated idioventricular rhythm after recovery from myocardial infarction. Angiology 1977; 28:579–582.

76. Krumholz HM, Goldberger AL. Reperfusion arrhythmias after thrombolysis: electrophysiologic tempest, or much ado about nothing. Chest 1991; 99:135S–140S.

77. Goldberg S, Greenspon AJ, Urban PL, et al. Reperfusion arrhythmia: a marker of restoration of antegrade flow during intracoronary thrombolysis for acute myocardial infarction. Am Heart J 1983; 105:26–32.

78. Cercek B, Horvat M. Arrhythmias with brief, high-dose intravenous streptokinase infusion in acute myocardial infarction. Eur Heart J 1985; 6:109–113.

79. Buckingham TA, Devine JE, Redd RM, Kennedy HL. Reperfusion arrhythmias during coronary reperfusion therapy in man: clinical and angiographic correlations. Chest 1986; 90:346–351.

80. Miller FC, Krucoff MW, Satler LF, et al. Ventricular arrhythmias during reperfusion. Am Heart J 1986; 112:928–932.

81. Cercek B, Lew AS, Laramee P, Shah PK, Peter TC, Ganz W. Time course and characteristics of ventricular arrhythmias after reperfusion in acute myocardial infarction. Am J Cardiol 1987; 60:214–218.

82. Gore JM, Ball SP, Corrao JM, Goldberg RJ. Arrhythmias in the assessment of coronary artery reperfusion following thrombolytic therapy. Chest 1988; 94:727–730.

83. Linnik W, Tintinalli JE, Ramos R. Associated reactions during and immediately after RTPA infusion. Ann Emerg Med 1989; 18:234–239.

84. Hohnloser SH, Zabel M, Kasper W, Meinertz T, Just H. Assessment of coronary artery patency after thrombolytic therapy: accurate prediction utilizing the combined analysis of three noninvasive markers. J Am Coll Cardiol 1991; 18:44–49.

85. Six AJ, Louwerenburg JH, Kingma JH, Robles de Medina EO, vanHemel NM. Predictive value of ventricular arrhythmias for patency of the infarct-related coronary artery after thrombolytic therapy. Br Heart J 1991; 66:143–146.

86. Zehender M, Utzolino S, Furtwangler A, Kasper W, Meinertz T, Just H. Time course and interrelation of reperfusion-induced ST changes and ventricular arrhythmias in acute myocardial infarction. Am J Cardiol 1991; 68:1138–1142.

87. Gressin V, Louvard Y, Pezzano M, Lardoux H. Holter recording of ventricular arrhythmias during intravenous thrombolysis for acute myocardial infarction. Am J Cardiol 1992; 69:152–159.

88. Doevendans PA, Gorgels AP, van der Zee R, Partouns J, Bar FW, Wellens HJJ. Electrocardiographic diagnosis of reperfusion during thrombolytic therapy in acute myocardial infarction. Am J Cardiol 1995; 75:1206–1210.

89. Gressin V, Gorgels AP, Louvard Y, Lardoux H, Bigelow RH. Is arrhythmogenicity related to the speed of reperfusion during thrombolysis for myocardial infarction? Eur Heart J 1993; 14:516–520.

90. Gorgels AP, Vos MA, Letsch IS, et al. Usefulness of the accelerated idioventricular rhythm as a marker for myocardial necrosis and reperfusion during thrombolytic therapy in acute myocardial infarction. Am J Cardiol 1988; 61:231–235.

91. Martini B, Nava A, Thiene G, et al. Accelerated idioventricular rhythm of infundibular origin in patients with a concealed form of arrhythmogenic right ventricular dysplasia. Br Heart J 1988; 59:564–571.

92. Rabbino MD, Dreifus LS, Likoff W. Cardiac arrhythmias following intracardiac surgery. Am J Cardiol 1961; 5:681–689.

93. Hoie J, Forfang K. Arrhythmias and conduction disturbances following aortic valve implantation. Scand J Thorac Cardiovasc Surg 1980; 14:177–183.

94. Kerr CR, Mason MA. Incidence and clinical significance of accelerated junctional rhythm following open heart surgery. Am Heart J 1985; 110:966–969.

95. Krongrad E. Postoperative arrhythmias in patients with congenital heart disease. Chest 1984; 85:107–113.

96. Nakagawa H, Beckman KJ, McClelland JH, et al. Radiofrequency catheter ablation of idiopathic left ventricular tachycardia guided by a Purkinje potential. Circulation 1993; 88:2607–2617.

97. MacLellan-Tobert SG, Porter CJ. Accelerated idioventricular rhythm: a benign arrhythmia in childhood. Pediatrics 1995; 96:122–125.

98. Seghaye MC, Duchateau J, Grabitz RG, et al. Histamine liberation related to cardiopulmonary bypass in children: possible relation to transient postoperative arrhythmias. J Thorac Cardiovasc Surg 1996; 111:971–981.

99. Goodman RM, Pick A. An unusual type of intermittent A-V dissociation in acute rheumatic myocarditis. Am Heart J 1961; 61:259–263.

100. Epstein MR, Saul JP, Fishberger SB, Triedman JK, Walsh EP. Spontaneous accelerated junctional rhythm: an unusual but useful observation prior to radiofrequency catheter ablation for atrioventricular node reentrant tachycardia in young patients. Pacing Clin Electrophysiol 1997; 20:1654–1661.

101. Shah PK, Cercek B, Lew AS, Ganz W. Angiographic validation of bedside markers of reperfustion. J Am Coll Cardiol 1993; 21:55–61.

102. Thakur RK, Klein GJ, Yee R, Stites HW. Junctional tachycardia: a useful marker during radiofrequency ablation for atrioventricular node reentrant tachycardia. J Am Coll Cardiol 1993; 22:1706–1710.

103. Jentzer JH, Goyal R, Williamson BD, et al. Analysis of

junctional ectopy during radiofrequency ablation of the slow pathway in patients with atrioventricular nodal reentrant tachycardia. Circulation 1994; 90:2820–2826.

104. Alison JF, Yeung-Lai-Wah JA, Schulzer M, Kerr CR. Characterization of junctional rhythm after atrioventricular node ablation. Circulation 1995; 91:84–90.

105. Epstein LM, Lesh MD, Griffin JC, Lee RJ, Scheinman MM. A direct midseptal approach to slow atrioventricular nodal pathway ablation. Pacing Clin Electrophysiol 1995; 18:57–64.

106. Nath S, DiMarco JP, Mounsey JP, Lobban JH, Haines DE. Correlation of temperature and pathophysiological effect during radiofrequency catheter ablation of the AV junction. Circulation 1995; 92:1188–1192.

107. Yu JC, Lauer MR, Young C, Liem LB, Hou C, Sung RJ. Localization of the origin of the atrioventricular junctional rhythm induced during selective ablation of slow-pathway conduction in patients with atrioventricular node reentrant tachycardia. Am Heart J 1996; 131:937–946.

108. Boyle NG, Anselme F, Monahan K, et al. Origin of junctional rhythm during radiofrequency ablation of atrioventricular nodal reentrant tachycardia in patients without structural heart disease. Am J Cardiol 1997; 80:575–580.

109. Zehender M, Meinertz T, Keul J, Just H. ECG variants and cardiac arrhythmias in athletes: clinical relevance and prognostic importance. Am Heart J 1990; 119:1378–1391.

110. Langhorne H, Phillips JH. Junctional rhythm and atrial contraction: a mechanism for systolic sound. Am Heart J 1992; 123:1699–1701.

111. Klein G, Peretz DI. Chronic accelerated idioventricular rhythm. Ann Intern Med 1975; 83:372–373.

112. Davidson RM. Chronic accelerated ventricular rhythm. J Electrocardiol 1976; 9:249–254.

113. Comerford TJ, Propert DB. Accelerated idioventricular rhythm inpatients without acute myocardial infarction. Angiology 1979; 30:768–775.

114. Gould L, Patel S, Gomes GI, Chokshi AB. Accelerated idioventricular rhythm in a young normal male. Angiology 1982; 33:738–742.

115. Waxman MB, Cupps CL, Cameron DA. Modulation of an idioventricular rhythm by vagal tone. J Am Coll Cardiol 1988; 11:1052–1060.

116. Lew DC, Keim SG, Curitis AB. Accelerated idioventricular rhythm detected during elective surgery in a healthy man. Clin Cardiol 1991; 14:772–774.

117. Navarro V, Nathan PE, Rosero H, Sacchi TJ. Accelerated idioventricular rhythm in pregnancy: a case report. Angiology 1993; 44:506–508.

118. Gaum WE, Biancaniello T, Kaplan S. Accelerated ventricular rhythm in childhood. Am J Cardiol 1979; 43:162–164.

119. Benchimol A, Bartall H, Desser KB. Accelerated ventricular rhythm and cocaine abuse. Anna Intern Med 1978; 88:519–520.

120. Jonsson S, O'Meara M, Young JB. Acute cocaine poisoning. Importance of treating seizures and acidosis. Am J Med 1983; 75:1061–1064.

121. Palileo EV, Bauernfeind RA, Swiryn SP, Wyndham CR, Rosen KM. Chronic nonparoxysmal junctional tachycardia. Chest 1981; 80:106–108.

122. Borgeat A, Chiolero R, Mosimann B, Freeman J. Accelerated idioventricular rhythm during flexible fiberoptic bronchoscopy. Crit Care Med 1987; 15:274–275.

123. Kernohan RJ, Froggatt P. Atrioventricular dissociation with prolonged QT interval and syncopal attacks in a 10-year-old boy. Br Heart J 1974; 36:516–519.

124. Nakagawa M, Hamaoka K, Okano S, Shiraishi I, Sawada T. Multiform accelerated idioventricular rhythm (AIVR) in a child with acute myocarditis. Clin Cardiol 1988; 11:853–855.

125. Scully RE, Mark EJ, McNeely WF, McNeely BU. Case records of the Massachusetts General Hospital. N Engl J Med 1992; 327:943–950.

126. Louvros N, Costeas FX. Atrioventricular dissociation with S-A interference (ventricular capture), A-V interference (atrial capture), and reciprocating beating: "incomplete" retrograde unidirectional A-V block. Am Heart J 1967; 73:240–244.

127. Walker WS, Winniford MD, Mauritson DR, Johnson SM, Hillis LD. Atrioventricular junctional rhythm in patients receiving oral verapamil therapy. JAMA 1983; 249:389–390.

128. Rothfeld EL, Zucker IR, Leff WA, Ritota MC. Coexisting paroxysmal ventricular tachycardia and idioventricular rhythm in acute myocardial infarction. J Electrocardiol 1973; 6:149–152.

129. Sclarovsky S, Strasberg B, Martonovich G, Agmon J. Ventricular rhythms with intermediate rates in acute myocardial infarction. Chest 1978; 74:180–182.

130. Schamroth L. Idioventricular tachycardia. J Electrocardiol 1968; 1:205–212.

131. Katz LN, Pick A. Clinical Electrocardiography. Part I. The Arrhythmias. Philadelphia: Lea & Febiger, 1956, p. 100.

132. Miller RA, Rodriguez-Coronel A. Congenital atrioventricular block. In Moss AJ, Adams FH (eds). Heart Disease in Infants, Children and Adolescents. Baltimore: Williams & Wilkins, 1968, p. 1045.

133. Patel A, Pumill R, Goldman D, Damato AN. Isorhythmic atrioventricular dissociation revisited. Am Heart J 1992; 124:823–829.

134. Marriott HJL. Atrioventricular synchronization and accrochage. Circulation 1956; 14:38–43.

135. Fletcher E, Morton P, Murtagh JG, Bekheit S. Atrioventricular dissociation with accrochage. Br Heart J 1971; 33:572–577.

136. Pick A. Aberrant ventricular conduction of escaped beats. Circulation 1956; 13:702–711.

137. Walsh TJ. Ventricular aberration of A-V nodal escape beats. Am J Cardiol 1962; 10:217–222.

138. Kistin AD. Atrioventricular junctional premature and escape beats with altered QRS and fusion. Circulation 1966; 34:740–751.

139. Kistin AD. Problems in the differentiation of ventricular arrhythmia from supraventricular arrhythmia with abnormal QRS. Prog Cardiovasc Dis 1966; 9:1–17.

140. Sherf L, James TN. The mechanism of aberration in late atrioventricular junctional beats. Am J Cardiol 1972; 29:529–539.

141. Massumi RA, Ertem GE, Vera Z. Aberrancy of junctional escape beats: evidence for origin in the fascicles of the left bundle branch. Am J Cardiol 1972; 29:351–359.

142. Massumi RA, DeMaria A, McFarland J, Amsterdam EA, Mason DT. Fascicular rhythms in myocardial infarction (MI): diagnostic significance. Circulation 1972; 89:45–46.

143. Josephson ME. Clinical Cardiac Electrophysiology. Techniques and Interpretations. 2nd ed. Philadelphia: Lea & Febiger, 1993, pp. 140–143.

144. Strasberg B, Kanakis C, Kehoe R, Wyndham C, Rosen KM. Similar echocardiographic wall motion abnormalities in left-side accelerated idioventricular rhythm and left-side preexcitation. Chest 1979; 75:380–381.

145. Schott A. Atrioventricular dissociation with and without interference. Prog Cardiovasc Dis 1960; 2:444–464.

146. Scherf D, Cohen J. The Atrioventricular Node and Selected Cardiac Arrhythmias. New York: Grune & Stratton, 1964, pp. 280–318.

147. Schamroth L, Friedberg HD. Significance of retrograde conduction in A-V dissociation. Br Heart J 1965; 27:896–901.

148. Bellet S. Clinical Disorders of the Heart Beat. Philadelphia: Lea & Febiger, 1971, p. 467.

149. Marriott HJL, Myerburg RJ. Recognition of cardiac arrhythmias. In Hurst JW (ed). The Heart, Arteries and Veins. 7th ed. New York: McGraw-Hill, 1990, p. 525.

150. Katz LN, Pick A. Clinical Electrocardiography. Part I. The Arrhythmias. Philadelphia: Lea & Febiger, 1956, pp. 6, 105.

151. Somlyo AP, Grayzel J. Left atrial arrhythmias. Am Heart J 1963; 65:68–76.

152. Massumi R, Tawakkol AA. Direct study of left atrial P waves. Am J Cardiol 1967; 20:331–340.

153. Harris BC, Shaver JA, Gray S, Kroetz FW, Leonard JJ. Left atrial rhythm. Circulation 1968; 37:1000–1014.

154. Massumi RA, Sarin RK, Tawakkol AA, Rios JC, Jackson H. Time sequence of right and left atrial depolarization as a guide to the origin of the P waves. Am J Cardiol 1969; 24:28–36.

155. Leon DF, Lancaster JF, Shaver JA, Kroetz FW, Leonard JJ. Right atrial ectopic rhythms: experimental production in man. Am J Cardiol 1970; 25:6–10.

156. Lown B, Kosowsky BD. Artifical cardiac pacemakers. N Engl J Med 1970; 283:971–977.

157. Piccolo E, Nava A, Furlanello F, Permutti B, Volta SD. Left atrial rhythm: vectorcardiographic study and electrophysiologic critical evaluation. Am Heart J 1970; 80:11–18.

158. Rutenberg HL, Soloff LA. Stimulation of "left atrial rhythm" by right atrial pacing. Am J Cardiol 1970; 26:427–431.

159. Waldo WL, Vitikainen KJ, Kaiser GA, Malm JR, Hoffman BF. The P wave and P-R interval. Circulation 1970; 42:653–671.

160. MacLean WAH, Karp RB, Kouchoukos NT, James TN, Waldo AL. P waves during ectopic atrial rhythms in man: a study utilizing atrial pacing with fixed electrodes. Circulation 1975; 52:426–434.

161. Waldo AL, MacLean WAH, Karp RB, Kouchoukos NT, James TN. Sequence of retrograde atrial activation of the human heart. Br Heart J 1977; 39:634–640.

162. Khalilullah M, Shrestha NK, Padmavati S. Left atrial rhythm in man: an experimental study. J Electrocardiol 1978; 11:375–378.

163. Scherf D, Harris R. Coronary sinus rhythm. Am Heart J 1946; 32:443–455.

164. Lown B, Ganong WF, Levine SA. The syndrome of short P-R interval, normal QRS complex and paroxysmal heart action. Circulation 1952; 5:693–706.

165. Eyring EJ, Spodick DH. Coronary nodal rhythm. Am J Cardiol 1960; 5:781–783.

166. Spodick DH, Colman R. Observations on coronary sinus rhythm and its mechanism. Am J Cardiol 1961; 7:198–203.

167. Hancock EW. Coronary sinus rhythm in sinus venosus defect and persistent left superior vena cava. Am J Cardiol 1964; 14:608–615.

168. Beder SD, Gillette PC, Garson A Jr, McNamara DG. Clinical confirmation of ECG criteria for left atrial rhythm. Am Heart J 1982; 103:848–852.

169. Mirowski M, Neill CA, Taussig HB. Left atrial ectopic rhythm in mirror-image dextrocardia and in normally placed malformed hearts: report of twelve cases with "dome and dart" P waves. Circulation 1963; 27:864–877.

170. Mirowski M. Left atrial rhythm: diagnostic criteria and differentiation from nodal arrhythmias. Am J Cardiol 1966; 17:203–210.

171. Mirowski M. Ectopic rhythms originating anteriorly in the left atrium: analysis of 12 cases with P wave inversion in all pericordial leads. Am Heart J 1967; 74:299–308.

172. Kastor JA. Abnormal atrial rhythms, an early interest of Michel Mirowski. Pacing Clin Electrophysiol 1991; 14:916–919.

173. Pick A, Langendorf R, Katz LN. A-V nodal tachycardia with block. Circulation 1961; 24:12–22.

174. Castellanos A, Lemberg L. The relationship between digitalis and A-V nodal tachycardia with block. Am Heart J 1963; 66:605–613.

175. Shmagranoff GL, Jick S. Simultaneous atrial and nodal tachycardia. Am Heart J 1957; 54:417–421.

176. Castellanos A, Azan L, Calvino JM. Simultaneous tachycardias. Am Heart J 1960; 59:358–373.

177. Chevalier RB, Fisch C. Dissociation of pacemakers located within the atrioventricular node. Am J Cardiol 1960; 5:564–565.

178. Jonas S, Richman SM. Double nodal rhythm with A-V dissociation. Am Heart J 1960; 60:811–816.

179. Halkin H, Kaplinsky E. Simultaneous tachycardias associated with acute myocardial infarction. Chest 1971; 60:394–396.

180. Wishner SH, Kastor JA, Yurchak PM. Double atrial and atrioventricular junctional tachycardia. N Engl J Med 1972; 287:552–553.

181. Jordan RM, McAnulty JH, Ritzmann L. Alternating atrial and ventricular tachycardia. Br Heart J 1979; 41:734–737.

182. Benson DW Jr, Gallagher JJ, Sterba R, Klein GJ, Armstrong BE. Catecholamine induced double tachycardia: case report in a child. Pacing Clin Electrophysiol 1980; 3:96–103.

183. Medina-Ravell V, Rozanski JJ, Castellanos A. His bundle recordings in double tachycardias not due to digitalis intoxication. Pacing Clin Electrophysiol 1982; 5:751–757.

184. Belhassen B, Pelleg A, Paredes A, Laniado S. Simultaneous A-V nodal reentrant and ventricular tachycardias. Pacing Clin Electrophysiol 1984; 7:325–331.

185. Eldar M, Belhassen B, Hod H, Schuger CD, Scheinman MM. Exercise-induced double (atrial and ventricular) tachycardia: a report of three cases. J Am Coll Cardiol 1989; 14:1376–1381.

186. Castellanos A Jr. Personal communication, 1992.

187. Scherf D, Cohen J. The Atrioventricular Node and Selected Cardiac Arrhythmias. New York: Grune & Stratton, 1964, pp. 47–124.

188. Bink-Boelkens MT, Velvis H, van der Heide JJ, Eygelaar A, Hardjowijono RA. Dysrhythmias after artrial surgery in children. Am Heart J 1983; 106:125–130.

189. Hartwell BL, Mark JB. Combinations of B-blockers and calcium channel blockers: a cause of malignant perioperative conduction disturbances? Anesth Analg 1986; 65:905–907.

190. Mirowski M. Left atrial rhythm. Am J Cardiol 1966; 17:299–308.

191. Mirowski M, Lau SH, Wit AL, et al. Ectopic right atrial rhythms: experimental and clinical data. Am Heart J 1971; 81:666–676.

192. Gold MR, Yurchak PM, Eagle KA. Personal Communication, 1992.

193. DeMots H, Brodeur MT, Rahimtoola SH. Concealed sinus rhythm: a cause of misdiagnosis of digitalis intoxication. Circulation 1974; 50:632–633.

194. Bellet S. Clinical Disorders of the Heart Beat. Philadelphia: Lea & Febiger, 1971, p. 898.

195. Vassalle M, Hoffman BF. The spread of sinus activation during potassium administration. Circulation Research 1965; 17:285–295.

196. Kennedy HL. Ambulatory Electrocardiography. Philadelphia: Lea & Febiger, 1981, pp. 107–111.

197. Taylor E, Effron M, Veltri EP. False positive signal-averaged ECG produced by junctional rhythm with retrograde P waves. Am Heart J 1992; 123:1701–1703.

198. Waldo AL, Vitikainen KJ, Harris PD, Malm JR, Hoffman BF. The mechanism of synchronization in isorhythmic A-V dissociation; some observations on the morphology and polarity of the P wave during retrograde capture of the atria. Circulation 1968; 38:880–898.

199. Levy MN, Edelstein J. The mechanism of synchronization in isorhythmic A-V dissociation. Circulation 1970; 42:689–699.

200. Rosen MR, Fisch C, Hoffman BF, Danilo P, Lovelace DE, Knoebel SB. Can accelerated atrioventricular junctional escape rhythms be explained by delayed after-depolarizations? Am J Cardiol 1980; 45:1272–1284.

201. Young ML, Mehta MB, Martinez RM, Wolff GS, Gelband H. Combined alpha-adrenergic blockade and radiofrequency ablation to treat junctional ectopic tachycardia successfully without atrioventricular block. Am J Cardiol 1993; 71:883–885.

202. Gavrilescu S, Luca C. His bundle rhythms with retrograde conduction to the atria. Br Heart J 1974; 36:468–474.

203. Watanabe Y, Nishimura M, Noda T, Habuchi Y, Tanaka H, Homma N. Atrioventricular junctional tachycardias. In Zipes DP, Jalife J (eds). Cardiac Electrophysiology. From Cell to Bedside. Philadelphia: W B Saunderes, 1990, pp. 564–570.

204. Gallagher JJ, Damato AN, Lau SH. Electrophysiologic studies during accelerated idioventricular rhythms. Circulation 1971; 44:671–677.

205. Wyndham CR, Dhingra RC, Smith T, Best D, Rosen KM. Concealed nonparoxysmal junctional tachycardia. Circulation 1979; 60:707–710.

206. Langendorf R. Concealed A-V conduction: the effect of blocked impulses on the formation and conduction of subsequent impulses. Am Heart J 1948; 35:542–552.

207. Langendorf R, Pick A. Concealed conduction: further evaluation of a fundamental aspect of propagation of the cardiac impulse. Circulation 1956; 13:381–399.

208. Hwang W, Langendorf R. Auriculoventricular nodal escape

in the presence of auricular fibrillation. Circulation 1950; 1:930–935.

209. Narula OS, Narula JT. Junctional pacemakers in man. Response to overdrive suppression with and without parasympathetic blockade. Circulation 1978; 57:880–889.

210. Breslow MJ, Evers AS, Lebowitz P. Successful treatment of accelerated junctional rhythm with propranolol: possible role of sympathetic stimulation in the genesis of this rhythm disturbance. Anesthesiology 1985; 62:180–182.

211. Kingma JH, van Gilst WH, Peels CH, Dambrink JH, Verheugt FW, Wielenga RP. Acute intervention with captopril during thrombolysis in patients with first anterior myocardial infarction: results from the captopril and thrombolysis study (CATS). Eur Heart J 1994; 15:898–907.

212. Santinelli V, Chiariello M, Condorelli M. Nonparoxysmal atrioventricular junctional rhythm. Eur Heart J 1984; 5:304–307.

213. Tenczer J, Littmann L, Rohla M, Fenyvesi T. The effects of overdrive pacing and lidocaine on atrioventricular junctional rhythm in man: the role of abnormal automaticity. Circulation 1985; 72:480–486.

214. Bertolet BD, Belardinelli L, Kerensky R, Hill JA. Adenosine blockade as primary therapy for ischemia-induced accelerated idioventricular rhythm: rationale and potential clinical application. Am Heart J 1994; 128:185–188.

215. Keefe DL, Williams S, Torres V, Flowers D, Somberg JC. Prophylactic tocainide or lidocaine in acute myocardial infarction. Am J Cardiol 1986; 57:527–531.

216. Cooper TB, MacLean WA, Waldo AL. Overdrive pacing for supraventricular tachycardia: a review of theoretical implications and therapeutic techniques. Pacing Clin Electrophysiol 1978; 1:196–221.

217. Pasternak RC, Braunwald E, Sobel BE. Acute myocardial infarction. In Braunwald E (ed). Heart Disease. A Textbook of Cardiovascular Medicine. 4th ed. Philadelphia: WB Saunders, 1992, p. 1245.

218. Myerburg RJ, Kessler KM. Clinical assessment and management of arrhythmias and conduction disturbances. In Hurst JW, (ed). The Heart, Arteries and Veins. 7th ed. New York: McGraw-Hill, 1990, pp. 544–545.

219. Denes P, Gillis AM, Pawitan Y, Kammerling JM, Wilhelmsen L, Salerno DM. Prevalence, characteristics and significance of ventricular premature complexes and ventricular tachycardia detected by 24-hour continuous electrocardiographic recording in the Cardiac Arrhythmia Suppression Trial. Am J Cardiol 1991; 68:887–896.

220. Kastor JA, Goldreyer BN, Moore EN, Spear JF. Re-entry: an important mechanism of cardiac arrhythmias. Cardiovasc Clin 1974; 6:111–135.

Ventricular
Premature Beats[1-12a]

Ventricular premature beats are almost ubiquitous among humans whether or not they have heart disease. Palpitations, the principal symptom ventricular premature beats produce, constitute one of our most familiar complaints. Easily recognized by the observer from the pulse or the electrocardiogram, ventricular beats seldom need treatment.

Ventricular premature beats have not been as much the subject of clinical electrophysiological study as have the tachyarrhythmias with which they are frequently associated. Most of the investigative work in recent decades has dealt with their

- Prevalence in different clinical settings, particularly coronary heart disease.
- Frequency and character on ambulatory and exercise electrocardiograms.
- Response to pharmacological agents.
- Prognostic significance.

DEFINITIONS
Beat, Contraction, Complex, or Depolarization

Clinical electrophysiologists have suggested that we discard the time-honored titles "ventricular premature *beats*" and "ventricular premature *contractions*" and refer to these abnormalities as "ventricular premature *depolarizations*."[13] Depolarization[b] describes an electrophysiologic event, whereas beat[c] and contraction[d] refer to mechanical events, which we do not see on the electrocardiogram. What we do see, it is argued, is an

electrical event, a depolarization, rendered in the form of a QRS complex.[14]

The logic is impeccable, but tradition and convenience dictate otherwise. "Depolarization" has six syllables, three more than "contraction," four more than "complex," and five more than "beat."[e] Furthermore, by using "beat," we acknowledge the clinical correlation between symptoms, physical findings, and electrocardiogram. I choose beat.[15-18f]

Next, which should come first, *ventricular* or *premature*? The beats originate in the ventricles; that is what most distinguishes them from other abnormal early beats. Their ventricular origin gives them particularly dangerous characteristics in certain patients. That they are usually premature seems of less significance; hence, *ventricular premature beats*.

Simple or Complex

Ventricular premature beats may be simple or complex. *Simple* ventricular premature beats occur by themselves, have one form, and are infrequently seen among the sinus beats. Ventricular premature beats are considered *complex*[g] if they occur in the T wave ("vulnerable phase") of the previous beat or when they are

- Repetitive (two or more consecutive ventricular beats).
- Bigeminal.
- Frequent.
- Multiform.

The designation *complex* is frequently assigned when their frequency is equal to or greater than 20 ventricular premature beats per hour,[4] but what constitutes frequent varies widely among reports. In reviewing the

---

[a]This chapter contains material from Chapter 13, "Ventricular Premature Complexes," by J. Thomas Bigger, Jr.[1] in the first edition of this book and from my earlier review of the subject.[2]

[b]A depolarization refers to only part of the event.[22] The more accurate electrophysiological term would be "premature depolarization-repolarization," a mouthful, to say the least.[18]

[c]From the Anglo-Saxon word *beaten*, meaning "to strike, throb, or pulsate." "What is better than a four-letter Anglo-Saxon word when it comes to punchy purity" (Henry J. L. Marriott, 1987).[18]

[d]From the Latin meaning "drawn together."

[e]"Short words are best and the old words when short are best of all" (Winston S. Churchill).[22]

[f]As do others.[15-18]

[g]Another reason to call them beats; *complex* ventricular premature *complexes* confuses further.

work in this field, one should bear in mind that what is frequent to one investigator is infrequent to another, and vice versa.[19]

Ectopy, Irritability, Extrasystole

The words "ectopy"[16, 20h] and "irritability"[21i] are occasionally applied to ventricular premature beats, as in "ventricular ectopic activity," or "ventricular irritability."[22] "Extrasystole" is less often used today, although electrocardiographers employed it frequently for premature beats in the past.[6, 18, 23–25j]

PREVALENCE

Premature beats, and ventricular premature beats in particular, are the most common arrhythmias in humans.[26–32k]

AGE AND GENDER

As Sir Thomas Lewis wrote:[33–36l]

> Premature beats have been recorded at all ages from a few weeks to old age. During the first decade they are rare. The incidence is actually heaviest between 50 and 70 years ... it becomes evident that they are essentially connected with advancing years.

The increasing rate of ventricular premature beats—simple, frequent, and complex—as people age[33] applies in the presence[37–51] or absence[44, 45, 52–62] of

heart disease. Men have more ventricular premature beats than women[63] at each decade of life.[56]

CLINICAL SETTINGS

People Without Apparent Heart Disease[m]

Fetuses, infants, and children. Fetuses, infants, and children without structural heart disease have had ventricular premature beats, as follows:[64–71]

- Twelve (0.35%) of 3,383 apparently healthy newborn infants from the Weymouth and Dorcester Maternity Hospital in England.[72]
- None of 134 full-term infants in their first 10 days of life.[73]
- Six (6%) of 100 healthy preterm or low birthweight infants.[74]
- Thirty-seven (8.2%) of 452 fetuses with ventricular or junctional beat.[69]
- Twenty-nine percent of 231 boys aged 10 to 16 years.[75, 76]

Adults. Few ventricular premature beats occur each day in healthy adults[55, 60, 62, 77–81] or in children.[82n] However, the arrhythmia persists in a majority of patients whose ventricular premature beats are recorded on two or more occasions, and some eventually show evidence of heart disease.[83]

With the use of extended electrocardiographic monitoring, ventricular premature beats appeared in the following fraction of several groups of healthy people:[37, 38, 52, 84–90o]

- Fifty-five (6.1%) of 904 subjects of different ages.[60–62, 77, 78, 91–93]
- None of 65 healthy adults during 2½ hours of automobile driving.[94]
- Eighty-six percent of 267 men and women, each of whom was at least 60 years of age.[34, 95–97]
- Seventy-six percent of healthy 85-year-old subjects.[98]
- Twenty percent of 101 healthy elderly subjects who had at least 10 ventricular premature beats per hour, both at the beginning and at the end of 5 years of study.[99]
- Frequent or complex ventricular premature beats in 35% of men older than 80 years without a history of myocardial infarction or angina in Malmo, Sweden.[100]

When the number of premature beats in subjects without heart disease rises to more than 100 per day, the prevalence of complex ventricular premature beats

---

[h]From the Greek *ek*, meaning "out of" and *topos* meaning "place," considered by David Spodick (1980) to be "An unfortunate neologism ... coined in ... the United States of America."[16, 20]

[i]An "Old chestnut ... analogous to an image of the short-tempered person who may be considered by his companions to be irritable" (David Spodick, 1984).[21]

[j]*Extra* from the Latin for "outside" + *systole* from the Greek for "contraction." The word still has its admirers.[23] However, writes Henry J. L. Marriott (1988), "Extrasystole is a Latin-Greek hybrid that means a systole arising outside ... the normal sinus pacemaker, and by usage has come to mean the sort of premature ectopic beat that is accurately coupled to and depends for its existence on the preceding beat."[25] The use of *extra* to mean "additional" beats is not what electrocardiographers in past decades meant when they used the word.[23]

[k]Except for sinus arrhythmia, bradycardia, and tachycardia, which are, in most cases, physiological events. Ventricular premature beats were the most frequently observed arrhythmia in the electrocardiograms of 50,000 consecutive patients seen at a busy Chicago teaching hospital.[28]

"The premature beat is almost universal. ... It is without doubt the commonest of all cardiac abnormalities; in fact, it is so frequent among otherwise normal individuals that it hardly deserves the name of abnormality" (Paul Dudley White, 1951).[27] "One of us (P.D.W.) has had premature beats, ventricular in nature as a rule, occurring ... perhaps every few days for at least 50 years."[31]

"A premature systole occurs in almost everyone at sometime or other" (Louis Katz and Alfred Pick, 1956).[29]

"Premature beats form the commonest of the cardiac arrhythmias and ventricular premature beats occur much more commonly than those arising in the atrioventricular node or elsewhere in the atria" (Charles K. Friedberg, 1966).[30]

[l]In a book published in 1949, 4 years after his death, Lewis, the leading cardiac physiologist of his time, defined many arrhythmias in humans for the first time. He died from his third myocardial infarction on March 17, 1945 at the age of 63.[36]

[m]"Extrasystoles in themselves are not signs of any specific injury to the heart, nor should a prognosis of any gravity be based on their appearance alone" (Sir James MacKenzie, 1913).[506]

"On the whole it is wise to assume that ectopic beats are innocent, and to judge organic disease on other grounds" (Paul Wood).[32]

[n]Greater than 10 per hour is distinctly unusual.

[o]The older literature described the frequency of ventricular premature beats[38] in healthy young people[37, 52, 84, 85, 88] and in elderly patients[86, 87, 89] from the standard electrocardiogram, which provided only a brief and inadequate period of observation.[90]

also increases.[101p] However, complex ventricular premature beats occur infrequently in most people without heart disease.[80, 102q] Multiform beats occur in 13%,[60–62, 77, 78, 81, 92, 93, 103r] couplets in 4%,[60–62, 78, 81, 103s] and bigeminy in 2%.[60, 62, 92t] In older people without obvious heart disease, the number of multiform beats rises to 25%[34, 95–97, 104] and couplets to 8%.[34, 95–97]

A few persons with frequent or complex beats appear otherwise healthy.[83, 105u] Well-trained athletes[106] have a similar number of ventricular premature beats, as do persons of approximately the same age who are in normal physical condition.[107–112v] One must keep in mind, however, that some healthy-appearing persons with simple and complex ventricular premature beats may have occult coronary or other forms of heart disease.[45, 58, 83, 113, 114] Gender does not affect the appearance of ventricular premature beats in people without heart disease.[60]

Coronary Heart Disease

Coronary heart disease is a factor during and after myocardial infarction.[66, 115–117]

Myocardial infarction. Ventricular premature beats[118, 119] develop in probably all,[120–148] and complex beats in most, patients during acute myocardial infarction[144] (Table 11.1). More and more complex ventricular premature beats occur in those patients who are older,[49] have more obstructed coronary arteries,[149] or have sustained more myocardial ischemia and damage as shown by

- A history of previous myocardial infarction or congestive heart failure.[49]
- Greater release of myocardial enzymes.[150–152]
- Greater ST segment elevation[153] or depression[154] in the electrocardiogram.
- A lower ejection fraction.[148, 149, 154, 155]

Reports differ on whether more ventricular premature beats[156–158] develop from transmural or from non-transmural (non–Q-wave) myocardial infarctions. More simple and complex ventricular premature beats appear after ischemic myocardium is successfully reperfused by thrombolysis than when thrombolysis is not administered or is unsuccessful.[152, 159–163] The incidence and severity of ventricular premature beats rise with higher polymorphic leukocyte activity.[164]

Ventricular beats occur in greatest frequency and complexity early in the course of myocardial in-

Table 11.1	DETECTION OF VENTRICULAR BEATS BY A COMPUTER AND BY CONVENTIONAL MONITORING IN 31 PATIENTS WITH MYOCARDIAL INFARCTION[a]	
Arrhythmia	Automated Detection (%)	Conventional Monitoring (%)
All beats	100	64.5
All complex beats	93.5	16.1
Multifocal	87.1	6.5
Consecutive	77.4	13
Bigeminy	25.8	9.7
R-on-T	13	3.2

[a]The observed incidence is significantly lower when the beats are counted by visual observation of monitors, manual review of electrocardiographic tapes, or Holter monitoring[120–132, 134, 135, 137–143, 145–148] than by a computer. Before monitoring was developed in the 1960s, most patients with myocardial infarction were thought not to have ventricular premature beats.[118, 119] (From Romhilt DW, Bloomfield SS, Chou T-C, Fowler NO. Unreliability of conventional electrocardiographic monitoring for arrhythmia detection in coronary care units. J Am Coll Cardiol 1973; 31:457–461. Reprinted with permission from the American College of Cardiology.)[144]

farction,[165, 166] particularly during the first hour,[140] decrease as the hours pass,[167] and continue to appear while patients recover from myocardial infarction both in the hospital and after they go home.[42, 57, 166, 168–198w] The incidence of these beats also increases after thrombolytic reperfusion of occluded coronary arteries.[199]

After myocardial infarction. About 36% of patients recovering from acute myocardial infarction have less than one ventricular premature beat per hour.[148] Twenty percent have frequent (>20 beats/hour)[148x] or repetitive beats[200] during convalescence.[y] The frequency of ventricular premature beats rises in those with a history of previous myocardial infarction,[42, 201] congestive heart failure,[201] and older age,[42, 201] but not because of the presence of ventricular beats[168, 173, 200, 201] during the acute process.

Greater ST segment depression[154] and decreased ejection fraction[154] predict the development of ventricular premature beats in patients after thrombolysis. However, thrombolysis itself does not increase,[154, 155,]

---

[p]One worker suggests that 200 ventricular premature beats per 24 hours should be considered the "normal" range in healthy subjects 40 to 79 years of age [author's quotation marks].[80]

[q]Although in one study, 33% of 73 patients found not to have heart disease by cardiac catheterization had complex beats on 24-hour recordings.[46]

[r]In 814 patients from nine series.[60–62, 77, 78, 81, 92, 93, 103]

[s]In 948 patients from six series.[60–62, 78, 81, 103]

[t]In 531 patients from three series.[60, 62, 92]

[u]More than three ventricular premature beats per minute.

[v]However, in one study 40 athletes had a greater, but not significantly greater (70% versus 55%), prevalence of ventricular ectopy than 40 healthy sedentary subjects.[111]

---

[w]In 725 patients who had sustained myocardial infarctions between 6 days and 2 years previously and had asymptomatic, untreated, ventricular premature beats:

- 16.2% had less than 10 beats per hour.
- 40.7% had 10 to 50 per hour.
- 15.8% had 50 to 100 per hour.
- 27.3% had greater than 100 per hour.

From the Cardiac Arrhythmia Suppression Trial (CAST), which included a minimum of 18 hours of analyzable data from ambulatory electrocardiography.[198]

[x]According to *Gruppo Italiano per lo Studio della Sopravvivenza nell'Infarto Miocardico* (GISSI-2 study) of 12,381 patients.[148]

[y]An earlier (1979) study suggested that 81% of patients had frequent, multiform, or repetitive ventricular premature beats.[183] The authors conclude that this surprisingly high incidence may have been due to the recordings' having been taken after discharge rather than when the patients were still in the hospital. Furthermore, no patients in this study were taking antiarrhythmic or beta-adrenergic–blocking drugs, and the investigators used a two-channel recording technique that they suggest may have increased the diagnosis of complex beats.[183]

[202, 203] and may decrease,[204] the incidence of ventricular premature beats recorded later during recovery from myocardial infarction, both before discharge from the hospital and subsequently.

While recovering from myocardial infarction, patients with complex ventricular premature beats are three times more likely than those without the beats to demonstrate this finding on subsequent recordings.[190] When ventricular premature beats occur at a rate of greater than 20 per hour, patients often have complex beats in the same recording and in records made 5 months later.[177] The incidence of serious ventricular arrhythmias is low in children who survive myocardial infarction, which is most often due to anomalous origin of the left coronary artery from the pulmonary artery.[205]

Chronic coronary heart disease. Patients with chronic coronary disease[40, 94, 206–208] have more premature beats than patients without heart disease.[208, 209]

Angina. Patients with angina, whether or not they have had myocardial infarctions, have more ventricular premature beats,[39, 210, 211] including complex beats,[210, 211] than patients without heart disease. Ventricular premature beats can develop in patients with silent ischemia,[212, 213] but the arrhythmia occurs more frequently during symptomatic than during asymptomatic ischemia.[213] According to one study,[214] the number of ventricular premature beats does not significantly increase during ST segment depressions recorded on Holter monitoring. Compared with patients having angina without arrhythmias, those with ventricular premature beats have more anginal episodes per day and greater and more prolonged ST segment depressions.[215]

Patients have more ventricular premature beats during angina

• When ventricular function is decreased.[211, 216, 217]
• If they have relatively frequent (>14/hour) beats at rest.[218, 219z]
• If the ST segments in the anterior electrocardiographic leads are transiently elevated.[220]

Prinzmetal's angina. Both simple and complex premature beats develop frequently during episodes of coronary vasospasm producing variant angina.[210, 221–239] Ventricular ectopy occurs

• In about 10% to 20% of episodes of variant angina[238] and more often during painful than asymptomatic episodes.[237]
• Less often when the daily frequency of ischemic episodes is high.[237]
• More often during the occlusive than the reperfusion phase.[235]

Patients with variant angina who develop ventricular ectopy during ergonovine-induced episodes are more likely to have such arrhythmias during spontaneous attacks.[240] The arrhythmias produced by ergonovine testing are more often caused by ischemia than by reperfusion.[240]

A history of myocardial infarction. Patients with prior myocardial infarctions have ventricular ectopic activity of a more advanced grade than those with angina alone.[241] They also have more ventricular premature beats

• Than if they have not had infarctions.[44, 49, 98, 242]
• If they have congestive heart failure.[49]
• If they take diuretics, regardless of indication.[242]

Resuscitation from cardiac arrest. Many patients who have been resuscitated from out-of-hospital ventricular fibrillation frequently have ventricular premature beats,[243] and those with complex beats are more likely to have a history of remote myocardial infarction or congestive heart failure than those without such beats.[192]

Risk factors. Men with risk factors for coronary heart disease such as hypertension, hyperlipidemia, diabetes, or at least 20 years of cigarette smoking have more multiform ventricular premature beats than patients without such factors.[208]

Valvular Heart Disease

Mitral valve prolapse. Although patients with mitral valve prolapse often have ventricular premature beats[244–248]—56% having at least one ventricular premature beat in 24 hours[91, 249–254aa]—they have no more simple or complex ventricular ectopy as a group than patients without heart disease.[253–257bb] In a series of 26 children with prolapse, 12 (46%) had ventricular premature beats; bigeminy was present in four, and the beats were multifocal in four.[258]

Aortic valve disease. Simple and complex ventricular premature beats that develop in patients with aortic valve disease[259–261cc] occur more often when the left ventricular ejection fraction is lower[259] or the peak systolic wall stress greater.[259] However, their occurrence is *not* related to

• The degree of regurgitation in patients with aortic insufficiency.[259, 260, 262]
• The presence of concomitant coronary heart disease.[260]

---

*aa*From 299 patients in six series.[91, 249–251, 253, 254] The presence of ventricular premature beats has been documented in other series of patients with prolapse.[252]

*bb*However, *some* patients with prolapse, including those who are older,[256, 257] have more mitral regurgitation,[256] or worse ventricular function, may have more simple and complex ventricular premature beats than healthy persons or patients with small amounts of prolapse.[253, 257] The presence of ventricular premature beats has also been noted in the older literature in patients with mitral regurgitation or incompetence.[255]

*cc*Ventricular premature beats appeared in 38 of 397 patients with aortic stenosis.[261]

---

*z*Although another investigator disagrees.[218]

- The transvalvular gradient in patients with aortic stenosis.[259, 260, 262]
- The type of valve lesion.[259, 262]

Cardiomyopathy and Myocarditis

Cardiomyopathy produces both simple and complex ventricular premature beats, particularly in ventricles with severely impaired function[46, 263–291] (Table 11.2). Simple and complex ventricular premature beats also develop in patients with myocardial inflammation.[292] The arrhythmia may persist after resolution of the acute illness.[292] Some children with ventricular beats, which are unusual in those with normal hearts, may have subclinical cardiomyopathy or myocarditis.[293]

Hypertension and Left Ventricular Hypertrophy

Patients with hypertension,[48, 50, 294–297] including those with isolated systolic hypertension,[45, 298] have more ventricular premature beats than normotensive persons. The relative risk for the occurrence of ventricular premature beats increases linearly with higher levels of diastolic blood pressure.[48]

Patients with left ventricular hypertrophy, whether produced by hypertension[51, 297, 299–303] or other causes,[304] have more simple and complex ventricular premature beats than hypertensive patients without hypertrophy[301, 302] or normotensive subjects.[298, 299, 301, 305dd] The number and complexity of ventricular premature beats are greater in obese than in lean patients with eccentric left ventricular hypertrophy.[306]

Age, the amount of left ventricular hypertrophy, and the volume and function of the left ventricle determine the frequency and severity of ventricular beats in patients with hypertension.[51] The prevalence of ventricular premature beats in patients with left ventricular hypertrophy from hypertension increases further when the left ventricle dilates.[307]

When left ventricular mass regresses in patients with mild to moderate hypertension and left ventricular hypertrophy, the incidence of ventricular premature beats decreases.[308] Treating hypertension with the diuretic chlorthalidone in doses adequate to decrease stroke and cardiovascular events and with potassium as

---

[dd]Although one report suggests that patients with electrocardiographic evidence of left ventricular hypertrophy have *fewer* ventricular premature beats than these without this finding.[298]

Table **11.2.** **CARDIOMYOPATHIES THAT PRODUCE VENTRICULAR PREMATURE BEATS**
Alcoholic cardiomyopathy[266]
Chagas cardiomyopathy[264, 291]
Dilated cardiomyopathy[280, 282, 284, 286, 289, 290a]
Familial amyloidosis[277]
Hypertrophic cardiomyopathy[267, 270–273, 279, 285, 287, 288]
Right ventricular dysplasia[274]
Sarcoid cardiomyopathy[268, 269, 276]

[a]Patients with dilated cardiomyopathy have, in general, more ventricular beats than those with coronary or valvular disease.[46]

needed does not increase the presence of ventricular premature beats.[309]

Pulmonary Disease

Patients with severe pulmonary disease develop ventricular premature beats,[310–322] particularly if left ventricular function is reduced.[322]

Congenital Heart Disease

Few patients with congenital heart disease have more ventricular premature beats than would be expected in healthy persons of similar age. The frequency of these beats grows, as in all people, with increasing age.[323ee] Ventricular premature beats may develop in both symptomatic and asymptomatic patients with congenital complete heart block.[304, 324]

Cardiac Surgery

Ventricular premature beats are among the most common arrhythmias that develop after coronary artery bypass surgery.[325] Some patients have more ventricular beats after than before such procedures, even in the absence of intraoperative myocardial infarction.[326]

Repetitive ventricular premature beats occur infrequently in patients with normal left ventricular ejection fractions after aortic valve replacement.[327] Those patients who develop both simple and complex ventricular beats after aortic valve replacement often have reduced left ventricular function.[328] However, the number and complexity of ventricular premature beats may decrease if the surgical procedure improves left ventricular function.[327] Ventricular premature beats have been reported to occur after operations to repair single ventricles (Fontan procedure), ventricular septal defect, Ebstein's anomaly of the tricuspid valve, and particularly tetralogy of Fallot.[329]

Tetralogy of Fallot. Simple or complex ventricular premature beats, which occur infrequently after uncomplicated surgical repair of tetralogy of Fallot,[330, 331] may develop in patients[332] who

- Are older when surgical repair is performed[323, 333–337] or have been followed longer.[334, 336–338ff]
- Have low left ventricular ejection fraction[339, 340] or cardiac index.[339]
- Have residual left-to-right shunts.[339, 341]
- Have syncope or presyncope.[337]
- Have the following right ventricular abnormalities: systolic hypertension,[334, 337, 339, 341–343ff] increased diastolic pressure,[341, 342] decreased ejection fraction,[334] or enlargement.[333, 342]

[ee]For example, only three of 35 young children, aged 1.2 to 7.7 (median, 4.3) years with uncorrected tetralogy of Fallot had ventricular premature beats; all beats were simple and occurred at a frequency of less than 10 during 24 hours of monitoring. Eight of 18 older patients, aged 13 to 43 (median, 28) years, had uniform ventricular premature beats, and five had frequent complex beats.[323]

[ff]One study did not find this variable to be important.[335]

- Were on cardiopulmonary bypass longer during the operation.[338]

However, the *grade* of ventricular arrhythmias does *not* correlate with

- Right ventricular pressure or ejection fraction.[332]
- The presence of complex beats before the operation.[323, 344–346]
- Development of conduction defects.[347]

Cardiac transplantation. Simple and complex ventricular premature beats develop in most patients[348–350] soon after cardiac transplantation and then decrease as time passes.[349] Long-term survivors have no more ventricular beats than do healthy individuals.[351]

Ventricular beats in transplant recipients do not necessarily indicate organ rejection,[349, 352] nor need their presence reflect advanced age of the donor[349] or the amount of time the transplanted heart was ischemic.[349, 352] Complex beats found in patients more than 70 days after cardiac transplantation may predict accelerated coronary atherosclerosis in the donor heart.[348]

Drugs

Many drugs and, in particular, antiarrhythmic drugs exert a "pro-arrhythmic effect," a drug's promotion of additional ventricular premature beats or more dangerous ventricular tachyarrhythmias.[gg] Fortunately, the incidence of pro-arrhythmia in patients with ventricular premature beats alone is low, 4% with flecainide,[353] for example.

Digitalis. Digitalis is infamous for causing ventricular premature beats and more advanced forms of ventricular ectopy when the drug is given in amounts that are toxic to patients with heart disease.[3, 354–360hh] Ventricular bigeminy and multiform and bidirectional beats are said to be characteristic.[357] Digitalis, however, does not appear to produce ventricular parasystole.[361] In subjects with normal hearts, atrioventricular conduction disturbances rather than ectopic beats are more likely to develop from digitalis intoxication.[358, 362ii]

Other drugs. Drugs, other than antiarrhythmic drugs and digitalis, incriminated in producing ventricular premature beats include

- Anthracyclines in cancer chemotherapy.[363]
- Aminophylline.[319, 364, 365]

- Atropine.[366]
- Azathioprine.[367]
- Catecholamines.[319, 368]
- Cocaine.[369–372]

Metabolic and Endocrine Disturbances

Hypokalemia. Hypokalemia,[373–380] usually produced by diuretic therapy, evokes ventricular premature beats in many patients with ischemic heart disease[381] and during myocardial infarction,[381, 382] and particularly in those with heart disease who are receiving digitalis,[383] even when digoxin levels are therapeutic.[384] However, hypokalemia does not appear to produce ventricular premature beats in patients with normal hearts or in those affected by mild or moderate hypertension,[385] so long as the potassium is not less than 3 mEq/L.[48, 309, 386–392jj] More ventricular premature beats appear when the potassium level is lower[302] and when patients have been taking diuretics for at least 2 years.[393kk] The severe hypokalemia that can develop in patients withdrawing from alcoholic intoxication probably helps to cause their ventricular beats.[394]

Hypomagnesemia. Hypomagnesemia,[374, 376, 379, 395] like hypokalemia often produced by diuretic therapy, may,[380, 396–400] or may not,[392] be associated with ventricular premature beats. Indeed, whether hypomagnesemia alone causes ventricular premature beats is uncertain because many patients with this disturbance also have hypokalemia[400] and, in some cases, digitalis intoxication.[399]

Chronic renal disease and hemodialysis. Simple and complex ventricular premature beats appear in patients with chronic renal disease soon after the beginning of and as many as 6 hours after hemodialysis.[401] Changes in serum potassium during dialysis seem greater in those patients with arrhythmias.[401]

Acromegaly. This disorder increases the presence of complex ventricular premature beats.[402]

Relation to Underlying Rate and Rhythm

In healthy subjects, the waking heart rate of the basic rhythm does not determine the frequency of ventricular ectopic beats,[37, 403–405] and the average heart rate of healthy people with numerous premature beats is the same as in those with infrequent beats.[37] Faster heart rates induced by exercise may increase[56ll] or decrease[105] the frequency of ventricular premature beats in healthy persons.

[gg]See Chapter 13, for a discussion and references on proarrhythmia.

[hh]Two contrasting opinions on this subject appeared several decades ago. David Scherf wrote in 1959: "The various digitalis glycosides abolish most atrial and ventricular extrasystoles provided they are not caused by digitalis."[3] The Boston physician and one of the founders of American cardiology, Paul Dudley White, who should know because he had premature beats "accentuated at the time of digitalis intoxication carried out experimentally in 1916,"[31] wrote in the fourth edition (1951) of his cardiology text: "Digitalis . . . much more often causes than dispels premature beats."[355] White's analysis more accurately reflects contemporary thinking about the subject.

[ii]Ventricular premature beats occurred in none of 48 children with accidental ingestion of digitalis; all but two had normal hearts.[362]

[jj]Although some workers disagree.[48, 380, 386, 387, 391] The importance of hypokalemia by itself in producing ventricular premature beats in a variety of clinical settings remains controversial.[375]

[kk]However, 20 patients with Barter syndrome (renal potassium wasting, hypokalemic alkalosis, hyperreninemia, and normal blood pressure) and presumably normal hearts whose mean serum potassium was 2.7 mmol/L (range, 2.3–3.3) did not develop more ventricular premature beats.

[ll]Despite a commonly held belief to the contrary.

Although heart rate does not affect the appearance of ventricular beats in most people with ventricular premature beats, tachycardia or bradycardia can enhance their development in some.[406, 407mm] Many, but not all, patients with heart disease and frequent chronic ventricular ectopy have more beats at faster heart rates.[366, 408, 409] Some have fewer or the same number of premature beats at faster rates.[408]

Circadian Effects

Simple and complex ventricular premature beats appear more frequently during the waking hours than during sleep[410–412] in most healthy persons[78, 93, 411, 413, 414] and in many,[411, 415–421] although not all,[422] patients with such heart diseases as stable coronary disease,[414] mitral valve prolapse,[249, 414] and hypertrophic cardiomyopathy.[418] The prevalence of ventricular premature beats is greatest during the early morning in patients with angina at rest.[423]

Although some investigators found that the rapid eye movement phase of sleep prompted the highest incidence of ventricular premature beats,[424] others suggested that the frequency of ectopic beats during sleep seems to relate more to the heart rate than to the level of arousal[418] or stage of sleep.[425] Some patients with chronic obstructive pulmonary disease have more ventricular premature beats, which can be diminished with oxygen, during sleep than when awake.[317] Ventricular premature beats also increase in sleeping patients whose left ventricular function is decreased and who have nocturnal hypoxia.[426]

Other patients with more premature beats during sleep may have a neurological disorder, such as cerebrovascular disease[427] or acute myocardial ischemia.[422] Usually, however, there are no significant differences in the presence or type of organic heart disease, hypertension, medicines, or electrocardiographic abnormalities in patients with increased ectopy during sleep.[427nn]

Stress and Autonomic Nervous System

Ventricular premature beats appear in some people during stress.[428–430oo] However, ventricular beats are not produced or increased during such experimental perturbation of the autonomic nervous system as head-up tilt to 70 degrees,[431pp] breath-holding, hyperventilation, carotid sinus massage, or the Valsalva maneuver, even

in patients with advanced grades of ventricular arrhythmias at rest.[430] Moreover, the autonomic nervous system is not required for the production of ventricular premature beats; the arrhythmia can develop in the denervated transplanted human heart.[432, 433] Vagal output, increased by a reflex reaction to the administration of phenylephrine, decreases the frequency of ventricular premature beats in some patients.[434, 435]

Caffeine and Alcohol

Although standard texts[15, 32, 436–438] state that caffeine—coffee is the usual culprit—produces ventricular premature beats, few experimental studies support this commonly held belief,[59qq] and many reports refute its significance,[56, 439–445rr] even in patients with recent myocardial infarctions[444] and in those at high risk of dangerous ventricular arrhythmias.[446]

Although ventricular premature beats are not the most frequent arrhythmia produced by ingestion of alcohol ("holiday heart syndrome"), they have been associated with the use of alcohol even in the absence of apparent cardiomyopathy.[447–449] Withdrawal from alcohol with the hypokalemia often associated with this condition produces ventricular beats in some patients.[394]

Procedures

Ventricular premature beats frequently develop during occlusion of coronary arteries[450] supplying ischemic regions during angioplasty.[451] The frequency of the beats is greater if the coronary occlusion being treated is mild rather than severe.[451] Gastroscopy can produce ventricular premature beats that disappear after the procedure is completed.[452–456]

Miscellaneous Factors

The following appear *not* to be associated with ventricular premature beats unless the heart is affected by some other abnormality[44, 363, 365, 453–468] (Table 11.3):

- Acute pericarditis.[469, 470]
- Cholesterol level.[44]
- Cigarette smoking.[56]

---

mmIn 201 patients with ventricular premature beats, tachycardia influenced their frequency in 28% and bradycardia in 24%; heart rate seemed to have no effect in 48%.[407]

nnAccording to a study in which 50 patients with more ventricular ectopy during sleep were compared with 50 subjects with more beats while awake. The members of each group were matched for age, sex, and 24-hour ventricular ectopic frequency.[427]

ooAlthough their appearance may be often related more to intrinsic heart disease than to the stress itself. In a series of 30 football and basketball coaches, only one coach with known coronary disease developed multifocal ventricular premature beats while being monitored during games in which their teams competed.[429]

ppAlthough according to G. Bourne, writing in 1927: "Posture has a definite effect. Standing causes an increase in the number of premature beats."[431]

qqHere is one. Of 7,311 middle-aged men with no history of heart disease or electrocardiographic abnormalities other than ventricular premature beats, those who drank at least nine cups of coffee per day were more than twice as likely to have ventricular premature beats as those who drank two cups or less per day, as detected on 2-minute electrocardiographic recordings.[59]

rrIn one study, total abstinence from coffee and smoking with reduction in alcohol intake and a physical conditioning program caused no significant change in the incidence of ventricular premature beats in 81 healthy men,[439] the writer (M.G. Myers, 1991) of a comprehensive review on the subject concludes: "Moderate ingestion of caffeine does not increase the frequency or severity of cardiac arrhythmias in normal persons, patients with ischemic heart disease, or those with pre-existing serious ventricular ectopy,"[444] and an editorialist (Thomas B. Graboys, 1983) suggests: "The physician should take care not to diminish life's pleasures when there is not sound basis to do so, lest he or she be deemed a modern-day Savonarola."[440]

Table 11.3	MISCELLANEOUS CAUSES OF VENTRICULAR PREMATURE BEATS

Cardiac tumors[458]
Cardiac irradiation[363]
Carbon monoxide[466, 468]
Diabetes mellitus[44]
Duchenne's muscular dystrophy[463, 467a]
Electrical injury[464]
Hyperventilation[457]
Sleep apnea[461, 462]
Smoking[44]
Systemic sclerosis (scleroderma)[453–456, 465]
Tuberous sclerosis[459]
Ventricular aneurysms[460]

[a]Particularly as the muscle disease progresses.

- Thyrotoxicosis, before, during, and after its treatment.[471–473]

SYMPTOMS

Palpitations[474–476ss] are the principal symptom produced by premature beats, and ventricular premature beats are the most common arrhythmia causing palpitations.[477] Contrary to most teaching,[15, 478] it is the premature beat itself, rather than the pause that follows or the sinus beat that terminates the pause, that most patients first notice.[436, 479tt]

Patients may observe ventricular premature beats more readily when resting or going to sleep. The absence of other distractions probably accounts for the increased awareness at this time.[480] Psychiatric and not cardiac abnormalities account for palpitations in many patients.[481–484] Premature beats can produce dizziness[485] and pain,[15] which may or may not be due to organic heart disease,[15] or no symptoms at all.[486, 487uu]

[ss]James Mackenzie wrote in 1908: "The most serious thing about these cases is that the consciousness of having an irregularity sometimes makes the patient introspective and depressed. He keeps feeling his pulse and communicates his doleful tale whenever he finds a sympathetic ear,"[474] and Paul Wood observed (1968): "The sensation seems to be caused by a radical change in the natural stroke action of the heart; it is the unusual movement of the heart within the thorax that is felt, not an increased force of cardiac contraction, nor more forcible valve closure."[475]

[tt]In the only objective study of this subject which I could find, the investigators synchronized the perceived sensation with the electrocardiogram. They concluded, "Without exception, it was found that the premature beat produced the subjective sensation" (E.M. Klein and T.G. Bidder 1946).[479] As usual, Paul Wood (1968) got it right: "It is usually said that it is not the ectopic beat which is felt but the strong beat following the compensatory pause. Anyone who has himself experienced ectopic palpitations is invited to question this. He may well beg to disagree: the quick beat, out-of-time, with the heart improperly filled, gives rise to the first sensation, and this alone may be felt; or it may be followed by a second sensation due to the beat of the overfilled heart after the pause. A run of ectopics makes it all too obvious that the quick beat is felt."[475]

Charles K. Friedberg's (1966) description is also quite apt: "The entire sequence of extrasystole, long pause, and strong beat produces an irregularity which evokes a distressing heart consciousness or palpitation which may be described as an oppression, fluttering, thumping, skipped beats, or a sinking feeling."[480]

[uu]Mackenzie observed: "Most patients are unconscious of the irregularity due to the extra-systole until their attention is called to it by the medical attendant."[474]

PHYSICAL EXAMINATION

Arterial and Venous Pulses

An irregularity in the pulse usually first alerts the examining physician to the presence of premature beats.[488–490] The pulse from the premature beat itself, however, may not be felt when the ectopic beat is very early, ventricular function is poor, or valvular obstruction is great. Palpating the pulse in a vessel closer to the heart, such as the carotid rather than the radial artery, is more likely to reveal a weak premature beat.[15]

A pulse stronger than that produced by the other sinus beats terminates the pause. This beat, which follows the compensatory pause, may be less full than the other sinus beats, however, in patients with hypertrophic cardiomyopathy.[491–494]

Single ventricular premature beats do not usually disrupt the basic rhythm of the heart, and the sinus beat that terminates the pause usually occurs when expected if the patient is in sinus rhythm.[vv] Pulsus alternans, a useful sign of poor ventricular function, can be produced by ventricular premature beats.[495, 496] In the jugular venous pulse, ventricular beats that are slightly premature produce large cannon A waves when right atrial contraction coincides with closure of the tricuspid valve.[497]

Heart Sounds

On auscultation, the examiner can usually hear the heart sounds of a premature beat, and its first sound is often louder than the first sound of the sinus beats.[498] Occasionally, only the first sound is heard.[15, 436ww]

A premature beat with the electrocardiographic form of right bundle branch block can produce wide splitting of the first and second heart sounds from delayed closure of the tricuspid and pulmonary valves.[499] Conversely, a premature beat with the appearance of left bundle branch block may produce reversed splitting of the first and second sounds from late closure of the mitral and aortic valves.[499] A ventricular premature beat can help one to differentiate between third and fourth heart sounds.[490]

Murmurs

By disrupting the regular rhythm, ventricular premature beats can assist one in differentiating between the systolic murmur of mitral regurgitation and aortic stenosis. Murmurs that originate from the left ventricular outflow tract, as in aortic stenosis, are softer after short intervals and louder after long periods[500] because their intensity depends in part on the volume of blood

---

[vv]This feature can be established by beating one's foot in time with the sinus rhythm. A premature beat occurs earlier than the tapping foot, but the next sinus beat coincides with the following foot tap.

[ww]"Infrequently, the premature beat occurs so early that there is not enough intraventricular pressure to raise the semi-lunar cusps and only a first heart sound is heard, sometimes very faintly, coming like a third heart sound or a reduplicated second sound of the preceding normal beat (frustrane contraction)" (Paul Dudley White, 1951).[15]

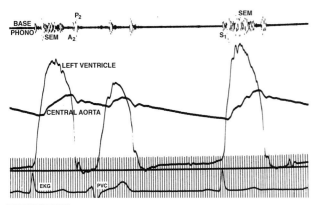

FIGURE 11.1 Effect of a ventricular premature beat on the intensity of a systolic murmur in a patient with aortic vascular stenosis. The murmur (SEM) is louder (**top**) during the beat that follows the pause after the premature beat (PVC in electrocardiogram (EKG) at **bottom**) than during the first sinus beat. The hemodynamic gradient across the obstruction is also greater in beat 3 than in beat 1 (**middle**). (Courtesy of James A. Shaver, M.D.)

flowing past the lesion (Fig. 11.1). The intensity of the murmur of mitral regurgitation, however, does not vary much with different beat-to-beat intervals.[500, 501] Consequently, in valvular, fixed subvalvular, and supravalvular aortic stenosis, the ventricular contraction after the compensatory pause produces a louder systolic murmur than does the premature beat or the sinus beats in the same patient.[493, 502] However, the intensity of the murmur may not increase after the compensatory pause in patients with hypertrophic cardiomyopathy.[502]

ELECTROCARDIOGRAPHY

In the electrocardiogram, the QRS complex of most ventricular premature beats[503–506]

- Is abnormally formed.
- Has a duration longer than that of the sinus beat.
- Is not preceded by a P wave.
- Appears earlier than the next beat conducted from the atria would have been expected to appear.
- Is usually followed by a compensatory pause.

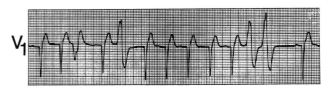

FIGURE 11.3 Repetitive and multiform ventricular premature beats. Just before the last sinus beat, we see two "back-to-back" ventricular premature beats. Beats 3 and 5 are also ventricular and have different forms.

Ventricular premature beats are more likely to occur in men with abnormal electrocardiograms than in those with tracings that are otherwise normal.[507]

Rate

Ventricular premature beats do not establish a rate by themselves because by definition they occur only alone or in couplets.

Rhythm

Ventricular premature beats momentarily interrupt the rhythm of the heart, but they do not usually change the fundamental rhythm. When the heart's rhythm is irregular, as during atrial fibrillation, ventricular premature beats are more likely to appear after longer intervals between the conducted beats, a phenomenon known as the "rule of bigeminy"[508] (Fig. 11.2).

Ventricular premature beats often occur in repetitive patterns as follows:

- Couplets: Two ventricular beats in a row (Fig. 11.3). More than two consecutive ventricular beats constitute ventricular tachycardia.
- Bigeminy[xx]: A supraventricular beat followed by a ventricular premature beat (Fig. 11.4).
- Trigeminy: Two supraventricular beats and one ventricular premature beat (Fig. 11.5) or, less frequently, one supraventricular beat, and two ventricular beats.
- Quadrigeminy: Three supraventricular beats followed by one ventricular beat (Fig. 11.6).

[xx]From the Latin *bi*, "occurring every two" and *geminus*, "twin."

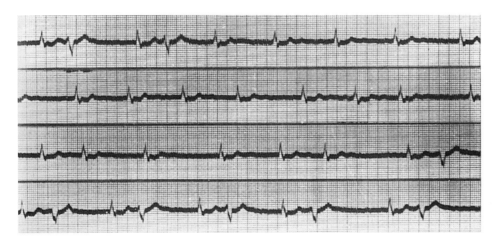

FIGURE 11.2 The rule of bigeminy. Ventricular bigeminal beats end after short postpremature beat intervals (**top**) and begin after long RR intervals (*end* of **third panel**). (Adapted from Langendorf R. Aberrant ventricular conduction. Am Heart J 1951; 41:700–707, with permission.)[1082]

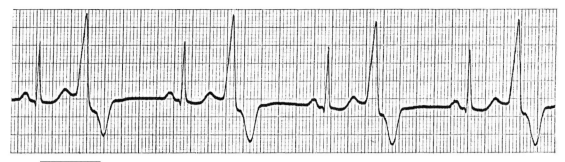

FIGURE 11.4   Ventricular bigeminy. Each conducted beat is followed by a ventricular premature beat.

The pause that follows most ventricular premature beats in patients with sinus rhythm is said to be *compensatory* because its length is such that the sinus beat following the blocked beat occurs on time. The duration of the compensatory pause is inversely related to length of the coupling interval; that is, the earlier the onset of the premature beat, the longer the postectopic interval.[509]

Ventricular premature beats that do not produce compensatory pauses are called *interpolated* beats[510] (Fig. 11.7).[yy] In the presence of an interpolated beat, the number of ventricular beats is one more than the number of sinus beats.

P Waves

P waves may or may not appear in association with ventricular premature beats during sinus rhythm. When a ventricular premature beat occurs during atrial depolarization, the P wave originating from the sinus node disappears within the larger and wider QRS complex of the premature beat. A P wave may be seen, however, if the premature beat begins after the P wave has been inscribed or is completed before the next sinus P wave is written.

The P wave is inverted in the inferior leads when a ventricular premature beat activates the atria by retrograde conduction (Fig. 11.8).[511–519] The prematurity of a ventricular beat can reveal the character of the atrial activity in patients with tachycardias[490] (Fig. 11.9). Atrial premature beats may occasionally induce ventricular premature beats.[520]

PR Interval

The PR interval of the next conducted beat can be *shortened* by a long pause produced by a premature beat,[521] and it may be *lengthened* by an interpolated ventricular premature beat,[521–523] by retrograde penetration of the atrioventricular node.[521] The PR intervals of one or several subsequent conducted beats may be prolonged by one ventricular premature beat.[522, 524]

QRS Complex

Duration. The duration of the QRS complex of most ventricular premature beats is at least 0.12 seconds, as befits their origin in the ventricle and abnormal activation of the ventricular myocardium. The duration of the QRS complexes of ventricular premature beats tends to lengthen as people age.[525]

Morphology. The morphology of ventricular premature beats is abnormal, and, although there may be some similarities, it differs from supraventricular beats with conduction disturbances such as right or left bundle branch block. The form, which is often constant over prolonged periods,[526, 527] depends on the state of the ventricles[404, 506, 528] (Table 11.4). Ventricular premature beats may have more than one form (see Fig. 11.3).

Another factor that may affect the morphology of a premature beat is its prematurity. The earlier the beat occurs, the more it must make its way through areas of varying refractoriness.[526zz]

[yy]Interpolated beats are true *extra*systoles, when one uses *extra* to mean "more than is due, usual or necessary."

[zz]Although this suggestion makes sense, I have found no experimental proof of it.

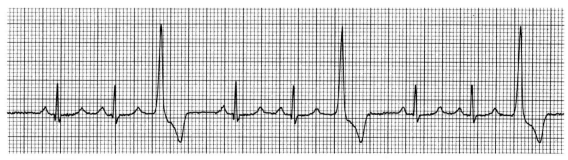

FIGURE 11.5   Ventricular trigeminy. One ventricular premature beat appears after every two sinus beats (lead V_5).

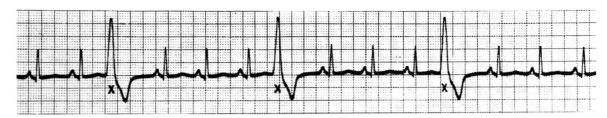

FIGURE 11.6   Ventricular quadrigeminy. Every fourth beat X is ventricular. (Adapted from Chung EK. Principles of Cardiac Arrhythmias. Baltimore: Williams & Wilkins, 1971, with permission.)[1083]

Site of origin. The form of the QRS complex suggests its site of origin within the ventricles[529–534] (Table 11.5).[aaa] Beats with the appearance of right bundle branch block often originate in the left ventricle (Fig. 11.10), and beats with the appearance of left bundle branch block often originate in the right ventricle (Fig. 11.11).

Heart disease is usually present in patients with left ventricular premature beats (right bundle branch block pattern), and it is frequently present in patients with right ventricular premature beats (left bundle branch block appearance).[535–538] The beats from patients without heart disease usually originate in the right ventricle.[105, 535, 537, 539bbb] The form of the QRS complexes of the ventricular premature beats correlates with the location of ST segment abnormalities of ischemia,[538] but in patients with chest pain, the site of origin of ventricular beats does not correlate with the presence or severity of coronary heart disease.[227]

Bundle of His and fascicular premature beats. Some beats arising in the ventricles have supraventricular or nearly supraventricular morphology because they arise within the bundle of His[540, 541ccc] or within the fascicular–bundle branch system.[540, 542–546] Like ventricular premature beats, the bundle of His and fascicular beats affect the heart's rhythm by producing compensatory pauses and slowing subsequent antegrade conduction by retrograde concealed conduction. These beats can discharge but not activate the ventricles and thus may be concealed from display on the electrocardiogram.[542, 544, 546–561]

In myocardial infarction. Q waves not present in the conducted beats of patients with myocardial infarction may appear in the ventricular premature beats and thereby reveal the presence of infarction when the morphology of sinus beats may not be diagnostic (Figs. 11.12 and 11.13).[490, 562–576ddd] The appearance of ventric-

---

[aaa]The correlation of site of origin with QRS morphology for single ventricular premature beats is based on "armchair reasoning"[534] and on artificial stimulation of the human ventricle at operation (first reported in the 1930s)[530, 531] or by pacing.[533] The origin of premature beats has also been estimated from studying the three-lead electrocardiogram, phonocardiogram, and arterial and venous pulses (reported in 1941).[532]

[bbb]This finding, which has become common knowledge, conflicts with a 1960 report, which found that in healthy subjects, three times as many ventricular premature beats originated from the left ventricle than the right ventricle.[37]

[ccc]Also called "mainstem extrasystoles."

[ddd]Morphological analysis of ventricular premature beats has a low sensitivity (29%), high specificity (97%), and high predictive value (86%) for the diagnosis of myocardial infarction.[576]

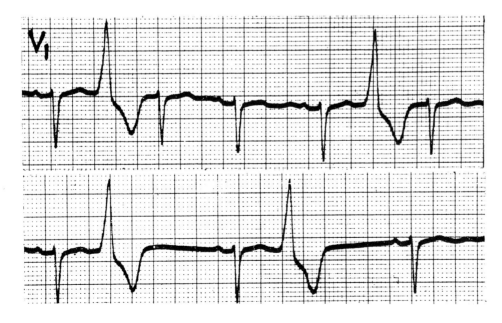

FIGURE 11.7   Interpolated ventricular premature beats. Two interpolated ventricular premature beats appear between two conducted beats. There is no compensatory pause, and the number of ventricular beats is the same as if no ventricular beats were present (**top**). For comparison (**bottom**), a similar ventricular premature beat appears followed by a compensatory pause; these beats are not interpolated, and the premature beats halve the number of ventricular beats. (Adapted from Marriott HJL. Practical Electrocardiography. 4th ed. Baltimore: Williams & Wilkins, 1968, with permission.)[1084]

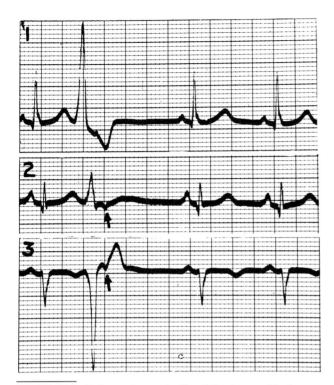

FIGURE 11.8 Retrograde conduction following ventricular premature beats. Compare the form of the P waves during sinus rhythm and after the ventricular beats. They are inverted (*arrows*) in leads 2 and 3 after the ventricular premature beats, a finding indicating ventriculoatrial conduction and activation of the atria from bottom to top. (Adapted from Marriott HJL. Practical Electrocardiography. 4th ed. Baltimore: Williams & Wilkins, 1968, with permission.)[1084]

ular premature beats produced by myocardial infarction correlates well with the location of the infarction but the morphology of *chronic* beats, not produced by the infarct itself, does not indicate the location of the damage.[577]

Of the conducted beats. When the conducted beats have abnormal rather than normal intraventricular conduction:

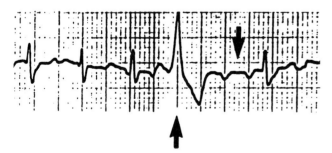

FIGURE 11.9 Ventricular premature beat revealing atrial rhythm. A ventricular premature beat (*upward arrow*) produces a pause in the ventricles of sufficient duration to expose the flutter waves (*downward arrow*) and to reveal the diagnosis of the underlying rhythm. (Adapted from Wang K, Hodges M. The premature ventricular complex as a diagnostic aid. Ann Intern Med 1992; 117:766–770, with permission.)[490]

Table 11.4	**DEPENDENCE OF THE MORPHOLOGY OF THE QRS COMPLEXES OF VENTRICULAR PREMATURE BEATS ON THE AMOUNT OF VENTRICULAR DISEASE**

Characteristics of QRS Complexes of Ventricular Premature Beats	Patients with No Heart Disease	Patients with Severe Myocardial Disease[a]
Size (amplitude in mm)	≥20[506]	≤10[506]
Width (msec)	120–160[506, 528]	≥160[404, 528]
Form	Smooth without notching[506, 528]	Notched and irregular[506]

[a]Producing dilated and globally hypokinetic left ventricles.

- Ventricular premature beats occur more frequently.[578]
- The longer the QRS duration of the sinus beats, the longer the duration of the premature beats.[578]
- The angle is greater between the QRS axis of the conducted beats and the ectopic beats.[578]
- The axis of the QRS complex of the premature beats may be directed away from the region of the bundle that is blocked, a finding suggesting that ventricular premature beats originate from the region of intraventricular conduction delay.[578]

The compensatory pause that follows a ventricular premature beat can allow the next conducted beat that has a rate-dependent bundle branch block or other intraventricular conduction defect to be conducted normally (Fig. 11.14).[490] The normally conducted beat may reveal useful diagnostic information that was normally hidden by the conduction abnormality.

Coupling intervals and parasystole. The period of time between the beginning of the QRS complex of a conducted beat that precedes a premature beat and the onset of the ventricular premature beat itself is known as the coupling interval.[403] Most ventricular premature beats have *fixed coupling*, in which the coupling interval varies little, if at all, during periods when the fundamental rhythm is relatively constant. Coupling intervals

- Usually shorten but may remain the same or inconsistently change when the sinus rate increases during exercise.[579eee]
- Lengthen when intraventricular conduction in the conducted beats is abnormal.[578, 580, 581]
- May vary in patients with multiform and repetitive beats.[582]
- May be used to calculate the prematurity index,[fff] which is inversely related to the heart rate in

---

[eee]In 32 of 60 patients, the coupling intervals decreased as the heart rate increased during exercise. In 16 patients, the coupling interval did not change throughout exercise, and in eight patients there was no consistent relationship between the coupling intervals and the heart rate.[579]

[fff]The ratio of the coupling interval between the preceding sinus beat and the premature beat divided by the QT interval of the preceding sinus complex.[583]

Table 11.5 ORIGIN OF VENTRICULAR PREMATURE BEATS

Location	Form of QRS Complexes		
	Lead V₁	*Leads V₂–V₆*	*Leads II, III, and aVF*
Left ventricle	Right bundle branch block		
Right ventricle	Left bundle branch block		
Apex		Negative (Q waves)	
Base		Positive (R waves)	
Posteroinferior			Left axis (< -30)
Anterior			Right axis ($> +100$)

(Data from references 530 to 534 and 1081.)

patients with myocardial infarction.[583] Accordingly, the premature index shortens at faster rates and lengthens at slower rates.

When the coupling intervals change, ventricular parasystole may be present.[6, 581, 584–616ggg] Parasystole[602] is recognized electrocardiographically by

---

ggg From the Greek *para,* meaning "beyond," "beside," or "against" + *systole* meaning "contraction." Parasystole has occupied the attention of many electrocardiographers over the years,[6, 584–611, 613, 615, 616] but it has not been the subject of invasive electrophysiological studies. The topic seems to be more an electrocardiographic curiosity than one of practical importance in the recognition and treatment of ventricular arrhythmias.

- Varying coupling intervals between the ectopic parasystolic beats and the conducted complexes. Fixed coupling, however, does occasionally occur in parasystole.[579, 617]
- Interectopic intervals that are equal to, or a multiple of, a common, minimal interval.
- Fusion beats.

Parasystolic beats,[618] which should appear in patients with the arrhythmia whenever the ventricles are excit-

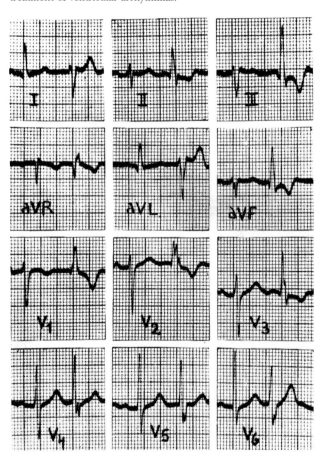

FIGURE 11.10 Ventricular premature beats with the form of right bundle branch block. These beats, one of which is shown following a sinus beat in each lead, more frequently occur in patients without structural heart disease. (Adapted from Rosenbaum MB. Classification of ventricular extrasystoles according to form. J Electrocardiol 1969; 2:289–297, with permission.)[634]

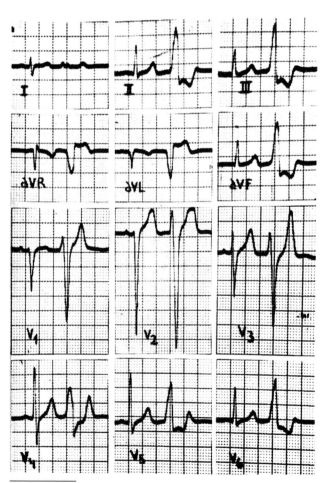

FIGURE 11.11 Ventricular premature beats with the form of left bundle branch block. Patients with these beats usually have structural heart disease. (Adapted from Rosenbaum MB. Classification of ventricular extrasystoles according to form. J Electrocardiol 1969; 2:289–297, with permission.)[634]

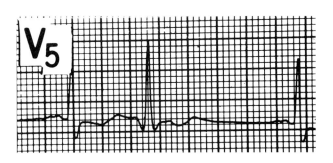

FIGURE 11.12 Ventricular premature beat revealing myocardial infarction. The patient had an extensive inferolateral myocardial infarction. Only the ventricular premature beat shows the Q wave from the infarction. (Adapted from Dash H, Ciotola TJ. Morphology of ventricular premature beats as an aid in the electrocardiographic diagnosis of myocardial infarction. Am J Cardiol 1983; 52:458–461, with permission.)[576]

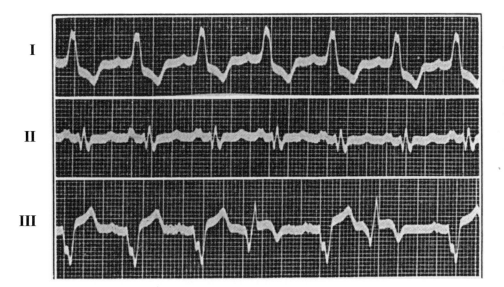

FIGURE 11.13 Ventricular premature beat revealing myocardial infarction in presence of left bundle branch block. In what may be the first report of this finding by William Dressler in 1943, ventricular premature beats (lead III) shows the Q waves from the infarction that are absent in the conducted beats. (Adapted from Dressler W. A case of myocardial infarction masked by bundle branch block but revealed by occasional premature ventricular beats. Am J Med Sci 1943; 206:361–363, with permission.)[562]

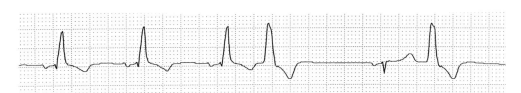

FIGURE 11.14 Ventricular premature beat revealing normal pattern in subsequent QRS complex. A ventricular premature beat (QRS complex 4) produces a compensatory pause of sufficient length to allow the right bundle branch to recover so that the beat 5 can be normally conducted without the right bundle branch block present in the other conducted beats (lead V₁). (Courtesy of Dr. C. William Hancock.)

able, may be intermittently,[585, 590, 593, 595, 597, 604, 611, 619, 620] rather than constantly, present.

Parasystole is detected uncommonly; it was found in only 0.3% of the electrocardiograms in 50,000 consecutive patients at a Chicago teaching hospital.[28] The arrhythmia, which occurs twice as frequently in men as in women,[602] also appears in children,[598, 599] including newborn.[621] Most,[579, 597] but not all,[37, 598, 599, 602, 607, 622] of the reported cases have occurred in patients with heart disease.

Concealed bigeminy and trigeminy. Reviews of long electrocardiographic tracings of patients with ventricular bigeminy have shown that the number of sinus beats between the intervals of bigeminy is frequently an odd number.[595, 623, 624] This observation has been explained by assuming that the source of the ventricular premature beats continues to discharge but does not activate the ventricular myocardium and consequently is *concealed* from being recorded in the electrocardiogram.[595, 620, 623, 625–629]

When trigeminy—one ventricular premature beat after two sinus beats—is present, the intervening beats of prolonged sinus rhythm frequently recur in even numbers. Concealed trigeminy may then be present.[630]

Electrical alternans. This condition may be diagnosed incorrectly when the ventricular premature beats in bigeminy occurs just after the P waves[631] (Fig. 11.15).

ST Segments and T Waves[hhh]

ST segments and T waves are characteristically abnormal after ventricular premature beats because abnormal ventricular depolarization produces abnormal ventricular repolarization. Ventricular arrhythmias are very unlikely to occur when the ST segments deviate less than 2 mm from the baseline in the absence of signs of severe myocardial damage 48 hours after the onset of the infarction.[632]

[hhh]See the chapters on ventricular tachycardia and ventricular fibrillation for discussions about the *R-on-T phenomenon*, which occurs when a ventricular premature beat appears during the "vulnerable phase" of the preceding T wave of the conducted beat.

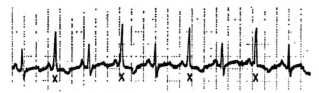

FIGURE 11.15 Ventricular bigeminy masquerading as electrical alternans. One makes the correct diagnosis by observing that the premature beats (X) occur slightly early and the PR intervals that precede them are slightly shorter than the normal PR intervals of the sinus beats (lead II). (Adapted from Chung DK, Chung EK. Ventricular bigeminy masquerading as total electrical alternans: in a case of probable tuberculous pericarditis. Am J Cardiol 1969;24:287–289, with permission.)[631]

Prinzmetal's variant angina. Alternation of the ST segments may precede the onset of ventricular premature beats during reperfusion after an episode of Prinzmetal's angina.[239] Prinzmetal's variant angina occurs

- Much more often during ST segment elevation than depression.[238]
- During the initial 2 to 3 minutes of ST segment deviation when its magnitude is increasing or maximal, according to one study,[238] or when the ST segment elevations are starting to return or have returned to baseline ("reperfusion period"), according to another.[237]
- Unrelated to the duration or magnitude of the ST segment deviation.[238]

Effects of Ventricular Premature Beats on the Morphology of Subsequent Beats

The T waves of the *sinus beats that follow the pauses* after ventricular premature beats may have abnormal contour, amplitude, or direction.[633–635] Such post-extrasystolic T waves changes occur more frequently after interpolated ventricular premature beats than after those followed by a fully compensatory pause.[635] Patients with post-extrasystolic T wave changes usually have intrinsic heart disease,[634, 636] whereas when they occur after *interpolated* premature beats, the patients frequently have no structural heart disease.[637iii] The QRS complexes as well as T waves of sinus beats after interpolated ventricular premature beats may also have abnormal morphology because of ventricular refractoriness produced by the interpolated beat.[635]

OTHER ELECTROCARDIOGRAPHIC STUDIES

Extended and Ambulatory (Holter) Monitoring

Duration of recording. The more electrocardiograms are taken or the longer the recordings are made, the more ventricular premature beats are detected.[26, 67, 79, 90, 170, 178, 415, 638–649] For example, in 160 survivors of myocardial infarction, 15% had ventricular premature beats on one electrocardiogram, but the number more than doubled to 34% when an average of four electrocardiograms was recorded.[170] When the same patients had ambulatory electrocardiographic records, the likelihood of finding ventricular premature beats rose to[170]

- Forty-three percent with one 12-hour record.
- Sixty-three percent with 24 hours of recording.
- Eighty percent with 48 to 60 hours.

In 66 patients, most of whom had coronary heart disease and no ventricular irritability on a 3-minute standard electrocardiogram, ventricular premature beats were detected in 27% during 10 hours of ambulatory monitoring.[645] However, the presence of ventricular premature beats in the standard electrocardiogram

---

[iii]In 8 of 26 (32%) patients.[637]

of patients who have had myocardial infarction correlates well with *repetitive* forms on the Holter recording.[183] No more than 1 hour of recording is needed to predict mortality from the appearance of ventricular premature beats.[650–652]

The likelihood of detecting at least one ventricular premature beat in several groups of patients who had had recent myocardial infarctions was

- Six percent to 15% with one standard electrocardiogram.[168, 169, 178, 653]
- Fifty-two percent with a 1-hour tape.[178]
- Fifty percent to 70% with a 6-hour tape.[43, 166]
- Seventy-eight percent with a 10-hour tape.[173]
- Fifty-two percent with a 24-hour tape.[180]

In patients with mitral valve prolapse, the recording of the electrocardiogram of 48 hours does not appear to increase the frequency or the complexity of the ventricular premature beats beyond what would appear in a 24-hour record,[647] but more such beats have been observed when 24 rather than 10 hours are examined.[91, 647]

The incidence of *complex* ventricular premature beats also tends to rise as longer periods of activity are monitored in patients who have had myocardial infarction, for example:

- Resting electrocardiogram, 2%.[169]
- One hour, 27%.[178]
- Six hours, 23% to 35%.[166]
- Ten hours, 37%.[653]
- Twenty-four hours, 39% to 43%.[90, 172]

Spontaneous variability. The number[285, 420, 421, 654–658] and complexity[658, 659] of ventricular premature beats vary greatly when similar periods of recording are compared within the same day,[660] and between days,[661] weeks,[661, 662] months,[657, 661, 662] or years.[661]*jjj* Left ventricular function does not affect the amount of spontaneous variability,[421, 663] but it is greater in patients

- When shorter periods are recorded.[655, 660, 664]
- When the interval between the recordings is longer.[661]
- Who have frequent ventricular premature beats.[665]
- Taking beta-blocking drugs.[663, 665]
- With coronary artery disease,[421] rather than no heart disease.[662]
- After myocardial infarction when compared with patients with stable coronary or other forms of heart disease.[663]
- With noncoronary rather than coronary heart disease.[665]

Miscellaneous factors. Symptoms, such as dizziness and syncope reported by patients in their diaries, correlate poorly with arrhythmias, including ventricular premature beats, detected on Holter monitoring.[468, 666] Many patients referred for Holter monitoring because of palpitations and similar symptoms have a psychiatric

disorder such as panic attacks.[481, 483] The number of ventricular premature beats does not significantly increase during ST segment depressions recorded on Holter monitoring.[214]

Computers programmed to detect ventricular premature beats reveal more abnormal beats than conventional electrocardiographic monitoring.[144] The accuracy of computers used for this purpose exceeds 95%.[667]

Heart Rate Variability

The variability of the heart rate, a measure of autonomic function, tends to be lower in patients with ventricular premature beats who have had myocardial infarction.[668] The components of heart rate variability controlled by parasympathetic sympathetic stimulation drop and those controlled by sympathetic influences rise just before repetitive ventricular premature beats begin.[669]

Exercise Electrocardiography*kkk*

Exercise may either increase or decrease the number of ventricular premature beats.[640, 670–681]

Subjects without heart disease. Ventricular premature beats appear in at least 11% of asymptomatic, apparently healthy adults during exercise testing[56, 67, 105, 507, 674, 682–689] or during vigorous sport.[690]*lll* The frequency of ventricular premature beats increases as subjects age[682] and as the heart rate rises from 120 to 150 beats per minute.[56] The number decreases during the recovery period after exercise in patients without heart disease.[56, 507, 674] Ectopic beats develop on exercise at slower rates in patients with cardiovascular disease than in healthy persons.[682]

Healthy children do not usually develop ventricular premature beats on exercise testing.[691] Exercise often causes ventricular premature beats to disappear in those without heart disease who have ectopic beats at rest[692] or at low levels of exercise.[331] The beats are suppressed when the heart rate exceeds about 140 to 150 beats per minute, but they return when the heart rate decreases. During the first 1 to 3 minutes after cessation of exercise, the frequency of ventricular premature beats may exceed the number observed at the beginning of the test.[692]

Angina and stable coronary heart disease. On treadmill or bicycle exercise, 22% to 56%*mmm* of patients with stable coronary heart disease have ventricular premature beats, including multiform beats,[209] significantly more often than patients without heart

---

*jjj*This characteristic must be taken into account when studying the effects of drugs designed to suppress ventricular beats.[285, 655–661, 663]

*kkk*Graded treadmill exercise is the usual technique now employed. However, arrhythmias are also produced by Master's two-step exercise test.[672]

*lll*The wide range of incidence probably reflects, among other factors, the presence or absence of nonclinical heart disease and the level of exercise achieved.

*mmm*The lower figure was observed in patients without any ventricular premature beats on their resting electrocardiograms.[687]

disease.[209, 241, 645, 653, 687, 693, 694]*nnn* Conversely, patients with simple ventricular premature beats on exercise are more likely to have coronary heart disease than those without the arrhythmia.[695]

When complex beats are observed, more coronary arteries tend to be involved and ventricular function is worse.[695] A strong correlation exists between the presence of ventricular premature beats during exercise and the appearance of ischemic electrocardiographic changes.[696] However, among adults evaluated for chest pain who have not yet had myocardial infarctions, exercise-induced ventricular premature beats less successfully predict the presence of coronary heart disease than do ST segment depressions greater than or equal to 1 mm.[697] The presence of ventricular premature beats on exercise testing predicts the future occurence of myocardial infarction, angina, or cardiac death.[698]*ooo*

Patients with coronary heart disease develop ventricular irritability when their heart rates reach about 130 beats per minute.[687] At faster rates, simple ventricular premature beats are suppressed with similar frequency in both patients with coronary disease and normal healthy persons,[687] and consequently, the disappearance of ventricular beats does not rule out the presence of coronary heart disease.[209] Complex ventricular premature beats, however, do not usually disappear at faster rates in either group.[687]

In patients with coronary heart disease, the frequency of both simple and complex ventricular beats rises as

- Left ventricular function becomes more abnormal.[684, 687, 699]
- More healed myocardial infarctions are present.[684]
- More coronary arteries are diseased.[699]*ppp*

The axis in the frontal plane of the QRS complexes of ventricular premature beats that develop during exercise in patients with coronary heart disease tends to be superior, to the left of −30°, whereas patients without heart disease tend to have a normal axis in their exercise-induced ectopic beats.[700]

Myocardial infarction. Ventricular premature beats are detected during exercise testing in up to 60% of patients who have recently sustained myocardial infarction,[653, 677, 701–712] and complex ventricular premature beats appear in as many as 40%.[704, 706, 710, 713] The number of simple and complex ventricular premature beats detected on exercise rises when tests are performed sequentially up to 11 weeks after the myocar-

dial infarction.[704] Ventricular premature beats tend to develop in patients with ischemic ST segment changes, but they do not correlate with exercise-induced angina.[704]

Unlike the patients with stable coronary heart disease, the extent of coronary artery disease[709] does not correlate with the incidence of ventricular premature beats that develop on exercise in patients who have had myocardial infarction. Neither has it been possible to relate ventricular premature beats in such patients to left ventricular function,*qqq* as revealed by

- Cardiomegaly or pulmonary vascular congestion in the roentgenogram after discharge.[711]
- Left ventricular ejection fraction.[709]
- Left ventricular failure in the coronary care unit or at the time of exercise.[711]

Ventricular premature beats do, however, occur more frequently after infarction in patients receiving digoxin,[711] a finding that may reflect myocardial factors, rather than effects of the drug itself. Holter monitoring shows that children who survive myocardial infarction have relatively few arrhythmias, including ventricular premature beats.[714]

Mitral valve prolapse. Patients with mitral valve prolapse have no more ventricular premature beats on exercise than normal individuals.[253]

Miscellaneous conditions. Exercise testing may also produce ventricular premature beats in patients with

- Congenital complete atrioventricular block,[715–717] in which more ectopic beats appear with increasing age and when the QRS complex is prolonged.[716]
- Uncomplicated hypertension who are taking diuretic monotherapy and who have more isolated ventricular premature beats, but no more frequent (>10% of beats) or complex ventricular ectopy while exercising than healthy, normotensive subjects.[718]
- Hypertrophic cardiomyopathy.[270]
- Occasionally, chronic obstructive pulmonary disease.[719]
- Scleroderma.[456]
- Tetralogy of Fallot after surgical repair.[331, 720, 721]

Spontaneous variability. The number or complexity of ventricular premature beats frequently differs in exercise tests taken in the same person,[439, 686] with or without heart disease, when the tests are separated by a rest period of as little as 45 minutes.[722] Reproducibility seems better at intervals of 1 to 5 days,[723] but not when months or years separate the tests.[507, 686]

Physical conditioning does not significantly change the frequency of ventricular beats despite the assumption that the number of beats may decrease in persons who have participated in a supervised exercise program designed to improve fitness and cardiovascular

---

*nnn*Isometric exercise may produce even more ventricular premature beats than dynamic exercise on a bicycle—35% versus 22% according to one study.[693]

*ooo*The annual incidence of new coronary events during a 5-year follow-up was as follows:[698]
- 1.7% among 1,067 patients without ventricular premature beats or ischemic ST segments changes.
- 6.4% in 758 patients with ventricular premature beats alone.
- 9.5% among 609 patients with ischemic ST segment changes alone.
- 11.4% in 569 patients with ventricular premature beats and ischemic ST segment changes.

*ppp*Another study questions this relationship.[697]

*qqq*The lack of correlation may be due to excluding from exercise those patients with poor left ventricular function or complex ventricular premature beats.[709, 711]

function.[507] In children, no differences appear in the incidence and character of ventricular beats produced during two exercise tests.[692]

Ambulatory Monitoring Versus Exercise Testing

Ambulatory monitoring usually reveals more ventricular premature beats,[207, 215, 241, 640, 647, 653, 712, 724] including multiform and repetitive patterns[241, 725, 726] (see Fig. 11.3) and the arrhythmias that cause syncope,[727] better than does exercise testing. However, because this is not always the case, both tests should be obtained when thoroughly evaluating ventricular arrhythmias.

Signal-averaged Electrocardiography

Late potentials in the signal-averaged electrocardiogram do not identify which patients will develop ventricular premature beats after myocardial infarction.[197]

ECHOCARDIOGRAPHY

Echocardiographic studies of patients with ventricular premature beats have revealed that

- Hypertension causes ventricular premature beats.[45, 48, 50, 295, 297, 298, 728]
- Left ventricular false tendons, detected echocardiographically, may produce ventricular premature beats.[729, 730]
- Men with left ventricular hypertrophy more often have ventricular premature beats than those without hypertrophy.[51, 297, 299, 301, 302]
- The association of ventricular premature beats with left ventricular hypertrophy is better predicted when the hypertrophy is determined by echocardiography than by electrocardiography.[304]
- Thickness or posterior displacement of the mitral valve may[256] or may not[257] correlate with increased numbers of complex ventricular arrhythmias in patients with mitral valve prolapse.
- Increased left ventricular volume, rather than depressed ejection fraction, relates to the presence of complex ventricular premature beats after myocardial infarction.[731]

CHEMISTRY

The more ventricular premature beats occur, the higher the levels of serum aspartate aminotransferase,[150] norepinephrine,[732] epinephrine,[732] free fatty acids,[733, 734] and creatine kinase[151] in patients during acute myocardial infarction.

PATHOLOGY

Some young patients with ventricular premature beats have microscopical structural heart disease despite normal cardiac anatomy and mechanical function. For example, in 26 patients, right ventricular endomyocardial biopsies revealed the following:[735]

- Normal myocardium in 10 (38%).
- Cellular hypertrophy, fibrosis, and degenerative changes in 11 (42%).
- Acute myocarditis in two (7%).
- Borderline myocarditis in one (3.5%).
- Vasculitis in one (3.5%).
- Right ventricular dysplasia in one (3.5%).

HEMODYNAMICS

The systolic pressure produced by a patient's ventricular premature beats is usually less than that produced by the sinus beats. Furthermore, the shorter the coupling interval of the ventricular premature beat to the preceding sinus beat, the less the systolic pressure produced by the premature beat.[509, 736, 737]

Whereas ventricular premature beats decrease stroke volume about 70% compared with sinus beats,[738] the stroke volume produced by the post-extrasystolic sinus beats is only about 18% greater than that produced by a sinus beat.[738] Thus, the extra volume produced by the post-extrasystolic sinus beat does not compensate for the loss produced by the premature beat.[738]

The systolic pressure generated during the post-ectopic interval is usually greater than that produced by the other sinus beats,[509, 737] except in infants less than 2 weeks old, who cannot raise the systolic pressure after the extra beat.[509] In patients with hypertrophic cardiomyopathy, however, the arterial pulse pressure produced by the sinus beat after the pause is often lower than from the normal beats because of increased dynamic obstruction of the left ventricular outflow tract produced by post-extrasystolic potentiation induced by the premature beat.[491, 492, 494, 502, 739]

Multifocal ventricular premature beats and ventricular bigeminal rhythm reduce the following:[737]

- Cardiac output.
- Central blood volume.
- Mean systemic pressure.
- Stroke volume and power.
- Ventricular power.

Mitral and tricuspid regurgitation may occur during the contraction produced by ventricular premature beats.[509, 737]

Evidence of early myocardial disease appears in some patients with ventricular premature beats and no clinically obvious structural heart disease. Hemodynamic studies reveal elevated left vetricular end-systolic and end-diastolic volume index and decreased mean velocity of circumferential fiber shortening.[740]

CLINICAL ELECTROPHYSIOLOGY

Identification from Bundle of His Electrograms

A bundle of His deflection, the low-amplitude H wave that appears between atrial and ventricular activation during sinus rhythm, does not precede the V wave produced by the depolarization[741] of a ventricular premature beat.[11, 741, 742] This occurs because the beat, which originates in the ventricle, in retrograde fashion

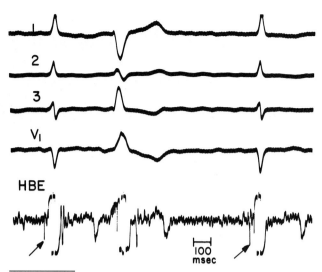

FIGURE 11.16 His bundle electrogram of ventricular premature beat during atrial fibrillation. In leads 1, 2, 3, and V₁, we see that the fundamental rhythm is atrial fibrillation. The first and third beats are conducted, and second beat is ectopic. The His bundle electrogram (HBE) shows that the second beat originates in the ventricles because it is not preceded by a His bundle deflection, as are conducted beats (arrows). The fibrillatory activity in the atrium produces the continuous low-amplitude deflections throughout the His bundle electrogram.

activates the bundle of His, the signal from which usually occurs during the large V wave whose amplitude hides the H wave (Fig. 11.16). Occasionally, the bundle of His is activated in retrograde fashion sufficiently late that an H deflection can be seen *after* the V wave.

Fascicular beats, those ventricular beats originating within the fascicles of the bundle branches close to the bundle of His,[743–745] may activate the bundle of His in retrograde fashion soon afterwards. In such cases, an H deflection can be seen *before* the V wave, but the HV interval is shorter than normal.[746] Bundle of His recordings may occasionally be needed to differentiate between supraventricular premature beats with aberrant conduction and ventricular premature beats.[rrr]

Concealed Conduction

Ventricular premature beats may affect the appearance of subsequent beats through concealed conduction in which the electrophysiological action of the premature beat is hidden from view and is revealed only by its effect on subsequent conduction or impulse formation.[747] This mechanism explains how interpolated ventricular premature beats that penetrate the atrioventricular node in retrograde fashion can prolong antegrade atrioventricular nodal conduction.[521, 523, 548, 549, 748, 749] Fascicular beats, whether manifest or concealed, may have a similar effect.[745]

Retrograde Conduction

The duration of retrograde conduction from the site of origin of the ventricular beat to the bundle of His (VH interval) depends on the following:[11, 543]

- Distance betweeen the two. Other factors being equal, the greater the spatial separation between the site of the ectopic beat and the bundle of His, the longer the conduction time as reflected in the VH interval.
- Speed of conduction. When retrograde conduction is slow even though the distance from the site of origin to the His bundle is short, the VH interval may be relatively long.
- Coupling interval. The duration of retrograde conduction from the site of the ventricular beat to the bundle of His increases as the coupling interval of the premature beat to the previous beat shortens.[750]

The simultaneous intranodal collision of supraventricular beats and ventricular beats may *facilitate* atrioventricular nodal conduction.[751]

Morphology of QRS Complexes

Ventricular premature beats with different forms are thought to originate in different regions of the ventricles. However, this is not always the case. The form of ectopic beats may change even though the origin is fixed in the presence of[752]

- Greater prematurity of the ectopic beat.
- Left ventricular wall motion abnormality.
- Prior myocardial infarction.
- Reduced left ventricular ejection fraction.

Programmed Stimulation

Some patients with complex ventricular premature beats, most often when the beats are multiform or bigeminal,[753] can be induced into sustained ventricular tachycardia or fibrillation during electrophysiological study.[753–756] Most,[sss] however, cannot. Furthermore, one cannot predict who will have these inducible arrhythmias on the basis of atherosclerotic heart disease, old myocardial infarction, or ejection fraction less than 40%.[754, 756]

Origin of Ventricular Premature Beats

Catheter mapping techniques[757, 758] and magnetocardiography[759] can locate the approximate site of ventricular premature beats that may originate from foci distant from the myocardial infarction[577] or in chronically diseased[760] myocardium.

[rrr]See Chapter 4 for the diagnosis of aberrantly conducted supraventricular beats versus ventricular beats.

[sss]Seventy-three percent in one series of 73 patients with various forms of heart disease and no clinical evidence of ventricular tachycardia, sudden death, or syncope.[754]

TREATMENT

Physical Maneuvers

Carotid sinus pressure may suppress[64, 761, 762] or enhance[763] the appearance of ventricular premature beats.

Drugs

Although each of the drugs described in this section will suppress ventricular premature beats, the cautious physician seldom prescribes them.[764–773] Most patients do not need specific treatment, and those who are treated with antiarrhythmic drugs often sustain annoying, if not life-threatening, side effects, including pro-arrhythmia and reduced ventricular function. Both these unwanted side effects more likely develop in the sickest patients, those patients whom cardiologists most want to treat.

Patients without heart disease. The anxiety that symptomatic ventricular premature beats can produce in patients without apparent heart disease can usually be relieved by a sympathetic review of the harmless nature of the problem.[32,ttt] Beta-blocking drugs may be prescribed for those patients who cannot tolerate the palpitations.

Cardiac arrhythmia suppression trial (CAST).[744] This trial established that long-term suppression of ventricular premature beats in asymptomatic or mildly symptomatic patients after myocardial infarction who have mild to moderate ventricular dysfunction (ejection fraction < 40%) does not prolong, and can reduce, survival.[198, 775–778uuu] In addition, death occurred more often in those patients in CAST who had faster heart rates, frequent ventricular premature beats, or non–Q-wave myocardial infarctions.[779]

CAST further revealed that, when compared with patients whose ventricular premature beats are difficult to suppress, those with easily suppressible beats are older and have[780]

- Average left ventricular ejection fraction.
- Heart failure less frequently.
- Myocardial infarction less often.
- Low risk of sudden death.
- More ventricular premature beats.

Although cardiologists do not know exactly how the drugs exerted their baleful effect on certain patients, further review of the CAST data suggests that the interaction between active ischemia and treatment with encainide or flecainide may have been responsible.[781]

In the past, the hope of increasing survival,[782, 783] supported by earlier studies,[784] led many physicians to suppress ventricular premature beats after myocardial infarction. CAST and other reports[785, 786] have taught us cardiologists not to "treat the electrocardiogram" that contains ventricular premature beats.[vvv] We do not yet know whether prescribing antiarrhythmic drugs will prolong survival in patients with forms of heart disease other than coronary disease or with clinical profiles different from those included in CAST.[www]

Amiodarone. Amiodarone,[787–790] a type III antiarrhythmic drug, decreases the number of,[791–805] and complexity of,[794–796, 798, 800, 803, 806, 807] ventricular premature beats in many patients

- After myocardial infarction.[800, 804]
- During exercise.[797]
- Who are unresponsive to other antiarrhythmic drugs.[795]
- With chronic chagasic myocarditis.[796]
- With reduced ventricular function.[804]
- With stable coronary heart disease.[797]

Amiodarone is more effective in suppressing ventricular premature beats than mexiletine or procainamide,[808] and, according to a meta-analysis, it may be more effective than all drugs in classes Ia, Ib, and II.[809] Some investigators have found,[799, 810] but others have not found,[795, 806] a relation between amiodarone's ability to suppress ventricular premature beats and the blood level of the drug or its deethylated metabolite.

Amiodarone reduces mortality in patients with previous myocardial infarction,[778] particularly during the first year after the infarction.[790, 803, 811–813] This effect has not yet been shown after 1 year probably because mortality is then low regardless of treatment.[804, 813]

Beta-adrenergic–blocking drugs. This class of drugs suppresses ventricular premature beats[194, 726, 764, 841–846] and decreases their degree of complexity[194, 726, 817, 827, 832, 839, 842, 844, 847, 848] in patients with many forms of heart disease,[726, 848] including

- Coronary heart disease after bypass surgery.[837, 849]
- Mitral valve prolapse.[850]
- Myocardial infarction both during the acute phase[194, 822, 825, 829, 832, 851xxx] and afterward.[822, 845, 852]

However, beta-blocking drugs do not decrease the number of ventricular ectopic beats produced by suc-

---

[ttt]As Paul Wood advised (1968): "Reassurance is important, and should be unconditional and convincing, for ectopic beats rarely constitute a complaint except in those prone to anxiety."[32]

[uuu]Although only three drugs were studied, encainide, flecainide, and moricizine, I assume that most other antiarrhythmic drugs will have similar effects in this setting. Amiodarone appears to be an important exception.[778]

[vvv]In the 1980s, before CAST was reported and despite warnings, 28% of cardiologists surveyed at university medical centers in the United States treated frequent ventricular premature beats, and 74% treated complex ventricular premature beats in asymptomatic patients convalescing from myocardial infarction.[1085] Even in 1990, when the first reports of CAST were appearing, many American cardiologists treated to suppress asymptomatic ventricular premature beats in patients with coronary heart disease and left ventricular dysfunction.[1086]

[www]Thus, CAST has greatly tempered our enthusiasm for treating ventricular premature beats with one or more of the antiarrhythmic drugs available. Of course, treating patients whose ventricular beats are associated with ventricular tachycardia or ventricular fibrillation is a different matter and is discussed in the chapters on those arrhythmias in this book.

[xxx]Although one study demonstrated that metoprolol does not reduce the incidence of ventricular premature beats during myocardial infarction.[831]

cessful thrombolysis.[163, 853] Whether the antiarrhythmic properties of beta-adrenergic–blocking drugs account for their well-known value in decreasing mortality after myocardial infarction is unknown.

Beta-blocking drugs decrease ventricular beats produced during exercise in many patients,[830, 841, 847] but they do not appear to affect significantly the frequency of ventricular premature beats in patients with hypertrophic cardiomyopathy during normal activities or when exercising.[272] Beta-adrenergic–blocking drugs are likely to decrease the frequency of ventricular premature beats in those patients in whom sleep also suppresses the arrhythmia.[854]

Beta-adrenergic–blocking drugs suppress ventricular premature beats more effectively when the beats are associated with faster underlying heart rates.[846] The importance of rate to this effect is supported by the reappearance of the ventricular beats in patients taking the drugs with rapid atrial pacing.[846]

This class of drugs is as effective as, or nearly as effective as, procainamide[847] and quinidine[726, 847] for suppressing ventricular premature beats and is better tolerated[726, 847] than either, but it is less effective than moricizine.[840, 855] Beta blockers given with procainamide and quinidine suppress ventricular premature beats better than either antiarrhythmic agent alone.[856] Beta-adrenergic–blocking drugs that have been shown to suppress ventricular premature beats include acebutolol,[726, 821, 822, 825, 828, 835, 837, 848, 857, 858] atenolol,[829, 832, 851] metoprolol,[831, 859] nadolol,[412, 833, 834, 841, 846, 854, 856] pindolol,[826] and propranolol.[242, 764, 818, 819, 824, 827, 836, 840, 850, 855]

Bretylium tosylate. This drug decreases ventricular premature beats, but it is seldom used now for this purpose.[860]

Calcium-channel–blocking drugs. Although a few reports[861–865] say that calcium-channel–blocking drugs reduce the presence of ventricular premature beats, the consensus[866] is that drugs of this class are relatively ineffective unless the ectopic beats are due to acute ischemia produced by coronary vasospasm. In these cases, the relief of the ischemia, rather than an antiarrhythmic action, suppresses the beats.[221, 231, 236, 867]

Corticosteroids. These drugs suppress ventricular premature beats in children with myocarditis.[868]

Digitalis. A few studies suggest that therapeutic doses of digitalis glycosides may decrease ventricular premature beats[869–873] in persons with normal left ventricular function,[872] although not in those with myocardial infarction.[874] However, digitalis is seldom prescribed specifically for this purpose.[yyy]

Digoxin-specific Fab antibody fragments. These agents eliminate ventricular premature beats produced by digitalis intoxication.[359, 360]

Disopyramide. A class I agent similar in action to procainamide and quinidine, disopyramide suppresses ventricular premature beats[764, 875–879] as effectively as quinidine,[880, 881] mexiletine,[882] and lidocaine when given intravenously,[883] but not as effectively as moricizine[884] or propafenone.[885, 886] Reports differ about whether[887] or not[876] disopyramide suppresses ventricular beats during myocardial infarction. The antiarrhythmic effects of disopyramide supplement those of mexiletine permitting effective treatment when both drugs are given together in lower, better tolerated doses.[888]

Encainide. A potent class IC antiarrhythmic agent, encainide reliably suppresses ventricular premature beats[882, 889–894] and is more effective and better tolerated than is quinidine.[890] However, the drug increases mortality when given to treat ventricular premature beats in asymptomatic or mildly symptomatic patients after myocardial infarction,[777] and it is no longer available in the United States.

Flecainide. Clinically and pharmacologically similar to encainide in many respects, flecainide is also very effective in suppressing ventricular premature beats[894–900] and is probably superior to quinidine[898, 901, 902] and disopyramide[879] for this purpose. Like encainide, flecainide increases mortality in asymptomatic and mildly symptomatic patients who are given the drug for suppression of ventricular premature beats after myocardial infarction.[777]

Lidocaine. Lidocaine[903,yyy] decreases ventricular premature beats in most patients with acute myocardial infarction[131, 139, 140, 577, 760, 904–912,zzz] and in other settings,[883] including during and after cardiac surgery.[913] Although usually given intravenously in a monitoring unit, lidocaine also suppresses ventricular premature beats when given intramuscularly so long as doses adequate to achieve therapeutic blood levels are given.[908, 909, 914–919]

Magnesium and potassium. Magnesium[376–379, 920, 921] and potassium,[373, 376, 378] when given to patients who are deficient in these cations, suppress ventricular premature beats that have been aroused by such electrolyte disturbances.[922, 923] Correction of hypokalemia or hypomagnesemia alone, however, may not be sufficient to eliminate ectopic beats produced by electrolyte deficiency from diuretic treatment.[376, 378, 396, 923] Furthermore, infusion of potassium in glucose can exacerbate the arrhythmia in hypokalemic patients when the metabolism of glucose further decreases the serum potassium.[924] Magnesium infusions may suppress ventricular premature beats[925] during myocardial infarction[926–928]

[yyy]The use of lidocaine to prevent ventricular tachyarrhythmias and cardiac arrest during acute myocardial infarction is discussed in Chapter 4.

[zzz]Data suggesting that lidocaine is relatively ineffective in decreasing ventricular premature beats in the first hours after onset of symptoms may have reflected the administration of inadequate doses.[140, 905, 908, 912] Other work has supported the early effectiveness of lidocaine.[910]

and in patients with congestive heart failure,[929] even when hypomagnesemia is not present.[930][aaaa]

Increasing the daily recommended minimal dietary intake of potassium or magnesium reduces the frequency of ventricular premature beats. This treatment, however, does not suppress repetitive tachyarrhythmias or relieve symptoms.[931]

Mexiletine. An antiarrhythmic drug with properties similar to lidocaine and tocainide, mexiletine suppresses ventricular premature beats in long-term[878, 888, 932–941] and acute clinical settings including myocardial infarction.[926, 933, 934, 942–944] Its efficacy is similar to, or better than, amiodarone,[808] disopyramide,[878, 882] procainamide,[808, 942] and quinidine,[941, 945–947] but not equal to its congener tocainide in individual patients. Combined therapy with mexiletine and quinidine[948] or mexiletine and disopyramide[888] can produce effective suppression of ventricular premature beats with fewer side effects than are produced from higher doses of either drug alone.

Moricizine. A class I antiarrhythmic agent, moricizine suppresses ventricular premature beats successfully in many patients.[840, 894, 949–958] The drug is more effective and has fewer side effects than disopyramide[959, 960] or propanolol,[840, 855] the addition of which does not enhance the effects of moricizine.[855] Moricizine, like encainide and flecainide, decreases survival in some patients who have asymptomatic or mildly symptomatic ventricular premature beats after myocardial infarction.[961]

Phenytoin. Phenytoin (diphenylhydantoin)[962–966] suppresses ventricular premature beats in many patients[764, 963, 967–971, bbbb] and was formerly prescribed for arrhythmias due to digitalis intoxication.[969, 972–974]

Procainamide. Like quinidine the classic type IA agent, procainamide successfully suppresses ventricular premature beats[975–977] that occur in patients with

• Acute myocardial infarction.[978–983]
• Prior myocardial infarction.[808, 942, 982–985]
• Cardiomyopathy.[838, 981–983]
• Chronic coronary heart disease including those with angina and previous myocardial infarctions.[838, 980, 982, 986]
• Exercise.[847, 981, 987]
• Hypertension.[838]
• No heart disease.[808, 981]

────────────

[aaaa]Potassium, given in a "polarizing solution" with glucose and insulin, has been purported to suppress ventricular premature beats during myocardial infarction, but this treatment has not achieved general acceptance.[930] A study performed 40 years ago suggested that potassium acts as a general antiarrhythmic drug and suppresses ventricular premature beats whether or not hypokalemia is present, the patient is receiving digitalis, or heart disease is present.[925]

[bbbb]Phenytoin gave more effective control of ventricular premature beats in 51 children than propranolol or quinidine,[764] and phenytoin has been recommended as the "drug of choice" for treating ventricular arrhythmias developing in children after surgery for congenital heart disease.[970]

Procainamide. This drug suppresses ventricular premature beats as effectively as quinidine,[847] propranolol,[847] and mexiletine,[808, 942] but not as effectively as amiodarone.[808] When given intravenously during acute myocardial infarction, procainamide suppresses ventricular premature beats as successfully as lidocaine.[979] When procainamide is administered with quinidine[988] or propafenone,[989] successful suppression can be achieved with smaller doses of each agent and less side effects in the case of quinidine than when either is given alone.[988]

Higher levels of procainamide in the blood are required to suppress ventricular premature beats in patients with chronic coronary heart disease than in those having acute myocardial infarction.[982] However, the drug can suppress early-cycle premature beats even when the total number is not reduced.[990]

Propafenone. This class IC antiarrhythmic drug, which also has slight beta-adrenergic–blocking effects, suppresses ventricular beats in many patients,[885, 886, 989, 991–1000] and it does so more effectively than disopyramide.[885, 886] Less propafenone is needed for equal suppression when given with procainamide or quinidine than when it is given alone.[989]

Quinidine. The first available class IA antiarrhythmic agent that is still employed, quinidine suppresses ventricular premature beats,[764, 901, 1001–1003] including early-cycle premature beats,[990] in patients with the following:

• Acute myocardial infarction.[145, 1004]
• Cardiomyopathy.[1005]
• Chronic coronary heart disease.[981, 988, 1002, 1005]
• Exercise.[1006]
• Hypertension.[1005]
• No heart disease.[981, 1002, 1005]

Quinidine is superior to tocainide,[1007] and equal to propafenone,[996] mexiletine,[947] and the beta-blocking agent acebutolol,[726, 835] in suppressing ventricular premature beats, but it is less effective than encainide[901, 1008, 1009] or flecainide.[902, 1005] Quinidine produces more side effects than flecainide[902] or acebutolol.[726] When given with procainamide,[988] propafenone,[989] or tocainide,[1010] quinidine suppresses these arrhythmias as effectively in lower doses and with fewer side effects.

More patients taking quinidine to suppress ventricular premature beats die than those taking flecainide, mexiletine, propafenone, or tocainide, presumably from the greater pro-arrhythmic effect of quinidine.[1011, 1012] However, quinidine can be safely initiated to outpatients with at least 30 ventricular premature beats per hour who have no evidence of such unstable clinical states as hypokalemia, digitalis toxicity, atrial fibrillation, or a prolonged QT interval.[1007]

Sotalol. Sotalol (d,l), a type III antiarrhythmic drug with beta-adrenergic blocking properties,[cccc] and d-sotalol, which has no beta-adrenergic–blocking

────────────

[cccc]Its type III antiarrhythmic properties may account for sotalol's superiority over propranolol.[843]

effects,[1013, 1014] suppress ventricular premature beats quite effectively.[816, 817, 830, 838, 839, 842–844, 1015–1019]

Tocainide. A class IB antiarrhythmic agent with properties similar to those of lidocaine and mexiletine, tocainide suppresses ventricular premature beats[820, 941, 1010, 1020–1028] in patients with a variety of cardiac abnormalities. Tocainide appears to be as safe as, but slightly less effective than, quinidine in suppressing ventricular premature beats.[1029] The antiarrhythmic effects of quinidine and tocainide, however, are additive; when given together, lower doses of either drug can be administered with greater effectiveness and fewer side effects than when one is used at a higher dose.[1010] The therapeutic effectiveness of tocainide or mexiletine does not predict the outcome with the other.[941]

Nonantiarrhythmic drug. Enalapril, an angiotensin-converting enzyme inhibitor, reduces the frequency of simple and complex ventricular premature beats in patients treated with this drug for congestive heart failure.[1030] The mechanism for this effect is unknown, but it may be due to the relief of the effects of congestive failure on the heart, rather than to specific antiarrhythmic action.

Surgery

Coronary artery bypass graft operations do not reduce the incidence of ventricular premature beats in most patients with chronic coronary heart disease.[694, 1031–1035] Surgical excision of a congenital right ventricular aneurysm cured a child of ventricular premature beats.[460]

Ablation

Ablating their origin with radiofrequency current delivered through electrode catheters can eliminate monomorphic ventricular premature beats in some patients.[757, 758, 1036–1038]

PROGNOSIS

People Without Heart Disease

The presence of *simple* ventricular premature beats does not increase the mortality of patients without heart disease.[53, 54, 67, 117, 695, 1039–1043] However, those relatively few healthy men with *frequent* (>33 ectopic beats/hour) or *complex* ventricular premature beats have a higher all-cause mortality than men without this arrhythmia.[1044dddd]

---

dddd Because these subjects are also more likely to have myocardial infarctions and to die of coronary heart disease, the investigators in the Framingham study who conducted this survey suggest that complex and frequent ventricular beats in this population may indicate the presence of subclinical coronary heart disease. Mortality is not increased in women with the arrhythmia, a finding possibly correlating with a lower incidence of coronary heart disease in the female population.[1044] An earlier study (1985), however, concluded that, "The long-term prognosis in asymptomatic healthy subjects with frequent and complex ventricular ectopy is similar to that of the healthy U.S. population and suggests no increased risk of sudden death."[1087]

In children with normal hearts, even couplets do not appear to affect prognosis.[1045] Ventricular premature beats in children disappear more often when they appear at night.[1046]

Coronary Heart Disease

During acute myocardial infarction. Because virtually all patients have ventricular premature beats during myocardial infarction, the prognostic significance of these beats during the acute event has been difficult to define. However, we do know that ventricular beats during the acute phase of the infarction do not reliably predict ventricular arrhythmias or death in patients after myocardial infarction.[26, 200, 1041, 1047–1049]

After myocardial infarction. The presence of ventricular premature beats after recovery from myocardial infarction[117, 191, 1050, 1051] increases mortality[173, 179, 189, 1052] for one[1053] and possibly two[195, 200, 1054] or more years after the acute event. Even one[174, 184, 652] or two[1055] ectopic beats per hour will raise the risk of death over that of patients who do not have them. Frequent and complex beats,[42, 43, 49, 170, 178, 179, 189–191, 194, 195, 1056–1059] but not parasystole,[170, 1060] increase the risk further.[1061–1065eeee] The development of ventricular premature beats on predischarge exercise testing provides further and possibly more predictive information about subsequent cardiac death than do the results of ambulatory monitoring.[712]

Although ventricular premature beats often occur in patients with reduced left ventricular function, which by itself helps to determine survival,[179, 193, 196, 1066–1071] ventricular beats independently predict premature death.[179, 195, 196, 1060ffff] When both ventricular beats and poor ventricular function are present, survival is reduced even further.[179, 196] Diminished cardiac function, quantitated by the left ventricular ejection fraction, more accurately predicts reduced survival during the first 6 months after myocardial infarction, whereas ventricular premature beats more reliably define mortality after 6 months.[195]

Chronic Cardiovascular Disease

Ventricular premature beats increase mortality in patients with heart disease in general,[1040] and particularly in those with chronic coronary disease even when unrelated to recent myocardial infarction.[39, 40, 53, 98, 100, 178, 695, 698, 1066, 1072, 1073] The mortality is higher in patients with chronic heart disease who also have

- Angina on effort even when they have not had myocardial infarction.[1074]
- Been resuscitated from out-of-hospital ventricular fibrillation and have complex ventricular premature beats subsequently[192] or have subtherapeutic levels of procainamide or quinidine.[785]

---

eeee Predicting the danger that ventricular premature beats present to patients with coronary heart disease has led investigators to develop categories of risk based on the electrocardiographic features of the beats.[1061–1065]
ffff Although possibly not when induced by exercise.[695, 1088]

- Received a transplanted heart and have complex ventricular premature beats.[348]
- Idiopathic dilated cardiomyopathy and persistent[280, 1075] or frequent complex[279, 289, 1073, 1076–1079] ventricular premature beats.
- Left ventricular hypertrophy and frequent (> 30 beats/min) or complex ventricular premature beats.[1080]
- Ventricular premature beats during exercise testing.[209]

The presence of ventricular premature beats does not predict which patients with repaired tetralogy of Fallot are at high risk of sudden death.[332]

Induction of Sustained Arrhythmias

The incidence of major arrhythmic events including cardiac arrest is very low in patients with high-grade ventricular ectopy in whom sustained ventricular tachycardia or ventricular fibrillation cannot be induced during electrophysiological study.[754–756] However, the prognosis may be worse for children with couplets and abnormal hearts in whom ventricular tachycardia can be induced than in children with normal hearts.[1045]

SUMMARY

The frequency of ventricular premature beats, the most common arrhythmia in humans, increases as we age. They occur more often in men than in women. Although present in many healthy persons, the beats are seldom complex (repetitive, bigeminal, frequent, or multiform). Ventricular premature beats occur in every patient with myocardial infarction and more frequently in those who have sustained more myocardial damage. Successful thrombolysis is often associated with additional simple and complex beats soon after therapy. Many patients have premature beats after recovery from myocardial infarction. Patients with angina pectoris have more ventricular premature beats than those without the condition, and both simple and complex beats frequently develop during episodes of coronary vasospasm.

Most patients with mitral valve prolapse have no more ventricular premature beats than patients without the lesion. Other conditions giving rise to ventricular premature beats include cardiomyopathy, hypertension, pulmonary disease, congenital heart disease, cardiac surgery, metabolic disturbances, alcohol consumption, and use of certain drugs. The time of day, whether one is awake or asleep, and stress also affect the frequency of ventricular premature beats.

Palpitations are the principal symptom produced by the arrhythmia, and the patient is usually aware of the premature beat itself as well as the strong sinus beat afterward. Principal physical findings include the premature beat in the pulse, the abnormality of the heart rhythm, cannon A waves, and variations in the heart sounds.

The form of the QRS complexes of ventricular premature beats is characteristically abnormal. The duration of these complexes is prolonged, and they are sometimes tall or deep. Ambulatory electrocardiographic monitoring best defines the frequency in character of premature beats in individual patients. The longer the recordings are made, up to a point, the more premature beats are detected. Spontaneous variability distorts analysis of the effects of treatment. Exercise can also expose premature beats. Clinical electrophysiological study can identify ventricular premature beats when the diagnosis is confused with aberrant conduction of supraventricular beats.

Few patients with ventricular premature beats require specific therapy. Although many antiarrhythmic drugs are effective, they can reduce ventricular function and may endanger the patient's life because of their proarrhythmic effect. Beta-blocking drugs can be helpful for a few patients with intolerable symptoms. Antiarrhythmic therapy does not prolong survival in patients with ventricular premature beats and myocardial infarction and may increase mortality. Coronary artery bypass graft surgery does not reduce the incidence of ventricular premature beats.

The prognosis is worse for patients with established coronary heart disease and ventricular premature beats than for those without the arrhythmia. When ventricular premature beats are present and ventricular function is diminished, survival is reduced further. Ventricular premature beats also increase mortality in patients with other forms of chronic heart disease including patients resuscitated from out-of-hospital ventricular fibrillation, those with cardiomyopathy, and those who have undergone cardiac transplantation.

REFERENCES

1. Bigger JT Jr. Ventricular premature complexes. In Kastor JA, (ed). Arrhythmias. Philadelphia: WB Saunders, 1994, pp. 310–335.
2. Kastor JA. Ventricular premature beats. Adv Intern Med 1983; 28:63–91.
3. Scherf D. The mechanism and treatment of extrasystoles. Prog Cardiovasc Dis 1959; 2:370–390.
4. Chung EK. Principles of Cardiac Arrhythmias. Baltimore: Williams & Wilkins, 1971, p. 312.
5. Zipes DP, Fisch C. Premature ventricular beats. Arch Intern Med 1971; 128:140–142.
6. Scherf D, Schott A. Extrasystoles and Allied Arrhythmias. 2nd ed. Chicago: Year Book Medical Publishers, 1973, pp. VII–IX.
7. Cobb LA, Werner JA. Antiarrhythmic therapy, ventricular premature depolarizations and sudden cardiac death: the tip of the iceberg. Circulation 1979; 59:864–865.
8. Guize L, Le Heuzey JY, Cabanis C, Chretien JM, Maurice P. Chronic ventricular extrasystoles: clinical aspects, prognosis, and indication for treatment. In Levy S, Scheinman MM (eds). Cardiac Arrhythmias. From Diagnosis to Therapy. Mount Kisco, NY: Futura Publishing Co., 1984, pp. 341–355.
9. Morganroth J. Premature ventricular complexes: diagnosis and indications for therapy. JAMA 1984; 252:673–676.
10. Garson A. Ventricular arrhythmias. In Gillette PC, Garson A Jr. (eds). Pediatric Arrhythmias. Electrophysiology and Pacing. Philadelphia: WB Saunders Company, 1990, pp. 427–432.
11. Josephson ME. Clinical Cardiac Electrophysiology. Techniques and Interpretations. 2nd ed. Philadelphia: Lea & Febiger, 1993, pp. 173–179.

12. Rubin AM, Morganroth J, Kowey PR. Ventricular premature depolarizations. In Podrid PJ, Kowey PR (eds). Cardiac Arrhythmia. Mechanisms, Diagnosis and Management. Baltimore: Williams & Wilkins, 1995, pp. 891–906.

13. Brugada P, Wellens HJJ. To beat or not to beat: arguments for use of the term ventricular premature depolarization. Am J Cardiol 1985; 55:1113–1114.

14. Roberts WC. I still prefer *ventricular premature complex*. Am J Cardiol 1985; 55:1117–1118.

15. White PD. Heart Disease. 4th ed. New York: Macmillan, 1951, pp. 866–877.

16. Spodick DH. Vogue words: ectopic language. JAMA 1978; 240:2439–2440.

17. Julian DG. A complex matter. Eur Heart J 1984; 5:513–514.

18. Marriott HJ. Depolarization, contraction, systole, complex, or beat? Take your choice, but may my sinus node go on beating. Heart Lung 1987; 16:117–119.

19. Lombardi F. Do we still need to count premature ventricular contractions? Eur Heart J 1995; 16:582–583.

20. Spodick DH. Ventricular ectopy. Br Heart J 1980; 43:367.

21. Spodick DH. Arrhythmias and sinus node dysfunction. JAMA 1984; 251:2513–2514.

22. Spodick DH. Cardiolocution. Am J Cardiol 1981; 48:973–974.

23. Schamroth L. Premature ventricular contraction or ventricular extrasystole? Am J Cardiol 1983; 51:1783–1784.

24. Schamroth L. North American malady: usage and meaning of "extrasystole." Heart Lung 1987; 16:119–121.

25. Marriott HJL. Practical Electrocardiography. 8th ed. Baltimore: Williams & Wilkins, 1988, p. 134.

26. Messineo FC. Ventricular ectopic activity: prevalence and risk. Am J Cardiol 1989; 64:53J–56J.

27. White PD. Heart Disease. 4th ed. New York: Macmillan, 1951, p. 866.

28. Katz LN, Pick A. Clinical Electrocardiography. Part I. The Arrhythmias. Philadelphia: Lea & Febiger, 1956, p. 43.

29. Katz LN, Pick A. Clinical Electrocardiography. Part I. The Arrhythmias. Philadelphia: Lea & Febiger, 1956, p. 159.

30. Friedberg CK. Diseases of the Heart. 3rd ed. Philadelphia: WB Saunders, 1966, pp. 496–511.

31. White PD, Donovan H. Hearts. Their Long Follow-up. Philadelphia: WB Saunders, 1967, pp. 250–251.

32. Anonymous. Paul Wood's Diseases of the Heart and Circulation. 3rd ed. Philadelphia, JB Lippincott, 1968, p. 256.

33. Sherman H, Sandberg S, Fineberg HV. Exponential increase in age-specific prevalence of ventricular dysrhythmia among males. J Chronic Dis 1982; 35:743–750.

34. Fleg JL. Ventricular arrhythmias in the elderly: prevalence, mechanisms, and therapeutic implications. Geriatrics 1988; 43:23–29.

35. Lewis T. Electrocardiography and Clinical Disorders of the Heart Beat. London: Shaw & Sons, 1949.

36. Hollman A. Sir Thomas Lewis. London: Springer Verlag, 1997.

37. Hiss RG, Averill KH, Lamb LE. Electrocardiographic findings in 67,375 asymptomatic subjects. III. Ventricular rhythms. Am J Cardiol 1960; 6:96–107

38. Okajima M, Scholmerich P, Simonson E. Frequency of premature beats in 715 healthy adult subjects. Minn Med 1960; 43:751–753.

39. Chiang BN, Perlman LV, Ostrander LD Jr, Epstein FH. Relationship of premature systoles to coronary heart disease and sudden death in the Tecumseh epidemiologic study. Ann Intern Med 1969; 70:1159–1166.

40. Hinkle LE, Carver ST, Argyros DC, Stevens M, Horvath J. The prognostic significance of ventricular premature contractions in healthy people and in people with coronary heart disease. Acta Cardiol 1974; 18:5–32.

41. Crow RS, Prineas RJ, Dias V, Taylor HL, Jacobs D, Blackburn H. Ventricular premature beats in a population sample: frequency and associations with coronary risk characteristics. Circulation 1975; 52:211–215.

42. Rehnqvist N, Lundman T, Sjogren A. Prognostic implications of ventricular arrhythmias registered before discharge and one year after acute myocardial infarction. Acta Med Scand 1978; 204:203–209.

43. Rehnqvist N. Ventricular arrhythmias after an acute myocardial infarction: prognostic weight and natural history. Eur J Cardiol 1978; 7:169–187.

44. Hennekens CH, Lown B, Rosner B, Grufferman S, Dalen J. Ventricular premature beats and coronary risk factors. Am J Epidemiol 1980; 112:93–99.

45. Kostis JB, McCrone K, Moreyra AE, Hosler M, Cosgrove N, Kuo PT. The effect of age, blood pressure and gender on the incidence of premature ventricular contractions. Angiology 1982; 33:464–473.

46. Uretz EF, Denes P, Ruggie N, Vasilomanolakis E, Messer JV. Relation of ventricular premature beats to underlying heart disease. Am J Cardiol 1984; 53:774–780.

47. Rajala S, Kaltiala K, Haavisto M, Mattila K. Prevalence of ECG findings in very old people. Eur Heart J 1984; 5:168–174.

48. Cohen JD, Neaton JD, Prineas RJ, Daniels KA. Diuretics, serum potassium and ventricular arrhythmias in the multiple risk factor intervention trial. Am J Cardiol 1987; 60:548–554.

49. Kostis JB, Byington R, Friedman LM, Goldstein S, Furberg C. Prognostic significance of ventricular ectopic activity in survivors of acute myocardial infarction. J Am Coll Cardiol 1987; 10:231–242.

50. Celentano A, Galderisi M, Mureddu GF, Garofalo M, Tammaro P, de Divitiis O. Arrhythmias, hypertensions and the elderly: Holter evaluation. J Hypertens Suppl 1988; 6:29–32.

51. Schmieder RE, Messerli FH. Determinants of ventricular ectopy in hypertensive cardiac hypertrophy. Am Heart J 1992; 123:89–95.

52. Hiss RG, Lamb LE. Electrocardiographic findings in 122,043 individuals. Circulation 1962; 25:947–961.

53. Desai DC, Hershberg PI, Alexander S. Clinical significance of ventricular premature beats in an outpatient population. Chest 1973; 64: 564–569.

54. Fisher FD, Tyroler HA. Relationship between ventricular premature contractions on routine electrocardiography and subsequent sudden death from coronary heart disease. Circulation 1973; 47:712–719.

55. Raftery EB, Cashman PM. Long-term recording of the electrocardiogram in a normal population. Postgrad Med J 1976; 52:32–38.

56. Ekblom B, Hartley LH, Day WC. Occurrence and reproducibility of exercise-induced ventricular ectopy in normal subjects. Am J Cardiol 1979; 43:35–40.

57. Lichstein E, Jonas S, Smith H Jr, Chadda KD, Gupta PK, Sudberg L. Characteristics of ventricular ectopic beats in patients with ventricular tachycardia: 24-hour Holter monitor study. Chest 1980; 77:731–735.

58. Kennedy HL, Pescarmona JE, Bouchard RJ, Goldberg RJ. Coronary artery status of apparently healthy subjects with frequent and complex ventricular ectopy. An Intern Med 1980; 92:179–185.

59. Prineas RJ, Jacobs DR Jr, Crow RS, Blackburn H. Coffee, tea and VPB. Chronic Dis 1980; 33:67–72.

60. Bethge KP, Bethge D, Meiners G, Lichtlen PR. Incidence and prognostic significance of ventricular arrhythmias in individuals without detectable heart disease. Eur Heart J 1983; 4:338–346.

61. Orth-Gomer K, Hogstedt C, Bodin L, Soderholm B. Frequency of extrasystoles in healthy male employees. Br Heart J 1986; 55:259–264.

62. Bjerregaard P, Sorensen KE, Molgaard H. Predictive value of ventricular premature beats for subsequent ischaemic heart disease in apparently healthy subjects. Eur Heart J 1991; 12:597–601.

63. Manolio TA, Furberg CD, Rautaharju PM, et al. Cardiac arrhythmias on 24-h ambulatory electrocardiography in older women and men: the cardiovascular health study. J Am Coll Cardiol 1994; 23:916–925.

64. Vlay SC, Reid PR. Ventricular ectopy: etiology, evaluation, and therapy. Am J Med 1982; 73:899–913.

65. Moss AJ. Clinical significance of ventricular arrhythmias in

patients with and without coronary artery disease. Prog Cardiovasc Dis 1980; 23:33–52.

66. Moss AJ. Detection, significance and management of VPBs in ambulatory patients. Cardiovasc Clin 1980; 11:143–158.

67. Barrett PA, Peter CT, Swan HJC, Singh BN, Mandel WJ. The frequency and prognostic significance of electrocardiographic abnormalities in clinically normal individuals. Prog Cardiovasc Dis 1981; 23:299–319.

68. Ruskin JN. Ventricular extrasystoles in healthy subjects. N Engl J Med 1985; 312:238–239.

69. Garson A. Jr. Ventricular arrhythmias. In Gillette PC, Garson A Jr. (eds). Pediatric Arrhythmias Electrophysiology and Pacing. Philadelphia: WB Saunders 1990, pp. 427–500.

70. Shenker L. Fetal cardiac arrhythmias. Obstet Gynecol Surv 1979; 34:561–572.

71. Stevens DC, Schreiner RL, Hurwitz RA, Gresham EL. Fetal and neonatal ventricular arrhythmia. Pediatrics 1979; 63:771–777.

72. Southall DP, Johnson AM, Shinebourne EA, Johnston PG, Vulliamy DG. Frequency and outcome of disorders of cardiac rhythm and conduction in a population of newborn infants. Pediatrics 1981; 68:58–66.

73. Southall DP, Richards J, Mitchell P, Brown DJ, Johnston PG, Shinebourne EA. Study of cardiac rhythm in healthy newborn infants. Br Heart J 1980; 43:14–20.

74. Southall DP, Richards J, Brown DJ, Johnston PG, de Swiet M, Shinebourne EA. 24-hour tape recordings of ECG and respiration in the newborn infant with findings related to sudden death and unexplained brain damage in infancy. Arch Dis Child 1980; 55:7–61.

75. Scott O, Williams GJ, Fiddler GI. Results of 24-hour ambulatory monitoring of electrocardiogram in 131 healthy boys aged 10 to 13 years. Br Heart J 1980; 44:304–308.

76. Dickinson DF, Scott O. Ambulatory electrocardiographic monitoring in 100 healthy teenage boys. Br Heart J 1984; 51:179–183.

77. Clarke JM, Hamer J, Shelton JR, Taylor S, Venning GR. The rhythm of the normal human heart. Lancet 1976; 1:508–512.

78. Brodsky M, Wu D, Denes P, Kanakis C, Rosen KM. Arrhythmias documented by 24-hour continuous electrocardiographic monitoring in 50 male medical students without apparent heart disease. Am J Cardiol 1977; 39:390–395.

79. Kennedy HL, Chandra V, Sayther KL, Caralis DG. Effectiveness of increasing hours of continuous ambulatory electrocardiography in detecting maximal ventricular ectopy: continuous 48 hour study of patients with coronary heart disease and normal subjects. Am J Cardiol 1978; 42:925–930.

80. Bjerregaard P. Premature beats in healthy subjects 40–79 years of age. Eur Heart J 1982; 3:493–503.

81. Takada H, Mikawa T, Murayama M, Sugai J, Yamamura Y. Range of ventricular ectopic complexes in healthy subjects studied with repeated ambulatory electrocardiographic recordings. Am J Cardiol 1989; 63:184–186.

82. Jacobsen JR, Garson A Jr, Gillette PC, McNamara DG. Premature ventricular contractions in normal children. J Pediatr 1978; 92:36–38.

83. Elkon KB, Swerdlow TA, Myburgh DP. Persistent ventricular ectopic beats: a long-term study. S Afr Med J 1977; 52:564–566.

84. Hall CG, Stewart LC, Manning GW. The electrocardiographic records of 2,000 R.C.A.F. aircrew. Can Med Assoc J 1942; 46:226–230.

85. Graybiel A, McFarland RA, Gates DC, Webster FA. Analysis of the electrocardiograms obtained from 1,000 young healthy aviators. Am Heart J 1944; 27:524–549.

86. McNamara RJ. A study of the electrocardiogram in persons over seventy. Geriatrics 1949; 4:150–160.

87. Wosika PH, Feldman E, Chesrow EJ, Myers GB. Unipolar precordial and limb lead electrocardiograms in the aged. Geriatrics 1950; 5:131–141.

88. Packard JM, Graettinger JS, Graybiel A. Analysis of the electrocardiograms obtained from 1,000 young healthy aviators: ten year follow-up. Circulation 1954; 10:384–400.

89. Gelfand ML. The octogenarian electrocardiogram. Geriatrics 1957; 12:156–161.

90. Federman J, Whitford JA, Anderson ST, Pitt A. Incidence of ventricular arrhythmias in first year after myocardial infarction. Br Heart J 1978; 40:1243–1250.

91. DeMaria AN, Amsterdam EA, Vismara LA, Neumann A, Mason DT. Arrhythmias in the mitral valve prolapse syndrome: prevalence, nature, and frequency. Ann Intern Med 1976; 84:656–660.

92. Kostis JB, McCrone K, Moreyra AE, et al. Premature ventricular complexes in the absence of identifiable heart disease. Circulation 1981; 63:1351–1356.

93. Sobotka PA, Mayer JH, Bauernfeind RA, Kanakis C Jr, Rosen KM. Arrhythmias documented by 24-hour continuous ambulatory electrocardiographic monitoring in young women without apparent heart disease. Am Heart J 1981; 101:753–759.

94. Bellet S, Roman L, Kostis J, Slater A. Continuous electrocardiographic monitoring during automobile driving: studies in normal subjects and patients with coronary disease. Am J Cardiol 1968; 22:856–862.

95. Glasser SP, Clark PI, Applebaum HJ. Occurrence of frequent complex arrhythmias detected by ambulatory monitoring: findings in an apparently healthy asymptomatic elderly population. Chest 1979; 75:565–568.

96. Camm AJ, Evans KE, Ward DE, Martin A. The rhythm of the heart in active elderly subjects. Am Heart J 1980; 99:598–603.

97. Kantelip JP, Sage E, Duchene-Marullaz P. Findings on ambulatory electrocardiographic monitoring in subjects older than 80 years. Am J Cardiol 1986; 57:398–401.

98. Ingerslev J, Bjerregaard P. Prevalence and prognostic significance of cardiac arrhythmias detected by ambulatory electrocardiography in subjects 85 years of age. Eur Heart J 1986; 7:570–575.

99. Martin A, Benbow LJ, Butrous GS, Leach C, Camm AJ. Five-year follow-up of 101 elderly subjects by means of long-term ambulatory cardiac monitoring. Eur Heart J 1984; 5:592–596.

100. Hedblad B, Janzon L, Johansson BW, Juul-Moller S. Survival and incidence of myocardial infarction in men with ambulatory ECG-detected frequent and complex ventricular arrhythmias: 10 year follow-up of the "men born 1914" study in Malmo, Sweden. Eur Heart J 1997; 18:1787–1795.

101. Montague TJ, Taylor PG, Stockton R, Roy DL, Smith ER. The spectrum of cardiac rate and rhythm in normal newborns. Pediatr Cardiol 1982; 2:33–38.

102. Manning GW. Electrocardiography in the selection of Royal Canadian Air Force aircrew. Circulation 1954; 10:401–412.

103. Romhilt DW, Chaffin C, Choi SC, Irby EC. Arrhythmias on ambulatory electrocardiographic monitoring in women without apparent heart disease. Am J Cardiol 1984; 54:582–586.

104. Clee MD, Smith N, McNeill GP, Wright DS. Dysrhythmias in apparently healthy elderly subjects. Age Ageing 1979; 8:173–176.

105. Kennedy HL, Underhill SJ. Frequent or complex ventricular ectopy in apparently healthy subjects: a clinical study of 25 cases. Am J Cardiol 1976; 38:141–148.

106. Huston TP, Puffer JC, Rodney WM. The athletic heart syndrome. N Engl J Med 1985; 313:24–32.

107. Hanne-Paparo N, Kellermann JJ. Long-term Holter ECG monitoring of athletes. Med Sci Sports Exerc 1981; 13:294–298.

108. Talan DA, Bauernfeind RA, Ashley WW, Kanakis C Jr, Rosen KM. Twenty-four hour continuous ECG recordings in long-distance runners. Chest 1982; 82:19–24.

109. Viitasalo MT, Kala R, Eisalo A. Ambulatory electrocardiographic recording in endurance athletes. Br Heart J 1982; 47:213–220.

110. Pilcher GF, Cook AJ, Johnston BL, Fletcher GF. Twenty-four-hour continuous electrocardiography during exercise and free activity in 80 apparently healthy runners. Am J Cardiol 1983; 52:859–861.

111. Palatini P, Maraglino G, Sperti G, et al. Prevalence and possible mechanisms of ventricular arrhythmias in athletes. Am Heart J 1985; 110:560–567.

112. Zehender M, Meinertz T, Keul J, Just H. ECG variants and cardiac arrhythmias in athletes: clinical relevance and prognostic importance. Am Heart J 1990; 119:1378–1391.

113. Horan MJ, Kennedy HL. Characteristics and prognosis of apparently healthy patients with frequent and complex ventricular ectopy: evidence for a relatively benign new syndrome with occult myocardial and/or coronary disease. Am Heart J 1981; 102:809–810.

114. Rabkin SW, Mathewson FA, Tate RB. Relationship of ventricular ectopy in men without apparent heart disease to occurrence of ischemic heart disease and sudden death. Am Heart J 1981; 101:135–142.

115. Bigger JT Jr, Dresdale FJ, Heissenbuttel RH, Weld FM, Wit AL. Ventricular arrhythmias in ischemic heart disease: mechanism, prevalence, significance, and management. Prog Cardiovasc Dis 1977; 19:255–300.

116. Campbell RWF, Julian DG. Incidence, prevalence and significance of ventricular ectopic activity in acute myocardial infarction. In Sandoe E, Julian DG, Bell JW (eds). Management of Ventricular Tachycardia. Role of Mexiletine. Amsterdam: Excerpta Medica, 1978, pp. 457–464.

117. Moss AJ. Clinical significance of ventricular arrhythmias in patients with and without coronary artery disease. Prog Cardiovasc Dis 1980; 23:33–52.

118. Master AM, Dack S, Jaffe HL. Disturbances of rate and rhythm in acute coronary artery thrombosis. Ann Intern Med 1937; 11:735–761.

119. Imperial ES, Carballo R, Zimmerman HA. Disturbances in rate, rhythm and conduction in acute myocardial infarction: a statistical study of 153 cases. Am J Cardiol 1960; 5:24–29.

120. Peel AAF, Semple T, Wang I, Lancaster WM, Dall JLG. A coronary prognostic index for grading the severity of infarction. Br Heart J 1962; 24:745–760.

121. Julian DG, Valentine PA, Miller GG. Disturbances of rate, rhythm and conduction in acute myocardial infarction: a prospective study of 100 consecutive unselected patients with the aid of electrocardiographic monitoring. Am J Med 1964; 37:915–927.

122. Meltzer LE, Kitchell JB. The incidence of arrhythmias associated with acute myocardial infarction. Prog Cardiovasc Dis 1966; 9:50–63.

123. Robinson JS, Sloman G, McRae C. Continuous electrocardiographic monitoring in the early stages after acute myocardial infarction. Med J Aust 1964; 1:427–432.

124. Spann JF, Moellering RC, Haber E, Wheeler EO. Arrhythmias in acute myocardial infarction: A study utilizing an electrocardiographic monitor for automatic detection and recording of arrhythmias. N Engl J Med 1964; 271:427–431.

125. Day HW. Effectiveness of an intensive coronary care area. Am J Cardiol 1965; 15:51–54.

126. Kurland GS, Pressman D. The incidence of arrhythmias in acute myocardial infarction studies with a constant monitoring system. Circulation 1965; 31:834–841.

127. Fluck DC, Olsen E, Pentecost BL, et al. Natural history and clinical significance of arrhythmias after acute cardiac infarction. Br Heart J 1967; 29:170–189.

128. Stock E, Goble A, Sloman G. Assessment of arrhythmias in myocardial infarction BMJ 1967; 2:719–723.

129. Langhorne WH. The coronary care unit: a year's experience in a community hospital. JAMA 1967; 201:92–95.

130. Lawrie DM, Goddard M, Greenwood TW, et al. A coronary care unit in the routine management of acute myocardial infarction. Lancet 1967; 2:109–114.

131. Lown B, Fakhro AM, Hood WB Jr, Thorn GW. The coronary care unit: new perspectives and directions. JAMA 1967; 199:188–198.

132. Lown B, Vasaux C, Hood WB Jr, Fakhro AM, Kaplinsky E, Roberge G. Unresolved problems in coronary care. Am J Cardiol 1967; 20:494–508.

133. MacMillan RL, Brown KWG, Peckham GB, Kahn O, Hutchison DB, Paton M. Changing perspectives in coronary care. Am J Cardiol 1967; 20:451–456.

134. Day HW. Acute coronary care: a five year report. Am J Cardiol 1968; 21:252–257.

135. Kimball JT, Killip T. Aggressive treatment of arrhythmias in acute myocardial infarction: procedures and results. Prog Cardiovasc Dis 1968; 10:483–504.

136. Norris RM. Acute coronary care. N Z Med J 1968; 67:470–476.

137. Wyman MG, Hammersmith L. Coronary care in the small community hospital. Dis Chest 1968; 53:584–591.

138. Lown B, Klein MD, Hershberg PI. Coronary and precoronary care. Am J Med 1969; 46:705–724.

139. Mogensen L. Ventricular tachyarrhythmias and lignocaine prophylaxis in acute myocardial infarction. Acta Med Scand 1970; 513:1–89.

140. Adgey AAJ, Geddes JS, Webb SW, et al. Acute phase of myocardial infarction. Lancet 1971; 2:501–504.

141. Chaturvedi NC, Shivalingappa G, Shanks B, et al. Myocardial infarction in the elderly. Lancet 1972; 1:280–282.

142. DeSanctis RW, Block P, Hutter AM Jr. Tachyarrhythmias in myocardial infarction. Circulation 1972; 45:681–702.

143. Skjaeggestad O. Arrhythmias in different types of acute coronary heart diseases. Acta Med Scand 1973; 193:299–302.

144. Romhilt DW, Bloomfield SS, Chou T-C, Fowler NO. Unreliability of conventional electrocardiographic monitoring for arrhythmia detection in coronary care units. Am J Cardiol 1973; 31:457–461.

145. Jones DT, Kostuk WJ, Gunton RW. Prophylactic quinidine for the prevention of arrhythmias after acute myocardial infarction. Am J Cardiol 1974; 33:655–660.

146. Vetter NJ, Julian DG. Comparison of arrhythmia computer and conventional monitoring in coronary-care unit. Lancet 1975; 1:1151–1154.

147. Campbell RW, Murrary A, Julian DG. Ventricular arrhythmias in first 12 hours of acute myocardial infarction: natural history study. Br Heart J 1981; 46:351–357.

148. Maggioni AP, Zuanetti G, Franzosi MG, et al. Prevalence and prognostic significance of ventricular arrhythmias after acute myocardial infarction in the fibrinolytic era: GISSI-2 results. Circulation 1993; 87:312–322.

149. Humphries JO, Taylor G, Baird M, Schulze RA, Pitt B, Griffith L. Ventricular irritability in the late hospital phase of acute myocardial infarction: relationship to left ventricular and coronary anatomy. In Sandoe E, Julian DG, Bell JW (eds). Management of Ventricular Tachycardia. Role of Mexiletine. Amsterdam: Excerpta Medica, 1978, pp. 487–496.

150. Chapman BL. Relation of cardiac complications to SGOT level in acute myocardial infarction. Br Heart J 1972; 34:890–896.

151. Roberts R, Husain A, Ambos HD, Oliver GC, Cox JR, Sobel BE. Relation between infarct size and ventricular arrhythmia. Br Heart J 1975; 37:1169–1175.

152. Gressin V, Louvard Y, Pezzano M, Lardoux H. Holter recording of ventricular arrhythmias during intravenous thrombolysis for acute myocardial infarction. Am J Cardiol 1992; 69:152–159.

153. Nielsen BL. ST-segment elevation in acute myocardial infarction: prognostic importance. Circulation 1973; 48:338–345.

154. Dorian P, Langer A, Morgan C, Casella L, Harris L, Armstrong P. Importance of ST-segment depression as a determinant of ventricular premature complex frequency after thrombolysis for acute myocardial infarction. Tissue plasminogen activator: Toronto (TPAT) study group. Am J Cardiol 1994; 74:419–423.

155. Marino P, Nidasio G, Golia G, et al. Frequency of predischarge ventricular arrhythmias in postmyocardial infarction patients depends on residual left ventricular pump performance and is independent of the occurrence of acute reperfusion: the GISSI-2 investigators. J Am Coll Cardiol 1994; 23:290–295.

156. Scheinman MM, Abbott JA. Clinical significance of transmural versus nontransmural electrocardiographic changes in patients with acute myocardial infarction. Am J Med 1973; 55:602–607.

157. Madias JE, Chahine RA, Gorlin R, Blacklow DJ. A comparison of transmural and nontransmural acute myocardial infarction. Circulation 1974; 49:498–507.

158. Thanavaro S, Krone RJ, Kleiger RE, et al. In-hospital prognosis of patients with first nontransmural and transmural infarctions. Circulation 1980; 61:29–33.

159. Cercek B, Lew AS, Laramee P, Shah PK, Peter TC, Ganz W. Time course and characteristics of ventricular arrhythmias after reperfusion in acute myocardial infarction. Am J Cardiol 1987; 60:214–218.

160. Alexopoulos D, Collins R, Adamopoulos S, Peto R, Sleight P. Holter monitoring of ventricular arrhythmias in a randomised, controlled study of intravenous streptokinase in acute myocardial infarction. Br Heart J 1991; 65:9–13.

161. Meinertz T, Treese N, Kasper W, et al. Determinants of prognosis in idiopathic dilated cardiomyopathy as determined by programmed electrical stimulation. Am J Cardiol 1985; 56:337–341.

162. Wilcox RG, Eastgate J, Harrison E, Skene AM. Ventricular arrhythmias during treatment with Alteplase (recombinant tissue plasminogen activator) in suspected acute myocardial infarction. Br Heart J 1991; 65:4–8.

163. Hohnloser SH, Zabel M, Olschewski M, Kasper W, Just H. Arrhythmias during the acute phase of reperfusion therapy for acute myocardial infarction: effects of beta-adrenergic blockage. Am Heart J 1992; 123:1530–1535.

164. Kuzuya T, Hoshida S, Suzuki K, et al. Polymorphonuclear leukocyte activity and ventricular arrhythmia in acute myocardial infarction. Am J Cardiol 1988; 62:868–872.

165. Talbot S. Prognostic importance of ventricular extrasystoles in acute myocardial infarction. Postgrad Med J 1977; 53:69–74.

166. Moss AJ, Davis HT, DeCamilla J, Bayer LW. Ventricular ectopic beats and their relation to sudden and nonsudden cardiac death after myocardial infarction. Circulation 1979; 60:998–1003.

167. Restieaux N, Bray C, Bullard H, et al. 150 patients with cardiac infarction treated in a coronary unit. Lancet 1967; 1:1285–1289.

168. Moss AJ, Schnitzler R, Green R, Decamilla J. Ventricular arrhythmias 3 weeks after acute myocardial infarction. Ann Intern Med 1971; 75:837–841.

169. Coronary Drug Project Research Group. Prognostic importance of premature beats following myocardial infarction: experience in the Coronary Drug Project. JAMA 1973; 223:1116–1124.

170. Kotler MN, Tabatznik B, Mower MM, Tominaga S. Prognostic significance of ventricular ectopic beats with respect to sudden death in the late postinfarction period. Circulation 1973; 47:959–966.

171. Kleiger RE, Martin TF, Miller JP, Oliver GC. Ventricular tachycardia and ventricular extrasystoles during the late recovery phase of myocardial infarction. Am J Cardiol 1974; 33:149.

172. Schulze RA Jr, Rouleau J, Rigo P, Bowers S, Strauss HW, Pitt B. Ventricular arrhythmias in the late hospital phase of acute myocardial infarction: relation to left ventricular function detected by gated cardiac blood pool scanning. Circulation 1975; 52:1006–1011.

173. Vismara LA, Amsterdam EA, Mason DT. Relation of ventricular arrhythmias in the late hospital phase of acute myocardial infarction to sudden death after hospital discharge. Am J Med 1975; 59:6–12.

174. Luria MH, Knoke JD, Margolis RM, Hendricks FH, Kuplic JB. Acute myocardial infarction: prognosis after recovery. Ann Intern Med 1976; 85:561–565.

175. Moss AJ, DeCamilla J, Davis HP, Bayer L. The early posthospital phase of myocardial infarction: prognostic stratification. Circulation 1976; 54:58–64.

176. Kennedy HL, Caralis DG, Khan MA, Poblete PF, Pescarmona JE. Ventricular arrhythmia 24 hours before and after maximal treadmill testing. Am Heart J 1977; 94:718–724.

177. Moss AJ, DeCamilla JJ, Davis HP, Bayer L. Clinical significance of ventricular ectopic beats in the early posthospital phase of myocardial infarction. Am J Cardiol 1977; 39:635–640.

178. Ruberman W, Weinblatt E, Goldberg JD, Frank CW, Shapiro S. Ventricular premature beats and mortality after myocardial infarction. N Engl J Med 1977; 297:750–757.

179. Schulze RA Jr, Strauss HW, Pitt B. Sudden death in the year following myocardial infarction: relation to ventricular premature contractions in the late hospital phase and left ventricular ejection fraction. Am J Med 1977; 62:192–199.

180. Bigger JT Jr, Heller CA, Wenger TL, Weld FM. Risk stratification after acute myocardial infarction. Am J Cardiol 1978; 42:202–210.

181. Rehnqvist N. Ventricular arrhythmias prior to discharge after acute myocardial infarction. Eur J Cardiol 1976; 4:63–70.

182. Rehnqvist N, Sjogren A. Ventricular arrhythmias prior to discharge and one year after acute myocardial infarction. Eur J Cardiol 1977; 5:425–442.

183. Lie KI, van Capelle FJ, Durrer D. Limitations of 24 hour ambulatory electrocardiographic recording in predicting coronary events after acute myocardial infarction. Am J Cardiol 1979; 44:1257–1262.

184. Luria MH, Knoke JD, Wachs JS, Luria MA. Survival after recovery from acute myocardial infarction: two and five year prognostic indices. Am J Med 1979; 67:7–14.

185. Federman J, Whitford JA, Anderson ST, Pitt A. The effect of a selective beta adrenergic blocking agent on ventricular arrhythmias in the first year following myocardial infarction. Aust N Z J Med 1980; 10:289–294.

186. DeCamilla JJ, Davis HT, Moss AJ. Frequency and complexity of ventricular ectopic beats in the posthospital phase of myocardial infarction. J Electrocardiol 1980; 13:125–134.

187. Moller M, Nielsen BL, Fabricius J. The spontaneous variation in the pattern of ventricular extrasystoles in patients recently recovered from an acute myocardial infarction. Clin Cardiol 1980; 3:106–110.

188. Morrison GW, Kumar EB, Portal RW, Aber CP. Cardiac arrhythmias 48 hours before, during, and 48 hours after discharge from hospital following acute myocardial infarction. B Heart J 1981; 45:500–511.

189. Ruberman W, Weinblatt E, Goldberg JD, Frank CW, Chaudhary BS, Shapiro S. Ventricular premature complexes and sudden death after myocardial infarction. Circulation 1981; 64:297–305.

190. Ruberman W, Weinblatt E, Frank CW, Goldberg JG, Shapiro S. Repeated 1 hour electrocardiographic monitoring of survivors of myocardial infarction at 6 month intervals: arrhythmia detection and relation to prognosis. Am J Cardiol 1981; 47:1197–1204.

191. Bigger JT Jr, Weld FM, Rolnitzky LM. Which postinfarction ventricular arrhythmias should be treated? Am Heart J 1982; 103:660–666.

192. Weaver WD, Cobb LA, Hallstrom AP. Ambulatory arrhythmias in resuscitated victims of cardiac arrest. Circulation 1982; 66:212–218.

193. Multicenter Post-Infarction Research Group. Risk stratification and survival after myocardial infarction. N Engl J Med 1983; 309:331–336.

194. Olsson G, Rehnqvist N. Ventricular arrhythmias during the first year after acute myocardial infarction: influence of long-term treatment with metoprolol. Circulation 1984; 69:1129–1134.

195. Bigger JT Jr, Fleiss JL, Kleiger R, Miller JP, Rolnitzky LM, Multicenter Post-Infarction Research Group. The relationships among ventricular arrhythmias, left ventricular dysfunction, and mortality in the 2 years after myocardial infarction. Circulation 1984; 69:250–258.

196. Mukharji J, Rude RE, Poole WK, et al. Risk factors for sudden death after acute myocardial infarction: two-year follow-up. Am J Cardiol 1984; 54:31–36.

197. Turitto G, Caref EB, Macina G, Fontaine JM, Ursell SN, el-Sherif N. Time course of ventricular arrhythmias and the signal average electrocardiogram in the post-infarction period: a prospective study of correlation. Br Heart J 1988; 60:17–22.

198. Cardiac Arrhythmia Suppression Trial (CAST) investigators. Preliminary report: effect of encainide and flecainide on mortality in a randomized trial of arrhythmia suppression after myocardial infarction. N Engl J Med 1989; 321:406–412.

199. Doevendans PA, Gorgels AP, van der Zee R, Partouns J, Bar

FW, Wellens HJJ. Electrocardiographic diagnosis of reperfusion during thrombolytic therapy in acute myocardial infaction. Am J Cardiol 1995; 75:1206–1210.

200. Bigger JT Jr, Fleiss JL, Rolnitzky LM, Multicenter Post-Infarction Research Group. Prevalence, characteristics and significance of ventricular tachycardia detected by 24-hour continuous electrocardiographic recordings in the late hospital phase of acute myocardial infarction. Am J Cardiol 1986; 58:1151–1160.

201. Connolly SJ, Cairns JA. Prevalence and predictors of ventricular premature complexes in survivors of acute myocardial infarction. CAMIAT pilot study groups. Canadian Amiodarone Myocardial Infarction Arrhythmia Trial. Am J Cardiol 1992; 69:408–411.

202. Pedretti R, Laporta A, Etro MD, et al. Influence of thrombolysis on signal-averaged electrocardiogram and late arrhythmic events after acute myocardial infarction. Am J Cardiol 1992; 69:866–872.

203. Statters DJ, Malik M, Redwood S, Hnatkova K, Staunton A, Camm AJ. Use of ventricular premature complexes for risk stratification after acute myocardial infarction in the thrombolytic era. Am J Cardiol 1996; 77:133–138.

204. Theroux P, Morissette D, Juneau M, de Guise P, Pelletier G, Waters DD. Influence of fibrinolysis and percutaneous transluminal coronary angioplasty on the frequency of ventricular premature complexes. Am J Cardiol 1989; 63:797–801.

205. Bhandari AK, Hong RA, Rahimtoola SH. Triggered activity as a mechanism of recurrent ventricular tachycardia. Br Heart J 1988; 59:501–505.

206. Taggart P, Gibbons D, Somerville W. Some effects of motor-car driving on the normal and abnormal heart. B Med J 1969; 4:130–134.

207. Poblete PF, Kennedy HL, Caralis DG. Detection of ventricular ectopy in patients with coronary heart disease and normal subjects by exercise testing and ambulatory electrocardiography. Chest 1978; 74:402–407.

208. Orth-Gomer K. Ventricular arrhythmias and risk indicators of ischemic heart disease. Acta Med Scand 1980; 207:283–289.

209. Murayama M, Shimomura K. Exercise and arrhythmia. Jpn Circ J 1979; 43:247–256.

210. Hinkle LE Jr, Carver ST, Stevens M. The frequency of asymptomatic disturbances of cardiac rhythm and conduction in middle-aged men. Am J Cardiol 1969; 24:629–650.

211. Calvert A, Lown B, Gorlin R. Ventricular premature beats and anatomically defined coronary heart disease. Am J Cardiol 1977; 39:627–634.

212. Ammon SE, Szlachcic J, Tubau JF, O'Kelly BF, Chin WL, Massie BM. Ventricular arrhythmias in asymptomatic hypertensives are associated with both silent ischemic and left ventricular hypertrophy. J Am Coll Cardiol 1992; 19:391A.

213. Turitto G, Zanchi E, Maddaluna A, Pellegrini A, Risa AL, Prati PL. Prevalence, time course and malignancy of ventricular arrhythmia during spontaneous ischemic ST-segment depression. Am J Cardiol 1989; 64:900–904.

214. Currie P, Saltissi S. Transient myocardial ischaemia after acute myocardial infarction does not induce ventricular arrhythmias. B Heart J 1993; 69:303–307.

215. Carboni GP, Lahiri A, Cashman PM, Raftery EB. Mechanisms of arrhythmias accompanying ST-segment depression on ambulatory monitoring in stable angina pectoris. Am J Cardiol 1987; 60:1246–1253.

216. Sharma SD, Ballantyne F, Goldstein S. The relationship of ventricular asynergy in coronary artery disease to ventricular premature beats. Chest 1974; 66:358–362.

217. Califf RM, Burks JM, Behar VS, Margolis JR, Wagner GS. Relationship among ventricular arrhythmias, coronary artery disease, and angiographic and electrocardiographic indicators of myocardial fibrosis. Circulation 1978; 57:725–732.

218. Hausmann D, Nikutta P, Trappe HJ, Daniel WG, Wenzlaff P, Lichtlen PR. Incidence of ventricular arrhythmias during transient myocardial ischemia in patients with stable coronary artery disease. J Am Coll Cardiol 1990; 16:49–54.

219. Stern S, Banai S, Keren A, Tzivoni D. Ventricular ectopic activity during myocardial ischemic episoldes in ambulatory patients. Am J Cardiol 1990; 65:412–416.

220. Plotnick GD, Fisher ML, Becker LC. Ventricular arrhythmias in patients with rest angina: correlation with ST segment changes and extent of coronary atherosclerosis. Am Heart J 1983; 105:32–36.

221. Heupler FA Jr. Coronary artery spasm: recognition and treatment. Cardiovasc Clin 1981; 12:29–41.

222. Prinzmetal M, Kennamer R, Merliss R, Wada T, Bor N. Angina pectoris: I. A variant form of angina pectoris. Am J Med 1959; 27:375–388.

223. Gianelly R, Mugler F, Harrison DC. Prinzmetal's variant of angina pectoris with only slight coronary atherosclerosis. Calif Med 1968; 108:129–132.

224. Selzer A, Langston M, Ruggeroli C, Cohn K. Clinical syndrome of variant angina with normal coronary arteriogram. N Engl J Med 1976; 295:1243–1347.

225. Wiener L, Kasparian H, Duca PR, et al. Spectrum of coronary arterial spasm: Clinical, angiographic and myocardial metabolic experience in 29 cases. Am J Cardiol 1976; 38:945–955.

226. Macalpin RN, Cabeen WR. The inside-out electrocardiographic stress test: a view from the left ventricular cavity. Angiology 1977; 28:384–393.

227. Bodenheimer MM, Banka VS, Helfant RH. Relation between the site of origin of ventricular premature complexes and the presence and severity of coronary artery disease. Am J Cardiol 1977; 40:865–869.

228. Heupler FA Jr, Proudfit WL, Razavi M, Shirey EK, Greenstreet R, Sheldon WC. Ergonovine maleate provocative test for coronary arterial spasm. Am J Cardiol 1978; 41:631–640.

229. Plotnick GD, Carliner NH, Fisher ML, DeFelice CE, Becker L. Rest angina with transient S-T segment elevation: correlation of clinical features with coronary anatomy. Am J Med 1978; 65:257–261.

230. Curry RC Jr, Pepine CJ, Sabom MB, Conti CR. Similarities of ergonovine-induced and spontaneous attacks of variant angina. Circulation 1979; 59:307–312.

231. Kerin NZ, Rubenfire M, Naini M, Wajszczuk WJ, Pamatmat A, Cascade PN. Arrhythmias in variant angina pectoris: relationship of arrhythmias to ST-segment elevation and R-wave changes. Circulation 1979; 60:1343–1350.

232. Waters DD, Theroux P, Szlachcic J, et al. Ergonovine testing in a coronary care unit. Am J Cardiol 1980; 46:922–930.

233. Buxton AE, Goldberg S, Harken A, Hirshfield J Jr, Kastor JA. Coronary-artery spasm immediately after myocardial revascularization: recognition and management. N Engl J Med 1981; 304:1249–1253.

234. Miller DD, Waters DD, Szlachcic J, Theroux P. Clinical characteristics associated with sudden death in patients with variant angina. Circulation 1982; 66:588–592.

235. Kerin NZ, Rubenfire M, Willens HJ, Rao P, Cascade PN. The mechanism of dysrhythmias in variant angina pectoris: occlusive versus reperfusion. Am Heart J 1983; 106:1332–1340.

236. Previtali M, Klersy C, Salerno JA, et al. Ventricular tachyarrhythmias in Prinzmetal's variant angina: clinical significance and relation to the degree and time course of S-T segment elevation. Am J Cardiol 1983; 52:19–25.

237. Araki H, Koiwaya Y, Nakagaki O, Nakamura M. Diurnal distribution of ST-segment elevation and related arrhythmias in patients with variant angina: a study by ambulatory ECG monitoring. Circulation 1983; 67:995–1000.

238. Gabliani GI, Winniford MD, Fulton KL, Johnson SM, Mauritson DR, Hillis LD. Ventricular ectopic activity with spontaneous variant angina: frequency and relation to transient ST segment deviation. Am Heart J 1985; 110:40–43.

239. Turitto G, el-Sherif N. Alternans of the ST segment in variant angina. Incidence, time course and relation to ventricular arrhythmias during ambulatory electrocardiographic recording. Chest 1988; 93:587–591.

240. Szlachcic J, Waters DD, Miller D, Theroux P. Ventricular arrhythmias during ergonovine-induced episodes of variant angina. Am Heart J 1984; 107:20–24.

241. Ryan M, Lown B, Horn H. Comparison of ventricular ectopic activity during 24-hour monitoring and exercise testing in patients with coronary heart disease. N Engl J Med 1975; 292:224–229.

242. Lichstein E, Morganroth J, Harrist R, Hubble E. Effect of propranolol on ventricular arrhythmia: the beta-blocker heart attack trial experience. Circulation 1983; 67:10.

243. Myerburg RJ, Briese FW, Conde C, Mallon SM, Liberthson RR, Castellanos A Jr. Long-term antiarrhythmic therapy in survivors of prehospital cardiac arrest: initial 18 months' experience. JAMA 1977; 238:2621–2624.

244. Swartz MH, Teichholz LE, Donoso E. Mitral valve prolapse: a review of associated arrhythmias. Am J Med 1977; 62:377–389.

245. Alpert JS. Association between arrhythmias and mitral valve prolapse. Arch Intern Med 1984; 144:2333–2334.

246. Kligfield P, Devereux RB. Arrhythmias in mitral valve prolapse. Clin Prog Electrophysiol Pacing 1985; 3:403–418.

247. Boudoulas H, Kligfield P, Wooley CF. Mitral valve prolapse: sudden death. In Boudoulas H, Wooley CF (eds). Mitral Valve Prolapse and the Mitral Valve Prolapse Syndrome. Mount Kisco, NY: Futura Publishing Co., 1988, pp. 591–605.

248. Pocock WA, Barlow JB. Postexercise arrhythmias in the billowing posterior mitral leaflet syndrome. Am Heart J 1970; 80:740–745.

249. Winkle RA, Lopes MG, Fitzgerald JW, Goodman DJ, Schroeder JS, Harrison DC. Arrhythmias in patients with mitral valve prolapse. Circulation 1975; 52:73–81.

250. Campbell RWF, Godman MG, Fiddler GI, Marquis RM, Julian DG. Ventricular arrhythmias in syndrome of balloon deformity of mitral valve: definition of possible high risk group. Br Heart J 1976; 38:1053–1057.

251. Jeresaty RM. Sudden death in the mitral valve prolapse-click syndrome. Am J Cardiol 1976; 37:317–318.

252. Kolibash AJ, Bush CA, Fontana MB, Ryan JM, Kilman J, Wooley CF. Mitral valve prolapse syndrome: analysis of 62 patients aged 60 years and older. Am J Cardiol 1983; 52:534–539.

253. Savage DD, Levy D, Garrison RJ, et al. Mitral valve prolapse in the general population. Dysrhythmias: the Framingham study. Am Heart J 1983; 106:582–586.

254. Kramer HM, Kligfield P, Devereux RB, Savage DD, Kramer-Fox R. Arrhythmias in mitral valve prolapse: effect of selection bias. Arch Intern Med 1984; 144:2360–2364.

255. Brigden W, Leatham A. Mitral incompetence. Br Heart J 1953; 15:55–73.

256. Zuppiroli A, Mori F, Favilli S, et al. Arrhythmias in mitral valve prolapse: relation to anterior mitral leaflet thickening, clinical variables, and color Doppler echocardiographic parameters. Am Heart J 1994; 128:919–927.

257. Babuty D, Cosnay P, Breuillac JC, et al. Ventricular arrhythmia factors in mitral valve proplase. PACE 1994; 17:1090–1099.

258. Kavey R-EW, Sondheimer HM, Blackman MS. Detection of dysrhythmia in pediatric patients with mitral valve prolapse. Circulation 1980; 62:582–587.

259. von Olshausen K, Schwarz F, Apfelbach J, Rohrig N, Kramer B, Kubler W. Determinants of the incidence and severity of ventricular arrhythmias in aortic valve disease. Am J Cardiol 1983; 51:1103–1109.

260. Klein RC. Ventricular arrhythmias in aortic valve disease: analysis of 102 patients. Am J Cardiol 1984; 53:1079–1083.

261. Lombard JT, Selzer A. Valvular aortic stenosis: a clinical and hemodynamic profile of patients. Ann Intern Med 1987; 106:292–298.

262. von Olshausen K, Witt T, Schmidt G, Meyer J. Ventricular tachycardia as a cause of sudden death in patients with aortic valve disease. Am J Cardiol 1987; 59:1214–1215.

263. Dec GW, Fuster V. Idiopathic dilated cardiomyopathy. N Engl J Med 1994; 331:1564–1575.

264. Rosenbaum MB, Alvarez AJ. The electrocardiogram in chronic chagasic myocarditis. Am Heart J 1955; 50:492–527.

265. Segal JP, Harvey WP, Gurel T. Diagnosis and treatment of primary myocardial disease. Circulation 1965; 32:837–844.

266. Bashour TT, Fahdul H, Cheng TO. Electrocardiographic abnormalities in alcoholic cardiomyopathy: a study of 65 patients. Chest 1975; 68:24–27.

267. Ingham RE, Rossen RM, Goodman DJ, Harrison DC. Treadmill arrhythmias in patients with idiopathic hypertrophic subaortic stenosis. Chest 1975; 68:759–764.

268. Roberts WC, McAllister HA Jr, Ferrans VJ. Sarcoidosis of the heart: a clinicopathologic study of 35 necropsy patients (group I) and review of 78 previously described necropsy patients (group II). Am J Med 1977; 63:86–108.

269. Silverman KJ, Hutchins GM, Bulkley BH. Cardiac sarcoid: a clinicopathologic study of 84 unselected patients with systemic sarcoidosis. Circulation 1978; 58:1204–1211.

270. Savage DD, Seides SF, Maron BJ, Myers DJ, Epstein SE. Prevalence of arrhythmias during 24-hour electrocardiographic monitoring and exercise testing in patients with obstructive and nonobstructive hypertrophic cardiomyopathy. Circulation 1979; 59:866–875.

271. Doi YL, McKenna WJ, Chetty S, Oakley CM, Goodwin JF. Prediction of mortality and serious ventricular arrhythmia in hypertrophic cardiomyopathy: an echocardiographic study. Br Heart J 1980; 44:150–157.

272. McKenna WJ, Chetty S, Oakley CM, Goodwin JF. Arrhythmia in hypertrophic cardiomyopathy: exercise and 48 hour ambulatory electrocardiographic assessment with and without beta adrenergic blocking therapy. Am J Cardiol 1980; 45:1–5.

273. Maron BJ, Savage DD, Wolfson JK, Epstein SE. Prognostic significance of 24 hour ambulatory electrocardiographic monitoring in patients with hypertrophic cardiomyopathy: a prospective study. Am J Cardiol 1981; 48:252–257.

274. Marcus FI, Fontaine GH, Guiraudon G, et al. Right ventricular dysplasia: a report of 24 adult cases. Circulation 1982; 65:384–398.

275. Huang SK, Messer JV, Denes P. Significance of ventricular tachycardia in idiopathic dilated cardiomyopathy: observations in 35 patients. Am J Cardiol 1983; 51:507–512.

276. Thunell M, Bjerle P, Stjernberg N. ECG abnormalities in patients with sarcoidosis. Acta Med Scand 1983; 213:115–118.

277. Eriksson P, Karp K, Bjerle P, Olofsson BO. Disturbances of cardiac rhythm and conduction in familial amyloidosis with polyneuropathy. Br Heart J 1984; 51:658–662.

278. Maskin CS, Siskind SJ, LeJemtel TH. High prevalence of nonsustained ventricular tachycardia in severe congestive heart failure. Am Heart J 1984; 107:896–901.

279. Meinertz T, Hofmann T, Kasper W, et al. Significance of ventricular arrhythmias in idiopathic dilated cardiomyopathy. Am J Cardiol 1984; 53:902–907.

280. Unverferth DV, Magorien RD, Moeschberger ML, Baker PB, Fetters JK, Leier CV. Factors influencing the one-year mortality of dilated cardiomyopathy. Am J Cardiol 1984; 54:147–152.

281. Vignola PA, Aonuma K, Swaye PS, et al. Lymphocytic myocarditis presenting as unexplained ventricular arrhythmias: diagnosis with endomyocardial biopsy and response to immunosuppression. J Am Coll Cardiol 1984; 4:812–819.

282. von Olshausen K, Schafer A, Mehmel HC, Schwarz F, Senges J, Kubler W. Ventricular arrhythmias in idiopathic dilated cardiomyopathy. Br Heart J 1984; 51:195–201.

283. Chakko CS, Gheorghiade M. Ventricular arrhythmias in severe heart failure: incidence, significance, and effectiveness of antiarrhythmic therapy. Am Heart J 1985; 109:497–504.

284. Holmes DR Jr, Danielson GK, Gersh BJ, et al. Surgical treatment of accessory atrioventricular pathways and symptomatic tachycardia in children and young adults. Am J Cardiol 1985; 55:1509–1512.

285. Mulrow JP, Healy MJ, McKenna WJ. Variability of ventricular arrhythmias in hypertrophic cardiomyopathy and implications for treatment. Am J Cardiol 1986; 58:615–618.

286. Neri R, Mestroni L, Salvi A, Camerini F. Arrhythmias in dilated cardiomyopathy. Postgrad Med J 1986; 62:593–597.

287. Maron BJ, Bonow RO, Cannon RO, Leon MB, Epstein SE. Hypertrophic cardiomyopathy: interrelations of clinical manifestations, pathophysiology, and therapy. N Engl J Med 1987; 316:780–789.

288. Maron BJ, Bonow RO, Cannon RO, Leon MB, Epstein SE. Hypertrophic cardiomyopathy: interrelations of clinical manifestations, pathophysiology, and therapy. N Engl J Med 1987; 316:844–852.

289. Hofmann T, Meinertz T, Kasper W, et al. Mode of death in idiopathic dilated cardiomyopathy: a multivariate analysis of prognostic determinants. Am Heart J 1988; 116:1455–1463.

290. Chen SC, Nouri S, Balfour I, Jureidini S, Appleton RS. Clinical profile of congestive cardiomyopathy in children. J Am Coll Cardiol 1990; 15:189–193.

291. Hagar JM, Rahimtoola SH. Chagas' heart disease in the United States. N Engl J Med 1991; 325:763–768.

292. Friedman RA, Kearney DL, Moak JP, Fenrich AL, Perry JC. Persistence of ventricular arrhythmia after resolution of occult myocarditis in children and young adults. J Am Coll Cardiol 1994; 24:780–783.

293. Wiles HB, Gillette PC, Harley RA, Upshur JK. Cardiomyopathy and myocarditis in children with ventricular ectopic rhythm. J Am Coll Cardiol 1992; 20:359–362.

294. Sideris DA. High blood pressure and ventricular arrhythmias. Eur Heart J 1993; 14:1548–1553.

295. Loaldi A, Pepi M, Agostoni PG, et al. Cardiac rhythm in hypertension assessed through 24 hour ambulatory electrocardiographic monitoring: effects of load manipulation with atenolol, verapamil, and nifedipine. Br Heart J 1983; 50:118–126.

296. Aronow WS, Epstein S, Schwartz KS, Koenigsberg M. Correlation of complex ventricular arrhythmias detected by ambulatory electrocardiographic monitoring with echocardiographic left ventricular hypertrophy in persons older than 62 years in a long-term health care facility. Am J Cardiol 1987; 60:730–732.

297. Mayet J, Shahi M, Poulter NR, Sever PS, Thom SA, Foale RA. Ventricular arrhythmias in hypertension: in which patients do they occur? J Hypertens 1995; 13:269–276.

298. James MA, Jones JV. Ventricular arrhythmia in untreated newly presenting hypertensive patients compared with matched normal population. J Hypertens 1989; 7:409–415.

299. Messerli FH, Ventura HO, Elizardi DJ, Dunn FG, Frohlich ED. Hypertension and sudden death: increased ventricular ectopic activity in left ventricular hypertropy. Am J Med 1984; 77:18–22.

300. Luque-Otero M, Perez-Casar F, Alcazar J, et al. Increased ventricular arrhythmias in hypertensive with left ventricular hypertrophy. J Hypertens 1986; 4:S66–S67.

301. McLenachan JM, Henderson E, Morris KI, Dargie HJ. Ventricular arrhythmias in patients with hypertensive left ventricular hypertrophy. N Engl J Med 1987; 317:787–792.

302. Siegel D, Cheitlin MD, Black DM, Seeley D, Hearst N, Hulley SB. Risk of ventricular arrhythmias in hypertensive men with left ventricular hypertrophy. Am J Cardiol 1990; 65:742–747.

303. Pringle SD, Dunn FG, Macfarlane PW, McKillop JH, Lorimer AR, Cobbe SM. Significance of ventricular arrhythmias in systemic hypertension with left ventricular hypertrophy. Am J Cardiol 1992; 69:913–917.

304. Levy D, Anderson KM, Savage DD, Balkus SA, Kannel WB, Castelli WP. Risk of ventricular arrhythmias in left ventricular hypertrophy: the Framingham heart study. Am J Cardiol 1987; 60:560–565.

305. Messerli FH, Glade LB, Ventura HO, et al. Diurnal variations of cardiac rhythm, arterial pressure, and urinary catecholamines in borderline and established essential hypertension. Am Heart J 1982; 104:109–114.

306. Messerli FH, Nunez BD, Ventura HO, Snyder DW. Overweight and sudden death: increased ventricular ectopy in cardiomyopathy of obesity. Arch Intern Med 1987; 147:1725–1728.

307. Bethge C, Motz W, von Hehn A, Strauer BE. Ventricular arrhythmias in hypertensive heart disease with and without heart failure. J Cardiovasc Pharmacol 1987; 10:S119–S128.

308. Gonzalez-Fernandez RA, Rivera M, Rodriguez PJ, et al. Prevalence of ectopic ventricular activity after left ventricular mass regression. Am J Hypertens 1993; 6:308–313.

309. Kostis JB, Lacy CR, Hall WD, et al. The effect of chlorthalidone on ventricular ectopic activity in patients with isolated systolic hypertension: the SHEP study group. Am J Cardiol 1994; 74:464–467.

310. Levine PA, Klein MD. Mechanisms of arrhythmias in chronic obstructive lung disease. Geriatrics 1976; 31:47–56.

311. Corazza LJ, Pastor BH. Cardiac arrhythmias in chronic cor pulmonale. N Engl J Med 1958; 259:862–865.

312. Thomas AJ, Valabhji P. Arrhythmia and tachycardia in pulmonary heart disease. Br Heart J 1969; 31:491–495.

313. Hudson LD, Kurt TL, Petty TL, Genton E. Arrhythmias associated with acute respiratory failure in patients with chronic airway obstruction. Chest 1973; 63:661–665.

314. Holford FD, Mithoefer JC. Cardiac arrhythmias in hospitalized patients with chronic obstructive pulmonary disease. Am Rev Respir Dis 1973; 108:879–885.

315. Kleiger RE, Senior RM. Longterm electrocardiographic monitoring of ambulatory patients with chronic airway obstruction. Chest 1974; 65:483–487.

316. Sideris DA, Katsadoros DP, Valianos G, Assioura A. Type of cardiac dysrhythmias in respiratory failure. Am Heart J 1975; 89:32–35.

317. Flick MR, Block AJ. Nocturnal vs diurnal cardiac arrhythmias in patients with chronic obstructive pulmonary disease. Chest 1979; 75:8–11.

318. Habibzadeh MA. Multifocal atrial tachycardia: a 66 month follow-up of 50 patients. Heart Lung 1980; 9:328–335.

319. Josephson GW, Kennedy HL, MacKenzie EJ, Gibson G. Cardiac dysrhythmias during the treatment of acute asthma: a comparison of two treatment regimens by a double blind protocol. Chest 1980; 78:429–435.

320. Tirlapur VG, Mir MA. Nocturnal hypoxemia and associated electrocardiographic changes in patients with chronic obstructive airways disease. N Engl J Med 1982; 306:125–130.

321. Shih HT, Webb CR, Conway WA, Peterson E, Tilley B, Goldstein S. Frequency and significance of cardiac arrhythmias in chronic obstructive lung disease. Chest 1988; 94:44–48.

322. Incalzi RA, Pistelli R, Fuso L, Cocchi A, Bonetti MG, Giordano A. Cardiac arrhythmias and left ventricular function in respiratory failure from chronic obstructive pulmonary disease. Chest 1990; 97:1092–1097.

323. Sullivan ID, Presbitero P, Gooch VM, Aruta E, Deanfield JE. Is ventricular arrhythmia in repaired tetralogy of Fallot an effect of operation or a consequence of the course of the disease? A prospective study. Br Heart J 1987; 58:40–44.

324. Sholler GF, Walsh EP. Congenital complete heart block in patients without anatomic cardiac defects. Am Heart J 1989; 118:1193–1198.

325. Angelini P, Feldman MI, Lufschanowski R, Leachman RD. Cardiac arrhythmias during and after heart surgery: diagnosis and management. Prog Cardiovasc Dis 1974; 16:469–495.

326. Michelson EL, Morganroth J, Mac Vaugh H III. Postoperative arrhythmias after coronary artery and cardiac valvular surgery detected by long-term electrocardiographic monitoring. Am Heart J 1979; 97:442–448.

327. von Olshausen K, Amann E, Hofmann M, Schwarz F, Mehmel HC, Kubler W. Ventricular arrhythmias before and late after aortic valve replacement. Am J Cardiol 1984; 54:142–146.

328. Gradman AH, Harbison MA, Berger HJ, et al. Ventricular arrhythmias late after aortic valve replacement and their relation to left ventricular performance. Am J Cardiol 1981; 48:824–831.

329. Stevenson WG, Klitzner T, Perloff JK. Electrophysiologic abnormalities: natural occurrence and postoperative residua and sequelae. In Perloff JK, Child JS (eds). Congenital Heart Disease in Adults. Philadelphia: WB Saunders, 1991, pp. 259–295.

330. Krongrad E. Postoperative arrhythmias in patients with congenital heart disease. Chest 1984; 85:107–113.

331. Joffe H, Georgakopoulos D, Celermajer DS, Sullivan ID, Deanfield JE. Late ventricular arrhythmia is rare after early repair of tetralogy of Fallot. J Am Coll Cardiol 1994; 23:1146–1150.

332. Cullen S, Celermajer DS, Franklin RC, Hallidie-Smith KA, Deanfield JE. Prognostic significance of ventricular arrhythmia after repair of tetralogy of Fallot: a 12-year prospective study. J Am Coll Cardiol 1994; 23:1151–1155.

333. Kavey RE, Blackman MS, Sondheimer HM. Incidence and severity of chronic ventricular dysrhythmias after repair of tetralogy of Fallot. Am Heart J 1982; 103:342–350.

334. Kobayashi J, Hirose H, Nakano S, Matsuda H, Shirakura R, Kawashima Y. Ambulatory electrocardiographic study of the frequency and cause of ventricular arrhythmia after correction of tetralogy of Fallot. Am J Cardiol 1984; 54:1310–1313.

335. Deanfield JE, McKenna WJ, Presbitero P, England D, Graham GR, Hallidie-Smith K. Ventricular arrhythmia in unrepaired and repaired tetralogy of Fallot: relation to age, timing of repair, and haemodynamic status. Br Heart J 1984; 52:77–81.

336. Gillette PC, Wampler DG, Garson A Jr, Zinner A, Ott DA, Cooley D. Treatment of atrial automatic tachycardia by ablation procedures. J Am Coll Cardiol 1985; 6:405–409.

337. Chandar JS, Wolff GS, Garson A Jr, et al. Ventricular arrhythmias in postoperative tetralogy of Fallot. Am J Cardiol 1990; 65:655–661.

338. Vaksmann G, Fournier A, Davignon A, Ducharme G, Houyel L, Fouron JC. Frequency and prognosis of arrhythmias after operative "correction" of tetralogy of Fallot. Am J cardiol 1990; 66:346–349.

339. Burns RJ, Liu PP, Druck MN, Seawright SJ, Williams WG, McLaughlin PR. Analysis of adults with and without complex ventricular arrhythmias after repair of tetralogy of Fallot. J Am Coll Cardiol 1984; 4:226–233.

340. Kavey RE, Thomas FD, Byrum CJ, Blackman MS, Sondheimer HM, Bove EL. Ventricular arrhythmias and biventricular dysfunction after repair of tetralogy of Fallot. J Am Coll Cardiol 1984; 4:126–131.

341. Garson A Jr, Nihill MR, McNamara DG, Cooley DA. Status of the adult and adolescent after repair of tetralogy of Fallot. Circulation 1979; 59:1232–1240.

342. Jack CM, Cleland J, Adgey AA. Successful surgical repair of a patent arterial duct (ductus arteriosus) in a 63-year-old woman. Int J Cardiol 1985; 8:335–338.

343. Wessel HU, Benson DW, Braunlin EA, Dunnigan A, Paul MH. Exercise response before and after termination of atrial tachycardia after congenital heart disease surgery. Circulation 1989; 80:106–111.

344. Quattlebaum TG, Varghese J, Neill CA, Donahoo JS. Sudden death among postoperative patients with tetralogy of Fallot: a follow-up study of 243 patients for an average of twelve years. Circulation 1976; 54:289–293.

345. Walsh EP, Rockenmacher S, Keane JF, Hougen TJ, Lock JE, Castaneda AR. Late results in patients with tetralogy of Fallot repaired during infancy. Circulation 1988; 77:1062–1067.

346. Presbitero P, Somerville J, Rabajoli F, Stone S, Conte MR. Corrected transposition of the great arteries without associated defects in adult patients: clinical profile and follow up. Br Heart J 1995; 74:57–59.

347. Deanfield JE, McKenna WJ, Hallidie-Smith KA. Detection of late arrhythmia and conduction disturbance after correction of tetralogy of Fallot. Br Heart J 1980; 44:248–253.

348. Romhilt DW, Doyle M, Sagar KB, et al. Prevalence and significance of arrhythmias in long-term survivors of cardiac transplantation. Circulation 1982; 66:1219–1222.

349. Scott CD, Dark JH, McComb JM. Arrhythmias after cardiac transplantation. Am J Cardiol 1992; 70:1061–1063.

350. Pietrucha A, Matysek J, Piwowarska W, et al. Analysis of circadian distribution of premature ventricular contractions in patients after heart transplantation. Pacing Clin Electrophysiol 1994; 17:2064–2067.

351. Alexopoulos D, Yusuf S, Bostock J, Johnston JA, Sleight P, Yacoub MH. Ventricular arrhythmias in long term survivors of orthotopic and heterotopic cardiac transplantation. Br Heart J 1988; 59:648–652.

352. Jacquet L, Ziady G, Stein K, et al. Cardiac rhythm disturbances early after orthotopic heart transplantation: prevalence and clinical importance of the observed abnormalities. J Am Coll Cardiol 1990; 16:832–837.

353. Morganroth J, Horowitz LN. Flecainide: its proarrhythmic effect and expected changes on the surface electrocardiogram. Am J Cardiol 1984; 53:89B–94B.

354. Vangt EJ, Wellens HJJ. The electrocardiogram in digitalis intoxication. In Wellens HJJ, Kulbertus HE (eds). What's New in Electrocardiography. Boston: Martinus Nijhoff, 1981, pp. 315–343.

355. White PD. Heart Disease. 4th ed. New York: Macmillan, 1951, p. 871.

356. Castellanos A, Lemberg L, Brown JP, Berkovits BV. An electrical digitalis tolerance test. Am J Med Sci 1967; 254:159/717–168/726.

357. Chung EK. Principles of Cardiac Arrhythmias. Baltimore: Williams & Wilkins, 1971, pp. 864–876.

358. Smith TW, Willerson JT. Suicidal and accidental digoxin ingestion: report of five cases with serum digoxin level correlations. Circulation 1971; 44:29–36.

359. Smith TW, Butler VP Jr, Haber E, et al. Treatment of life-threatening digitalis intoxication with digoxin-specific Fab antibody fragments. N Engl J Med 1982; 307:1357–1400.

360. Wenger TL, Butler VP Jr, Haber E, Smith TW. Treatment of 63 severely digitalis-toxic patients with digoxin-specific antibody fragments. J Am Coll Cardiol 1985; 5:118A–123A.

361. Chung EK. Principles of Cardiac Arrhythmias. Baltimore: Williams & Wilkins Company, 1971, p. 372.

362. Fowler RS, Rathi L, Keith JD. Accidental digitalis intoxication in children. J Pediatr 1964; 64:188–200.

363. Larsen RL, Jakacki RI, Vetter VL, Meadows AT, Silber JH, Barber G. Electrocardiographic changes and arrhythmias after cancer therapy in children and young adults. Am J Cardiol 1992; 70:73–77.

364. Dutt AK, de Soyza ND, Au WY, Hargis JL, Tuck RL. The effect of aminophylline on cardiac rhythm in advanced chronic obstructive pulmonary disease: correlation with serum theophylline levels. Eur J Respir Dis 1983; 64:264–270.

365. Greenberg A, Piraino BH, Kroboth PD, Weiss J. Severe theophylline toxicity: role of conservative measures, antiarrhythmic agents, and charcoal hemoperfusion. Am J Med 1984; 76:854–860.

366. Zipes DP, Knoebel SB. Rapid rate-dependent ventricular ectopy: adverse responses to atropine-induced rate increase. Chest 1972; 62:255–258.

367. Little RE, Kay GN, Epstein AE, et al. Arrhythmias after orthotopic cardiac transplantation: prevalence and determinants during initial hospitalization and late follow-up. Circulation 1989; 80:140–146.

368. Banner AS, Sunderrajan EV, Agarwal MK, Addington WW. Arrhythmogenic effects of orally administered bronchodilators. Arch Intern Med 1979; 139:434–437.

369. Orr D, Jones I. Anaesthesia for laryngoscopy: a comparison of the cardiovascular effects of cocaine and lignocaine. Anaesthesia 1968; 23:194–202.

370. Isner JM, Estes NA III, Thompson PD, et al. Acute cardiac events temporally related to cocaine abuse. N Engl J Med 1986; 315:1438–1443.

371. Kloner RA, Hale S, Alker K, Rezkalla S. The effects of acute and chronic cocaine use on the heart. Circulation 1992; 85:407–419.

372. Warner EA. Cocaine abuse. Ann Intern Med 1993; 119:226–235.

373. Pick A. Arrhythmias and potassium in man. Am Heart J 1966; 72:295–306.

374. Hollifield JW. Thiazide treatment of hypertension: effects of thiazide diuretics on serum potassium, magnesium, and ventricular ectopy. Am J Med 1986; 80:8–12.

375. Papademetriou V. Diuretics, hypokalemia, and cardiac arrhythmias: a critical analysis. Am Heart J 1986; 111:1217–1224.

376. Hollifield JW. Electrolyte disarray and cardiovascular disease. Am J Cardiol 1989; 63:21B–26B.

377. Roden DM. Magnesium treatment of ventricular arrhythmias. Am J Cardiol 1989; 63:43G–46G.

378. Seelig M. Cardiovascular consequences of magnesium deficiency and loss: pathogenesis, prevalence and manifestations—magnesium and chloride loss in refractory potassium repletion. Am J Cardiol 1989; 63:4G–21G.

379. Tzivoni D, Keren A. Suppression of ventricular arrhythmias by magnesium. Am J Cardiol 1990; 65:1397–1399.

380. Tsuji H, Venditti FJ Jr, Evans JC, Larson MG, Levy D. The associations of levels of serum potassium and magnesium with ventricular premature complexes (the Framingham heart study). Am J Cardiol 1994; 74:232–235.

381. Stewart DE, Ikram H, Espiner EA, Nicholls MG. Arrhythmogenic potential of diuretic induced hypokalaemia in patients with mild hypertension and ischaemic heart disease. Br Heart J 1985; 54:290–297.

382. Nordrehaug JE, Johannessen KA, von der Lippe G. Serum potassium concentration as a risk factor of ventricular arrhythmias early in acute myocardial infarction. Circulation 1985; 71:645–649.

383. Davidson S, Surawicz B. Ectopic beats and atrioventricular conduction disturbances: in patients with hypopotassemia. Arch Intern Med 1967; 120:280–285.

384. Steiness E, Olesen KH. Cardiac arrhythmias induced by hypokalaemia and potassium loss during maintenance digoxin therapy. Br Heart J 1976; 38:167–172.

385. Lief PD, Belizon I, Matos J, Bank N. Diuretic-induced hypokalemia does not cause ventricular ectopy in uncomplicated essential hypertension. Kidney Int 1984; 25:203.

386. Holland OB, Nixon JV, Kuhnert L. Diuretic-induced ventricular ectopic activity. Am J Med 1981; 70:762–768.

387. Hollifield JW, Slaton PE. Thiazide diuretics, hypokalemia and cardiac arrhythmias. Acta Med Scand Suppl 1981; 647:67–73.

388. Papademetriou V, Fletcher R, Khatri IM, Freis ED. Diuretic-induced hypokalemia in uncomplicated systemic hypertension: effect of plasma potassium correction on cardiac arrhythmias. Am J Cardiol 1983; 52:1017–1022.

389. Madias JE, Madias NE, Gavras HP. Nonarrhythmogenicity of diuretic-induced hypokalemia: its evidence in patients with uncomplicated hypertension. Arch Intern Med 1984; 144:2171–2176.

390. Papademetriou V, Price M, Notargiacomo A, Gottdiener J, Fletcher RD, Freis ED. Effect of diuretic therapy on ventricular arrhythmias in hypertensive patients with or without left ventricular hypertrophy. Am Heart J 1985; 110:595–599.

391. Holland OB, Kuhnert L, Pollard J, Padia M, Anderson RJ, Blomqvist G. Ventricular ectopic activity with diuretic therapy. Am J Hypertens 1988; 1:380–385.

392. Siegel D, Black DM, Seeley DG, Hulley SB. Circadian variation in ventricular arrhythmias in hypertensive men. Am J Cardiol 1992; 69:344–347.

393. Medical Research Council Working Party on Mild to Moderate Hypertension. Ventricular extrasystoles during thiazide treatment: substudy of MRC mild hypertension trial. BMJ 1983; 287:1249–1253.

394. Vetter WR, Cohn LH, Reichgott M. Hypokalemia and electrocardiographic abnormalities during acute alcohol withdrawal. Arch Intern Med 1967; 120:536–541.

395. Iseri LT, Freed J, Bures AR. Magnesium deficiency and cardiac disorders. Am J Med 1975; 58:837–846.

396. Dyckner T, Wester PO. Ventricular extrasystoles and intracellular electrolytes before and after potassium and magnesium infusions in patients on diuretic treatment. Am Heart J 1979; 97:12–18.

397. Dyckner T. Serum magnesium in acute myocardial infarction: relation to arrhythmias. Acta Med Scand 1980; 207:59–66.

398. Rector WG Jr, DeWood MA, Williams RV, Sullivan JF. Serum magnesium and copper levels in myocardial infarction. Am J Med Sci 1981; 281:25–29.

399. Hollifield JW. Potassium and magnesium abnormalities: diuretics and arrhythmias in hypertension. Am J Med 1984; 77:28–32.

400. Kafka H, Langevin L, Armstrong PW. Serum magnesium and potassium in acute myocardial infarction. Influence on ventricular arrhythmias. Arch Intern Med 1987; 147:465–469.

401. Abe S, Yoshizawa M, Nakanishi N, et al. Electrocardiographic abnormalities in patients receiving hemodialysis. Am Heart J 1996; 131:1137–1144.

402. Kahaly G, Olshausen KV, Mohr-Kahaly S, et al. Arrhythmia profile in acromegaly. Eur Heart J 1992; 13:51–56.

403. Coumel P. Rate dependence and adrenergic dependence of arrhythmias. Am J Cardiol 1989; 64:41J–45J.

404. Berliner K, Huppert VF. Ventricular premature systoles occurring at rapid heart rates. Cardiologia 1951; 9:153–162.

405. Berliner K, Huppert VF. Benign ventricular premature systoles. Cardiologia 1955; 24:184–191.

406. Tsumabuki S, Ito M, Arita M, Saikawa T, Ito S. Day-to-day variation of the frequency of ventricular premature contractions depends on variation of heart rates. Jpn Circ J 1988; 52:1231–1239.

407. Pitzalis MV, Mastropasqua F, Massari F, et al. Dependency of premature ventricular contractions on heart rate. Am Heart J 1997; 133:153–161.

408. Winkle RA. The relationship between ventricular ectopic beat frequency and heart rate. Circulation 1982; 66:439–446.

409. Acanfora D, De Caprio L, Di Palma A, et al. Relationship between ventricular ectopic beat frequency and heart rate: study in patients with severe arrhythmias. Am Heart J 1993; 125:1022–1029.

410. Canada WB, Woodward W, Lee G, et al. Circadian rhythm of hourly ventricular arrhythmia frequency in man. Angiology 1983; 34:274–282.

411. Lanza GA, Cortellessa MC, Rebuzzi AG, et al. Reproducibility in circadian rhythm of ventricular premature complexes. Am J Cardiol 1990; 66:1099–1106.

412. Pitzalis MV, Mastropasqua F, Massari F, et al. Effects of nadolol and its combination with atrial pacing on rate-enhanced ventricular premature complexes. Am J Cardiol 1996; 78:1178–1179.

413. Lown B, Tykocinski M, Garfein A, Brooks P. Sleep and ventricular premature beats. Circulation 1973; 48:691–701.

414. Pickering TG, Miller NE. Learned voluntary control of heart rate and rhythm in two subjects with premature ventricular contractions. Br Heart J 1977; 39:152–159.

415. Lopes MG, Runge P, Harrison DC, Schroeder JS. Comparison of 24 versus 12 hours of ambulatory ECG monitoring. Chest 1975; 67:269–273.

416. Gradman AH, Bell PA, Debusk RF. Sudden death during ambulatory monitoring. Clinical and electrocardiographic correlations: report of a case. Circulation 1977; 55:210–211.

417. Pickering TG, Goulding L, Cobern BA. Diurnal variations in ventricular ectopic beats and heart rate. Cardiovasc Med 1977; 2:1013–1022.

418. Pickering TG, Johnston J, Honour AJ. Comparison of the effects of sleep, exercise and autonomic drugs on ventricular extrasystoles, using ambulatory monitoring of electrocardiogram and electroencephalogram. Am J Med 1978; 65:575–583.

419. Winkle RA. Circadian variation in ventricular ectopic activity. In Sandoe E, Julian DG, Bell JW (eds). Management of Ventricular Tachycardia. Role of Mexiletine. Amsterdam: Excerpta Medica, 1978, pp. 165–169.

420. Steinbach K, Glogar D, Weber H, Joskowicz G, Kaindl F. Frequency and variability of ventricular premature contractions: the influence of heart rate and circadian rhythms. Pacing Clin Electrophysiol 1982; 5:38–51.

421. Raeder EA, Hohnloser SH, Graboys TB, Podrid PJ, Lampert S, Lown B. Spontaneous variability and circadian distribution of ectopic activity in patients with malignant ventricular arrhythmia. J Am Coll Cardiol 1988; 12:656–661.

422. Smith R, Johnson L, Rothfeld D, Zir L, Tharp B. Sleep and cardiac arrhythmias. Arch Intern Med 1972; 130:751–753.

423. Saito D, Matsuno S, Haraoka S. The daily profile of ventricular premature beats in the patients with ischemic heart disease. Jpn Circ J 1987; 51:208–216.

424. Rosenblatt G, Hartmann E, Zwilling GR. Cardiac irritability during sleep and dreaming. J Psychosom Res 1973; 17:129–134.

425. Orr WC, Stahl ML, Whitsett T, Langevin E. Physiological sleep patterns and cardiac arrhythmias. Am Heart J 1979; 97:128–129.

426. Cripps T, Rocker G, Stradling J. Nocturnal hypoxia and arrhythmias in patients with impaired left ventricular function. Br Heart J 1992; 68:382–386.

427. Rosenberg MJ, Uretz E, Denes P. Sleep and ventricular arrhythmias. Am Heart J 1983; 106:703–709.

428. Dreifus LS, Watanabe Y. Tension, drugs, and premature systoles. Am Heart J 1965; 70:291–294.

429. Gazes PC, Sovell BF, Dellastatious JW. Continuous radioelectrocardiographic monitoring of football and basketball coaches during games. Am Heart J 1969; 78:509–512.

430. Lown B, DeSilva RA. Roles of psychologic stress and autonomic nervous system changes in provocation of ventricular premature complexes. Am J Cardiol 1978; 41:979–985.

431. Bourne G. An attempt at the clinical classification of premature ventricular beats. Q J Med 1927; April:219–243.

432. Schroeder JS, Berke DK, Graham AF, Rider AK, Harrison DC. Arrhythmias after cardiac transplantation. Am J Cardiol 1974; 33:604–607.

433. Mason JW, Stinson EB, Harrison DC. Autonomic nervous system and arrhythmias: studies in the transplanted denervated human heart. Cardiology 1976; 61:75–87.

434. Weiss T, Lattin GM, Engelman K. Vagally mediated suppression of premature ventricular contractions in man. Am Heart J 1975; 89:700–707.

435. Facchini M, De Ferrari GM, Bonazzi O, Weiss T, Schwartz PJ. Effect of reflex vagal activation on frequency of ventricular premature complexes. Am J Cardiol 1991; 68:349–354.

436. Friedberg CK. Diseases of the Heart. Philadelphia: WB Saunders, 1966, p. 539.

437. Rall TW. Drugs used in the treatment of asthma: the methylxanthines, cromolyn sodium, and other agents. In Gilman AG, Rall TW, Nies AS, Taylor P (eds). The Pharmacological Basis of Therapeutics. 8th ed. New York: Pergamon Press, 1990, pp. 629–630.

438. Zipes DP. Specific arrhythmias: diagnosis and treatment. In Braunwald E (ed). Heart Disease. A Textbook of Cardiovascular Medicine. 5th ed. Philadelphia: WB Saunders, 1997, pp. 675–677.

439. DeBacker G, Jacobs D, Prineas R, et al. Ventricular premature contractions: a randomized non-drug intervention trial in normal men. Circulation 1979; 59:762–769.

440. Graboys TB, Lown B. Coffee, arrhythmias, and common sense. N Engl J Med 1983; 308:835–837.

441. Myers MG, Harris L, Leenen FH, Grant DM. Caffeine as a possible cause of ventricular arrhythmias during the healing phase of acute myocardial infarction. Am J Cardiol 1987; 59:1024–1028.

442. Newcombe PF, Renton KW, Rautaharju PM, Spencer CA, Montague TJ. High-dose caffeine and cardiac rate and rhythm in normal subjects. Chest 1988; 94:90–94.

443. Chelsky LB, Cutler JE, Griffith K, Kron J, McClelland JH, McAnulty JH. Caffeine and ventricular arrhythmias: an electrophysiological approach. JAMA 1990; 264:2236–2240.

444. Myers MG. Caffeine and cardiac arrhythmias. Ann Intern Med 1991; 114:147–150.

445. Newby DE, Neilson JM, Jarvie DR, Boon NA. Caffeine restriction has no role in the management of patients with symptomatic idiopathic ventricular premature beats. Heart 1996; 76:355–357.

446. Graboys TB, Blatt CM, Lown B. The effect of caffeine on ventricular ectopic activity in patients with malignant ventricular arrhythmia. Arch Intern Med 1989; 149:637–639.

447. Singer K, Lundberg WB. Ventricular arrhythmias associated with the ingestion of alcohol. Ann Intern Med 1972; 77:247–248.

448. Ettinger PO, Wu CF, De La Cruz C Jr, Weisse AB, Ahmed SS, Regan TJ. Arrhythmias and the "holiday heart": alcohol-associated cardiac rhythm disorders. Am Heart J 1978; 95:555–562.

449. Greenspon AJ, Schaal SF. The "holiday heart": electrophysiologic studies of alcohol effects in alcoholics. Ann Intern Med 1983; 98:135–139.

450. Airaksinen KE, Huikuri HV. Antiarrhythmic effect of repeated coronary occlusion during balloon angioplasty. J Am Coll Cardiol 1997; 29:1035–1038.

451. Airaksinen KEJ, Ikaheimo MJ, Huikuri HV. Stenosis severity and the occurrence of ventricular ectopic activity during acute coronary occlusion during balloon angioplasty. Am J Cardiol 1995; 76:346–349.

452. Levy N, Abinader E. Continuous electrocardiographic monitoring with Holter electrocardiocorder throughout all stages of gastroscopy. Am J Dig Dis 1977; 22:1091–1096.

453. Roberts NK, Cabeen WR Jr, Moss J, Clements PJ, Furst DE. The prevalence of conduction defects and cardiac arrhythmias in progressive systemic sclerosis. Ann Intern Med 1981; 94:38–40.

454. Clements PJ, Furst DE, Cabeen W, Tashkin D, Paulus HE, Roberts N. The relationship arrhythmias and conduction disturbances to other manifestations of cardiopulmonary disease in progressive systemic sclerosis (PSS). Am J Med 1981; 71:38–46.

455. Ferri C, Bernini L, Bongiorni MG, et al. Noninvasive evaluation of cardiac dysrhythmias, and their relationship with multisystemic symptoms, in progressive systemic sclerosis patients. Arthritis Rheum 1985; 28:1259–1266.

456. Follansbee WP, Curtiss EI, Rahko PS, et al. The electrocardiogram in systemic sclerosis (scleroderma): study of 102 consecutive cases with functional correlations and review of the literature. Am J Med 1985; 79:183–192.

457. Lamb LE, Dermksian G, Sarnoff CA. Significant cardiac arrhythmias induced by common respiratory maneuvers. Am J Cardiol 1958; 2:563–571.

458. Harvey WP. Clinical aspects of cardiac tumors. Am J Cardiol 1968; 21:328–343.

459. Taylor TR. Tuberous sclerosis presenting as cardiac arrhythmia. Br Heart J 1968; 30:132–134.

460. Tomisawa M, Onouchi Z, Goto M, Nakata K, Mizukawa K, Kusunoki T. Right ventricular aneurysm with ventricular premature beats. Br Heart J 1974; 36:1182–1185.

461. Tilkian AG, Guilleminault C, Schroeder JS, Lehrman KL, Simmons FB, Dement WC. Sleep-induced apnea syndrome: prevalence of cardiac arrhythmias and their reversal after tracheostomy. Am J Med 1977; 63:348–358.

462. Imaizumi T. Arrhythmias in sleep apnea. Am Heart J 1980; 100:513–516.

463. Perloff JK. Cardiac rhythm and conduction in Duchenne's muscular dystrophy: a prospective study of 20 patients. J Am Coll Cardiol 1984; 3:1263–1268.

464. Jensen PJ, Thomsen PE, Bagger JP, Norgaard A, Baandrup U. Electrical injury causing ventricular arrhythmias. Br Heart J 1987; 57:279–283.

465. Kostis JB, Seibold JR, Turkevich D, et al. Prognostic importance of cardiac arrhythmias in systemic sclerosis. Am J Med 1988; 84:1007–1015.

466. Sheps DS, Herbst MC, Hinderliter AL, et al. Production of arrhythmias by elevated carboxyhemoglobin in patients with coronary artery disease. Ann Intern Med 1990; 113:343–351.

467. Yanagisawa A, Miyagawa M, Yotsukura M, et al. The prevalence and prognostic significance of arrhythmias in Duchenne type muscular dystrophy. Am Heart J 1992; 124:1244–1250.

468. Dahms TE, Younis LT, Wiens RD, Zarnegar S, Byers SL, Chaitman BR. Effects of carbon monoxide exposure in patients with documented cardiac arrhythmias. J Am Coll Cardiol 1993; 21:442–450.

469. Spodick DH. Arrhythmias during acute pericarditis: a prospective study of 100 consecutive cases. JAMA 1976; 235:39–41.

470. Spodick DH. Frequency of arrhythmias in acute pericarditis determined by Holter monitoring. Am J Cardiol 1984; 53:842–845.

471. Northcote RJ, MacFarlane P, Kesson CM, Ballantyne D. Continuous 24-hour electrocardiography in thyrotoxicosis before and after treatment. Am Heart J 1986; 112:339–344.

472. von Olshausen K, Bischoff S, Kahaly G, et al. Cardiac arrhythmias and heart rate in hyperthyroidism. Am J Cardiol 1989; 63:930–933.

473. Polikar R, Feld GK, Dittrich HC, Smith J, Nicod P. Effect of thyroid replacement therapy on the frequency of benign atrial and ventricular arrhythmias. J Am Coll Cardiol 1989; 14:999–1002.

474. Mackenzie J. The extra-systole: a contribution to the functional pathology of the primitive cardiac tissue. Part II. Q J Med 1907; 1:481–490.

475. Anonymous. Paul Wood's Diseases of the Heart and Circulation. 3rd ed. Philadelphia: JB Lippincott, 1968, pp. 17–18.

476. Zimetbaum P, Josephson ME. Evaluation of patients with palpitations. N Engl J Med 1998; 338:1369–1373.

477. Lochen ML, Snaprud T, Zhang W, Rasmussen K. Arrhythmias in subjects with and without a history of palpitations: the TROMSO study. Eur Heart J 1994; 15:345–349.

478. Braunwald E. Examination of the patient: the history. In Braunwald E (ed). Heart Disease. A Textbook of Cardiovascular Medicine. 5th ed. Philadelphia: WB Saunders, 1997, p. 9.

479. Kline EM, Bidder TG. A study of the subjective sensations associated with extrasystoles. Am Heart J 1946; 31:254–259.

480. Friedberg CK. Diseases of the Heart. 3rd ed. Philadelphia: WB Saunders, 1966, p. 506.

481. Barsky AJ, Cleary PD, Coeytaux RR, Ruskin JN. Psychiatric disorders in medical outpatients complaining of palpitations. J Gen Intern Med 1994; 9:306–313.

482. Barsky AJ, Cleary PD, Coeytaux RR, Ruskin JN. The clinical course of palpitations in medical outpatients. Arch Intern Med 1995; 155:1782–1788.

483. Barsky AJ, Cleary PD, Sarnie MK, Ruskin JN. Panic disorder, palpitations, and the awareness of cardiac activity. J Nerv Ment Dis 1994; 182:63–71.

484. Weber BE, Kapoor WN. Evaluation and outcomes of patients with palpitations. Am J Med 1996; 100:138–148.

485. Van Durme JP. Tachyarrhythmias and transient cerebral ischemic attacks. Am Heart J 1975; 89:538–540.

486. Clark PI, Glasser SP, Spoto E Jr. Arrhythmias detected by ambulatory monitoring: lack of correlation with symptoms of dizziness and syncope. Chest 1980; 77:722–725.

487. Zeldis SM, Levine BJ, Michelson EL, Morganroth J. Cardiovascular complaints: correlation with cardiac arrhythmias on 24-hour electrocardiographic monitoring. Chest 1980; 78:456–461.

488. Levine SA, Harvey WP. Clinical Auscultation of the Heart. Philadelphia: WB Saunders, 1959, pp. 148–151.

489. Marriott HJ. Bedside recognition of cardiac arrhythmias. Geriatrics 1975; 30:55–63.

490. Wang K, Hodges M. The premature ventricular complex as a diagnostic aid. Ann Intern Med 1992; 117:766–770.

491. Brockenbrough EC, Braunwald E, Morrow AG. A hemodynamic technic for the detection of hypertrophic subaortic stenosis. Circulation 1961; 23:189–194.

492. Ross J Jr, Braunwald E, Gault JH, Mason DT, Morrow AG. The mechanism of the intraventricular pressure gradient in idiopathic hypertrophic subaortic stenosis. Circulation 1966; 34:558–578.

493. Schweizer W, Burkart F. The diagnostic value of premature beats. Cardiology 1966; 48:236–242.

494. Pollock SG. Images in clinical medicine: pressure tracings in obstructive cardiomyopathy. N Engl J Med 1994; 331:238.

495. Cohn KE, Sandler H, Hancock EW. Mechanisms of pulsus alternans. Circulation 1967; 36:372–380.

496. Hada Y, Wolfe C, Craige E. Pulsus alternans determined by biventricular simultaneous systolic time intervals. Circulation 1982; 65:617–626.

497. Perloff JK. Physical Examination of the Heart and Circulation. 2nd ed. Philadelphia: WB Saunders, 1990, pp. 128–129.

498. Cossio P, Dambrosi RG, Warnford-Thomson HF. The first heart sound in auricular and ventricular extrasystoles. Br Heart J 1947; 9:275–282.

499. Haber E, Leathem A. Splitting of heart sounds from ventricular asynchrony in bundle-branch block, ventricular ectopic beats, and artificial pacing. Br Heart J 1965; 27:691–696.

500. Lembo NJ, Dell'Italia LJ, Crawford MH, O'Rourke RA. Bedside diagnosis of systolic murmurs. N Engl J Med 1988; 318:1572–1578.

501. Karliner JS, O'Rourke RA, Kearney DJ, Shabetai R. Haemodynamic explanation of why the murmur of mitral regurgitation is independent of cycle length. Br Heart J 1973; 35:397–401.

502. Kramer DS, French WJ, Criley JM. The postextrasystolic murmur response to gradient in hypertrophic cardiomyopathy. Ann Intern Med 1986; 104:772–776.

503. Katz LN, Pick A. Clinical Electrocardiography. Part I. The Arrhythmias. Philadelphia: Lea & Febiger, 1956, pp. 169–172.

504. Schamroth L, Dove E. The Wenckebach phenomenon in sino-atrial block. Br Heart J 1966; 28:350–358.

505. Schamroth L. The physiological basis of ectopic ventricular rhythm: a unifying concept. S Afr Med J 1971; 45:3–26.

506. Schamroth L. Ventricular extrasystoles, ventricular tachycardia, and ventricular fibrillation: clinical-electrocardiographic considerations. Prog Cardiovasc Dis 1980; 23:13–32.

507. Blackburn H, Taylor HL, Hamrell B, Buskirk E, Nicholas WC, Thorsen RD. Premature ventricular complexes induced by stress testing: their frequency and response to physical conditioning. Am J Cardiol 1973; 31:441–449.

508. Langendorf R, Pick A, Winternitz M. Mechanisms of intermittent ventricular bigeminy. I. Appearance of ectopic beats dependent upon length of the ventricular cycle, the "rule of bigeminy." Circulation 1955; 11:422–430.

509. Arcilla RA, Lind J, Zetterqvist P, Oh W, Gessner IH. Hemodynamic features of extrasystoles in newborn and older infants. Am J Cardiol 1966; 18:191–199.

510. Scherf D, Schott A. Extrasystoles and Allied Arrhythmias. 2nd ed. Chicago: Year Book Medical Publishers, 1973, pp. 154–171.

511. Kistin AD, Landowne M. Retrograde conduction from premature ventricular contractions, a common occurrence in the human heart. Circulation 1951; 3:738–751.

512. Bussan R, Torin S, Scherf D. Retrograde conduction of ventricular extrasystoles to the atria. Am J Med Sci 1955; 230:293–298.

513. Schott A. Upper atrio-ventricular nodal beats precipitated by ventricular extrasystoles with retrograde conduction. Br Heart J 1955; 17:247–254.

514. Kistin AD. Mechanisms determining reciprocal rhythm initiated by ventricular premature systoles: multiple pathways of conduction. Am J Cardiol 1959; 3:365–383.

515. Kistin AD. Retrograde conduction to the atria in ventricular tachycardia. Circulation 1961; 24:236–249.

516. Schamroth L, Rosenzweig D. Reciprocal ventricular extrasystoles. Br Heart J 1962; 24:805–808.

517. Kistin AD. Multiple pathways of conduction and reciprocal rhythm with interpolated ventricular premature systoles. Am Heart J 1963; 65:162–179.

518. Schamroth L, Yoshonis KF. Mechanisms in reciprocal rhythm. Am J Cardiol 1969; 24:224–233.

519. Mirowski M, Tabatznik B. The spatial characteristics of atrial activation in ventriculo-atrial excitation. Chest 1970; 57:9–17.

520. Myerburg RJ, Sung RJ, Gerstenblith G, Mallon SM, Castellanos A Jr. Ventricular ectopic activity after premature atrial beats in acute myocardial infarction. Br Heart J 1977; 39:1033–1037.

521. Haft JI, Levites R, Gupta PK. Effects of ventricular premature contractions on atrioventricular conduction: studies with His bundle electrography. Am J Cardiol 1973; 32:794–798.

522. Katz LN, Langendorf R, Cole SL. An unusual effect of interpolated ventricular premature systoles. Am Heart J 1944; 28:167–176.

523. Camous JP, Baudouy M, Guarino L, Gibelin P, Patouraux G, Guiran JB. Effects of an interpolated premature ventricular

contraction on the AV conduction of the subsequent premature atrial depolarization: an apparent facilitation. J Electrocardiol 1980; 13:353–357.

524. Langendorf R. Ventricular premature systoles with postponed compensatory pause. Am Heart J 1953; 46:401–404.

525. Huppert VF, Berliner K. The intraventricular conduction time (QRS duration) of ventricular premature systoles. Cardiologia 1955; 27:87–96.

526. Childers RW. Usefulness of extrasystoles in cardiac diagnosis and prognosis. Med Clin North Am 1966; 50:51–71.

527. Myburgh DP, van Gelder AL. The nature of ventricular ectopic beats in chronic ischaemic heart disease. S Afr Med J 1974; 48:1067–1071.

528. Moulton KP, Medcalf T, Lazzara R. Premature ventricular complex morphology: a marker for left ventricular structure and function. Circulation 1990; 81:1245–1251.

529. Josephson ME. The origin of premature ventricular complexes: role and limitations of the 12-lead electrocardiogram. Int J Cardiol 1982; 2:87–90.

530. Barker PS, Macleod AG, Alexander J. The excitatory process observed in the exposed human heart. Am Heart J 1930; 5:720–742.

531. Marvin HM, Oughterson AW. The form of premature beats resulting from direct stimulation of the human ventricles. Am Heart J 1932; 7:471–476.

532. Castex MR, Battro A, Gonzalez R. Diagnosis of the site of origin of ventricular extrasystoles in human beings. Arch Intern Med 1941; 67:76–90.

533. Swanick EJ, LaCamera F Jr, Marriott HJ. Morphologic features of right ventricular ectopic beats. Am J Cardiol 1972; 30:888–891.

534. Rosenbaum MB. Classification of ventricular extrasystoles according to form. J Electrocardiol 1969; 2:289–297.

535. Manning GW, Ahuja SP, Gutierrez MR. Electrocardiographic differentiation between ventricular ectopic beats from subjects with normal and diseased hearts. Acta Cardiol 1968; 23:462–470.

536. Talbot S. Measuring ventricular extrasystoles. J Electrocardiol 1975; 8:325–331.

537. Lewis S, Kanakis C, Rosen KM, Denes P. Significance of site of origin of premature ventricular contractions. Am Heart J 1979; 97:159–164.

538. Tsuji Y, Watanabe Y. Electrocardiographic ischemic ST-T changes and ventricular premature systoles. Int J Cardiol 1982; 2:73–86.

539. Sharma PR, Chung EK. Clinical implication of surface morphology of ventricular premature contractions. J Electrocardiol 1980; 13:331–336.

540. Marriott HJ, Nizet PM. Main-stem extrasystoles with aberrant ventricular conduction mimicking ventricular extrasystoles. Am J Cardiol 1967; 19:755–757.

541. Massumi RA. Interpolated His bundle extrasystoles: an unusual cause of tachycardia. Am J Med 1970; 49:265–270.

542. Lindsay AE, Schamroth L. Atrioventricular junctional parasystole with concealed conduction simulating second degree atrioventricular block. Am J Cardiol 1973; 31:397–399.

543. Massumi RA, Hilliard G, Demaria A, et al. Paradoxic phenomenon of premature beats with narrow QRS in the presence of bundle-branch block. Circulation 1973; 47:543–553.

544. Nasrallah AT, Gillette PC, Mullins CE, Nihill MR, McNamara DG. Concealed His bundle extrasystoles in congenital heart disease. Am J Cardiol 1975; 35:288–292.

545. Curtiss EI, Heibel RH, Shaver JA. Mobitz II atrioventricular block due to infra-Hisian block and bundle branch extrasystoles. J Electrocardiol 1976; 9:181–186.

546. Castellanos A, Sung RJ, Mallon SM, Ghahramani A, Moleiro F, Myerburg RJ. His bundle electrocardiography in manifest and concealed right bundle branch extrasystoles. Am Heart J 1977; 94:307–315.

547. Langendorf R, Mehlman JS. Blocked (nonconducted) A-V nodal premature systoles imitating first and second degree A-V block. Am Heart J 1947; 34:500–506.

548. Rosen KM, Rahimtoola SH, Gunnar RM. Pseudo A-V block secondary to premature nonpropagated His bundle depolarizations: documentation by His bundle electrocardiography. Circulation 1970; 42:367–373.

549. Cannom DS, Gallagher JJ, Goldreyer BN, Damato AN. Concealed bundle of His extrasystoles simulating nonconducted atrial premature beats. Am Heart J 1972; 83:777–779.

550. Eugster GS, Godfrey CC, Brammell HL, Pryor R. Pseudo A-V block associated with A-H and H-V conduction defects. Am Heart J 1973; 85:789–796.

551. Lightfoot PR, Sasse L, Mandel WJ, Hayakawa H. His bundle electrograms in healthy adolescents with persistent second degree A-V block. Chest 1973; 63:358–362.

552. Castellanos A, Befeler B, Myerburg RJ. Pseudo AV block produced by concealed extrasystoles arising below the bifurcation of the His bundle. Br Heart J 1974; 36:457–461.

553. Kerin N, Edelstein J, Louridas G, Goldberg LB. Direct and incomplete concealed Wenckebach phenomenon in the left bundle-branch system. J Electrocardiol 1975; 8:179–183.

554. Bonner AJ, Zipes DP. Lidocaine and His bundle extrasystoles: His bundle discharge conducted with functional right or left bundle-branch block, or blocked entirely (concealed). Arch Intern Med 1976; 136:700–704.

555. Childers RW. The junctional premature beat: an instructional exercise in modes of concealment. J Electrocardiol 1976; 9:85–88.

556. Fisch C, Zipes DP, McHenry PL. Electrocardiographic manifestations of concealed junctional ectopic impulses. Circulation 1976; 53:217–223.

557. Abrams J, Dykstra JR. Pseudo A-V block secondary to concealed junctional extrasystoles: case report and review of the literature. Am J Med 1977; 63:434–440.

558. Donzeau JP, Bernadet P, Bounhoure JP, Calazel P. His bundle block and concealed His bundle premature depolarization. Eur J Cardiol 1979; 9:13–20.

559. Freeman G, Hwang MH, Danoviz J, Moran JF, Gunnar RM. Exercise induced "Mobitz type II" second degree AV block in a patient with chronic bifascicular block (right bundle branch block and left anterior hemiblock). J Electrocardiol 1984; 17:409–412.

560. Wang K, Salerno DM. Pseudo AV block secondary to concealed premature His bundle depolarizations. Am Heart J 1991; 121:1236–1237.

561. Geelen P, Malacky T, Lorga A, Manios E, Brugada P. The valve of an electrophysiological study in a clear-cut case. Pacing Clin Electrophysiol 1996; 19:1643–1645.

562. Dressler W. A case of myocardial infarction masked by bundle branch block but revealed by occasional premature ventricular beats. Am J Med Sci 1943; 206:361–363.

563. Simonson E, Enzer N, Goodman JS. Coronary insufficiency, revealed by ectopic nodal and ventricular beats in the presence of left bundle branch block. Am J Med Sci 1945; 209:349–355.

564. Myers GB. Other QRS-T patterns that may be mistaken for myocardial infarction. IV. Alteration in blood potassium; myocardial ischemia; subepicardial myocarditis; distortion associated with arrhythmias. Circulation 1950; 2:75–93.

565. Katz KH, Berk MS, Mayman CI. Acute myocardial infarction revealed in an isolated premature ventricular beat. Circulation 1958; 18:897–901.

566. Silverman JJ, Salomon S. Myocardial infarction pattern disclosed by ventricular extrasystoles. Am J Cardiol 1959; 4:695–697.

567. Bisteni A, Medrano GA, Sodi-Pallares D. Ventricular premature beats in the diagnosis of myocardial infarction. Br Heart J 1961; 23:521–532.

568. Cohen J. Acute myocardial infarction early and objectively diagnosed through ventricular extrasystoles. Am J Cardiol 1961; 7:882–885.

569. Soloff LA. Ventricular premature beats diagnostic of myocardial disease. Am J Med Sci 1961; 242:315–319.

570. Anttonen V-M, Leskinen E, Meurman L, Oka M, Raunio H. The diagnostic value of unipolar precordial patterns of ventricular premature beats in myocardial infarction. Acta Med Scand 1962;387:1–65.

571. Szilagyi N, Ginsburg M. Acute myocardial infarction revealed in the presence of right bundle branch block and ventricular extrasystoles. Am J Cardiol 1962; 9:632–638.

572. Benchimol A, Lasry JE, Carvalho FR. The ventricular premature contraction. Its place in the diagnosis of ischemic heart disease. Am Heart J 1963; 65:334–339.

573. Freundlich J, Kavanagh-Gray D. The significance of ventricular premature beats in the diagnosis of septal infarction. Can Med Assoc J 1964; 91:1145–1148.

574. Martinez A. Aberrant ventricular conduction in the diagnosis of myocardial infarction. Am J Cardiol 1964; 14:352–356.

575. Lichtenberg SB, Schwartz MJ, Case RB. Value of premature ventricular contraction morphology in the detection of myocardial infarction. J Electrocardiol 1980; 13:167–171.

576. Dash H, Ciotola TJ. Morphology of ventricular premature beats as an aid in the electrocardiographic diagnosis of myocardial infarction. Am J Cardiol 1983; 52:458–461.

577. Sclarovsky S, Strasberg B, Lahav M, Lewin RF, Agmon J. Premature ventricular contractions in acute myocardial infarction: correlation between their origin and the location of infarction. J Electrocardiol 1979; 12:157–161.

578. Watanabe Y, Pamintuan JC, Dreifus LS. Role of intraventricular conduction disturbances in ventricular premature systoles. Am J Cardiol 1973; 32:188–195.

579. Michelson EL, Morganroth J, Spear JF, Kastor JA, Josephson ME. Fixed coupling: different mechanisms revealed by exercise-induced changes in cycle length. Circulation 1978; 58:1002–1009.

580. Talbot S. Significance of coupling intervals of ventricular extrasystoles. Cardiology 1974; 59:231–243.

581. Talbot S, Dreifus LS. Characteristics of ventricular extrasystoles and their prognostic importance: a reappraisal of their method of classification. Chest 1975; 67:665–674.

582. Kessler KM, McAuliffe D, Chakko CS, Castellanos A, Myerburg RJ. Multiform ventricular complexes: a transitional arrhythmia form? Am Heart J 1989; 118:441–444.

583. Yusuf S, Lopez R, Sleight P. Heart rate and ectopic prematurity in relation to sustained ventricular arrhythmias. Br Heart J 1980; 44:233–239.

584. Mack I, Langendorf R. Factors influencing the time of appearance of premature systoles (including a demonstration of cases with ventricular premature systoles due to re-entry but exhibiting variable coupling). Circulation 1950; 1:910–921.

585. Scherf D, Boyd LJ. Three unusual cases of parasystole. Am Heart J 1950; 39:650–663.

586. Scherf D, Schott A. Coupled extrasystoles and automatic ventricular rhythms. Am Heart J 1951; 41:291–298.

587. Mueller P, Baron B. Clinical studies on parasystole. Am Heart J 1953; 45:441–447.

588. Pick A. Parasystole. Circulation 1953; 8:243–252.

589. Golbey M, Ladopulos CP, Roth FH, Scherf D. Changes of ventricular impulse formation during carotid pressure in man. Circulation 1954; 10:735–741.

590. Langendorf R, Pick A. Mechanisms of intermittent ventricular bigeminy. II. Parasystole, and parasystole or re-entry with conduction disturbance. Circulation 1955; 11:431–439.

591. Katz LN, Pick A. Clinical Electrocardiography. Part I. The Arrhythmias. Philadelphia: Lea & Febiger, 1956, pp. 178–184.

592. Heinz RE, Eldridge FL. Ventricular parasystole in a five-year-old child. Am Heart J 1957; 53:624–627.

593. Scherf D, Schott A, Reid EC, Chamsal DG. Intermittent parasystole. Cardiologia 1957; 30:217–228.

594. Rossi P, Motolese M, Passaro G. Idioventricular parasystole with exit block in a subject with complete atrioventricular dissociation. Am Heart J 1959; 57:775–781.

595. Schamroth L, Marriott HJL. Intermittent ventricular parasystole with observations on its relationship to extrasystolic bigeminy. Am J Cardiol 1961; 7:799–809.

596. Scherf D, Bornemann C. Parasystole with a rapid ventricular center. Am Heart J 1961; 62:320–331.

597. Castellanos A, Mayer JW, Lemberg L. Intermittent parasystole with disturbance in impulse formation and impulse conduction. Acta Cardiol 1962; 17:49–58.

598. Schwartz NL, Marriott HJL. Unusual dysrhythmia in a normal child: ventricular parasystole of high septal or junctional origin. Am J Cardiol 1962; 10:302–305.

599. Scherf D, Choi KH, Bahadori A, Orphanos RP. Parasystole. Am J Cardiol 1963; 12:527–538.

600. Surawicz B, MacDonald MG. Ventricular ectopic beats with fixed and variable coupling: Incidence, clinical significance and factors influencing the coupling interval. Am J Cardiol 1964; February:198–208.

601. Chung K-Y, Walsh TJ, Massie E. Ventricular parasystolic tachycardia. Br Heart J 1965; 27:392–400.

602. Chung EK. Principles of Cardiac Arrhythmias. Baltimore: Williams & Wilkins, 1971, pp. 361–377.

603. Watanabe Y. Reassessment of parasystole. Am Heart J 1971; 81:451–466.

604. Cohen H, Langendorf R, Pick A. Intermittent parasystole: mechanism of protection. Circulation 1973; 48:761–774.

605. el-Sherif N, Samet P. Multiform ventricular ectopic rhythm: evidence for multiple parasystolic activity. Circulation 1975; 51:492–505.

606. Furuse A, Shindo G, Makuuchi H, et al. Apparent suppression of ventricular parasystole by cardiac pacing. Jpn Heart J 1979; 20:843–851.

607. Kuo CS, Surawicz B. Coexistence of ventricular parasystole and ventricular couplets: mechanism and clinical significance. Am J Cardiol 1979; 44:435–441.

608. Castellanos A, Alatriste VM, Sung RJ, Sheps DS, Myerburg RJ. A search for modulation in intermittent ventricular parasystole. Pacing Clin Electrophysiol 1980; 3:73–83.

609. Jalife J, Antzelevitch C, Moe GK. The case for modulated parasystole. Pacing Clin Electrophysiol 1982; 5:911–926.

610. Nau GJ, Aldariz AE, Acunzo RS, et al. Modulation of parasystolic activity by nonparasystolic beats. Circulation 1982; 66:462–469.

611. Castellanos A, Luceri RM, Moleiro F, et al. Annihilation, entrainment and modulation of ventricular parasystolic rhythms. Am J Cardiol 1984; 54:317–322.

612. Lanza GA, Lucente M, Rebuzzi AG, Spagnolo A, Dulcimascolo C, Manzoli U. Ventricular parasystole: a chronobiologic study. Pacing Clin Electrophysiol 1986; 9:860–867.

613. Oreto G, Satullo G, Luzza F, et al. "Irregular" ventricular parasystole: the influence of sinus rhythm on a parasystolic focus. Am Heart J 1988; 115:121–133.

614. Robles de Medina EO, Delmar M, Sicouri S, Jalife J. Modulated parasystole as a mechanism of ventricular ectopic activity leading to ventricular fibrillation. Am J Cardiol 1989; 63:1326–1332.

615. Castellanos A, Moleiro F, Interian A Jr, Myerburg RJ. A different approach to the analysis of pure ventricular parasystole. Chest 1995; 107:1463–1464.

616. Castellanos A, Saoudi N, Moleiro F, Myerburg RJ. Parasystole. In Zipes DP, Jalife J (eds). Cardiac Electrophysiology. From Cell to Bedside. 2nd ed. Philadelphia: WB Saunders, 1995, pp. 942–954.

617. Langendorf R, Pick A. Parasystole with fixed coupling. Circulation 1967; 35:304–315.

618. Steffens TG, Gettes LS. Parasystole. Cardiovasc Clin 1974; 6:99–110.

619. Steffens TG. Intermittent ventricular parasystole due to entrance block failure. Circulation 1971; 44:442–445.

620. Kinoshita S. Concealed ventricular extrasystoles due to interference and due to exit block. Circulation 1975; 52:230–237.

621. Blanchard WB, Bucciarelli RL, Miller BL. Ventricular parasystole in a newborn infant. J Electrocardiol 1979; 12:427–429.

622. Myburgh DP, Lewis BS. Ventricular parasystole in healthy hearts. Am Heart J 1971; 82:307–311.

623. Schamroth L, Dubb A. Escape-capture bigeminy: mechanisms in S-A block, A-V block, and reversed reciprocal rhythm. Br Heart J 1965; 27:667–669.

624. Schamroth L. Concealed extrasystoles and the rule of bigeminy. Cardiologia 1965; 46:51–58.

625. Friedberg HD. Concealed extrasystoles. Am J Cardiol 1969; 24:283–286.

626. Levy MN, Adler DS, Levy JR. Three variants of concealed bigeminy. Circulation 1975; 51:646–655.

627. Levy MN, Kerin N, Eisenstein I. A subvariant of concealed bigeminy. J Electrocardiol 1977; 10:225–232.

628. Kinoshita S. Mechanisms of ventricular parasystole. Circulation 1978; 58:715–722.

629. Kerin NZ, Rubenfire M, Stoler R, Levy MN. Concealed ventricular premature complexes in a population sample. Am J Cardiol 1986; 57:392–397.

630. Levy MN, Mori I, Kerin N. Two variants of concealed trigeminy. Am Heart J 1977; 93:183–188.

631. Chung DK, Chung EK. Ventricular bigeminy masquerading as total electrical alternans: in a case of probable tuberculous pericarditis. Am J Cardiol 1969; 23:287–289.

632. Wilson C, Pantridge JF. ST-segment displacement and early hospital discharge in acute myocardial infarction. Lancet 1973; 2:1284–1288.

633. Scherf D. Alterations in the form of the T waves with changes in heart rate. Am Heart J 1944; 28:332–347.

634. Levine HD, Lown B, Streeper RB. The clinical significance of postextrasystolic T-wave changes. Circulation 1952; 6:538–548.

635. Chung EK. Principles of Cardiac Arrhythmias. Baltimore: Williams & Wilkins, 1971, pp. 315–316.

636. Mann RH, Burchell HB. The significance of T-wave inversion in sinus beats following ventricular extrasystoles. Am Heart J 1954; 47:504–513.

637. Robitaille GA, Phillips JH Jr. A study of the postextrasystolic T wave changes associated with interpolated premature ventricular beats. Am J Med Sci 1965; 250:315–323.

638. Iyengar R, Castellanos A Jr, Spence M. Continuous monitoring of ambulatory patients with coronary disease. Prog Cardiovasc Dis 1971; 13:392–404.

639. Bleifer SB, Bleifer DJ, Hansmann DR, Sheppard JJ, Harold HL. Diagnosis of occult arrhythmias by Holter electrocardiography. Prog Cardiovasc Dis 1974; 16:569–599.

640. Lown B, Calvert AF, Armington R, Ryan M. Monitoring for serious arrhythmias and high risk of sudden death. Circulation 1975; 52(Suppl III):III-189–III-198.

641. Harrison DC, Fitzgerald JW, Winkle RA. Ambulatory electrocardiography for diagnosis and treatment of cardiac arrhythmias. N Engl J Med 1976; 294:373–380.

642. Romero CA Jr. Holter monitoring in the diagnosis and management of cardiac rhythm disturbances. Med Clin North Am 1976; 60:299–313.

643. Harrison DC, Fitzgerald JW, Winkle RA. Contribution of ambulatory electrocardiographic monitoring to antiarrhythmic management. Am J Cardiol 1978; 41:996–1004.

644. Coumel P. Ambulatory electrocardiographic monitoring and the management of arrhythmias: precision versus inflexibility. Br Heart J 1983; 49:201–204.

645. Kosowsky BD, Lown B, Whiting R, Guiney T. Occurrence of ventricular arrhythmias with exercise as compared to monitoring. Circulation 1971; 44:826–832.

646. Ryden L, Waldenstrom A, Homberg S. The reliability of intermittent ECG sampling in arrhythmia detection. Circulation 1975; 52:540–545.

647. Winkle RA, Goodman DJ, Popp RL. Simultaneous echocardiographic phonocardiographic recordings at rest and during amyl nitrite administration in patients with mitral valve prolapse. Circulation 1975; 51:522–529.

648. DeMaria AN, Vera Z, Neumann A, Mason DT. Alterations in ventricular contraction pattern in the Wolff-Parkinson-White syndrome: detection by echocardiography. Circulation 1976; 53:249–257.

649. Vismara LA, Pratt C, Price JE, Miller RR, Amsterdam EA, Mason DT. Correlation of the standard electrocardiogram and continuous ambulatory monitoring in the detection of ventricular arrhythmias in coronary patients. J Electrocardiol 1977; 10:299–304.

650. Davis BR, Friedman LM, Lichstein E. Are 24 hours of ambulatory Ecg monitoring necessary for a patient after infarction? Am Heart J 1988; 115:83–91.

651. Connolly SJ, Cairns JA. Comparison of one-, six- and 24-hour ambulatory electrocardiographic monitoring for ventricular arrhythmia as a predictor of mortality in survivors of acute myocardial infarction: CAMIAT pilot study group. Canadian Amiodarone Myocardial Infarction Arrhythmia Trial. Am J Cardiol 1992; 69:308–313.

652. Petretta M, Bianchi V, Pulcino A, et al. Continuous electrocardiographic monitoring for more than one hour does not improve the prognostic value of ventricular arrhythmias in survivors of first acute myocardial infarction. Am J Cardiol 1994; 73:139–142.

653. Crawford M, O'Rourke RA, Ramakrishna N, Henning H, Ross J Jr. Comparative effectiveness of exercise testing and continuous monitoring for detecting arrhythmias in patients with previous myocardial infarction. Circulation 1974; 50:301–305.

654. Janssen MJ, Swenne CA, Manger Cats V, van Bemmel JH, Bruschke AV. Autonomic, ischaemic, circadian and rhythmic factors as causes of the spontaneous variability of ventricular arrhythmias. Eur Heart J 1995; 16:674–681.

655. Morganroth J, Michelson EL, Horowitz LN, Josephson ME, Pearlman AS, Dunkman WB. Limitations of routine long-term electrocardiographic monitoring to assess ventricular ectopic frequency. Circulation 1978; 58:408–414.

656. Pratt CM, Delclos G, Wierman AM, et al. The changing base line of complex ventricular arrhythmias: a new consideration in assessing long-term antiarrhythmic drug therapy. N Engl J Med 1985; 313:1444–1449.

657. Toivonen L. Spontaneous variability in the frequency of ventricular premature complexes over prolonged intervals and implications for antiarrhythmic treatment. Am J Cardiol 1987; 60:608–612.

658. Schmidt G, Ulm K, Barthel P, Goedel-Meinen L, Jahns G, Baedeker W. Spontaneous variability of simple and complex ventricular premature contractions during long time intervals in patients with severe organic heart disease. Circulation 1988; 78:296–301.

659. Michelson EL, Morganroth J. Spontaneous variability of complex ventricular arrhythmias detected by long-term electrocardiographic recording. Circulation 1980; 61:690–695.

660. Winkle RA. Antiarrhythmic drug effect mimicked by spontaneous variability of ventricular ectopy. Circulation 1978; 57:1116–1121.

661. Anastasiou-Nana M, Menlove RL, Nanas JN, Anderson JL. Changes in spontaneous variability of ventricular ectopic activity as a function of time in patients with chronic arrhythmias. Circulation 1988; 78:286–295.

662. Pratt CM, Slymen DJ, Wierman AM, et al. Analysis of the spontaneous variability of ventricular arrhythmias: consecutive ambulatory electrocardiographic recordings of ventricular tachycardia. Am J Cardiol 1985; 56:67–72.

663. Pratt CM, Theroux P, Slymen D, et al. Spontaneous variability of ventricular arrhythmias in patients at increased risk for sudden death after acute myocardial infarction: consecutive ambulatory electrocardiographic recordings of 88 patients. Am J Cardiol 1987; 59:278–283.

664. Poblete PF, Pescarmona JE, Kennedy HL, Gillilan RE. Hour to hour vs day to day variation of ventricular ectopic beats. Circulation 1979; 59 and 60(Suppl II):II-188.

665. Anderson JL, Anastasiou-Nana M, Menlove RL, Moreno FL, Nanas JN, Barker AH. Spontaneous variability in ventricular ectopic activity during chronic antiarrhythmic therapy. Circulation 1990; 82:830–840.

666. Barsky AJ, Cleary PD, Barnett MC, Christiansen CL, Ruskin JN. The accuracy of symptom reporting by patients complaining of palpitations. Am J Med 1994; 97:214–221.

667. Shah PM, Arnold JM, Haberern NA, Bliss DT, McClelland KM, Clarke WB. Automatic real time arrhythmia monitoring in the intensive coronary care unit. Am J Cardiol 1977; 39:701–708.

668. Farrell TG, Odemuyiwa O, Bashir Y, et al. Prognostic value of baroreflex sensitivity testing after acute myocardial infarction. Br Heart J 1992; 67:129–137.

669. Hayashi H, Fujiki A, Tani M, Mizumaki K, Shimono M,

Inoue H. Role of sympathovagal balance in the initiation of idiopathic ventricular tachycardia originating from right ventricular outflow tract. PACE 1997; 20:2371–2377.

670. Gooch AS, Mcconnell D. Analysis of transient arrhythmias and conduction disturbances occurring during submaximal treadmill exercise testing. Prog Cardiovasc Dis 1970; 13:293–307.

671. Gooch AS. Exercise testing for detecting changes in cardiac rhythm and conduction. Am J Cardiol 1972; 30:741–746.

672. Master AM. Cardiac arrhythmias elicited by the two-step exercise test. Am J Cardiol 1973; 32:766–771.

673. DeMaria AN, Vera Z, Amsterdam EA, Mason DT, Massumi RA. Disturbances of cardiac rhythm and conduction induced by exercise: diagnostic, prognostic and therapeutic implications. Am J Cardiol 1974; 33:732–736.

674. Jelinek MV, Lown B. Exercise stress testing for exposure of cardiac arrhythmia. Prog Cardiovasc Dis 1974; 16:497–522.

675. Goldschlager N, Cohn K, Goldschlager A. Exercise-related ventricular arrhythmias. Mod Concepts Cardiovasc Dis 1979; 67–72.

676. Halpern SW, Mandel WJ. The significance of exercise-induced ventricular arrhythmias. Chest 1980; 77:1–2.

677. Cohn PF. Current concepts: the role of noninvasive cardiac testing after an uncomplicated myocardial infarction. N Engl Med 1983; 309:90–93.

678. Coumcl P, Zimmermann M, Funck Brentano C. Exercise test: arrhythmogenic or antiarrhythmic? Rate-dependency vs. adrenergic-dependency of tachyarrhythmias. Eur Heart J 1987; 8:7–15.

679. Podrid PJ, Graboys TB, Lampert S, Blatt C. Exercise stress testing for exposure of arrhythmias. Circulation 1987; 75(Suppl III):III-60–III-68.

680. Podrid PJ, Venditti FJ, Levine PA, Klein MD. The role of exercise testing in evaluation of arrhythmias. Am J Cardiol 1988; 62:24H–33H.

681. Pitzalis MV, Mastropasqua F, Massari F, et al. Heart rate dependency of premature ventricular contractions: correlation between electrocardiographic monitoring and exercise-related patterns. Eur Heart J 1997; 18:1642–1648.

682. McHenry MM. Factors influencing longevity in adults with congenital complete heart block. Am J Cardiol 1972; 29:416–421.

683. Beard EF, Owen CA. Cardiac arrhythmias during exercise testing in healthy men. Aerospace Med 1973; 44:286–289.

684. Goldschlager N, Cake D, Cohn K. Exercise-induced ventricular arrhythmias in patients with coronary artery disease: their relation to angiographic findings. Am J Cardiol 1973; 31:434–440.

685. Froelicher VF Jr, Thomas MM, Pillow C, Lancaster MC. Epidemiologic study of asymptomatic men screened by maximal treadmill testing for latent coronary artery disease. Am J Cardiol 1974; 34:770–776.

686. Faris JV, McHenry PL, Jordan JW, Morris SN. Prevalence and reproducibility of exercise-induced ventricular arrhythmias during maximal exercise testing in normal men. Am J Cardiol 1976; 37:617–622.

687. McHenry PL, Morris SN, Kavalier M, Jordan JW. Comparative study of exercise-induced ventricular arrhythmias in normal subjects and patients with documented coronary artery disease. Am J Cardiol 1976; 37:609–616.

688. Viitasalo MT, Kala R, Eisalo A, Halonen PI. Ventricular arrhythmias during exercise testing, jogging, and sedentary life: a comparative study of healthy physically active men, healthy sedentary men, and men with previous myocardial infarction. Chest 1979; 76:21–26.

689. Whinnery JE. Dysrhythmia comparison in apparently healthy males during and after treadmill and acceleration stress testing. Am Heart J 1983; 105:732–737.

690. Northcote RJ, MacFarlane P, Ballantyne D. Ambulatory electrocardiography in squash players. Br Heart J 1983; 50:372–377.

691. Thapar MK, Strong WB, Miller MD, Leatherbury L, Salehbhai M. Exercise electrocardiography of healthy black children. Am J Dis Child 1978; 132:592–595.

692. Rozanski JJ, Dimich I, Steinfeld L. Kupersmith J. Maximal exercise stress testing in evaluation of arrhythmias in children: results and reproducibility. Am J Cardiol 1979; 43:951–956.

693. Atkins JM, Matthews OA, Blomqvist CG, Mullins CB. Incidence of arrhythmias induced by isometric and dynamic exercise. Br Heart J 1976; 38:465–471.

694. Lehrman KL, Tilkian AG, Hultgren HN, Fowles RE. Effect of coronary arterial bypass surgery on exercise-induced ventricular arrhythmias: long-term follow-up of a prospective randomized study. Am J Cardiol 1979; 44:1056–1061.

695. Califf RM, McKinnis RA, McNeer JF, et al. Prognostic value of ventricular arrhythmias associated with treadmill exercise testing in patients studied with cardiac catheterization for suspected ischemic heart disease. J Am Coll Cardiol 1983; 2:1060–1067.

696. Vedin JA, Wilhelmsson CE, Wilhelmsen L, Bjure J, Ekstrom-Jodal B. Relation of resting and exercise-induced ectopic beats to other ischemic manifestations and to coronary risk factors: men born in 1913. Am J Cardiol 1972; 30:25–31.

697. Nair CK, Aronow WS, Sketch MH, et al. Diagnostic and prognostic significance of exercise-induced premature ventricular complexes in men and women: a four year follow-up. J Am Coll Cardiol 1983; 1:1201–1206.

698. Udall JA, Ellestad MH. Predictive implications of ventricular premature contractions associated with treadmill stress testing. Circulation 1977; 56:985–989.

699. Helfant RH, Pine R, Kabde V, Banka VS. Exercise-related ventricular premature complexes in coronary heart disease: correlations with ischemia and angiographic severity. Ann Intern Med 1974; 80:589–592.

700. Mardelli TJ, Morganroth J, Dreifus LS. Superior QRS axis of ventricular premature complexes: an additional criterion to enhance the sensitivity of exercise stress testing. Am J Cardiol 1980; 45:236–243.

701. Miller WP. Cardiac arrhythmias and conduction disturbances in the sleep apnea syndrome: prevalence and significance. Am J Med 1982; 73:317–321.

702. Ericsson M, Granath A, Ohlsen P, Sodermark T, Volpe U. Arrhythmias and symptoms during treadmill testing three weeks after myocardial infarction in 100 patients. Br Heart J 1973; 35:787–790.

703. Granath A, Sodermark T, Winge T, Volpe U, Zetterquist S. Early work load tests for evaluation of long-term prognosis of acute myocardial infarction. Br Heart J 1977; 39:758–765.

704. Markiewicz W, Houston N, DeBusk RF. Exercise testing soon after myocardial infarction. Circulation 1977; 56:26–31.

705. Smith JW, Dennis CA, Gassmann A, et al. Exercise testing three weeks after myocardial infarction. Chest 1979; 75:12–16.

706. Theroux P, Waters DD, Halphen C, Debaisieux JC, Mizgala HF. Prognostic value of exercise testing soon after myocardial infarction. N Engl J Med 1979; 301:341–345.

707. Davidson DM, DeBusk RF. Prognostic value of a single exercise test 3 weeks after uncomplicated myocardial infarction. Circulation 1980; 61:236–242.

708. Starling MR, Crawford MH, Kennedy GT, O'Rourke RA. Exercise testing early after myocardial infarction: predictive value for subsequent unstable angina and death. Am J Cardiol 1980; 46:909–914.

709. Fuller CM, Raizner AE, Verani MS, et al. Early post-myocardial infarction treadmill stress testing: an accurate predictor of multivessel coronary disease and subsequent cardiac events. Ann Intern Med 1981; 94:734-739.

710. Starling MR, Crawford MH, Kennedy GT, O'Rourke RA. Treadmill exercise tests predischarge and six weeks post-myocardial infarction to detect abnormalities of known prognostic value. Ann Intern Med 1981; 94:721–727.

711. Weld FM, Chu KL, Bigger JT Jr, Rolnitzky LM. Risk stratification with low-level exercise testing 2 weeks after acute myocardial infarction. Circulation 1981; 64:306–314.

712. Henry RL, Kennedy GT, Crawford MH. Prognostic value of exercise-induced ventricular ectopic activity for mortality after acute myocardial infarction. Am J Cardiol 1987; 59:1251–1255.

713. Ibsen H, Kjoller E, Styperek J, Pedersen A. Routine exercise ECG three weeks after acute myocardial infarction. Acta Med Scand 1975; 198:463–469.

714. Celermajer DS, Sholler GF, Howman-Giles R, Celermajer JM. Myocardial infarction in childhood: clinical analysis of 17 cases and medium term follow up of survivors. Br Heart J 1991; 65:332–336.

715. Ikkos D, Hanson JS. Response to exercise in congenital complete atrioventricular block. Circulation 1960; 22:538–590.

716. Winkler RB, Freed MD, Nadas AS. Exercise-induced ventricular ectopy in children and young adults with complete heart block. Am Heart J 1980; 99:87–92.

717. Karpawich PP, Gillette PC, Garson A Jr, Hesslein PS, Porter CB, McNamara DG. Congenital complete atrioventricular block: clinical and electrophysiologic predictors of need for pacemaker insertion. Am J Cardiol 1981; 48:1098–1102.

718. Bause GS, Fleg JL, Lakatta EG. Exercise-induced arrhythmias in diuretic-treated patients with uncomplicated systemic hypertension. Am J Cardiol 1987; 59:874–877.

719. Cheong TH, Magder S, Shapiro S, Martin JG, Levy RD. Cardiac arrhythmias during exercise in severe chronic obstructive pulmonary disease. Chest 1990; 97:793–797.

720. James FW, Kaplan S, Schwartz DC, Chou TC, Sandker MJ, Naylor V. Response to exercise in patients after total surgical correction of tetralogy of Fallot. Circulation 1976; 54:671–679.

721. Garson A Jr., Gillette PC, Gutgesell HP, McNamara DG. Stress-induced ventricular arrhythmia after repair of tetralogy of Fallot. Am J Cardiol 1980; 46:1006–1012.

722. Sheps DS, Ernst JC, Briese FR, et al. Decreased frequency of exercise-induced ventricular ectopic activity in the second of two consecutive treadmill tests. Circulation 1977; 55:892–895.

723. Sami M, Kraemer H, DeBusk RF. Reproducibility of exercise-induced ventricular arrhythmia after myocardial infarction. Am J Cardiol 1979; 43:724–730.

724. Goldberg AD, Raftery EB, Cashman PM. Ambulatory electrocardiographic records in patients with transient cerebral attacks or palpitation. BMJ 1975; 4:569–571.

725. Simoons M, Lap C, Pool J. Heart rate levels and ventricular ectopic activity during cardiac rehabilitation. Am Heart J 1980; 100:9–14.

726. Shapiro W, Park J, Koch GG. Variability of spontaneous and exercise-induced ventricular arrhythmias in the absence and presence of treatment with acebutolol or quinidine. Am J Cardiol 1982; 49:445–454.

727. Boudoulas H, Schaal SF, Lewis RP, Robinson JL. Superiority of 24-hour outpatient monitoring over multistage exercise testing for the evaluation of syncope. J Electrocardiol 1979; 12:103–108.

728. Kostis JB, Lacy CR, Shindler DM, et al. Frequency of ventricular ectopic activity in isolated systolic systemic hypertension. Am J Cardiol 1992; 69:557–559.

729. Suwa M, Hirota Y, Nagao H, Kino M, Kawamura K. Incidence of the coexistence of left ventricular false tendons and premature ventricular contractions in apparently healthy subjects. Circulation 1984; 70:793–798.

730. Suwa M, Hirota Y, Kaku K, et al. Prevalence of the coexistence of left ventricular false tendons and premature ventricular complexes in apparently healthy subjects: a prospective study in the general population. J Am Coll Cardiol 1988; 12:910–914.

731. Popovic AD, Neskovic AN, Pavlovski K, et al. Association of ventricular arrhythmias with left ventricular remodelling after myocardial infarction. Heart 1997; 77:423–427.

732. Jewitt DE, Reid D, Thomas M, Mercer CJ, Valori C, Shillingford JP. Free noradrenaline and adrenaline excretion in relation to the development of cardiac arrhythmias and heart-failure in patients with acute myocardial infarction. Lancet 1969; 1:635–641.

733. Oliver MF, Kurien VA, Greenwood TW. Relation between serum-free-fatty acids and arrhythmias and death after acute myocardial infarction. Lancet 1968; 1:710–714.

734. Rutenberg HL, Soloff LA. Serum-free-fatty-acids and arrhythmias after acute myocardial infarction. Lancet 1970; 1:198.

735. Di Biase M, Chiddo A, Caruso G, Tritto M, Marchese A, Rizzon P. Ventricular premature beats in young subjects without evidence of cardiac disease: histological findings. Euro Heart J 1992; 13:732–737.

736. Oturo C. Hemodynamics of cardiac arrhythmias. Jpn Circ J 1962; 26:237–244.

737. Ferrer MI, Harvey RM. Some hemodynamic aspects of cardiac arrhythmias in man: a clinico-physiologic correlation. Am Heart J 1964; 68:153–165.

738. Cohn K, Kryda W. The influence of ectopic beats and tachyarrhythmias on stroke volume and cardiac output. J Electrocardiol 1981; 14:207–218.

739. Pierce GE, Morrow AG, Braunwald E. Idiopathic hypertrophic subaortic stenosis. III. Intraoperative studies of the mechanism of obstruction and its hemodynamic consequences. Circulation 1964; 29 and 30(Suppl IV):IV-152–IV-213.

740. Kennedy HL, Pescarmona JE, Bouchard RJ, Goldberg RJ, Caralis DG. Objective evidence of occult myocardial dysfunction in patients with frequent ventricular ectopy without clinically apparent heart disease. Am Heart J 1982; 104:57–65.

741. Damato AN, Lau SH. Clinical value of the electrogram of the conduction system. Prog Cardiovasc Dis 1970; 13:119–140.

742. Goldreyer BN. Intracardiac electrocardiography in the analysis and understanding of cardiac arrhythmias. Ann Inter Med 1972; 77:117–136.

743. Castellanos A Jr., O'Brien H, Castillo CA, Myerburg RJ, Beffler B. Contribution of His bundle recordings to analysis of abnormal beats with right bundle-branch block–superior axis pattern. Br Heart J 1972; 34:795–799.

744. Massumi RA, Mason DT, Vera Z, Miller R, Amsterdam EA. Fascicular rhythm: morphologic features and protean manifestations. Postgrad Med 1973; 53:95–102.

745. Nalos PC, Mandel WJ, Gang ES, Cain RP, Massumi RA, Peter T. Intermittent fascicular extrasystoles producing pseudo AV block: electrophysiologic effects of beta agonists and antagonists. Pacing Clin Electrophysiology 1987; 10:1160–1167.

746. Castillo C, Castellanos A Jr, Agha AS, Myerburg R. Significance of His bundle recordings with short H-V intervals. Chest 1971; 60:142–150.

747. Langendorf R. How everything started in clinical electrophysiology. In Brugada P, Wellens HJJ (eds). Cardiac Arrhythmias: Where to Go from Here? Mount Kisco, NY: Futura Publishing Co., 1987, pp. 715–722.

748. Nasrallah AT, Gillette PC, Mullins CE. Congenital and surgical atrioventricular block within the His bundle. Am J Cardiol 1975; 36:914–920.

749. Ezri MD, Huang SK, Messer JV, Denes P. Electrophysiologic observations of concealed ventricular depolarizations due to amiodarone. Am Heart J 1982; 104:169–172.

750. Josephson ME, Kastor JA. His-Purkinje conduction during retrograde stress. J Clin Invest 1978; 61:171–177.

751. Shenasa M, Denker S, Mahmud R, Lehmann M, Gilbert CJ, Akhtar M. Atrioventricular nodal conduction and refractoriness after intranodal collision from antegrade and retrograde impulses. Circulation 1983; 67:651–660.

752. Booth DC, Popio KA, Gettes LS. Multiformity if induced unifocal ventricular premature beats in human subjects: electrocardiographic and angiographic correlations. Am J Cardiol 1982; 49:1643–1653.

753. Gradman AH, Batsford WP, Rieur EC, Leon L, Van Zetta AM. Ambulatory electrocardiographic correlates of ventricular inducibility during programmed electrical stimulation. J Am Coll Cardiol 1985; 5:1087–1093.

754. Gomes JAC, Hariman RI, Kang PS, el-Sherif N, Chowdhry I, Lyons J. Programmed electrical stimulation in patients with high-grade ventricular ectopy: electrophysiologic findings and prognosis for survival. Circulation 1984; 70:43–51.

755. Zheutlin TA, Roth H, Chua W, et al. Programmed electrical stimulation to determine the need for antiarrhythmic therapy in patients with complex ventricular ectopic activity. Am Heart J 1986; 111:860–867.

756. Kharsa MH, Gold RL, Moore H, Yazaki Y, Haffajee CI, Alpert JS. Long-term outcome following programmed electrical stimulation in patients with high-grade ventricular ectopy. Pacing Clin Electrophysiol 1988; 11:603–609.

757. Gumbrielle T, Bourke JP, Furniss SS. Is ventricular ectopy a legitimate target for ablation? Br Heart J 1994; 72:492–494.

758. Zhu DW, Maloney JD, Simmons TW, et al. Radiofrequency catheter ablation for management of symptomatic ventricular ectopic activity. J Am Coll Cardiol 1995; 26:843–849.

759. Fenici R, Melillo G. Magnetocardiography: ventricular arrhythmias. Eur Heart J 1993; 14:53–60.

760. Spracklen FHN, Kimerling JJ, Besterman EMM, Litchfield JW. Use of lignocaine in treatment of cardiac arrhythmias. BMJ 1968; 1:89–91.

761. Mitchell LB. Treatment of ventricular arrhythmias after recovery from myocardial infarction. Annu Rev Med 1994; 45:119–138.

762. Cope RL. Suppressive effect of carotid sinus stimulation on premature ventricular beats in certain instances. Am J Cardiol 1959; 4:314–320.

763. Scherf D, Cohen J, Rafailzadeh M. Excitatory effects of carotid sinus pressure: enhancement of ectopic impulse formation and of impulse conduction. Am J Cardiol 1966; 17:240–252.

764. Garson A Jr, Gillette PC. Treatment of chronic ventricular dysrhythmias in the young. Pacing Clin Electrophysiol 1981; 4:658–669.

765. Gumbrielle T, Campbell RW. Pharmacological therapy of arrhythmias complicating dilated cardiomyopathy: implications of the arrhythmogenic substrate. Eur Heart J 1993; 14:103–106.

766. Roden DM. Risks and benefits of antiarrhythmic therapy. N Engl J Med 1994; 331:785–791.

767. Campbell RW. Should post-infarction asymptomatic ventricular arrhythmias be treated? Eur Heart J 1995; 16:46–48.

768. Sleight P. Should post-infarction asymptomatic ventricular arrhythmias be treated? The need for caution. Eur Heart J 1995; 16:49.

769. Landers MD, Reiter MJ. General principles of antiarrhythmic therapy for ventricular tachyarrhythmias. Am J Cardiol 1997; 80:31G–44G.

770. Singh BN. Controlling cardiac arrhythmias: an overview with a historical perspective. Am J Cardiol 1997; 80:4G–15G.

771. Prystowsky EN, Packer D. Nonpharmacologic treatment of supraventricular tachycardia. Am J Cardiol 1988; 62:74L–77L.

772. Pratt CM, Eaton T, Francis M, et al. The inverse relationship between baseline left ventricular ejection fraction and outcome of antiarrhythmic therapy: a dangerous imbalance in the risk-benefit ratio. Am Heart J 1989; 118:433–440.

773. Buxton AE. Antiarrhythmic drugs: good for premature ventricular complexes but bad for patients? Ann Intern Med 1992; 116:420–422.

774. Myerburg RJ, Mitrani R, Interian A, Castellanos A. Interpretation of outcomes of antiarrhythmic clinical trials: design features and population impact. Circulation 1998; 97:1514–1521.

775. Morganroth J, Bigger JT Jr. Pharmacologic management of ventricular arrhythmias after the Cardiac Arrhythmia Suppression Trial. Am J Cardiol 1990; 65:1497–1503.

776. Akhtar M, Breithardt G, Camm AJ, et al. CAST and beyond. Implications of the Cardiac Arrhythmia Suppression Trial: task force of the Working Group on Arrhythmias of the European Society of Cardiology. Circulation 1990; 81:1123–1127.

777. Echt DS, Liebson PR, Mitchell LB, et al. Mortality and morbidity in patients receiving encainide, flecainide, or placebo: the Cardiac Arrhythmia Suppression Trial. N Engl J Med 1991; 324:781–788.

778. Cairns JA, Connolly SJ, Roberts R, Gent M. Randomised trial of outcome after myocardial infarction in patients with frequent or repetitive ventricular premature depolarisations: CAMIAT. Canadian Amiodarone Myocardial Infarction Arrhythmia Trial Investigators. Lancet 1997; 349:675–682.

779. Anderson JL, Platia EV, Hallstrom A, et al. Interaction of baseline characteristics with the hazard of encainide, flecainide, and moricizine therapy in patients with myocardial infarction. Circulation 1994; 90:2843–2852.

780. Goldstein S, Brooks MM, Ledingham R, et al. Association between ease of suppression of ventricular arrhythmia and survival. Circulation 1995; 91:79–83.

781. Greenberg HM, Dwyer EM Jr, Hochman JS, Steinberg JS, Echt DS, Peters RW. Interaction of ischaemia and encainide/flecainide treatment: a proposed mechanism for the increased mortality in CAST I. Br Heart J 1995; 74:631–635.

782. Warnowicz MA, Denes P. Chronic ventricular arrhythmias: comparative drug effectiveness and toxicity. Prog Cardiovasc Dis 1980; 23:225–236.

783. Whiting RB. Ventricular premature contractions: which should be treated? Arch Intern Med 1980; 140:1423–1426.

784. Hoffmann A, Schutz E, White R, Follath F, Burckhardt D. Suppression of high-grade ventricular ectopic activity by antiarrhythmic drug treatment as a marker for survival in patients with chronic coronary artery disease. Am Heart J 1984; 107:1103–1108.

785. Myerburg RJ, Conde C, Sheps DS, et al. Antiarrhythmic drug therapy in survivors of prehospital cardiac arrest: comparison of effects on chronic ventricular arrhythmias and recurrent cardiac arrest. Circulation 1979; 59:855–863.

786. Hine LK, Laird NM, Hewitt P, Chalmers TC. Meta-analysis of empirical long-term antiarrhythmic therapy after myocardial infraction. JAMA 1989; 262:3037–3040.

787. Mason JW. Amiodarone. N Engl J Med 1987; 316:455–466.

788. Cairns JA, Connolly SJ, Roberts R, Gent M. Amiodarone for patients with ventricular premature depolarizations after myocardial infarction: is it safe to stop treatment at one year? Circulation 1993; 87:637–639.

789. Nademanee K, Singh BN, Stevenson WG, Weiss JN. Amiodarone and post-MI patients. Circulation 1993; 88:764–774.

790. Teo KK, Yusuf S, Furberg CD. Effects of prophylactic antiarrhythmic drug therapy in acute myocardial infarction: an overview of results from randomized controlled trials. JAMA 1993; 270:1589–1595.

791. Nademanee K, Hendrickson JA, Cannom DS, Goldreyer BN, Singh BN. Control of refractory life-threatening ventricular tachyarrhythmias by amiodarone. Am Heart J 1981; 101:759-768.

792. Podrid PJ, Lown B. Amiodarone therapy in symptomatic, sustained refractory atrial and ventricular tachyarrhythmias. Am Heart J 1981; 101:374–379.

793. Greene HL, Graham EL, Werner JA, et al. Toxic and therapeutic effects of amiodarone in the treatment of cardiac arrhythmias. J Am Coll Cardiol 1983; 2:1114–1128.

794. Nademanee K, Singh BN, Hendrickson J, et al. Amiodarone in refractory life-threatening ventricular arrhythmias. Ann Intern Med 1983; 98:577–584.

795. Collaborative Group for Amiodarone Evaluation. Multicenter controlled observation of a low-dose regimen of amiodarone for treatment of severe ventricular arrhythmias. Am J Cardiol 1984; 53:1564–1569.

796. Chiale PA, Halpern MS, Nau GJ, et al. Efficacy of amiodarone during long-term treatment of malignant ventricular arrhythmias in patients with chronic chagasic myocarditis. Am Heart J 1984; 107:656–665.

797. Kaski JC, Girotti LA, Elizari MV, et al. Efficacy of amiodarone during long-term treatment of potentially dangerous ventricular arrhythmias in patients with chronic stable ischemic heart disease. Am Heart J 1984; 107:648–655.

798. Marchlinski FE, Buxton AE, Flores BT, Doherty JU, Waxman HL, Josephson ME. Value of Holter monitoring in identifying risk for sustained ventricular arrhythmia recurrence on amiodarone. Am J Cardiol 1985; 55:709–712.

799. Escoubet B, Coumel P, Poirier JM, et al. Suppression of arrhythmias within hours after a single oral dose of amiodarone and relation to plasma and myocardial concentrations. Am J Cardiol 1985; 55:696–702.

800. Hockings BE, George T, Mahrous F, Taylor RR, Hajar HA.

Effectiveness of amiodarone on ventricular arrhythmias during and after acute myocardial infarction. Am J Cardiol 1987; 60:967–970.

801. Cairns JA, Connolly SJ, Gent M, Roberts R. Post-myocardial infarction mortality in patients with ventricular premature depolarizations: Canadian Amiodarone Myocardial Infarction Arrhythmia Trial pilot study. Circulation 1991; 84:550–557.

802. Nicklas JM, McKenna WJ, Stewart RA, et al. Prospective, double-blind, placebo-controlled trial of low-dose amiodarone in patients with severe heart failure and asymptomatic frequent ventricular ectopy. Am Heart J 1991; 122:1016–1021.

803. Ceremuzynski L, Kleczar E, Krzeminska-Pakula M, et al. Effect of amiodarone on mortality after myocardial infarction: a double-blind, placebo-controlled, pilot study. J Am Coll Cardiol 1992; 20:1056–1062.

804. Navarro-Lopez F, Cosin J, Marrugat J, Guindo J, Bayes de Luna A. Comparison of the effects of amiodarone versus metoprolol on the frequency of ventricular arrhythmias and on mortality after acute myocardial infarction. SSSD investigators: Spanish Study on Sudden Death. Am J Cardiol 1993; 72:1243–1248.

805. Singh SN, Fletcher RD, Fisher SG, et al. Amiodarone in patients with congestive heart failure and asymptomatic ventricular arrhythmia: survival trial of antiarrhythmic therapy in congestive heart failure. N Engl J Med 1995; 333:77–82.

806. Mostow ND, Rakita L, Vrobel TR, Noon DL, Blumer J. Amiodarone: correlation of serum concentration with suppression of complex ventricular ectopic activity. Am J Cardiol 1984; 54:569–574.

807. Leak D. Intravenous amiodarone in the treatment of refractory life-threatening cardiac arrhythmias in the critically ill patient. Am Heart J 1986; 111:456–462.

808. Nademanee K, Feld G, Hendrickson J, et al. Mexiletine: double-blind comparison with procainamide in PVC suppression and open-label sequential comparison with amiodarone in life-threatening ventricular arrhythmias. Am Heart J 1985; 110:923–931.

809. Salerno DM, Gillingham KJ, Berry DA, Hodges M. A comparison of antiarrhythmic drugs for the suppression of ventricular ectopic depolarizations: a meta-analysis. Am Heart J 1990; 120:340–353.

810. Rotmensch HH, Belhassen B, Swanson BN, et al. Steady-state serum amiodarone concentrations: relationships with antiarrhythmic efficacy and toxicity. Ann Intern Med 1984; 101:462–469.

811. Burkart F, Pfisterer M, Kiowski W, Follath F, Burckhardt D. Effect of antiarrhythmic therapy on mortality in survivors of myocardial infarction with asymptomatic complex ventricular arrhythmias: Basel Antiarrhythmic Study of Infarct Survival (BASIS). J Am Coll Cardiol 1990; 16:1711–1718.

812. Cairns JA, Connolly SJ, Roberts R, Gent M. Canadian Amiodarone Myocardial Infarction Arrhythmia Trial (CAMIAT): rationale and protocol. CAMIAT investigators. Am J Cardiol 1993; 72:87F–94F.

813. Pfisterer ME, Kiowski W, Brunner H, Burckhardt D, Burkart F. Long-term benefit of 1-year amiodarone treatment for persistent complex ventricular arrhythmias after myocardial infarction. Circulation 1993; 87:309–311.

814. Jewitt DE, Singh BN. Special article: the role of beta-adrenergic blockade in myocardial infarction. Prog Cardiovasc Dis 1974; 16:421–438.

815. Frishman WH, Furberg CD, Friedewald WT. Beta-adrenergic blockade for survivors of acute myocardial infarction. N Engl J Med 1984; 310:830–837.

816. Ruffy R. Sotalol. J Cardiovasc Electrophysiol 1993; 4:89–98.

817. Hohnloser SH, Woosley RL. Sotalol. N Engl J Med 1994; 331:31–38.

818. Schamroth L. Immediate effects of intravenous propranolol on various cardiac arrhythmias. Am J Cardiol 1966; 18:438–443.

819. Sloman G, Stannard M. Beta-adrenergic blockade and cardiac arrhythmias. BMJ 1967; 4:508–512.

820. Winkle RA, Meffin PJ, Fitzgerald JW, Harrison DC. Clinical efficacy and pharmacokinetics of a new orally effective antiarrhythmic, tocainide. Circulation 1976; 54:885–889.

821. Gradman AH, Winkle RA, Fitzgerald JW, et al. Suppression of premature ventricular contractions by acebutolol. Circulation 1977; 55:785–791.

822. Ahumada GG, Karlsberg RP, Jaffe AS, Ambos HD, Sobel BE, Roberts R. Reduction of early ventricular arrhythmia by acebutolol in patients with acute myocardial infarction. Br Heart J 1979; 41:654–659.

823. Aronow WS, Turbow M, Lurie M, Whittaker K, Van Camp S. Treatment of premature ventricular complexes with acebutolol. Am J Cardiol 1979; 43:106–108.

824. Woosley RL, Kornhauser D, Smith R, et al. Suppression of chronic ventricular arrhythmias with propranolol. Circulation 1979; 60:819–827.

825. de Soyza N, Kane JJ, Murphy ML, Laddu AR, Doherty JE, Bissett JK. The long-term suppression of ventricular arrhythmia by oral acebutolol in patients with coronary artery disease. Am Heart J 1980; 100:631–638.

826. Podrid PJ, Lown B. Pindolol for ventricular arrhythmia. Am Heart J 1982; 104:491–496.

827. Hansteen V. Beta blockade after myocardial infarction: the Norwegian propranolol study in high-risk patients. Circulation 1983; 67(Suppl I):I-57–I-60.

828. Lui HK, Lee G, Dhurandhar R, et al. Reduction of ventricular ectopic beats with oral acebutolol: a double-blind, randomized crossover study. Am Heart J 1983; 105:722–726.

829. Rossi PRF, Yusuf S, Ramsdale D, Furze L, Sleight P. Reduction of ventricular arrhythmias by early intravenous atenolol in suspected acute myocardial infarction. BMJ 1983; 286:506–510.

830. Stroobandt R, Kesteloot H. Efficacy of intravenous sotalol on ventricular arrhythmias occurring during maximal exercise stress testing. Arch Int Pharmacodyn Ther 1983; 264:290–297.

831. Ryden L, Ariniego R, Arnman K, et al. A double-blind trial of metoprolol in acute myocardial infarction: effects on ventricular tachyarrhythmias. N Engl J Med 1983; 308:614–618.

832. Yusuf S, Sleight P, Rossi P, et al. Reduction in infarct size, arrhythmias and chest pain by early intravenous beta blockade in suspected acute myocardial infarction. Circulation 1983; 67:132–141.

833. Coumel P, Escoubet B, Attuel P. Beta-blocking therapy in atrial and ventricular tachyarrhythmias: experience with nadolol. Am Heart J 1984; 108:1098–1108.

834. Nademanee K, Schleman MM, Singh BN, Morganroth J, Reid PR, Stritar JA. Beta-adrenergic blockade by nadolol in control of ventricular tachyarrhythmias. Am Heart J 1984; 108:1109–1115.

835. Chandraratna PA. Comparison of acebutolol with propranolol, quinidine, and placebo: results of three multicenter arrhythmia trials. Am Heart J 1985; 109:1198–1204.

836. Matangi MF, Neutze JM, Graham KJ, Hill DG, Kerr AR, Barratt-Boyes BG. Arrhythmia prophylaxis after aorta-coronary bypass: the effect of minidose propranolol. J Thorac Cardiovasc Surg 1985; 89:439–443.

837. Materne P, Larbuisson R, Collignon P, Limet R, Kulbertus H. Prevention by acebutolol of rhythm disorders following coronary bypass surgery. Int J Cardiol 1985; 8:275–286.

838. Lidell C, Rehnqvist N, Sjogren A, Yli-Uotila RJ, Ronnevik PK. Comparative efficacy of oral sotalol and procainamide in patients with chronic ventricular arrhythmias: a multicenter study. Am Heart J 1985; 109:970–975.

839. Anderson JL, Askins JC, Gilbert EM, et al. Multicenter trial of sotalol for suppression of frequent, complex ventricular arrhythmias: a double-blind, randomized, placebo-controlled evaluation of two doses. J Am Coll Cardiol 1986; 8:752–762.

840. Pratt CM, Butman SM, Young JB, Knoll M, English LD. Antiarrhythmic efficacy of ethmozine (moricizine HCl) compared with disopyramide and propranolol. Am J Cardiol 1987; 60:52F–58F.

841. Sung RI, Olukotun AY, Baird CL, Huycke EC. Efficacy and safety of oral nadolol for exercise-induced ventricular arrhythmias. Am J Cardiol 1987; 60:15D–20D.

842. Singh SN, Chen YW, Cohen A, et al. Relation between ventricular function and antiarrhythmic responses to sotalol. Am J Cardiol 1989; 64:943–945.

843. Deedwania PC. Suppressant effects of conventional beta blockers and sotalol on complex and repetitive ventricular premature complexes. Am J Cardiol 1990; 65:43A–50A.

844. Anastasiou-Nana MI, Gilbert EM, Miller RH, et al. Usefulness of d, l sotalol for suppression of chronic ventricular arrhythmias. Am J Cardiol 1991; 67:511–516.

845. Kennedy HL, Brooks MM, Barker AH, et al. Beta-blocker therapy in the Cardiac Arrhythmia Suppression Trial: CAST investigators. Am J Cardiol 1994; 74:674–680.

846. Pitzalis MV, Mastropasqua F, Massari F, Totaro P, Di Maggio M, Rizzon P. Holter-guided identification of premature ventricular contractions susceptible to suppression by beta-blockers. Am Heart J 1996; 131:508–515.

847. Winkle RA, Gradman AH, Fitzgerald JW. Antiarrhythmic drug effect assessed from ventricular arrhythmia reduction in the ambulatory electrocardiogram and treadmill test: comparison of propranolol, procainamide and quinidine. Am J Cardiol 1978; 42:473–480.

848. de Soyza N, Shapiro W, Chandraratna PA, Aronow WS, Laddu AR, Thompson CH. Acebutolol therapy for ventricular arrhythmia: a randomized placebo-controlled double-blind multicenter study. Circulation 1982; 65:1129–1133.

849. Matangi MF, Strickland J, Garbe GJ, et al. Atenolol for the prevention of arrhythmias following coronary artery bypass grafting. Can J Cardiol 1989; 5:229–234.

850. Winkle RA, Lopes MG, Goodman DJ, Fitzgerald JW, Schroeder JS, Harrison DC. Propranolol for patients with mitral valve prolapse. Am Heart J 1977; 93:422–427.

851. Van de Werf F, Janssens L, Brzostek T, et al. Short-term effects of early intravenous treatment with a beta-adrenergic blocking agent or a specific bradycardiac agent in patients with acute myocardial infarction receiving thrombolytic therapy. J Am Coll Cardiol 1993; 22:407–416.

852. Hansteen V, Endresen K, Hellemann H, et al. Comparative effects of long-acting and conventional propranolol on stress-induced angina pectoris and on frequency of ventricular premature beats. Br J Clin Pharmacol 1984; 17:579–584.

853. Heidbuchel H, Tack J, Vanneste L, Ballet A, Ector H, Van de Werf F. Significance of arrhythmias during the first 24 hours of acute myocardial infarction treated with alteplase and effect of early administration of a β-blocker or a bradycardiac agent on their incidence. Circulation 1994; 89:1051-1059.

854. Pitzalis MV, Mastropasqua F, Massari F, Totaro P, Scrutinio D, Rizzon P. Sleep suppression of ventricular arrhythmias: a predictor of beta-blocker efficacy. Eur Heart J 1996; 17:917–925.

855. Butman SM, Knoll ML, Gardin JM. Comparison of ethmozine to propranolol and the combination for ventricular arrhythmias. Am J Cardiol 1987; 60:603–607.

856. Deedwania PC, Olukotun AY, Kupersmith J, Jenkins P, Golden P. Beta blockers in combination with class I antiarrhythmic agents. Am J Cardiol 1987; 60:21D–26D.

857. Aronow WS, Van Camp S, Turbow M, Whittaker K, Lurie M. Acebutolol in supraventricular arrhythmias. Clin Pharmacol Ther 1979; 25:149–153.

858. de Soyza N. Acebutolol for premature ventricular contractions: short- and long-term effects. Am Heart J 1985; 109:1205–1209.

859. Olsson G, Rehnqvist N, Sjogren A, Erhardt L, Lundman T. Long-term treatment with metoprolol after myocardial infarction: effect on 3 year mortality and morbidity. J Am Coll Cardiol 1985; 5:1428–1437.

860. Romhilt DW, Bloomfield SS, Lipicky RJ, Welch RM, Fowler NO. Evaluation of bretylium tosylate for the treatment of premature ventricular contractions. Circulation 1972; 45:800–807.

861. Antman EM, Stone PH, Muller JE, Braunwald E. Calcium channel blocking agents in the treatment of cardiovascular disorders. I: Basic and clinical electrophysiologic effects. Ann Intern Med 1980; 93:875–885.

862. Opie LH. Drugs and the heart. III. Calcium antagonists. Lancet 1980; 1:806–810.

863. Schamroth L, Krikler DM, Garrett C. Immediate effects of intravenous verapamil in cardiac arrhythmias. BMJ 1972; 1:660–662.

864. Pickering TG, Goulding L. Supression of ventricular extrasystoles by perhexiline. Br Heart J 1978; 40:851–855.

865. Messerli FH, Nunez BD, Nunez MM, Garavaglia GE, Schmieder RE, Ventura HO. Hypertension and sudden death: disparate effects of calcium entry blocker and diuretic therapy on cardiac dysrhythmias. Arch Intern Med 1989; 149:1263–1267.

866. Bigger JT Jr, Hoffman BF. Antiarrhythmic drugs. In Gilman AG, Rall TW, Nies AS, Taylor P (eds). The Pharmacological Basis of Therapeutics. 8th ed. New York: Pergamon Press, 1990, pp. 840–873.

867. Szlachcic J, Tubau JF, O'Kelly B, Ammon S, Massie BM. Influence of therapy on silent ischemia and ventricular arrhythmias in hypertensive patients. J Cardiovasc Pharmacol 1991; 18:106–108.

868. Balaji S, Wiles HB, Sens MA, Gillette PC. Immunosuppressive treatment for myocarditis and borderline myocarditis in children with ventricular ectopic rhythm. Br Heart J 1994; 72:354–359.

869. De Mey C, Snoeck J. Review of the use of digitalis glycosides in ventricular dysrhythmia. Acta Cardiol 1980; 35:153–165.

870. Scherf D, Schott A. Extrasystoles and Allied Arrhythmias. 2nd ed. Chicago: Year Book Medical Publishers, 1973, pp. 317–318.

871. Lown B, Graboys TB, Podrid PJ, Cohen BH, Stockman MB, Gaughan CE. Effect of a digitalis drug on ventricular premature beats. N Engl J Med 1977; 296:301–306.

872. Gradman AH, Cunningham M, Harbison MA, Berger HJ, Zaret BL. Effects of oral digoxin on ventricular ectopy and its relation to left ventricular function. Am J Cardiol 1983; 51:765–769.

873. Podrid P, Lown B, Zielonka J, Holman BL. Effects of acetyl-strophanthidin on left ventricular function and ventricular arrhythmias. Am Heart J 1984; 107:882–887.

874. Morrison J, Coromilas J, Robbins M, et al. Digitalis and myocardial infarction in man. Circulation 1980; 62:8–16.

875. Koch-Weser J. Disopyramide. N Engl J Med 1979; 300:957–962.

876. Morady F, Scheinman MM, Desai J. Disopyramide. Ann Intern Med 1982; 96:337–343.

877. Deano DA, Wu D, Mautner RK, Sherman RH, Ehsani AI, Rosen KM. The antiarrhythmic efficacy of intravenous therapy with disopyramide phosphate. Chest 1977; 71:597–606.

878. Trimarco B, Volpe M, Ricciardelli B, et al. Disopyramide and mexiletine: which is the agent of choice in the long term-oral treatment of lidocaine-responsive arrhythmias? Efficacy comparison in a randomized trial. Arch Int Pharmacodyn Ther 1980; 248:251–259.

879. Kjekshus J, Bathen J, Orning OM, Storstein L. A double-blind, crossover comparison of flecainide acetate and disopyramide phosphate in the treatment of ventricular premature complexes. Am J Cardiol 1984; 53:72B–78B.

880. Kimura E, Mashima S, Tanaka T. Clinical evaluation of antiarrhythmic effects of disopyramide by multiclinical controlled double-blind methods. Int J Clin Pharmacol Ther Toxicol 1980; 18:338–343.

881. Morady F, Kou WH, Kadish AH, et al. Antagonism of quinidine's electrophysiologic effects by epinephrine in patients with ventricular tachycardia. J Am Coll Cardiol 1988; 12:388–394.

882. Breithardt G, Seipel L, Lersmacher J, Abendroth RR. Comparative study of the antiarrhythmic efficacy of mexiletine and disopyramide in patients with chronic ventricular arrhythmias. J Cardiovasc Pharmacol 1982; 4:276–284.

883. Sbarbaro JA, Rawling DA, Fozzard HA. Suppression of ventricular arrhythmias with intravenous disopyramide and lidocaine: efficacy comparison in a randomized trial. Am J Cardiol 1979; 44:513–520.

884. Pratt CM, Luck JC, Mann DE, Wyndham CR. Investigational antiarrhythmic drugs for the treatment of ventricular rhythm disturbances. Cardiol Clin 1984; 2:35–46.

885. Naccarella F, Bracchetti D, Palmieri M, Cantelli I, Bertaccini P, Ambrosioni E. Comparison of propafenone and disopyramide for treatment of chronic ventricular arrhythmias: placebo-controlled, double-blind, randomized crossover study. Am Heart J 1985; 109:833–840.

886. Jonason T, Ringqvist I, Bandh S, et al. Propafenone versus disopyramide for treatment of chronic symptomatic ventricular arrhythmias: a multicenter study. Acta Med Scand 1988; 223:515–523.

887. Jennings G, Jones MS, Besterman EM, Model DG, Turner PP, Kidner PH. Oral disopyramide in prophylaxis of arrhythmias following myocardial infarction. Lancet 1976; 1:51–54.

888. Kim SG, Mercando AD, Tam S, Fisher JD. Combination of disopyramide and mexiletine for better tolerance and additive effects for treatment of ventricular arrhythmias. J Am Coll Cardiol 1989; 13:659–664.

889. Roden DM, Duff HJ, Primm RK, Kronenberg MW, Woosley RL. Control of ventricular preexcitation and associated arrhythmias by encainide. Am Heart J 1981; 102:794–797.

890. Sami M, Mason JW, Peters F, Harrison DC. Clinical electrophysiologic effects of encainide, a newly developed antiarrhythmic agent. Am J Cardiol 1979; 44:526–532.

891. DiBianco R, Fletcher RD, Cohen AI, et al. Treatment of frequent ventricular arrhythmia with encainide: assessment using serial ambulatory electrocardiograms, intracardiac electrophysiologic studies, treadmill exercise tests, and radionuclide cineangiographic studies. Circulation 1982; 65:1134–1147.

892. Duff HJ, Roden DM, Carey EL, Wang T, Primm RK, Woosley RL. Spectrum of antiarrhythmic response to encainide. Am J Cardiol 1985; 56:887–891.

893. Morganroth J, Pool P, Miller R, Hsu PH, Lee I, Clark DM. Dose-response range of encainide for benign and potentially lethal ventricular arrhythmias. Am J Cardiol 1986; 57:769–774.

894. Cardiac Arrhythmia Pilot Study investigators: effects of encainide, flecainide, imipramine and moricizine on ventricular arrhythmias during the year after acute myocardial infarction. Am J Cardiol 1988; 61:501–509.

895. Roden DM, Woosley RL. Drug therapy: flecainide. N Engl J Med 1986; 315:36–41.

896. Anderson JL, Stewart JR, Perry BA, et al. Oral flecainide acetate for the treatment of ventricular arrhythmias. N Engl J Med 1981; 305:473–477.

897. Duff HJ, Roden DM, Maffucci RJ, et al. Suppression of resistant ventricular arrhythmias by twice daily dosing with flecainide. Am J Cardiol 1981; 48:1133–1140.

898. Hodges M, Haugland JM, Granrud G, et al. Suppression of ventricular ectopic depolarizations by flecainide acetate, a new antiarrhythmic agent. Circulation 1982; 65:879–885.

899. Abitol H, Califano JE, Abate C, Beilis P, Castellanos H. Use of flecainide acetate in the treatment of premature ventricular contractions. Am Heart J 1983; 105:227–230.

900. Morganroth J, Anderson JL, Gentzkow GD. Classification by type of ventricular arrhythmia predicts frequency of adverse cardiac events from flecainide. J Am Coll Cardiol 1986; 8:607–615.

901. Anonymous. Flecainide versus quinidine for treatment of chronic ventricular arrhythmias: a multicenter clinical trial. Circulation 1983; 67:1117–1123.

902. Salerno DM, Hodges M, Granrud G, Sharkey P. Comparison of flecainide with quinidine for suppression of chronic stable ventricular ectopic depolarizations: a double-blind randomized study in ambulatory outpatients. Ann Intern Med 1983; 98:455–460.

903. Gunnar RM, Bourdillon PD, Dixon DW, et al. ACC/AHA guidelines for the early management of patients with acute myocardial infarction: a report of the American College of Cardiology/American Heart Association Task Force on assessment of diagnostic and therapeutic cardiovascular procedures (subcommittee to develop guidelines for the early management of patients with acute myocardial infarction). Circulation 1990; 82:664–707.

904. Jewitt DE, Kishon Y, Thomas M. Lignocaine in the management of arrhythmias after acute myocardial infarction. Lancet 1968; 1:266–270.

905. Bennett MA, Wilner JM, Pentecost BL. Controlled trial of lignocaine in prophylaxis of ventricular arrhythmias complicating myocardial infarction. Lancet 1970; 2:909–911.

906. Chopra MP, Thadani U, Portal RW, Aber CP. Lignocaine therapy for ventricular ectopic activity after acute myocardial infarction: a double-blind trial. BMJ 1971; 3:668–670.

907. Pitt A, Lipp H, Anderson ST. Lignocaine given prophylactically to patients with acute myocardial infarction. Lancet 1971; 1:612–616.

908. Darby S, Cruickshank JC, Bennett MA, Pentecost BL. Trial of combined intramuscular and intravenous lignocaine in prophylaxis of ventricular tachyarrhythmias. Lancet 1972; 1:817–819.

909. Fehmers MC, Dunning AJ. Intramuscularly and orally administered lidocaine in the treatment of ventricular arrhythmias in acute myocardial infarction. Am J Cardiol 1972; 29:514–519.

910. Goldreyer BN, Wyman MG. The effect of first hour hospitalization in myocardial infarction. Circulation 1974; 50(Suppl III):III-121.

911. Lie KI, Wellens HJJ, van Capelle FJ, Durrer D. Lidocaine in the prevention of primary ventricular fibrillation: a double-blind, randomized study of 212 consecutive patients. N Engl J Med 1974; 291:1324–1326.

912. Harrison DC. Should lidocaine be administered routinely to all patients after acute myocardial infarction? Circulation 1978; 58:581–584.

913. Harrison DC, Sprouse JH, Morrow AG. The antiarrhythmic properties of lidocaine and procaine amide: clinical and physiologic studies of their cardiovascular effects in man. Circulation 1963; 28:486–491.

914. Bellet S, Roman L, Kostis JB, Fleischmann D. Intramuscular lidocaine in the therapy of ventricular arrhythmias. Am J Cardiol 1971; 27:291–293.

915. Ryden L, Waldenstrom A, Ehn L, Holmberg S, Husaini M. Comparison between effectiveness of intramuscular and intravenous lignocaine on ventricular arrhythmia complicating acute myocardial infarction. Br Heart J 1973; 35:1124–1131.

916. Alderman EL, Kerber RE, Harrison DC. Evaluation of lidocaine resistance in man using intermittent large-dose infusion techniques. Am J Cardiol 1974; 34:342–349.

917. Singh JB, Kocot SL. A controlled trial of intramuscular lidocaine in the prevention of premature ventricular contractions associated with acute myocardial infarction. Am Heart J 1976; 91:430–436.

918. Sheridan DJ, Crawford L, Rawlins MD, Julian DG. Antiarrhythmic action of lignocaine in early myocardial infarction: plasma levels after combined intramuscular and intravenous administration. Lancet 1977; 1:824–825.

919. Wennerblom B, Holmberg S, Wedel H. The effect of a mobile coronary care unit on mortality in patients with acute myocardial infarction or cardiac arrest outside hospital. Eur Heart J 1982; 3:504–515.

920. Wester PO. Magnesium: effect on arrhythmias. Int J Cardiol 1986; 12:181–183.

921. Keren A, Tzivoni D. Magnesium therapy in ventricular arrhythmias. Pacing Clin Electrophysiol 1990; 13:937–945.

922. Fisch C, Shields JP, Ridolfo SA, Feigenbaum H. Effect of potassium on conduction and ectopic rhythms in atrial fibrillation treated with digitalis. Circulation 1958; 18:98–106.

923. Dyckner T, Wester PO. Ventricular extrasystoles and intracellular electrolytes in hypokalemic patients before and after correction of the hypokalemia. Acta Med Scand 1978; 204:375–379.

924. Kunin AS, Surawicz B, Sims EAH. Decrease in serum potassium concentrations and appearance of cardiac arrhythmias during infusion of potassium with glucose in potassium-depleted patients. N Engl J Med 1962; 266:228–233.

925. Bettinger JC, Surawicz B, Bryfogle JW, Anderson BN, Bellet S. The effect of intravenous administration of potassium chloride on ectopic rhythms, ectopic beats and disturbances in A-V conduction. Am J Med 1956; 21:521–533.

926. Smith LF, Heagerty AM, Bing RF, Barnett DB. Intravenous infusion of magnesium sulphate after acute myocardial infarction: effects on arrhythmias and mortality. Int J Cardiol 1986; 12:175–183.

927. Abraham AS, Rosenmann D, Kramer M, et al. Magnesium in the prevention of lethal arrhythmias in acute myocardial infarction. Arch Intern Med 1987; 147:753–755.

928. Shechter M, Hod H, Marks N, Behar S, Kaplinsky E, Rabinowitz B. Beneficial effect of magnesium sulfate in acute myocardial infarction. Am J Cardiol 1990; 66:271–274.

929. Gottlieb SS, Fisher ML, Pressel MD, Patten RD, Weinberg M, Greenberg N. Effects of intravenous magnesium sulfate on arrhythmias in patients with congestive heart failure. Am Heart J 1993; 125:1645–1650.

930. Fletcher GF, Hurst JW, Schlant RC. "Polarizing" solutions in patients with acute myocardial infarction: a double-blind study with negative results. Am Heart J 1968; 75:319–324.

931. Zehender M, Meinertz T, Faber T, et al. Antiarrhythmic effects of increasing the daily intake of magnesium and potassium in patients with frequent ventricular arrhythmias: Magnesium in Cardiac Arrhythmias (MAGICA) Investigators. J Am Coll Cardiol 1997; 29:1028–1034.

932. Campbell RW. Mexiletine. N Engl J Med 1987; 316:29–34.

933. Campbell NP, Kelly JG, Shanks RG, Chaturvedi NC, Strong JE, Pantridge JF. Mexiletine (KO 1173) in the management of ventricular dysrhythmias. Lancet 1973; 2:404–407.

934. Talbot RG, Nimmo J, Julian DG, Clark RA, Neilson JM, Prescott LF. Treatment of ventricular arrhythmias with mexiletine (KO 1173). Lancet 1973; 2:399–404.

935. Talbot RG, Julian DG, Prescott LF. Long-term treatment of ventricular arrhythmias with oral mexiletine. Am Heart J 1976; 91:58–65.

936. Campbell NP, Pantridge JF, Adgey AA. Long-term oral antiarrhythmic therapy with mexiletine. Br Heart J 1978; 40:796–801.

937. Podrid PJ, Lown B. Mexiletine for ventricular arrhythmias. Am J Cardiol 1981; 47:895–902.

938. Mehta J, Conti CR. Mexiletine, a new antiarrhythmic agent, for treatment of premature ventricular complexes. Am J Cardiol 1982; 49:455–460.

939. Breithardt G, Borggrefe M, Karbenn U, Abendroth RR, Yeh HL, Seipel L. Prevalence of late potentials in patients with and without ventricular tachycardia: correlation with angiographic findings. Am J Cardiol 1982; 49:1932–1937.

940. Rutledge JC, Harris F, Amsterdam EA. Clinical evaluation of oral mexiletine therapy in the treatment of ventricular arrhythmias. J Am Coll Cardiol 1985; 6:780–784.

941. Hession M, Blum R, Podrid PJ, Lampert S, Stein J, Lown B. Mexiletine and tocainide: does response to one predict response to the other? J Am Coll Cardiol 1986; 7:338–343.

942. Campbell RWF, Dolder MA, Prescott LF, Talbot RG, Murray A, Julian DG. Comparison of procainamide and mexiletine in prevention of ventricular arrhythmias after acute myocardial infarction. Lancet 1975; 1:1257–1260.

943. Campbell RW, Dolder MA, Prescott LF, Talbot RG, Murray A, Julian DG. Ventricular arrhythmias after acute myocardial infarction treated with procainamide or mexiletine. Postgrad Med J 1977; 53:150–153.

944. Chamberlain DA, Jewitt DE, Julian DG, Campbell RW, Boyle DM, Shanks RG. Oral mexiletine in high-risk patients after myocardial infarction. Lancet 1980; 2:1324–1327.

945. Singh JB, Rasul AM, Shah A, Adams E, Flessas A, Kocot SL. Efficacy of mexiletine in chronic ventricular arrhythmias compared with quinidine: a single-blind, randomized trial. Am J Cardiol 1984; 53:84–87.

946. Stein J, Podrid PJ, Lampert S, Hirsowitz G, Lown B. Long-term mexiletine for ventricular arrhythmia. Am Heart J 1984; 107:1091–1098.

947. Morganroth J. Comparative efficacy and safety of oral mexiletine and quinidine in benign or potentially lethal ventricular arrhythmias. Am J Cardiol 1987; 60:1276–1281.

948. Duff HJ, Roden D, Primm RK, Oates JA, Woosley RL. Mexiletine in the treatment of resistant ventricular arrhythmias: enhancement of efficacy and reduction of dose-related side effects by combination with quinidine. Circulation 1983; 67:1124–1128.

949. Morganroth J, Pearlman AS, Dunkman WB, Horowitz LN, Josephson ME, Michelson EL. Ethmozin: a new antiarrhythmic agent developed in the USSR. Efficacy and tolerance. Am Heart J 1979; 98:621–628.

950. Clyne CA, Estes NA III, Wang PJ. Moricizine. N Engl J Med 1992; 327:255–260.

951. Podrid PJ, Lyakishev A, Lown B, Mazur N. Ethmozin, a new antiarrhythmic drug for suppressing ventricular premature complexes. Circulation 1980; 61:450–457.

952. Pratt CM, Yepsen SC, Taylor AA, et al. Ethmozine suppression of single and repetitive ventricular premature depolarizations during therapy: documentation of efficacy and long-term safety. Am Heart J 1983; 106:85–91.

953. Morganroth J, Pratt CM, Kennedy HL, et al. Efficacy and tolerance of ethmozine (moricizine HCl) in placebo-controlled trials. Am J Cardiol 1987; 60:48F–51F.

954. Smetnev AS, Shugushev KK, Rosenshtraukh LV. Clinical, electrophysiologic and antiarrhythmic efficacy of moricizine HCl. Am J Cardiol 1987; 60:40F–44F.

955. Kennedy HL, Sprague MK, Homan SM, et al. Natural history of potentially lethal ventricular arrhythmias in patients treated with long-term antiarrhythmic drug therapy. Am J Cardiol 1989; 64:1289–1297.

956. Horowitz LN. Efficacy of moricizine in malignant ventricular arrhythmias. Am J Cardiol 1990; 65:41D–46D.

957. Podrid PJ, Beau SL. Antiarrhythmic drug therapy for congestive heart failure with focus on moricizine. Am J Cardiol 1990; 65:56D–64D.

958. Morganroth J, Bigger JT Jr. Overview: moricizine: can it meet the challenge? Am J Cardiol 1990; 65:1D–2D.

959. Mann DE, Luck JC, Herre JM, et al. Electrophysiologic effects of ethmozin in patients with ventricular tachycardia. Am Heart J 1984; 107:674–679.

960. Pratt CM, Podrid PJ, Seals AA, et al. Effects of ethmozine (moricizine HCl) on ventricular function using echocardiographic, hemodynamic and radionuclide assessments. Am J Cardiol 1987; 60:73F–78F.

961. Cardiac Arrhythmia Suppression Trial II investigators. Effect of the antiarrhythmic agent moricizine on survival after myocardial infarction. N Engl J Med 1992; 327:227–233.

962. Ruthen GC. Antiarrhythmic drugs. IV. Diphenylhydantoin in cardiac arrhythmias. Am Heart J 1965; 70:275–278.

963. Mercer EN, Osborne JA. The current status of diphenylhydantoin in heart disease. Ann Intern Med 1967; 67:1084–1107.

964. Dreifus LS, Watanabe Y. Current status of diphenylhydantoin. Am Heart J 1970; 80:709–713.

965. Atkinson AJ Jr, Davison R. Diphenylhydantoin as an antiarrhythmic drug. Annu Rev Med 1974; 25:99–113.

966. Wit AL, Rosen MR, Hoffman BF. Electrophysiology and pharmacology of cardiac arrhythmias. VIII. Cardiac effects of diphenylhydantoin. Am Heart J 1975; 90:397–404.

967. Bernstein H, Gold H, Lang TW, Pappelbaum S, Bazika V, Corday E. Sodium diphenylhydantoin in the treatment of recurrent cardiac arrhythmias. JAMA 1965; 191:695–697.

968. Conn RD. Diphenylhydantoin sodium in cardiac arrhythmias. N Engl J Med 1965; 272:277–282.

969. Rosen M, Lisak R, Rubin IL. Diphenylhydantoin in cardiac arrhythmias. Am J Cardiol 1967; 20:674–678.

970. Kavey RE, Blackman MS, Sondheimer HM. Phenytoin therapy for ventricular arrhythmias occurring late after surgery for congenital heart disease. Am Heart J 1982; 104:794–798.

971. Garson A Jr, Kugler JD, Gillette PC, Simonelli A, McNamara DG. Control of late postoperative ventricular arrhythmias

with phenytoin in young patients. Am J Cardiol 1980; 46:290–294.

972. Bigger JT Jr, Schmidt DH, Kutt H. Relationship between the plasma level of diphenylhydantoin sodium and its cardiac antiarrhythmic effects. Circulation 1968; 38:363–374.

973. Bashour FA, Edmonson RE, Gupta DN, Prati R. Treatment of digitalis toxicity by diphenylhydantoin (Dilantin). Dis Chest 1968; 53:263–270.

974. Rumack BH, Wolfe RR, Gilfrich H. Phenytoin (diphenylhydantoin) treatment of massive digoxin overdose. Br Heart J 1974; 36:405–408.

975. Kayden HJ, Brodie BB, Steele JM. Procaine amide: a review. Circulation 1957; 25:118–126.

976. Berry K, Garlett EL, Bellet S, Gefter WI. Use of pronestyl in the treatment of ectopic rhythms: treatment of ninety-eight episodes in seventy-eight patients. Am J Med 1951; October:431–441.

977. Kayden HJ, Steele JM, Mark LC, Brodie BB. The use of procaine amide in cardiac arrhythmias. Circulation 1951; 4:13–22.

978. Koch-Weser J, Klein SW, Foo-Canto LL, Kastor JA, DeSanctis RW. Antiarrhythmic prophylaxis with procainamide in acute myocardial infarction. N Engl J Med 1969; 281:1253–1260.

979. Miller RR, Hilliard G, Lies JE, et al. Hemodynamic effects of procainamide in patients with acute myocardial infarction and comparison with lidocaine. Am J Med 1973; 55:161–168.

980. Giardina EG, Heissenbuttel RH, Bigger JT Jr. Intermittent intravenous procaine amide to treat ventricular arrhythmias: correlation of plasma concentration with effect on arrhythmia, electrocardiogram, and blood pressure. Ann Intern Med 1973; 78:183–193.

981. Jelinek MV, Lohrbauer L, Lown B. Antiarrhythmic drug therapy for sporadic ventricular ectopic arrhythmias. Circulation 1974; 49:659–666.

982. Myerburg RJ, Kessler KM, Kiem I, et al. Relationship between plasma levels of procainamide, suppression of premature ventricular complexes and prevention of recurrent ventricular tachycardia. Circulation 1981; 64:280–290.

983. Kessler KM, McAuliffe D, Kozlovskis P, et al. QRS morphology-dependent pharmacodynamics in multiform ventricular ectopic activity. Am J Cardiol 1988; 61:563–569.

984. Giardina EG, Bigger JT Jr. Procaine amide against re-entrant ventricular arrhythmias: lengthening R-V intervals of coupled ventricular premature depolarization as an insight into the mechanism of action of procaine amide. Circulation 1973; 48:959–970.

985. Kosowsky BD, Taylor J, Lown B, Ritchie RF. Long-term use of procaine amide following acute myocardial infarction. Circulation 1973; 47:1204–1210.

986. Giardina EG, Bigger JT Jr. Effect of procainamide and lidocaine on total electrical systole of ventricular premature depolarizations. Am J Med 1975; 59:405–410.

987. Gey GO, Levy RH, Fisher L, Pettet G, Bruce RA. Plasma concentration of procainamide and prevalence of exertional arrhythmias. Ann Intern Med 1974; 80:718–722.

988. Kim SG, Seiden SW, Matos JA, Waspe LE, Fisher JD. Combination of procainamide and quinidine for better tolerance and additive effects for ventricular arrhythmias. Am J Cardiol 1985; 56:84–88.

989. Klein RC, Huang SK, Marcus FI, et al. Enhanced antiarrhythmic efficacy of propafenone when used in combination with procainamide or quinidine. Am Heart J 1987; 114:551–558.

990. Krone RJ, Miller JP, Kleiger RE, Clark KW, Oliver GC. The effectiveness of antiarrhythmic agents on early-cycle premature ventricular complexes. Circulation 1981; 63:664–669.

991. Funck-Brentano C, Kroemer HK, Lee JT, Roden DM. Propafenone. N Engl J Med 1990: 322:518–525.

992. de Soyza N, Terry L, Murphy ML, et al. Effect of propafenone in patients with stable ventricular arrhythmias. Am Heart J 1984; 108:285–289.

993. Naccarella F, Bracchetti D, Palmieri M, Marchesini B, Ambrosioni E. Propafenone for refractory ventricular arrhythmias: correlation with drug plasma levels during long-term treatment. Am J Cardiol 1984; 54:1008–1014.

994. Salerno DM, Granrud G, Sharkey P, Asinger R, Hodges M. A controlled trial of propafenone for treatment of frequent and repetitive ventricular premature complexes. Am J Cardiol 1984; 53:77–83.

995. Podrid PJ, Cytryn R, Lown B. Propafenone: noninvasive evaluation of efficacy. Am J Cardiol 1984; 54:53D–59D.

996. Dinh HA, Murphy ML, Baker BJ, deSoyza N, Franciosa JA. Efficacy of propafenone compared with quinidine in chronic ventricular arrhythmias. Am J Cardiol 1985; 55:1520–1524.

997. Dinh H, Baker BJ, de Soyza N, Murphy ML. Sustained therapeutic efficacy and safety of oral propafenone for treatment of chronic ventricular arrhythmias: a 2-year experience. Am Heart J 1988; 115:92–96.

998. Singh BN, Kaplinsky E, Kirsten E, Guerrero J. Effects of propafenone on ventricular arrhythmias: double-blind parallel, randomized, placebo-controlled dose-ranging study. Am Heart J 1988; 116:1542–1551.

999. Nielsen H, Sorum C, Rasmussen V, Madsen JK, Hansen JF. Propafenone versus quinidine slow-release for the treatment of chronic ventricular arrhythmias. Acta Cardiol 1990; 45:359–363.

1000. Zehender M, Hohnloser S, Geibel A, et al. Short-term and long-term treatment with propafenone: determinants of arrhythmia suppression, persistence of efficacy, arrhythmogenesis, and side effects in patients with symptoms. Br Heart J 1992; 67:491–497.

1001. Grace AA, Camm AJ. Quinidine. N Engl J Med 1998; 338:35–45.

1002. Gaughan CE, Lown B, Lanigan J, Voukydis P, Besser HW. Acute oral testing for determining antiarrhythmic drug efficacy. I. Quinidine. Am J Cardiol 1976; 38:677–684.

1003. Carliner NH, Fisher ML, Crouthamel WG, Narang PK, Plotnick GD. Relation of ventricular premature beat suppression to serum quinidine concentration determined by a new and specific assay. Am Heart J 1980; 100:483–489.

1004. Bloomfield SS, Romhilt DW, Chou TC, Fowler NO. Quinidine for prophylaxis of arrhythmias in acute myocardial infarction. N Engl J Med 1971; 285:979–986.

1005. Hodges M, Salerno DM, Granrud G. Flecainide versus quinidine: results of a multicenter trial. Am J Cardiol 1984; 53:66B–71B.

1006. Winkle RA, Meffin PJ, Harrison DC. Long-term tocainide therapy for ventricular arrhythmias. Circulation 1978; 57:1008–1016.

1007. Morganroth J, Horowitz LN. Incidence of proarrhythmic effects from quinidine in the outpatient treatment of benign or potentially lethal ventricular arrhythmias. Am J Cardiol 1985; 56:585–587.

1008. Sami M, Harrison DC, Kraemer H, Houston N, Shimasaki C, DeBusk RF. Antiarrhythmic efficacy of encainide and quinidine: validation of a model for drug assessment. Am J Cardiol 1981; 48:147–156.

1009. Morganroth J, Somberg JC, Pool PE, et al. Comparative study of encainide and quinidine in the treatment of ventricular arrhythmias. J Am Coll Cardiol 1986; 7:9–16.

1010. Kim SG, Mercando AD, Fisher JD. Combination of tocainide and quinidine for better tolerance and additive effects in patients with coronary artery disease. J Am Coll Cardiol 1987; 9:1369–1374.

1011. Morganroth J, Goin JE. Quinidine-related mortality in the short-to-medium-term treatment of ventricular arrhythmias: a meta-analysis. Circulation 1991; 84:1977–1983.

1012. Salerno DM. Quinidine: worse than adverse? Circulation 1991; 84:2196–2198.

1013. Soyka LF, Wirtz C, Spangenberg RB. Clinical safety profile of sotalol in patients with arrhythmias. Am J Cardiol 1990; 65:74A–81A.

1014. Hohnloser SH, Meinertz T, Stubbs P, et al. Efficacy and safety of d-sotalol, a pure class III antiarrhythmic compound, in patients with symptomatic complex ventricular ectopy: results of a multicenter, randomized, double-blind, placebo-controlled dose-finding study. Circulation 1995; 92:1517–1525.

1015. Prakash R, Parmley WW, Allen HN, Matloff JM. Effect of sotalol on clinical arrhythmias. Am J Cardiol 1972; 29:397–400.

1016. Wang T, Bergstrand RH, Thompson KA, et al. Concentration-dependent pharmacologic properties of sotalol. Am J Cardiol 1986; 57:1160–1165.

1017. Anastasiou-Nana MI, Anderson JL, Askins JC, Gilbert EM, Nanas JN, Menlove RL. Long-term experience with sotalol in the treatment of complex ventricular arrhythmias. Am Heart J 1987; 114:288–296.

1018. Kienzle MG, Martins JB, Wendt DJ, Constantin L, Hopson R, McCue ML. Enhanced efficacy of oral sotalol for sustained ventricular tachycardia refractory to type I antiarrhythmic drugs. Am J Cardiol 1988; 61:1012–1017.

1019. Hohnloser SH, Zabel M, Krause T, Just H. Short- and long-term antiarrhythmic and hemodynamic effects of d, l-sotalol in patients with symptomatic ventricular arrhythmias. Am Heart J 1992; 123:1220–1224.

1020. Morganroth J, Nestico PF, Horowitz LN. A review of the uses and limitations of tocainide: a class Ib antiarrhythmic agent. Am Heart J 1985; 110:856–863.

1021. Roden DM, Woosley RL. Drug therapy: tocainide. N Engl J Med 1986; 315:41–45.

1022. Woosley RL, McDevitt DG, Nies AS, Smith RF, Wilkinson GR, Oates JA. Suppression of ventricular ectopic depolarizations by tocainide. Circulation 1977; 56:980–984.

1023. Bastian BC, Macfarlane PW, McLauchlan JH, et al. III. Chronic tocainide therapy studies: a prospective randomized trial of tocainide in patients following myocardial infarction. Am Heart J 1980; 100:1017–1022.

1024. Roden DM, Reele SB, Higgins SB, et al. Tocainide therapy for refractory ventricular arrhythmias. Am Heart J 1980; 100:15–22.

1025. Haffajee CI, Alpert JS, Dalen JE. Tocainide for refractory ventricular arrhythmias of myocardial infarction. Am Heart J 1980; 100:1013–1016.

1026. LeWinter MM, Engler RL, Karliner JS. Tocainide therapy for treatment of ventricular arrhythmias: assessment with ambulatory electrocardiographic monitoring and treadmill exercise. Am J Cardiol 1980; 45:1045–1052.

1027. Nyquist O, Forssell G, Nordlander R, Schenck-Gustafsson K. Hemodynamic and antiarrhythmic effects of tocainide in patients with acute myocardial infarction. Am Heart J 1980; 100:1000–1005.

1028. Podrid PJ, Lown B. Tocainide for refractory symptomatic ventricular arrhythmias. Am J Cardiol 1982; 49:1279–1286.

1029. Morganroth J, Oshrain C, Steele PP. Comparative efficacy and safety of oral tocainide and quinidine for benign and potentially lethal ventricular arrhythmias. Am J Cardiol 1985; 56:581–585.

1030. Webster MW, Fitzpatrick MA, Nicholls MG, Ikram H, Wells JE. Effect of enalapril on ventricular arrhythmias in congestive heart failure. Am J Cardiol 1985; 56:566–569.

1031. Tilkian AG, Pfeifer JF, Barry WH, Lipton MJ, Hultgren HN. The effect of coronary bypass surgery on exercise-induced ventricular arrhythmias. Am Heart J 1976; 92:707–714.

1032. Guinn GA, Mathur VS. Ambulatory, nocturnal and exercise arrhythmias in coronary artery disease: a prospective randomized study to assess the influence of aorto-coronary bypass surgery. Am J Cardiol 1977; 39:270.

1033. Graboys TB, Lown B, Collins JJ, Cohn LH. Does coronary revascularization reduce the prevalence of ventricular ectopic activity? Am J Cardiol 1978; 41:401.

1034. Leutenegger F, Giger G, Fuhr P, et al. Evaluation of aortocoronary venous bypass grafting for prevention of cardiac arrhythmias. Am Heart J 1979; 98:15–19.

1035. de Soyza N, Thenabadu PN, Murphy ML, Kane JJ, Doherty JE. Ventricular arrhythmia before and after aorto-coronary bypass surgery. Int J Cardiol 1981; 1:123–130.

1036. Wellens HJJ. Radiofrequency catheter ablation of benign ventricular ectopic beats: a therapy in search of a disease? J Am Coll Cardiol 1995; 26:850–851.

1037. Gursoy S, Brugada J, Souza O, Steurer G, Andries E, Brugada P. Radiofrequency ablation of symptomatic but benign ventricular arrhythmias. Pacing Clin Electrophysiol 1992; 15:738–741.

1038. Merino JL, Jimenez-Borreguero J, Peinado R, Merino SV, Sobrino JA. Unipolar mapping and magnetic resonance imaging of "idiopathic" right ventricular outflow tract ectopy. J Cardiovasc Electrophysiol 1998; 9:84–87.

1039. Anderson MH. Risk Assessment of Ventricular Tachyarrhythmias. Armonk, NY: Futura Publishing Co., 1995.

1040. Rodstein M, Wolloch L, Gubner RS. Mortality study of the significance of extrasystoles in an insured population. Circulation 1971; 44:617–625.

1041. Peter T, Hamamoto H, Jordon J, Platt M, Mandel W. Indications for antiarrhythmic therapy as prophylaxis against sudden death. Cardiovasc Clin 1980; 11:249–266.

1042. Crow R, Prineas R, Blackburn H. The prognostic significance of ventricular ectopic beats among the apparently healthy. Am Heart J 1981; 101:244–248.

1043. Moss AJ. Asymptomatic ventricular arrhythmias in healthy persons: smoke or smoke screen? Ann Intern Med 1992; 117:1053–1054.

1044. Bikkina M, Larson MG, Levy D. Prognostic implications of asymptomatic ventricular arrhythmias: the Framingham heart study. Ann Intern Med 1992; 117:990–996.

1045. Paul T, Marchal C, Garson A Jr. Ventricular couplets in the young: prognosis related to underlying substrate. Am Heart J 1990; 119:577–582.

1046. Tsuji A, Nagashima M, Hasegawa S, et al. Long-term follow-up of idiopathic ventricular arrhythmias in otherwise normal children. Jpn Circ J 1995; 59:654–662.

1047. Moss AJ. Profile of high risk in people known to have coronary heart disease: a review. Circulation 1975; 52(Suppl III):III-147–III-154.

1048. Vismara LA, Vera Z, Foerster JM, Amsterdam EA, Mason DT. Identification of sudden death risk factors in acute and chronic coronary artery disease. Am J Cardiol 1977; 39:821–828.

1049. Moss AJ, Goldstein S, Greene W, DeCamilla J. Prehospital precursors of ventricular arrhythmias in acute myocardial infarction. Arch Intern Med 1972; 129:756–762.

1050. Scheidt S. Ventricular premature complexes as villains: still an important part of the problem. J Am Coll Cardiol 1987; 10:243–245.

1051. Moss AJ, Benhorin J. Prognosis and management after a first myocardial infarction. N Engl J Med 1990; 322:743–753.

1052. Khattar RS, Basu SK, Raval U, Senior R, Lahiri A. Prognostic value of predischarge exercise testing, ejection fraction, and ventricular ectopic activity in acute myocardial infarction treated with streptokinase. Am J Cardiol 1996; 78:136–141.

1053. Hallstrom AP, Bigger JT Jr, Roden D, et al. Prognostic significance of ventricular premature depolarizations measured 1 year after myocardial infarction in patients with early postinfarction asymptomatic ventricular arrhythmia. J Am Coll Cardiol 1992; 20:259–264.

1054. Anonymous. The prognostic importance of the electrocardiogram after myocardial infarction: experience in the coronary drug project. Ann Intern Med 1972; 77:677–689.

1055. Kostis JB, Wilson AC. Increased mortality is associated with even very low frequency ventricular ectopic activity in survivors of myocardial infarction. Circulation 1990; 82(Suppl III):III-139.

1056. Moss AJ, DeCamilla J, Engstrom F, Hoffman W, Odoroff C, Davis H. The posthospital phase of myocardial infarction: identification of patients with increased mortality risk. Circulation 1974; 49:460–466.

1057. Moss AJ. Factors influencing prognosis after myocardial infarction. Curr Probl Cardiol 1979; 4:6–53.

1058. Rapaport E, Remedios P. The high risk patient after recovery from myocardial infarction: recognition and management. J Am Coll Cardiol 1983; 1:391–400.

1059. Denes P, Gillis AM, Pawitan Y, Kammerling JM, Wilhelmsen L, Salerno DM. Prevalence, characteristics and significance of ventricular premature complexes and ventricular tachycardia detected by 24-hour continuous electrocardiographic recording in the Cardiac Arrhythmia Suppression Trial. Am J Cardiol 1991; 68:887–896.

1060. Tabatznik B. Ambulatory monitoring in the late post-myocardial infarction period. Postgrad Med J 1976; 52:56–59.

1061. Lown B, Wolf M. Approaches to sudden death from coronary heart disease. Circulation 1971; 44:130–142.

1062. Bigger JT Jr, Wenger TL, Heissenbuttel RH. Limitations of the Lown grading system for study of human ventricular arrhythmias. Am Heart J 1977; 93:727–729.

1063. Bigger JT Jr, Weld FM. Analysis of prognostic significance of ventricular arrhythmias after myocardial infarction: shortcomings of Lown grading system. Br Heart J 1981; 45:717–724.

1064. Bigger JT Jr, Weld FM. Shortcomings of the Lown grading system for observational or experimental studies in ischemic heart disease. Am Heart J 1980; 100:1081–1088.

1065. Myerburg RJ, Kessler KM, Luceri RM, et al. Classification of ventricular arrhythmias based on parallel hierarchies of frequency and form. Am J Cardiol 1984; 54:1355–1358.

1066. Hammermeister KE, DeRouen TA, Dodge HT. Variables predictive of survival in patients with coronary disease: selection by univariate and multivariate analyses from the clinical, electrocardiographic, exercise, arteriographic, and quantitative angiographic evaluations. Circulation 1979; 59:421–430.

1067. Taylor GJ, Humphries JO, Mellits ED, et al. Predictors of clinical course, coronary anatomy and left ventricular function after recovery from acute myocardial infarction. Circulation 1980; 62:960–970.

1068. Califf RM, McKinnis RA, Burks J, et al. Prognostic implications of ventricular arrhythmias during 24 hour ambulatory monitoring in patients undergoing cardiac catheterization for coronary artery disease. Am J Cardiol 1982; 50:23–31.

1069. de Feyter PJ, van Eenige MJ, Dighton DH, Visser FC, de Jong J, Roos JP. Prognostic value of exercise testing, coronary angiography and left ventriculography 6–8 weeks after myocardial infarction. Circulation 1982; 66:527–536.

1070. Marchlinski FE, Buxton AE, Waxman HL, Josephson ME. Identifying patients at risk of sudden death after myocardial infarction: value of the response to programmed stimulation, degree of ventricular ectopic activity and severity of left ventricular dysfunction. Am J Cardiol 1983; 52:1190–1196.

1071. White HD, Norris RM, Brown MA, Brandt PW, Whitlock RM, Wild CJ. Left ventricular end-systolic volume as the major determinant of survival after recovery from myocardial infarction. Circulation 1987; 76:44–51.

1072. Chiang BN, Perlman LV, Fulton M, Ostrandep LD Jr, Epstein FH. Predisposing factors in sudden cardiac death in Tecumseh, Michigan: a prospective study. Circulation 1970; 41:31–37.

1073. Holmes J, Kubo SH, Cody RJ, Kligfield P. Arrhythmias in ischemic and nonischemic dilated cardiomyopathy: prediction of mortality by ambulatory electrocardiography. Am J Cardiol 1985; 55:146–151.

1074. Ruberman W, Weinblatt E, Goldberg JD, Frank CW, Shapiro S, Chaudhary BS. Ventricular premature complexes in prognosis of angina. Circulation 1980; 61:1172–1182.

1075. Shugoll GI, Bowen PJ, Moore JP, Lenkin ML. Follow-up observations and prognosis in primary myocardial disease. Arch Intern Med 1972; 129:67–72.

1076. Kron J, Hart M, Schual-Berke S, Niles NR, Hosenpud JD, McAnulty JH. Idiopathic dilated cardiomyopathy: role of programmed electrical stimulation and Holter monitoring in predicting those at risk of sudden death. Chest 1988; 93:85–90.

1077. Romeo F, Pelliccia F, Cianfrocca C, Cristofani R, Reale A. Predictors of sudden death in idiopathic dilated cardiomyopathy. Am J Cardiol 1989; 63:138–140.

1078. Stewart RA, McKenna WJ, Oakley CM. Good prognosis for dilated cardiomyopathy without severe heart failure or arrhythmia. Q J Med 1990; 74:309–318.

1079. De Maria R, Gavazzi A, Caroli A, Ometto R, Biagini A, Camerini F. Ventricular arrhythmias in dilated cardiomyopathy as an independent prognostic hallmark: Italian Multicenter Cardiomyopathy Study (SPIC) group. Am J Cardiol 1992; 69:1451–1457.

1080. Bikkina M, Larson MG, Levy D. Asymptomatic ventricular arrhythmias and mortality risk in subjects with left ventricular hypertrophy. J Am Coll Cardiol 1993; 22:1111–1116.

1081. Josephson ME, Waxman HL, Cain ME, Gardner MJ, Buxton AE. Ventricular activation during ventricular endocardial pacing. II. Role of pace-mapping to localize origin of ventricular tachycardia. Am J Cardiol 1982; 50:11–22.

1082. Langendorf R. Aberrant ventricular conduction. Am Heart J 1951; 41:700–707.

1083. Chung EK. Principles of Cardiac Arrhythmias. Baltimore: Williams & Wilkins, 1971, p. 313.

1084. Marriott HJL. Practical Electrocardiography. 4th ed. Baltimore: Williams & Wilkins, 1968, p. 95.

1085. Vlay SC. How the university cardiologist treats ventricular premature beats: a nationwide survey of 65 university medical centers. Am Heart J 1985; 110:904–912.

1086. Morganroth J, Bigger JT Jr, Anderson JL. Treatment of ventricular arrhythmias by United States cardiologists: a survey before the Cardiac Arrhythmia Suppression Trial results were available. Am J Cardiol 1990; 65:40–48.

1087. Kennedy HL, Whitlock JA, Sprague MK, Kennedy LJ, Buckingham TA, Goldberg RJ. Long-term follow-up of asymptomatic healthy subjects with frequent and complex ventricular ectopy. N Engl J Med 1985; 312:193–197.

1088. Nair CK, Thomson W, Aronow WS, Pagano T, Ryschon K, Sketch MH. Prognostic significance of exercise-induced complex ventricular arrhythmias in coronary artery disease with normal and abnormal left ventricular ejection fraction. Am J Cardiol 1984; 54:1136–1138.

Ventricular Tachycardia[1-12a]

Investigators did not at first attack the mysteries of ventricular tachycardia after the method for recording electrical activity from the bundle of His was published in 1969[13] and opened the era of clinical cardiac electrophysiology. Atrioventricular block, supraventricular tachycardia, the Wolff-Parkinson-White syndrome, and sinus node disease first occupied their attention. The ventricles, the soul of the heart, seemed off limits—at least for a few years.

The first article describing the induction of ventricular tachycardia by programmed stimulation appeared from the Netherlands in 1972.[14] Six years later, American investigators entered the field,[15] and, subsequently, few topics in the field have been so vigorously studied. In short order, the reentrant nature of most cases of ventricular tachycardia was established in its most common setting—the patient with chronic coronary heart disease. Cardiologists learned that ventricular tachycardia is not one arrhythmia but rather a family of arrhythmias affecting patients differently, having different electrocardiographic forms and driven by mechanisms other than reentry. The terms "sustained" and "nonsustained," "monomorphic," and "polymorphic" came into use, distinctions not previously emphasized.

New methods of treatment quickly followed. Cardiologists learned how to administer antiarrhythmic drugs based on their electrophysiological effects on the arrhythmia. Surgical operations and catheter ablation to eliminate the electrophysiological source of the tachycardia followed. By the 1980s, and particularly in the past decade, the implantable cardioverter-defibrillator, now the definitive, albeit most expensive, method of silently interrupting the paroxysms and preventing cardiac arrest, took over. Although the large volume of electrophysiological literature would suggest other-wise, all this work is devoted to an arrhythmia that is a relatively infrequent affliction, although of supreme importance to the patient in whom it develops.

SOME ADVANCES SINCE THE FIRST EDITION OF THIS BOOK

- Description of the circadian pattern of paroxysmal ventricular tachycardia.
- Value of QT interval dispersion and heart rate variability in selecting patients likely to develop ventricular tachycardia.
- Realization that idiopathic ventricular tachycardia may often be due to subtle pathology requiring magnetic resonance imaging or biopsy to define.
- Better understanding of the electrophysiology of idiopathic ventricular tachycardia, now thought to be due to triggered activity in many cases.
- Tendency toward greater use of implantable cardioverter-defibrillators and less use of drugs selected with electrophysiological study to treat the arrhythmia.
- Application of catheter ablation with radiofrequency current to treat some cases of ventricular tachycardia including many in patients without structural heart disease.

PREVALENCE

Ventricular tachycardia is an uncommon arrhythmia.[b] It was the diagnosis in

- None of more than 100,000 standard electrocardiograms taken on apparently healthy subjects.[16-18]
- One (0.56%) of every 1,800 electrocardiograms

---

[a]This chapter includes material from Chapter 14, "Sustained Ventricular Tachycardia," by Mark E. Josephson and David J. Callans,[1] and Chapter 15, "Transient Ventricular Tachycardia," by Alfred E. Buxton,[2] in the first edition of this book.

[b]A fact that clinical electrophysiologists may find difficult to accept because ventricular tachycardia is one of the most frequent diagnoses of patients referred to them.

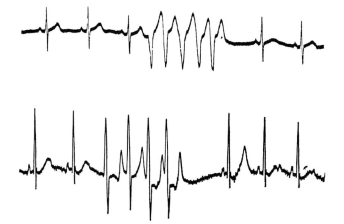

FIGURE 12.1 **Transient ventricular tachycardia** from a Holter monitor recording of an asymptomatic patient. (From Hinkle LE Jr, Carver ST, Stevens M. The frequency of asymptomatic disturbances of cardiac rhythm and conduction in middle-aged men. Am J Cardiol 1969; 24:629–650, with permission.)[1366]

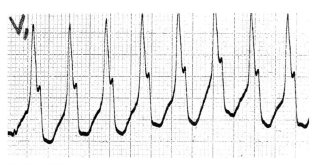

FIGURE 12.2 **Recurrent sustained ventricular tachycardia.** A typical example with the pattern of right bundle branch block in which the first positive deflection is taller than the second in lead V_1. The patient presented to an emergency department with this arrhythmia, which was cardioverted to sinus rhythm. (From Kastor JA. Ventricular tachycardia. Clin Cardiol 1989; 12:586–599, with permission.)[7]

taken at the Boston City Hospital in the 20 years preceding 1943.[19c]

- Eighty (0.16%) of 50,000 consecutive patients whose electrocardiograms were taken at the Michael Reese Hospital in Chicago before 1956.[20d]
- Ten (1.1%) of 922 apparently healthy, exercising subjects whose average age was 54 years.[21]

AGE, GENDER, AND INHERITANCE

Ventricular tachycardia occurs at all ages. The greatest incidence coincides with the time of life when patients develop coronary heart disease, its most common cause. For example:

- The average age of 107 cases collected from 1915 to 1948 at a Boston teaching hospital was 54.8 years;[22] two-thirds were male.
- In a more recently reported series (1985) of 113 patients collected at a San Francisco center known for its clinical electrophysiological work, the mean age was 57 ± 15 years.[23]
- Only 1 of 922 apparently healthy men and women aged 21 to 96 years (mean, 54 ± 16 years) who developed ventricular tachycardia on exercise was younger than 65 years in another series.[21]

---

[c]Admittedly, in the early days of electrocardiography.
[d]For comparison, the incidence of atrial fibrillation in the same hospital at this time was 11.7%.[20]

In patients 65 years of age or older, transient ventricular tachycardia occurs in 4% of women and 10% of men when monitored for 24 hours.[24] Ventricular tachycardia, although rare, does occur in children[25–27] and neonates.[28] Ventricular tachycardia in children must be carefully differentiated from other regular tachycardias with wide QRS complexes.[29]

CATEGORIES

Ventricular tachycardia can be considered in several categories.

By Duration

- *Transient,* also called *unsustained* or *nonsustained* (Fig. 12.1 and Table 12.1),[30–33e] in which the arrhythmia lasts no longer than 30 seconds.
- *Sustained* (Fig. 12.2), in which the paroxysms last more than 30 seconds or, if less, require immediate treatment to prevent cardiovascular collapse.
- *Incessant,* in which the arrhythmia is present much of the time.

By Electrocardiographic Appearance

- *Monomorphic ventricular tachycardia,* in which each of the QRS complexes has identical or nearly identical

---

[e]I prefer the specifically descriptive word "transient" to the more frequently used "nonsustained" or "unsustained," both of which describe one form of ventricular tachycardia in terms of another.

| Table 12.1 | CATEGORIES OF VENTRICULAR TACHYCARDIA DEFINED BY ELECTROCARDIOGRAPHIC APPEARANCE AND BY WHETHER EMERGENCY TREATMENT FOR CARDIOVASCULAR DETERIORATION IS REQUIRED |

Type of Ventricular Tachycardia	Minimum Number of Consecutive Ventricular Beats	Duration of Tachycardia
Transient (nonsustained or unsustained)	3	No longer than 30 sec and without cardiovascular deterioration
Sustained	—	More than 30 sec, or if less, with cardiovascular deterioration
Incessant[a]	—	Most of the time

[a]The proportion of time that ventricular tachycardia must be present to qualify for the description "incessant" varies from 50%[1374] to more than 90%.[251]

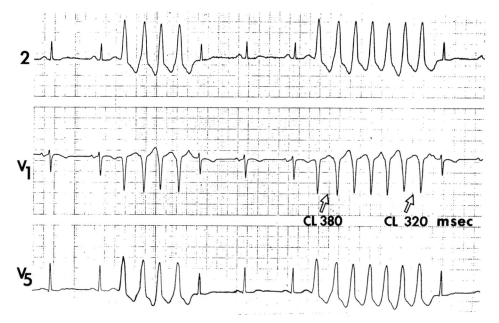

2

V₁

CL 380   CL 320 msec

V₅

FIGURE 12.3 **Repetitive mono-morphic ventricular tachycardia** in a patient without structural heart disease. Shown are two bursts of transient ventricular tachycardia, the rates of which increase during the second paroxysm; cycle lengths (CL) decrease from 380 to 320 milliseconds. Notice the pattern of left bundle branch block with a normal axis in the frontal plane, the characteristic form of the electrocardiogram of these patients during ventricular tachycardia. (From Carlson RW, Geheb MA. Principles and Practice of Medical Intensive Care. Philadelphia: WB Saunders, 1993, with permission.)

form. An unusual variant is *repetitive monomorphic ventricular tachycardia* characterized by short, recurring paroxysms (Fig. 12.3)[34f] of monomorphic tachycardia among periods of sinus rhythm and ventricular premature beats with the same form as the ventricular tachycardia. Most patients with this arrhythmia are young and have no, as yet recognized, structural heart disease.[35, 36g]

- *Polymorphic ventricular tachycardia,* in which the morphology (form) of the QRS complexes changes (Fig. 12.4).[h]
- *Ventricular parasystolic tachycardia,* a diagnosis assigned occasionally in the past but seldom employed now.[37–39] Cases with slower rates are

currently seen as examples of accelerated idioventricular rhythm.[i]

By the Presence or Absence of Heart Disease

- *With* heart disease, most often coronary or cardiomyopathic.
- *Without* structural heart disease or *idiopathic.*

By Electrophysiological Mechanism

- *Reentry,* by far the most frequent mechanism and characteristic of most cases of ventricular tachycardia in patients with coronary heart disease and cardiomyopathy.
- *Triggered activity,* thought to be the mechanism of repetitive monomorphic ventricular tachycardia and paroxysmal stress-induced or exercise-induced

[f]The number of discrete episodes of ventricular tachycardia ranged from 10 to 10,000 per day in 1 series of 11 patients.[34]

[g]Sir James Parkinson (the second name of the Wolff-Parkinson-White syndrome) and Cornelio Papp may have been the first to describe this arrhythmia.[35] No discernible structural heart disease could be found, at least by the techniques then available (1947), in their patients who had recurrent bursts of both ventricular and supraventricular tachycardias.

[h]See Chapter 13.

[i]See Chapter 9.

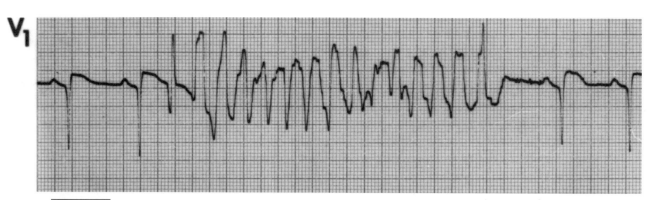

V₁

FIGURE 12.4 **Polymorphic ventricular tachycardia,** identified by the nonuniform morphology of the QRS complexes.

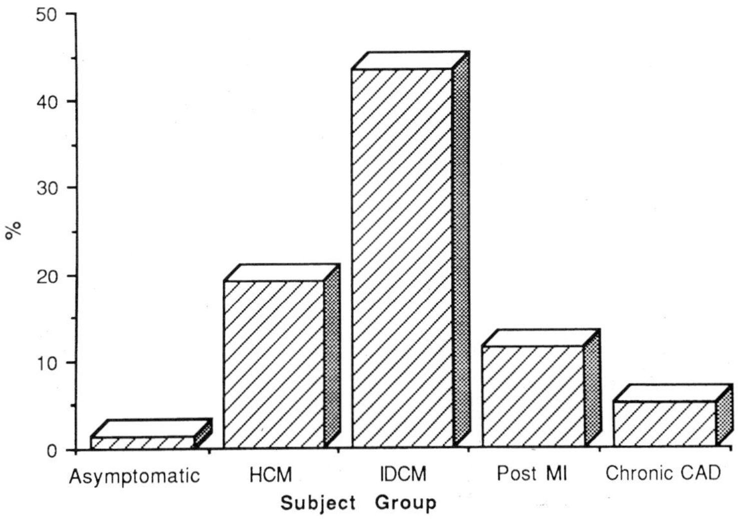

FIGURE 12.5 **Prevalance of transient ventricular tachycardia** (*vertical axis*) in patients who have no symptoms of heart disease, hypertrophic cardiomyopathy (HCM), idiopathic dilated cardiomyopathy (IDCM), recent myocardial infarction (MI), and chronic coronary artery disease (CAD). (From Buxton AE. Transient ventricular tachycardia. In Kastor JA (ed). Arrhythmias. Philadelphia: WB Saunders, 1994, pp. 363–375, with permission.)[2]

ventricular tachycardia usually found in patients without structural heart disease.[40–43j]

- *Automaticity,* the cause of accelerated idioventricular rhythm, which is sometimes incorrectly called "slow ventricular tachycardia," and the rare ventricular tachycardia that originates from the posterior fascicle of the left bundle branch in patients without structural heart disease.

SETTING[44, 45]

Coronary Heart Disease[46]

The most common cause of ventricular tachycardia is coronary heart disease[44–46] (Fig. 12.5) which was present in 74% of patients in the Boston series[22] and in 72% in the San Francisco series (Table 12.2).[23]

Acute myocardial infarction.[47, 48k] Primary sustained and transient ventricular tachycardia develops in 3.7%

---

[j]And in one patient (so far) with mitral valve prolapse and ventricular tachycardia.[43]

[k]Defined as occurring "in patients with acute myocardial infarction in the absence of obvious heart failure or hypotension."[48]

Table 12.2	**ETIOLOGY OF HEART DISEASES IN PATIENTS WITH VENTRICULAR TACHYCARDIA FROM TWO CITIES IN TWO SERIES 35 YEARS APART**

	Boston	**San Francisco**
Year	1950	1985
Number of patients	107	113
Etiology of Heart Disease		
Coronary heart disease	74%	72%
Hypertension	—	9%
Rheumatic heart disease	8%	—
Congestive cardiomyopathy	—	6%
No heart disease	12%	10%
Other	6%	4%

(Data from references 22 and 23.)

of patients during myocardial infarction (Fig. 12.6).[48l] They are more frequently male, are younger than the age of 60 years, and do not have angina.[48] Many of the other features listed here that characterize those patients who develop ventricular tachycardia during myocardial infarction are recognized as indicating larger amounts of myocardial damage.[48]

- Angiographically documented proximal stenosis of the left anterior descending coronary artery.[49]
- Anterior infarctions.[49]
- Bifascicular bundle branch block.[50]
- Greater ST segment elevations.[51]

---

[l]From a combined study published in 1992 from 13 Israeli hospitals of 4,339 patients, 162 of whom developed ventricular tachycardia during myocardial infarction after arriving at the hospital.[48]

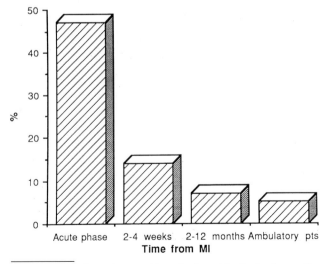

FIGURE 12.6 **Prevalance of transient ventricular tachycardia** (*vertical axis*) in patients with coronary artery disease at different times after beginning of myocardial infarction (MI) (*horizontal axis*). (From Buxton AE. Transient ventricular tachycardia. In Kastor JA (ed). Arrhythmias. Philadelphia: WB Saunders, 1994, pp. 363–375, with permission.)[2]

- High levels of lactic dehydrogenase,[48, 52] serum aspartic transaminase,[53] or creatine kinase.[49, 50]
- Higher Killip class.[50]
- More episodes of accelerated idioventricular rhythm.[54]
- More single and coupled ventricular premature beats.[54]
- Prolonged initial corrected QT intervals.[49]
- Right ventricular infarctions.[55]
- Scintigraphic evidence of hypoperfusion of the interventricular septum.[49]
- Successful thrombolysis[56–60] in which the artery causing the infarction has opened. The arrhythmia presumably derives from the arrhythmogenic effects of reperfusion, although the appearance of ventricular tachycardia cannot be taken as proof that the vessel has opened.[61]

Most episodes of ventricular tachycardia occur soon after symptoms of myocardial infarction develop, usually within the first 12 hours.[48] The arrhythmia is more often sustained than transient in women and in those patients who have had less angina and higher lactic acid dehydrogenase levels.[48]

Fifty percent of patients with *sustained* ventricular tachycardia during myocardial infarction develop ventricular fibrillation, 57% lose consciousness, 21% have sustained hypotension, and 11% die.[48] Compared with patients without the arrhythmia, those with sustained ventricular tachycardia more often have atrial fibrillation, atrioventricular block, cardiogenic shock, and a higher mortality.[48]

Compared with patients who develop ventricular fibrillation during myocardial infarction, those with sustained monomorphic ventricular tachycardia have[50]

- Higher creatine kinase–MB activity.
- Higher Killip class.
- Worse prognosis.

Of 96 children, aged 1 day to 16 years, who suffered acute myocardial infarction, sustained ventricular tachycardia developed in eight, and transient ventricular tachycardia, occurred in eight.[62]

After myocardial infarction. Between 11% and 22% of patients develop ventricular tachycardia toward the end of, or after discharge from hospitalization, for myocardial infarction.[63–67] The paroxysms, which are more often transient than sustained,[64–66]

- Are self-limiting.[64]
- Develop more often in those who have more frequent ventricular premature beats.[65, 66]
- Last for only three beats in 30% of the cases.[65, 66]
- Occur infrequently during sleep.[64]
- Occur more often after than during the acute event.[64]
- Seldom produce symptoms.[64]

Ventricular tachycardia appears more often after myocardial infarction in those patients who, during the infarction, had atrial[54, 68] and ventricular[54, 68, 69] premature beats, atrial fibrillation,[65, 66] intraventricular

conduction defects,[68] bundle branch blocks,[70] ventricular tachycardia,[64–66] or ventricular fibrillation.[64–66] These patients frequently are older,[65, 66] have multivessel coronary disease,[71] less, not more, angina than those who do not have the arrhythmia,[72] and such evidence of severe myocardial damage as follows:

- Cardiomegaly and left ventricular hypertrophy.[68]
- Congestive heart failure.[65, 66, 68]
- Ejection fractions[71] of less than 30%.[65, 66]
- Higher peak enzyme levels.[68]
- Previous infarctions.[65, 66]
- Need for digitalis, diuretics, or antiarrhythmic drugs.[65, 66]
- Transmural, often anterior,[71] rather than subendocardial infarctions.[64]

Most patients with *sustained* ventricular tachycardia after myocardial infarction are more likely to have had other myocardial infarctions and more complicated courses during the first 48 hours of the infarction,[70] including

- Bundle branch, particularly right[73] bundle branch, block.
- Impaired left ventricular function.[73]
- Transmural anterior[73] more often than transmural inferior infarctions and transmural more often than non–Q-wave infarctions.

No clinical, angiographic or hemodynamic clues distinguish who will develop drug-refractory sustained ventricular tachycardia within 4 months from those who will first develop the arrhythmia after 1 year following the myocardial infarction.[74] Transient ventricular tachycardia occurs less often in survivors of myocardial infarction who have had effective thrombolysis.[75] Ventricular tachycardia seldom appears in children who survive myocardial infarction, which is most often due to anomalous origin of the left coronary artery from the pulmonary artery.[40]

Angina. A few patients develop ventricular tachycardia during ischemia provoked by exercise.[76–81] Ventricular tachycardia also develops during silent ischemia[82] and during coronary vasospasm (Prinzmetal's angina),[83–87] whether or not[88, 89] pain is present. The arrhythmia occurs during both ischemic[86, 87, 89] and reperfusion[85, 86, 89] phases of Prinzmetal's angina.

Aneurysms. Aneurysms of the left ventricle frequently accompany sustained ventricular tachycardia in patients with coronary heart disease and occasionally with other illnesses.[72, 76, 90–110] However, the incidence of ventricular aneurysms among patients with ventricular tachycardia due to myocardial infarction appears to have decreased with the use of thrombolysis and acute angioplasty. Furthermore, sustained ventricular tachycardia occurs in only about 3% of patients with aneurysms.[111m]

---

[m]As reported from the Cardiac Arrhythmia Suppression Trial (CAST).[111]

Hypertension

Transient ventricular tachycardia occurs more often in patients with the electrocardiographic and echocardiographic diagnosis of left ventricular hypertrophy from hypertension than in those without hypertrophy.[112, 113]

Cardiomyopathy

Patients with idiopathic congestive cardiomyopathy[114, 115] frequently have transient ventricular tachycardia.[25, 116–118n] The arrhythmia occurs more often in those who are older[118] and whose congestive heart failure is severe.[119] Sustained ventricular tachycardia occurs much less frequently.[120, 121o]

Ventricular tachycardia may rarely, like supraventricular tachycardias more frequently, produce cardiomyopathy.[122–128p]

Hypertrophic cardiomyopathy. Transient ventricular tachycardia appears not infrequently in patients with hypertrophic cardiomyopathy,[129–136] particularly in those with left ventricular dilatation.[137] However, transient ventricular tachycardia in these patients does not correspond with the degree of left ventricular hypertrophy, outflow tract gradient, or dysfunction.[138] The development of sustained monomorphic ventricular tachycardia may require an apical aneurysm in patients with hypertrophic cardiomyopathy and normal coronary arteries.[136]

Arrhythmogenic right ventricular dysplasia. An unusual cardiomyopathy primarily affecting the right ventricle,[139–142] it often presents, even in young athletes during sports,[143] as sustained ventricular tachycardia.[143–156]

Other cardiomyopathies. Occasionally, cardiac sarcoidosis may produce sustained ventricular tachycardia.[157] Left ventricular function is reduced in most of these patients. Some have no pulmonary or other systemic involvement with the disease. Ventricular tachycardia may complicate "focal myocardial degeneration"[158] and Becker muscular dystrophy.[159]

Valvular Heart Disease

Rheumatic heart disease is seldom now the cause of ventricular tachycardia in the United States; none had this diagnosis in a series reported in 1985.[23] Formerly, rheumatic heart disease was the cause in as many as

15% of cases.[22] Whether mild or moderate mitral valve prolapse, by itself,[23, 25, 116, 117, 160–167] produces ventricular tachycardia has not been established.

Congenital Heart Disease

Transient and sustained ventricular tachycardia occurs in association with

- Atrialized right ventricle in Ebstein's anomaly of the tricuspid valve.[168]
- Congenitally corrected transposition of the great arteries.[169]

Surgery

Cardiac operations can produce ventricular tachycardia, usually transient, occasionally sustained, after coronary artery bypass grafting[170–180] or valvular surgery.[181] The incidence increases in patients with more extensive revascularization.[172]

When sustained monomorphic ventricular tachycardia occurs for the first time after surgical revascularization, the source is usually old ventricular scars or regions of newly reperfused myocardial tissue.[182] The patients who develop this arrhythmia usually have

- A healed infarction.[182]
- Reduced preoperative left ventricular function.[182]
- *No* perioperative infarction.[182]

Ventricular tachycardia may also follow

- Apical aneurysms produced by the sumps inserted to vent left ventricles during surgery.[183]
- Conventional ventricular aneurysmectomy.[184]
- Repair of tetralogy of Fallot.[185–191]
- Valve replacement.[173, 176, 177, 181, 192]

Ventricular tachycardia sustained in a bundle branch may first appear after valvular surgery[181] or successful surgical treatment of a *different* ventricular tachycardia.[193]

Drugs

Many drugs, including those used to treat the arrhythmia, can cause ventricular tachycardia ("pro-arrhythmic" effect).[q] Digitalis infrequently precipitates ventricular tachycardia.[22]

No Structural Heart Disease[194–199r]

Ventricular tachycardia develops in patients who have no clinical heart disease other than the arrhythmia.[36, 117, 149, 194–225] Such patients constituted 10% of the patients in the San Francisco series[23] and 12% in the older Boston series.[22, 226, 227] These patients are usually younger than those with coronary heart disease,[149, 201, 203, 207–209, 212, 214, 216, 218s] although the arrhythmia may have

---

[n]In 21 (60%) of 35 consecutively studied patients with idiopathic dilated cardiomyopathy.[118] The number of beats varied from 3 to 46 (average, 8). The average age of the patients with ventricular tachycardia was 55 years, and it was 47 years in those without ventricular tachycardia.

[o]Congestive cardiomyopathy was the diagnosis in 6% of the San Francisco series of patients with sustained ventricular tachycardia.[23]

[p]This phenomenon developed in a 77-year-old man with repetitive monomorphic ventricular tachycardia and no significant coronary heart disease. After ablation of the site of origin of the arrhythmia in the right ventricular outflow tract, his symptoms resolved, and his left ventricular ejection fraction rose to 51%.[127]

---

[q]See Chapter 13.

[r]See elsewhere for a more comprehensive list of pertinent references.[194, 196]

[s]The average age was 36 years in a series of 52 patients.[149]

been present for years before the patient is evaluated. The tachycardia in patients without structural heart disease can be transient, sustained, or incessant,[149, 228] and it is often provoked by,[207, 209, 216, 218, 229] but can also be suppressed by,[213] exercise.

Some patients with ventricular tachycardia and no clinically evident structural heart disease have subtle abnormalities of myocardial function,[215, 228, 230, 231] abnormal findings on magnetic resonance imaging[232, 233] or pathological changes in ventricular endocardial tissue.[226, 234] Thus, their presentation with ventricular tachycardia may constitute the first manifestation of cardiomyopathy,[228] including arrhythmogenic right ventricular dysplasia,[215, 235, 236] myocarditis,[230, 231] or other types of pathological features that cardiologists cannot as yet define.[227] Children at all ages occasionally develop idiopathic ventricular tachycardia.[25, 116, 164, 228, 237–247]

Children[28]

No structural heart disease[238, 243] is found in about half[246] of those few infants and children who develop ventricular tachycardia.[28] Cardiomyopathy and myocarditis account for most of the rest.[246] Rarely, ventricular tumors,[244, 248–250] usually hamartomas,[251] produce ventricular tachycardia in children. Most children with primary cardiac tumors, however, do not require specific treatment for arrhythmias.[252] Cocaine, used by the mother, produced ventricular tachycardia in a newborn.[253]

Circadian Effects

Implantable cardioverter-defibrillators detect and treat life-threatening ventricular arrhythmias such as sustained ventricular tachycardia most frequently in the morning,[254–257] on Mondays, and to a lesser extent on Fridays.[258] Weekends are particularly free of the arrhythmias that produce defibrillator shocks.[258] Antiarrhythmic[259] and beta-adrenergic–blocking[258, 260] drugs eliminate the hourly[259, 260] and day-to-day[258] circadian pattern. Ambulatory monitoring reveals that transient ventricular tachycardia also occurs most often early in the morning[261] and more frequently when patients who have recovered from myocardial infarction are awake.[262*t*]

Miscellaneous Conditions

Ventricular tachycardia is also associated with several other conditions (Table 12.3).[116, 203, 231, 263–279]

OTHER ARRHYTHMIAS

Ventricular Premature Beats

Ventricular premature beats, often frequent and complex, are frequently recorded in patients who will have

---

*The longest paroxysms of ventricular tachycardia in one study lasted for 18 beats; the average rate was 137 beats per minute (range, 100–250 beats/min).[262]

Table 12.3	**MISCELLANEOUS CONDITIONS IN WHICH VENTRICULAR TACHYCARDIA OCCURS**

Alcohol[265]
Labor and delivery[263]
Inspiration, which may produce,[267, 274] and expiration, which may convert,[274] the arrhythmia
Liquid protein diet[266]
Long-duration space flight[279]
Myocarditis,[116, 231, 276, 277] including that due to Lyme disease[278]
Pacemakers inserted to treat other arrhythmias[268, 270, 273]
Pulmonary artery catheterization performed at the bedside[269]
Sleep apnea[264, 272]
Tobacco and coffee,[a] which may or may not affect its occurrence[203, 271]
Trauma[275*b*]

---

[a]In one electrophysiological study, transient ventricular tachycardia was induced by programmed ventricular stimulation in 2 of 19 subjects who drank coffee or received infusions of caffeine citrate.[271]

[b]Ventricular tachycardia developed after a soccer ball struck an athlete's chest, the first indication that he has arrhythmogenic right ventricular dysplasia.[150]

---

or have had ventricular tachycardia.[280–302] The morphology of the QRS complexes that precede the onset of ventricular tachycardia is usually similar to, if not the same as, that of the tachyarrhythmia.[303, 304]

Double Tachycardia

Ventricular tachycardia can occasionally constitute one of the arrhythmias in patients who also have atrial tachycardias, a combination known as double or simultaneous tachycardia.[*u*]

Ventricular Fibrillation

Although the final arrhythmia of most patients dying suddenly with cardiac disease is ventricular fibrillation, ventricular tachycardia often precedes it. At the beginning of a potentially fatal arrhythmia, acute ischemia tends to produce ventricular fibrillation, whereas chronic coronary disease usually first produces ventricular tachycardia.

SYMPTOMS

Most episodes of transient ventricular tachycardia do not produce symptoms.[305] It is usually patients with sustained ventricular tachycardia who report the symptoms most associated with paroxysmal ventricular tachycardia. However, contrary to the impression of many physicians that sustained ventricular tachycardia always produces severe symptoms, some patients with the arrhythmia have few complaints during a paroxysm.[23] Thus, the absence of severe symptoms may lead incorrectly to the diagnosis of supraventricular tachycardia.

---

[u]See Chapter 9 for a discussion of double tachycardia.

The symptoms produced by ventricular tachycardia are[23v]

- Palpitations in 57%.
- Chest pain in 27%, and, as expected, more often in patients with coronary heart disease.
- Dyspnea in 25%, which, however, does not occur more frequently in patients with congestive heart failure than in those without failure.
- Weakness in 6%.
- Nausea in 3%.
- Sweating in 3%.
- Flushing in 2%.

Cerebral symptoms,[23] which 65% of patients with sustained ventricular tachycardia experience, include

- Slight lightheadedness in 35%.
- Near syncope in 15%.
- Syncope in 15%.

Syncope is more likely due to ventricular tachycardia or atrioventricular block than to neurocardiogenic influences in patients who are male, who are more than 54 years of age, and who have had less than three episodes of fainting with warning symptoms lasting less than 6 seconds.[306] Symptoms that suggest that ventricular tachycardia or atrioventricular block is *not* the cause include palpitations, blurred vision, warmth, sweating, and lightheadedness before the faint and nausea, warmth, sweating, or fatigue after syncope.[306]

Ventricular tachyarrhythmias account for most episodes of syncope or near-syncope in patients with sustained ventricular tachycardia induced in the electrophysiology laboratory and left ventricular dysfunction.[307] Transient or sustained ventricular tachycardia can usually be established at electrophysiological study in patients with syncope who have had surgical correction of tetralogy of Fallot even though no spontaneous episodes have been documented.[308]

Effects of Heart Rate and Ventricular Function on Symptoms

The heart rate during ventricular tachycardia tends to be faster in patients who have symptoms,[23, 164] including syncope.[23, 164, 309, 310] For example:

- 222 ± 38 beats per minute in those with symptoms versus 159 ± 17 beats per minute in those without symptoms.[228w]
- 224 ± 29 beats per minute in patients with syncope, 191 ± 38 beats per minute with near syncope, 170 ± 26 beats per minute with lightheadedness, and 163 ± 31 beats per minute with no cerebral symptoms.[23x] However, many patients whose heart rates during ventricular tachycardia exceed 200 beats per minute do not faint.[23]

Patients with congestive heart failure are more likely to faint and to have at least some cerebral symptoms than those without heart failure.[23] Ventricular function does not determine who will faint from ventricular tachycardia, at least during electrophysiological study.[309] One should keep in mind that patients with ventricular tachycardia due to structural heart disease often faint because the arrhythmia changes to ventricular fibrillation.[310]

Exercise

When a drug slows the heart rate during ventricular tachycardia to less than 200 beats per minute, patients who fainted during the arrhythmia before taking the drug no longer do so when the arrhythmia recurs.[309, 311–314] Most episodes of transient ventricular tachycardia occur during ordinary activity.[315] However, exercise can produce the arrhythmia,[316y] usually transient, sometimes sustained in patients with and without structural heart disease.

Coronary heart disease. Those patients who develop ventricular tachycardia during angina provoked by exercise often have severe coronary disease with obstructions of the left main coronary artery or the proximal segment of the left anterior coronary artery.[81] Many also have right coronary disease as well.[81] When coronary artery bypass graft surgery relieves ischemia, exercise may no longer produce the arrhythmia.[76, 77] However, exercise need not provoke clinical ischemia in patients with coronary heart disease to start ventricular tachycardia,[317] which can be sustained.[206] Exercise suppresses ventricular tachycardia in those few patients with repetitive monomorphic ventricular tachycardia who have coronary heart disease.[210]

Cardiomyopathy. Exercise may induce sustained and transient ventricular tachycardia in patients with dilated and hypertrophic cardiomyopathy,[78, 154, 318] arrhythmogenic right ventricular dysplasia,[146, 148, 149, 319] and chronic chagasic cardiomyopathy.[320]

Patients who are apparently healthy or have no structural heart disease. Asymptomatic, transient ventricular tachycardia appears in apparently healthy persons when exercising.[21, 194, 203z] Symptomatic ventricular tachycardia, usually transient, occasionally sustained, may also appear during exercise in patients without structural heart disease.[78, 149, 204, 205, 216, 229, 321–323] These patients often come to medical attention because of exercise-related symptoms even though they are asymptomatic when not exercising and are without ventricular tachycardia during extended monitoring.[321]

Exercise may also expose repetitive monomorphic

---

[v]From the San Francisco study of 113 patients with ventricular tachycardia. Patients whose arrhythmia occurred during myocardial infarction or who had been resuscitated from out-of-hospital cardiac arrest were excluded from this study.

[w]In 24 young patients without clinical heart disease other than the arrhythmia.[228]

[x]In 113 patients with sustained ventricular tachycardia.[23]

[y]Which is unrelated to plasma norepinephrine, the levels of which are similar whether or not the arrhythmia is induced by exercise.[316]

[z]In 10 of 922 subjects, each of whom with one exception at peak exercise.[21] The longest paroxysm lasted 6 beats in this series.[21] In another study of six patients, three had less rise in systolic blood pressure than predicted for the heart rate achieved during exercise.[203]

ventricular tachycardia[210, 219] and may suppress the ventricular tachycardia that originates in the right ventricular outflow tract.[213] Both these tachycardias usually occur in patients without structural heart disease.

Exercise can exacerbate or suppress ventricular tachycardia in children without structural heart disease.[242] In general, exercise tends to increase the degree of arrhythmia in symptomatic children with ventricular tachycardia and decrease the arrhythmia in children without symptoms.[164] Children with exercise-induced ventricular tachycardia are often asymptomatic.[242aa]

PHYSICAL EXAMINATION[bb]
Characteristic Physical Signs[cc]

The physical signs of ventricular tachycardia are produced by:[22, 324]

- Rapid heart rate.
- Regular rhythm.
- Atrioventricular dissociation.
- Reduced cardiac output.

Rapid heart rate and regular rhythm. Rapidity is, by definition, a feature of all tachyarrhythmias and is not, by itself, helpful in making the diagnosis. Ventricular tachycardia, however, usually feels regular or almost regular to the examiner, and this feature can help one to eliminate diagnoses of atrial fibrillation, multifocal atrial tachycardia, and some cases of atrial flutter. The absence of respiratory sinus arrhythmia reduces the likelihood of confusing relatively slow ventricular tachycardia with sinus tachycardia. Rarely, only one heart sound may be heard with each beat, a feature that can lead the examiner to conclude that the heart rate is half the actual rate.[22]

Atrioventricular dissociation. In ventricular tachycardia, the sequence of atrial and ventricular contraction may be abnormal. This dissociation produces characteristic physical signs that should be sought at the bedside of each patient with a tachyarrhythmia. They include

- Variation of the systolic blood pressure.[325]
- Irregular large ("cannon") A waves in the jugular venous pulse from right atrial contraction against a closed tricuspid valve. The A waves have a slower rate than the waves of ventricular contraction.[326, 327]

- Changing amplitude of the first heart sound.[327]
- Varying intensity of systolic murmurs, unrelated to respiration.

Examination of patients with other regular tachycardias such as atrial and supraventricular tachycardia, atrial flutter (when regular), and sinus tachycardia does not reveal the findings of atrioventricular dissociation, thereby eliminating most cases of ventricular tachycardia. One must keep in mind, however, that because the atria and ventricles are sometimes associated in ventricular tachycardia (through retrograde conduction), absence of the physical signs of dissociation does not rule out the arrhythmia.[327]

Reduced cardiac output. Pallor, sweating, weak pulse, distant heart sounds, and hypotension characterize the patient whose ventricular tachycardia severely decreases cardiac function. These signs, which in varying degrees of intensity characterize many patients with sustained ventricular tachycardia, are not present in all patients.[23]

Carotid Sinus Pressure

Ventricular tachycardia rarely slows or converts to sinus rhythm in response to carotid sinus pressure, as do many of the supraventricular tachyarrhythmias. However, because carotid sinus pressure does not affect all supraventricular tachycardias, ventricular tachycardia may still not be the only arrhythmia present when carotid sinus pressure has no effect.

Extra Sounds

Extra, multiple, low-frequency "staccato-type"[328] sounds may occasionally be heard at the apex of the heart in ventricular tachycardia.

ELECTROCARDIOGRAM

One makes the electrocardiographic diagnosis of ventricular tachycardia from the presence of three or more consecutive ventricular beats.[329dd]

Duration

Before contemporary treatment was available, episodes of sustained ventricular tachycardia persisted for as long as 35[330] and 62 days.[331] The mean duration of 1,102 episodes of spontaneous, sustained ventricular tachycardia recorded more recently with ambulatory electrocardiography was 13.9 ± 76.6 minutes, with a range of 30 seconds to 16.4 hours.[332]

[aa]Symptoms were present in only 8 of 26 children with ventricular tachycardia.[242]

[bb]The physical examination of patients with tachyarrhythmias is frequently overlooked, an unwise omission because physicians and other health care workers must occasionally attend patients when an electrocardiographic recorder is not available. As observed in 1950, "There are bedside methods available which will enable the physician to suspect the diagnosis of paroxysmal ventricular tachycardia in most cases and even to make a fairly reliable diagnosis in many instances without the aid of the electrocardiograph."[22]

[cc]In making the diagnosis of a regular tachycardia of uncertain origin, variation in the loudness of the first heart sound and the appearance of the jugular venous pulse are the most helpful signs. The characteristics of the arterial pulse are of little value.[324]

[dd]Despite reviewing the literature and asking several authorities, I have not found the origin of the three-beat requirement for the diagnosis of ventricular tachycardia. The statement that "ventricular tachycardia is said to be present if *six* or more consecutive ventricular premature contractions appear" (italics mine)[329] has not been generally accepted.

Rate

The minimum heart rate for ventricular tachycardia is 100 beats per minute.[67][ee] Different reports give different values for the spontaneous mean rate in the different types of ventricular tachycardia:

- *Sustained:* 179 ± 37 beats per minute in 113 patients with various forms of heart disease[23] and 183 beats per minute in 20 patients without structural heart disease.[149]
- *Transient:* 121 ± 34 beats per minute in 92 patients with transient[ff] ventricular tachycardia after myocardial infarction[66] and 178 beats per minute in 21 patients without structural heart disease.[149]
- *Incessant:* 190 beats per minute in 11 patients without structural heart disease.[149]

In 40 infants and young children, the median maximum rate was 214 beats per minute (range, 152–375 beats/min).[246] The rate of the patient's sinus rhythm does not relate to the rate of the ventricular tachycardia.[333, 334] Ventricular tachycardias that occur soon after myocardial infarction tend to have faster rates than those that develop later.[74]

The rate of ventricular tachycardia is faster in patients with dilated cardiomyopathy during the day than at night.[335]

Rhythm

Although the rhythm of ventricular tachycardia seems regular on casual inspection of the electrocardiogram, it is often slightly irregular.[336] This irregularity is greater.[337]

- Soon after the arrhythmia begins and decreases as the paroxysm progresses.
- Throughout the paroxysm when the variability is high during the first 20 beats.
- When the rate of the ventricular tachycardia is slow, especially during the first 20 to 30 beats of the tachycardia; afterward, the variability seems unrelated to the rate.

P Waves

The P waves of atrial activation may or may not be found, even with careful inspection of the electrocardiogram during ventricular tachycardia. The faster the ventricular rate, the less likely are P waves to be visible, lost within the large and frequent QRS complexes and T waves.

When P waves can be seen, one should observe their relation to the QRS complexes and their form, particularly in the inferior electrocardiographic leads. Three patterns may be discerned (Table 12.4):[327, 338–340]

- *Atrioventricular dissociation.* In this pattern, which

Table 12.4	**ATRIOVENTRICULAR RELATIONSHIPS DURING VENTRICULAR TACHYCARDIA**
Atrioventricular Relationship	**100 Patients**
Atrioventricular dissociation	51
1:1 ventriculoatrial conduction	28
Partial atrioventricular dissociation	13
Other	8

(From Wellens HJJ, Bar FW, Vanagt EJ, Brugada P, Farre J. The differentiation between ventricular tachycardia and supraventricular tachycardia with aberrant conduction; the value of the 12-lead electrocardiogram. In Wellens HJJ, Kulbertus HE. [eds]. What's New in Electrocardiography. The Hague: Martinus Nijhoff, 1981, pp. 184–199, with permission.)[340]

occurs in about half of cases, the P waves have the form of sinus rhythm, and their rhythm is unrelated to that of the QRS complexes (Fig. 12.7). Of course, the atria may have another rhythm such as atrial fibrillation, atrial flutter, or atrial tachycardia, but the important concept is that neither the ventricles nor the atria control the rhythm of each other. Atrioventricular dissociation during ventricular tachycardia can occur even when the ventricular rate exceeds 200 beats per minute.

- *1:1 ventriculoatrial conduction.* Now, each QRS complex is followed by a P wave,[341] which is inverted in the inferior electrocardiographic leads because of retrograde atrial activation (see Fig. 12.7). This pattern, which is characteristic of supraventricular tachycardia, occurs in 25% to 30% of cases of ventricular tachycardia, more frequently than is generally believed.
- *Partial ventriculoatrial conduction.* Some of the ventricular impulses traverse the atrioventricular conduction system in retrograde fashion through different amount of block. The P waves are inconstantly present—some disappear, hidden in the QRS complexes. The atrial rhythm is difficult to discern in the midst of this irregularity.

QRS Complex

The duration of the QRS complexes of ventricular tachycardia is usually at least 0.12 second, the classic definition. Fascicular tachycardias,[342] which originate within the ventricles and below the bundle of His, may have slightly narrower QRS complexes.[128, 278, 343, 344] In infants, the width of the QRS complexes during ventricular tachycardia ranges from 0.06 to 0.11 second.[8] As children age, the QRS complexes widen; they often last more than 0.09 second in children older than 3 years.[8]

The form (morphology) of the QRS complexes during the tachycardia is similar, by definition, during a paroxysm of monomorphic ventricular tachycardia. However, the QRS complexes can take different forms[gg] in the same patient during different paroxysms.[345–348] This is more likely to occur in patients who have had several previous myocardial infarctions,

---

[ee]The number varies in different reports. I prefer the recommendations of the investigators of the Cardiac Arrhythmia Suppression Trial (CAST) for a minimum of 100 beats per minute for ventricular tachycardia and less than 100 beats per minute for accelerated idioventricular rhythm.[67]

[ff]Includes two patients with sustained ventricular tachycardia.[66]

[gg]Called pleomorphism, from the Greek *pleo,* meaning "more," + *morph,* meaning "form."

VT with 1:1 V-A Conduction   VT without V-A Conduction

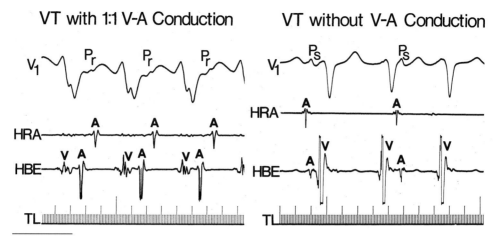

FIGURE 12.7   Ventriculoatrial, (V-A) conduction during ventricular tachycardia (VT). With 1:1 retrograde conduction during ventricular tachycardia **(left)**, each ventricular beat produces a retrograde P wave (P$_r$) in the surface electrocardiogram. The P waves of sinus rhythm (P$_s$) have their own rhythm at 100 beats per minute in the absence of ventriculoatrial conduction **(right)** and are unaffected by the ventricular arrhythmia at a rate of 150 beats per minute. (V$_1$, surface lead; HRA and HBE, intracardiac recordings from the high right atrium (HRA) and the region of the bundle of His (HBE); V, activation of the ventricles; A, activation of the atria; Tl, time lines.) (From Kastor JA, Horowitz LN, Harken AH, Josephson ME. Clinical electrophysiology of ventricular tachycardia. N Engl J Med 1981; 304:1004–1020, reprinted, by permission, from the New England Journal of Medicine.)[548]

particularly when relatively recent,[74] or were taking different antiarrhythmic drugs when the ventricular tachycardias were recorded.[347]

The QRS complexes of ventricular tachycardia often look like right or left bundle branch block, and this feature relates to the location of its origin in the ventricles and the cause of the tachycardia. Rarely, when bundle branch block is present during sinus rhythm, the QRS complexes can appear similar in ventricular tachycardia and in sinus rhythm.[349]

Right bundle branch block. Patients whose ventricular tachycardia has the appearance of right bundle branch block more often are older,[350] male,[350] and have structural, most often coronary, heart disease (see Fig. 12.2; Fig. 12.8).[210, 350, 351] However, a few have no structural heart disease, and this group includes patients

with idiopathic sustained left ventricular tachycardia.[196, 208, 214, 220, 225, 344, 352–354] The QRS complexes of ventricular tachycardia in infants usually have the appearance of right bundle branch block with left axis deviation.[8]

Left bundle branch block. Clinical observations show that most patients whose ventricular tachycardia looks like left bundle branch block, often with inferior axis in the electrocardiographic frontal plane, tend to be younger[216, 350] and female,[350] and many, although not all,[351, 356] have no apparent structural heart disease (Fig. 12.9).[149, 205, 208, 210, 216, 219, 221, 228, 350, 351, 353, 355, 357, 358] However, in patients with coronary disease, and this group constitutes many, if not most, who come to electrophysiological study, ventricular tachycardia with the form of left bundle branch block starts in the left

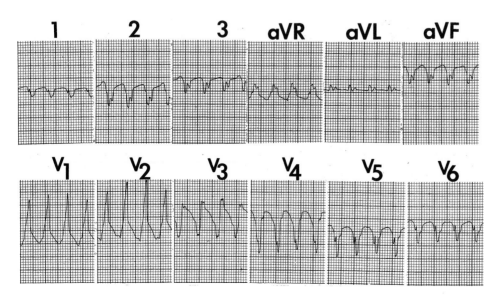

FIGURE 12.8   Ventricular tachycardia with the morphology of right bundle branch block. Criteria supporting the diagnosis of ventricular tachycardia over aberrant conduction in this case include prolonged duration of the QRS complexes to 0.16 second, superior frontal plane axis, monophasic R wave in V$_1$, and R wave to S wave ratio of less than one in lead V$_6$. Ventriculoatrial conduction cannot be assessed because P waves are not clearly seen. (From Josephson ME, Callans DJ. Sustained ventricular tachycardia. In Kastor JA (ed). Arrhythmias. Philadelphia: WB Saunders, 1994, pp. 336–362, with permission.)[1]

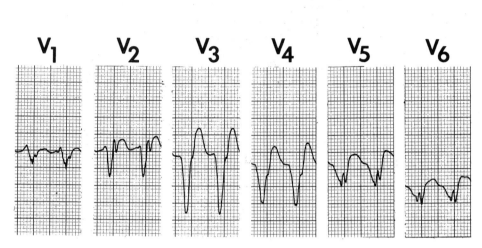

FIGURE 12.9 Ventricular tachycardia with the morphology of left bundle branch block. Criteria supporting the diagnosis of ventricular tachycardia include broad R wave in V_1 and V_2, notching of the S wave in V_2, prolonged duration from the onset of the QRS complex to the nadir of the S wave in leads V_1 and V_2, and Q wave in V_6. (From Josephson ME, Callans DJ. Sustained ventricular tachycardia. In Kastor JA (ed). Arrhythmias. Philadelphia: WB Saunders, 1994, pp. 336–362, with permission.)[1]

ventricle or in the adjacent interventricular septum.[359] Others with left bundle branch block morphology have severe myocardial disease,[356] such as dilated cardiomyopathy and sustained bundle branch reentrant ventricular tachycardia[360] or arrhythmogenic right ventricular dysplasia.[148, 149, 356]

Myocardial infarction versus no structural heart disease. The QRS complexes of patients with ventricular tachycardia who have had myocardial infarction usually have the form of right bundle branch block. The QRS complexes of these patients tend to have a longer duration and a lower amplitude than the complexes of those with the arrhythmia who have no structural heart disease (Table 12.5). The electrocardiograms of patients with ventricular tachycardia and previous myo-

cardial infarction[361] often have QR patterns in leads other than a VR or a QS pattern in leads V_5 or V_6 and abnormal axes. The electrocardiograms of those with idiopathic ventricular tachycardia do not have such QR or QS patterns, and their axes are more often normal.[362hh]

Epsilon waves. These waves are ripples in the first portion of the ST segments in the right precordial leads of the electrocardiograms of some patients with arrhythmogenic right ventricular dysplasia; they reflect delayed activation of the diseased ventricle (Fig. 12.10).[145]

[hh]Abnormal axes: with myocardial infarction; 74%, idiopathic, 25%.[362]

Table 12.5	APPEARANCE OF QRS COMPLEXES DURING VENTRICULAR TACHYCARDIA IN PATIENTS WITH PREVIOUS MYOCARDIAL INFARCTION OR WITH NO STRUCTURAL HEART DISEASE (IDIOPATHIC)			
Etiology	Number of Patients in Study	Width of QRS Complexes	Sum of Amplitude of QRS Complexes in Unipolar Limb Leads	Axis in Frontal Plane
Myocardial infarction	100	171 ± 32 msec	2.6 ± 0.8 mV	Usually abnormal
Idiopathic	70	135 ± 11 msec	4.3 ± 1.3 mV	Usually normal

(From Coumel P, Leclercq JF, Attuel P, Maisonblanche P. The QRS morphology in post-myocardial infarction ventricular tachycardia: a study of 100 tracings compared with 70 cases of idiopathic ventricular tachycardia. Eur Heart J 1984; 5:792–805, with permission.)[362]

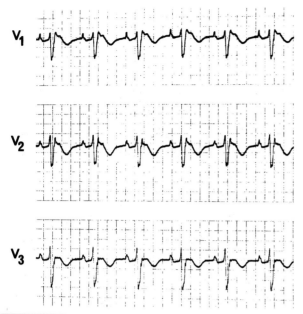

FIGURE 12.10 Postexcitation or "epsilon waves" in a patient with arrhythmogenic right ventricular dysplasia. Ripples in the first portion of the ST segments can be seen in the right precordial leads of some patients with arrhythmogenic right ventricular dysplasia. They reflect representing delayed activation of abnormal tissue in the right ventricle. (The electrocardiogram was recorded at double sensitivity of 0.5 mV/cm.) (From Marcus FI, Fontaine GH, Guiraudon G, et al. Right ventricular dysplasia: a report of 24 adult cases. Circulation 1982; 65:384–398, by permission of the American Heart Association, Inc.)[145]

ST Segment, T Wave, and QT Interval

As in bundle branch block, the ST segments and T waves are always abnormal in ventricular tachycardia. ST segments are more elevated[51] and the initial corrected QT interval is longer[49] in those patients who develop, than in those who do not develop, ventricular tachycardia during myocardial infarction.

Ventricular tachycardia seldom starts as a consequence of the "R-on-T phenomenon" (Fig. 12.11). The arrhythmia rarely begins when the first ventricular beat appears in the T wave of the previous beat.[54, 64–66, 160, 305, 333, 334] Furthermore, the coupling interval[ii] during

---

[ii]The coupling interval is the time between the beginning of the QRS complexes of the last sinus beat and a ventricular premature beat or the first ventricular beat of a paroxysm of ventricular tachycardia.

myocardial infarction is no different from the coupling interval of isolated ventricular premature beats unassociated with a bout of ventricular tachycardia.[54]

Morphology during sinus rhythm. The ST segments are often depressed and the T waves are inverted in the inferior and lateral leads during sinus rhythm in patients with idiopathic ventricular tachycardia.[305] These changes may reflect early cardiac disease as yet undefined. When sinus rhythm returns, the T waves may temporarily remain abnormally inverted from as yet unknown effects of the tachycardia (Fig. 12.12).[363jj]

Ventricular Tachycardia Versus Supraventricular Tachycardia[kk]

Ventricular tachycardia is the mechanism of most tachycardias with wide QRS complexes.[364–373] Nevertheless, electrocardiographic readers reach an incorrect more often than a correct diagnosis.[372, 373] Physicians often decide, wrongly, that the arrhythmia is supraventricular tachycardia with aberrant ventricular conduction from bundle branch block or, less often, antegrade conduction in an accessory pathway (Wolff-Parkinson-White syndrome). However, by considering the clinical situation and carefully inspecting the 12-lead electrocardiogram, one can make the correct diagnosis in about 90% of cases.[340, 373–376] Reaching a correct diagnosis increases the likelihood of a favorable outcome for the patient.[372]

To increase success, one should examine and measure intervals in each of the 12 leads, not rely on monitoring lead MCL₁, which is an unsuitable substitute for lead V₁, and exercise caution in reaching a definite diagnosis if the rate of the tachycardia exceeds 190 beats per minute.[376] A stepwise approach reduces

---

[jj]Ventricular tachycardia, rather than supraventricular tachycardia, as reported, was probably the culprit in a case published in 1969 of post-tachycardia T-wave changes.[363]

[kk]Before clinical electrophysiological studies were developed, electrocardiographers thought and wrote extensively about the differential diagnosis of ventricular tachycardia versus supraventricular tachycardia with aberrancy, a topic of much theoretical and clinical importance.[364, 365, 367] With the availability of intracardiac recordings to locate the tachyarrhythmia and programmed stimulation to induce the arrhythmia during study, investigators could then conclusively define which tachyarrhythmia was which. What follows is based on the data from those electrophysiological studies.

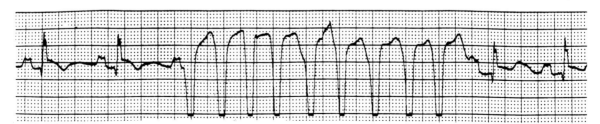

FIGURE 12.11 **Absence of R-on-T phenomenon** at the beginning of a paroxysm of repetitive monomorphic ventricular tachycardia in a 56-year-old patient with a previous myocardial infarction. Notice that the first complex of the tachycardia begins after a long coupling interval from the previous sinus beat. This illustration was prepared from a Holter monitor recording. (From Buxton AE. Transient ventricular tachycardia. In Kastor JA (ed). Arrhythmias. Philadelphia: WB Saunders, 1994, pp. 363–375, with permission.)[2]

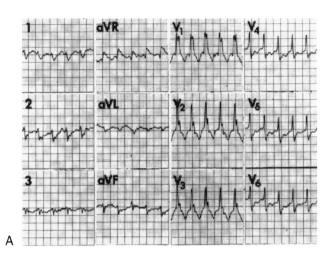

A

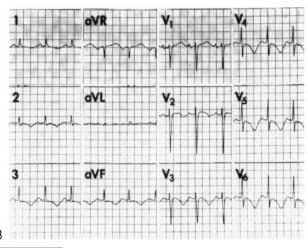

B

FIGURE 12.12 Post-tachycardia repolarization abnormalities. Abnormal ST-segment and T-wave abnormalities persist **(B)** after spontaneous termination of ventricular tachycardia at a rate of 150 beats per minute **(A)** in a patient without structural heart disease. (From Josephson ME, Callans DJ. Sustained ventricular tachycardia. In Kastor JA (ed). Arrhythmias. Philadelphia: WB Saunders, 1994, pp. 336–362, with permission.)[1]

the likelihood of making the wrong diagnosis, according to one group.[377]

Clinical information. Ventricular tachycardia is more likely when the patient has a history of complex ventricular premature beats and ventricular disease,[375] such as myocardial infarction, ventricular aneurysm, or cardiomyopathy, and is the appropriate age for severe heart disease. One is struck by how often physicians ignore these obvious clues.[375] The wrong diagnosis is frequently made, and supraventricular tachycardia with aberrancy is the one usually incorrectly chosen.[375ll] Conversely, physicians may wrongly choose ventricular tachycardia by assuming that only that arrhythmia produces hypotension or shock.[378]

[ll]I am convinced that physicians often favor a diagnosis of supraventricular tachycardia, regardless of the signs pointing to ventricular tachycardia, because of their understandable desire to assign the patient what they consider to be the less dangerous arrhythmia.

General electrocardiographic clues. Ventricular tachycardia is favored when (Table 12.6)

- *Width of the QRS complex exceeds 160 milliseconds.* Almost all tachycardias with this finding, except those in patients with bundle branch block during sinus rhythm, are ventricular. If one uses width greater than 140 milliseconds, according to one report,[376] supraventricular tachycardia will be the diagnosis in one-third of cases.
- *Atrioventricular dissociation is present* (see Fig. 12.7). This finding appears in about 50% of patients with ventricular tachycardia and, when observed, confirms the diagnosis. The relationship between atria and ventricles is usually 1:1 in supraventricular tachycardia with aberrancy.
- *Concordance,* similarity of the form of the QRS complexes in each of the six precordial leads, is an infrequent but diagnostic finding (Fig. 12.13).
- *Fusion beats* are present (Figs. 12.14 and 12.15). This time-honored finding is uncommon.[340mm]

Right bundle branch block form of the QRS complex. Ventricular tachycardia is favored when

- Left axis deviation is present.[nn]
- In lead V_1, the R waves are monophasic or biphasic.
- In lead V_6, the initial septal Q wave is absent.
- In lead V_6, the S wave is larger than the R wave.

Left bundle branch block form of the QRS complex. Observation of the QRS complexes helps in the diag-

---

[mm]Fusion and capture beats were seen in only 5 of 100 patients with electrophysiologically proven ventricular tachycardia.[340]

[nn]Ventricular tachycardia: 59% of 35 patients. Supraventricular tachycardia: 4% of 69 patients with right bundle branch block aberrancy and 13% of 31 patients with left bundle branch block aberrancy.[340]

Table 12.6	**CLUES IN REGULAR TACHYCARDIAS WITH WIDE QRS COMPLEXES THAT FAVOR VENTRICULAR TACHYCARDIA MORE THAN SUPRAVENTRICULAR TACHYCARDIA WITH ABERRANCY**

Presence of	
QRS complexes with duration greater than 160 msec	
Atrioventricular dissociation	
Concordance	
Fusion beats	

Form of QRS Complexes	
Right Bundle Branch Block	*Left Bundle Branch Block*
Left axis deviation	Leads V_1 and V_2: Notching in downstroke of S wave
Lead V_1: Monophasic or biphasic R waves	Leads V_1 and V_2: Greater than 60 msec from onset of QRS complex to nadir of S wave
Lead V_6: Absent septal Q wave	Lead V_6: Q wave of any size
Lead V_6: S wave > R wave	—

(Data from references 340, 375 to 377, 379, and 384.)

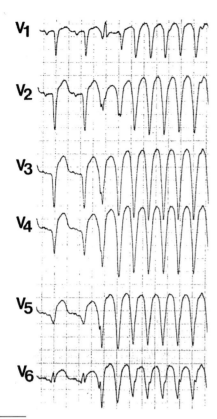

FIGURE 12.13 Concordance. All the beats of ventricular tachycardia in leads V_1 to V_6 have a similar appearance. This finding is known as concordance and appears in some examples of ventricular tachycardia. (From Wellens HJJ, Bar FW, Vanagt EJ, Brugada P, Farre J. The differentiation between ventricular tachycardia and supraventricular tachycardia with aberrant conduction: the value of the 12-lead electrocardiogram. In Wellens HJJ, Kulbertus HE (eds). What's New In Electrocardiography. The Hague: Martinus Nijhoff, 1981, pp. 184–199, with permission.)[340]

nosis,[379] except in patients with no structural heart disease, in whom the criteria have low sensitivity:[380]

- In leads V_1 or V_2, one sees notching on the downstroke of the S wave.
- In leads V_1 or V_2, the time from the onset of the QRS complex to the nadir of the S wave is greater than 60 milliseconds.
- In leads V_1 or V_2, the duration (width) of the R wave is greater than 30 milliseconds (Fig. 12.16); preexisting left bundle branch block diminishes the sensitivity of this finding.[381]
- In lead V_6, there is a Q wave of any size; this is the only one of the four criteria that occurs more frequently in patients who have had myocardial infarction.

Patients with intraventricular conduction defect during sinus rhythm. Most of the clues described earlier favoring ventricular tachycardia are present in many, but not all, patients with an intraventricular conduction defect during sinus rhythm.[382] Furthermore, in patients with preexisting bundle branch block,[383]

- If the QRS complexes are identical during sinus

rhythm and tachycardia, the arrhythmia is supraventricular.
- When the form of the QRS complexes differs during sinus rhythm and tachycardia, the arrhythmia is ventricular.

Unhelpful differences

Rate. Although the average rate of supraventricular tachycardia exceeds that of ventricular tachycardia, the overlap is too great for this finding to help in deciding the nature of the arrhythmia.[340, 384]

QRS complex. Triphasic R waves in lead V_1 are seen in both ventricular and supraventricular tachycardia.[340, 384] However, the triphasic QRS complex with the "classic" form of rsR′, in which the S wave reaches below the baseline, favors supraventricular tachycardia. *Left axis deviation* of greater than −30 degrees during ventricular tachycardia with the form of left bundle branch block does not add to the differential diagnosis.[379]

Alternation of the height and depth of the QRS complex by greater than 0.1 mV, which is best seen in leads V_2 and V_3, occurs in 39% of the electrocardiograms of patients during ventricular tachycardia. This finding, which also occurs during supraventricular tachycardia, does not differentiate between the two arrhythmias.[385]

Onset of Ventricular Tachycardia[oo]

The heart rate increases just before ventricular tachycardia begins.[54, 64, 281, 357, 386, 387pp] The cycle lengths of the first beats of ventricular tachycardia vary.[388] Some of the RR intervals of the rhythm preceding the onset of monomorphic ventricular tachycardia vary in a short-long-short sequence.[389]

The first ventricular beat of a paroxysm of sustained monomorphic ventricular tachycardia usually

- Is single.[390qq]
- Has the same form as the other beats of the paroxysm.[304, 390rr]
- Has a *long*, not a short, coupling interval to the previous supraventricular beat.[390, 391]

However, whether a paroxysm of ventricular tachycardia will begin is *not* dependent on

- The coupling interval between the last sinus beat and the first ventricular beat.[54, 65]
- The number and complexity of ventricular

[oo]Sustained monomorphic ventricular tachycardia has been divided into two forms on the basis of the morphology of the premature beats that initiate the tachycardia.[304] In type I, the episode of spontaneous ventricular tachycardia is preceded by one or more premature beats whose morphology is different from that of the tachycardia. In type II, the premature beat has the same form as the tachycardia.

[pp]Refuting earlier work that found no change in sinus rhythm before ventricular tachycardia.[54, 64]

[qq]Eleven of 16 episodes of ventricular tachycardia in one study began after a single ventricular premature beat, three episodes after 2 premature beats, and two episodes after 5 beats.[390rr]

[rr]In 92% of 1,102 episodes of spontaneous ventricular tachycardia in the Electrophysiologic Study Versus Electrocardiographic Monitoring (ESVEM) Trial.[304]

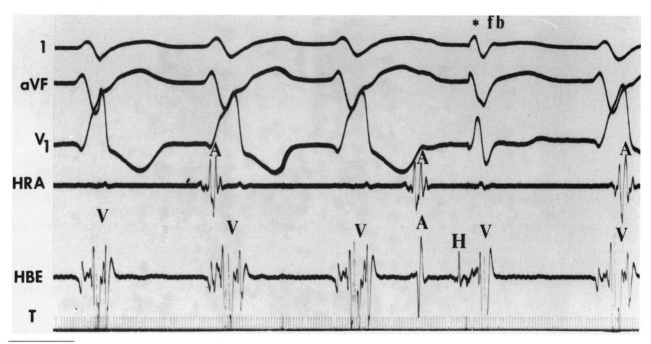

FIGURE 12.14 **Fusion beat during ventricular tachycardia.** The arrhythmia is ventricular tachycardia with the form of right bundle branch and retrograde ventriculoatrial block. The fourth QRS complex (* fb) is a fusion beat merging contours of the QRS complexes from the beats of the tachycardia and sinus rhythm. Notice that the QRS complex of the fusion beat is narrower than those of the tachycardia and is preceded by a sinus P wave with a PR interval similar to that during sinus rhythm (not shown). Intracardiac records are from the high right atrium (HRA) and the bundle of His (HBE); electrograms are from the atrium (A), bundle of His (H), and ventricle (V). T, time lines. (From Josephson ME, Callans DJ. Sustained ventricular tachycardia. In Kastor JA (ed). Arrhythmias. Philadelphia: WB Saunders, 1994, pp. 336–362, with permission.)[1]

premature beats in the hour preceding onset of ventricular tachycardia in patients with coronary heart disease and hypertrophic cardiomyopathy.[334]

During myocardial infarction. The rate of ventricular tachycardia during myocardial infarction is usually 140 to 180 beats per minute, but it tends to be faster during sinus tachycardia.[392] Ventricular premature beats precede some, but not all, episodes of ventricular

tachycardia during myocardial infarction (Table 12.7).[291, 392]

Repetitive idiopathic monomorphic ventricular tachycardia. When this unusual form of ventricular tachycardia begins in patients without structural heart disease, the coupling interval between the last sinus beat and the first ventricular beat is longer when a paroxysm of ventricular tachycardia begins than when an isolated ventricular premature beat appears.[393] Fur-

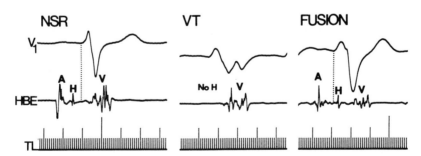

FIGURE 12.15 **Fusion beat during ventricular tachycardia.** The tachyarrhythmia produces the first portion of the QRS complex (V$_1$) of the fusion beat **(right)**, and the sinus beat, produces the latter portion from atrioventricular conduction. The intracardiac electrogram from the bundle of His (HBE) shows that the bundle (H) discharges normally between atrial (A) and ventricular (V) activation during sinus rhythm (NSR, **left**), within the QRS complex and therefore invisibly during ventricular tachycardia (VT, **middle**), and during the early portion of the QRS complex in the fusion beat **(right)**. (From Kastor JA, Horowitz LN, Harken AH, Josephson ME. Clinical electrophysiology of ventricular tachycardia. N Engl J Med 1981; 304:1004–1020, reprinted, by permission, from the New England Journal of Medicine.)[548]

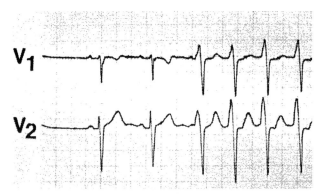

FIGURE 12.16 Width of the R wave in ventricular tachycardia. In patients whose ventricular tachycardia has the form of left bundle branch block, the R wave in lead V_1 during the arrhythmia (beats 3–6) is typically wider and taller than the R wave in sinus rhythm (first two beats). This recording also illustrates how the arrhythmia characteristically begins spontaneously (beat 3) after a relatively long interval from the previous sinus beat. (From Wellens HJJ, Bar FW, Vanagt EJ, Brugada P, Farre J. The differentiation between ventricular tachycardia and supraventricular tachycardia with aberrant conduction: the value of the 12-lead electrocardiogram. In Wellens HJJ, Kulbertus HE (eds). What's New in Electrocardiography. The Hague: Martinus Nijhoff, 1981, pp. 184–199, with permission.)[340]

thermore, when the heart rate is fast, paroxysms of ventricular tachycardia are more likely to appear than are isolated ventricular premature beats[393] and, when ventricular tachycardia does appear, to last longer.[393]

Right ventricular dysplasia. Increasing heart rate characterizes the onset of ventricular tachycardia in patients with right ventricular dysplasia:[387]

- The sinus rate for the 15 beats preceding the arrhythmia is greater than before isolated ventricular premature beats.
- The first cycle of the ventricular tachycardia is shorter than that during runs or couplets.
- The second cycle of the arrhythmia is shorter than during runs.[387]

Termination of Ventricular Tachycardia

Spontaneous termination of ventricular tachycardia is associated with the following:

Table 12.7	**APPEARANCE OF VENTRICULAR PREMATURE BEATS (%) DURING 10 MINUTES AND 1 MINUTE BEFORE THE ONSET OF VENTRICULAR TACHYCARDIA DURING MYOCARDIAL INFARCTION**	
Ventricular Premature Beats	10 min	1 min
None	24	60
Multifocal	30	10
Couplets	24	9
Early	12	3

(From Bluzhas J, Lukshiene D. Ventricular tachycardia in myocardial infarction: relation to heart rate and premature ventricular contractions. Eur Heart J 1985; 6:745–750, with permission.)[392]

- Transient shortening of the duration of the QRS complexes.[394]
- Impingement of the QT_p[ss] on the cycle length[tt] of the arrhythmia.[394]
- Paradoxical prolongation of the QT_p after abrupt shortening of the cycle length of the arrhythmia.[394]

Greater beat-to-beat variation of the cycle lengths, QT intervals, and duration of the QRS complexes accompany the end of ventricular tachycardia in patients not taking drugs or receiving ineffective treatment.[394]

OTHER ELECTROCARDIOGRAPHIC STUDIES
Ambulatory (Holter) Recordings

Extended electrocardiographic recordings have been used to study patients who have ventricular tachycardia and[305, 333, 334, 387, 395–399]

- Are being evaluated for treatment with antiarrhythmic drugs.[400–404]
- Dizziness or syncope.[405, 406]
- Hypertension.[113]
- Idiopathic congestive cardiomyopathy,[118] hypertrophic obstructive cardiomyopathy,[132–134, 136, 138] and arrhythmogenic right ventricular dysplasia.[387, 407]
- Myocardial infarction, both during[54] and afterward.[59, 64–66, 68, 69, 75, 408–413]
- Recent cardiac surgery,[172, 185, 186, 191] including operations for ventricular tachycardia.[414, 415]
- Repetitive monomorphic ventricular tachycardia.[34, 393]
- Ventricular aneurysms.[72, 409]
- Heart rate variability being studied.[357, 416–421]

Heart Rate Variability

The normal variability of the sinus rate in patients with coronary heart disease including previous myocardial infarction and sustained ventricular tachycardia decreases[417, 419, 422–424] during the hour preceding the onset of the arrhythmia.[418] The low to high ratio is often increased,[422] largely from a decreasing high-frequency component, during the 6- to 8-minute period before the onset of paroxysms in repetitive monomorphic ventricular tachycardia.[357, 416, 422uu] Although the variability of the heart rate is abnormal in some patients during ischemia and transient ventricular tachycardia,[420] this finding does not predict which patients will develop stable monomorphic ventricular tachycardia.[421]

The components of heart rate variability controlled by parasympathetic sympathetic stimulation drop and sympathetic influences rise just before ventricular tachycardia originating in the right ventricular outflow

[ss]QT_p is the duration of ventricular repolarization measured from the onset of the QRS complex to the peak of the T wave.[394]

[tt]Cycle length is the duration (usually measured in milliseconds) between QRS complexes.

[uu]Others have found different results in their patients with transient and sustained ventricular tachycardia.[416, 422]

tract begins.[425] The high-frequency component of heart rate variability is significantly decreased, and the relation of QT interval to heart rate variability is significantly altered in patients with idiopathic ventricular tachycardia as compared with healthy persons.[426]

Signal-averaged Electrocardiography

Low-amplitude electrocardiographic signals filtered from extraneous activity by computer processing may be detected just after the QRS complex in many patients with ventricular tachycardia[427–459] (Fig. 12.17).[vv] Regions of ventricular myocardium in which activation is slower than normal produce these signals, often called ventricular late potentials. The more the left ventricle is damaged, the greater is the likelihood that late potentials can be recorded.[460, 461]

After myocardial infarction. About 35% of patients with myocardial infarction develop ventricular late po-

---

[vv]See elsewhere[438, 440–443, 445–459, 1367] for technical aspects of late potentials.

tentials.[412, 413, 462–468ww] Patients with inferior infarctions seem to develop late potentials more often than those with anterior infarctions.[412]

Late potentials develop soon after myocardial infarction begins; they are present within 3 hours of the development of chest pain in some patients without prior infarctions.[466] However, patients who develop ventricular tachycardia within the first 48 hours after onset of the infarction do not usually have late potentials.[413] If late potentials do not develop within 4 weeks, they are unlikely ever to appear from that infarction.[469]

Late potentials disappear in about half those patients who had them soon after infarction and did not develop ventricular tachycardia.[469] Successful thrombolysis of coronary artery occlusions during myocardial infarction reduces the incidence of ventricular late potentials,[470, 471] more likely from patency of the infarct-related coronary artery than from changes in global left ventricular function.[471] Patients with ventricular

---

[ww]From seven series of 889 patients.[412, 413, 463–466] The incidence ranged from 24% to 58%. Different recording techniques account for part of the variation. Alteration of early activation from myocardial infarction can also be detected with signal-averaging techniques.[468] These findings may relate to the subsequent occurrence of ventricular tachycardia.

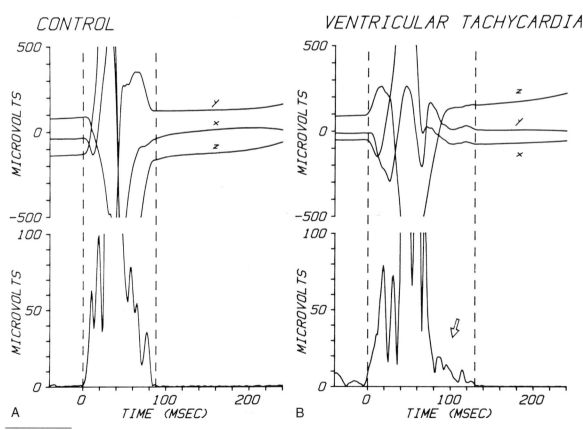

FIGURE 12.17 **Late potentials** *(arrow)* in the signal averaged electrocardiogram recorded during sinus rhythm distinguish patients with **(A)** from patients without **(B)** recurrent sustained ventricular tachycardia. The signals have been greatly amplified and processed by a computer. The amplitude in microvolts is on the vertical axis, and the time in milliseconds is on the horizontal axis. (Adapted from Simson MB. Use of signals in the terminal QRS complex to identify patients with ventricular tachycardia after myocardial infarction. Circulation 1981; 64:235–242, by permission of the American Heart Association, Inc.)[435]

aneurysms produced by myocardial infarction frequently have late potentials.[409, 437, 460]

The risk of developing sustained ventricular arrhythmias or sudden death rises[472] by six times[473] in patients with previous myocardial infarction if they have abnormal signal-averaged electrocardiograms. About 15% of patients with late potentials from myocardial infarction develop documented sustained ventricular tachycardia,[412xx] and most survivors of acute myocardial infarction who develop ventricular tachycardia have late potentials.[463, 469, 474, 475] Late potentials independently predict the development of sustained ventricular tachycardia after myocardial infarction,[409, 411, 476, 477] and they do so with greater power than the peak rate of ventricular premature beats[yy] or the presence of ventricular aneurysm.[409] However, ventricular late potentials that are only temporarily present[466] do not predict the appearance of ventricular tachycardia.[413, 469]

Cardiomyopathy. Patients with dilated cardiomyopathy more often have late potentials than patients without heart disease, and those with cardiomyopathy and sustained ventricular tachycardia are much more likely to have late potentials than those without the arrhythmia.[120, 478, 479zz] Furthermore, more patients with dilated cardiomyopathy have late potentials than patients with chronic myocarditis, hypertrophic cardiomyopathy, or hypertension.[432]

Late potentials are recorded in some, but not all, patients with arrhythmogenic right ventricular dysplasia and recurrent sustained ventricular tachycardia.[407, 480–482] In the absence of bundle branch block, the more abnormal the signal-averaged electrocardiogram, the greater is the enlargement of the right ventricle.[482]

Cardiac surgery. Late potentials increase the risk of having serious ventricular arrhythmias after coronary artery bypass graft surgery.[483] Late potentials predict which patients who have had right ventriculotomy for repair of congenital heart disease (most often tetralogy of Fallot) will have ventricular tachycardia induced at electrophysiological study.[484] However, late potentials cannot distinguish whether the induced ventricular tachycardia will be sustained or transient.[484]

When electrophysiological study demonstrates that endocardial resection and/or encircling ventriculotomy has successfully prevented induction of sustained ventricular tachycardia, late potentials, present before the operation, can usually no longer be recorded.[485–488] Late potentials may persist, however, even when the surgery has successfully suppressed the arrhythmia.[486]

No structural heart disease. No late potentials appear in the signal-averaged electrocardiogram of most patients without clinically apparent structural heart disease who have sustained ventricular tachycardia.[194, 209, 434, 489aaa] However, some of these patients who have ventricular disease established from myocardial biopsy have late potentials.[490]

About 50% of patients with idiopathic ventricular tachycardia and normal left ventricular function in one study had late potentials.[491] Biopsies of the right ventricles of these patients showed fibrous tissue, and clinical evaluation revealed "subclinical right ventricular abnormalities,"[491] providing further evidence that pathological features, yet to be fully understood, may cause what we now call idiopathic ventricular tachycardia.

Syncope. The presence of late potentials in patients with syncope suggests that ventricular tachycardia may have caused the fainting.[492–495] Ventricular tachycardia is unusual in patients with syncope who do not have late potentials.

Effects of antiarrhythmic drugs. Most antiarrhythmic drugs do not affect the presence of late potentials, even when the drugs suppress the clinical appearance or electrophysiological induction of the arrhythmia.[496, 497bbb] Consequently, late potentials, recorded while patients are taking antiarrhythmic drugs, do not predict future ventricular tachycardia with the same accuracy as when the recordings were made while the patients are not taking the drugs.[444]

Ventricular tachycardia versus cardiac arrest. The duration of late potentials is greater and their amplitude is smaller in patients with ventricular tachycardia than in those who have sustained cardiac arrest.[475]

Body Surface Electrocardiographic Mapping

This technique reveals abnormalities in patients with ventricular arrhythmias including ventricular tachycardia,[498] helps to determine efficacy of drugs in patients with ventricular tachycardia,[499] and can distinguish when right ventricular tachycardia is idiopathic or arises from arrhythmogenic right ventricular dysplasia.[155, 500] Principal component analysis of the ST and T waves reveals abnormalities not detected by electrocardiograms in patients with arrhythmogenic right ventricular dysplasia.[501]

Abnormalities of QT Interval and U Waves

QT dispersion. Differences of the QT interval among electrocardiographic leads predict which pa-

---

[xx]The incidence of ventricular tachycardia in patients with myocardial infarction and late potentials, although similar to the 15% figure, varies in different reports.[464, 468] The differences among the studies reporting such data are due, in particular, to different technical criteria for late potentials and the length of time the patients were followed after the infarction producing the late potentials.

[yy]When greater than 100 beats per hour.[409]

[zz]In a study of 41 patients with nonischemic congestive cardiomyopathy, 83% with sustained ventricular tachycardia had late potentials, and 14% without ventricular tachycardia had late potentials.[120]

[aaa]None of 17 young patients with idiopathic ventricular tachycardia confirmed by normal coronary angiography had late potentials.[434] By use of technically sophisticated fast Fourier transform analysis, abnormal high-frequency components of the electrocardiogram can be detected in some patients with idiopathic ventricular tachycardia.[1368]

[bbb]The drug sotalol, however, can shorten or lengthen the duration of the signal-averaged electrocardiogram.[497]

tients with damaged left ventricles from myocardial infarction will develop ventricular tachycardia,[477, 502–505] but the test does not discriminate in this respect among patients with dilated cardiomyopathy.[417, 421, 503, 506–508] Algorithms that combine QT dispersion with the signal-averaged electrocardiogram[509] or the duration of the QRS complexes[510] predict sensitively which patients will develop spontaneous or inducible ventricular tachyarrhythmias. QT interval dispersion is greater when ventricular tachycardia can be induced during electrophysiological study,[511] and it is shorter in patients when antiarrhythmic drugs suppress inducible sustained ventricular tachycardia than in those still inducible.[512]

T-wave alternans. The form of the T waves alternates in some patients with ventricular tachycardia and other serious ventricular arrhythmias.[153, 514] Exercise[515, 516] reveals these electrocardiographic abnormalities at the microvolt level. Ventricular tachycardia can more likely be induced in the electrophysiology laboratory in patients who have T-wave alternans.[515]

Post-extrasystolic T-wave and U-wave abnormalities. Patients without long QT syndrome who develop ventricular tachycardia and ventricular fibrillation may have post-extrasystolic U-wave but not T-wave abnormalities.[517]

ECHOCARDIOGRAPHY

Suprasternal M-mode echocardiography can demonstrate atrioventricular dissociation during ventricular tachycardia.[518] Furthermore, echocardiograms show that

- Higher left ventricular mass characterizes patients with left ventricular hypertrophy from hypertension who will have more transient ventricular tachycardia.[113]
- The occurrence of ventricular tachycardia in patients with hypertrophic obstructive cardiomyopathy is not related to the degree of left ventricular hypertrophy,[519ccc] outflow tract gradient, or dysfunction.[138]
- Patients with idiopathic ventricular tachycardia have several abnormalities of the right ventricle.[227, 520–522]

Transesophageal echocardiography permits continuous monitoring of the position of electrode catheters during radiofrequency current ablation of ventricular tachycardia.[523–526] Transthoracic and transesophageal two-dimensional echocardiography reveals false tendons in the left ventricles of patients with idiopathic left ventricular tachycardia,[527, 528] features that different investigators postulate may,[527, 528] or may not,[529] cause the arrhythmia in these patients.

RADIOLOGY

Computed tomography and magnetic resonance imaging reveal structural abnormalities of the ventri-

cles[530] and of the right ventricular outflow tract, not evident from other imaging techniques, in many patients with idiopathic ventricular tachycardia.[232, 233, 531] The locations of the right ventricular abnormalities do not correlate closely with the specific sites of origin of the arrhythmia.[233]

HEMODYNAMICS

Left ventricular function[ddd] drops, sometimes to low levels, during ventricular tachycardia in patients who have structural heart disease.[409–411, 461, 464, 532–534] The systemic blood pressure falls precipitously when ventricular tachycardia begins, but it usually rises and stabilizes, except in patients with syncope. In a hemodynamic study of 40 patients, the blood pressure of those who fainted fell to 36 ± 8 mm Hg within 5 seconds after onset of ventricular tachycardia, but it decreased to only 50 ± 9 mm Hg in those who did not faint.[534] Neither ventricular function nor the form of the QRS complexes determines whether patients with ventricular tachycardia induced at electrophysiological study will faint.[534, 535eee]

In another study of 20 patients, the left ventricular mean systolic pressure decreased from 123 ± 19 mm Hg in sinus rhythm to 61 ± 24 mm Hg when ventricular tachycardia was induced during electrophysiological study.[536] Left ventricular end-diastolic pressure did not change in the patients evaluated in this study.[536] Hemodynamic values during sinus rhythm in patients who have ventricular tachycardia and no structural heart disease are, as expected, usually normal.[203]

PATHOLOGY

Compared with diseased hearts from patients without ventricular tachycardia, those with ventricular tachycardia demonstrate more old and larger infarcts, more hydropic change in the endocardium, and greater areas where the subendocardium is spared, including regions of uniform contour with thickness of no more than 1 mm.[537]

Healed Myocardial Infarction

Endocardial tissue resected during cardiac surgery in patients with ventricular tachycardia from healed myocardial infarctions and, in some cases, ventricular aneurysms contains viable, although abnormal, tissue that may give rise to the reentrant substrate for ventricular tachycardia.[538, 539] The findings include the following:[538]

[ccc]According to the most recent data. Other studies have found more ventricular tachycardia when hypertrophy is greater.[519]

[ddd]Measured by the ejection fraction, cardiac index, or cineangiography. Some of the patients in studies reporting decreased left ventricular function also had cardiac arrest, but sustained ventricular tachycardia was probably an important feature in each case. Other factors contributing to the symptoms include rapid rate, drop in blood pressure, loss of atrioventricular synchrony, reflux through mitral and tricuspid valves, decreased coronary perfusion, and myocardial ischemia.[532]

[eee]However, pacing different sites in the left and right ventricles suggests that the site of origin of ventricular tachycardia may affect left ventricular performance.[535]

- Bundles of myocardial fibers embedded in dense fibrous tissue that extend to the margins of the surgical resections.
- Purkinje tissues with normal ultrastructure.
- Normal and abnormal muscle cells, the abnormal cells characterized by loss of contractile elements, aggregates of dilated sarcoplasmic reticulum, and osmiophilic dense bodies.
- Intact sarcolemma and evenly dispersed nuclear chromatin, a finding suggesting that the cells are still viable.

Action potentials recorded from excised endocardial tissue of patients with previous myocardial infarction and ventricular tachycardia may be only slightly abnormal or may show reduced amplitude or slow upstrokes.[539]

No Structural Heart Disease

Microscopic abnormalities appear in the myocardial biopsies of many and possibly most patients with ventricular tachycardia and no clinically apparent heart disease.[234, 490, 520, 522] For example, right ventricular endocardial biopsies taken from 12 patients with ventricular tachycardia or fibrillation and no clinically established structural heart disease showed such histological abnormalities in 11 as[226]

- Myocardial cell hypertrophy in seven.
- Interstitial fibrosis in five.
- Endocardial fibrosis in five.
- Myocardial changes in one.
- Increased cellularity in one.
- Acute lymphocytic myocarditis in one.

Another study reported that endomyocardial biopsies of the right ventricular septum are usually normal in patients with idiopathic ventricular tachycardia from the right ventricular outflow tract, whereas the biopsies show abnormal tissue in most patients with arrhythmogenic right ventricular dysplasia.[540]

ELECTROPHYSIOLOGY

Recognition

The His bundle electrogram from a patient during ventricular tachycardia is dominated by large V waves, one for each QRS complex and not preceded by H waves from the bundle of His as in supraventricular tachycardia and other supraventricular arrhythmias (Fig. 12.18).[368, 384, 541–558] The bundle is activated in retrograde fashion, and the H deflection usually hidden within the V wave. When ventricular tachycardia originates in the fascicles of the bundle branch system,[342] an arrhythmia called fascicular tachycardia, the H wave may precede the QRS complex,[343, 559] but the HV interval is usually shorter than normal.

The relation between the A waves and the HV complexes depends on the extent that atrioventricular dissociation is present (see Fig. 12.7):

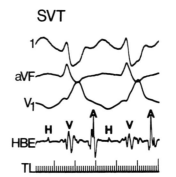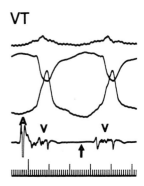

FIGURE 12.18   Ventricular tachycardia (VT) versus supraventricular tachycardia (SVT).   The His bundle electrogram (HBE) reveals the mechanism of the two arrhythmias. Notice that in supraventricular tachycardia, an H deflection precedes each QRS complex, whereas in ventricular tachycardia, the H deflection is absent, buried within the V wave of ventricular activation. The QRS complexes in ventricular tachycardia (**right**) are characteristic with left axis deviation and one broad positive deflection in lead V₁. (From Kastor JA, Horowitz LN, Harken AH, Josephson ME. Clinical electrophysiology of ventricular tachycardia. N Engl J Med 1981; 304:1004–1020, reprinted, by permission, from the New England Journal of Medicine.)[548]

- If the atrial and ventricular rhythms beat independently of each other, the A wave and HV complex will not relate to each other.
- If 1:1 ventriculoatrial conduction occurs, then each V wave will be followed at an unchanging interval by an A wave, often better seen under these circumstances in the record taken from the intra-atrial electrode. Because the bundle of His is activated in retrograde fashion by the ventricles, the H wave follows the beginning of ventricular activation and is usually obscured by the large V wave.
- Mixtures of these two patterns appear when the atria are intermittently activated from the ventricles.

By atrial pacing, one may produce a supraventricular rhythm with different QRS complexes than the intrinsic tachycardia and thereby establish the arrhythmia as ventricular.[560]

Electrophysiological Basis of Ventricular Tachycardia

Ventricular tachycardia in adults is usually sustained by localized[561] *reentry* within damaged endocardial tissue with abnormal conduction and refractoriness.[562, 563*fff*] These are the patients with previous myocardial infarctions and cardiomyopathy with whom physicians are most familiar. Reentry can also cause ventricular tachycardia in infants[564] and children.[243]

Triggered activity[565] is probably the mechanism in most patients with no obvious structural heart disease who have repetitive monomorphic ventricular tachycardia and paroxysmal, exercise-induced ventricular tachycardia.[41, 42, 224] Triggered activity may also account

---

*fff*Subepicardial microreentry may account for some ventricular tachycardias.[563]

for some cases of ventricular tachycardia due to digitalis toxicity.[566]

Induction

Ventricular tachycardia, like other reentrant arrhythmias, can be started by programmed stimulation in the electrophysiology laboratory (Fig. 12.19). The rate of the induced tachycardia is faster in survivors of cardiac arrest than in patients who present with syncope or palpitations.[567]

Electrophysiological techniques.[ggg] To induce ventricular tachycardia, the clinical electrophysiologist places electrode catheters in the ventricles and then introduces electrical stimuli from a computer-controlled stimulator.[568] The induction of ventricular tachycardia can be facilitated by the use of

- *Different ventricular pacing rates* (basic cycle lengths):[hhh] A faster[210, 569–573] and, occasionally, a slower[574] pacing rate will increase the likelihood of inducing the arrhythmia. However, introducing premature stimuli when the basic cycle length is 300 milliseconds is not superior to 400 milliseconds.[575] Most recurrent sustained ventricular tachycardias can be started, without using premature beats, if the pacing rate is sufficiently rapid ("burst pacing").[209, 214, 576, 577]
- *"Short-to-long" ventricular pacing* in which the last interval before the premature beat is longer than the basic cycle length.[578–580]
- *More premature stimuli:*[576, 577, 579, 581–586] One or two premature beats will induce ventricular tachycardia in most susceptible patients (88% in one series).[587] One premature beat usually suffices when the rate of the ventricular tachycardia does not exceed about 175 beats per minute[576, 588] or the origin of the tachycardia is nearby, usually in the same ventricle where the pacing is being conducted.[588] Extra premature beats more successfully induce ventricular tachycardia than faster pacing rates.[570, 573]
- *Different pacing locations:* Pacing the ventricles at locations other than the right ventricular apex, the usual location, such as the left ventricle and elsewhere in the right ventricle,[589] can increase the likelihood of inducing sustained ventricular tachycardia.[574, 577, 580, 588, 590–592] Using more than two ventricular premature beats at the apex, however, is

more effective.[593, 594] Extra beats plus increasing pacing strength will often eliminate the necessity of pacing at a different location.[595] Ventricular tachycardia can also be induced by stimulating through epicardial electrodes inserted during cardiac surgery.[596]
- *Greater current strength* of the pacing stimuli can slightly increase the likelihood of inducing ventricular tachycardia, but not as effectively as the use of additional premature beats.[593, 597–599iii]
- *Isoproterenol* by itself or in association with pacing can increase the likelihood of inducing sustained ventricular tachycardia, particularly in patients with structurally normal hearts.[210, 214, 216, 323, 593, 600–603]
- *Antiarrhythmic drugs* may facilitate the induction of ventricular tachycardia[604, 605] and occasionally may convert transient ventricular tachycardia to sustained ventricular tachycardia.[604, 606, 607]

Sustained ventricular tachycardia. A period of ventricular pacing followed by one or more premature extrastimuli induces sustained monomorphic ventricular tachycardia with similar electrocardiographic form, axis, and rate[390, 608] as the spontaneous arrhythmia[304, 609] in most patients with coronary disease who have had sustained ventricular tachycardia and in a few with transient ventricular tachycardia (see Fig. 12.19).[14, 15, 583, 587, 609–615] Atrial premature beats,[616] atrial tachycardia,[617] atrial pacing,[207, 209, 323, 618, 619] and single ventricular premature beats[616, 619] also occasionally induce sustained ventricular tachycardia. The arrhythmia, however, can seldom be started while the patient is in sinus rhythm.[15]

The RR intervals vary immediately after the tachycardia is induced.[620]

Transient ventricular tachycardia. This arrhythmia can be induced in about half the patients who have spontaneous episodes of this arrhythmia,[621iii] and this includes some patients without structural heart disease.[622–624kkk] However, transient ventricular tachycardia is less likely to be induced than is sustained ventricular tachycardia in patients who have been resuscitated from ventricular fibrillation and who have had clinical episodes of sustained ventricular tachycardia or fibrillation.[625lll] Among those with asymptomatic transient ventricular tachycardia, inducibility rises if the patient has both an ejection fraction of less than 40% and coronary heart disease.[626]

Sustained ventricular tachycardia can occasionally be induced in patients who have spontaneous transient

---

[ggg]The failure of some investigators to induce ventricular tachycardia early in the electrophysiological study of the arrhythmia was probably due to undeveloped understanding of these technical considerations.[568]

[hhh]Clinical electrophysiologists refer to the ventricular pacing interval as the "basic cycle length" and the paced beats with the code "V1"; hence, the ventricular beats of the basic cycle length are "V1-V1." The electrocardiographic artifacts produced by the pacing stimuli are labeled "S," and the pacing signals producing the basic cycle length are "S1-S1." The induced premature beats are called "V2, V3," etc., and the stimuli that drive them "S2, S3," etc. Thus, the coupling interval of a single stimulated premature ventricular beat is "V1-V2" and the interval programmed into the pacing computer is "S1-S2." "S1-S2-S3-S4" and "V1-V2-V3-V4" indicate a more complex stimulation sequence with three premature beats.

[iii]Pacing with increased current at the site of origin of the ventricular tachycardia can *reduce* the ability of premature beats at the right ventricular apex to start the arrhythmia.[598]

[jjj]Fifty-two (63%) of 83 patients in one series[622] and 22 (55%) of 40 in another.[1369]

[kkk]Transient ventricular tachycardia can be started even with simple induction techniques in about 10% of patients with Wolff-Parkinson-White syndrome and no clinical evidence of ventricular tachycardia.[623]

[lll]Sixty-one percent (41 of 66 patients) with transient ventricular tachycardia, 89% (81 of 91 patients) with sustained ventricular tachycardia, and 66% (69 of 104 patients) with ventricular fibrillation.[625]

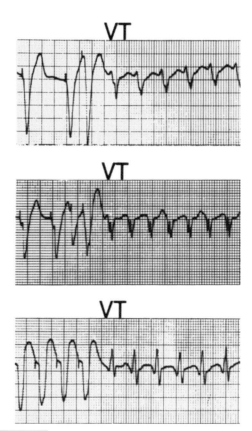

FIGURE 12.19 Starting ventricular tachycardia (VT) by programmed stimulation and continuous pacing. One **(top)** or two **(middle)** ventricular premature stimuli introduced at the appropriate time institute paroxysms of ventricular tachycardia. In some cases, rapid ventricular pacing, in this case at 170 beats per minute, is required to start the arrhythmia. (From Kastor JA, Horowitz LN, Harken AH, Josephson ME. Clinical electrophysiology of ventricular tachycardia. N Engl J Med 1981; 304:1004–1020, reprinted, by permission, from the New England Journal of Medicine.)[548]

ventricular tachycardia.[621, 622, 627, 628mmm] Such patients almost always have structural heart disease,[621, 624, 628–631] such as coronary disease with ventricular aneurysms[622] or dilated cardiomyopathy.[479] Their heart rates during spontaneous transient ventricular tachycardia are almost always slower than during induced sustained ventricular tachycardia.[399] No electrocardiographic characteristics of transient ventricular tachycardia predict whether patients with this arrhythmia can be induced into sustained ventricular tachycardia.[632]

Ventricular tachycardia can seldom be induced in patients with spontaneous episodes of transient ventricular tachycardia, no late potentials, and ejection fractions of 40% or more.[633] Such patients do not need electrophysiologic study for risk stratification.[633]

The administration of antiarrhythmic drugs can facilitate the induction of sustained ventricular tachycardia in some patients in whom only transient ventricular tachycardia could be induced when no drug was taken.[606] Inducibility varies as time passes.[634] When the ability to induce ventricular tachycardia decreases, the

likelihood that the patient will suffer a clinical episode of the arrhythmia also decreases and vice versa.[634]

Patients with coronary heart disease. Sustained ventricular tachycardia can almost always be induced in patients with previous myocardial infarction and a history of the arrhythmia, except during the first 24 hours of the acute infarction.[610] Programmed stimulation induces sustained ventricular tachycardia in 22% of survivors of myocardial infarction complicated by angina, heart failure, or transient ventricular tachycardia.[635] Left ventricular aneurysm and Lown grade 4B ventricular beating select those patients most likely to be inducible into sustained monomorphic ventricular tachycardia after myocardial infarction.[636]

Certain clinical characteristics,[637] particularly the combined presence of established coronary disease, especially myocardial infarction,[584] a history of sustained ventricular tachycardia,[584] and a left ventricular ejection fraction of less than 30%, predict that ventricular tachycardia can be induced better than data derived from ambulatory electrocardiography.[638]

Survivors of myocardial infarction most likely to benefit from electrophysiological study and therapy based on its results have[639]

- Ejection fraction less than 40%.
- Prolonged filtered duration of QRS complexes in signal-averaged electrocardiograms.
- Two or more runs of transient ventricular tachycardia per period of ambulatory monitoring.
- Reduced heart rate variability.

Administering streptokinase reduces the likelihood that ventricular tachycardia can be induced after the infarction.[640]

Patients with cardiomyopathy.[114] Sustained ventricular tachycardia can often be induced in patients with idiopathic cardiomyopathy who have, but not in those without,[641] the clinical arrhythmia.[642, 643] Sustained ventricular tachycardia can be induced in only a few patients with transient ventricular tachycardia.[479, 644nnn] The value of such studies in these patients is limited.[641, 645–647] The arrhythmia can also be induced in most patients with spontaneous sustained ventricular tachycardia who have arrhythmogenic right ventricular dysplasia[146, 407] and sarcoid cardiomyopathy.[157]

Patients who have had cardiac surgery. Sustained ventricular tachycardia can be induced in some patients with the arrhythmia when it develops after coronary artery bypass grafting.[179, 182] The arrhythmia may appear after correction of tetralogy of Fallot.[187] Induction of ventricular tachycardia correlates in these patients with the presence of ventricular premature beats and ventricular tachycardia on ambulatory monitoring[189] and with abnormally long duration of the QRS complex.[648] Induced sustained ventricular tachycardia relates to all forms of spontaneous ventricular prema-

---

[mmm]Fifteen (18%) of 83 patients.[622]

[nnn]Thirteen percent in one series of 80 patients with idiopathic cardiomyopathy and transient ventricular tachycardia.[479]

ture beats, and induced transient polymorphic ventricular tachycardia relates to complex ventricular premature beats.[189] Ventricular tachycardia cannot be induced in asymptomatic patients with normal 24-hour ambulatory electrocardiographic records and normal right ventricular pressures.[189]

Patients with trauma. Ventricular tachycardia can occasionally be induced in patients with right ventricular trauma.[275]

Patients with exercise-induced ventricular tachycardia. Electrophysiological induction of sustained ventricular tachycardia in patients whose arrhythmia appears during exercise can be facilitated by infusing isoproterenol.[205, 218, 323, 649–651]

Patients with syncope of uncertain cause. Sustained ventricular tachycardia can be induced in 11% and transient ventricular tachycardia in 15% of patients with syncope of uncertain cause[652–657ooo] and in a somewhat larger proportion of patients if they have bundle branch block[658ppp] or bifascicular block.[659qqq] Sustained ventricular tachycardia cannot be induced, however, in patients who faint and have no structural heart disease or history of tachyarrhythmias.[660]

One can predict whether an electrophysiological study will reveal an abnormality such as ventricular tachycardia in patients with syncope by the presence of (in descending order of predicting power) the following:[657rrr]

- Bundle branch block.
- Coronary heart disease.
- Injury related to loss of consciousness.
- Left ventricular ejection fraction equal to or less than 40%.
- Male gender.
- Remote myocardial infarction.
- Use of type I antiarrhythmic drugs.

Transient and sustained ventricular tachycardia can be induced in patients with syncope who have had surgery to correct tetralogy of Fallot even in the absence of any other clinical evidence for the arrhythmias.[308]

Patients with mitral valve prolapse. No relation exists between inducibility and prognosis in patients with mitral value prolapse even though ventricular arrhythmias can be induced more often in them than in persons without structural heart disease.[473]

Patients with left ventricular hypertrophy from hypertension. More transient ventricular tachycardia can be induced in these patients than in those without hypertrophy.[661]

Patients without structural heart disease.[194, 196, 199] The ventricular tachycardia that occurs in patients without structural heart disease is usually not due to reentry, but rather, it is presumed, to triggered activity that is mediated by cyclic adenosine monophosphate.[662sss] Exercise often promotes and isoproterenol facilitates the induction of *sustained* monomorphic ventricular tachycardia in these patients.[149, 205, 207, 209, 212, 214, 218, 220, 313, 322, 352, 651] However, exercise can sometimes suppress repetitive monomorphic ventricular tachycardia, another electrocardiographic form of the arrhythmia in patients with structurally normal hearts, that develops at rest and can usually be induced by one or more of the standard techniques.[210, 219, 224]

Even though they lack other features of reentry, these ventricular tachycardias can be induced in many cases by ventricular burst pacing, sometimes with premature extrastimuli,[149, 209, 210, 216, 221, 228, 229, 322, 647, 649, 660] and even by atrial pacing, a rarely effective method of induction in the common form of ventricular tachycardia due to reentry.[ttt]

Most of the ventricular tachycardias ascribed to triggered activity originate in the right ventricular outflow tract,[41, 42, 425, 663, 664] and they have the electrocardiographic appearance of left bundle branch block and right axis deviation. A few start elsewhere in the right or left ventricle.[40, 128, 220]

The relatively few ventricular tachycardias in patients without structural heart disease that reentry causes originate in the fascicles of the left bundle branch[665] or in the Purkinje network.[666] The electrocardiograms of those that arise in the posterior fascicle[559]—by far the more frequent location—have the appearance of right bundle branch block and left axis deviation. The axis is rightward (inferior) in the few starting in the anterior fascicle.[667] Most of the ventricular tachycardias in these patients respond to adenosine, verapamil, and beta-adrenergic–blocking drugs.

Subjects without documented or suspected ventricular arrhythmias. Programmed ventricular stimulation with one or two premature beats seldom induces sustained ventricular tachycardia in patients without a history of the arrhythmia.[584, 609, 612] Those in whom ventricular tachycardia can be induced with one or two premature beats presumably have the electrophysiological substrate for the arrhythmia, and some will have spontaneous episodes in the future.[609, 668] Accordingly, one is not surprised that, in some patients with ventricular aneurysms and no history of the spontaneous arrhythmia, ventricular tachycardia can be induced at electrophysiological study.[669]

Some patients with no history of ventricular arrhythmias may develop them when stimulated with three or four premature beats[583, 587, 658, 670, 671] at the right and left ventricular apices. This testing produces in subjects

---

ooo Among 429 patients from six series:[652, 654–657, 1370] sustained ventricular tachycardia in 49 patients and transient ventricular tachycardia in 64 patients.

ppp Eight (25%) of 32 patients.[1371]

qqq Three (23%) of 13 patients.[659]

rrr This study did not evaluate the importance of signal-averaged electrocardiograms or T-wave alternans.[657]

sss Patients without structural heart disease constitute about 10% of those studied in, at least, one busy electrophysiology laboratory.[662]

ttt Atrial pacing induces the arrhythmia in about 15% of patients with ventricular tachycardia due to triggered activity, but only 1% to 2% of patients with reentrant ventricular tachycardia.[662]

both with and without heart disease ventricular arrhythmias such as[587, 658, 670]

- One to five intraventricular reentry beats.
- Transient monomorphic and polymorphic ventricular tachycardia, usually in patients with structural heart disease.
- Rarely, sustained ventricular tachycardia and ventricular fibrillation.[670*uuu*]

These results, which do not predict that the patients will develop such arrhythmias, are considered "nonspecific responses" to aggressive ventricular stimulation.[583, 587]

Induced versus spontaneous onset. Ventricular tachycardia begins differently when spontaneous or induced in the electrophysiological laboratory.[390]

- Single ventricular premature beats more often start spontaneous ventricular tachycardia than can single paced beats induce ventricular tachycardia.
- The form of the first ventricular premature beat of a spontaneous episode is similar to that of the tachycardia, whereas the stimulated ventricular premature beat usually has a different form than has the arrhythmia that it induces.
- The coupling interval of the ventricular premature beat to the previous sinus beat in spontaneous episodes is long, whereas the interval between the last of a train of paced ventricular beats and the ventricular premature beat needed to induce in the electrophysiological laboratory is short.

Signal-averaged electrocardiography. The presence of late potentials predicts, more effectively than 24-hour ambulatory electrocardiography,[494] that sustained ventricular tachycardia can be induced in patients with the following:

- Coronary heart disease,[672, 673] and, in such patients, more effectively than left ventricular ejection fraction, ventricular aneurysm, or a history of myocardial infarction.[672]
- Idiopathic dilated cardiomyopathy.[121, 479]
- Unexplained syncope.[492, 494, 495]
- Transient ventricular tachycardia,[674] regardless of the length of the episodes[675] or the cause of the heart disease. However, whereas late potentials predict inducibility in patients with transient ventricular tachycardia and *inferior* myocardial infarction, they do not so predict in patients with this arrhythmia and *anterior* myocardial infarction. Probably, the signal-averaged electrocardiogram does not clearly display delayed activation of the anterior wall, which occurs relatively early in the QRS complex.[630, 676]
- High-grade ventricular arrhythmias such as 10 or more ventricular premature beats per hour or ventricular couplets.[677]

Inducibility is unlikely in a patient who has a normal signal-averaged electrocardiogram despite the presence of transient ventricular tachycardia or high-grade ventricular arrhythmias.[677] Late potentials usually disappear when surgical endocardial resection and aneurysmectomy prevent induction of sustained ventricular tachycardia,[436, 485, 486, 488] but they persist when antiarrhythmic drugs[436, 444, 496] or electrical ablation[678] prevent its induction. The coupling intervals required to induce sustained ventricular tachycardia are longer in patients with, than in patients without, late potentials.[679]

Selection of drugs. During the 1970s and 1980s, clinical electrophysiologists developed methods for selecting, in the laboratory, which drugs would best suppress sustained ventricular tachycardia.[547, 680–695] Implantable cardioverter-defibrillators have, to a great extent, superseded this process because large studies have shown that the devices treat the arrhythmia and prolong life more successfully than do drugs, even drugs chosen by electrophysiology testing. Consequently, this review has more historical interest than practical application for the primary treatment of ventricular tachycardia.

A drug or combination of drugs will usually suppress spontaneous sustained and transient ventricular tachycardia if it prevents induction of the arrhythmia by programmed stimulation in the electrophysiology laboratory (Fig. 12.20).[397, 398, 607, 621, 627, 631, 692, 694, 696–732*vvv*] The levels of the drug in the blood must be similar in the laboratory and the clinic for the method to predict reliably whether the drug will be effective. Conversely, if the drug does not suppress the ventricular tachycardia in the laboratory, the arrhythmia will probably recur after discharge.

The technique identifies drugs that best suppress the arrhythmia in patients with

- Coronary heart disease when the ejection fraction is equal to or more than 30%.[733]
- Dilated cardiomyopathy.[734]
- No structural heart disease.[149, 209]
- Repair of tetralogy of Fallot.[715]
- Short corrected QT interval.[723, 735*www*]

A series[117, 606, 698, 699, 701, 725] or combinations[736–739] of drugs can also be tested in this manner.[740*xxx*]

---

*uuu*None of the patients with ventricular fibrillation, in one group, had spontaneous arrhythmias, and all were well at an average of 14 months after they were studied.[670]

*vvv*The Electrophysiologic Study Versus Electrocardiographic Monitoring (ESVEM) investigation found that ambulatory monitoring predicts antiarrhythmic drug efficacy more often than electrophysiological study,[726] an issue that investigators have long debated.[397, 398, 694, 712, 1372] However, according to ESVEM, there is no significant difference in the success of drug treatment when selected by ambulatory monitoring or electrophysiological study.[727, 730] Electrophysiological study, as expected, is the more expensive technique.[729] The growing use of implantable cardioverter-defibrillators has reduced the amount of electrophysiological drug testing for patients with ventricular tachycardia.

*www*When measured during ventricular pacing at a cycle length of 400 milliseconds. Other technical features may, or may not, help to identify which subjects are likely to respond favorably.[723, 735]

*xxx*Sequential testing is usually carried out in the electrophysiological laboratory by inserting electrode catheters each day the test is performed. Such studies can be conducted, however, with a multiprogrammable permanently implanted pacemaker.[740]

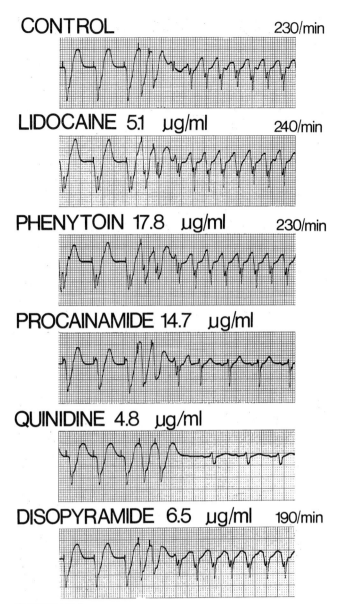

CONTROL   230/min

LIDOCAINE 5.1 μg/ml   240/min

PHENYTOIN 17.8 μg/ml   230/min

PROCAINAMIDE 14.7 μg/ml

QUINIDINE 4.8 μg/ml

DISOPYRAMIDE 6.5 μg/ml   190/min

FIGURE 12.20 Electrophysiological drug testing. In each of the panels, programmed stimulation tries to induce ventricular tachycardia. In the presence of no drug **(top)** and after administration of lidocaine, phenytoin, and disopyramide, the arrhythmia can still be induced. Procainamide and quinidine prevent induction and would probably suppress spontaneous development of the arrhythmia in this patient. (From Kastor JA, Horowitz LN, Harken AH, Josephson ME. Clinical electrophysiology of ventricular tachycardia. N Engl J Med 1981; 304:1004–1020, reprinted, by permission, from the New England Journal of Medicine.)[548]

Despite pharmacological similarities among drugs of a particular electrophysiologic type, the response to one drug to programmed stimulation does not necessarily predict the response to other drugs of the same type.[741–744] Adding a seond type Ia drug, such as procainamide or quinidine,[737] to a patient already receiving a type Ia drug or amiodarone[738] does not significantly decrease the inducibility of ventricular tachycardia. Congestive heart failure reduces the likelihood that a class Ia drug such as procainamide and a class Ib drug such as mexiletine given together will

successfully suppress inducible sustained ventricular tachycardia.[745] These patients respond better to a class III drug such as sotalol.[745]

Greater ventricular refractoriness improves, and slower intraventricular conduction worsens, the ability of a drug to suppress the inducibility of ventricular tachycardia or ventricular fibrillation.[746] This relationship can be expressed in the ratio of the effective refractory period to the duration of the QRS complex determined during ventricular pacing; the greater the ratio, the greater is the likelihood of suppression.[746]

Serial drug testing is not reliable in guiding antiarrhythmic drug treatmnt in patients with valvular heart disease and ventricular tachyarrhythmias.[747] Women, rather than men, are more likely to respond to drugs given for ventricular tachycardia at electrophysiological evaluation, as are patients with fewer obstructed coronary arteries and fewer arrhythmic episodes.[708] QT interval dispersion is likely to be shorter and infarct-related arteries open in patients whose sustained ventricular tachycardia can be suppressed by antiarrhythmic drugs compared with those still inducible.[512]

Reproducibility. The electrophysiological techniques required to induce sustained monomorphic ventricular tachycardia change little when studies are conducted within minutes of each other[748] and even, in many cases, after months have elapsed.[614, 749–752] However, the rate and the electrocardiographic form of the ventricular tachycardia induced by programmed stimulation, which are similar when the studies are conducted soon after each other,[748] may change when longer periods of time elapse between studies.[748, 751, 753–755] Furthermore, different techinques may be needed to induce the same ventricular tachycardia in the same patient at different times. This is most likely when

- More than one premature beat is required to induce the arrhythmia.[582, 753, 756]
- The rate of the ventricular tachycardia is 250 beats per minute or more.[756]
- The ventricular tachycardia induced is transient or polymorphic rather than sustained.[756]

Termination

Most episodes of sustained ventricular tachycardia can be terminated with single[14, 574, 588] or double ventricular extrastimuli (Fig. 12.21)[588] or by ventricular pacing.[588, 757–761] A single stimulus is usually effective when the tachycardia is relatively slow (≤175 beats/min) or when the stimulus is applied in the ventricle where the tachycardia originates.[588, 762–764yyy] Programmed extrastimuli, regardless of the number, are usually ineffective when the rate of the tachycardia exceeds 200 beats per minute.[765] In such cases, rapid pacing or

---

yyy Double stimuli also terminate more effectively when the rate of the ventricular tachycardia is slow.[762] More sophisticated criteria have been developed to explain and predict when termination by pacing will occur.[763, 764]

SINGLE VPD

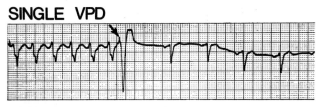

UNDERDRIVE PACING

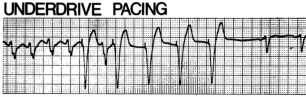

FIGURE 12.21 Stopping ventricular tachycardia with pacing. A single paced premature beat (VPD, ventricular premature depolarization) stops a burst of sustained ventricular tachycardia **(top)**. Underdrive pacing the ventricles at the relatively slow rate of 88 per minute also stops the arrhythmia **(bottom)**. These techniques tend to be effective when the rate of the tachycardia is relatively slow, 145 per minute in this case. (From Kastor JA, Horowitz LN, Harken AH, Josephson ME. Clinical electrophysiology of ventricular tachycardia. N Engl J Med 1981; 304:1004–1020, reprinted, by permission, from the New England Journal of Medicine.)[548]

cardioversion is needed.[765] Atrial pacing is rarely effective.[588, 616]

The likelihood of successful termination can be increased by raising the amount of current above the conventional level, which equals twice that required to capture the ventricles during diastole ("twice diastolic threshold").[766] Ventricular tachycardia can also be stopped in some cases by stimulating the ventricles with single impulses[767] or groups of rapid stimuli[768] delivered with power so low that no propagated signal producing a QRS complex appears ("subthreshold pacing").

Antiarrhythmic drugs that slow the rate of ventricular tachycardia can facilitate,[757, 762] or interfere with,[765] the efficacy of termination by pacing. Ventricular tachycardia not due to reentry, which includes most patients with exercise induced ventricular tachycardia, cannot be suppressed even by rapid pacing.[313, 650]

Acceleration. Introduction of extrastimuli and, particularly, rapid pacing can accelerate the tachycardia so that cardioversion must be used.[769, 770] Subthreshold pacing, when effective, converts without accelerating the arrhythmia.[768]

Changes at termination. The cycle length (the interval between the QRS complexes) may vary just before the arrhythmia terminates.[771] Antiarrhythmic drugs can increase this pre-termination variability.[771] The form of the QRS complexes does not usually change at the time of conversion.[771]

Mapping

One can locate the origin and study the sequence of depolarization of ventricular tachycardia in humans by several techniques:[561, 589, 772–782zzz]

---

zzzIncluding such devices as a transatrial balloon,[779] specially constructed mesh-covered balloons with silver bead electrodes,[777] or orthogonal electrode array.[781]

- Recording from intracardiac electrode catheters (Fig. 12.22).
- Recording from the surface or through the myocardium during cardiac surgery.[778–780, 782–790]
- Pace mapping, in which correlation is sought between the electrocardiogram produced by spontaneous ventricular tachycardia and pacing at the presumed origin of the arrhythmia and elsewhere.[213, 791–797]
- Epicardial mapping in the electrophysiology laboratory with a steerable catheter introduced into the pericardial space.[798, 799]
- Magnetocardiography.[800]
- The CARTO electroanatomical mapping system.[801]

Origin. Ventricular tachycardia originates in the left ventricle when the QRS complexes have the appearance of right bundle branch block.[359] Beats with the form of left bundle branch block start in the right ventricle,[359] except in patients with coronary disease, in whom they start in the left ventricle or the adjacent interventricular septum.[359] The origin of the arrhythmia is usually at the periphery of a resting thallium defect and at the border of ventricular aneurysms in patients with this pathological process.[783, 791–794, 802–804]

Most electrophysiologists estimate where ventricular tachycardia originates in patients with coronary heart disease by inspecting lead V_1 for the general morphology of the QRS complexes and the inferior and lateral leads for further localization. Accordingly, in many patients with coronary heart disease, ventricular tachycardia with right bundle branch block morphology starts in the left ventricular free wall, and that with the form of left bundle branch block starts in the interventricular septum. When the QRS complexes are

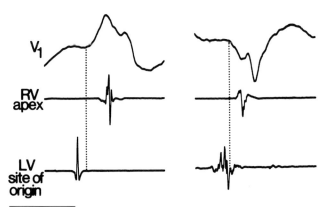

FIGURE 12.22 Endocardial mapping of ventricular tachycardia. Two tachycardias, one with QRS complexes resembling right bundle branch block **(left)** and the other resembling left bundle branch block **(right)** both originate in the left ventricle (LV) in this patient with coronary heart disease. The intracardiac electrogram from the site of origin precedes, and the electrogram from the right ventricular (RV) apex follows, the onset of the beat in both cases. The endocardial signal from the site of origin **(right)** is characteristically broad and fragmented. (TL, time lines of 10 milliseconds.) (From Kastor JA, Horowitz LN, Harken AH, Josephson ME. Clinical electrophysiology of ventricular tachycardia. N Engl J Med 1981; 304:1004–1020, reprinted, by permission, from the New England Journal of Medicine.)[548]

predominantly negative in leads II, III, and aVF, the tachycardia starts in the inferior portion of the ventricle, and when the complexes are positive, it starts in the anterior part of the ventricle. Leads V_5 and V_6 can indicate whether the origin is apical (negative QRS complexes) or basal (positive QRS complexes). The site can be localized further to the anterior or posterior portions of the left ventricle and to the inferior or superior aspects of the interventricular septum (Table 12.8).[359, 805, 806] Radionuclide gated studies can approximate the origin of ventricular tachycardia, determined more precisely with electrophysiological techniques.[741]

Idiopathic ventricular tachycardia. This arrhythmia[663] originates in the *right* ventricle,[149, 151, 209, 221] specifically in the right ventricular outflow tract,[151, 209, 213, 221, 797, 807] in 50%[149] to 75%[662] of patients with ventricular tachycardia and no structural heart disease. This form of ventricular tachycardia, which is often due to triggered automaticity, responds to adenosine.[808–810] Repetitive monomorphic ventricular tachycardia also originates in the right ventricular outflow tract, as does exercise-induced ventricular tachycardia in patients without structural heart disease.[205]

Other causes of ventricular tachycardia in the right ventricle include

- Arrhythmogenic right ventricular dysplasia, as one would expect.[146]
- Surgical correction of tetralogy of Fallot (outflow tract and occasionally inflow-septal area).[151, 187, 525]
- Cardiac trauma.[275]

Idiopathic sustained ventricular tachycardia, including an occasional case of repetitive monomorphic ventricular tachycardia,[353] sometimes originates in the *left* ventricle.[214, 220, 225, 354, 811, 812] Exercise and catecholamines often precipitate these tachycardias, which are most often due to reentry; they usually respond to verapamil but not to adenosine.[528, 666, 808, 809, 813, 814] The electrocardiograms show right bundle branch block and left axis deviation.

One authority suggests that left ventricular tachycardia should be considered in three types:[812]

- Intrafascicular tachycardia, which originates near the apex of the left ventricle in the region of the left posterior fascicle, is due to reentry,[559] and responds to verapamil.[811]
- Adenosine-sensitive tachycardia originating from deep within the intraventricular septum and probably due to triggered activity. This form also responds to verapamil.
- Propranolol-sensitive tachycardia, which responds electrophysiologically like an automatic arrhythmia.

Pleomorphism. Pleomorphism of the QRS complexes[345, 347, 348] can occur in the absence of changes in the origin as determined from endocardial recordings.[345] As the morphology and axis of the QRS complexes shift during ventricular tachycardia, however, the time of activation changes at the right ventricular apex, the site where electrodes for pacing and defibrillators are frequently implanted.[815]

Activation. Endocardial activation during ventricular tachycardia in most patients with coronary heart disease spreads centrifugally from the site of origin, which is less than 6 cm.[74] The endocardium is activated before the epicardium,[816] but it is mostly epicardial activation that determines the configuration of the surface electrocardiogram.[817] Although the sequence of activation on the epicardial surface, which begins about 10 milliseconds after the onset of the QRS complex,[816] closely matches the pattern of endocardial activation,[817] epicardial activation does not identify the site of origin of the tachycardia.[816] Epicardial activation is delayed in regions of ventricular akinesis and dyskinesis but not hypokinesis.[818]

Electrograms. The form of the electrical activity recorded from intracardiac electrode catheters during sinus rhythm reflects the health of the adjacent myocardium. Signals from ischemic and infarcted tissues, including ventricular aneurysms,[786, 819–822] have reduced amplitude and are fragmented and prolonged (Fig. 12.23). Conduction is often slower than normal in these regions.[823]

During sinus rhythm, abnormal signals appear in endocardial recordings from patients with a history of sustained ventricular tachycardia.[824, 825aaaa] Abnormal signals are also recorded in those patients with transient ventricular tachycardia who can be induced into sustained ventricular tachycardia[622] but not in persons with normal electrocardiograms.[821, 826] Abnormal elec-

Form of QRS Complexes	Origin of Ventricular Tachycardia
Table 12.8 ELECTROCARDIOGRAPHIC PATTERNS USEFUL IN DIFFERENTIATING ANTERIOR FROM POSTERIOR SITES OF ORIGIN IN THE LEFT VENTRICLE OF SUSTAINED VENTRICULAR TACHYCARDIA IN PATIENTS WITH CORONARY HEART DISEASE[a]	
Right bundle branch block plus:	
Q wave in leads I, V_6	Anterior left ventricle
R wave in leads I, V_1–V_6	Posterior left ventricle
Left bundle branch block plus:	
Q wave in leads I, V_6	Anterior left ventricle
R wave in leads I, V_2, V_3, V_6	Posterior left ventricle
Q wave in leads I, V_6, superior axis	Inferior aspect of anterior interventricular septum
Inferior, rightward axis	Superior aspect of anterior interventricular septum

[a]More detailed systems for correlating electrocardiographic findings with the origin of ventricular tachycardia are described in references 805 and 806.

(From Josephson ME, Horowitz LN, Waxman HL, et al. Sustained ventricular tachycardia: role of the 12-lead electrocardiogram in localizing site of origin. Circulation 1981; 64:257–272, by permission of the American Heart Association, Inc.)

aaaaWith sophisticated techniques, one can differentiate between the abnormal electrograms recorded during sinus rhythm and ventricular tachycardia in the same patient from the same endocardial location.[825]

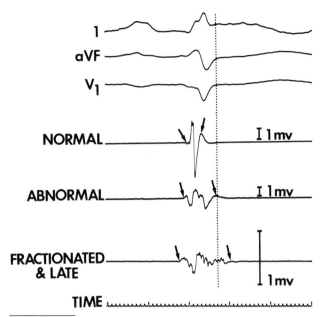

FIGURE 12.23 Endocardial electrograms recorded from normal and abnormal regions of the left ventricle of a patient with ventricular tachycardia. Three surface electrocardiogram leads are shown above three intracardiac bipolar recordings from different left ventricular sites. Electrograms recorded from areas of normal myocardium are sharp monophasic or biphasic deflections with high amplitude. In contrast, electrograms recorded from structurally abnormal myocardium have less amplitude, longer duration, and many components. The most abnormal electrograms are called fractionated and are seen mostly in patients with coronary artery disease and inducible ventricular tachycardia. (The QRS complexes end at the dashed vertical line, and the *arrows* show the beginning and end of the local electrical activity.) (From Cassidy DM, Vassallo JA, Buxton AE, Doherty JU, Marchlinski FE, Josephson ME. The value of catheter mapping during sinus rhythm to localize site of origin of ventricular tachycardia. Circulation 1984; 69:1103–1110, by permission of the American Heart Association, Inc.)[830]

trograms are likely to be found in akinetic but not in normal or hypokinetic regions of the left ventricle.[827]

Electrograms recorded from patients with cardiomyopathy, including those with sustained ventricular tachycardia, are relatively normal.[828] The duration of the electrograms does not correlate with the rate or the cycle length of the tachycardia.[829]

The electrograms recorded during *sinus rhythm* at the site of origin of ventricular tachycardia often, but not always, have lower amplitude and longer duration than elsewhere in the ventricle.[830] The prevalence of severely abnormal electrograms in patients with extensive myocardial disease prevents their use to locate the site of origin of the tachycardia.[831, 832] The extent of abnormal endocardial electrograms is greater in patients with ventricular tachycardia than in patients who have had cardiac arrest.[475]

Continuous local electrical activity persisting throughout the cardiac cycle[588] can be recorded in some patients during sustained ventricular tachycardia who have previous myocardial infarction or arrhythmogenic right ventricular dysplasia, although not in patients with idiopathic sustained ventricular tachycardia.[593] The electrograms during sinus rhythm are abnormal at the sites where continuous activity is recorded during ventricular tachycardia.[593]

Signal-averaged electrocardiograms. Late potentials recorded from the signal-averaged electrocardiogram correspond to delayed, fragmented signals recorded during endocardial,[833] but not epicardial, mapping.[834] By comparing the maximal amplitude of late potentials in the right-sided and left-sided leads, one can map the origin of the late potentials to the right or left ventricle.[835] Late potentials can also be recorded from endocardial electrodes and can help to locate where to apply radiofrequency current in ablating ventricular tachycardia.[836]

Bundle Branch Reentry

In some patients with ventricular tachycardia, the arrhythmia is sustained within the His bundle, right and left bundle branches, and transseptal ventricular muscle.[837–845] These patients with bundle branch reentrant ventricular tachycardia*bbbb* often have dilated cardiomyopathy, either idiopathic or from coronary heart disease. Their ejection fractions are usually markedly reduced.[360, 846, 847]*cccc* Consequently, they frequently present with syncope or cardiac arrest. A few, however, have no structural heart disease[847] or have had surgery for valvular disease.[181]

Entrainment and Resetting[776, 796, 848, 849]

By pacing the ventricles slightly faster than the rate of ventricular tachycardia, the arrhythmia, which now assumes a slightly different morphology, can be entrained and will follow the pacing stimulus.[562, 563, 796, 849–864] When the pacer is turned off, the intrinsic ventricular tachycardia resumes. The form of the QRS complexes is identical to that of the spontaneous arrhythmias when the entrainment is *concealed* because, it is presumed, the pacing occurs within the reentrant circuit.[865] When premature beats are introduced from within the reentrant circuit, the timing of the tachycardia can be reset without disrupting the arrhythmia.[763, 851, 854, 855, 863, 866–872] Entrainment and resetting have provided electrophysiologists with much theoretical information about the reentrant nature of ventricular tachycardia.[776, 873–879]

Sympathetic Activity

Regional sympathetic denervation can be demonstrated in patients with or without heart disease who have ventricular tachycardia but not in those with normal hearts and no ventricular tachycardia.[880]

---

*bbbb*Bundle branch reentry accounts for 6% of patients with sustained ventricular tachycardia treated at a center with a particular interest in the arrhythmia.[846]

*cccc*The ejection fraction was 23.2% (range, 14%–65%) in 45 patients with bundle branch reentrant ventricular tachycardia.[360, 847]

TREATMENT[194, 881–890]

Each patient with sustained ventricular tachycardia should be referred to a center with a team of experienced clinical electrophysiologists so that the most appropriate treatment program can be developed. None should be treated empirically.

Most patients with *transient* ventricular tachycardia, including those with repetitive monomorphic ventricular tachycardia, need no treatment or electrophysiological evaluation if their arrhythmia produces few, if any, symptoms and *their ventricular function is normal.* As for patients who have troublesome ventricular premature beats and normal ventricular function, beta-adrenergic–blocking drugs can be given to reduce symptoms. Other antiarrhythmic drugs should not be prescribed empirically. Their side effects can be disabling and even fatal.

No patient should drive a vehicle for at least 1 month after hospitalization for ventricular tachycardia, when the hazard for recurrence is greatest. Caution dictates, moreover, that most patients should not drive for another 6 months because dangerous events may occur during that time. Afterward, in the absence of recurrences, the likelihood that an arrhythmia will interfere with driving is low.[891]*dddd*

Physical Maneuvers

Actions that stimulate vagal function such as carotid sinus pressure[22] or the Valsalva maneuver seldom convert ventricular tachycardia to sinus rhythm, a negative observation of some value in distinguishing supraventricular from ventricular tachycardia. However, a few patients with exercise-induced ventricular tachycardia[212, 223, 323] and some others without coronary heart disease or congestive heart failure[892] respond to one or more of these maneuvers.

One or more blows to the chest,[893–895] even when administered by the patient,[896] can occasionally convert ventricular tachycardia to sinus rhythm (Fig. 12.24).[897]*eeee* Vigorous coughing may also produce sinus rhythm.[898]

Drugs[691, 899–906]

Adenosine.[358, 907] Adenosine does not affect the arrhythmia in most patients with ventricular tachycar-

---

*dddd*The authors of a study of 501 survivors of ventricular tachycardia and fibrillation also conclude: "Individualized recommendations should be allowed because the accident rate for patients who actually suffer sudden death is low."[891]

*eeee*Chest thump accelerated the rate of ventricular tachycardia in three patients receiving digitalis. After the drug was discontinued, chest thump reverted two of the patients to sinus rhythm and did not accelerate the rate of the ventricular tachycardia in the other.[897]

dia.[908, 909] It may, however, convert the arrhythmia to sinus rhythm[212] in patients without structural heart disease when the arrhythmia is not due to reentry and

- Occurs predominantly during stress or exertion.[221, 651]
- Has the form of left bundle branch block and inferior axis from origin in the right ventricular outflow tract,[809] and occasionally right bundle branch block from the left ventricle.[220, 323, 651]
- Produces no abnormal findings in the signal-averaged electrocardiogram.[221]
- Arises in the free wall of the pulmonary infundibulum[221] and, occasionally, adjacent to the outflow tract of the left ventricle.[651]

Adenosine may also convert an occasional case of ventricular tachycardia due to reentry in the bundle branches.[844]

Amiodarone.[689, 910–916] Amiodarone converts ventricular tachycardia to sinus rhythm and suppresses recurrent sustained ventricular tachycardia in many patients whose arrhythmia is refractory to other antiarrhythmic drugs,[152, 218, 404, 706, 716, 917–934]*ffff* including those with arrhythmogenic right ventricular dysplasia[152, 935–937] and hypertrophic cardiomyopathy.[938] Amiodarone, given prophylactically, reduces the appearance of ventricular tachycardia after coronary artery bypass graft surgery.[939]

Amiodarone suppresses transient ventricular tachycardia,[940, 941] and it may prolong survival of patients with this arrhythmia and decreased left ventricular function.[941] Amiodarone slows the rate of ventricular tachycardia, even when it does not convert the arrhythmia or prevent its induction,[642, 936, 942–944] and more so than does sotalol, a drug with similar electropharmacological properties.[945]

The patients in whom amiodarone suppresses induction of ventricular tachycardia seldom have spontaneous episodes when taking the drug afterward.[946–953] However, some patients in whom induction cannot be achieved are also free of clinical ventricular tachycardia, which is less often the case with other antiarrhythmic drugs.[936, 942, 946, 947, 951, 954]

Amiodarone seldom suppresses the induction of ventricular tachycardia in patients whose ventricular tachycardia has not been suppressed by class IA agents[944] or by sotalol.[955] Furthermore, adding the type

---

*ffff*The combination of amiodarone and flecainide controlled ventricular tachycardia in each of three infants in whom treatment with one of the drugs was ineffective.[934]

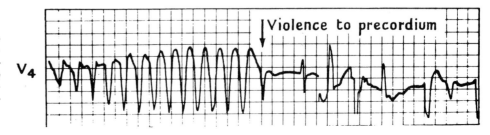

FIGURE 12.24 Conversion of ventricular tachycardia by "thumpversion," or "violence to precordium," as the author of one article so expressively puts it. (Reproduced from a slide in my collection, source unknown.)

IA agents quinidine or procainamide, although slowing the rate further and improving hemodynamic tolerance, does not assist amiodarone in preventing induction of ventricular tachycardia.[738, 956]

Amiodarone, given intravenously, is particularly useful in suppressing incessant[916, 953] and recurrent sustained ventricular tachycardia in adults,[937, 957–964] even when hypotensive,[965] and in children.[966] Compared with bretylium, amiodarone is as effective and does not produce as much hypotension.[963] Although oral loading can also achieve good therapeutic results in patients with frequent episodes of ventricular tachycardia,[967] intravenous loading shortens the time until control of the arrhythmia is achieved and lowers the cumulative dose required.[968] Abolition of complex and frequent ventricular premature beats by amiodarone predicts the drug's control of sustained ventricular tachycardia.[969]

The likelihood of dying suddenly during follow-up is high in patients taking amiodarone if electrophysiological study produces cardiovascular collapse or other severe symptoms. However, nonfatal ventricular tachycardia is the more likely future event if electrophysiological study produces only moderate symptoms.[947]

Aprindine.[970] Aprindine and the related drug moxaprindine[971] convert incessant ventricular tachycardia when given intravenously. Intravenous aprindine helps predict the subsequent response to the oral drug.[972]

Atropine. By increasing the sinus rate, atropine temporarily suppresses ventricular tachycardia in some patients. The drug is seldom used for this purpose now.[973]

Bretylium tosylate.[974, 975] Bretylium tosylate can suppress recurrent ventricular tachycardia refractory to other antiarrhythmic drugs.[976–981] The drug, however, is seldom used today.

Beta-adrenergic–blocking drugs. Beta blockers do not convert or suppress the appearance or induction of monomorphic ventricular tachycardia in most patients,[205, 218, 982, 983] but they seem to render noninducible some patients still inducible after taking type I antiarrhythmic drugs.[984] Beta blockers suppress the inducibility of patients with catecholamine-dependent, exercise-induced ventricular tachycardia,[216, 218, 313, 649, 985, 986gggg] and they suppress noninducible ventricular tachycardia in many patients with arrhythmogenic right ventricular dysplasia.[152] Beta-adrenergic–blocking drugs alone have not as yet been shown to suppress the spontaneous appearance of non–catecholamine-dependent sustained ventricular tachycardia.

Calcium-channel–blocking drugs. Verapamil only occasionally suppresses or converts ventricular tachycardia,[987, 988] and then usually in those relative few patients with structurally normal hearts whose arrhythmia is due to mechanisms other than reentry, such as triggered activity, and is often provoked by exercise. In many of these patients, the drug slows the rate[126, 225, 323, 989, 990] and may prevent the induction of the arrhythmia and reduce its spontaneous appearance.[207, 208, 211, 212, 214, 220, 229, 313, 343, 344, 649, 651, 985, 989–997hhhh] Diltiazem has a similar effect.[996] However, verapamil, given intravenously to patients with wide-complex tachycardias under the mistaken impression that the arrhythmia is supraventricular, can produce severe hemodynamic deterioration[372] and loss of consciousness.[998]

Captopril. Given to patients during thrombolytic treatment for first myocardial infarctions, captopril decreases the incidence of transient ventricular tachycardia.[999]

Corticosteroids. Corticosteroids may assist the recovery of those few patients whose ventricular tachycardia is caused by myocarditis proven by myocardial biopsy.[227]

Dipyridamole. An adenosine transport inhibitor, dipyridamole terminates the arrhythmia in some patients with exercise-induced sustained ventricular tachycardia.[323]

Flecainide. A type IC antiarrhythmic drug, flecainide can suppress ventricular tachycardia in some patients without structural heart disease.[245, 995] The combination of amiodarone and flecainide controlled ventricular tachycardia in each of three infants in whom treatment with one of the drugs was ineffective.[934]

Disopyramide. A type IA antiarrhythmic agent like procainamide and quinidine, disopyramide slows the rate of ventricular tachycardia[757, 1000, 1001] and, when given intravenously in adequate doses, it converts sustained ventricular tachycardia[757, 1000, 1002] and suppresses transient ventricular tachycardia.[1002] Disopyramide prevents spontaneous recurrence when taken orally in amounts shown to be effective in preventing induction at electrophysiological study.[1000]

Ibutilide. A new class III antiarrhythmic drug, ibutilide suppresses induction of monomorphic sustained ventricular tachycardia in some patients with coronary heart disease.[1003]

Isoproterenol. Isoproterenol reduces the slowing of the rate of ventricular tachycardia produced by many antiarrhythmic drugs.[1004] Like atropine, isoproterenol may help to suppress ventricular tachycardia temporarily by increasing the sinus rate.[973]

Lidocaine. Contrary to general belief, lidocaine seldom converts recurrent, sustained ventricular tachycar-

---

gggg Although one report disagrees. Beta-adrenergic–blocking drugs failed to prevent induction of ventricular tachycardia in 75% of 37 patients in this series with exercise-related ventricular tachycardia.[218]

hhhh In a few of these patients, verapamil exacerbates the arrhythmia.[229]

dia to sinus rhythm.[1005–1010][iiii] However, lidocaine does convert and suppress transient and possibly sustained ventricular tachycardia during acute myocardial infarction.[1011–1013] There is no clinical advantage in administering lidocaine to patients undergoing coronary artery bypass graft surgery even though the drug in this setting may decrease the incidence of transient ventricular tachycardia.[1014][jjjj] Lidocaine infrequently prevents induction of sustained ventricular tachycardia in the electrophysiological laboratory.[1008, 1015]

Mexiletine. While slowing the rate of the arrhythmia,[1016, 1017] mexiletine is relatively ineffective in suppressing induction of sustained ventricular tachycardia.[400, 703, 1015, 1018] The drug works better on transient ventricular tachycardia.[1018] The ability of mexiletine to suppress ventricular tachycardia in the electrophysiological laboratory increases when it is combined with other antiarrhythmic drugs.[739, 1019] Mexiletine reduces the spontaneous appearance of ventricular tachycardia,[703] as recorded on ambulatory monitoring in patients in whom ventricular tachycardia can still be induced in the electrophysiological laboratory.[403]

Moricizine. Moricizine suppresses spontaneous episodes of transient ventricular tachycardia in about 60% of cases.[1020] Although the drug slows the rate of sustained ventricular tachycardia,[1021] moricizine prevents induction of the arrhythmia in few patients.[1021–1023]

Phenylephrine. Phenylephrine occasionally converts ventricular tachycardia, thus eliminating the diagnostic value of the drug in distinguishing between ventricular and supraventricular arrhythmias.[1024]

Procainamide. Procainamide slows the rate[860, 871, 956, 1025–1029] of sustained ventricular tachycardia, thereby reducing or relieving many of the symptoms produced by the arrhythmia.[1027] The drug also terminates ventricular tachycardia[604, 1010] in most patients[kkkk] when given in adequate doses.[1028]

The amount infused to stop ventricular tachycardia, however, is usually inadequate to prevent induction of the arrhythmia. Larger doses are needed for this purpose,[1027, 1029][llll] as much as 500 to 1500 mg orally every 4 hours often required to prevent spontaneous episodes.[1027] The blood levels of the drug required to prevent induction predict the blood levels and the dosage needed to secure relief of spontaneous episodes in most patients.[1027] When procainamide does not prevent induction of the arrhythmia, adding quini-

dine or disopyramide does not prevent induction.[737] Procainamide and other type I agents are rarely effective in treating inducible and noninducible ventricular tachycardia in patients with arrhythmogenic right ventricular dysplasia.[152]

Propafenone. Propafenone slows the rate of,[1030, 1031] and reduces recurrences of, transient and sustained ventricular tachycardia[1031–1033] in children[1034, 1035] as well as in adults. The drug suppresses induction of ventricular tachycardia in a few patients,[1031] and it may reduce recurrences of spontaneous paroxysms even when it does not prevent induction of the arrhythmia in the electrophysiological laboratory.[1030] Of concern is a report that incessant ventricular tachycardia can be induced in some patients with ventricular dysfunction being treated with propafenone for ventricular tachycardia or fibrillation.[1036]

Quinidine.[1037] Quinidine was the first antiarrhythmic drug found effective for treating ventricular tachycardia.[22] Like many antiarrhythmic drugs, quinidine slows the rate of the arrhythmia,[739] and it renders ventricular tachycardia uninducible at electrophysiological study with similar efficacy as procainamide.[1038] However, quinidine is seldom used today for conversion and is increasingly less often given to maintain sinus rhythm. Both the intravenous and oral preparations are associated with troublesome side effects, and more satisfactory drugs are available.

Sotalol (d,l).[911, 913, 1039–1042] Sotalol converts ventricular tachycardia[1009] and suppresses induction of sustained ventricular tachycardia,[709, 714, 720, 721, 731, 995, 1043–1054] both orally and intravenously,[1044] with success similar to that of amiodarone, another type III agent,[945, 1055] in many patients, including some refractory to procainamide.[720, 1052, 1056] The similarity of these drugs, both type III agents, means that some patients whose ventricular tachycardia cannot be suppressed by sotalol will respond similarly to amiodarone.[955]

Sotalol suppresses recurrences of spontaneous ventricular tachycardia[709, 728, 995, 1057] more effectively than six other antiarrhythmic drugs[1051, 1058–1060][mmmm] but no more effectively than metoprolol.[1054] Sotalol is also preferable to flecainide and verapamil in treating ventricular tachycardia in many patients with structurally normal hearts.[1061]

Sotalol and amiodarone are particularly effective in treating the arrhythmia in patients without structural heart disease,[215] some of whose ventricular tachycardia is induced by exercise,[218] and in those with arrhythmogenic right ventricular dysplasia.[152] Sotalol decreases the speed and increases the variability of the heart rate during ventricular tachycardia induced during electrophysiological study.[1062]

Sotalol decreases the rate of ventricular tachycardia[955, 1044, 1053] further when added to procainamide or

---

[iiii]Lidocaine converted only 10 (8%) of 125 patients with stable spontaneous or induced sustained ventricular tachycardia to sinus rhythm.[1008]

[jjjj]Before more effective methods were developed, lidocaine was given by continuous intravenous infusion to suppress ventricular tachycardia in an occasional patient.[1006]

[kkkk]In 14 (93%) of 15 patients after administration at 50 mg per minute of 100 to 1080 mg; median dose 600 mg.[1028]

[llll]One thousand to 2500 mg in one study.[1027] However, doses that prevent inducibility of the predominant ventricular tachycardia may not prevent induction of ventricular tachycardias with different forms and different, often faster, rates.[1029]

[mmmm]Imipramine, mexiletine, procainamide, propafenone, pirmenol, and quinidine. One group questions some technical features of the study that led to this conclusion.[1060]

quinidine[1063] and it prolongs refractoriness further when used with procainamide.[1064] Occasionally, sotalol, which contains beta-adrenergic–blocking properties, decreases the sinus rate so much that permanent pacemaking is needed.[1065]

Sotalol (d). The isomer of *d,l* sotalol with no beta-adrenergic–blocking effects, this drug acutely and chronically suppresses sustained ventricular tachycardia.[1066] However, *d*-sotalol is no longer available for use because of its proarrhythmic effects.[1067, 1068nnnn]

Tocainide. A class IB antiarrhythmic drug like lidocaine, tocainide reduces the likelihood of ventricular tachycardia developing during myocardial infarction better than does lidocaine.[1069] Tocainide, however, does not affect the incidence of spontaneous symptomatic ventricular tachycardia[1070] after myocardial infarction and suppresses the induction of sustained ventricular tachycardia due to coronary heart disease in a few patients refractory to other agents.[1015]

Other drugs. Drugs that have been found relatively or totally ineffective for treating or preventing treating ventricular tachycardia include

• Corticosteroids for sarcoid heart disease.[157, 1071]
• Phenytoin.[1072]
• Potassium.[22oooo]

Cardioversion

External cardioversion terminates ventricular tachycardia in most patients.[1072–1079pppp] Less power is required to convert ventricular tachycardia, usually a reentrant arrhythmia, than atrial fibrillation or ventricular fibrillation. However, because 200 joules will convert almost all cases of ventricular tachycardia, electrophysiologists frequently choose this amount during electrophysiological studies.[1080] External cardioversion, often required during electrophysiological studies in patients with ventricular tachycardia, seldom, if ever, damages the heart. Creatine phospokinase-B is infrequently elevated after such shocks.[1081, 1082]

Bradyarrhythmias, sometimes requiring temporary pacing, supraventricular arrhythmias, or transient ventricular tachycardia frequently occur after cardioversion of ventricular tachycardia.[1080, 1083] Antiarrhythmic drugs increase the incidence of post-cardioversion bradycardia.[1080, 1083] The amount of potassium and magnesium in the blood frequently decreases after ventricular tachycardia is successfully cardioverted, presumably an effect of the hypotension associated with the arrhythmia.[1084]

Pacing

Pacing with bursts or extrastimuli from the atria[374, 1085–1090] and the ventricles[696, 1087, 1091–1104] has been clinically employed to terminate and suppress such ventricular arrhythmias as multiple ventricular premature beats, transient and sustained monomorphic ventricular tachycardia, and polymorphic ventricular tachycardia. When the arrhythmias persist and drugs fail to suppress them, pacemakers can be implanted permanently in the atria or ventricles.[1097, 1103, 1105–1124] Such units discharge continuously or, if intermittently, can be activated automatically or by the patient when the arrhythmia appears.

Pacemakers, although employed occasionally from the mid 1960s, are seldom used by themselves today to treat patients with ventricular tachyarrhythmias, except as required for associated bradyarrhythmias.[570, 697, 699, 762, 765, 769, 770, 1125qqqq] Pacing function is incorporated in all contemporary implantable cardioverter-defibrillators, which can then be programmed to convert ventricular tachycardia with extrastimuli or bursts of ventricular beats.[256, 1126]

Implantable Cardioverter-Defibrillators[rrrr]

Implantation of cardioverter-defibrillators has increasingly become the definitive treatment of *sustained* ventricular tachycardia, at least in the United States. When cost is not a consideration, most patients with sustained ventricular tachycardia receive these devices if their arrhythmias cannot be cured by revascularization, with catheter ablation, or, in a few cases, with antiarrhythmic drugs. Cardioverter-defibrillators convert most clinical episodes of the arrhythmia with pacing, thereby eliminating many of the painful shocks administered before the units incorporated this feature.[1127, 1128]

Implantable cardioverter-defibrillators are indicated for few patients with *transient* ventricular tachycardia. However, their use is growing when this arrhythmia occurs in patients with increased risk of cardiac arrest. For example, implantable cardioverter-defibrillators have been shown to reduce mortality by as much as 50% in patients with documented transient ventricular tachycardia not producing syncope, prior Q-wave myocardial infarction, and[1129–1131ssss]

• Left ventricular ejection fraction less than 35%.
• New York Heart Association classification I, II, or III.
• Ventricular arrhythmias inducible during electrophysiological study and unsuppressible with procainamide.

---

nnnnAs revealed in the Survival with Oral *d*-Sotalol (SWORD) Study.[1068]

ooooExcept in the presence of hypokalemia with, in particular, digitalis toxicity.

ppppExternal cardioversion terminated 93 (97%) of 96 episodes of ventricular tachycardia as reported from six series in the mid-1960s when the technique was first applied.[1074–1078, 1373] Its use in emergency departments, however, is significantly less frequent than depicted on television.[1079]

qqqqRapid pacing for conversion, often at rates faster than that of the ventricular tachycardia, can occasionally increase the rate of the tachycardia.[570, 697, 699, 762, 765, 769, 770, 1125] Such a development can produce cardiac arrest, which can be fatal in the absence of an implantable cardioverter-defibrillator.

rrrrSee Chapter 14 for a comprehensive discussion of the use of implantable cardioverter-defibrillators for treating life-threatening ventricular tachyarrhythmias.

ssssAccording to MADIT (Multicenter Automatic Defibrillator Implantation Trial).[1129]

• No indications for coronary revascularization.

Implantable cardioverter-defibrillators and the newer antiarrhythmic drugs have, for the most part, superseded antiarrhythmic surgery for treatment of recurrent sustained ventricular tachycardia.[1132]

Catheter Ablation

Applying radiofrequency current[810, 1133–1156] or direct current shock[811, 1135, 1157–1162] through electrode catheters can interrupt the reentrant circuit or region of triggered activity,[40, 810] which sustains ventricular tachycardia, and can eliminate the arrhythmia's spontaneous occurrence and inducibility in the electrophysiological laboratory.[40, 787, 1163tttt] Operators should try to ablate all hemodynamically tolerated ventricular tachycardias because of the high rate of recurrence of unablated tachycardias.[1155]

Clinical electrophysiologists use detailed endocardial activation, pace[795, 797, 811, 836, 1164] and entrainment mapping during sinus rhythm and ventricular tachycardia to locate the regions where application of current is most likely to be effective. Investigators are exploring the value of transesophageal echocardiography to monitor the position of the electrode catheters continuously.[523–526]

Ablation performed *after* the implantation of cardioverter-defibrillators can eliminate or reduce the frequency of paroxysms of sustained ventricular tachycardia in patients whose arrhythmia recurs frequently.[1165]

Coronary heart disease. Ablation, with shock[1138, 1161, 1166–1170] or radiofrequency current[836, 1151, 1161, 1171–1175] successfully suppresses ventricular tachycardia produced by coronary heart disease and myocardial infarction. The value of ablation is supported by the observation that the number of discharges from implantable cardioverter-defibrillators decreases after ablation of the sites of ventricular tachycardia.[1175]

However, ablation provides extended relief to a smaller proportion of patients with congenital heart disease than for those less commonly encountered cases without structural heart disease or with bundle branch reentry.[1166, 1172, 1176–1179] Even when ablation successfully prevents further episodes of one ventricular tachycardia, other tachycardias originating from non-ablated locations may arise. Consequently, clinically successful treatment requires ablating as many sites as possible.

Thus, ablating ventricular tachycardia is palliative rather than curative in the majority of patients with coronary heart disease, who often continue to require additional antiarrhythmic treatment.[1172, 1178, 1179uuuu] The left ventricular endocardium is the usual site for ablation of ventricular tachycardia in patients with coronary heart disease; occasionally, however, the arrhythmia is best treated in the septal surface of the right ventricle.[1180]

Bundle branch reentry. Because the arrhythmia is sustained within anatomically discrete structures, ablation, usually applied to the right,[360, 841, 842, 846, 1152, 1181–1187] and occasionally the left,[1181, 1182] bundle branch, is particularly effective in eliminating the tachycardia despite the severe myocardial disease that afflicts many of these patients.[1152] Most, however, have advanced cardiomyopathy, and many have other ventricular tachycardias[1185] sustained within the diseased myocardium in addition to the bundle branches. Atrioventricular block is a well-recognized complication of the procedure.

Cardiomyopathy. Ventricular tachycardia can be ablated in some patients with hypertrophic[901, 1188] and right ventricular cardiomyopathy.[1189] However, ablation alone achieves complete prevention in only a minority of those so treated.[1190] Surgical[122] or catheter ablation[122, 125] of the arrhythmia can cure the cardiomyopathy induced by the arrhythmia. Epicardial ablation can suppress some cases of ventricular tachycardia in patients with Chagas disease.[799]

After repair of tetralogy of Fallot. The right ventricular outflow tract is usually the site at which ventricular tachycardia originates in these patients. Current applied in this location often ablates the arrhythmia.[525, 1191–1195]

No structural heart disease. Ablation with radiofrequency and direct current eliminates ventricular tachycardia, often exercise and catecholamine sensitive, in most patients without structural heart disease.[199, 1196–1198] The current can be successfully applied to loci in both the right[124, 524, 664, 795, 1137, 1199–1210] and left[40, 220, 354, 528, 529, 667, 795, 810, 811, 813, 1203, 1204, 1209–1224] ventricles and in children[1210] as well as adults.[vvvv] The right ventricular outflow tract is the usual site for ablating repetitive monomorphic ventricular tachycardia, but in a few patients, the arrhythmia, starting in the left ventricle,[353, 1162] including the fascicles,[811, 1221] can be successfully ablated.

Complications. Complications from ablating ventricular tachycardia include

• Chronic occlusion of the left main coronary artery.[1225]
• Pericardial tamponade.[1154]
• Third-degree atrioventricular block.[1226]

Angioplasty

Coronary angioplasty can cure ventricular tachycardia in the few patients whose ventricular tachycardia is due to ischemia.[80, 1227]

---

tttt Radiofrequency current is the favored electrical source now. Sites of ventricular tachycardia have also been ablated chemically with transcoronary ethanol[1163] and during open-heart surgery with electric shock.[40, 787]

uuuu Among the best results were reported in a series of 136 patients with coronary heart disease and sustained ventricular tachycardia.[1178] Ablation rendered the tachycardias uninducible in 102 (75%) of the patients. Of 97 who were closely followed, ventricular tachycardia recurred in 16 (16%).

vvvv Ablation of the slow atrioventricular nodal pathway in a patient with both left ventricular and supraventricular tachycardia eliminated both arrhythmias.[1214]

Surgery

Several surgical operations have been developed to treat patients with recurrent sustained ventricular tachycardia.[773, 1228-1247] Postoperative electrophysiological studies demonstrate the success of the procedures by showing that the arrhythmia is no longer inducible. The operative mortality is low when performed by experienced surgical and electrophysiological teams on stable patients. Many patients die, however, when surgery is attempted on an emergency basis in those who may be in cardiogenic shock.[1248, 1249]

Because antiarrhythmic operations do not prevent cardiac arrest in all patients, implantable cardioverter-defibrillators may also be implanted for further protection.[1250] Wider application of implantable defibrillators has, at least in the United States, reduced the number of these operations performed on patients with coronary heart disease and sustained ventricular tachycardia.[1132]

Subendocardial and epicardial resection and ablation. Surgical excision,[778, 786, 1132, 1251-1284] reconstruction and endoaneurysmorrhaphy,[1079, 1285] or ablation with cold (cryoablation)[1257, 1268, 1270, 1271, 1273, 1286-1292] or laser (photocoagulation)[563, 1293-1298] of the tissues that support the reentrant arrhythmia cures many patients of recurrent sustained ventricular tachycardia. In most, but not all, reports, mapping in the electrophysiology laboratory or the operating room locates the origin of the arrhythmia which may be close to or, in some cases, relatively distant from that of the target arrhythmia.[1267, 1299]*wwww* The source of each of the arrhythmias must be excised or ablated to cure patients who have ventricular tachycardias with more than one QRS morphology.[805, 1249]

Subendocardial resection does not affect the presence or severity of ventricular premature beats, and persistence of these beats does not predict whether ventricular tachycardia will be inducible after surgery.[414, 1300] Left bundle branch block sometimes appears after resection in the inferoposterobasal region of the left ventricle, but complete heart block is seldom a complication of the procedure.[1301]

When spontaneous recurrences and inducibility in the electrophysiological laboratory[1300]*xxxx* continue after subendocardial resection, patients often have

- A history of cardiac arrest requiring resuscitation.[1302]
- Incomplete mapping of the tachycardia.[1302]
- Myocardial infarction within the past 2 months.[1302]
- QRS complexes during ventricular tachycardia with right bundle branch block morphology.[1262]
- Origin of the arrhythmia in the inferior wall.[1262, 1269]

Mitral valve repair or replacement is sometimes indi-

cated when ventricular tachycardia develops in patients with mitral regurgitation.[1303] Even when competent, the valve may need to be replaced when the tachycardia originates in the papillary muscle.[1303]

Ventricular tachycardia can arise from damaged subepicardial myocardium. Consequently, surgeons and clinical electrophysiologists also map the epicardium in some cases to locate the origin and guide the resection or ablation.[275, 563, 1286, 1297, 1304, 1305]

Encircling endocardial ventriculotomy. In this operation, which does not require mapping, the surgeon performs a transmural ventriculotomy perpendicular to the ventricular wall and at the edge of the region of myocardial fibrosis.[1257, 1261, 1271, 1274, 1306-1308] The incision separates the diseased from the healthy myocardium, thereby preventing arrhythmias in the abnormal portion from activating the functioning myocardium.*yyyy*

Coronary artery bypass grafting. Coronary revascularization alone seldom cures ventricular tachycardia[415, 1309-1311] because the arrhythmia is usually due to reentry within permanently fibrosed endocardium and not transient ischemia. However, when ischemia is the cause, ventricular tachycardia and ventricular fibrillation with cardiac arrest[1312] often respond to coronary surgery.[83, 1313-1315] Accordingly, the function and anatomy of the coronary circulation should often be evaluated during the workup of patients with sustained ventricular tachycardia.

Patients with coronary heart disease. Treating sustained ventricular tachycardia with subendocardial resection guided by electrophysiological mapping gives the best results in patients with coronary heart disease and healed myocardial infarctions.[1249]*zzzz* Many of these patients have ventricular aneurysms, which are usually excised during the operation. The arrhythmia, however, seldom arises within the aneurysm but rather in the abnormal subendocardium surrounding it.

Before electrophysiologic studies were developed, cardiac surgeons excised ventricular aneurysms in the hope that the procedure would eliminate dangerous ventricular arrhythmias.[76, 93, 96-101, 105-109] Some of the reports described favorable results,[90-92, 95, 102-104, 108] but without programmed stimulation, investigators could not establish proof of suppression.[106, 109]*aaaaa* Furthermore, direct comparison of simple aneurysmectomy

---

*wwww*The "target" arrhythmia is the one the surgeon seeks to ablate. It is usually the spontaneous arrhythmia or the principal one induced during electrophysiological study.

*xxxx*However, ventricular tachycardia no longer occurs spontaneously in some patients in whom the arrhythmia can still be induced.[1300]

*yyyy*It is difficult to compare the relative effectiveness of subendocardial resection versus encircling endocardial ventriculotomy, in part, because different groups favor one procedure over the other. To my reading of the reports, the clinical results appear similar.

*zzzz*Ventricular tachycardia could no longer be induced in 35 of 41 survivors of subendocardial resection, only one of whom required antiarrhythmic drugs on discharge. Each of 39 patients operated on electively survived; four of six additional patients operated on an emergency basis died.[1249] Refinements in mapping and operative technique used in these cases partly account for the high rate of noninducibility.

*aaaaa*After analyzing with Holter monitoring and exercise testing the results of simple resection of saccular ventricular aneurysms without electrophysiological support in 106 patients, the authors[106] concluded, "Aneurysmectomy does not abolish ventricular tachyarrhythmias. . . ."[106]

versus aneurysmectomy guided by electrophysiological techniques establishes that aneurysmectomy alone does not cure ventricular tachycardia.[1255] Sustained ventricular tachycardia after myocardial infarction has been successfully treated by photocoagulating the epicardium with an yttrium-aluminum-garnet (YAG) laser during coronary artery bypass graft surgery.[1316]

Cardiomyopathy. Cardiac operations have not been particularly successful in treating ventricular tachycardia when it occurs in the setting of idiopathic cardiomyopathy.[1317, 1318] However, the ventricular tachycardia produced by arrhythmogenic right ventricular dysplasia can be suppressed surgically[148] by functionally isolating the right ventricular free wall where the arrhythmia originates from the remainder of the chamber with a full-thickness ventriculotomy.[1318–1320]

Tetralogy of Fallot. Sustained ventricular tachycardia that develops in a few patients after surgical repair of tetralogy of Fallot can be cured by excising the origin, which mapping usually locates to the region of the ventriculotomy scar in the right ventricular outflow tract.[1321, 1322]

Patients without structural heart disease. Cardiac surgery for sustained ventricular tachycardia in this group of patients is seldom successful.[1317, 1318]

Miscellaneous conditions. Cardiac surgery guided by electrophysiological mapping has also been employed to cure the occasional case of sustained or incessant ventricular tachycardia due to

- Ventricular aneurysms in a patient with hypertrophic cardiomyopathy[1323] and in others of unknown causes.[1317, 1318]
- Ebstein's anomaly of the tricuspid valve.[168]*bbbbb*
- Left ventricular false tendon.[527]*ccccc*
- Myocardial hamartomas[251, 1289, 1324] and other rare tumors,[1324, 1325] which cause many of the few cases of incessant ventricular tachycardia not due to surgery for congenital heart disease that develop in infants and young children.[244]
- Sarcoid heart disease.[1295]
- Scleroderma.[1286]
- Trauma.[1326]

General anesthesia. General anesthesia can suppress ventricular tachycardia.[1327]

PROGNOSIS

The prognosis of most patients with ventricular tachycardia was grave in the middle of the twentieth century.[22, 1328–1330]*ddddd*

---

*bbbbb*Intraoperative ablation obliterated the origin of the arrhythmia in the septal wall of the atrialized right ventricle in a patient with Ebstein's anomaly.[168]

*ccccc*A cause not accepted by all.[529]

*ddddd*His certain and accurate prediction that a favorite professor with ventricular tachycardia would soon die inspired Michel Mirowski to develop the implantable cardioverter-defibrillator.[1329, 1330]

- Twenty-eight (64%) of 42 patients whose ventricular tachycardia complicated myocardial infarction were dead within 1 month.
- Ten (42%) of 24 patients with ventricular tachycardia and "coronary sclerosis" (presumably, chronic coronary disease) were dead within 6 months after the first episode of the arrhythmia.
- Thirteen patients without structural heart disease, however, had a "very favorable prognosis."[22] Eight of 11 were alive and well from 9 to 21 years after the first attack, and in some, the paroxysms ceased spontaneously.

More recent studies confirm that ventricular tachycardia usually reduces survival, but in predicting mortality, ventricular function more than the arrhythmia separates the quick from the dead.

Factors Influencing Survival

Reduced ventricular function. The prognosis of patients with ventricular tachycardia, regardless of the etiology of the heart disease, depends foremost on ventricular function,[1331] whether determined by

- Left ventricular ejection fraction.[411, 624, 639, 1332–1335]
- New York Heart Association[69, 1336] or Killip[1337] classification.
- Severity of heart failure.[1336]
- The presence of Q waves or multiple previous infarctions in the electrocardiogram.[1337]

Coronary artery disease. Sudden cardiac death and total mortality in patients with hemodynamically stable sustained ventricular tachycardia are higher in those with multivessel coronary heart disease.[1284]

Electrophysiological induction.[671] Electrophysiological induction of ventricular tachycardia predicts shorter survival.[668, 1338–1340] Induction of the arrhythmia is, according to one report,[1341] the single best predictor of the subsequent occurrence of spontaneous ventricular tachycardia and sudden death in survivors of myocardial infarction. This finding predicts better than[1341]

- High-grade ectopy in ambulatory electrocardiogram.
- Late potentials in signal-averaged electrocardiogram.
- Positive exercise test.
- Reduced left ventricular ejection fraction from gated blood pool scan.

The probability of surviving for 1 year is significantly lower in patients with high-grade ventricular premature beats in whom ventricular tachycardia and ventricular fibrillation can be induced.[1342] The risk of dying suddenly increases seven times in patients who develop transient ventricular tachycardia and both inducible sustained ventricular tachycardia and an ejection fraction of 40% or less.[210]

In patients with dilated cardiomyopathy, initiation of sustained ventricular tachycardia or ventricular fibrillation does not predict subsequent sudden death.[647] Furthermore, even when tachyarrhythmias cannot be induced at electrophysiological study, patients with spontaneous ventricular tachycardia may still have recurrences, particularly if their ejection fraction is reduced[1335] or they have cardiomyopathy.[210] Those in whom therapy does not suppress induction of ventricular tachycardia live less long than those for whom adequate therapy can be developed.[1336, 1343] Induction of transient or sustained ventricular tachycardia or ventricular fibrillation in survivors of cardiac arrest independently predicts a potentially fatal recurrence.[1344]

Signal-averaged electrocardiogram. Fatal cardiac arrest is more likely to occur in patients who have late potentials on their signal-averaged electrocardiograms, many of whom have had spontaneous ventricular tachycardia.[411, 464, 465, 1340]

Exercise. Patients who have recovered from myocardial infarction and have spontaneous ventricular tachycardia reproduced by exercise testing and not due to ischemia have a high incidence of cardiac arrest.[317eeeee]

Treatment with drugs.[fffff] Mortality decreases in patients with ventricular tachycardia producing syncope or hemodynamic compromise when treatment with drugs suppresses high-grade ventricular ectopy on ambulatory monitoring[1331, 1345, 1346] and exercise testing.[1331, 1345] The risk of sudden cardiac death, but not total mortality, in patients with hemodynamically stable sustained ventricular tachycardia treated with antiarrhythmic drugs selected by electrophysiological study is low.[1284ggggg]

Treatment with metoprolol and with electrophysiologically guided antiarrhythmic therapy provides similar outcomes in patients with sustained ventricular arrhythmias.[724] Amiodarone decreases mortality during the first year after myocardial infarction in patients with asymptomatic transient ventricular tachycardia.[940] Occasionally, even incessant ventricular tachycardia spontaneously resolves and thus permits discontinuing treatment with antiarrhythmic drugs.[1347]

Coronary Heart Disease

During myocardial infarction. The 1-year prognosis of patients who have *transient* ventricular tachycardia during myocardial infarction is no worse than that of those who do not. Primary *sustained* ventricular tachycardia during myocardial infarction, however, carries a worse in-hospital[48, 50] and 2-month[1348] prognosis but not during the next year.[48]

After myocardial infarction. The prognosis of patients with transient ventricular tachycardia after recov-

ery from myocardial infarction seems worse than in those without the arrhythmia.[69, 1337hhhhh] Patients with the most severe underlying heart disease die sooner,[69, 1349iiiii] even if the electrophysiological study is negative.[1349] An ejection fraction of less than 30% predicts mortality better during the first 6 months after myocardial infarction, but ventricular arrhythmias predict better after 6 months.[1350]

The prognosis is worse for patients with sustained ventricular tachycardia occurring between 3 and 90 days after myocardial infarction who have[1351]

• Anterior myocardial infarction.
• Multivessel coronary disease.
• Three or more episodes of ventricular tachycardia.

Induction of sustained monomorphic ventricular tachycardia in survivors of myocardial infarction at particularly high risk of sudden death (those with left ventricular ejection fraction less than 41%, late potentials, or spontaneous complex ventricular arrhythmias) selects those most likely to suffer cardiac death or other arrhythmic events.[1352]

The prognosis of patients with sustained ventricular tachycardia is worse if they have had previous myocardial infarctions than if they have right ventricle dysplasia or no structural heart disease[1353] and, surprisingly, if the rate of ventricular tachycardia after myocardial infarction is slower.[1284]

Patients with transient ventricular tachycardia in whom sustained ventricular tachycardia cannot be induced have a relatively low probability of dying suddenly,[630, 1354] as do those in whom drugs can prevent the induction of sustained ventricular tachycardia.[630] The mortality is higher in patients with transient ventricular tachycardia who are elderly[1355] and have

• Cardiomyopathy.[396]
• Congestive heart failure.[396]
• Sustained ventricular tachycardia that can be persistently induced at electrophysiological study.[628, 630, 711, 1354]

When ventricular tachycardia or fibrillation complicates the course of myocardial infarction in children, the mortality rises from 59% to 80%.[62]

Angina. Ventricular tachycardia induced in patients with unstable angina predicts sudden death insensitively and nonspecifically.[1356]

Cardiomyopathy

Complex ventricular arrhythmias, including transient ventricular tachycardia, increase mortality in patients with both ischemic and nonischemic dilated cardiomyopathy.[1357] Normal signal-averaged electrocardiograms,[479] failure to induce sustained ventricular tachy-

---

eeeeeSix of 17 patients (35%).[317]
fffffThe data in this paragraph were collected before large, definitive studies established the superiority of implantable cardioverter-defibrillators for treating patients with sustained ventricular tachyarrhythmias. See Chapter 14 for further information.
ggggg2.4% per year in patients followed for 3 years.[1284]

hhhhhEleven of 132 patients (87%) without ventricular tachycardia were alive within 48 months, whereas 11 of 66 (75%) with ventricular tachycardia died.[69] The longest paroxysm of ventricular tachycardia in 47% of the patients was only 3 beats.[69]
iiiiiAs measured by their New York Heart Association functional classifications[69] or their left ventricular ejection fractions.[1349]

cardia,[210, 479] and empiric antiarrhythmic therapy[643] do not always imply a benign outcome in patients with idiopathic cardiomyopathy and sustained ventricular tachycardia.[643] However, the prognosis is favorable in these patients when drugs suppress induction of the arrhythmia.[643, 734]

Ventricular tachycardia, detected by ambulatory monitoring in patients with hypertrophic cardiomyopathy, identifies those at high risk of sudden death.[132] Patients with sustained ventricular tachycardia and arrhythmogenic right ventricular dysplasia generally have a favorable outcome.[407]

Congestive Heart Failure[1358, 1359]

Transient ventricular tachycardia predicts worse overall mortality in,[1360] and more sudden death of, patients with congestive heart failure, as would be expected because such patients have severely reduced left ventricular ejection fractions.[1361] The longer the duration of the longest episode of ventricular tachycardia on an ambulatory electrocardiographic tracing in patients with congestive heart failure due to nonischemic cardiomyopathy, the worse is the prognosis.[1362]

Hypertension

Transient ventricular tachycardia worsens the prognosis of patients with hypertension who have neither symptomatic coronary heart disease nor left ventricular dysfunction.[1363]

No Structural Heart Disease

Survival in patients with sustained or transient ventricular tachycardia and no structural heart disease is excellent even when such arrhythmias can be induced in the electrophysiological laboratory.[149, 194, 209, 322, 1364] However, the mortality when these patients are followed for many years[228]iiiii suggests that, in some cases, underlying, as yet undetected, heart disease such as cardiomyopathy may be present.[228, 236]

The cardiac morbidity and mortality are not increased in patients with asymptomatic transient ventricular tachycardia produced on exercise testing.[21]

After Cardiac Surgery

Sustained ventricular tachycardia occurs rarely for the first time after coronary artery bypass grafting.[170] When it does occur, the complication implies a poor prognosis for those patients who develop it, probably because the arrhythmia often indicates that intraoperative or postoperative acute myocardial infarction has occurred.[170] If the left ventricular ejection fraction is normal, however, complex ventricular arrhythmias, including transient ventricular tachycardia, after coronary artery bypass graft surgery do not worsen the prognosis.[174]

---

iiiiiThirteen percent over 8 years in 1 series of 24 young patients.[228]

Children

The prognosis for infants with ventricular tachycardia is excellent if the arrhythmia can be controlled by treatment.[246, 1365] In general, the outlook is good for children with the arrhythmia who are[246]

- Asymptomatic.
- Have no progressive myocardial disease.
- Survive for more than 6 months after diagnosis.

SUMMARY

Ventricular tachycardia is an uncommon arrhythmia that occurs more frequently in men than women. The arrhythmia appears briefly (transient ventricular tachycardia) or persistently (sustained or incessant ventricular tachycardia). The most common cause is chronic coronary heart disease, and many of these patients had ventricular aneurysms before the development of thrombolysis and acute angioplasty during myocardial infarction. Ventricular tachycardia also occurs in patients with cardiomyopathy, rheumatic heart disease, or no evidence of structural heart disease and occasionally in association with a variety of other cardiac conditions. Exercise induces ventricular tachycardia particularly in patients without structural heart disease.

Most episodes of ventricular tachycardia are transient and do not produce symptoms. Patients aware of the arrhythmia usually complain of rapid heart action. Chest pain, dyspnea, weakness, and neurological symptoms, including fainting, can also appear. The most characteristic physical finding is a rapid heart rate of an apparently regular tachyarrhythmia. Irregular, large A waves in the neck veins and changing intensity of the first heart sound, the systolic blood pressure, and systolic murmurs identify atrioventricular dissociation, which is characteristic of about half the cases of sustained ventricular tachycardia.

The electrocardiogram shows a rapid, sometimes slightly irregular, tachycardia with QRS complexes of greater than normal width and having the appearance of either right or left bundle branch block. The complexes may have constant (monomorphic) or changing (polymorphic) form. P waves identify atrioventricular dissociation when present. The arrhythmia can be differentiated from atrial or supraventricular tachycardia with aberrant conduction in most cases through the clinical history and physical examination and by careful review of the electrocardiogram. Ventricular tachycardia is the diagnosis when the width of the QRS complexes exceeds 0.14 second, or when atrioventricular dissociation, concordance, or fusion beat is present. Other specific features of the QRS complexes favor ventricular tachycardia. Late potentials are frequently seen during sinus rhythm in the signal-averaged electrocardiogram of patients with sustained ventricular tachycardia.

Many patients have severe hemodynamic distress during sustained and incessant ventricular tachycardia that produces many of the symptoms they observe. Hypotension and decreased ventricular function are frequent. Pathological ventricular endocardial tissue provides the substrate for the arrhythmia in those cases with structural heart disease.

Electrophysiological study shows that ventricular tachycardia is sustained most frequently by reentry and occasionally by triggered activity or automaticity. Ventricular pacing by programmed stimulation induces the arrhythmia in most patients with spontaneous sustained ventricular tachycardia. The efficacy of many antiarrhythmic drugs can be assessed by their ability to prevent induction. Sustained ventricular tachycardia can be induced in some symptomatic patients with transient ventricular tachycardia. Programmed stimulation often terminates ventricular tachycardia.

Intravenous antiarrhythmic drugs and electric shock convert most episodes of spontaneous sustained or incessant ventricular tachycardia. Long-term treatment should be developed through electrophysiological study, which usually leads to implantation of implantable cardioverter-defibrillators in patients with sustained ventricular tachycardia. Most patients with transient ventricular tachycardia do not require specific treatment unless they have severe symptoms or reduced ventricular function.

The prognosis of patients with recurrent ventricular tachycardia depends primarily on their ventricular function. Consequently, survival is excellent in those with transient or sustained ventricular tachycardia and no structural heart disease, but it worsens as ventricular function deteriorates from myocardial infarctions, cardiomyopathy, or other diseases.

REFERENCES

1. Josephson ME, Callans DJ. Sustained ventricular tachycardia. In Kastor JA (ed). Arrhythmias. Philadelphia: WB Saunders, 1994, pp. 336–362.
2. Buxton AE. Transient ventricular tachycardia. In Kastor JA (ed). Arrhythmias. Philadelphia: WB Saunders, 1994, pp. 363–375.
3. Josephson ME. Ventricular Tachycardia. Mechanisms and Management. Mount Kisco, NY: Futura Publishing Co., 1982.
4. Buxton AE, Josephson ME. Ventricular tachycardia: 1983. PACE 1984; 7:96–108.
5. Josephson ME, Wellens HJJ. Tachycardias. Mechanisms, Diagnosis, Treatment. Philadelphia: Lea & Febiger, 1984.
6. McGovern B, Schoenfeld MH, Ruskin JN, Garan H, Yurchak JN. Ventricular tachycardia: historical perspective. PACE 1986; 9:449–462.
7. Kastor JA. Ventricular tachycardia. Clin Cardiol 1989; 12:586–599.
8. Garson A Jr. Ventricular arrhythmias. In Gillette PC, Garson A Jr (eds). Pediatric Arrhythmias: Electrophysiology and Pacing. Philadelphia: WB Saunders, 1990, pp. 427–500.
9. Prystowsky EN, Klein GJ. Ventricular tachycardia. In Prystowsky EN, Klein GJ (eds). Cardiac Arrhythmias. An Integrated Approach for the Clinician. New York: McGraw-Hill, 1994, pp. 155–177.
10. Prystowsky EN, Klein GJ. Sustained monomorphic ventricular tachycardia. In Prystowsky EN, Klein GJ (eds). Cardiac Arrhythmias. An Integrated Approach for the Clinician. New York: McGraw-Hill, 1994, pp. 179–210.
11. Mandel WJ. Sustained monomorphic ventricular tachycardia. In Podrid PJ, Kowey PR (eds). Cardiac Arrhythmia.
Mechanisms, Diagnosis and Management. Baltimore: Williams & Wilkins, 1995, pp. 919–935.
12. Sodowick BC, Buxton AE. Clinical significance of nonsustained ventricular tachycardia. In Podrid PJ, Kowey PR (eds). Cardiac Arrhythmia. Mechanisms, Diagnosis and Management. Baltimore: Williams & Wilkins, 1995, pp. 907–918.
13. Scherlag BJ, Lau SH, Helfant RH, Berkowitz WD, Stein E, Damato AN. Catheter technique for recording His bundle activity in man. Circulation 1969; 39:13–18.
14. Wellens HJJ, Schuilenburg RM, Durrer D. Electrical stimulation of the heart in patients with ventricular tachycardia. Circulation 1972; 46:216–226.
15. Josephson ME, Horowitz LN, Farshidi A, Kastor JA. Recurrent sustained ventricular tachycardia. I. Mechanisms. Circulation 1978; 57:431–440.
16. Packard JM, Graettinger JS, Graybiel A. Analysis of the electrocardiograms obtained from 1,000 young healthy aviators: ten year follow-up. Circulation 1954; 10:384–400.
17. Hiss RG, Lamb LE. Electrocardiographic findings in 122,043 individuals. Circulation 1962; 25:947–961.
18. Ostrander LD Jr, Brandt RL, Kjelsberg MO, Epstein FH. Electrocardiographic findings among the adult population of a total natural community, Tecumseh, Michigan. Circulation 1965; 31:888–898.
19. Williams C, Ellis LB. Ventricular tachycardia: an analysis of thirty-six cases. Arch Intern Med 1943; 71:137–156.
20. Katz LN, Pick A. Clinical Electrocardiography. Part I. The Arrhythmias. Philadelphia: Lea & Febiger, 1956, p. 43.
21. Fleg JL, Lakatta EG. Prevalence and prognosis of exercise-induced nonsustained ventricular tachycardia in apparently healthy volunteers. Am J Cardiol 1984; 54:762–764.
22. Armbrust CA, Levine SA. Paroxysmal ventricular tachycardia: a study of one hundred and seven cases. Circulation 1950; 1:28–40.
23. Morady F, Shen EN, Bhandari A, Schwartz AB, Scheinman MM. Clinical symptoms in patients with sustained ventricular tachycardia. West J Med 1985; 142:341–344.
24. Manolio TA, Furberg CD, Rautaharju PM, et al. Cardiac arrhythmias on 24-h ambulatory electrocardiography in older women and men: the cardiovascular health study. J Am Coll Cardiol 1994; 23:916–925.
25. Radford DJ, Izukawa T, Rowe RD. Evaluation of children with ventricular arrhythmias. Arch Dis Child 1977; 52:345–353.
26. Van Hare GF, Stanger P. Ventricular tachycardia and accelerated ventricular rhythm presenting in the first month of life. Am J Cardiol 1991; 67:42–45.
27. Pfammatter JP, Paul T, Kallfelz HC. Recurrent ventricular tachycardia in asymptomatic young children with an apparently normal heart. Eur J Pediatr 1995; 154:513–517.
28. Perry JC. Ventricular tachycardia in neonates. Pacing Clin Electrophysiol 1997; 20:2061–2064.
29. Benson DWJ, Smith WM, Dunnigan A, Sterba R, Gallagher JJ. Mechanisms of regular, wide QRS tachycardia in infants and children. Am J Cardiol 1982; 49:1778–1788.
30. Mitra RL, Buxton AE. The clinical significance of nonsustained ventricular tachycardia. J Cardiovasc Electrophysiol 1993; 4:490–496.
31. Buxton AE. Nonsustained ventricular tachycardia: clinical significance and mechanisms. In Josephson ME, Wellens HJJ (eds). Tachycardias. Mechanisms and Management. Mount Kisco, NY: Futura Publishing Co., 1993, pp. 257–272.
32. Pires LA, Huang SKS. Nonsustained ventricular tachycardia: identification and management of high-risk patients. Am Heart J 1993; 126:189–200.
33. Kinder C, Tamburro P, Kopp D, Kall J, Olshansky B, Wilber D. The clinical significance of nonsustained ventricular tachycardia: current perspectives. PACE 1994; 17:637–664.
34. Rahilly GT, Prystowsky EN, Zipes DP, Naccarelli GV, Jackman WM, Heger JJ. Clinical and electrophysiologic findings in patients with repetitive monomorphic ventricular tachycardia and otherwise normal electrocardiogram. Am J Cardiol 1982; 50:459–468.
35. Parkinson J, Papp C. Repetitive paroxysmal tachycardia. Br Heart J 1947; 9:241–262.

36. Cass RM. Repetitive tachycardia: a review of 40 cases with no demonstrable heart disease. Am J Cardiol 1967; 19:597–602.

37. Chung K-Y, Walsh TJ, Massie E. Ventricular parasystolic tachycardia. Br Heart J 1965; 27:392–400.

38. Roelandt J, Schamroth L. Parasystolic ventricular tachycardia: observations on differential stimulus threshold as possible mechanism for exit block. Br Heart J 1971; 505–527.

39. Jacobson LB. Spontaneous ventricular parasystole initiating ventricular tachycardia. J Electrocardiol 1973; 6:63–70.

40. Bhandari AK, Hong RA, Rahimtoola SH. Triggered activity as a mechanism of recurrent ventricular tachycardia. Br Heart J 1988; 59:501–505.

41. Sakurai M, Nishiono T, Yoshida I, Kato N, Yasuda H. Mechanisms of chronic recurrent idiopathic ventricular tachycardia. Jpn Circ J 1988; 52:272–279.

42. Nakagawa H, Mukai J, Nagata K, et al. Early afterdepolarizations in a patient with idiopathic monomorphic right ventricular tachycardia. Pacing Clin Electrophysiol 1993; 16:2067–2072.

43. Wilde AA, Duren DR, Hauer RN, et al. Mitral valve prolapse and ventricular arrhythmias: observations in a patient with a 20-year history. J Cardiovasc Electrophysiol 1997; 8:307–316.

44. Lown B, Temte JV, Arter WJ. Ventricular tachyarrhythmias: clinical aspects. Circulation 1973; 47:1364–1381.

45. Breithardt G, Borggrefe M, Podczeck A. Has the clinical presentation of ventricular tachycardia changed? In Breithardt G, Borggrefe M, Zipes DP (eds). Nonpharmacological Therapy of Tachyarrhythmias. Mount Kisco, NY: Futura Publishing Co., 1987, pp. 51–63.

46. Callans DJ, Josephson ME. Ventricular tachycardias in the setting of coronary artery disease. In Zipes DP, Jalife J (eds). Cardiac Electrophysiology. From Cell to Bedside. 2nd ed. Philadelphia: WB Saunders, 1995, pp. 732–743.

47. DeSanctis RW, Block P, Hutter AM Jr. Tachyarrhythmias in myocardial infarction. Circulation 1972; 45:681–702.

48. Eldar M, Sievner Z, Goldbourt U, Reicher-Reiss H, Kaplinsky E, Behar S. Primary ventricular tachycardia in acute myocardial infarction: clinical characteristics and mortality: the SPRINT study group. Ann Intern Med 1992; 117:31–36.

49. Taylor GJ, Crampton RS, Gibson RS, Stebbins PT, Waldman MTG, Beller GA. Prolonged QT interval at onset of acute myocardial infarction in predicting early phase ventricular tachycardia. Am Heart J 1981; 102:16–24.

50. Cinca J, Blanch P, Blanco J, Figueras J, Brotons C, Soler-Soler J. Predisposing factors and prognostic value of sustained monomorphic ventricular tachycardia in the early phase of acute myocardial infarction. J Am Coll Cardiol 1996; 28:1670–1676.

51. Nielsen BL, Dalsgaard P, Nielsen JS, Thayssen P, Thygesen K. ST-segment elevation in acute myocardial infarction: correlation between ST-segment elevation and the serum enzyme values. Dan Med Bull 1975; 22:113–119.

52. Herlitz J, Hjalmarson A, Swedberg K, Waagstein F, Holmberg S, Waldenstrom J. Relationship between infarct size and incidence of severe ventricular arrhythmias in a double-blind trial with metoprolol in acute myocardial infarction. Int J Cardiol 1984; 6:47–60.

53. Chapman BL. Relation of cardiac complications to SGOT level in acute myocardial infarction. Br Heart J 1972; 34:890–896.

54. de Soyza N, Bissett JK, Kane JJ, Murphy ML, Doherty JE. Ectopic ventricular prematurity and its relationship to ventricular tachycardia in acute myocardial infarction in man. Circulation 1974; 50:529–533.

55. Zehender M, Kasper W, Kauder E, et al. Right ventricular infarction as an independent predictor of prognosis after acute inferior myocardial infarction. N Engl J Med 1993; 328:981–988.

56. Miller FC, Krucoff MW, Satler LF, et al. Ventricular arrhythmias during reperfusion. Am Heart J 1986; 112:928–932.

57. Wilcox RG, Eastgate J, Harrison E, Skene AM. Ventricular arrhythmias during treatment with alteplase (recombinant tissue plasminogen activator) in suspected acute myocardial infarction. Br Heart J 1991; 65:4–8.

58. Six AJ, Louwerenburg JH, Kingma JH, Robles de Medina EO, van Hemel NM. Predictive value of ventricular arrhythmias for patency of the infarct-related coronary artery after thrombolytic therapy. Br Heart J 1991; 66:143–146.

59. Gressin V, Louvard Y, Pezzano M, Lardoux H. Holter recording of ventricular arrhythmias during intravenous thrombolysis for acute myocardial infarction. Am J Cardiol 1992; 69:152–159.

60. Solomon SD, Ridker PM, Antman EM. Ventricular arrhythmias in trials of thrombolytic therapy for acute myocardial infarction: a meta-analysis. Circulation 1993; 88:2575–2581.

61. Berger PB, Ruocco NA, Ryan TJ, Frederick MM, Podrid PJ. Incidence and significance of ventricular idiopathic tachycardia and fibrillation in the absence of hypotension or heart failure in acute myocardial infarction treated with recombinant tissue-type plasminogen activator: results from the Thrombolysis in Myocardial Infarction (TIMI) Phase II Trial. J Am Coll Cardiol 1993; 22:1773–1779.

62. Johnsrude CL, Towbin JA, Cecchin F, Perry JC. Postinfarction ventricular arrhythmias in children. Am Heart J 1995; 129:1171–1177.

63. Andresen D, Bruggemann T, Behrens S, Ehlers C. Risk of ventricular arrhythmias in survivors of myocardial infarction. Pacing Clin Electrophysiol 1997; 20:2699–2705.

64. Moller M, Nielsen BL, Fabricius J. Paroxysmal ventricular tachycardia during repeated 24-hour ambulatory electrocardiographic monitoring of postmyocardial infarction patients. Br Heart J 1980; 43:447–453.

65. Bigger JT Jr, Weld FM, Rolnitzky LM. Prevalence, characteristics and significance of ventricular tachycardia (three or more complexes) detected with ambulatory electrocardiographic recording in the late hospital phase of acute myocardial infarction. Am J Cardiol 1981; 48:815–823.

66. Bigger JT Jr, Fleiss JL, Rolnitzky LM, Multicenter Post-Infarction Research Group. Prevalence, characteristics and significance of ventricular tachycardia detected by 24-hour continuous electrocardiographic recordings in the late hospital phase of acute myocardial infarction. Am J Cardiol 1986; 58:1151–1160.

67. Denes P, Gillis AM, Pawitan Y, et al. Prevalence, characteristics and significance of ventricular premature complexes and ventricular tachycardia detected by 24-hour continuous electrocardiographic recording in the Cardiac Arrhythmia Suppression Trial. Am J Cardiol 1991; 68:887–896.

68. Kleiger RE, Miller JP, Thanavaro S, Province MA, Martin TF, Oliver GC. Relationship between clinical features of acute myocardial infarction and ventricular runs 2 weeks to 1 year after infarction. Circulation 1981; 63:64–70.

69. Anderson KP, DeCamilla J, Moss AJ. Clinical significance of ventricular tachycardia (3 beats or longer) detected during ambulatory monitoring after myocardial infarction. Circulation 1978; 57:890–897.

70. Marchlinski FE, Waxman HL, Buxton AE, Josephson ME. Sustained ventricular tachyarrhythmias during the early postinfarction period: electrophysiologic findings and prognosis for survival. J Am Coll Cardiol 1983; 2:240–250.

71. Kleiman RB, Miller JM, Buxton AE, Josephson ME, Marchlinski FE. Prognosis following sustained ventricular tachycardia occurring early after myocardial infarction. Am J Cardiol 1988; 62:528–533.

72. Cohen M, Wiener I, Pichard A, Holt J, Smith H Jr, Gorlin R. Determinants of ventricular tachycardia in patients with coronary artery disease and ventricular aneurysm: clinical, hemodynamic, and angiographic factors. Am J Cardiol 1983; 51:61–64.

73. Braat SH, de Zwaan C, Brugada P, Wellens HJJ. Value of left ventricular ejection fraction in extensive anterior infarction to predict development of ventricular tachycardia. Am J Cardiol 1983; 52:686–689.

74. Miller JM, Marchlinski FE, Harken AH, Hargrove WC, Josephson ME. Subendocardial resection for sustained ventricular tachycardia in the early period after acute myocardial infarction. Am J Cardiol 1985; 55:980–984.

75. Theroux P, Morissette D, Juneau M, de Guise P, Pelletier G, Waters DD. Influence of fibrinolysis and percutaneous transluminal coronary angioplasty on the frequency of ventricular premature complexes. Am J Cardiol 1989; 63:797–801.

76. Bryson AL, Parisi AF, Schechter E, Wolfson S. Life-threatening ventricular arrhythmias induced by exercise: cessation after coronary bypass surgery. Am J Cardiol 1973; 32:995–999.

77. Talbot S, Kilpatrick D, Krikler D, Oakley CM. Ventricular tachycardia due to cardiac ischaemia: assessment by exercise electrocardiography. BMJ 1978; 2:733–736.

78. Mokotoff DM, Quinones MA, Miller RR. Exercise-induced ventricular tachycardia: clinical features, relation to chronic ventricular ectopy, and prognosis. Chest 1980; 77:10–16.

79. Baltazar R, Mower MM, Salomon J, Labib A. Exertional ventricular tachycardia. Am Heart J 1981; 101:354–355.

80. Molajo AO, Summers GD, Bennett DH. Effect of percutaneous transluminal coronary angioplasty on arrhythmias complicating angina. Br Heart J 1985; 54:375–377.

81. Berntsen RF, Gunnes P, Rasmussen K. Pattern of coronary artery disease in patients with ventricular tachycardia and fibrillation exposed by exercise-induced ischemia. Am Heart J 1995; 129:733–738.

82. Pedersen F, Pietersen A, Sandoe E. Silent myocardial ischaemia and life threatening ventricular arrhythmias. Ann Clin Res 1988; 20:404–409.

83. Nordstrom LA, Lillehei JP, Adicoff A, Sako Y, Gobel FL. Coronary artery surgery for recurrent ventricular arrhythmias in patients with variant angina. Am Heart J 1975; 89:236–241.

84. Kerin NZ, Rubenfire M, Naini M, Wajszczuk WJ, Pamatmat A, Cascade PN. Arrhythmias in variant angina pectoris: relationship of arrhythmias to ST-segment elevation and R-wave changes. Circulation 1979; 60:1343–1350.

85. Kerin NZ, Rubenfire M, Willens HJ, Rao P, Cascade PN. The mechanism of dysrhythmias in variant angina pectoris: occlusive versus reperfusion. Am Heart J 1983; 106:1332–1340.

86. Previtali M, Klersy C, Salerno JA, et al. Ventricular tachyarrhythmias in Prinzmetal's variant angina: clinical significance and relation to the degree and time course of S-T segment elevation. Am J Cardiol 1983; 52:19–25.

87. Szlachcic J, Waters DD, Miller D, Theroux P. Ventricular arrhythmias during ergonovine-induced episodes of variant angina. Am Heart J 1984; 107:20–24.

88. Gorfinkel HJ, Inglesby TV, Lansing AM, Goodin RR. ST-segment elevation, transient left-posterior hemiblock, and recurrent ventricular arrhythmias unassociated with pain. Ann Intern Med 1973; 79:795–799.

89. Myerburg RJ, Kessler KM, Mallon SM, et al. Life-threatening ventricular arrhythmias in patients with silent myocardial ischemia due to coronary artery spasm. N Engl J Med 1992; 326:1451–1455.

90. Couch OA. Cardiac aneurysm with ventricular tachycardia and subsequent excision of aneurysm: case report. Circulation 1959; 10:251–253.

91. Hunt D, Sloman G, Westlake G. Ventricular aneurysmectomy for recurrent tachycardia. Br Heart J 1969; 31:264–266.

92. Magidson O. Resection of postmyocardial infarction ventricular aneurysms for cardiac arrhythmias. Dis Chest 1969; 56:211–218.

93. Ritter ER. Intractable ventricular tachycardia due to ventricular aneurysm with surgical cure. Ann Intern Med 1969; 71:1155–1157.

94. Maloy WC, Arrants JE, Sowell BF, Hendrix GH. Left ventricular aneurysm of uncertain etiology with recurrent ventricular arrhythmias. N Engl J Med 1971; 285:662–663.

95. Schlesinger Z, Lieberman Y, Neufeld HN. Ventricular aneurysmectomy for severe rhythm disturbances. J Thorac Cardiovasc Surg 1971; 61:602–604.

96. Thind GS, Blakemore WS, Zinsser HF. Ventricular aneurysmectomy for the treatment of recurrent ventricular tachyarrhythmia. Am J Cardiol 1971; 27:690–694.

97. Lull RJ, Dunn BE, Gregoratos G, Cox WA, Fisher GW. Ventricular aneurysm due to cardiac sarcoidosis with surgical cure of refractory ventricular tachycardia. Am J Cardiol 1972; 30:282–287.

98. Wardekar A, Son B, Gosaynie CD, Bercu B. Recurrent ventricular tachycardia successfully treated by excision of ventricular aneurysm. Chest 1972; 62:505–508.

99. Basta LL, Takeshita A, Theilen EO, Ehrenhaft JL. Aneurysmectomy in treatment of ventricular and supraventricular tachyarrhythmias in patients with postinfarction and traumatic ventricular aneurysms. Am J Cardiol 1973; 32:693–699.

100. Graham AF, Miller DC, Stinson EB, Daily PO, Fogarty TJ, Harrison DC. Surgical treatment of refractory life-threatening ventricular tachycardia. Am J Cardiol 1973; 32:909–912.

101. Poblete PF, Mendez AM, Zubiate P, Gray R, Kay JH. Surgery for ventricular tachycardia unresponsive to medical treatment. Chest 1973; 64:574–578.

102. Kenaan G, Mendez AM, Zubiate P, Gray R, Kay JH. Surgery for ventricular tachycardia unresponsive to medical treatment. Chest 1973; 64:574–578.

103. Welch TG, Fontana ME, Vasko JS. Aneurysmectomy for recurrent ventricular tachyarrhythmias. Am Heart J 1973; 85:685–688.

104. Winkle RA, Alderman EL, Fitzgerald JW, Harrison DC. Treatment of recurrent symptomatic ventricular tachycardia. Ann Intern Med 1976; 85:1–7.

105. Ricks WB, Winkle RA, Shumway NE, Harrison DC. Surgical management of life-threatening ventricular arrhythmias in patients with coronary artery disease. Circulation 1977; 56:38–42.

106. Sami M, Chaitman BR, Bourassa MG, Charpin D, Chabot M. Long term follow-up of aneurysmectomy for recurrent ventricular tachycardia or fibrillation. Am Heart J 1978; 96:303–308.

107. Buda AJ, Stinson EB, Harrison DC. Surgery for life-threatening ventricular tachyarrhythmias. Am J Cardiol 1979; 44:1171–1177.

108. Wald RW, Waxman MB, Corey PN, Gunstensen J, Goldman BS. Management of intractable ventricular tachyarrhythmias after myocardial infarction. Am J Cardiol 1979; 44:329–336.

109. Mason JW, Stinson EB, Winkle RA, et al. Surgery for ventricular tachycardia: efficacy of left ventricular aneurysm resection compared with operation guided by electrical activation mapping. Circulation 1982; 65:1148–1155.

110. Miller JM, Vassallo JA, Kussmaul WG III, et al. Anterior left ventricular aneurysm: factors associated with the development of sustained ventricular tachycardia. J Am Coll Cardiol 1988; 12:375–382.

111. Hochman JS, Brooks MM, Morris M, Ahmad T, CAST Investigators. Prognostic significance of left ventricular aneurysm in the Cardiac Arrhythmia Suppression Trial (CAST) population. Am Heart J 1994; 127:824–832.

112. Aronow WS, Epstein S, Schwartz KS, Koenigsberg M. Correlation of complex ventricular arrhythmias detected by ambulatory electrocardiographic monitoring with echocardiographic left ventricular hypertrophy in persons older than 62 years in a long-term health care facility. Am J Cardiol 1987; 60:730–732.

113. McLenachan JM, Henderson E, Morris KI, Dargie HJ. Ventricular arrhythmias in patients with hypertensive left ventricular hypertrophy. N Engl J Med 1987; 317:787–792.

114. Brachmann J, Hilbel T, Grunig E, Benz A, Haass M, Kubler W. Ventricular arrhythmias in dilated cardiomyopathy. PACE 1997; 20:2714–2718.

115. Roelke M, Ruskin JN. Dilated cardiomyopathy: ventricular arrhythmias and sudden death. In Zipes DP, Jalife J (eds). Cardiac Electrophysiology. From Cell to Bedside. 2nd ed. Philadelphia: WB Saunders, 1995, pp. 744–753.

116. Pedersen DH, Zipes DP, Foster PR, Troup PJ. Ventricular tachycardia and ventricular fibrillation in a young population. Circulation 1979; 60:988–997.

117. Naccarelli GV, Prystowsky EN, Jackman WM, Heger JJ, Rahilly GT, Zipes DP. Role of electrophysiologic testing in

managing patients who have ventricular tachycardia unrelated to coronary artery disease. Am J Cardiol 1982; 50:165–171.

118. Huang SK, Messer JV, Denes P. Significance of ventricular tachycardia in idiopathic dilated cardiomyopathy: observations in 35 patients. Am J Cardiol 1983; 51:507–512.

119. Maskin CS, Siskind SJ, LeJemtel TH. High prevalence of nonsustained ventricular tachycardia in severe congestive heart failure. Am Heart J 1984; 107:896–901.

120. Poll DS, Marchlinski FE, Falcone RA, Josephson ME, Simson MB. Abnormal signal-averaged electrocardiograms in patients with nonischemic congestive cardiomyopathy: relationship to sustained ventricular tachyarrhythmias. Circulation 1985; 72:1308–1313.

121. Turitto G, Ahuja RK, Bekheit S, Caref EB, Ibrahim B, el-Sherif N. Incidence and prediction of induced ventricular tachyarrhythmias in idiopathic dilated cardiomyopathy. Am J Cardiol 1994; 73:770–773.

122. Fyfe DA, Gillette PC, Crawford FA Jr, Kline CH. Resolution of dilated cardiomyopathy after surgical ablation of ventricular tachycardia in a child. J Am Coll Cardiol 1987; 9:231–234.

123. Rakovec P, Lajovic J, Dolenc M. Reversible congestive cardiomyopathy due to chronic ventricular tachycardia. Pacing Clin Electrophysiol 1989; 12:542–545.

124. Jaggarao NS, Nanda AS, Daubert JP. Ventricular tachycardia induced cardiomyopathy: improvement with radiofrequency ablation. Pacing Clin Electrophysiol 1996; 19:505–508.

125. Singh B, Kaul U, Talwar KK, Wasir HS. Reversibility of "tachycardia induced cardiomyopathy" following the cure of idiopathic left ventricular tachycardia using radiofrequency energy. Pacing Clin Electrophysiol 1996; 19:1391–1392.

126. Ma JS, Kim BJ, Cho JG. Verapamil responsive incessant ventricular tachycardia resulting in severe ventricular dysfunction in a young child: successful management with oral verapamil. Heart 1997; 77:286–287.

127. Vijgen J, Hill P, Biblo LA, Carlson MD. Tachycardia-induced cardiomyopathy secondary to right ventricular outflow tract ventricular tachycardia: improvement of left ventricular systolic function after radiofrequency catheter ablation of the arrhythmia. J Cardiovasc Electrophysiol 1997; 8:445–450.

128. Anselme F, Boyle N, Josephson M. Incessant fascicular tachycardia: a cause of arrhythmia induced cardiomyopathy. PACE 1998; 21:760–763.

129. Fananapazir L, McAreavey D, Epstein ND. Hypertrophic cardiomyopathy. In Zipes DP, Jalife J (eds). Cardiac Electrophysiology. From Cell to Bedside. 2nd ed. Philadelphia: WB Saunders 1995, pp. 769–779.

130. Kuck KH. Arrhythmias in hypertrophic cardiomyopathy. PACE 1997; 20:2706–2713.

131. Doi YL, McKenna WJ, Chetty S, Oakley CM, Goodwin JF. Prediction of mortality and serious ventricular arrhythmia in hypertrophic cardiomyopathy: an echocardiographic study. Br Heart J 1980; 44:150–157.

132. Maron BJ, Savage DD, Wolfson JK, Epstein SE. Prognostic significance of 24 hour ambulatory electrocardiographic monitoring in patients with hypertrophic cardiomyopathy: a prospective study. Am J Cardiol 1981; 48:252–257.

133. Frank MJ, Watkins LO, Prisant LM, Stefadouros MA, Abdulla AM. Potentially lethal arrhythmias and their management in hypertrophic cardiomyopathy. Am J Cardiol 1984; 53:1608–1613.

134. Mulrow JP, Healy MJ, McKenna WJ. Variability of ventricular arrhythmias in hypertrophic cardiomyopathy and implications for treatment. Am J Cardiol 1986; 58:615–618.

135. Maron BJ, Bonow RO, Cannon RO, Leon MB, Epstein SE. Hypertrophic cardiomyopathy: interrelations of clinical manifestations, pathophysiology, and therapy. N Engl J Med 1987; 316:780–789.

136. Alfonso F, Frenneaux MP, McKenna WJ. Clinical sustained uniform ventricular tachycardia in hypertrophic cardiomyopathy: association with left ventricular apical aneurysm. Br Heart J 1989; 61:178–181.

137. Lorenzoni R, Gistri R, Cecchi F, et al. Syncope and ventricular arrhythmias in hypertrophic cardiomyopathy are not related to the derangement of coronary microvascular function. Eur Heart J 1997; 18:1946–1950.

138. Dritsas A, Gilligan D, Sbarouni E, Oakley CM, Nihoyannopoulos P. Influence of left ventricular hypertrophy and function on the occurrence of ventricular tachycardia in hypertrophic cardiomyopathy. Am J Cardiol 1992; 70:913–916.

139. Fontaine G. "Dysplasia" rehabilitated. Eur Heart J 1990; 11:678.

140. McLay JS, Norris A, Campbell RW, Kerr F. Arrhythmogenic right ventricular dysplasia: an uncommon cause of ventricular tachycardia in young and old? Br Heart J 1993; 69:158–160.

141. Fontaine G, Fontaliran F, Lascault G, Aouate P, Tonet J, Frank R. Arrhythmogenic right ventricular dysplasia. In Zipes DP, Jalife J (eds). Cardiac Electrophysiology. From Cell to Bedside. 2nd ed. Philadelphia: WB Saunders, 1995, pp. 754–769.

142. Fontaine G, Fontaliran F, Frank R. Arrhythmogenic right ventricular cardiomyopathies: clinical forms and main differential diagnoses. Circulation 1998; 97:1532–1535.

143. Furlanello F, Bettini R, Bertoldi A, et al. Arrhythmia patterns in athletes with arrhythmogenic right ventricular dysplasia. Eur Heart J 1989; 10:16–19.

144. Dungan WT, Garson A Jr, Gillette PC. Arrhythmogenic right ventricular dysplasia: a cause of ventricular tachycardia in children with apparently normal hearts. Am Heart J 1981; 102:745–750.

145. Marcus FI, Fontaine GH, Guiraudon G, et al. Right ventricular dysplasia: a report of 24 adult cases. Circulation 1982; 65:384–398.

146. Solomon SL, Van Osdol KD, Massumi A, Warda M, Hall RJ. Exercise-induced right ventricular tachycardia and arrhythmogenic right ventricular dysplasia: electrophysiologic and therapeutic considerations. Texas Heart Inst J 1983; 10:351–357.

147. Blomstrom-Lundqvist C, Sabel KG, Olsson SB. A long term follow up of 15 patients with arrhythmogenic right ventricular dysplasia. Br Heart J 1987; 58:477–488.

148. Leclercq JF, Coumel P. Characteristics, prognosis and treatment of the ventricular arrhythmias of right ventricular dysplasia. Eur Heart J 1989; 10:61–67.

149. Lemery R, Brugada P, Janssen J, Cheriex E, Dugernier T, Wellens HJJ. Nonischemic sustained ventricular tachycardia: clinical outcome in 12 patients with arrhythmogenic right ventricular dysplasia. J Am Coll Cardiol 1989; 14:96–105.

150. Leor J, Glikson M, Vered Z, Kaplinsky E, Motro M. Ventricular tachycardia after soccer ball blow to the chest: first manifestation of arrhythmogenic right ventricular dysplasia in two brothers. Am J Med 1990; 89:687–688.

151. Hoch DH, Rosenfeld LE. Tachycardias of right ventricular origin. Cardiol Clin 1992; 10:151–164.

152. Wichter T, Borggrefe M, Haverkamp W, Chen X, Breithardt G. Efficacy of antiarrhythmic drugs in patients with arrhythmogenic right ventricular disease: results in patients with inducible and noninducible ventricular tachycardia. Circulation 1992; 86:29–37.

153. Dalal P, Fujisic K, Hupart P, Schwietzer P. Arrhythmogenic right ventricular dysplasia: a review. Cardiology 1994; 85:361–369.

154. Marcus FI, Fontaine G. Arrhythmogenic right ventricular dysplasia/cardiomyopathy: a review. Pacing Clin Electrophysiol 1995; 18:1298–1314.

155. Peeters HA, Sippens Groenewegen A, Schoonderwoerd BA, et al. Body-surface QRST integral mapping: arrhythmogenic right ventricular dysplasia versus idiopathic right ventricular tachycardia. Circulation 1997; 95:2668–2676.

156. Furlanello F, Bertoldi A, Dallago M, et al. Cardiac arrest and sudden death in competitive athletes with arrhythmogenic right ventricular dysplasia. PACE 1998; 21:331–335.

157. Winters SL, Cohen M, Greenberg S, et al. Sustained ventricular tachycardia associated with sarcoidosis: assessment of the underlying cardiac anatomy and the prospective utility of programmed ventricular stimulation, drug therapy and an implantable antitachycardia device. J Am Coll Cardiol 1991; 18:937–943.

158. Haese WH, Maron BJ, Mirowski M, Rowe RD, Hutchins GM.

Peculiar focal myocardial degeneration and fatal ventricular arrhythmias in a child. N Engl J Med 1972; 287:180–181.

159. Negri SM, Cowan MD. Becker muscular dystrophy with bundle branch reentry ventricular tachycardia. J Cardiovasc Electrophysiol 1998; 9:652–654.

160. Campbell RWF, Godman MG, Fiddler GI, Marquis RM, Julian DG. Ventricular arrhythmias in syndrome of balloon deformity of mitral valve: definition of possible high risk group. Br Heart J 1976; 38:1053–1057.

161. Wei JY, Bulkley BH, Schaeffer AH, Greene HL, Reid PR. Mitral-valve prolapse syndrome and recurrent ventricular tachyarrhythmias: a malignant variant refractory to conventional drug therapy. Ann Intern Med 1978; 89:6–9.

162. Engel TR, Meister SG, Frankl WS. Ventricular extrastimulation in the mitral valve prolapse syndrome: evidence for ventricular reentry. J Electrocardiology 1978; 11:137–142.

163. Kavey R-EW, Sondheimer HM, Blackman MS. Detection of dysrhythmia in pediatric patients with mitral valve prolapse. Circulation 1980; 62:582–587.

164. Rocchini AP, Chun PKC, Dick M. Ventricular tachycardia in children. Am J Cardiol 1981; 47:1091–1097.

165. Kligfield P, Hochreiter C, Kramer H, et al. Complex arrhythmias in mitral regurgitation with and without mitral valve prolapse: contrast to arrhythmias in mitral valve prolapse without mitral regurgitation. Am J Cardiol 1985; 55:1545–1549.

166. Babuty D, Cosnay P, Breuillac JC, et al. Ventricular arrhythmia factors in mitral valve prolapse. Pacing Clin Electrophysiol 1994; 17:1090–1099.

167. Kosmas CE, Dalessandro DA, Langieri G, et al. Monomorphic right ventricular tachycardia in a patient with mitral valve prolapse. Pacing Clin Electrophysiol 1996; 19:509–513.

168. Lo H-M, Lin F-Y, Jong Y-S, Tseng Y-Z, Wu T-L. Ebstein's anomaly with ventricular tachycardia: evidence for the arrhythmogenic role of the atrialized ventricle. Am Heart J 1989; 117:959–962.

169. Fontaine JM, Kamal BM, Sokil AB, Wolf NM. Ventricular tachycardia: a life-threatening arrhythmia in a patient with congenitally corrected transposition of the great arteries. J Cardiovasc Electrophysiol 1998; 9:517–522.

170. Pires LA, Wagshal AB, Lancey R, Huang SK. Arrhythmias and conduction disturbances after coronary artery bypass graft surgery: epidemiology, management, and prognosis. Am Heart J 1995; 129:799–808.

171. Angelini P, Feldman MI, Lufschanowski R, Leachman RD. Cardiac arrhythmias during and after heart surgery: diagnosis and management. Prog Cardiovasc Dis 1974; 16:469–495.

172. Michelson EL, Morganroth J, MacVaugh H III. Postoperative arrhythmias after coronary artery and cardiac valvular surgery detected by long-term electrocardiographic monitoring. Am Heart J 1979; 97:442–448.

173. Kron IL, DiMarco JP, Harman PK, et al. Unanticipated postoperative ventricular tachyarrhythmias. Ann Thorac Surg 1984; 38:317–322.

174. Rubin DA, Nieminski KE, Monteferrante JC, Mage T, Reed GE, Herman MV. Ventricular arrhythmias after coronary artery bypass graft surgery: incidence, risk factors and long-term prognosis. J Am Coll Cardiol 1985; 6:307–310.

175. Topol EJ, Lerman BB, Baughman KL, Platia EV, Griffith LSC. De novo refractory ventricular tachyarrhythmias after coronary revascularization. Am J Cardiol 1986; 57:57–59.

176. Sapin PM, Woelfel AK, Foster JR. Unexpected ventricular tachyarrhythmias soon after cardiac surgery. Am J Cardiol 1991; 68:1099–1100.

177. Tam SK, Miller JM, Edmunds LH Jr. Unexpected, sustained ventricular tachyarrhythmias after cardiac operations. J Thorac Cardiovasc Surg 1991; 102:883–889.

178. Smith RC, Leung JM, Keith FM, Merrick S, Mangano DT. Ventricular dysrhythmias in patients undergoing coronary artery bypass graft surgery: incidence, characteristics, and prognostic importance. Am Heart J 1992; 123:73–81.

179. Costeas XF, Schoenfeld MH. Usefulness of electrophysiologic studies for new-onset sustained ventricular tachyarrhythmias shortly after coronary artery bypass grafting. Am J Cardiol 1993; 72:1291–1294.

180. Azar RR, Berns E, Seecharran B, Veronneau J, Lippman N, Kluger J. De novo monomorphic and polymorphic ventricular tachycardia following coronary artery bypass grafting. Am J Cardiol 1997; 80:76–78.

181. Narasimhan C, Jazayeri MR, Sra J, et al. Ventricular tachycardia in valvular heart disease: facilitation of sustained bundle-branch reentry by valve surgery. Circulation 1997; 96:4307–4313.

182. Saxon LA, Wiener I, Natterson PD, Laks H, Drinkwater D, Stevenson WG. Monomorphic versus polymorphic ventricular tachycardia after coronary artery bypass grafting. Am J Cardiol 1995; 75:403–405.

183. Weesner KM, Byrum CJ, Dick M, Rocchini AP, Behrendt DM, Hees P. Ventricular tachycardia associated with a left ventricular apex sump aneurysm in an adolescent. Am Heart J 1983; 105:334–336.

184. Curtis JL, Foster JR, Gettes LS, Simpson RJ Jr, Woelfel A. Initial presentation of sustained ventricular tachycardia after resection of left ventricular aneurysm. Am J Cardiol 1986; 58:560–561.

185. Deanfield JE, McKenna WJ, Hallidie-Smith KA. Detection of late arrhythmia and conduction disturbance after correction of tetralogy of Fallot. Br Heart J 1980; 44:248–253.

186. Kavey RE, Blackman MS, Sondheimer HM. Incidence and severity of chronic ventricular dysrhythmias after repair of tetralogy of Fallot. Am Heart J 1982; 103:342–350.

187. Kugler JD, Pinsky WW, Cheatham JP, Hofschire PJ, Mooring PK, Fleming WH. Sustained ventricular tachycardia after repair of tetralogy of Fallot: new electrophysiologic findings. Am J Cardiol 1983; 51:1137–1143.

188. Krongrad E. Postoperative arrhythmias in patients with congenital heart disease. Chest 1984; 85:107–113.

189. Chandar JS, Wolff GS, Garson A Jr, et al. Ventricular arrhythmias in postoperative tetralogy of Fallot. Am J Cardiol 1990; 65:655–661.

190. Stevenson WG, Klitzner T, Perloff JK. Electrophysiologic abnormalities: natural occurrence and postoperative residua and sequelae. In Perloff JK, Child JS (eds). Congenital Heart Disease in Adults. Philadelphia: WB Saunders, 1991, pp. 259–295.

191. Cullen S, Celermajer DS, Franklin RC, Hallidie-Smith KA, Deanfield JE. Prognostic significance of ventricular arrhythmia after repair of tetralogy of Fallot: a 12-year prospective study. J Am Coll Cardiol 1994; 23:1151–1155.

192. Gradman AH, Harbison MA, Berger HJ, et al. Ventricular arrhythmias late after aortic valve replacement and their relation to left ventricular performance. Am J Cardiol 1981; 48:824–831.

193. Skanes AC, Green MS, Tang AS. A case of wide complex tachycardia after ventricular tachycardia surgery. Pacing Clin Electrophysiol 1997; 20:356–358.

194. Brooks R, Burgess JH. Idiopathic ventricular tachycardia: a review. Medicine 1988; 67:271–294.

195. Campbell RW. Ventricular rhythm disturbances in the normal heart. Eur Heart J 1992; 13:139–143.

196. Belhassen B, Viskin S. Idiopathic ventricular tachycardia and fibrillation. J Cardiovasc Electrophysiol 1993; 4:356–368.

197. Bhadha K, Marchlinski FE, Iskandrian AS. Ventricular tachycardia in patients without structural heart disease. Am Heart J 1993; 126:1194–1198.

198. Wellens HJJ, Rodriguez LM, Smeets JL. Ventricular tachycardia in structurally normal hearts. In Zipes DP, Jalife J (eds). Cardiac Electrophysiology. From Cell to Bedside. 2nd ed. Philadelphia: WB Saunders, 1995, pp. 780–788.

199. Bourke JP, Doig JC. Ventricular Tachyarrhythmias in the Normal Heart. Armonk, NY: Futura Publishing Co. 1998.

200. Froment R, Gallavardin L, Cahen P. Paroxysmal ventricular tachycardia: a clinical classification. B Heart J 1953; 15:172–178.

201. Adams CW. Functional paroxysmal ventricular tachycardia. Am J Cardiol 1962; 9:215–222.

202. Lesch M, Lewis E, Humphries JO, Ross RS. Paroxysmal

ventricular tachycardia in the absence of organic heart disease: report of a case and review of the literature. Ann Intern Med 1967; 66:950–960.

203. Chapman JH, Schrank JP, Crampton RS. Idiopathic ventricular tachycardia: an intracardiac electrical, hemodynamic and angiographic assessment of six patients. Am J Med 1975; 59:470–480.

204. Wu D, Kou H-C, Hung J-S. Exercise-triggered paroxysmal ventricular tachycardia: a repetitive rhythmic activity possibly related to afterdepolarization. Ann Intern Med 1981; 95:410–414.

205. Palileo EV, Ashley WW, Swiryn S, et al. Exercise provocable right ventricular outflow tract tachycardia. Am Heart J 1982; 104:185–193.

206. Sung RJ, Shen EN, Morady F, Scheinman MM, Hess D, Botvinick EH. Electrophysiologic mechanisms of exercise-induced sustained ventricular tachycardia. Am J Cardiol 1983; 51:525–530.

207. German LD, Packer DL, Bardy GH, Gallagher JJ. Ventricular tachycardia induced by atrial stimulation in patients without symptomatic cardiac disease. Am J Cardiol 1983; 52:1202–1207.

208. Lin F-C, Finley D, Rahimtoola SH, Wu D. Idiopathic paroxysmal ventricular tachycardia with a QRS pattern of right bundle branch block and left axis deviation: a unique clinical entity with specific properties. Am J Cardiol 1983; 52:95–100.

209. Buxton AE, Waxman HL, Marchlinski FE, Simson MB, Cassidy D, Josephson ME. Right ventricular tachycardia: clinical and electrophysiologic characteristics. Circulation 1983; 68:917–927.

210. Buxton AE, Marchlinski FE, Doherty JU, et al. Repetitive, monomorphic ventricular tachycardia: clinical and electrophysiologic characteristics in patients with and patients without organic heart disease. Am J Cardiol 1984; 54:997–1002.

211. Belhassen B, Shapira I, Pelleg A, Copperman I, Kauli N, Laniado S. Idiopathic recurrent sustained ventricular tachycardia responsive to verapamil: an ECG-electrophysiologic entity. Am Heart J 1984; 108:1034–1037.

212. Lerman BB, Belardinelli L, West A, Berne RM, DiMarco JP. Adenosine-sensitive ventricular tachycardia: evidence suggesting cyclic AMP-mediated triggered activity. Circulation 1986; 74:270–280.

213. Holt PM, Wainwright RJ, Curry PV. Right ventricular outflow tract tachycardias in patients without apparent structural heart disease. Int J Cardiol 1986; 10:99–110.

214. Ohe T, Shimomura K, Aihara N, et al. Idiopathic sustained left ventricular tachycardia: clinical and electrophysiologic characteristics. Circulation 1988; 77:560–568.

215. Proclemer A, Ciani R, Feruglio GA. Right ventricular tachycardia with left bundle branch block and inferior axis morphology: clinical and arrhythmological characteristics in 15 patients. Pacing Clin Electrophysiol 1989; 12:977–989.

216. Ritchie AH, Kerr CR, Qi A, Yeung-Lai-Wah JA. Nonsustained ventricular tachycardia arising from the right ventricular outflow tract. Am J Cardiol 1989; 64:594–598.

217. Stevenson WG, Nademanee K, Weiss JN, Wiener I. Treatment of catecholamine-sensitive right ventricular tachycardia by endocardial catheter ablation. J Am Coll Cardiol 1990; 16:752–755.

218. Seixas T, Brugada P, Brugada J, et al. Clinical and electrophysiologic characteristics of exercise-related idiopathic ventricular tachycardia. Am J Cardiol 1991; 68:897–900.

219. Seixas T, Brugada P, Brugada J, et al. The electrocardiographic, clinical, and electrophysiologic spectrum of idiopathic monomorphic ventricular tachycardia. Am Heart J 1992; 124:746–753.

220. DeLacey WA, Nath S, Haines DE, Barber MJ, DiMarco JP. Adenosine and verapamil-sensitive ventricular tachycardia originating from the left ventricle: radiofrequency catheter ablation. PACE 1992; 15:2240–2244.

221. Wilber DJ, Baerman J, Olshansky B, Kall J, Kopp D. Adenosine-sensitive ventricular tachycardia: clinical

characteristics and response to catheter ablation. Circulation 1993; 87:126–134.

222. Gill JS, Blaszyk K, Ward DE, Camm AJ. Verapamil for the suppression of idiopathic ventricular tachycardia of left bundle branch block-like morphology. Am Heart J 1993; 126:1126–1133.

223. Lerman BB. Response of nonreentrant catecholamine-mediated ventricular tachycardia to endogenous adenosine and acetylcholine: evidence for myocardial receptor-mediated effects. Circulation 1993; 87:382–390.

224. Lerman BB, Stein K, Engelstein ED, et al. Mechanism of repetitive monomorphic ventricular tachycardia. Circulation 1995; 92:421–429.

225. Ohe T, Aihara N, Kamakura S, Kurita T, Shimizu W, Shimomura K. Long-term outcome of verapamil-sensitive sustained left ventricular tachycardia in patients without structural heart disease. J Am Coll Cardiol 1995; 25:54–58.

226. Sugrue DD, Holmes DR, Gersh BJ, et al. Cardiac histologic findings in patients with life-threatening ventricular arrhythmias of unknown origin. J Am Coll Cardiol 1984; 4:952–957.

227. Orlov MV, Brodsky MA, Allen BJ, Winters RJ, Orlov YSK. Spectrum of right heart involvement in patients with ventricular tachycardia unrelated to coronary artery disease or left ventricular dysfunction. Am Heart J 1993; 126:1348–1356.

228. Deal BJ, Miller SM, Scagliotti D, Prechel D, Gallastegui JL, Hariman RJ. Ventricular tachycardia in a young population without overt heart disease. Circulation 1986; 73:1111–1118.

229. Gill JS, Hunter GJ, Gane G, Camm AJ. Heterogeneity of the human myocardial sympathetic innervation: in vivo demonstration by iodine 123-labeled meta-iodobenzylguanidine scintigraphy. Am Heart J 1993; 126:390–398.

230. Vignola PA, Aonuma K, Swaye PS, et al. Lymphocytic myocarditis presenting as unexplained ventricular arrhythmias: diagnosis with endomyocardial biopsy and response to immunosuppression. J Am Coll Cardiol 1984; 4:812–819.

231. Wiles HB, Gillette PC, Harley RA, Upshur JK. Cardiomyopathy and myocarditis in children with ventricular ectopic rhythm. J Am Coll Cardiol 1992; 20:359–362.

232. Globits S, Kreiner G, Frank H, et al. Significance of morphological abnormalities detected by MRI in patients undergoing successful ablation of right ventricular outflow tract tachycardia. Circulation 1997; 96:2633–2640.

233. Markowitz SM, Litvak BL, Ramirez de Arellano EA, Markisz JA, Stein KM, Lerman BB. Adenosine-sensitive ventricular tachycardia: right ventricular abnormalities delineated by magnetic resonance imaging. Circulation 1997; 96:1192–1200.

234. Strain JE, Grose RM, Factor SM, Fisher JD. Results of endomyocardial biopsy in patients with spontaneous ventricular tachycardia but without apparent structural heart disease. Circulation 1983; 68:1171–1181.

235. Nava A, Thiene G, Canciani B, et al. Clinical profile of concealed form of arrhythmogenic right ventricular cardiomyopathy presenting with apparently idiopathic ventricular arrhythmias. Int J Cardiol 1992; 35:195–206.

236. Tada H, Ohe T, Yutani C, et al. Sudden death in a patient with apparent idiopathic ventricular tachycardia. Jpn Circ J 1996; 60:133–136.

237. Dimich I, Steinfeld L, Richman R, Lasser R. Treatment of recurrent paroxysmal ventricular tachycardia. Am Heart J 1970; 79:811–815.

238. Hernandez A, Strauss A, Kleiger RE, Goldring D. Idiopathic paroxysmal ventricular tachycardia in infants and children. J Pediatr 1975; 86:182–188.

239. Steffens TG, Pierce PL, Zegerius RJ. Multiple ventricular premature beats in five adolescents. Eur J Cardiol 1978; 8:177–184.

240. Bergdahl DM, Stevenson JG, Kawabori I, Guntheroth WG. Prognosis in primary ventricular tachycardia in the pediatric patient. Circulation 1980; 62:897–901.

241. Vetter VL, Josephson ME, Horowitz LN. Idiopathic recurrent

sustained ventricular tachycardia in children and adolescents. Am J Cardiol 1981; 47:315–322.

242. Fulton DR, Chung KJ, Tabakin BS, Keane JF. Ventricular tachycardia in children without heart disease. Am J Cardiol 1985; 55:1328–1331.

243. Noh CI, Gillette PC, Case CL, Zeigler VL. Clinical and electrophysiological characteristics of ventricular tachycardia in children with normal hearts. Am Heart J 1990; 120:1326–1333.

244. Zeigler VL, Gillette PC, Crawford FA Jr, Wiles HB, Fyfe DA. New approaches to treatment of incessant ventricular tachycardia in the very young. J Am Coll Cardiol 1990; 16:681–685.

245. Case CL, Gillette PC. Treatment of ventricular arrhythmias in children without structural heart disease with class Ic agents as guided by invasive electrophysiology. Am J Cardiol 1990; 66:1265–1266.

246. Davis AM, Gow RM, McCrindle BW, Hamilton RM. Clinical spectrum, therapeutic management, and follow-up of ventricular tachycardia in infants and young children. Am Heart J 1996; 131:186–191.

247. Lopes LM, Cha SC, Scanavacca MI, Tuma-Calil VML, Zugaib M. Fetal idiopathic ventricular tachycardia with nonimmune hydrops: benign course. Pediatr Cardiol 1996; 17:192–193.

248. Caldwell PD, Ricketts HJ, Dillard DH, Guntheroth WG. Ventricular tachycardia in a child: an indication for angiocardiography? Am Heart J 1974; 88:777–781.

249. Engle MA, Ebert PA, Redo SF. Recurrent ventricular tachycardia due to resectable cardiac tumor: Report of two cases in two-years-olds in heart failure. Circulation 1974; 50:1052–1057.

250. Enbergs A, Borggrefe M, Kurlemann G, et al. Ventricular tachycardia caused by cardiac rhabdomyoma in a young adult with tuberous sclerosis. Am Heart J 1996; 132:1263–1265.

251. Garson A Jr, Smith RT Jr, Moak JP, et al. Incessant ventricular tachycardia in infants: myocardial hamartomas and surgical cure. J Am Coll Cardiol 1987; 10:619–626.

252. Muhler EG, Kienast W, Turniski-Harder V, von Bernuth G. Arrhythmias in infants and children with primary cardiac tumors. Eur Heart J 1994; 15:915–921.

253. Geggel RL, McInerny J, Estes NA III. Transient neonatal ventricular tachycardia associated with maternal cocaine use. Am J Cardiol 1989; 63:383–384.

254. Lampert R, Rosenfeld L, Batsford W, Lee F, McPherson C. Circadian variation of sustained ventricular tachycardia in patients with coronary artery disease and implantable cardioverter-defibrillators. Circulation 1994; 90:241–247.

255. Tofler GH, Gebara OC, Mittleman MA, et al. Morning peak in ventricular tachyarrhythmias detected by time of implantable cardioverter/defibrillator therapy: the CPI investigators. Circulation 1995; 92:1203–1208.

256. Fries R, Heisel A, Nikoloudakis N, Jung J, Schafers HJ, Schieffer H. Antitachycardia pacing in patients with implantable cardioverter-defibrillators: inverse circadian variation of therapy success and acceleration. Am J Cardiol 1997; 80:1487–1489.

257. Nanthakumar K, Newman D, Paquette M, Greene M, Rakovich G, Dorian P. Circadian variation of sustained ventricular tachycardia in patients subject to standard adrenergic blockade. Am Heart J 1997; 134:752–757.

258. Peters RW, McQuillan S, Resnick SK, Gold M. Increased Monday incidence of life-threatening ventricular arrhythmias: experience with a third-generation implantable defibrillator. Circulation 1996; 94:1346–1349.

259. Wood MA, Simpson PM, London WB, et al. Circadian pattern of ventricular tachyarrhythmias in patients with implantable cardioverter-defibrillators. J Am Coll Cardiol 1995; 25:901–907.

260. Behrens S, Ehlers C, Bruggemann T, et al. Modification of the circadian pattern of ventricular tachyarrhythmias by beta-blocker therapy. Clin Cardiol 1997; 20:253–257.

261. Valkama JO, Huikuri HV, Linnaluoto MK, Takkunen JT. Circadian variation of ventricular tachycardia in patients with coronary arterial disease. Int J Cardiol 1992; 34:173–178.

262. Lucente M, Rebuzzi AG, Lanza GA, et al. Circadian variation of ventricular tachycardia in acute myocardial infarction. Am J Cardiol 1988; 62:670–674.

263. Spritzer RC, Seldon M, Mattes LM, Donoso E, Friedberg CK. Serious arrhythmias during labor and delivery in women with heart disease. JAMA 1970; 211:1005–1007.

264. Tilkian AG, Guilleminault C, Schroeder JS, Lehrman KL, Simmons FB, Dement WC. Sleep-induced apnea syndrome: prevalence of cardiac arrhythmias and their reversal after tracheostomy. Am J Med 1977; 63:348–358.

265. Greenspon AJ, Stang JM, Lewis RP, Schaal SF. Provocation of ventricular tachycardia after consumption of alcohol. N Engl J Med 1979; 301:1049–1050.

266. Lantigua RA, Amatruda JM, Biddle TL, Forbes GB, Lockwood DH. Cardiac arrhythmias associated with a liquid protein diet for the treatment of obesity. N Engl J Med 1980; 303:735–738.

267. Waxman MB, Staniloff H, Wald RW. Respiratory and vagal modulation of ventricular tachycardia. J Electrocardiol 1981; 14:83–90.

268. Scheibelhofer W, Glogar D, Probst P, Mlczoch J, Kaindl F. Induction of ventricular tachycardia by pacemaker programming. PACE 1982; 5:587–592.

269. Sprung CL, Pozen RG, Rozanski JJ, Pinero JR, Eisler BR, Castellanos A. Advanced ventricular arrhythmias during bedside pulmonary artery catheterization. Am J Med 1982; 72:203–208.

270. Tommaso C, Belic N, Brandfonbrener M. Asynchronous ventricular pacing: a rare cause of ventricular tachycardia. PACE 1982; 5:561–563.

271. Dobmeyer DJ, Stine RA, Leier CV, Greenberg R, Schaal SF. The arrhythmogenic effects of caffeine in human beings. N Engl J Med 1983; 308:814–816.

272. Guilleminault C, Connolly SJ, Winkle RA. Cardiac arrhythmia and conduction disturbances during sleep in 400 patients with sleep apnea syndrome. Am J Cardiol 1983; 52:490–494.

273. Luceri RM, Ramirez AV, Castellanos A, Zaman L, Thurer RJ, Myerburg RJ. Ventricular tachycardia produced by a normally functioning AV sequential demand (DVI) pacemaker with "committed" ventricular stimulation. J Am Coll Cardiol 1983; 1:1177–1179.

274. Belhassen B, Webb C, Shapira I, Miller H, Laniado S. Unusual features of ventricular tachycardia during respiration and exercise in arrhythmogenic right ventricular dysplasia. Am J Cardiol 1984; 54:1368–1371.

275. Kong C-W, Kertes P, Vohra J. Traumatic right ventricular tachycardia. Am Heart J 1984; 108:1357–1360.

276. Tubman TR, Craig B, Mulholland HC. Ventricular tachycardia associated with coxsackie B4 virus infection. Acta Paediatr Scand 1990; 79:572–575.

277. Ino T, Okubo M, Akimoto K, et al. Corticosteroid therapy for ventricular tachycardia in children with silent lymphocytic myocarditis. J Pediatr 1995; 126:304–308.

278. Greenberg YJ, Brennan JJ, Rosenfeld LE. Lyme myocarditis presenting as fascicular tachycardia with underlying complete heart block. J Cardiovasc Electrophysiol 1997; 8:323–324.

279. Fritsch-Yelle JM, Leuenberger UA, D'Aunno DS, et al. An episode of ventricular tachycardia during long-duration spaceflight. Am J Cardiol 1998; 81:1391–1392.

280. Lown B, Wolf M. Approaches to sudden death from coronary heart disease. Circulation 1971; 44:130–142.

281. Bleifer SB, Karpman HL, Sheppard JJ, Bleifer DJ. Relation between premature ventricular complexes and development of ventricular tachycardia. Am J Cardiol 1973; 31:400–403.

282. Chiang BN, Perlman LV, Ostrander LD Jr, Epstein FH. Relationship of premature systoles to coronary heart disease and sudden death in the Tecumseh epidemiologic study. Ann Intern Med 1969; 70:1159–1166.

283. Bennett MA, Pentecost BL. Warning of cardiac arrest due to ventricular fibrillation and tachycardia. Lancet 1972; 2:1351–1352.

284. Coronary Drug Project Research Group. Prognostic importance of premature beats following myocardial

infarction: experience in the coronary drug project. JAMA 1973; 223:1116–1124.

285. Kotler MN, Tabatznik B, Mower MM, Tominaga S. Prognostic significance of ventricular ectopic beats with respect to sudden death in the late postinfarction period. Circulation 1973; 47:959–966.

286. Hinkle LE, Carver ST, Argyros DC, Stevens M, Horvath J. The prognostic significance of ventricular premature contractions in healthy people and in people with coronary heart disease. Acta Cardiol 1974; 18:5–32.

287. Ruberman W, Weinblatt E, Goldberg JD, Frank CW, Shapiro S. Ventricular premature beats and mortality after myocardial infarction. N Engl J Med 1977; 297:750–757.

288. Schulze RA Jr, Strauss HW, Pitt B. Sudden death in the year following myocardial infarction: relation to ventricular premature contractions in the late hospital phase and left ventricular ejection fraction. Am J Med 1977; 62:192–199.

289. Boudoulas H, Dervenagas S, Schaal SF, Lewis RP, Dalamangas G. Malignant premature ventricular beats in ambulatory patients. Ann Intern Med 1979; 91:723–726.

290. Moss AJ, Davis HT, DeCamilla J, Bayer LW. Ventricular ectopic beats and their relation to sudden and nonsudden cardiac death after myocardial infarction. Circulation 1979; 60:998–1003.

291. Yusuf S, Lopez R, Sleight P. Heart rate and ectopic prematurity in relation to sustained ventricular arrhythmias. Br Heart J 1980; 44:233–239.

292. Ruberman W, Weinblatt E, Goldberg JD, Frank CW, Chaudhary BS, Shapiro S. Ventricular premature complexes and sudden death after myocardial infarction. Circulation 1981; 64:297–305.

293. Bigger JT Jr, Weld FM. Analysis of prognostic significance of ventricular arrhythmias after myocardial infarction: shortcomings of Lown grading system. Br Heart J 1981; 45:717–724.

294. Califf RM, McKinnis RA, Burks J, et al. Prognostic implications of ventricular arrhythmias during 24 hour ambulatory monitoring in patients undergoing cardiac catheterization for coronary artery disease. Am J Cardiol 1982; 50:23–31.

295. Nikolic G, Bishop RL, Singh JB. Sudden death recorded during Holter monitoring. Circulation 1982; 66:218–225.

296. Multicenter Post-Infarction Research Group. Risk stratification and survival after myocardial infarction. N Engl J Med 1983; 309:331–336.

297. Olson HG, Lyons KP, Troop P, Butman SM, Piters KM. Prognostic implications of complicated ventricular arrhythmias early after hospital discharge in acute myocardial infarction: a serial ambulatory electrocardiography study. Am Heart J 1984; 108:1221–1228.

298. Gomes JAC, Hariman RI, Kang PS, el-Sherif N, Chowdhry I, Lyons J. Programmed electrical stimulation in patients with high-grade ventricular ectopy: electrophysiologic findings and prognosis for survival. Circulation 1984; 70:43–51.

299. Mukharji J, Rude RE, Poole K, et al. Risk factors for sudden death after acute myocardial infarction: two-year follow-up. Am J Cardiol 1984; 54:31–36.

300. Meinertz T, Hofmann T, Kasper W, el al. Significance of ventricular arrhythmias in idiopathic dilated cardiomyopathy. Am J Cardiol 1984; 53:902–907.

301. Romeo F, Pelliccia F, Cianfrocca C, Cristofani R, Reale A. Predictors of sudden death in idiopathic dilated cardiomyopathy. Am J Cardiol 1989; 63:138–140.

302. Maggioni AP, Zuanetti G, Franzosi MG, et al. Prevalence and prognostic significance of ventricular arrhythmias after acute myocardial infarction in the fibrinolytic era: GISSI-2 results. Circulation 1993; 87:312–322.

303. Anderson KP, Lux RA, Dustman T. Comparison of QRS morphologies of spontaneous premature ventricular complexes and ventricular tachycardia induced by programmed stimulation. Am Heart J 1990; 119:1302–1311.

304. Anderson KP, Walker R, Dustman T, Fuller M, Mori M, ESVEM Investigators. Spontaneous sustained ventricular tachycardia in the Electrophysiologic Study Versus Electrocardiographic Monitoring (ESVEM) Trial. J Am Coll Cardiol 1995; 26:489–496.

305. Winkle RA, Derrington DC, Schroeder JS. Characteristics of ventricular tachycardia in ambulatory patients. Am J Cardiol 1977; 39:487–492.

306. Calkins H, Shyr Y, Frumin H, Schork A, Morady F. The value of the clinical history in the differentiation of syncope due to ventricular tachycardia, atrioventricular block, and neurocardiogenic syncope. Am J Med 1995; 98:365–373.

307. Militianiu A, Salacata A, Seibert K, et al. Implantable cardioverter defibrillator utilization among device recipients presenting exclusively with syncope or near-syncope. J Cardiovasc Electrophysiol 1997; 8:1087–1097.

308. Garson A Jr, Porter C-B J, Gillette PC, McNamara DG. Induction of ventricular tachycardia during electrophysiologic study after repair of tetralogy of Fallot. J Am Coll Cardiol 1983; 1:1493–1502.

309. Hamer AW, Rubin SA, Peter T, Mandel WJ. Factors that predict syncope during ventricular tachycardia in patients. Am Heart J 1984; 107:997–1005.

310. Tanabe T, Goto Y. Evaluation of ventricular tachycardia with respect to syncope in patients with old myocardial infarction, dilated cardiomyopathy and no overt heart disease. Jpn Circ J 1990; 54:1297–1303.

311. Gooch AS, McConnell D. Analysis of transient arrhythmias and conduction disturbances occurring during submaximal treadmill exercise testing. Prog Cardiovasc Dis 1970; 13:293–307.

312. Vlay SC. Catecholamine-sensitive ventricular tachycardia. Am Heart J 1987; 114:455–461.

313. Sung RJ, Huycke EC, Lai W-T, Tseng C-D, Chu H, Keung EC. Clinical and electrophysiologic mechanisms of exercise-induced ventricular tachyarrhythmias. PACE 1988; 11:1347–1357.

314. Sung RJ, Lauer MR. Exercise-induced cardiac arrhythmias. In Zipes DP, Jalife J (eds). Cardiac Electrophysiology. From Cell to Bedside. 2nd ed. Philadelphia: WB Saunders, 1995, pp. 1013–1023.

315. Winkle RA, Derrington DC, Schroeder JS. Characteristics of ventricular tachycardia in ambulatory patients. Am J Cardiol 1977; 39:487–492.

316. Sokoloff NM, Spielman SR, Greenspan AM, et al. Plasma norepinephrine in exercise-induced ventricular tachycardia. J Am Coll Cardiol 1986; 8:11–17.

317. O'Hara GE, Brugada P, Rodriguez L-M, et al. Incidence, pathophysiology and prognosis of exercise-induced sustained ventricular tachycardia associated with healed myocardial infarction. Am J Cardiol 1992; 70:875–878.

318. Sung RJ, Shen EN, Morady F, Scheinman MM, Hess D, Botvinick EH. Electrophysiologic mechanism of exercise-induced sustained ventricular tachycardia. Am J Cardiol 1983; 51:525–530.

319. Belhassen B, Webb C, Shapira I, Miller H, Laniado S. Unusual features of ventricular tachycardia during respiration and exercise in arrhythmogenic right ventricular dysplasia. Am J Cardiol 1984; 54:1368–1371.

320. de Paola AA, Gomes JA, Terzian AB, Miyamoto MH, Martinez Fo EE. Ventricular tachycardia during exercise testing as a predictor of sudden death in patients with chronic chagasic cardiomyopathy and ventricular arrhythmias. Br Heart J 1995; 74:293–295.

321. Woelfel A, Foster JR, Simpson RJ Jr, Gettes LS. Reproducibility and treatment of exercise-induced ventricular tachycardia. Am J Cardiol 1984; 53:751–756.

322. Brodsky MA, Orlov MV, Winters RJ, Allen BJ. Determinants of inducible ventricular tachycardia in patients with clinical ventricular tachyarrhythmia and no apparent structural heart disease. Am Heart J 1993; 126:1113–1120.

323. Kobayashi Y, Kikushima S, Tanno K, Kurano K, Baba T, Katagiri T. Sustained left ventricular tachycardia terminated by dipyridamole: cyclic AMP-mediated triggered activity as a possible mechanism. PACE 1994; 17:377–385.

324. Garratt CJ, Griffith MJ, Young G, et al. Value of physical signs in the diagnosis of ventricular tachycardia. Circulation 1994; 90:3103–3107.

325. Wilson WS, Judge RD, Siegel JH. A simple diagnostic sign in ventricular tachycardia. N Engl J Med 1964; 270:446–448.

326. Prinzmetal M, Kellogg F. On the significance of the jugular pulse in the clinical diagnosis of ventricular tachycardia. Am Heart J 1934; 9:370–377.

327. Massumi RA, Tawakkol AA, Kistin AD. Reevaluation of electrocardiographic and bedside criteria for diagnosis of ventricular tachycardia. Circulation 1967; 36:628–636.

328. Harvey WP, Corrado MA. Multiple sounds in paroxysmal ventricular tachycardia. N Engl J Med 1957; 257:325–327.

329. Chung EK. Principles of Cardiac Arrhythmias. Baltimore: Williams & Wilkins, 1971, p. 312.

330. Trever RW. Ventricular tachycardia of thirty-five days' duration: report of a case reverted by direct current external electric countershock. Ann Intern Med 1963; 59:732–737.

331. Kilpatrick TR, Moore CB, Maza E. Drug-resistant ventricular tachycardia of 62 days' duration. JAMA 1966; 197:762–766.

332. Anderson KP, Walker R, Dustman T, Fuller M, Mori M. Spontaneous sustained ventricular tachycardia in the Electrophysiologic Study Versus Electrocardiographic Monitoring (ESVEM) Trial. J Am Coll Cardiol 1995; 26:489–496.

333. Swerdlow B, Axelrod P, Kolman B, Perry D, Mark R. Ambulatory ventricular tachycardia: characteristics of the initiating beat. Am Heart J 1983; 106:1326–1331.

334. Suyama A, Anan T, Araki H, Takeshita A, Nakamura M. Prevalence of ventricular tachycardia in patients with different underlying heart disease: a study by Holter ECG monitoring. Am Heart J 1986; 112:44–51.

335. Manolis AG, Katsivas A, Lazaris E, Koutsogeogis D, Louvros N. Circadian modulation of ventricular tachycardia cycle length variability in ICD patients with dilated cardiomyopathy. PACE 1997; 20:203–207.

336. Garcia-Alberola A, Yli-Mayry S, Block M, et al. RR interval variability in irregular monomorphic ventricular tachycardia and atrial fibrillation. Circulation 1996; 93:295–300.

337. Volosin KJ, Beauregard L-AM, Fabiszewski R, Mattingly H, Waxman HL. Spontaneous changes in ventricular tachycardia cycle length. J Am Coll Cardiol 1991; 17:409–414.

338. Kistin AD. Retrograde conduction to the atria in ventricular tachycardia. Circulation 1961; 24:236–249.

339. Kistin AD, Tawakkol A, Massumi RA. Atrial rhythm in ventricular tachycardia occurring during cardiac catheterization. Circulation 1967; 35:10–14.

340. Wellens HJJ, Bar FW, Vanagt EJ, Brugada P, Farre J. The differentiation between ventricular tachycardia and supraventricular tachycardia with aberrant conduction: the value of the 12-lead electrocardiogram. In Wellens HJJ, Kulbertus HE (eds). What's New in Electrocardiography. The Hague: Martinus Nijhoff, 1981, pp. 184–199.

341. Evans GL, Charles MA, Thornsvard CT. Ventricular tachycardia with retrograde conduction: Simplified diagnostic approach. Br Heart J 1974; 36:512–515.

342. Gonzalez RP, Scheinman MM, Lesh MD, Helmy I, Torres V, Van Hare GF. Clinical and electrophysiologic spectrum of fascicular tachycardias. Am Heart J 1994; 128:147–156.

343. Ward DE, Nathan AW, Camm AJ. Fascicular tachycardia sensitive to calcium antagonists. Eur Heart J 1984; 5:896–905.

344. Andrade FR, Eslami M, Elias J, et al. Diagnostic clues from the surface Ecg to identify idiopathic (fascicular) ventricular tachycardia: correlation with electrophysiologic findings. J Cardiovasc Electrophysiol 1996; 7:2–8.

345. Josephson ME, Horowitz LN, Farshidi A, Spielman SR, Michelson EL, Greenspan AM. Recurrent sustained ventricular tachycardia. IV. Pleomorphism. Circulation 1979; 3:459–468.

346. Ross DL, Hamer AW, Vohra JK, Sloman JG, Hunt D. Multiform ventricular tachycardia. Pacing Clin Electrophysiol 1980; 3:24–37.

347. Wilber DJ, Davis MJ, Rosenbaum M, Ruskin JN, Garan H. Incidence and determinants of multiple morphologically distinct sustained ventricular tachycardias. J Am Coll Cardiol 1987; 10:583–591.

348. Tai Y-T, Lee KL-F. Pleomorphic ventricular tachycardia with antegrade His-bundle activation: elucidation by multiple His-bundle recordings. J Cardiovasc Electrophysiol 1994; 5:350–355.

349. Ross DL, Vohra JK, Sloman JG. Similar QRS morphology in sinus rhythm and ventricular tachycardia. PACE 1979; 2:486–489.

350. Pietras RJ, Mautner R, Denes P, et al. Chronic recurrent right and left ventricular tachycardia: comparison of clinical, hemodynamic and angiographic findings. Am J Cardiol 1977; 40:32–37.

351. Lewis S, Kanakis C, Rosen KM, Denes P. Significance of site of origin of premature ventricular contractions. Am Heart J 1979; 97:159–164.

352. Aizawa Y, Chinushi M, Kitazawa H, et al. Spatial orientation of the reentrant circuit of idiopathic left ventricular tachycardia. Am J Cardiol 1995; 76:316–319.

353. Callans DJ, Menz V, Schwartzman D, Gottlieb CD, Marchlinski FE. Repetitive monomorphic tachycardia from the left ventricular outflow tract: electrocardiographic patterns consistent with a left ventricular site of origin. J Am Coll Cardiol 1997; 29:1023–1027.

354. Wen MS, Yeh SJ, Wang CC, Lin FC, Wu D. Successful radiofrequency ablation of idiopathic left ventricular tachycardia at a site away from the tachycardia exit. J Am Coll Cardiol 1997; 30:1024–1031.

355. Nibley C, Wharton JM. Ventricular tachycardias with left bundle branch block morphology. Pacing Clin Electrophysiol 1995; 18:334–356.

356. Reiter MJ, Smith WM, Gallagher JJ. Clinical spectrum of ventricular tachycardia with left bundle branch morphology. Am J Cardiol 1983; 51:113–121.

357. Fei L, Statters DJ, Hnatkova K, Poloniecki J, Malik M, Camm AJ. Change of autonomic influence on the heart immediately before the onset of spontaneous idiopathic ventricular tachycardia. J Am Coll Cardiol 1994; 24:1515–1522.

358. Lerman BB, Stein KM, Markowitz SM. Adenosine-sensitive ventricular tachycardia: a conceptual approach. J Cardiovasc Electrophysiol 1996; 7:559–569.

359. Josephson ME, Horowitz LN, Waxman HL, et al. Sustained ventricular tachycardia: role of the 12-lead electrocardiogram in localizing site of origin. Circulation 1981; 64:257–272.

360. Blanck Z, Jazayeri M, Dhala A, Deshpande S, Sra J, Akhtar M. Bundle branch reentry: a mechanism of ventricular tachycardia in the absence of myocardial or valvular dysfunction. J Am Coll Cardiol 1993; 22:1713–1722.

361. Rodriguez LM. Observations on the QRS complex in post-infarction and non-ischemic ventricular tachycardias. In Rodriguez LM (ed). New Observations on Cardiac Arrhythmias. Maastricht: Universitaire Pers Maastricht, 1994, pp. 79–95.

362. Coumel P, Leclercq JF, Attuel P, Maisonblanche P. The QRS morphology in post-myocardial infarction ventricular tachycardia: a study of 100 tracings compared with 70 cases of idiopathic ventricular tachycardia. Eur Heart J 1984; 5:792–805.

363. Kernohan RJ. Post-paroxysmal tachycardia syndrome. Br Heart J 1969; 31:803–806.

364. Langendorf R. Differential diagnosis of ventricular paoxysmal tachycardia. In Anonymous (ed). Experimental Medicine and Surgery. Brooklyn Medical Press, 1950, pp. 228–239.

365. Pick A, Langendorf R. Differentiation of supraventricular and ventricular tachycardia. Prog Cardiovasc Dis 1960; 2:391.

366. Kistin AD. Problems in the differentiation of ventricular arrhythmia from supraventricular arrhythmia with abnormal QRS. Prog Cardiovasc Dis 1966; 9:1–17.

367. Marriott HJL. Differential diagnosis of supraventricular and ventricular tachycardia. Geriatrics 1970; 91:25.

368. Akhtar M. Electrophysiologic bases for wide QRS complex tachycardia. PACE 1983; 6:81–98.

369. Barold SS. Bedside diagnosis of wide QRS tachycardia. PACE 1995; 18:2109–2115.

370. Garratt CJ, Griffith MJ. Electrocardiographic Diagnosis of Tachycardias. Armonk, NY: Futura Publishing Co., 1994.

371. Levy S. Differentiating SVT from VT: a personal viewpoint. Eur Heart J 1994; 15:31–38.

372. Stewart RB, Bardy GH, Greene HL. Wide complex tachycardia: misdiagnosis and outcome after emergent therapy. Ann Intern Med 1986; 104:766–771.

373. Akhtar M, Shenasa M, Jazayeri M, Caceres J, Tchou PJ. Wide QRS complex tachycardia: reappraisal of a common clinical problem. Ann Intern Med 1988; 109:905–912.

374. Wellens HJJ, Bar FW, Lie KI. The value of the electrocardiogram in the differential diagnosis of a tachycardia with a widened QRS complex. Am J Med 1978; 64:27–33.

375. Dancy M, Camm AJ, Ward D. Misdiagnosis of chronic recurrent ventricular tachycardia. Lancet 1985; 2:320–323.

376. Drew BJ, Scheinman MM. ECG criteria to distinguish between aberrantly conducted supraventricular tachycardia and ventricular tachycardia: practical aspects for the immediate care setting. Pacing Clin Electrophysiol 1995; 18:2194–2208.

377. Brugada P, Brugada J, Smeets J, Andries EW. A new approach to the differential diagnosis of a regular tachycardia with a wide QRS complex. Circulation 1991; 83:1649–1659.

378. Morady F, Baerman JM, DiCarlo LA Jr, DeBuitleir M, Krol RB, Wahr DW. A prevalent misconception regarding wide-complex tachycardias. JAMA 1985; 254:2790–2792.

379. Kindwall KE, Brown J, Josephson ME. Electrocardiographic criteria for ventricular tachycardia in wide complex left bundle branch block morphology tachycardias. Am J Cardiol 1988; 61:1279–1283.

380. Griffith MJ, de Belder MA, Linker NJ, Ward DE, Camm AJ. Difficulties in the use of electrocardiographic criteria for the differential diagnosis of left bundle branch block pattern tachycardia in patients with a structurally normal heart. Eur Heart J 1992; 13:478–483.

381. Kremers MS, Black WH, Wells PJ, Solodyna M. Effect of preexisting bundle branch block on the electrocardiographic diagnosis of ventricular tachycardia. Am J Cardiol 1988; 62:1208–1212.

382. Alberca T, Almendral J, Sanz P, Almazan A, Cantalapiedra JL, Delcan JL. Evaluation of the specificity of morphological electrocardiographic criteria for the differential diagnosis of wide QRS complex tachycardia in patients with intraventricular conduction defects. Circulation 1997; 96:3527–3533.

383. Dongas J, Lehmann MH, Mahmud R, Denker S, Soni J, Akhtar M. Value of preexisting bundle branch block in the electrocardiographic differentiation of supraventricular from ventricular origin of wide QRS tachycardia. Am J Cardiol 1985; 55:717–721.

384. Wellens HJJ, Bar FWHM, Lie KI. The value of the electrocardiogram in the differential diagnosis of a tachycardia with a widened QRS complex. Am J Med 1978; 64:27–33.

385. Kremers MS, Miller JM, Josephson ME. Electrical alternans in wide complex tachycardias. Am J Cardiol 1985; 56:305–308.

386. Inoue T, Koumatsu K, Ito M, Arita M, Saikawa T. Heart rate-dependent alteration of the frequency and coupling interval of ventricular arrhythmias as measured by 24-hour ECG monitoring. Jpn Circ J 1991; 55:942–950.

387. Leclercq JF, Potenza S, Maison-Blanche P, Chastang C, Coumel P. Determinants of spontaneous occurrence of sustained monomorphic ventricular tachycardia in right ventricular dysplasia. J Am Coll Cardiol 1996; 28:720–724.

388. Vinet A, Cardinal R, LeFranc P, et al. Cycle length dynamics and spatial stability at the onset of postinfarction monomorphic ventricular tachycardias induced in patients and canine preparations. Circulation 1996; 93:1845–1859.

389. Meyerfeldt U, Schirdewan A, Wiedemann M, et al. The mode of onset of ventricular tachycardia: a patient-specific phenomenon. Eur Heart J 1997; 18:1956–1965.

390. Berger MD, Waxman HL, Buxton AE, Marchlinski FE, Josephson ME. Spontaneous compared with induced onset of sustained ventricular tachycardia. Circulation 1988; 78:885–892.

391. Kinoshita S, Kato Y, Kawasaki T, Okimori K. Ventricular tachycardia initiated by late-coupled ventricular extrasystoles: the concept of longitudinal dissociation in the microreentry pathway. Am Heart J 1982; 103:1090–1095.

392. Bluzhas J, Lukshiene D. Ventricular tachycardia in myocardial infarction: relation to heart rate and premature ventricular contractions. Eur Heart J 1985; 6:745–750.

393. Zimmermann M, Maisonblanche P, Cauchemez B, Leclercq J-F, Coumel P. Determinants of the spontaneous ectopic activity in repetitive monomorphic idiopathic ventricular tachycardia. J Am Coll Cardiol 1986; 7:1219–1227.

394. Duff HJ, Mitchell LB, Gillis AM, et al. Electrocardiographic correlates of spontaneous termination of ventricular tachycardia in patients with coronary artery disease. Circulation 1993; 88:1054–1062.

395. Romero CA Jr. Holter monitoring in the diagnosis and management of cardiac rhythm disturbances. Med Clin North Am 1976; 60:299–313.

396. Follansbee WP, Michelson EL, Morganroth J. Nonsustained ventricular tachycardia in ambulatory patients: characteristics and association with sudden cardiac death. Ann Intern Med 1980; 92:741–747.

397. Platia EV, Reid PR. Comparison of programmed electrical stimulation and ambulatory electrocardiographic (Holter) monitoring in the management of ventricular tachycardia and ventricular fibrillation. J Am Coll Cardiol 1984; 4:493–500.

398. Kim SG, Felder SD, Figura I, Johnston DR, Mercando AD, Fisher JD. Prognostic value of the changes in the mode of ventricular tachycardia induction during therapy with amiodarone or amiodarone and a class 1a antiarrhythmic agent. Am J Cardiol 1987; 59:1314–1318.

399. Kim SG. The management of patients with life-threatening ventricular tachyarrhythmias: programmed stimulation or Holter monitoring (either or both)? Circulation 1987; 76:1–5.

400. Heger JJ, Nattel S, Rinkenberger RL, Zipes DP. Mexiletine therapy in 15 patients with drug-resistant ventricular tachycardia. Am J Cardiol 1980; 45:627–632.

401. Pratt CM, Slymen DJ, Wierman AM, et al. Analysis of the spontaneous variability of ventricular arrhythmias: consecutive ambulatory electrocardiographic recordings of ventricular tachycardia. Am J Cardiol 1985; 56:67–72.

402. Veltri EP, Griffith LS, Platia EV, Guarnieri T, Reid PR. The use of ambulatory monitoring in the prognostic evaluation of patients with sustained ventricular tachycardia treated with amiodarone. Circulation 1986; 74:1054–1060.

403. Kim SG, Seiden SW, Felder SD, Waspe LE, Fisher JD. Is programmed stimulation of value in predicting the long-term success of antiarrhythmic therapy for ventricular tachycardias? N Engl J Med 1986; 315:356–362.

404. Kim SG, Felder SD, Figura I, Johnston DR, Waspe LE, Fisher JD. Value of Holter monitoring in predicting long-term efficacy and inefficacy of amiodarone used alone and in combination with class 1a antiarrhythmic agents in patients with ventricular tachycardia. J Am Coll Cardiol 1987; 9:169–174.

405. Van Durme JP. Tachyarrhythmias and transient cerebral ischemic attacks. Am Heart J 1975; 89:538–540.

406. Aronow WS. Usefulness of the resting electrocardiogram in the elderly. Comprehensive Therapy 1992; 18:11–16.

407. Lemery R, Brugada P, Della Bella P, et al. Predictors of long-term success during closed-chest catheter ablation of the atrioventricular junction. Eur Heart J 1989; 10:826–832.

408. de Soyza N, Meacham D, Murphy ML, Kane JJ, Doherty JE, Bissett JK. Evaluation of warning arrhythmias before paroxysmal ventricular tachycardia during acute myocardial infarction in man. Circulation 1979; 60:814–818.

409. Kanovsky MS, Falcone RA, Dresden CA, Josephson ME, Simson MB. Identification of patients with ventricular tachycardia after myocardial infarction: signal-averaged electrocardiogram, Holter monitoring, and cardiac catheterization. Circulation 1984; 70:264–270.

410. Gomes JA, Winters SL, Stewart D, Horowitz S, Milner M, Barreca P. A new noninvasive index to predict sustained

ventricular tachycardia and sudden death in the first year after myocardial infarction: based on signal-averaged electrocardiogram, radionuclide ejection fraction and Holter monitoring. J Am Coll Cardiol 1987; 10:349–357.

411. Kuchar DL, Thorburn CW, Sammel NL. Prediction of serious arrhythmic events after myocardial infarction: signal-averaged electrocardiogram, Holter monitoring and radionuclide ventriculography. J Am Coll Cardiol 1987; 9:531–538.

412. Gomes JA, Winters SL, Martinson M, Machac J, Stewart D, Targonski A. The prognostic significance of quantitative signal-averaged variables relative to clinical variables, site of myocardial infarction, ejection fraction and ventricular premature beats: a prospective study. J Am Coll Cardiol 1989; 13:377–384.

413. el-Sherif N, Ursell SN, Bekheit S, et al. Prognostic significance of the signal-averaged ECG depends on the time of recording in the postinfarction period. Am Heart J 1989; 118:256–264.

414. Herling IM, Horowitz LN, Josephson ME. Ventricular ectopic activity after medical and surgical treatment for recurrent sustained ventricular tachycardia. Am J Cardiol 1980; 45:633–639.

415. de Soyza N, Thenabadu PN, Murphy ML, Kane JJ, Doherty JE. Ventricular arrhythmia before and after aorto-coronary bypass surgery. Int J Cardiol 1981; 1:123–130.

416. Hohnloser SH, Klingenheben T, van de Loo A, Hablawetz E, Just H, Schwartz PJ. Reflex versus tonic vagal activity as a prognostic parameter in patients with sustained ventricular tachycardia or ventricular fibrillation. Circulation 1994; 89:1068–1073.

417. Perkiomaki JS, Koistinen MJ, Yli-Mayry S, Huikuri HV. Dispersion of QT interval in patients with and without susceptibility to ventricular tachyarrhythmias after previous myocardial infarction. J Am Coll Cardiol 1995; 26:174–179.

418. Huikuri HV, Seppanen T, Koistinen MJ, et al. Abnormalities in beat-to-beat dynamics of heart rate before the spontaneous onset of life-threatening ventricular tachyarrhythmias in patients with prior myocardial infarction. Circulation 1996; 93:1836–1844.

419. Makikallio TH, Seppanen T, Airaksinen KE, et al. Dynamic analysis of heart rate may predict subsequent ventricular tachycardia after myocardial infarction. Am J Cardiol 1997; 80:779–783.

420. van Boven AJ, Jukema JW, Crijns HJ, Lie KI. Heart rate variability profiles in symptomatic coronary artery disease and preserved left ventricular function: relation to ventricular tachycardia and transient myocardial ischemia. Regression Growth Evaluation Statin Study (REGRESS). Am Heart J 1995; 130:1020–1025.

421. Perkiomaki JS, Huikuri HV, Koistinen JM, Makikallio T, Castellanos A, Myerburg RJ. Heart rate variability and dispersion of QT interval in patients with vulnerability to ventricular tachycardia and ventricular fibrillation after previous myocardial infarction. J Am Coll Cardiol 1997; 30:1331–1338.

422. Huikuri HV, Valkama JO, Airaksinen J, et al. Frequency domain measures of heart rate variability before the onset of nonsustained and sustained ventricular tachycardia in patients with coronary artery disease. Circulation 1993; 87:1220–1228.

423. Huikuri HV, Koistinen MJ, Yli-Mayry S, et al. Impaired low-frequency oscillations of heart rate in patients with prior acute myocardial infarction and life-threatening arrhythmias. Am J Cardiol 1995; 76:56–60.

424. Valkama JO, Huikuri HV, Koistinen MJ, Yli-Mayry S, Airaksinen KE, Myerburg RJ. Relation between heart rate variability and spontaneous and induced ventricular arrhythmias in patients with coronary artery disease. J Am Coll Cardiol 1995; 25:437–443.

425. Hayashi H, Fujiki A, Tani M, Mizumaki K, Shimono M, Inoue H. Role of sympathovagal balance in the initiation of idiopathic ventricular tachycardia originating from right ventricular outflow tract. PACE 1997; 20:2371–2377.

426. Fei L, Gill JS, Katritsis D, Camm AJ. Abnormal autonomic

modulation of QT interval in patients with idiopathic ventricular tachycardia associated with clinically normal hearts. Br Heart J 1993; 69:311–314.

427. Ideker RE, Mirvis DM, Smith WM. Late, fractionated potentials. Am J Cardiol 1985; 55:1614–1621.

428. Breithardt G, Borggrefe M. Pathophysiological mechanisms and clinical significance of ventricular late potentials. Eur Heart J 1986; 7:364–385.

429. Gomes JA, Winters SL, Ip J. Signal averaging of the surface QRS complex: practical applications. J Cardiovasc Electrophysiol 1991; 2:316–330.

430. Almendral J, Ormaetxe J, Delcan JL. Idiopathic ventricular tachycardia and fibrillation: incidence, prognosis, and therapy. PACE 1992; 15:627–630.

431. Winters SL, Goldman DS, Banas JS Jr. Prognostic impact of late potentials in nonischemic dilated cardiomyopathy: potential signals for the future. Circulation 1993; 87:1405–1407.

432. Vester EG, Strauer BE. Ventricular late potentials: state of the art and future perspectives. Eur Heart J 1994; 15 (Suppl C):34–48.

433. Simson MB. Signal-averaged electrocardiography. In Zipes DP, Jalife J (eds). Cardiac Electrophysiology. From Cell to Bedside. 2nd ed. Philadelphia: WB Saunders, 1995, pp. 1038–1048.

434. Fauchier JP, Fauchier L, Babuty D, Cosnay P. Time-domain signal-averaged electrocardiogram in nonischemic ventricular tachycardia. Pacing Clin Electrophysiol 1996; 19:231–244.

435. Simson MB. Use of signals in the terminal QRS complex to identify patients with ventricular tachycardia after myocardial infarction. Circulation 1981; 64:235–242.

436. Rozanski JJ, Mortara D, Myerburg RJ, Castellanos A. Body surface detection of delayed depolarizations in patients with recurrent ventricular tachycardia and left ventricular aneurysm. Circulation 1981; 63:1172–1178.

437. Breithardt G, Becker R, Seipel L, Abendroth R-R, Ostermeyer J. Non-invasive detection of late potentials in man: a new marker for ventricular tachycardia. Eur Heart J 1981; 2:1–11.

438. Cain ME, Ambos HD, Witkowski FX, Sobel BE. Fast-fourier transform analysis of signal-averaged electrocardiograms for identification of patients prone to sustained ventricular tachycardia. Circulation 1984; 69:711–720.

439. Freedman RA, Gillis AM, Keren A, Soderholm-Difatte V, Mason JW. Signal-averaged electrocardiographic late potentials in patients with ventricular fibrillation or ventricular tachycardia: correlation with clinical arrhythmia and electrophysiologic study. Am J Cardiol 1985; 55:1350–1353.

440. Lindsay BD, Ambos HD, Schechtman KB, Cain ME. Improved selection of patients for programmed ventricular stimulation by frequency analysis of signal-averaged electrocardiograms. Circulation 1986; 73:675–683.

441. Haberl R, Jilge G, Pulter R, Steinbeck G. Comparison of frequency and time domain analysis of the signal-averaged electrocardiogram in patients with ventricular tachycardia and coronary artery disease: methodologic validation and clinical relevance. J Am Coll Cardiol 1988; 12:150–158.

442. Lindsay BD, Markham J, Schechtman KB, Ambos HD, Cain ME. Identification of patients with sustained ventricular tachycardia by frequency analysis of signal-averaged electrocardiograms despite the presence of bundle branch block. Circulation 1988; 77:122–130.

443. Machac J, Weiss A, Winters SL, Barecca P, Gomes JA. A comparative study of frequency domain and time domain analysis of signal-averaged electrocardiograms in patients with ventricular tachycardia. J Am Coll Cardiol 1988; 11:284–296.

444. Nalos PC, Gang ES, Mandel WJ, et al. Utility of the signal-averaged electrocardiogram in patients presenting with sustained ventricular tachycardia or fibrillation while on an antiarrhythmic drug. Am Heart J 1988; 115:108–114.

445. Haberl R, Jilge G, Pulter R, Steinbeck G. Spectral mapping of the electrocardiogram with Fourier transform for

identification of patients with sustained ventricular tachycardia and coronary artery disease. Eur Heart J 1989; 10:316–322.

446. Pierce DL, Easley AR Jr, Windle JR, Engel TR. Fast Fourier transformation of the entire low amplitude late QRS potential to predict ventricular tachycardia. J Am Coll Cardiol 1989; 14:1731–1740.

447. Steinberg JS, Bigger JT Jr. Importance of the endpoint of noise reduction in analysis of the signal-averaged electrocardiogram. Am J Cardiol 1989; 63:556–560.

448. Branyas NA, Cassidy DM, Cain ME. Periodicity of global ventricular activation of sinus beats in patients with coronary artery disease and sustained ventricular tachycardia. Am J Cardiol 1991; 68:901–908.

449. Kelen GJ, Henkin R, Starr AM, Caref EB, Bloomfield D, el-Sherif N. Spectral turbulence analysis of the signal-averaged electrocardiogram and its predictive accuracy for inducible sustained monomorphic ventricular tachycardia. Am J Cardiol 1991; 67:965–975.

450. Hood MA, Pogwizd SM, Peirick J, Cain ME. Contribution of myocardium responsible for ventricular tachycardia to abnormalities detected by analysis of signal-averaged ECGs. Circulation 1992; 86:1888–1901.

451. Kinoshita O, Kamakura S, Ohe T, et al. Spectral analysis of signal-averaged electrocardiograms in patients with idiopathic ventricular tachycardia of left ventricular origin. Circulation 1992; 85:2054–2059.

452. Hoher M, Axmann J, Eggeling T, Kochs M, Weismuller P, Hombach V. Beat-to-beat variability of ventricular late potentials in the unaveraged high resolution electrocardiogram: effects of antiarrhythmic drugs. Eur Heart J 1993; 14:33–39.

453. Kavesh NG, Cain ME, Ambos D, Arthur RM. Enhanced detection of distinguishing features in signal-averaged electrocardiograms from patients with ventricular tachycardia by combined spatial and spectral analyses of entire cardiac cycle. Circulation 1994; 90:254–263.

454. Makijarvi M, Montonen J, Toivonen L, Leinio M, Siltanen P, Katila T. High-resolution and signal-averaged electrocardiography to separate post-myocardial infarction patients with and without ventricular tachycardia. Eur Heart J 1994; 15:189–199.

455. Englund A, Andersson M, Bergfeldt L. Spectral turbulence analysis of the signal-averaged electrocardiogram for predicting inducible sustained monomorphic ventricular tachycardia in patients with and without bundle branch block. Eur Heart J 1995; 16:1936–1942.

456. Okin PM, Stein KM, Lippman N, Lerman BB, Kligfield P. Performance of the signal-averaged electrocardiogram: relation to baseline QRS duration. Am Heart J 1995; 129:932–940.

457. Christiansen EH, Frost L, Molgaard H, Nielsen TT, Pedersen AK. Noise in the signal-averaged electrocardiogram and accuracy for identification of patients with sustained monomorphic ventricular tachycardia after myocardial infarction. Eur Heart J 1996; 17:911–916.

458. Gatzoulis KA, Carlson MD, Biblo LA, et al. Time domain analysis of the signal averaged electrocardiogram in patients with a conduction defect or a bundle branch block. Eur Heart J 1995; 16:1912–1919.

459. Lander P, Gomis P, Goyal R, et al. Analysis of abnormal intra-QRS potentials: improved predictive value for arrhythmic events with the signal-averaged electrocardiogram. Circulation 1997; 95:1386–1393.

460. Breithardt G, Borggrefe M, Karbenn U, Abendroth R-R, Yeh H-L, Seipel L. Prevalence of late potentials in patients with and without ventricular tachycardia: correlation with angiographic findings. Am J Cardiol 1982; 49:1932–1937.

461. Breithardt G, Borggrefe M, Quantius B, Karbenn U, Seipel L. Ventricular vulnerability assessed by programmed ventricular stimulation in patients with and without late potentials. Circulation 1983; 68:275–281.

462. Borggrefe M, Fetsch T, Martinez-Rubio A, Makijarvi M, Breithardt G. Prediction of arrhythmia risk based on signal-averaged ECG in postinfarction patients. PACE 1997; 20:2566–2576.

463. Breithardt G, Schwarzmaier J, Borggrefe M, Haerten K, Seipel L. Prognostic significance of late ventricular potentials after acute myocardial infarction. Eur Heart J 1983; 4:487–495.

464. Zimmermann M, Adamec R, Simonin P, Richez J. Prognostic significance of ventricular late potentials in coronary artery disease. Am Heart J 1985; 109:725–732.

465. Kuchar DL, Kelly RP, Thorburn CW. High-frequency analysis of the surface electrocardiograms of patients with supraventricular tachycardia: accurate identification of atrial activation and determination of the mechanism of tachycardia. Circulation 1986; 74:1016–1026.

466. McGuire M, Kuchar D, Ganis J, Sammel N, Thorburn C. Natural history of late potentials in the first ten days after acute myocardial infarction and relation to early ventricular arrhythmias. Am J Cardiol 1988; 61:1187–1190.

467. Cripps T, Bennett ED, Camm AJ, Ward DE. High gain signal averaged electrocardiogram combined with 24 hour monitoring in patients early after myocardial infarction for bedside prediction of arrhythmic events. Br Heart J 1988; 60:181–187.

468. Kienzle MG, Falcone RA, Simson MB. Alterations in the initial portion of the signal-averaged QRS complex in acute myocardial infarction with ventricular tachycardia. Am J Cardiol 1988; 61:99–103.

469. Denniss AR, Ross DL, Richards DA, Uther JB. Changes in ventricular activation time on the signal-averaged electrocardiogram in the first year after acute myocardial infarction. Am J Cardiol 1987; 60:580–583.

470. Gang ES, Lew AS, Hong M, Wang FZ, Siebert CA, Peter T. Decreased incidence of ventricular late potentials after successful thrombolytic therapy for acute myocardial infarction. N Engl J Med 1989; 321:712–716.

471. Zimmermann M, Adamec R, Ciaroni S, Malbois F, Tieche R. Reduction in the frequency of ventricular late potentials after acute myocardial infarction by early thrombolytic therapy. Am J Cardiol 1991; 67:697–703.

472. Zimmerman M, Sentici A, Adamec R, Metzger J, Mermillod B, Rutishauser W. Long-term prognostic significance of ventricular late potentials after a first acute myocardial infarction. Am Heart J 1997; 134:1019–1028.

473. Rosenthal ME, Hamer A, Gang ES, Oseran DS, Mandel WJ, Peter T. The yield of programmed ventricular stimulation in mitral valve prolapse patients with ventricular arrhythmias. Am Heart J 1985; 110:970–976.

474. Denes P, Santarelli P, Hauser RG, Uretz EF. Quantitative analysis of the high-frequency components of the terminal portion of the body surface QRS in normal subjects and in patients with ventricular tachycardia. Circulation 1983; 67:1129–1138.

475. Vaitkus PT, Kindwall KE, Marchlinski FE, Miller JM, Buxton AE, Josephson ME. Differences in electrophysiological substrate in patients with coronary artery disease and cardiac arrest or ventricular tachycardia. Insights from endocardial mapping and signal-averaged electrocardiography. Circulation 1991; 84:672–678.

476. Buckingham TA, Ghosh S, Homan SM, et al. Independent value of signal-averaged electrocardiography and left ventricular function in identifying patients with sustained ventricular tachycardia with coronary artery disease. Am J Cardiol 1987; 59:568–572.

477. Puljevic D, Smalcelj A, Durakovic Z, Goldner V. QT dispersion, daily variations, QT interval adaptation and late potentials as risk markers for ventricular tachycardia. Eur Heart J 1997; 18:1343–1349.

478. Winters SL, Ip J, Deshmukh P, et al. Determinants of induction of ventricular tachycardia in nonsustained ventricular tachycardia after myocardial infarction and the usefulness of the signal-averaged electrocardiogram. Am J Cardiol 1993; 72:1281–1285.

479. Turitto G, Ahuja RK, Caref EB, el-Sherif N. Risk stratification for arrhythmic events in patients with nonischemic dilated cardiomyopathy and nonsustained ventricular tachycardia: role of programmed ventricular stimulation and the signal-averaged electrocardiogram. J Am Coll Cardiol 1994; 24:1523–1528.

480. Oselladore L, Nava A, Buja G, et al. Signal-averaged electrocardiography in familial form of arrhythmogenic right ventricular cardiomyopathy. Am J Cardiol 1995; 75:1038–1041.

481. Kinoshita O, Fontaine G, Rosas F, et al. Time- and frequency-domain analyses of the signal-averaged ECG in patients with arrhythmogenic right ventricular dysplasia. Circulation 1995; 91:715–721.

482. Mehta D, Goldman M, David O, Gomes JA. Value of quantitative measurement of signal-averaged electrocardiographic variables in arrhythmogenic right ventricular dysplasia: correlation with echocardiographic right ventricular cavity dimensions. J Am Coll Cardiol 1996; 28:713–719.

483. Frielingsdorf J, Gerber AE, Laske A, Bertel O. Influence of coronary artery bypass grafting on ventricular late potentials as a predictive factor for ventricular arrhythmias during short- and long-term follow-up. Eur Heart J 1995; 16:660–666.

484. Stelling JA, Danford DA, Kugler JD, et al. Late potentials and inducible ventricular tachycardia in surgically repaired congenital heart disease. Circulation 1990; 82:1690–1696.

485. Breithardt G, Seipel L, Ostermeyer J, et al. Effects of antiarrhythmic surgery on late ventricular potentials recorded by precordial signal averaging in patients with ventricular tachycardia. Am Heart J 1982; 104:996–1003.

486. Marcus NH, Falcone RA, Harken AH, Josephson ME, Simson MB. Body surface late potentials: effects of endocardial resection in patients with ventricular tachycardia. Circulation 1984; 70:632–637.

487. Kertes PJ, Glabus M, Murray A, Julian DG, Campbell RWF. Delayed ventricular depolarization: correlation with ventricular activation and relevance to ventricular fibrillation in acute myocardial infarction. Eur Heart J 1984; 5:974–983.

488. Denniss AR, Johnson DC, Richards DA, Ross DL, Uther JB. Effect of excision of ventricular myocardium on delayed potentials detected by the signal-averaged electrocardiogram in patients with ventricular tachycardia. Am J Cardiol 1987; 59:591–595.

489. Gomes JA. The arrhythmic substrate in patients without overt heart disease. J Am Coll Cardiol 1989; 14:380–381.

490. Mehta D, McKenna WJ, Ward DE, Davies MJ, Camm AJ. Significance of signal-averaged electrocardiography in relation to endomyocardial biopsy and ventricular stimulation studies in patients with ventricular tachycardia without clinically apparent heart disease. J Am Coll Cardiol 1989; 14:372–379.

491. La Vecchia L, Ometto R, Bedogni F, et al. Ventricular late potentials, interstitial fibrosis, and right ventricular function in patients with ventricular tachycardia and normal left ventricular function. Am J Cardiol 1998; 81:790–792.

492. Gang ES, Peter T, Rosenthal ME, Mandel WJ, Lass Y. Detection of late potentials on the surface electrocardiogram in unexplained syncope. Am J Cardiol 1986; 58:1014–1020.

493. Kuchar DL, Thorburn CW, Sammel NL. Late potentials detected after myocardial infarction: natural history and prognostic significance. Circulation 1986; 74:1280–1289.

494. Winters SL, Stewart D, Gomes JA. Signal averaging of the surface QRS complex predicts inducibility of ventricular tachycardia in patients with syncope of unknown origin: a prospective study. J Am Coll Cardiol 1987; 10:775–781.

495. Steinberg JS, Prystowsky E, Freedman RA, et al. Use of signal-averaged electrocardiogram for predicting inducible ventricular tachycardia in patients with unexplained syncope: relation to clinical variables in multivariate analysis. J Am Coll Cardiol 1994; 23:99–106.

496. Denniss AR, Ross DL, Richards DA, et al. Effect of antiarrhythmic therapy on delayed potentials detected by the signal-averaged electrocardiogram in patients with ventricular tachycardia after acute myocardial infarction. Am J Cardiol 1986; 58:261–265.

497. Freedman RA, Karagounis LA, Steinberg JS. Effects of sotalol on the signal-averaged electrocardiogram in patients with sustained ventricular tachycardia: relation to suppression of inducibility and changes in tachycardia cycle length. J Am Coll Cardiol 1992; 20:1213–1219.

498. Gardner MJ, Montague TJ, Armstrong CS, Horacek BM, Smith ER. Vulnerability to ventricular arrhythmia: assessment by mapping of body surface potential. Circulation 1986; 73:684–692.

499. Mitchell LB, Hubley-Kozey CL, Smith ER, et al. Electrocardiographic body surface mapping in patients with ventricular tachycardia: assessment of utility in the identification of effective pharmacological therapy. Circulation 1992; 86:383–393.

500. Fontaine G, Aouate P, Fontaliran F. Repolarization and the genesis of cardiac arrhythmias: role of body surface mapping. Circulation 1997; 95:2600–2602.

501. De Ambroggi L, Aime E, Ceriotti C, Rovida M, Negroni S. Mapping of ventricular repolarization potentials in patients with arrhythmogenic right ventricular dysplasia: principal component analysis of the ST-T waves. Circulation 1997; 96:4314–4318.

502. Higham PD, Campbell RW. QT dispersion. Br Heart J 1994; 71:508–510.

503. Pye M, Quinn AC, Cobbe SM. QT interval dispersion: a non-invasive marker of susceptibility to arrhythmia in patients with sustained ventricular arrhythmias? Br Heart J 1994; 71:511–514.

504. Zaidi M, Robert A, Fesler R, Derwael C, Brohet C. Dispersion of ventricular repolarisation: a marker of ventricular arrhythmias in patients with previous myocardial infarction. Heart 1997; 78:371–375.

505. Oikarinen L, Viitasalo M, Toivonen L. Dispersions of the QT interval in postmyocardial infarction patients presenting with ventricular tachycardia or with ventricular fibrillation. Am J Cardiol 1998; 81:694–697.

506. Barr CS, Naas A, Freeman M, Lang CC, Struthers AD. QT dispersion and sudden unexpected death in chronic heart failure. Lancet 1994; 343:327–329.

507. Glancy JM, Garratt CJ, Woods KL, de Bono DP. QT dispersion and mortality after myocardial infarction. Lancet 1995; 345:945–948.

508. Grimm W, Steder U, Menz V, Hoffman J, Maisch B. QT dispersion and arrhythmic events in idiopathic dilated cardiomyopathy. Am J Cardiol 1996; 78:458–461.

509. Goldner B, Brandspiegel HZ, Horwitz L, Jadonath R, Cohen TJ. Utility of QT dispersion combined with the signal-averaged electrocardiogram in detecting patients susceptible to ventricular tachyarrhythmia. Am J Cardiol 1995; 76:1192–1194.

510. Cohen TJ, Goldner B, Merkatz K, Jadonath R, Adler H, Ehrlich JC. A simple electrocardiographic algorithm for detecting ventricular tachycardia. PACE 1997; 20:2412–2418.

511. Lee KW, Okin PM, Kligfield P, Stein KM, Lerman BB. Precordial QT dispersion and inducible ventricular tachycardia. Am Heart J 1997; 134:1005–1013.

512. Gillis AM, Traboulsi M, Hii JTY, et al. Antiarrhythmic drug effects on QT interval dispersion in patients undergoing electropharmacologic testing for ventricular tachycardia and fibrillation. Am J Cardiol 1998; 81:588–593.

513. Verrier RL, Stone PH. Exercise stress testing for T wave alternans to expose latent electrical instability. J Cardiovasc Electrophysiol 1997; 8:994–997.

514. Rosenbaum DS, Jackson LE, Smith JM, Garan H, Ruskin JN, Cohen RJ. Electrical alternans and vulnerability to ventricular arrhythmias. N Engl J Med 1994; 330:235–241.

515. Estes NAM, Michaud G, Zipes DP, et al. Electrical alternans during rest and exercise as predictors of vulnerability to ventricular arrhythmias. Am J Cardiol 1997; 80:1314–1318.

516. Hohnloser SH, Klingenheben T, Zabel M, Li YG, Albrecht P, Cohen RJ. T wave alternans during exercise and atrial pacing in humans. J Cardiovasc Electrophysiol 1997; 8:987–993.

517. Viskin S, Heller K, Barron HV, et al. Postextrasystolic U wave augmentation, a new marker of increased arrhythmic risk in patients without the long QT syndrome. J Am Coll Cardiol 1996; 28:1746–1752.

518. Ruckel A, Kasper W, Treese N, Henkel B, Pop T, Meinertz T. Atrioventricular dissociation detected by suprasternal M-mode echocardiography: a clue to the diagnosis of ventricular tachycardia. Am J Cardiol 1984; 54:561–563.

519. Spirito P, Watson RM, Maron BJ. Relation between extent of left ventricular hypertrophy and occurrence of ventricular tachycardia in hypertrophic cardiomyopathy. Am J Cardiol 1987; 60:1137–1142.

520. Morgera T, Salvi A, Alberti E, Silvestri F, Camerini F. Morphological findings in apparently idiopathic ventricular tachycardia. An echocardiographic haemodynamic and histologic study. Eur Heart J 1985; 6:323–334.

521. Foale RA, Nihoyannopoulos P, Ribeiro P, et al. Right ventricular abnormalities in ventricular tachycardia of right ventricular origin: relation to electrophysiological abnormalities. Br Heart J 1986; 56:45–54.

522. Mehta D, Odawara H, Ward DE, McKenna WJ, Davies MJ, Camm AJ. Echocardiographic and histologic evaluation of the right ventricle in ventricular tachycardias of left bundle branch block morphology without overt cardiac abnormality. Am J Cardiol 1989; 63:939–944.

523. Saxon LA, Stevenson WG, Fonarow GC, et al. Transesophageal echocardiography during radiofrequency catheter ablation of ventricular tachycardia. Am J Cardiol 1993; 72:658–661.

524. Gill JS, de Belder M, Ward DE. Right ventricular outflow tract ventricular tachycardia associated with an aneurysmal malformation: use of transesophageal echocardiography during low-energy, direct-current ablation. Am Heart J 1994; 128:620–623.

525. Jadonath RL, Schwartzman DS, Preminger MW, Gottlieb CD, Marchlinski FE. Utility of the 12-lead electrocardiogram in localizing the origin of right ventricular outflow tract tachycardia. Am Heart J 1995; 130:1107–1113.

526. Stevenson WG. Ventricular tachycardia after myocardial infarction: from arrhythmia surgery to catheter ablation. J Cardiovasc Electrophysiol 1995; 6:942–950.

527. Suwa M, Yoneda Y, Nagao H, et al. Surgical correction of idiopathic paroxysmal ventricular tachycardia possibly related to left ventricular false tendon. Am J Cardiol 1989; 64:1217–1220.

528. Thakur RK, Klein GJ, Sivaram CA, et al. Anatomic substrate for idiopathic left ventricular tachycardia. Circulation 1996; 93:497–501.

529. Lin FC, Wen MS, Wang CC, Yeh SJ, Wu D. Left ventricular fibromuscular band is not a specific substrate for idiopathic left ventricular tachycardia. Circulation 1996; 93:525–528.

530. Klersy C, Raisaro A, Salerno JA, Montemartini C, Campani R. Arrhythmogenic right and left ventricular disease: evaluation by computed tomography and nuclear magnetic resonance imaging. Eur Heart J 1989; 10:33–36.

531. Carlson MD, White RD, Trohman RG, et al. Right ventricular outflow tract ventricular tachycardia: detection of previously unrecognized anatomic abnormalities using cine magnetic resonance imaging. J Am Coll Cardiol 1994; 24:720–727.

532. Steinbach KK, Merl O, Frohner K, et al. Hemodynamics during ventricular tachyarrhythmias. Am Heart J 1994; 127:1102–1106.

533. Josephson ME, Horowitz LN, Spielman SR, Greenspan AM. Electrophysiologic and hemodynamic studies in patients resuscitated from cardiac arrest. Am J Cardiol 1980; 46:948–955.

534. Hamer AW, Zaher CA, Peter T, Mandel WJ. Verapamil effects in AV node reentry tachycardia with intermittent supra-Hisian AV block. Am Heart J 1984; 107:431–439.

535. Raichlen JS, Links JM, Reid PR. Effect of electrical activation site on left ventricular performance in ventricular tachycardia patients with coronary heart disease. Am J Cardiol 1985; 55:84–88.

536. Saksena S, Ciccone JM, Craelius W, Pantopoulos D, Rothbart ST, Werres R. Studies on left ventricular function during sustained ventricular tachycardia. J Am Coll Cardiol 1984; 4:501–508.

537. Bolick DR, Hackel DB, Reimer KA, Ideker RE. Quantitative analysis of myocardial infarct structure in patients with ventricular tachycardia. Circulation 1986; 74:1266–1279.

538. Fenoglio JJ, Pham TC, Harken AH, Horowitz LN, Josephson ME, Wit AL. Recurrent sustained ventricular tachycardia:

structure and ultrastructure of subendocardial regions in which tachycardia originates. Circulation 1983; 68:518–533.

539. de Bakker JMT, Van Capelle FJL, Janse MJ, et al. Reentry as a cause of ventricular tachycardia in patients with chronic ischemic heart disease: electrophysiologic and anatomic correlation. Circulation 1988; 77:589–606.

540. Peters S, Davies MJ, McKenna WJ. Diagnostic value of endomyocardial biopsies of the right ventricular septum in arrhythmias originating from the right ventricle. Jpn Heart J 1996; 37:195–202.

541. Castellanos A Jr, Myerburg RJ, Craparo K, Befeler B, Agha AS. Factors regulating ventricular rates during atrial flutter and fibrillation in preexcitation (Wolff-Parkinson-White) syndrome. Br Heart J 1973; 35:811–816.

542. Wellens HJJ, Lie KI. Ventricular tachycardia: The value of programmed electrical stimulation. In Krikler DM, Goodwin JF (eds). Cardiac Arrhythmias. The Modern Electrophysiological Approach. London: WB Saunders, 1975, pp. 182–194.

543. Wellens HJJ. Pathophysiology of ventricular tachycardia in man. Arch Intern Med 1975; 135:473–479.

544. Scheinman MM. Induction of ventricular tachycardia: a promising new technique or clinical electrophysiology gone awry? Circulation 1978; 58:998–999.

545. Josephson ME, Horowitz LN. Recurrent ventricular tachycardia: an electrophysiologic approach. Med Clin North Am 1979; 63:53–71.

546. Josephson ME, Horowitz LN. Electrophysiologic approach to therapy of recurrent sustained ventricular tachycardia. Am J Cardiol 1979; 43:631–642.

547. Josephson ME, Kastor JA, Horowitz LN. Electrophysiologic management of recurrent ventricular tachycardia in acute and chronic ischemic heart disease. Cardiovascular Clinics 1980; 35–55.

548. Kastor JA, Horowitz LN, Harken AH, Josephson ME. Clinical electrophysiology of ventricular tachycardia. N Engl J Med 1981; 304:1004–1020.

549. Horowitz LN, Spielman SR, Greenspan AM, Josephson ME. Mechanisms in the genesis of recurrent ventricular tachyarrhythmias as revealed by clinical electrophysiologic studies. Ann N Y Acad Sci 1982; 382:116–135.

550. Graboys TB. The stampede to stimulation: numerators and denominators revisited relative to electrophysiologic study of ventricular arrhythmias. Am Heart J 1982; 103:1089–1090.

551. Surawicz B. Intracardiac extrastimulation studies: How to? Where? By whom? Circulation 1982; 65:428–431.

552. Wiener I. Current applications of clinical electrophysiologic study in the diagnosis and treatment of cardiac arrhythmias. Am J Cardiol 1982; 49:1287–1292.

553. Waldo AL, Akhtar M, Brugada P, et al. The minimally appropriate electrophysiologic study for the initial assessment of patients with documented sustained monomorphic ventricular tachycardia. J Am Coll Cardiol 1985; 6:1174–1177.

554. Josephson ME, Almendral JM, Buxton AE, Marchlinski FE. Mechanisms of ventricular tachycardia. Circulation 1987; 75 (Suppl II):II-141–II-147.

555. Weiss JN, Nademanee K, Stevenson WG, Singh B. Ventricular arrhythmias in ischemic heart disease. Ann Intern Med 1991; 114:784–797.

556. Josephson ME. Clinical Cardiac Electrophysiology. Techniques and Interpretations. Philadelphia: Lea & Febiger, 1993, pp. 417–615.

557. ACC/AHA Task Force Report. Guidelines for clinical intracardiac electrophysiological and catheter ablation procedures. Circulation 1995; 92:673–691.

558. Akhtar M, Jazayeri MR, Sra J, Dhala A, Deshpande S, Blanck Z. Electrophysiology of wide QRS tachycardia. In Josephson ME, Wellens HJJ (eds). Tachycardias. Mechanisms and Management. Mount Kisco, NY: Futura Publishing Co., 1993, pp. 215–235.

559. Tai YT, D'Onofrio A, Bourke JP, Campbell RW. Left posterior fascicular tachycardia due to localized microreentry. Eur Heart J 1990; 11:949–953.

560. Easley RM Jr, Goldstein S. Differentiation of ventricular

tachycardia from junctional tachycardia with aberrant conduction: the use of competitive atrial pacing. Circulation 1968; 37:1015–1019.

561. Josephson ME, Horowitz LN, Farshidi A, Spear JF, Kastor JA, Moore EN. Recurrent sustained ventricular tachycardia II. Endocardial mapping. Circulation 1978; 57:440–447.

562. Okumura K, Olshansky B, Henthorn RW, Epstein AE, Plumb VJ, Waldo AL. Demonstration of the presence of slow conduction during sustained ventricular tachycardia in man: use of transient entrainment of the tachycardia. Circulation 1987; 75:369–378.

563. Littmann L, Svenson RH, Gallagher JJ, et al. Functional role of the epicardium in postinfarction ventricular tachycardia: observations derived from computerized epicardial activation mapping, entrainment, and epicardial laser photoablation. Circulation 1991; 83:1577–1591.

564. Gaum WE, Schwartz DC, Kaplan S. Ventricular tachycardia in infancy: evidence for a reentrant mechanism. Circulation 1980; 62:401–406.

565. Rosen MR, Reder RF. Does triggered activity have a role in the genesis of cardiac arrhythmias? Ann Intern Med 1981; 94:794–801.

566. Wieland JM, Marchlinski FE. Electrocardiographic response of digoxin-toxic fascicular tachycardia to Fab fragments: implications for tachycardia mechanism. Pacing Clin Electrophysiol 1986; 9:727–738.

567. Saxon LA, Uretz EF, Denes P. Significance of the clinical presentation in ventricular tachycardia/fibrillation. Am Heart J 1989; 118:695–701.

568. Denes P, Wyndham CR, Rosen KM. Intractable paroxysmal tachycardia caused by a concealed retrogradely conducting Kent bundle: demonstration by epicardial mapping and cure of tachycardias by surgical interruption of the His bundle. Br Heart J 1976; 38:758–763.

569. Estes NAM III, Garan H, McGovern B, Ruskin JN. Influence of drive cycle length during programmed stimulation on induction of ventricular arrhythmias: analysis of 403 patients. Am J Cardiol 1986; 57:108–112.

570. Gillis AM, Winkle RA, Echt DS. Role of extrastimulus prematurity and intraventricular conduction time in inducing ventricular tachycardia or ventricular fibrillation secondary to coronary artery disease. Am J Cardiol 1987; 60:590–595.

571. Breithardt G, Borggrefe M, Podczeck A, Budde T. Influence of the cycle length of basic drive on induction of sustained ventricular tachycardia associated with coronary artery disease. Am J Cardiol 1987; 60:1306–1310.

572. Summitt J, Rosenheck S, Kou WH, Schmaltz S, Kadish AH, Morady F. Effect of basic drive cycle length on the yield of ventricular tachycardia during programmed ventricular stimulation. Am J Cardiol 1990; 65:49–52.

573. Ho DSW, Cooper MJ, Richards DAB, Uther JB, Yip ASB, Ross DL. Comparison of number of extrastimuli versus change in basic cycle length for induction of ventricular tachycardia by programmed ventricular stimulation. J Am Coll Cardiol 1993; 22:1711–1717.

574. Wellens HJJ, Duren DR, Lie KI. Observations on mechanisms of ventricular tachycardia in man. Circulation 1976; 54:237–244.

575. Lee CS, Wan SH, Cooper MJ, Ross DL. Lack of benefit of very short basic drive train cycle length or repetition of extrastimulus coupling intervals for induction of ventricular tachycardia. J Cardiovasc Electrophysiol 1998; 9:574–581.

576. Doherty JU, Kienzle MG, Waxman HL, Buxton AE, Marchlinski FE, Josephson ME. Relation of mode of induction and cycle length of induced ventricular tachycardia: analysis of 104 patients. Am J Cardiol 1983; 52:60–64.

577. Morady F, Shapiro W, Shen E, Sung RJ, Scheinman MM. Programmed ventricular stimulation in patients without spontaneous ventricular tachycardia. Am Heart J 1984; 107:875–882.

578. Denker S, Lehmann M, Mahmud R, Gilbert C, Akhtar M. Facilitation of ventricular tachycardia induction with abrupt changes in ventricular cycle length. Am J Cardiol 1984; 53:508–515.

579. Rosenfeld LE, McPherson CA, Kennedy EE, Stark SI, Batsford WP. Ventricular tachycardia induction: comparison of triple extrastimuli with an abrupt change in ventricular drive cycle length. Am Heart J 1986; 111:868–874.

580. Simonson JS, Gang ES, Mandel W, Peter T. Increasing the yield of ventricular tachycardia induction: a prospective, randomized comparative study of the standard ventricular stimulation protocol to a short-to-long protocol and a new two-site protocol. Am Heart J 1991; 121:68–76.

581. Buxton AE. The use of multiple extrastimuli during programmed ventricular stimulation: how many should be used? Int J Cardiol 1985; 7:86–91.

582. Kudenchuk PJ, Kron J, Walance CG, et al. Reproducibility of arrhythmia induction with intracardiac electrophysiologic testing: patients with clinical sustained ventricular tachyarrhythmias. J Am Coll Cardiol 1986; 7:819–828.

583. Mann DE, Luck JC, Griffin JC, et al. Induction of clinical ventricular tachycardia using programmed stimulation: value of third and fourth extrastimuli. Am J Cardiol 1983; 52:501–506.

584. Swerdlow CD, Bardy GH, McAnulty J, et al. Determinants of induced sustained arrhythmias in survivors of out-of-hospital ventricular fibrillation. Circulation 1987; 76:1053–1060.

585. Hummel JD, Strickberger SA, Daoud E, et al. Results and efficiency of programmed ventricular stimulation with four extrastimuli compared with one, two, and three extrastimuli. Circulation 1994; 90:2827–2832.

586. Koller BS, Karasik PE, Solomon AJ, Franz MR. Relation between repolarization and refractoriness during programmed electrical stimulation in the human right ventricle: implications for ventricular tachycardia induction. Circulation 1995; 91:2378–2384.

587. Brugada P, Wellens HJJ. Standard diagnostic programmed electrical stimulation protocols in patients with paroxysmal recurrent tachycardias. Pacing Clin Electrophysiol 1984; 7:1121–1128.

588. Josephson ME, Horowitz LN, Farshidi A. Continuous local electrical activity: a mechanism of recurrent ventricular tachycardia. Circulation 1978; 57:659–665.

589. Michelson EL, Spielman SR, Greenspan AM, Farshidi A, Horowitz LN, Josephson ME. Electrophysiologic study of the left ventricle: indications and safety. Chest 1979; 75:592–596.

590. Robertson JF, Cain ME, Horowitz LN, et al. Anatomic and electrophysiologic correlates of ventricular tachycardia requiring left ventricular stimulation. Am J Cardiol 1981; 48:263–268.

591. Doherty JU, Kienzle MG, Buxton AE, Marchlinski FE, Waxman HL, Josephson ME. Discordant results of programmed ventricular stimulation at different right ventricular sites in patients with and without spontaneous sustained ventricular tachycardia: a prospective study of 56 patients. Am J Cardiol 1984; 54:336–342.

592. Martinez-Rubio A, Stachowitz A, Borggrefe M, et al. Comparison of the results of programmed ventricular stimulation from the right ventricular apex and outflow tract: a randomized, prospective study. Eur Heart J 1995; 16:1234–1243.

593. Brugada P, Wellens HJJ. Comparison in the same patient of two programmed ventricular stimulation protocols to induce ventricular tachycardia. Am J Cardiol 1985; 55:380–383.

594. Kudenchuk PJ, Kron J, Walance C, McAnulty JH. Limited value of programmed electrical stimulation from multiple right ventricular pacing sites in clinically sustained ventricular fibrillation or ventricular tachycardia associated with coronary artery disease. Am J Cardiol 1988; 61:303–308.

595. Oseran DS, Gang ES, Hamer AW, et al. Mode of stimulation versus response: validation of a protocol for induction of ventricular tachycardia. Am Heart J 1985; 110:646–651.

596. Dailey SM, Kay GN, Epstein AE, McGiffin DC, Kirklin JK, Plumb VJ. Comparison of endocardial and epicardial programmed stimulation for the induction of ventricular tachycardia. J Am Coll Cardiol 1989; 13:1608–1612.

597. Morady F, Dicarlo LA Jr, Liem LB, Krol RB, Baerman JM. Effects of high stimulation current on the induction of ventricular tachycardia. Am J Cardiol 1985; 56:73–78.

598. Marchlinski FE. Characterization of oscillations in ventricular refractoriness in man after an abrupt increment in heart rate. Circulation 1987; 75:550–556.

599. Hook BG, Marchlinski FE, Josephson ME, Buxton AE. Effect of high-current stimulation in patients with sustained ventricular tachycardia rendered noninducible by antiarrhythmic drugs. Am J Cardiol 1992; 70:752–757.

600. Reddy CP, Gettes LS. Use of isoproterenol as an aid to electric induction of chronic recurrent ventricular tachycardia. Am J Cardiol 1979; 44:705–713.

601. Freedman RA, Swerdlow CD, Echt DS, Winkle RA, Soderholm-Difatte V, Mason JW. Facilitation of ventricular tachyarrhythmia induction by isoproterenol. Am J Cardiol 1984; 54:765–770.

602. Olshansky B, Martins JB. Usefulness of isoproterenol facilitation of ventricular tachycardia induction during extrastimulus testing in predicting effective chronic therapy with beta-adrenergic blockade. Am J Cardiol 1987; 59:573–577.

603. Jazayeri MR, Van Wyhe G, Avitall B, McKinnie J, Tchou P, Akhtar M. Isoproterenol reversal of antiarrhythmic effects in patients with inducible sustained ventricular tachyarrhythmias. J Am Coll Cardiol 1989; 14:705–711.

604. Kang PS, Gomes JA, el-Sherif N. Procainamide in the induction and perpetuation of ventricular tachycardia in man. Pacing Clin Electrophysiol 1982; 5:311–322.

605. Welch WJ, Strasberg B, Coelho A, Rosen KM. Sustained macroreentrant ventricular tachycardia. Am Heart J 1982; 104:166–169.

606. Rinkenberger RL, Prystowsky EN, Jackman WM, Naccarelli GV, Heger JJ, Zipes DP. Drug conversion of nonsustained ventricular tachycardia to sustained ventricular tachycardia during serial electrophysiologic studies: identification of drugs that exacerbate tachycardia and potential mechanisms. Am Heart J 1982; 103:177–184.

607. Buxton AE, Waxman HL, Marchlinski FE, Josephson ME. Electropharmacology of nonsustained ventricular tachycardia: effects of class I antiarrhythmic agents, verapamil and propranolol. Am J Cardiol 1984; 53:738–744.

608. Zaim BR, Zaim SH, Rankin AC, McGovern BA, Garan H, Ruskin JN. Comparison of cycle lengths between induced and spontaneous sustained ventricular tachycardia during concordant antiarrhythmic therapy associated with healed myocardial infarction. Am J Cardiol 1996; 77:202–204.

609. Vandepol CJ, Farshidi A, Spielman SR, Greenspan AM, Horowitz LN, Josephson ME. Incidence and clinical significance of induced ventricular tachycardia. Am J Cardiol 1980; 45:725–731.

610. Wellens HJJ, Janse MJ, Van Dam RT, et al. Epicardial mapping and surgical treatment in Wolff-Parkinson-White syndrome type A. Am Heart J 1974; 88:69–78.

611. Livelli FD Jr, Bigger JT Jr, Reiffel JA, et al. Response to programmed ventricular stimulation: sensitivity, specificity and relation to heart disease. Am J Cardiol 1982; 50:452–458.

612. Richards DA, Cody DV, Denniss AR, Russell PA, Young AA, Uther JB. A new protocol of programmed stimulation for assessment of predisposition to spontaneous ventricular arrhythmias. Eur Heart J 1983; 4:376–382.

613. Stevenson WG, Brugada P, Waldecker B, Zehender M, Wellens HJJ. Clinical, angiographic, and electrophysiologic findings in patients with aborted sudden death as compared with patients with sustained ventricular tachycardia after myocardial infarction. Circulation 1985; 76:1146–1152.

614. Stevenson WG, Brugada P, Kersschot I, et al. Electrophysiologic characteristics of ventricular tachycardia or fibrillation in relation to age of myocardial infarction. Am J Cardiol 1986; 57:387–391.

615. Kim SG, Mercando AD, Fisher JD. Comparison of the characteristics of nonsustained ventricular tachycardia on Holter monitoring and sustained ventricular tachycardia observed spontaneously or induced by programmed stimulation. Am J Cardiol 1987; 60:288–292.

616. Wellens HJJ, Bar FW, Farre J, Ross DL, Wiener I, Vanagt EJ. Initiation and termination of ventricular tachycardia by

supraventricular stimuli: incidence and electrophysiologic determinants as observed during programmed stimulation of the heart. Am J Cardiol 1980; 46:576–582.

617. Roy D, Brugada P, Bar FW, Wellens HJJ. Repetitive responses to ventricular extrastimuli: incidence and significance in patients without organic heart disease. Eur Heart J 1983; 4:79–85.

618. Zipes DP, Foster PR, Troup PJ, Pedersen DH. Atrial induction of ventricular tachycardia: reentry versus triggered automaticity. Am J Cardiol 1979; 44:1–8.

619. Friedman PL, Brugada P, Kuck K-H, Bar FWHM, Wellens HJJ. Initiation of ventricular tachycardia by interpolated ventricular premature depolarizations. Am J Cardiol 1981; 48:967–972.

620. Anastasiou-Nana MI, Anderson JL, Askins JC, Gilbert EM, Nanas JN, Menlove RL. Long-term experience with sotalol in the treatment of complex ventricular arrhythmias. Am Heart J 1987; 114:288–296.

621. Klein RC, Machell C. Use of electrophysiologic testing in patients with nonsustained ventricular tachycardia: prognostic and therapeutic implications. J Am Coll Cardiol 1989; 14:155–161.

622. Buxton AE, Waxman HL, Marchlinski FE, Josephson ME. Electrophysiologic studies in nonsustained ventricular tachycardia: relation to underlying heart disease. Am J Cardiol 1983; 52:985–991.

623. Milstein S, Sharma AD, Klein GJ. Nonclinical ventricular tachycardia in the Wolff-Parkinson-White syndrome. Pacing Clin Electrophysiol 1985; 8:678–683.

624. Sulpizi AM, Friehling TD, Kowey PR. Value of electrophysiologic testing in patients with nonsustained ventricular tachycardia. Am J Cardiol 1987; 59:841–845.

625. Schoenfeld MH, McGovern B, Garan H, Kelly E, Grant G, Ruskin JN. Determinants of the outcome of electrophysiologic study in patients with ventricular tachyarrhythmias. J Am Coll Cardiol 1985; 6:298–306.

626. Hammill SC, Trusty JM, Wood DL, et al. Influence of ventricular function and presence or absence of coronary artery disease on results of electrophysiologic testing for asymptomatic nonsustained ventricular tachycardia. Am J Cardiol 1990; 65:722–728.

627. Podrid PJ, Schoeneberger A, Lown B, et al. Use of nonsustained ventricular tachycardia as a guide to antiarrhythmic drug therapy in patients with malignant ventricular arrhythmia. Am Heart J 1983; 105:181–188.

628. Wilber DJ, Olshansky B, Moran JF, Scanlon PJ. Electrophysiological testing and nonsustained ventricular tachycardia: use and limitations in patients with coronary artery disease and impaired ventricular function. Circulation 1990; 82:350–358.

629. Veltri EP, Platia EV, Griffith LSC, Reid PR. Programmed electrical stimulation and long-term follow-up in asymptomatic, nonsustained ventricular tachycardia. Am J Cardiol 1985; 56:309–314.

630. Buxton AE, Marchlinski FE, Flores BT, Miller JM, Doherty JU, Josephson ME. Nonsustained ventricular tachycardia in patients with coronary artery disease: role of electrophysiologic study. Circulation 1987; 75:1178–1185.

631. Manolis AS, Estes NAM III. Value of programmed ventricular stimulation in the evaluation and management of patients with nonsustained ventricular tachycardia associated with coronary artery disease. Am J Cardiol 1990; 65:201–205.

632. Buxton AE, Lee KL, DiCarlo L, et al. Nonsustained ventricular tachycardia in coronary artery disease: relation to inducible sustained ventricular tachycardia: MUSTT investigators. Ann Intern Med 1996; 125:35–39.

633. Turitto G, Fontaine JM, Ursell S, Caref EB, Bekheit S, el-Sherif N. Risk stratification and management of patients with organic heart disease and nonsustained ventricular tachycardia: role of programmed stimulation, left ventricular ejection fraction, and the signal-averaged electrocardiogram. Am J Med 1990; 88:35N–41N.

634. Gillis AM, Sheldon RS, Wyse DG, et al. Long-term reproducibility of ventricular tachycardia induction in patients with implantable cardioverter/defibrillators: serial noninvasive studies. Circulation 1995; 91:2605–2613.

635. Bhandari AK, Widerhorn J, Sager PT, et al. Prognostic significance of programmed ventricular stimulation in patients surviving complicated acute myocardial infarction: a prospective study. Am Heart J 1992; 124:87–96.

636. Iesaka Y, Nogami A, Aonuma K, et al. Prognostic significance of sustained monomorphic ventricular tachycardia induced by programmed ventricular stimulation using up to triple extrastimuli in survivors of acute myocardial infarction. Am J Cardiol 1990; 65:1057–1063.

637. Vorperian VR, Gittelsohn AM, Veltri EP. Predictors of inducible sustained ventricular tachyarrhythmias in patients with coronary artery disease. J Am Coll Cardiol 1989; 13:637–645.

638. Pratt CM, Thornton BC, Magro SA, Wyndham CRC. Spontaneous arrhythmia detected on ambulatory electrocardiographic recording lacks precision in predicting inducibility of ventricular tachycardia during electrophysiologic study. J Am Coll Cardiol 1987; 10:97–104.

639. Pedretti R, Etro MD, Laporta A, Braga SS, Caru B. Prediction of late arrhythmic events after acute myocardial infarction from combined use of noninvasive prognostic variables and inducibility of sustained monomorphic ventricular tachycardia. Am J Cardiol 1993; 71:1131–1141.

640. Bourke JP, Young AA, Richards DAB, Uther JB. Reduction in incidence of inducible ventricular tachycardia after myocardial infarction by treatment with streptokinase during infarct evolution. J Am Coll Cardiol 1990; 16:1703–1710.

641. Meinertz T, Treese N, Kasper W, et al. Determinants of prognosis in idiopathic dilated cardiomyopathy as determined by programmed electrical stimulation. Am J Cardiol 1985; 56:337–341.

642. Poll DS, Marchlinski FE, Buxton AE, Doherty JU, Waxman HL, Josephson ME. Sustained ventricular tachycardia in patients with idiopathic dilated cardiomyopathy: electrophysiologic testing and lack of response to antiarrhythmic drug therapy. Circulation 1984; 70:451–456.

643. Poll DS, Marchlinski FE, Buxton AE, Josephson ME. Usefulness of programmed stimulation in idiopathic dilated cardiomyopathy. Am J Cardiol 1986; 58:992–997.

644. Stamato NJ, O'Connell JB, Murdock DK, Moran JF, Loeb HS, Scanlon PJ. The response of patients with complex ventricular arrhythmias secondary to dilated cardiomyopathy to programmed electrical stimulation. Am Heart J 1986; 112:505–508.

645. Geibel A, Brugada P, Zehender M, Stevenson W, Waldecker B, Wellens HJJ. Value of programmed electrical stimulation using a standardized ventricular stimulation protocol in hypertrophic cardiomyopathy. Am J Cardiol 1987; 60:738–739.

646. Gonska BD, Bethge KP, Kreuzer H. Programmed ventricular stimulation in coronary artery disease and dilated cardiomyopathy: influence of the underlying heart disease on the results of electrophysiologic testing. Clin Cardiol 1987; 10:294–304.

647. Chen X, Shenasa M, Borggrefe M, et al. Role of programmed ventricular stimulation in patients with idiopathic dilated cardiomyopathy and documented sustained ventricular tachyarrhythmias: inducibility and prognostic value in 102 patients. Eur Heart J 1994; 15:76–82.

648. Balaji S, Lau YR, Case CL, Gillette PC. QRS prolongation is associated with inducible ventricular tachycardia after repair of tetralogy of Fallot. Am J Cardiol 1997; 80:160–163.

649. Wu D, Hung JS, Kuo CT. Determinants of sustained slow pathway conduction and relation to reentrant tachycardia in patients with dual atrioventricular nodal transmission. Am Heart J 1981; 101:521–528.

650. Sung RJ. Incessant supraventricular tachycardia. Pacing Clin Electrophysiol 1983; 6:1306–1326.

651. Yeh SJ, Wen MS, Wang CC, Lin FC, Wu D. Adenosine-sensitive ventricular tachycardia from the anterobasal left ventricle. J Am Coll Cardiol 1997; 30:1339–1345.

652. DiMarco JP, Garan H, Harthorne JW, Ruskin JN. Intracardiac electrophysiologic techniques in recurrent syncope of unknown cause. Ann Intern Med 1981; 95:542–548.

653. Morady F, Scheinman MM. The role and limitations of electrophysiologic testing in patients with unexplained syncope. Int Cardiol 1983; 4:229–234.

654. Akhtar M, Shenasa M, Denker S, Gilbert CJ, Rizwi N. Role of cardiac electrophysiologic studies in patients with unexplained recurrent syncope. PACE 1983; 6:192–201.

655. Olshansky B, Mazuz M, Martins JB. Significance of inducible tachycardia in patients with syncope of unknown origin: a long-term follow-up. J Am Coll Cardiol 1985; 5:216–223.

656. Doherty JU, Pembrook-Rogers D, Grogan EW, et al. Electrophysiologic evaluation and follow-up characteristics of patients with recurrent unexplained syncope and presyncope. Am J Cardiol 1985; 55:703–708.

657. Krol RB, Morady F, Flaker GC, et al. Electrophysiologic testing in patients with unexplained syncope: clinical and noninvasive predictors of outcome. J Am Coll Cardiol 1987; 10:358–363.

658. Morady F, Higgins J, Peters RW, et al. Electrophysiologic testing in bundle branch block and unexplained syncope. Am J Cardiol 1984; 54:587–591.

659. Ezri M, Lerman BB, Marchlinski FE, Buxton AE, Josephson ME. Electrophysiologic evaluation of syncope in patients with bifascicular block. Am Heart J 1983; 106:693–697.

660. Silka MJ, Kron J, Cutler JE, McAnulty JH. Analysis of programmed stimulation methods in the evaluation of ventricular arrhythmias in patients 20 years old and younger. Am J Cardiol 1990; 66:826–830.

661. Coste P, Clementy J, Besse P, Bricaud H. Left ventricular hypertrophy and ventricular dysrhythmic risk in hypertensive patients: evaluation by programmed electrical stimulation. J Hypertens Suppl 1988; 6:S116–S118.

662. Lerman BB. Personal communication, 1996.

663. Lerman BB, Stein KM, Markowitz SM. Idiopathic right ventricular outflow tract tachycardia: a clinical approach. Pacing Clin Electrophysiol 1996; 19:2120–2137.

664. Chinushi M, Aizawa Y, Ohhira K, et al. Repetitive ventricular responses induced by radiofrequency ablation for idiopathic ventricular tachycardia originating from the outflow tract of the right ventricle. PACE 1998; 21:669–678.

665. Kottkamp H, Chen X, Hindricks G, Willems S, Borggrefe M, Breithardt G. Radiofrequency catheter ablation of idiopathic left ventricular tachycardia: further evidence for microentry as the underlying mechanism. J Cardiovasc Electrophysiol 1994; 5:268–273.

666. Lai LP, Lin JL, Hwang JJ, Huang SKS. Entrance site of the slow conduction zone of verapamil-sensitive idiopathic left ventricular tachycardia: evidence supporting macroreentry in the Purkinje system. J Cardiovasc Electrophysiol 1998; 9:184–190.

667. Bogun F, el-Atassi R, Daoud E, Man KC, Strickberger SA, Morady F. Radiofrequency ablation of idiopathic left anterior fascicular tachycardia. J Cardiovasc Electrophysiol 1995; 6:1113–1116.

668. Denniss AR, Richards DA, Cody DV, et al. Prognostic significance of ventricular tachycardia and fibrillation induced at programmed stimulation and delayed potentials detected on the signal-averaged electrocardiograms of survivors of acute myocardial infarction. Circulation 1986; 74:731–745.

669. Woelfel A, Foster JR, Rowe WW, Jain A, Gettes LS. Induction of ventricular tachycardia in patients with left ventricular aneurysms and no history of arrhythmia. Am J Cardiol 1988; 62:814–816.

670. Brugada P, Dassen WR, Braat S, Gorgels AP, Wellens HJJ. Value of the ajmaline-procainamide test to predict the effect of long-term oral amiodarone on the anterograde effective refractory period of the accessory pathway in the Wolff-Parkinson-White syndrome. Am J Cardiol 1983; 52:70–72.

671. Waspe LE, Seinfeld D, Ferrick A, Kim SG, Matos JA, Fisher JD. Prediction of sudden death and spontaneous ventricular tachycardia in survivors of complicated myocardial infarction: value of the response to programmed stimulation using a maximum of three ventricular extrastimuli. J Am Coll Cardiol 1985; 5:1292–1301.

672. Nalos PC, Gang ES, Mandel WJ, Ladenheim ML, Lass Y,

Peter T. The signal-averaged electrocardiogram as a screening test for inducibility of sustained ventricular tachycardia in high risk patients: a prospective study. J Am Coll Cardiol 1987; 9:539–548.

673. Denniss AR, Cody DV, Russell PA, Young AA, Ross DL, Uther JB. Correlation between signal-averaged electrocardiogram and programmed stimulation in patients with and without spontaneous ventricular tachyarrhythmias. Am J Cardiol 1987; 59:586–590.

674. Winters SL, Ip J, Deshmukh P, et al. Determinants of induction of ventricular tachycardia in nonsustained ventricular tachycardia after myocardial infarction and the usefulness of the signal-averaged electrocardiogram. Am J Cardiol 1993; 72:1281–1285.

675. Turitto G, Fontaine JM, Ursell SN, Caref EB, Henkin R, el-Sherif N. Value of the signal-averaged electrocardiogram as a predictor of the results of programmed stimulation in nonsustained ventricular tachycardia. Am J Cardiol 1988; 61:1272–1278.

676. Buxton AE, Britton N, Simson MB. Application of the signal-averaged electrocardiogram in patients with nonsustained ventricular tachycardia after myocardial infarction: implications for prediction of sudden cardiac death. J Electrocardiol 1988; 21(Suppl): S40–S45.

677. Winters SL, Stewart D, Targonski A, Gomes JA. Role of signal averaging of the surface QRS complex in selecting patients with nonsustained ventricular tachycardia and high grade ventricular arrhythmias for programmed ventricular stimulation. J Am Coll Cardiol 1988; 12:1481–1487.

678. Twidale N, Hazlitt HA, Berbari EJ, et al. Late potentials are unaffected by radiofrequency catheter ablation in patients with ventricular tachycardia. Pacing Clin Electrophysiol 1994; 17:157–165.

679. Martinez-Rubio A, Shenasa M, Borggrefe M, Chen X, Benning F, Breithardt G. Electrophysiologic variables characterizing the induction of ventricular tachycardia versus ventricular fibrillation after myocardial infarction: relation between ventricular late potentials and coupling intervals for the induction of sustained ventricular tachyarrhythmias. J Am Coll Cardiol 1993; 21:1624–1631.

680. Fisher JD. Ventricular tachycardia: practical and provocative electrophysiology. Circulation 1978; 58:1000–1001.

681. Horowitz LN, Josephson ME, Kastor JA. Intracardiac electrophysiologic studies as a method for the optimization of drug therapy in chronic ventricular arrhythmia. Prog Cardiovasc Dis 1980; 23:81–98.

682. Horowitz LN, Spielman SR, Greenspan SR, Josephson ME. Role of programmed stimulation in assessing vulnerability to ventricular arrhythmias. Am Heart J 1982; 103:604–610.

683. Horowitz LN. Electrophysiologic testing of antiarrhythmic therapy. Drug Intell Clin Pharm 1982; 16:284–290.

684. Prystowsky EN. Electrophysiologic testing in patients with ventricular tachycardia: past performance and future expectations. J Am Coll Cardiol 1983; 1:558–560.

685. Breithardt G, Abendroth R-R, Borggrefe M, Yeh HL, Haerten K, Seipel L. Prevalence and clinical significance of the repetitive ventricular response during sinus rhythm in coronary disease patients. Am Heart J 1984; 107:229–236.

686. Wellens HJJ, Brugada P, Stevenson WG. Programmed electrical stimulation of the heart in patients with life-threatening ventricular arrhythmias: what is the significance of induced arrhythmias and what is the correct stimulation protocol? Circulation 1985; 72:1–7.

687. Reddy CP, Chen TJ, Guillory WR. Electrophysiologic studies in selection of antiarrhythmic agents: use with ventricular tachycardia. PACE 1986; 9:756–763.

688. Anderson JL, Mason JW. Testing the efficacy of antiarrhythmic drugs. N Engl J Med 1986; 315:391–393.

689. Fisher JD, Kim SG, Waspe LE, Johnston DR. Amiodarone: value of programmed electrical stimulation and Holter monitoring. Pacing Clin Electrophysiol 1986; 9:422–435.

690. Gottlieb C, Josephson ME. The preference of programmed stimulation-guided therapy for sustained ventricular arrhythmias. In Brugada P, Wellens HJJ (eds). Cardiac Arrhythmias. Where To Go From Here? Mount Kisco, NY: Futura Publishing Co., 1987, pp. 421–434.

691. Fisher JD, Mercando AD, Kim SG. Prospective criteria for the selection of therapy for ventricular tachycardia and ventricular fibrillation. In Brugada P, Wellens HJJ (eds). Cardiac Arrhythmias. Where To Go From Here? Mount Kisco, NY: Futura Publishing Co., 1987, pp. 471–482.

692. Marchlinski FE. Sorting out the mechanisms of antiarrhythmic drug action. J Am Coll Cardiol 1990; 16:1238–1239.

693. Peter CT, Helfant RH. Postinfarction ventricular tachycardia and fibrillation: reassessing the role of drug therapy and approach to the high risk patient. J Am Coll Cardiol 1990; 16:531–532.

694. Ward DE, Camm AJ. Dangerous ventricular arrhythmias: can we predict drug efficacy? N Engl J Med 1993; 329:498–499.

695. Wellens HJJ. Significance of sustained ventricular arrhythmias in patients with valvular heart disease (editorial; comment). Circulation 1997; 96:386–387.

696. Hartzler GO, Maloney JD. Programmed ventricular stimulation in management of recurrent ventricular tachycardia. Mayo Clin Proc 1977; 52:731–741.

697. Fisher JD, Cohen HL, Mehra R, Altschuler H, Escher DJW, Furman S. Cardiac pacing and pacemakers. II. Serial electrophysiologic-pharmacologic testing for control of recurrent tachyarrhythmias. Am Heart J 1977; 93:658–668.

698. Horowitz LN, Josephson ME, Farshidi A, Spielman SR, Michelson EL, Greenspan AM. Recurrent sustained ventricular tachycardia. III. Role of the electrophysiologic study in selection of antiarrhythmic regimens. Circulation 1978; 58:986–997.

699. Mason JW, Winkle RA. Electrode-catheter arrhythmia induction in the selection and assessment of antiarrhythmic drug therapy for recurrent ventricular tachycardia. Circulation 1978; 58:971–985.

700. Mason JW, Winkle RA. Accuracy of the ventricular tachycardia-induction study for predicting long-term efficacy and inefficacy of antiarrhythmic drugs. N Engl J Med 1980; 303:1073–1077.

701. Breithardt G, Seipel L, Abendroth R-R, Loogen F. Serial electrophysiological testing of antiarrhythmic drug efficacy in patients with recurrent ventricular tachycardia. Eur Heart J 1980; 1:11–24.

702. Denes P, Wu D, Wyndham C, et al. Chronic longterm electrophysiologic study of paroxysmal ventricular tachycardia. Chest 1980; 77:478–487.

703. DiMarco JP, Garan H, Ruskin JN. Mexiletine for refractory-ventricular arrhythmias: results using serial electrophysiologic testing. Am J Cardiol 1981; 47:131–138.

704. Swerdlow CD, Blum J, Winkle RA, Griffin JC, Ross DL, Mason JW. Decreased incidence of antiarrhythmic drug efficacy at electrophysiologic study associated with the use of a third extrastimulus. Am Heart J 1982; 104:1004–1011.

705. Benditt DG, Benson DW, Klein GJ, Pritzker MR, Kriett JM, Anderson RW. Prevention of recurrent sudden cardiac arrest: role of provocative electropharmacologic testing. J Am Coll Cardiol 1983; 2:418–425.

706. Horowitz LN, Spielman SR, Greenspan AM, Webb CR, Kay HR. Ventricular arrhythmias: use of electrophysiologic studies. Am Heart J 1983; 106:881–886.

707. Spielman SR, Schwartz JS, McCarthy DM, et al. Predictors of the success or failure of medical therapy in patients with chronic recurrent sustained ventricular tachycardia: a discriminant analysis. J Am Coll Cardiol 1983; 1:401–408.

708. Swerdlow CD, Gong G, Echt DS, et al. Clinical factors predicting successful electrophysiologic-pharmacologic study in patients with ventricular tachycardia. J Am Coll Cardiol 1983; 1:409–417.

709. Senges J, Lengfelder W, Jauernig R, et al. Electrophysiologic testing in assessment of therapy with sotalol for sustained ventricular tachycardia. Circulation 1984; 69:577–584.

710. Greenspan AM, Spielman SR, Webb CR, Sokoloff NM, Rae AP, Horowitz LN. Efficacy of combination therapy with mexiletine and a type Ia agent for inducible ventricular tachyarrhythmias secondary to coronary artery disease. Am J Cardiol 1985; 56:277–284.

711. Platia EV, Reid PR. Nonsustained ventricular tachycardia

during programmed ventricular stimulation: criteria for a positive test. Am J Cardiol 1985; 56:79–83.

712. Kim SS, Lal R, Ruffy R. Treatment of paroxysmal reentrant supraventricular tachycardia with flecainide acetate. Am J Cardiol 1986; 58:80–85.

713. Lombardi F, Stein J, Podrid PJ, Graboys TB, Lown B. Daily reproducibility of electrophysiologic test results in malignant ventricular arrhythmia. Am J Cardiol 1986; 57:96–101.

714. Steinbeck G, Bach P, Haberl R. Electrophysiologic and antiarrhythmic efficacy of oral sotalol for sustained ventricular tachyarrhythmias: evaluation by programmed stimulation and ambulatory electrocardiogram. J Am Coll Cardiol 1986; 8:949–958.

715. Deal BJ, Scagliotti D, Miller SM, Gallastegui JL, Hariman RJ, Levitsky S. Electrophysiologic drug testing in symptomatic ventricular arrhythmias after repair of tetralogy of Fallot. Am J Cardiol 1987; 59:1380–1385.

716. Lavery D, Saksena S. Management of refractory sustained ventricular tachycardia with amiodarone: a reappraisal. Am Heart J 1987; 113:49–56.

717. Mitchell LB, Duff HJ, Manyari DE, Wyse DG. A randomized clinical trial of the noninvasive and invasive approaches to drug therapy of ventricular tachycardia. N Engl J Med 1987; 317:1681–1687.

718. Waller TJ, Kay HR, Spielman SR, Kutalek SP, Greenspan AM, Horowitz LN. Reduction in sudden death and total mortality by antiarrhythmic therapy evaluated by electrophysiologic drug testing: criteria of efficacy in patients with sustained ventricular tachyarrhythmia. J Am Coll Cardiol 1987; 10:83–89.

719. Borggrefe M, Trampisch H-J, Breithardt G. Reappraisal of criteria for assessing drug efficacy in patients with ventricular tachyarrhythmias: complete versus partial suppression of inducible arrhythmias. J Am Coll Cardiol 1988; 12:140–149.

720. Gonzalez R, Scheinman MM, Herre JM, Griffin JC, Sauve MJ, Sharkey H. Usefulness of sotalol for drug-refractory malignant ventricular arrhythmias. J Am Coll Cardiol 1988; 12:1568–1572.

721. Jordaens LJ, Palmer A, Clement DL. Low-dose oral sotalol for monomorphic ventricular tachycardia: effects during programmed electrical stimulation and follow-up. Eur Heart J 1989; 10:218–226.

722. ESVEM Investigators. The ESVEM trial. Electrophysiologic study versus electrocardiographic monitoring for selection of antiarrhythmic therapy of ventricular tachyarrhythmias. Circulation 1989; 79:1354–1360.

723. Gillis AM, Wyse DG, Duff HJ, Mitchell LB. Drug response at electropharmacologic study in patients with ventricular tachyarrhythmias: the importance of ventricular refractoriness. J Am Coll Cardiol 1991; 17:914–920.

724. Steinbeck G, Andresen D, Bach P, et al. A comparison of electrophysiologically guided antiarrhythmic drug therapy with beta-blocker therapy in patients with symptomatic, sustained ventricular tachyarrhythmias. N Engl J Med 1992; 327:987–992.

725. Kudenchuk PJ, Halperin B, Kron J, Walance CG, Griffith KK, McAnulty JH. Serial electropharmacologic studies in patients with ischemic heart disease and sustained ventricular tachyarrhythmias: when is drug testing sufficient? Am J Cardiol 1993; 72:1400–1405.

726. ESVEM Investigators. Determinants of predicted efficacy of antiarrhythmic drugs in the Electrophysiologic Study Versus Electrocardiographic Monitoring Trial. Circulation 1993; 87:323–329.

727. Mason JW. A comparison of electrophysiologic testing with Holter monitoring to predict antiarrhythmic-drug efficacy for ventricular tachyarrhythmias. N Engl J Med 1993; 329:445–451.

728. Kuhlkamp V, Mermi J, Mewis C, Braun U, Seipel L. Long-term efficacy of d/l sotalol in patients with sustained ventricular tachycardia refractory to class I antiarrhythmic drugs. Eur Heart J 1995; 16:1625–1631.

729. Omoigui NA, Marcus FI, Mason JW, et al. Cost of initial therapy in the Electrophysiological Study Versus ECG Monitoring Trial (ESVEM). Circulation 1995; 91:1070–1076.

730. Reiter MJ, Mann DE, Reiffel JE, Hahn E, Hartz V, ESVEM Investigators. Significance and incidence of concordance of drug efficacy predictions by Holter monitoring and electrophysiological study in the ESVEM trial. Circulation 1995; 91:1988–1995.

731. Haverkamp W, Martinez-Rubio A, Hief C, et al. Efficacy and safety of d,l-sotalol in patients with ventricular tachycardia and in survivors of cardiac arrest. J Am Coll Cardiol 1997; 30:487–495.

732. Mitchell LB, Sheldon RS, Gillis AM, et al. Definition of predicted effective antiarrhythmic drug therapy for ventricular tachyarrhythmias by the electrophysiologic study approach: randomized comparison of patient response criteria. J Am Coll Cardiol 1997; 30:1346–1353.

733. Meissner MD, Kay HR, Horowitz LN, Spielman SR, Greenspan AM, Kutalek SP. Relation of acute antiarrhythmic drug efficacy to left ventricular function in coronary artery disease. Am J Cardiol 1988; 61:1050–1055.

734. Rae AP, Spielman SR, Kutalek SP, Kay HR, Horowitz LN. Electrophysiologic assessment of antiarrhythmic drug efficacy for ventricular tachyarrhythmias associated with dilated cardiomyopathy. Am J Cardiol 1987; 59:291–295.

735. Gold RL, Haffajee CI, Alpert JS. Electrophysiologic and clinical factors influencing response to class Ia antiarrhythmic agents in patients with inducible sustained monomorphic ventricular tachycardia. Am Heart J 1986; 112:9–13.

736. Ross DL, Sze DY, Keefe DL, et al. Antiarrhythmic drug combinations in the treatment of ventricular tachycardia. Circulation 1982; 66:1205–1210.

737. Duffy CE, Swiryn S, Bauernfeind RA, Strasberg B, Palileo E, Rosen KM. Inducible sustained ventricular tachycardia refractory to individual class I drugs: effect of adding a second class I drug. Am Heart J 1983; 106:450–458.

738. Marchlinski FE, Buxton AE, Miller JM, Vassallo JA, Flores BT, Josephson ME. Amiodarone versus amiodarone and a type Ia agent for treatment of patients with rapid ventricular tachycardia. Circulation 1986; 74:1037–1043.

739. Bonavita GJ, Pires LA, Wagshal AB, et al. Usefulness of oral quinidine-mexiletine combination therapy for sustained ventricular tachyarrhythmias as assessed by programmed electrical stimulation when quinidine monotherapy has failed. Am Heart J 1994; 127:847–851.

740. Menozzi C, Brignole M, Monducci I, Lolli G. Noninvasive serial electrophysiological testing using an implanted pacemaker for management of recurrent ventricular tachycardia. PACE 1986; 9:589–593.

741. Swiryn S, Bauernfeind RA, Strasberg B, et al. Prediction of response to class I antiarrhythmic drugs during electrophysiologic study of ventricular tachycardia. Am Heart J 1982; 104:43–50.

742. Wyse DG, Mitchell LB, Duff HJ. Procainamide, disopyramide and quinidine: discordant antiarrhythmic effects during crossover comparison in patients with inducible ventricular tachycardia. J Am Coll Cardiol 1987; 9:882–889.

743. Gonzalez R, Arriagada D, Corbalan R, Chamorro G, Fajuri A, Rodriguez JA. Role of programmed electrical stimulation of the heart in risk stratification post-myocardial infarction. Pacing Clin Electrophysiol 1988; 11:283–288.

744. Pires LA, Wagshal SB, Greene TO, Mittleman RS, Huang SKS. Usefulness of the response to intravenous procainamide during electrophysiologic study in predicting the response to oral quinidine in patients with inducible sustained monomorphic ventricular tachycardia associated with coronary artery disease. Am J Cardiol 1993; 72:908–910.

745. Khalighi K, Peters RW, Feliciano Z, Shorofsky SR, Gold MR. Comparison of class Ia/Ib versus class III antiarrhythmic drugs for the suppression of inducible sustained ventricular tachycardia associated with coronary artery disease. Am J Cardiol 1997; 80:591–594.

746. Karagounis LA, Anderson JL, Allen A, Osborn JS. Electrophysiologic effects of antiarrhythmic drug therapy in the prediction of successful suppression of induced ventricular tachycardia. Am Heart J 1995; 129:343–349.

747. Martinez-Rubio A, Schwammenthal Y, Schwammenthal E, et

al. (Patients with valvular heart disease presenting with sustained ventricular tachyarrhythmias or syncope): results of programmed ventricular stimulation and long-term follow-up. Circulation 1997; 96:500–508.

748. Cooper MJ, Koo CC, Skinner MP, et al. Comparison of immediate versus day to day variability of ventricular tachycardia induction by programmed stimulation. J Am Coll Cardiol 1989; 13:1599–1607.

749. Schoenfeld MH, McGovern B, Garan H, Ruskin JN. Long-term reproducibility of responses to programmed cardiac stimulation in spontaneous ventricular tachyarrhythmias. Am J Cardiol 1984; 54:564–568.

750. Roy D, Marchand E, Theroux P, et al. Long-term reproducibility and significance of provokable ventricular arrhythmias after myocardial infarction. J Am Coll Cardiol 1986; 8:32–39.

751. Rosenbaum MS, Wilber DJ, Finkelstein D, Ruskin JN, Garan H. Immediate reproducibility of electrically induced sustained monomorphic ventricular tachycardia before and during antiarrhythmic therapy. J Am Coll Cardiol 1991; 17:133–138.

752. Mann DE, Hartz V, Hahn EA, Reiter MJ, ESVEM Investigators. Effect of reproducibility of baseline arrhythmia induction on drug efficacy predictions and outcome in the Electrophysiologic Study Versus Electrocardiographic Monitoring (ESVEM) Trial. Am J Cardiol 1997; 80:1448–1452.

753. McPherson CA, Rosenfeld LE, Batsford WP. Day-to-day reproducibility of responses to right ventricular programmed electrical stimulation: implications for serial drug testing. Am J Cardiol 1985; 55:689–695.

754. Beckman KJ, Velasco CE, Krafchek J, Lin H-T, Magro SA, Wyndham CRC. Significant variability in the mode of ventricular tachycardia induction and its implications for interpretation of acute drug testing. Am Heart J 1988; 116:718–725.

755. Cooper MJ, Hunt LJ, Richards DA, Denniss AR, Uther JB, Ross DL. Effect of repetition of extrastimuli on sensitivity and reproducibility of mode of induction of ventricular tachycardia by programmed stimulation. J Am Coll Cardiol 1988; 11:1260–1267.

756. Volgman AS, Zheutlin TA, Mattioni TA, Parker MA, Kehoe RF. Reproducibility of programmed electrical stimulation responses in patients with ventricular tachycardia or fibrillation associated with coronary artery disease. Am J Cardiol 1992; 70:758–763.

757. Camm J, Ward D, Spurrell RA. The effect of intravenous disopyramide phosphate on recurrent paroxysmal tachycardias. Br J Clin Pharmacol 1979; 8:441–449.

758. Saksena S, Greenberg E, Ferguson D. Prospective reimbursement for state-of-the-art medical practice: the case for invasive electrophysiologic evaluation. Am J Cardiol 1985; 55:963–967.

759. Gillis AM, Leitch JW, Sheldon RS, et al. A prospective randomized comparison of autodecremental pacing to burst pacing in device therapy for chronic ventricular tachycardia secondary to coronary artery disease. Am J Cardiol 1993; 72:1146–1151.

760. Kantoch MJ, Green MS, Tang AS. Randomized cross-over evaluation of two adaptive pacing algorithms for the termination of ventricular tachycardia. Pacing Clin Electrophysiol 1993; 16:1664–1672.

761. Callans DJ, Hook BG, Mitra RL, Josephson ME. Characterization of return cycle responses predictive of successful pacing-mediated termination of ventricular tachycardia. J Am Coll Cardiol 1995; 25:47–53.

762. Naccarelli GV, Zipes DP, Rahilly GT, Heger JJ, Prystowsky EN. Influence of tachycardia cycle length and antiarrhythmic drugs on pacing termination and acceleration of ventricular tachycardia. Am Heart J 1983; 105:1–5.

763. Gottlieb CD, Rosenthal ME, Stamato NJ, et al. A quantitative evaluation of refractoriness within a reentrant circuit during ventricular tachycardia: relation to termination. Circulation 1990; 82:1289–1295.

764. Aizawa M, Aizawa Y, Chinushi M, Takahashi K, Shibata A. Conductive property of the zone of slow conduction of reentrant ventricular tachycardia and its relation to pacing induced terminability. PACE 1994; 17:46–55.

765. Roy D, Waxman HL, Buxton AE, et al. Termination of ventricular tachycardia: role of tachycardia cycle length. Am J Cardiol 1982; 50:1346–1350.

766. Waxman MB, Sharma AD, Cameron DA, Huerta F, Wald RW. Reflex mechanisms responsible for early spontaneous termination of paroxysmal supraventricular tachycardia. Am J Cardiol 1982; 49:259–272.

767. Ruffy R, Friday KJ, Southworth WF. Termination of ventricular tachycardia by single extrastimulation during the ventricular effective refractory period. Circulation 1983; 67:457–459.

768. Shenasa M, Cardinal R, Kus T, Savard P, Fromer M, Page P. Termination of sustained ventricular tachycardia by ultrarapid subthreshold stimulation in humans. Circulation 1988; 78:1135–1143.

769. Gardner MJ, Waxman HL, Buxton AE, Cain ME, Josephson ME. Termination of ventricular tachycardia: evaluation of a new pacing method. Am J Cardiol 1982; 50:1338–1344.

770. Waldecker B, Brugada P, Zehender M, Stevenson W, Dulk KD, Wellens HJJ. Importance of modes of electrical termination of ventricular tachycardia for the selection of implantable antitachycardia devices. Am J Cardiol 1986; 57:150–155.

771. Callans DJ, Marchlinski FE. Characterization of spontaneous termination of sustained ventricular tachycardia associated with coronary artery disease. Am J Cardiol 1991; 67:50–54.

772. Gallagher JJ, Kasell JH, Cox JL, Smith WM, Ideker RE. Techniques of intraoperative electrophysiologic mapping. Am J Cardiol 1982; 49:221–240.

773. Josephson ME, Horowitz LN, Spielman SR, Waxman HL, Greenspan AM. Role of catheter mapping in the preoperative evaluation of ventricular tachycardia. Am J Cardiol 1982; 49:207–220.

774. Miller JM, Josephson ME. Intraoperative mapping ventricular tachycardia: utility and pitfalls. Int J Cardiol 1985; 8:173–175.

775. Doig JC, Saito J, Harris L, et al. Ventricular tachycardia in ischaemic heart disease: insights into the mechanisms from cardiac mapping and implications for patient management. Eur Heart J 1995; 16:1027–1035.

776. Stevenson WG, Friedman PL, Sager PT, et al. Exploring postinfarction reentrant ventricular tachycardia with entrainment mapping. J Am Coll Cardiol 1997; 29:1180–1189.

777. Downar E, Harris L, Mickleborough LL, Shaikh N, Parson ID. Endocardial mapping of ventricular tachycardia in the intact human ventricle: evidence for reentrant mechanisms. J Am Coll Cardiol 1988; 11:783–791.

778. Mickleborough LL, Harris L, Downar E, Parson I, Gray G. A new intraoperative approach for endocardial mapping of ventricular tachycardia. J Thorac Cardiovasc Sur 1988; 95:271–280.

779. Mickleborough LL, Usui A, Downar E, Harris L, Parson I, Gray G. Transatrial balloon technique for activation mapping during operations for recurrent ventricular tachycardia. J Thorac Cardiovasc Surg 1990; 99:227–232.

780. Chung MK, Pogwizd SM, Miller DP, Cain ME. Three-dimensional mapping of the initiation of nonsustained ventricular tachycardia in the human heart. Circulation 1997; 95:2517–2527.

781. Fisher WG, Bacon ME, Swartz JF. Use of an orthogonal electrode array to identify the successful ablation site in right ventricular outflow tract tachycardia. Pacing Clin Electrophysiol 1997; 20:2188–2192.

782. Pogwizd SM, Chung MK, Cain ME. Termination of ventricular tachycardia in the human heart: insights from three-dimensional mapping of nonsustained and sustained ventricular tachycardias. Circulation 1997; 95:2528–2540.

783. Josephson ME, Horowitz LN, Spielman SR, Greenspan AM, VandePol C, Harken AH. Comparison of endocardial catheter mapping with intraoperative mapping of ventricular tachycardia. Circulation 1980; 61:395–404.

784. Klein H, Karp RB, Kouchoukos NT, Zorn GL, James TN, Waldo AL. Intraoperative electrophysiologic mapping of the ventricles during sinus rhythm in patients with a previous myocardial infarction: identification of the electrophysiologic substrate of ventricular arrhythmias. Circulation 1982; 66:847–853.

785. Downar E, Parson ID, Mickleborough LL, Cameron DA, Yao LC, Waxman MB. On-line epicardial mapping of intraoperative ventricular arrhythmias: initial clinical experience. J Am Coll Cardiol 1984; 4:703–714.

786. Wiener I, Mindich B, Pitchon R. Fragmented endocardial electrical activity in patients with ventricular tachycardia: a new guide to surgical therapy. Am Heart J 1984; 107:86–90.

787. Downar E, Mickleborough L, Harris L, Parson I. Intraoperative electrical ablation of ventricular arrhythmias: a "closed heart" procedure. J Am Coll Cardiol 1987; 10:1048–1059.

788. Kaltenbrunner W, Cardinal R, Dubuc M, et al. Epicardial and endocardial mapping of ventricular tachycardia in patients with myocardial infarction: is the origin of the tachycardia always subendocardially localized? Circulation 1991; 84:1058–1071.

789. Pogwizd SM, Hoyt RH, Saffitz JE, Corr PB, Cox JL, Cain ME. Reentrant and focal mechanisms underlying ventricular tachycardia in the human heart. Circulation 1992; 86:1872–1887.

790. Downar E, Saito J, Doig JC, et al. Endocardial mapping of ventricular tachycardia in the intact human ventricle. III. Evidence of multiuse reentry with spontaneous and induced block in portions of reentrant path complex. J Am Coll Cardiol 1995; 25:1591–1600.

791. Josephson ME, Waxman HL, Cain ME, Gardner MJ, Buxton AE. Ventricular activation during ventricular endocardial pacing. II. Role of pace-mapping to localize origin of ventricular tachycardia. Am J Cardiol 1982; 50:11–22.

792. Holt PM, Smallpeice C, Deverall PB, Yates AK, Curry PVL. Ventricular arrhythmias: a guide to their localisation. Br Heart J 1985; 53:417–430.

793. Kuchar DL, Ruskin JN, Garan H. Electrocardiographic localization of the site of origin of ventricular tachycardia in patients with prior myocardial infarction. J Am Coll Cardiol 1989; 13:893–900.

794. SippensGroenewegen A, Spekhorst H, van Hemel NM, et al. Localization of the site of origin of postinfarction ventricular tachycardia by endocardial pace mapping: body surface mapping compared with the 12-lead electrocardiogram. Circulation 1993; 88:2290–2306.

795. Coggins DL, Lee RJ, Sweeney J, et al. Radiofrequency catheter ablation as a cure for idiopathic tachycardia of both left and right ventricular origin. J Am Coll Cardiol 1994; 23:1333–1341.

796. Stevenson WG, Sager PT, Friedman PL. Entrainment techniques for mapping atrial and ventricular tachycardias. J Cardiovasc Electrophysiol 1995; 6:201–216.

797. Movsowitz C, Schwartzman D, Callans DJ, et al. Idiopathic right ventricular outflow tract tachycardia: narrowing the anatomic location for successful ablation. Am Heart J 1996; 131:930–936.

798. Sosa E, Scanavacca M, d'Avila A, Pilleggi F. A new technique to perform epicardial mapping in the electrophysiology laboratory. J Cardiovasc Electrophysiol 1996; 7:531–536.

799. Sosa E, Scanavacca M, d'Avila A, et al. Endocardial and epicardial ablation guided by nonsurgical transthoracic epicardial mapping to treat recurrent ventricular tachycardia. J Cardiovasc Electrophysiol 1998; 9:229–239.

800. Fenici R, Melillo G. Magnetocardiography: ventricular arrhythmias. Eur Heart J 1993; 14:53–60.

801. Stevenson WG, Delacretaz E, Friedman PL, Ellison KE. Identification and ablation of macroreentrant ventricular tachycardia with the CARTO electroanatomical mapping system. PACE 1998; 21:1448–1456.

802. McFarland TM, McCarthy DM, Makler PT, Josephson ME. Relation between site of origin of ventricular tachycardia and relative left ventricular myocardial perfusion and wall motion. Am J Cardiol 1983; 51:1329–1333.

803. Miller JM, Harken AH, Hargrove WC, Josephson ME. Pattern of endocardial activation during sustained ventricular tachycardia. J Am Coll Cardiol 1985; 6:1280–1287.

804. Stevenson WG, Sager PT, Natterson PD, Saxon LA, Middlekauff HR, Wiener I. Relation of pace mapping QRS configuration and conduction delay to ventricular tachycardia reentry circuits in human infarct scars. J Am Coll Cardiol 1995; 26:481–488.

805. Waspe LE, Brodman R, Kim SG, et al. Activation mapping in patients with coronary artery disease with multiple ventricular tachycardia configurations: occurrence and therapeutic implications of widely separate apparent sites of origin. J Am Coll Cardiol 1985; 5:1075–1086.

806. Miller JM, Marchlinski FE, Buxton AE, Josephson ME. Relationship between the 12-lead electrocardiogram during ventricular tachycardia and endocardial site of origin in patients with coronary artery disease. Circulation 1988; 4:759–766.

807. Klug D, Ferracci A, Molin F, et al. Body surface potential distributions during idiopathic ventricular tachycardia. Circulation 1995; 91:2002–2009.

808. Griffith MJ, Garratt CJ, Rowland E, Ward DE, Camm AJ. Effects of intravenous adenosine on verapamil-sensitive "idiopathic" ventricular tachycardia. Am J Cardiol 1994; 73:759–764.

809. Ng KS, Wen MS, Yeh SJ, Lin FC, Wu D. The effects of adenosine on idiopathic ventricular tachycardia. Am J Cardiol 1994; 74:195–197.

810. Diker E, Tezcan K, Ozdemir M, Goksel S. Adenosine sensitive left ventricular tachycardia. PACE 1998; 21:134–136.

811. Lau CP. Radiofrequency ablation of fascicular tachycardia: efficacy of pace-mapping and implications on tachycardia origin. Int J Cardiol 1994; 46:255–265.

812. Lerman BB, Stein KM, Markowitz SM. Mechanisms of idiopathic left ventricular tachycardia. J Cardiovasc Electrophysiol 1997; 8:571–583.

813. Nakagawa H, Beckman KJ, McClelland JH, et al. Radiofrequency catheter ablation of idiopathic left ventricular tachycardia guided by a Purkinje potential. Circulation 1993; 88:2607–2617.

814. Zivin A, Goyal R, Daoud E, Man KC, Strickberger SA, Morady F. Idiopathic left ventricular tachycardia with left and right bundle branch block configurations. J Cardiovasc Electrophysiol 1997; 8:441–444.

815. Almendral JM, Grogan EW, Cassidy DM, et al. Timing of the right ventricular apical electrogram during sustained ventricular tachycardia: relation to surface QRS morphology and potential clinical implications. Am J Cardiol 1984; 54:1003–1007.

816. Horowitz LN, Josephson ME, Harken AH. Epicardial and endocardial activation during sustained ventricular tachycardia in man. Circulation 1980; 61:1227–1238.

817. Harris L, Downar E, Mickleborough L, et al. Activation sequence of ventricular tachycardia: endocardial and epicardial mapping studies in the human ventricle. J Am Coll Cardiol 1987; 10:1040–1047.

818. Wiener I, Mindich B, Pitchon R, et al. Epicardial activation in patients with coronary artery disease: effects of regional contraction abnormalities. Circulation 1982; 65:154–160.

819. Josephson ME, Wit AL. Fractionated electrical activity and continuous electrical activity: fact or artifact? Circulation 1984; 70:529–532.

820. Wiener I, Mindich B, Pitchon R. Determinants of ventricular tachycardia in patients with ventricular aneurysms: results of intraoperative epicardial and endocardial mapping. Circulation 1982; 65:856–861.

821. Untereker WJ, Spielman SR, Waxman HL, Horowitz LN, Josephson ME. Ventricular activation in normal sinus rhythm: abnormalities with recurrent sustained tachycardia and a history of myocardial infarction. Am J Cardiol 1985; 55:974–979.

822. Miller WE, Kennedy GT, Ruberg SJ, O'Rourke RA, Crawford MH. Hemodynamic effects of a constant intravenous infusion of piroximone in patients with severe congestive heart failure. J Cardiovasc Pharmacol 1988; 12:72–77.

823. Stevenson WG, Weiss JN, Wiener I, et al. Fractionated endocardial electrograms are associated with slow conduction in humans: evidence from pace-mapping. J Am Coll Cardiol 1989; 13:369–376.

824. Waxman HL, Sung RJ. Significance of fragmented ventricular electrograms observed using intracardiac recording techniques in man. Circulation 1980; 62:1349–1356.

825. Langberg JJ, Gibb WJ, Auslander DM, Griffin JC. Identification of ventricular tachycardia with use of the morphology of the endocardial electrogram. Circulation 1988; 77:1363–1369.

826. Cassidy DM, Vassallo JA, Marchlinski FE, Buxton AE, Untereker WJ, Josephson ME. Endocardial mapping in humans in sinus rhythm with normal left ventricles: activation patterns and characteristics of electrograms. Circulation 1984; 70:37–42.

827. Wiener I, Mindich B, Pitchon R. Endocardial activation in patients with coronary artery disease: effects of regional contraction abnormalities. Am Heart J 1984; 107:1146–1152.

828. Cassidy DM, Vassallo JA, Miller JM, et al. Endocardial catheter mapping in patients in sinus rhythm: relationship to underlying heart disease and ventricular arrhythmias. Circulation 1986; 4:645–652.

829. Cassidy DM, Vassallo JA, Buxton AE, Doherty JU, Marchlinski FE, Josephson ME. Catheter mapping during sinus rhythm: relation of local electrogram duration to ventricular tachycardia cycle length. Am J Cardiol 1985; 55:713–716.

830. Cassidy DM, Vassallo JA, Buxton AE, Doherty JU, Marchlinski FE, Josephson ME. The value of catheter mapping during sinus rhythm to localize site of origin of ventricular tachycardia. Circulation 1984; 69:1103–1110.

831. Kienzle MG, Miller J, Falcone RA, Harken A, Josephson ME. Intraoperative endocardial mapping during sinus rhythm: relationship to site of origin of ventricular tachycardia. Circulation 1984; 70:957–965.

832. Vassallo JA, Cassidy D, Simson MB, Buxton AE, Marchlinski FE, Josephson ME. Relation of late potentials to site of origin of ventricular tachycardia associated with coronary heart disease. Am J Cardiol 1985; 55:985–989.

833. Simson MB, Untereker WJ, Spielman SR, et al. Relation between late potentials on the body surface and directly recorded fragmented electrograms in patients with ventricular tachycardia. Am J Cardiol 1983; 51:105–112.

834. Josephson ME, Simson MB, Harken AH, Horowitz LN, Falcone RA. The incidence and clinical significance of epicardial late potentials in patients with recurrent sustained ventricular tachycardia and coronary artery disease. Circulation 1982; 66:1199–1204.

835. Ohe T, Konoe A, Shimizu A, et al. Differentiation between late potentials of right ventricular and of left ventricular origin. Am J Cardiol 1989; 64:37–41.

836. Harada T, Stevenson WG, Kocovic DZ, Friedman PL. Catheter ablation of ventricular tachycardia after myocardial infarction: relation of endocardial sinus rhythm late potentials to the reentry circuit. J Am Coll Cardiol 1997; 30:1015–1023.

837. Reddy CP, Slack JD. Recurrent sustained ventricular tachycardia: report of a case with His-bundle branches reentry as the mechanism. Eur J Cardiol 1980; 11:23–31.

838. Lloyd EA, Zipes DP, Heger JJ, Prystowsky EN. Sustained ventricular tachycardia due to bundle branch reentry. Am Heart J 1982; 104:1095–1097.

839. Touboul P, Kirkorian G, Atallah G, Moleur P. Bundle branch reentry: a possible mechanism of ventricular tachycardia. Circulation 1983; 67:674–680.

840. Akhtar M, Denker S, Lehmann MH, Mahmud R. Macro-reentry within the His Purkinje system. PACE 1983; 6:1010–1025.

841. Blanck Z, Akhtar M. Ventricular tachycardia due to sustained bundle branch reentry: diagnostic and therapeutic considerations. Clin Cardiol 1993; 16:619–622.

842. Tchou P, Mehdirad AA. Bundle branch reentry ventricular tachycardia. Pacing Clin Electrophysiol 1995; 18:1427–1437.

843. Simons GR, Sorrentino RA, Zimerman LI, Wharton JM, Natale A. Bundle branch reentry tachycardia and possible sustained interfascicular reentry with a shared unusual induction pattern. J Cardiovasc Electrophysiol 1996; 7:44–50.

844. Rubenstein DS, Burke MC, Kall JG, Kinder CA, Kopp DE, Wilber DJ. Adenosine-sensitive bundle branch reentry. J Cardiovasc Electrophysiol 1997; 8:80–88.

845. Oreto G, Smeets JL, Rodriguez LM, Timmermans C, Wellens HJJ. Wide complex tachycardia with atrioventricular dissociation and QRS morphology identical to that of sinus rhythm: a manifestation of bundle branch reentry. Heart 1996; 76:541–547.

846. Caceres J, Jazayeri M, McKinnie J, et al. Sustained bundle branch reentry as a mechanism of clinical tachycardia. Circulation 1989; 79:256–270.

847. Blanck Z, Dhala A, Deshpande S, Sra J, Jazayeri M, Akhtar M. Bundle branch reentrant ventricular tachycardia: cumulative experience in 48 patients. J Cardiovasc Electrophysiol 1993; 4:253–262.

848. Waldo AL, Olshansky B, Okumura K, Henthorn RW. Current perspective on entrainment of tachyarrhythmias. In Brugada P, Wellens HJJ (eds). Cardiac Arrhythmias. Where To Go From Here? Mount Kisco, NY: Futura Publishing Co., 1987, pp. 171–189.

849. Frazier DW, Stanton MS. Resetting and transient entrainment of ventricular tachycardia. Pacing Clin Electrophysiol 1995; 18:1919–1946.

850. MacLean WAH, Plumb VJ, Waldo AL. Transient entrainment and interruption of ventricular tachycardia. PACE 1981; 4:358–366.

851. Inoue H, Inoue K, Matsuo H, Kuwaki K, Shirai T, Murao S. Resetting of tachycardia cycle by single and double ventricular extrastimuli in recurrent sustained ventricular tachycardia. PACE 1984; 7:3–9.

852. Waldo AL, Henthorn RW, Plumb VJ, MacLean WAH. Demonstration of the mechanism of transient entrainment and interruption of ventricular tachycardia with rapid atrial pacing. J Am Coll Cardiol 1984; 3:422–430.

853. Almendral JM, Gottlieb C, Marchlinski FE, Buxton AE, Doherty JU, Josephson ME. Entrainment of ventricular tachycardia by atrial depolarizations. Am J Cardiol 1985; 56:298–304.

854. Almendral JM, Stamato NJ, Rosenthal ME, Marchlinski FE, Miller JM, Josephson ME. Resetting response patterns during sustained ventricular tachycardia: relationship to the excitable gap. Circulation 1986; 74:722–730.

855. Almendral JM, Rosenthal ME, Stamato NJ, et al. Analysis of the resetting phenomenon in sustained uniform ventricular tachycardia: incidence and relation to termination. J Am Coll Cardiol 1986; 8:294–300.

856. Okumura K, Matsuyama K, Miyagi H, Tsuchiya T, Yasue H. Entrainment of idiopathic ventricular tachycardia of left ventricular origin with evidence for reentry with an area of slow conduction and effect of verapamil. Am J Cardiol 1988; 62:727–732.

857. Almendral JM, Gottlieb CD, Rosenthal ME, et al. Entrainment of ventricular tachycardia: explanation for surface electrocardiographic phenomena by analysis of electrograms recorded within the tachycardia circuit. Circulation 1988; 77:569–580.

858. Henthorn RW, Okumura K, Olshansky B, Plumb VJ, Hess PG, Waldo AL. A fourth criterion for transient entrainment: the electrogram equivalent of progressive fusion. Circulation 1988; 77:1003–1012.

859. Waldo AL, Henthorn RW. Use of transient entrainment during ventricular tachycardia to localize a critical area in the reentry circuit for ablation. PACE 1989; 12:231–244.

860. Kay GN, Epstein AE, Plumb VJ. Preferential effect of procainamide on the reentrant circuit of ventricular tachycardia. J Am Coll Cardiol 1989; 14:382–390.

861. Aizawa Y, Niwano S, Chinushi M, et al. Incidence and mechanism of interruption of reentrant ventricular tachycardia with rapid ventricular pacing. Circulation 1992; 85:589–595.

862. Aizawa Y, Naitoh N, Kitazawa H, et al. Frequency of

presumed reentry with an excitable gap in sustained ventricular tachycardia unassociated with coronary artery disease. Am J Cardiol 1993; 72:916–921.

863. Callans DJ, Hook BG, Josephson ME. Comparison of resetting and entrainment of uniform sustained ventricular tachycardia: further insights into the characteristics of the excitable gap. Circulation 1993; 87:1229–1238.

864. Olshansky B, Moreira D, Waldo AL. Characterization of double potentials during ventricular tachycardia. Studies during transient entrainment. Circulation 1993; 87:373–381.

865. Morady F, Kadish A, Rosenheck S, et al. Concealed entrainment as a guide for catheter ablation of ventricular tachycardia in patients with prior myocardial infarction. J Am Coll Cardiol 1991; 17:678–689.

866. Rosenthal ME, Stamato NJ, Almendral JM, et al. Influence of the site of stimulation on the resetting phenomenon in ventricular tachycardia. Am J Cardiol 1986; 58:970–976.

867. Stamato NJ, Rosenthal ME, Almendral JM, Josephson ME. The resetting response of ventricular tachycardia to single and double extrastimuli: implications for an excitable gap. Am J Cardiol 1987; 60:596–601.

868. Rosenthal ME, Stamato NJ, Almendral JM, Gottlieb CD, Josephson ME. Resetting of ventricular tachycardia with electrocardiographic fusion: incidence and significance. Circulation 1988; 77:581–588.

869. Stevenson WG, Weiss JN, Wiener I, et al. Resetting of ventricular tachycardia: implications for localizing the area of slow conduction. J Am Coll Cardiol 1988; 11:522–529.

870. Rosenthal ME, Stamato NJ, Almendral JM, Gottlieb CD, Josephson ME. Coupling intervals of ventricular extrastimuli causing resetting of sustained ventricular tachycardia secondary to coronary artery disease: relation to subsequent termination. Am J Cardiol 1988; 61:770–774.

871. Stamato NJ, Frame LH, Rosenthal ME, Almendral JM, Gottlieb CD, Josephson ME. Procainamide-induced slowing of ventricular tachycardia with insights from analysis of resetting response patterns. Am J Cardiol 1989; 63:1455–1461.

872. Kay GN, Epstein AE, Plumb VJ. Resetting of ventricular tachycardia by single extrastimuli: relation to slow conduction within the reentrant circuit. Circulation 1990; 81:1507–1519.

873. Aizawa Y, Funazaki T, Takahashi M, et al. Entrainment of ventricular tachycardia in arrhythmogenic right ventricular tachycardia. Pacing Clin Electrophysiol 1991; 14:1606–1613.

874. Yamabe H, Okumura K, Tsuchiya T, Yasue H. Demonstration of entrainment and presence of slow conduction during ventricular tachycardia in arrhythmogenic right ventricular dysplasia. Pacing Clin Electrophysiol 1994; 17:172–178.

875. Okumura K, Yamabe H, Tsuchiya T, Tabuchi T, Iwasa A, Yasue H. Characteristics of slow conduction zone demonstrated during entrainment of idiopathic ventricular tachycardia of left ventricular origin. Am J Cardiol 1996; 77:379–383.

876. Sarter BH, Schwartzman D, Callans DJ, Gottlieb CD, Marchlinski FE. Bundle branch reentry ventricular tachycardia: an investigation of the circuit with resetting. J Cardiovasc Electrophysiol 1996; 7:1082–1085.

877. Hadjis TA, Harada T, Stevenson WG, Friedman PL. Effect of recording site on postpacing interval measurement during catheter mapping and entrainment of postinfarction ventricular tachycardia. J Cardiovasc Electrophysiol 1997; 8:398–404.

878. Hadjis TA, Stevenson WG, Harada T, Friedman PL, Sager P, Saxon LA. Preferential locations for critical reentry circuit sites causing ventricular tachycardia after inferior wall myocardial infarction. J Cardiovasc Electrophysiol 1997; 8:363–370.

879. Nishizaki M, Arita M, Sakurada H, et al. Demonstration of Purkinje potential during idiopathic left ventricular tachycardia: a marker for ablation site by transient entrainment. PACE 1997; 20:3004–3007.

880. Mitrani RD, Klein LS, Miles WM, et al. Regional cardiac sympathetic denervation in patients with ventricular tachycardia in the absence of coronary artery disease. J Am Coll Cardiol 1993; 22:1344–1353.

881. Kastor JA. How should refractory ventricular tachycardia be treated? Am J Cardiol 1979; 44:1213–1216.

882. Akhtar M. Management of ventricular tachyarrhythmias. II. JAMA 1982; 247:1178–1181.

883. Myerburg RJ, Zaman L, Kessler KM, Castellanos A. Evolving concepts of management of stable and potentially lethal arrhythmias. Am Heart J 1982; 103:615–622.

884. Akhtar M. Management of ventricular tachyarrhythmias. I. JAMA 1982; 247:671–674.

885. Campbell RW. Treatment and prophylaxis of ventricular arrhythmias in acute myocardial infarction. Am J Cardiol 1983; 52:55C–59C.

886. Brugada P, Lemery R, Talajic M, Della Bella P, Wellens HJJ. Treatment of patients with ventricular tachycardia or ventricular fibrillation: first lessons from the "parallel study." In Brugada P, Wellens HJJ (eds). Cardiac Arrhythmias. Where To Go From Here? Mount Kisco, NY: Futura Publishing Co., 1987, pp. 457–470.

887. Fisher JD, Brodman RF, Kim SG, Ferrick KJ, Roth JA. VT/VF: 60/60 protection. PACE 1990; 13:218–222.

888. Bocker D, Breithardt G, Block M, Borggrefe M. Management of patients with ventricular tachyarrhythmias: does an optimal therapy exist? PACE 1994; 17:559–570.

889. Mitchell LB. Treatment of ventricular arrhythmias after recovery from myocardial infarction. Annu Rev Med 1994; 45:119–138.

890. Trappe HJ, Pfitzner P, Figuth HG, Wenzlaff P, Kielblock B, Klein H. Nonpharmacological therapy of ventricular tachyarrhythmias: observations in 554 patients. Pacing Clin Electrophysiol 1994. 17:2172–2177.

891. Larsen GC, Stupey MR, Walance CG, et al. Recurrent cardiac events in survivors of ventricular fibrillation or tachycardia: implications for driving restrictions. JAMA 1994; 271:1335–1339.

892. Waxman MB, Wald RW, Finley JP, Bonet JF, Downar E, Sharma AD. Valsalva termination of ventricular tachycardia. Circulation 1980; 62:843–851.

893. Bornemann C, Scherf D. Paroxysmal ventricular tachycardia abolished by a blow to the precordium. Dis Chest 1969; 56:83–84.

894. Pennington JE, Taylor J, Lown B. Chest thump for reverting ventricular tachycardia. N Engl J Med 1970; 283:1192–1195.

895. Befeler B, Aranda JM. Termination of ventricular tachycardia by a chest thump over the area of paradoxical pulsation. Am Heart J 1977; 94:773–775.

896. Conner D, Shander D, Deegan C, Craddock D, Wolf PS, Baum RS. Self-administered chest thump for cardioversion of recurrent ventricular tachycardia. Chest 1978; 78:877.

897. Sclarovsky S, Kracoff OH, Agmon J. Acceleration of ventricular tachycardia induced by a chest thump. Chest 1981; 80:596–599.

898. Wei JY, Greene HL, Weisfeldt ML. Cough-facilitated conversion of ventricular tachycardia. Am J Cardiol 1980; 45:174–176.

899. Andresen D, Bruggemann T, Ehlers C, Behrens S. Management and prophylaxis of life-threatening arrhythmias: recent achievements. Eur Heart J 1995; 16:20–23.

900. Kim SG. Evolution of the management of malignant ventricular tachyarrhythmias: the roles of drug therapy and implantable defibrillators. Am Heart J 1995; 130:1144–1150.

901. Blanck Z, Akhtar M. Therapy of ventricular tachycardia in patients with nonischemic cardiomyopathies. J Cardiovasc Electrophysiol 1996; 7:671–683.

902. Link MS, Homoud M, Foote CB, Wang PJ, Estes NAM III. Antiarrhythmic drug therapy for ventricular arrhythmias: current perspectives. J Cardiovasc Electrophysiol 1996; 7:653–670.

903. Haverkamp W, Eckardt L, Borggrefe M, Breithardt G. Drugs versus devices in controlling ventricular tachycardia, ventricular fibrillation, and recurrent cardiac arrest. Am J Cardiol 1997; 80:67G–73G.

904. Landers MD, Reiter MJ. General principles of antiarrhythmic therapy for ventricular tachyarrhythmias. Am J Cardiol 1997; 80:31G–44G.

905. Reiffel JA. Prolonging survival by reducing arrhythmic death: pharmacologic therapy of ventricular tachycardia and fibrillation. Am J Cardiol 1997; 80:45G–55G.

906. Singh BN. Controlling cardiac arrhythmias: an overview with a historical perspective. Am J Cardiol 1997; 80:4G–15G.

907. DiMarco JP. Electrophysiology of adenosine. J Cardiovasc Electrophysiol 1990; 1:340–348.

908. Griffith MJ, Linker NJ, Ward DE, Camm AJ. Adenosine in the diagnosis of broad complex tachycardia. Lancet 1988; 1:672–675.

909. Sharma AD, Klein GJ, Yee R. Intravenous adenosine triphosphate during wide QRS complex tachycardia: safety, therapeutic efficacy, and diagnostic utility. Am J Med 1990; 88:337–343.

910. Mason JW. Amiodarone. N Engl J Med 1987; 316:455–466.

911. Nora M, Zipes DP. Empiric use of amiodarone and sotalol. Am J Cardiol 1993; 72:62F–69F.

912. Nademanee K, Singh BN, Stevenson WG, Weiss JN. Amiodarone and post-MI patients. Circulation 1993; 88:764–774.

913. Singh BN, Ahmed R. Class III antiarrhythmic drugs. Curr Opin Cardiol 1994; 9:12–22.

914. Podrid PJ. Amiodarone: reevaluation of an old drug. Ann Intern Med 1995; 122:689–700.

915. Desai AD, Chun S, Sung RJ. The role of intravenous amiodarone in the management of cardiac arrhythmias. Ann Intern Med 1997; 127:294–303.

916. Kowey PR, Marinchak RA, Rials SJ, Filart RA. Intravenous amiodarone. J Am Coll Cardiol 1997; 29:1190–1198.

917. Ward DE, Camm AJ, Wang R, Dymond D, Spurrell RA. Suppression of long-standing incessant ventricular tachycardia by amiodarone. J Electrocardiol 1980; 13:193–198.

918. Podrid PJ, Lown B. Amiodarone therapy in symptomatic, sustained refractory atrial and ventricular tachyarrhythmias. Am Heart J 1981; 101:374–379.

919. Kaski JC, Girotti LA, Messuti H, Rutitzky B, Rosenbaum MB. Long-term management of sustained, recurrent, symptomatic ventricular tachycardia with amiodarone. Circulation 1981; 64:273–279.

920. Nademanee K, Hendrickson JA, Cannom DS, Goldreyer BN, Singh BN. Control of refractory life-threatening ventricular tachyarrhythmias by amiodarone. Am Heart J 1981; 101:759–768.

921. Waxman HL, Groh WC, Marchlinski FE, et al. Amiodarone for control of sustained ventricular tachyarrhythmia: clinical and electrophysiologic effects in 51 patients. Am J Cardiol 1982; 50:1066–1074.

922. Fogoros RN, Anderson KP, Winkle RA, Swerdlow CD, Mason JW. Amiodarone: clinical efficacy and toxicity in 96 patients with recurrent, drug-refractory arrhythmias. Circulation 1983; 68:88–94.

923. Haffajee CI, Love JC, Canada AT, Lesko LJ, Asdourian G, Alpert JS. Clinical pharmacokinetics and efficacy of amiodarone for refractory tachyarrhythmias. Circulation 1983; 67:1347–1355.

924. Greene HL, Graham EL, Werner JA, et al. Toxic and therapeutic effects of amiodarone in the treatment of cardiac arrhythmias. J Am Coll Cardiol 1983; 2:1114–1128.

925. Heger JJ, Prystowsky EN, Zipes DP. Clinical efficacy of amiodarone in treatment of recurrent ventricular tachycardia and ventricular fibrillation. Am Heart J 1983; 106:887–894.

926. Peter T, Hamer A, Mandel WJ, Weiss D. Evaluation of amiodarone therapy in the treatment of drug-resistant cardiac arrhythmias: long-term follow-up. Am Heart J 1983; 106:943–950.

927. Garson A Jr, Gillette PC, McVey P, et al. Amiodarone treatment of critical arrhythmias in children and young adults. J Am Coll Cardiol 1984; 4:749–755.

928. Kaski JC, Girotti LA, Elizari MV, et al. Efficacy of amiodarone during long-term treatment of potentially dangerous ventricular arrhythmias in patients with chronic stable ischemic heart disease. Am Heart J 1984; 107:648–655.

929. Collaborative Group for Amiodarone Evaluation. Multicenter controlled observation of a low-dose regimen of amiodarone for treatment of severe ventricular arrhythmias. Am J Cardiol 1984; 53:1564–1569.

930. Chiale PA, Halpern MS, Nau GJ, et al. Efficacy of amiodarone during long-term treatment of malignant ventricular arrhythmias in patients with chronic chagasic myocarditis. Am Heart J 1984; 107:656–665.

931. Hockings BEF, George T, Mahrous F, Taylor RR, Hajar HA. Effectiveness of amiodarone on ventricular arrhythmias during and after acute myocardial infarction. Am J Cardiol 1987; 60:967–970.

932. Myers M, Peter T, Weiss D, et al. Benefit and risks of long-term amiodarone therapy for sustained ventricular tachycardia/fibrillation: minimum of three-year follow-up in 145 patients. Am Heart J 1990; 119:8–14.

933. Ceremuzynski L, Kleczar E, Krzeminska-Pakula M, et al. Effect of amiodarone on mortality after myocardial infarction: a double-blind, placebo-controlled, pilot study. J Am Coll Cardiol 1992; 20:1056–1062.

934. Fenrich AL, Jr., Perry JC, Friedman RA. Flecainide and amiodarone: combined therapy for refractory tachyarrhythmias in infancy. J Am Coll Cardiol 1995; 25:1195–1198.

935. Heger JJ, Prystowsky EN, Jackman WM, et al. Clinical efficacy and electrophysiology during long-term therapy for recurrent ventricular tachycardia or ventricular fibrillation. N Engl J Med 1981; 305:539–544.

936. Nademanee K, Hendrickson J, Kannan R, Singh BN. Antiarrhythmic efficacy and electrophysiologic actions of amiodarone in patients with life-threatening ventricular arrhythmias: potent suppression of spontaneously occurring tachyarrhythmias versus inconsistent abolition of induced ventricular tachycardia. Am Heart J 1982; 103:950–959.

937. Morady F, DiCarlo LA, Krol RB, Baerman JM, de Buitleir M. Acute and chronic effects of amiodarone on ventricular refractoriness, intraventricular conduction and ventricular tachycardia induction. J Am Coll Cardiol 1986; 7:148–157.

938. McKenna WJ, Oakley CM, Krikler DM, Goodwin JF. Improved survival with amiodarone in patients with hypertrophic cardiomyopathy and ventricular tachycardia. Br Heart J 1985; 53:412–416.

939. Butler J, Harriss DR, Sinclair M, Westaby S. Amiodarone prophylaxis for tachycardias after coronary artery surgery: a randomised, double blind, placebo controlled trial. Br Heart J 1993; 70:56–60.

940. Burkart F, Pfisterer M, Kiowski W, Follath F, Burckhardt D, Jordi S. Effect of antiarrhythmic therapy on mortality in survivors of myocardial infarction with asymptomatic complex ventricular arrhythmias: Basel Antiarrhythmic Study of Infarct Survival (BASIS). J Am Coll Cardiol 1990; 16:1711–1718.

941. Kerin NZ, Frumin H, Faitel K, Aragon E, Rubenfire M. Survival of patients with nonsustained ventricular tachycardia and impaired left ventricular function treated with low-dose amiodarone. J Clin Pharmacol 1991; 31:1112–1117.

942. Hamer AW, Finerman WB Jr, Peter T, Mandel WJ. Disparity between the clinical and electrophysiologic effects of amiodarone in the treatment of recurrent ventricular tachyarrhythmias. Am Heart J 1981; 102:992–1000.

943. Marchlinski FE, Flores B, Miller JM, Gottlieb CD, Hargrove WC III. Relation of the intraoperative defibrillation threshold to successful postoperative defibrillation with an automatic implantable cardioverter defibrillator. Am J Cardiol 1988; 62:393–398.

944. Ferrick KJ, Singh S, Roth JA, Kim SG, Fisher JD. Prediction of electrophysiologic study results in patients treated with amiodarone. Am Heart J 1995; 129:496–501.

945. Man KC, Williamson BD, Niebauer M, et al. Electrophysiologic effects of sotalol and amiodarone in patients with sustained monomorphic ventricular tachycardia. Am J Cardiol 1994; 74:1119–1123.

946. McGovern B, Garan H, Malacoff RF, et al. Long-term clinical outcome of ventricular tachycardia or fibrillation treated with amiodarone. Am J Cardiol 1984; 53:1558–1563.

947. Horowitz LN, Greenspan AM, Spielman SR, et al. Usefulness

of electrophysiologic testing in evaluation of amiodarone therapy for sustained ventricular tachyarrhythmias associated with coronary heart disease. Am J Cardiol 1985; 55:367–371.

948. Kadish AH, Buxton AE, Waxman HL, Flores B, Josephson ME, Marchlinski FE. Usefulness of electrophysiologic study to determine the clinical tolerance of arrhythmia recurrences during amiodarone therapy. J Am Coll Cardiol 1987; 10:90–96.

949. Kim SS, Lal R, Ruffy R. Paroxysmal nonreentrant supraventricular tachycardia due to simultaneous fast and slow pathway conduction in dual atrioventricular node pathways. J Am Coll Cardiol 1987; 10:456–461.

950. Schmitt C, Brachmann J, Waldecker B, Rizos I, Senges J, Kubler W. Amiodarone in patients with recurrent sustained ventricular tachyarrhythmias: results of programmed electrical stimulation and long-term clinical outcome in chronic treatment. Am Heart J 1987; 114:279–283.

951. Yazaki Y, Haffajee CI, Gold RL, Bishop RL, Alpert JS. Electrophysiologic predictors of long-term clinical outcome with amiodarone for refractory ventricular tachycardia secondary to coronary artery disease. Am J Cardiol 1987; 60:293–297.

952. Strasberg B, Kusniec J, Zlotikamien B, Mager A, Sclarovsky S. Long-term follow-up of postmyocardial infarction patients with ventricular tachycardia or ventricular fibrillation treated with amiodarone. Am J Cardiol 1990; 66:673–678.

953. Kowey PR, Marinchak RA, Rials SJ, Rubin AM, Smith L. Electrophysiologic testing in patients who respond acutely to intravenous amiodarone for incessant ventricular tachyarrhythmias. Am Heart J 1993; 125:1628–1632.

954. Waxman HL, Cain ME, Greenspan AM, Josephson ME. Termination of ventricular tachycardia with ventricular stimulation: salutary effect of increased current strength. Circulation 1982; 65:800–804.

955. Martinez-Rubio A, Shenasa M, Chen X, Wichter T, Breithardt G, Borggrefe M. Response to sotalol predicts the response to amiodarone during serial drug testing in patients with sustained ventricular tachycardia and coronary artery disease. Am J Cardiol 1994; 73:357–360.

956. Marchlinski FE, Buxton AE, Josephson ME, Schmitt C. Predicting ventricular tachycardia cycle length after procainamide by assessing cycle length-dependent changes in paced QRS duration. Circulation 1983; 79:39–46.

957. Hariman RJ, Gomes JA, Kang PS, el-Sherif N. Effects of intravenous amiodarone in patients with inducible repetitive ventricular responses and ventricular tachycardia. Am Heart J 1984; 107:1109–1117.

958. Mostow ND, Rakita L, Vrobel TR, Noon D, Blumer J. Amiodarone: intravenous loading for rapid suppression of complex ventricular arrhythmias. J Am Coll Cardiol 1984; 4:97–104.

959. Helmy I, Herre JM, Gee G, et al. Use of intravenous amiodarone for emergency treatment of life-threatening ventricular arrhythmias. J Am Coll Cardiol 1988; 12:1015–1022.

960. Klein RC, Machell C, Rushforth N, Standefur J. Efficacy of intravenous amiodarone as short-term treatment for refractory ventricular tachycardia. Am Heart J 1988; 115:96–101.

961. Schutzenberger W, Leisch F, Kerschner K, Harringer W, Herbinger W. Clinical efficacy of intravenous amiodarone in the short term treatment of recurrent sustained ventricular tachycardia and ventricular fibrillation. Br Heart J 1989; 62:367–371.

962. Williams ML, Woelfel A, Cascio WE, Simpson RJ Jr, Gettes LS, Foster JR. Intravenous amiodarone during prolonged resuscitation from cardiac arrest. Ann Intern Med 1989; 110:839–842.

963. Kowey PR, Levine JH, Herre JM, et al. Randomized, double-blind comparison of intravenous amiodarone and bretylium in the treatment of patients with recurrent, hemodynamically destabilizing ventricular tachycardia or fibrillation. Circulation 1995; 92:3255–3263.

964. Scheinman MM, Levine JH, Cannom DS, et al. Dose-ranging study of intravenous amiodarone in patients with life-threatening ventricular tachyarrhythmias. Circulation 1995; 92:3264–3272.

965. Levine JH, Massumi A, Scheinman MM, et al. Intravenous amiodarone for recurrent sustained hypotensive ventricular tachyarrhythmias. Intravenous amiodarone multicenter trial group. J Am Coll Cardiol 1996; 27:67–75.

966. Perry JC, Knilans TK, Marlow D, Denfield SW, Fenrich AL, Friedman RA. Intravenous amiodarone for life-threatening tachyarrhythmias in children and young adults. J Am Coll Cardiol 1993; 22:95–98.

967. Russo AM, Beauregard LM, Waxman HL. Oral amiodarone loading for the rapid treatment of frequent, refractory, sustained ventricular arrhythmias associated with coronary artery disease. Am J Cardiol 1993; 72:1395–1399.

968. Kerin NZ, Blevins RD, Frumin H, Faitel K, Rubenfire M. Intravenous and oral loading versus oral loading alone with amiodarone for chronic refractory ventricular arrhythmias. Am J Cardiol 1985; 55:89–91.

969. Marchlinski FE, Buxton AE, Flores BT, Doherty JU, Waxman HL, Josephson ME. Value of Holter monitoring in identifying risk for sustained ventricular arrhythmia recurrence on amiodarone. Am J Cardiol 1985; 55:709–712.

970. Strasberg B, Palileo E, Prechel D, et al. Ventricular tachycardia: prediction of response to oral aprindine with intravenous aprindine. Am J Cardiol 1981; 47:676–682.

971. Waleffe A, Mary-Rabine L, Kulbertus HE. Study of moxaprindine with programmed electrical stimulation of the heart in patients with reentrant tachyarrhythmias. Am J Cardiol 1980; 45:640–647.

972. Strasberg B, Swiryn S, Bauernfeind RU, Palileo E, Scagli-otti D, Duffy CE, Rosen KM. Retrograde dual atrioventricular nodal pathways. Am J Cardiol 1981; 48:639–646.

973. Lyon LJ, Donoso E, Friedberg CK. Temporary control of ventricular arrhythmias by drug-induced sinus tachycardia. Arch Intern Med 1969; 123:436–438.

974. Koch-Weser J. Drug therapy: bretylium. N Engl J Med 1979; 300:473–477.

975. Heissenbuttel RH, Bigger JT Jr. Bretylium tosylate: a newly available antiarrhythmic drug for ventricular arrhythmias. Ann Intern Med 1979; 91:229–238.

976. Bacaner MB. Treatment of ventricular fibrillation and other acute arrhythmias with bretylium tosylate. Am J Cardiol 1968; 21:530–543.

977. Macalpin RN, Zalis EG, Kivowitz CF. Prevention of recurrent ventricular tachycardia with oral bretylium tosylate. Ann Intern Med 1970; 72:909–912.

978. Terry G, Vellani CW, Higgins MR, Doig A. Bretylium tosylate in treatment of refractory ventricular arrhythmias complicating myocardial infarction. Br Heart J 1970; 32:21–25.

979. Bernstein JG, Koch-Weser J. Effectiveness of bretylium tosylate against refractory ventricular arrhythmias. Circulation 1972; 45:1024–1034.

980. Cohen HC, Gozo EG Jr, Langendorf R, et al. Response of resistant ventricular tachycardia to bretylium: relation to site of ectopic focus and location of myocardial disease. Circulation 1973; 47:331–340.

981. Holder DA, Sniderman AD, Fraser G, Fallen EL. Experience with bretylium tosylate by a hospital cardiac arrest team. Circulation 1977; 55:541–544.

982. Ryden L, Ariniego R, Arnman K, et al. A double-blind trial of metoprolol in acute myocardial infarction. N Engl J Med 1983; 308:614–618.

983. Huikuri HV, Cox M, Interian A, et al. Efficacy of intravenous propranolol for suppression of inducibility of ventricular tachyarrhythmias with different electrophysiologic characteristics in coronary artery disease. Am J Cardiol 1989; 64:1305–1309.

984. Brodsky MA, Chough SP, Allen BJ, Capparelli EV, Orlov MV, Caudillo G. Adjuvant metoprolol improves efficacy of class I antiarrhythmic drugs in patients with inducible sustained monomorphic ventricular tachycardia. Am Heart J 1992; 124:629–635.

985. Sung RJ, Keung EC, Nguyen NX, Huycke EC. Effects of b-

adrenergic blockade on verapamil-responsive and verapamil-irresponsive sustained ventricular tachycardias. J Clin Invest 1988; 81:688–699.

986. Brodsky MA, Orlov MV, Allen BJ, Orlov YSK, Wolff L, Winters R. Clinical assessment of adrenergic tone and responsiveness to β-blocker therapy in patients with symptomatic ventricular tachycardia and no apparent structural heart disease. Am Heart J 1996; 131:51–58.

987. Mason JW, Swerdlow CD, Mitchell LB. Efficacy of verapamil in chronic, recurrent ventricular tachycardia. Am J Cardiol 1983; 51:1614–1617.

988. Jordaens L, Weyne A, Clement D. Ventricular tachycardia during exercise treated by verapamil. Int J Cardiol 1986; 11:9–15.

989. Kasanuki H, Ohnishi S, Tanaka E, Hirosawa K. Idiopathic sustained ventricular tachycardia responsive to verapamil: clinical electrocardiographic and electrophysiologic considerations. Jpn Circ J 1986; 50:109–118.

990. Kasanuki H, Ohnishi S, Hosoda S. Differentiation and mechanisms of prevention and termination of verapamil-sensitive sustained ventricular tachycardia. Am J Cardiol 1989; 64:46J–49J.

991. Belhassen B, Rotmensch HH, Laniado S. Response of recurrent sustained ventricular tachycardia to verapamil. Br Heart J 1981; 46:679–682.

992. Sung RJ, Shapiro WA, Shen EN, Morady F. Effects of verapamil on ventricular tachycardias possibly caused by reentry, automaticity, and triggered activity. J Clin Invest 1983; 72:350–360.

993. Klein GJ, Millman PJ, Yee R. Recurrent ventricular tachycardia responsive to verapamil. Pacing Clin Electrophysiol 1984; 7:938–948.

994. Belhassen B, Pelleg A. Electrophysiologic effects of adenosine triphosphate and adenosine on the mammalian heart: clinical and experimental aspects. J Am Coll Cardiol 1984; 4:414–424.

995. Gill JS, Mehta D, Ward DE, Camm AJ. Efficacy of flecainide, sotalol, and verapamil in the treatment of right ventricular tachycardia in patients without overt cardiac abnormality. Br Heart J 1992; 68:392–397.

996. Gill JS, Ward DE, Camm AJ. Comparison of verapamil and diltiazem in the suppression of idiopathic ventricular tachycardia. Pacing Clin Electrophysiol 1992; 15:2122–2126.

997. Lee KL, Lauer MR, Young C, et al. Spectrum of electrophysiologic and electropharmacologic characteristics of verapamil-sensitive ventricular tachycardia in patients without structural heart disease. Am J Cardiol 1996; 77:967–973.

998. Buxton AE, Marchlinski FE, Doherty JU, Flores B, Josephson ME. Hazards of intravenous verapamil for sustained ventricular tachycardia. Am J Cardiol 1987; 59:1107–1110.

999. Kingma JH, van Gilst WH, Peels CH, Dambrink JH, Verheugt FW, Wielenga RP. Acute intervention with captopril during thrombolysis in patients with first anterior myocardial infarction: results from the Captopril and Thrombolysis Study (CATS). Eur Heart J 1994; 15:898–907.

1000. Benditt DG, Pritchett ELC, Wallace AG, Gallagher JJ. Recurrent ventricular tachycardia in man: evaluation of disopyramide therapy by intracardiac electrical stimulation. Eur J Cardiol 1979; 9:255–276.

1001. Lerman BB, Waxman HL, Buxton AE, Josephson ME. Disopyramide: evaluation of electrophysiologic effects and clinical efficacy in patients with sustained ventricular tachycardia or ventricular fibrillation. Am J Cardiol 1983; 51:759–764.

1002. Deano DA, Wu D, Mautner RK, Sherman RH, Ehsani AI, Rosen KM. The antiarrhythmic efficacy of intravenous therapy with disopyramide phosphate. Chest 1977; 71:597–606.

1003. Wood MA, Stambler BS, Ellenbogen KA, et al. Suppression of inducible ventricular tachycardia by ibutilide in patients with coronary artery disease. Am Heart J 1998; 135:1048–1054.

1004. Markel ML, Miles WM, Luck JC, Klein LS, Prystowsky EN. Differential effects of isoproterenol on sustained ventricular

tachycardia before and during procainamide and quinidine antiarrhythmic drug therapy. Circulation 1993; 87:783–792.

1005. Josephson ME. Lidocaine and sustained monomorphic ventricular tachycardia: fact or fiction. Am J Cardiol 1996; 78:82–83.

1006. Markel ML, Zipes DP, Bailey JC. Continuous lidocaine infusion in an ambulatory patient with recurrent ventricular tachycardia. Am Heart J 1986; 112:184–186.

1007. Armengol RE, Graff J, Baerman JM, Swiryn S. Lack of effectiveness of lidocaine for sustained, wide QRS complex tachycardia. Ann Emerg Med 1989; 18:254–257.

1008. Nasir N, Taylor A, Doyle TK, Pacifico A. Evaluation of intravenous lidocaine for the termination of sustained monomorphic ventricular tachycardia in patients with coronary artery disease with or without healed myocardial infarction. Am J Cardiol 1994; 74:1183–1186.

1009. Ho DS, Zecchin RP, Richards DA, Uther JB, Ross DL. Double-blind trial of lignocaine versus sotalol for acute termination of spontaneous sustained ventricular tachycardia. Lancet 1994; 344:18–23.

1010. Gorgels AP, van den Dool A, Hofs A, et al. Comparison of procainamide and lidocaine in terminating sustained monomorphic ventricular tachycardia. Am J Cardiol 1996; 78:43–46.

1011. Spracklen FHN, Kimerling JJ, Besterman EMM, Litchfield JW. Use of lignocaine in treatment of cardiac arrhythmias. BMJ 1968; 1:89–91.

1012. Jewitt DE, Kishon Y, Thomas M. Lignocaine in the management of arrhythmias after acute myocardial infarction. Lancet 1968; Feb:266–270.

1013. Mogensen L. Ventricular tachyarrhythmias and lignocaine prophylaxis in acute myocardial infarction. Acta Med Scand 1970; 513:1–89.

1014. Johnson RG, Goldberger AL, Thurer RL, Schwartz M, Sirois C, Weintraub RM. Lidocaine prophylaxis in coronary revascularization patients: a randomized, prospective trial. Ann Thorac Surg 1993; 55:1180–1184.

1015. Reiter MJ, Easley AR, Mann DE. Efficacy of class Ib (lidocaine-like) antiarrhythmic agents for prevention of sustained ventricular tachycardia secondary to coronary artery disease. Am J Cardiol 1987; 59:1319–1324.

1016. Campbell RW. Mexiletine. N Engl J Med 1987; 316:29–34.

1017. Aizawa Y, Chinushi M, Kitazawa H, et al. Discrepant effects of mexiletine on cycle length of ventricular tachycardia and on the effective refractory period in the area of slow conduction. Heart 1996; 75:281–286.

1018. Whitford EG, McGovern B, Schoenfeld MH, et al. Long-term efficacy of mexiletine alone and in combination with class Ia antiarrhythmic drugs for refractory ventricular arrhythmias. Am Heart J 1988; 115:360–366.

1019. Waspe LE, Waxman HL, Buxton AE, Josephson M. Mexiletine for control of drug-resistant ventricular tachycardia: clinical and electrophysiologic results in 44 patients. Am J Cardiol 1983; 51:1175–1181.

1020. Horowitz LN. Efficacy of moricizine in malignant ventricular arrhythmias. Am J Cardiol 1990; 65:41D–46D.

1021. Bhandari AK, Lerman R, Ehrlich S, et al. Electrophysiological evaluation of moricizine in patients with sustained ventricular tachyarrhythmias: low efficacy and high incidence of proarrhythmia. PACE 1993; 16:1853–1861.

1022. Mann DE, Luck JC, Herre JM, et al. Electrophysiologic effects of ethmozin in patients with ventricular tachycardia. Am Heart J 1984; 107:674–679.

1023. Powell AC, Gold MR, Brooks R, Garan H, Ruskin JN, McGovern BA. Electrophysiologic response to moricizine in patients with sustained ventricular arrhythmias. Ann Intern Med 1992; 116:382–387.

1024. Waxman MB, Downar E, Berman ND, Felderhof CH. Phenylephrine (neo-synephrine) terminated ventricular tachycardia. Circulation 1974; 50:656–664.

1025. Engel TR, Gonzalez AC, Meister SG, Frankl WS. Effect of procainamide on induced ventricular tachycardia. Clin Pharmacol Ther 1978; 24:274–282.

1026. Engel TR, Meister SG, Luck JC. Modification of ventricular tachycardia by procainamide in patients with coronary artery disease. Am J Cardiol 1980; 46:1033–1038.

1027. Greenspan AM, Horowitz LN, Spielman SR, Josephson ME. Large dose procainamide therapy for ventricular tachyarrhythmia. Am J Cardiol 1980; 46:453–462.

1028. Callans DJ, Marchlinski FE. Dissociation of termination and prevention of inducibility of sustained ventricular tachycardia with infusion of procainamide: evidence for distinct mechanisms. J Am Coll Cardiol 1992; 19:111–117.

1029. Grimm W, Cho J-G, Marchlinski FE. Effects of incremental doses of procainamide in patients with sustained uniform ventricular tachycardia. J Cardiovasc Electrophysiol 1994; 5:313–322.

1030. Chilson DA, Heger JJ, Zipes DP, Browne KF, Prystowsky EN. Electrophysiologic effects and clinical efficacy of oral propafenone therapy in patients with ventricular tachycardia. J Am Coll Cardiol 1985; 5:1407–1413.

1031. Budde T, Borggrefe M, Podczeck A, Martinez-Rubio A, Breithardt G. Acute and long-term efficacy of oral propafenone in patients with ventricular tachyarrhythmias. J Cardiovasc Pharmacol 1991; 18:254–260.

1032. Naccarella F, Bracchetti D, Palmieri M, Marchesini B, Ambrosioni E. Propafenone for refractory ventricular arrhythmias: correlation with drug plasma levels during long-term treatment. Am J Cardiol 1984; 54:1008–1014.

1033. Kowey PR, Stohler JL, Friehling TD, Marinchak RA. Propafenone in the treatment of patients with malignant ventricular tachyarrhythmias. Can J Cardiol 1991; 7:175–180.

1034. Guccione P, Drago F, Di Donato RM, et al. Oral propafenone therapy for children with arrhythmias: efficacy and adverse effects in midterm follow-up. Am Heart J 1991; 122:1022–1027.

1035. Beaufort-Krol GCM, Bink-Boelkens MTE. Oral propafenone as treatment for incessant supraventricular and ventricular tachycardia in children. Am J Cardiol 1993; 72:1213–1214.

1036. Stavens CS, McGovern B, Garan H, Ruskin JN. Aggravation of electrically provoked ventricular tachycardia during treatment with propafenone. Am Heart J 1985; 110:24–29.

1037. Grace AA, Camm AJ. Quinidine. N Engl J Med 1998; 338:35–45.

1038. Holzberger PT, Greenberg ML, Paicopolis MC, Ozahowski TP, Ho PC, O'Connor GT. Prospective comparison of intravenous quinidine and intravenous procainamide in patients undergoing electrophysiologic testing. Am Heart J 1998; 136:49–56.

1039. Soyka LF, Wirtz C, Spangenberg RB. Clinical safety profile of sotalol in patients with arrhythmias. Am J Cardiol 1990; 65:74A–81A.

1040. Campbell RWF, Furniss SS. Practical considerations in the use of sotalol for ventricular tachycardia and ventricular fibrillation. Am J Cardiol 1993; 72:80A–85A.

1041. Aliot E, Sadoul N, de Chillou C. Effects of sotalol and d-sotalol on ventricular tachycardia and fibrillation induced by programmed electrical stimulation. Eur Heart J 1993; 14:H74–H77.

1042. Hohnloser SH, Woosley RL. Sotalol. N Engl J Med 1994; 331:31–38.

1043. Kienzle MG, Martins JB, Wendt DJ, Constantin L, Hopson R, McCue ML. Enhanced efficacy of oral sotalol for sustained ventricular tachycardia refractory to type I antiarrhythmic drugs. Am J Cardiol 1988; 61:1012–1017.

1044. Kopelman HA, Woosley RL, Lee JT, Roden DM, Echt DS. Electrophysiologic effects of intravenous and oral sotalol for sustained ventricular tachycardia secondary to coronary artery disease. Am J Cardiol 1988; 61:1006–1011.

1045. Singh SN, Cohen A, Chen YW, et al. Sotalol for refractory sustained ventricular tachycardia and nonfatal cardiac arrest. Am J Cardiol 1988; 62:399–402.

1046. Kuchar DL, Garan H, Venditti FJ, et al. Usefulness of sotalol in suppressing ventricular tachycardia or ventricular fibrillation in patients with healed myocardial infarcts. Am J Cardiol 1989; 64:33–36.

1047. Ruder MA, Ellis T, Lebsack C, Mead RH, Smith NA, Winkle RA. Clinical experience with sotalol in patients with drug-refractory ventricular arrhythmias. J Am Coll Cardiol 1989; 13:145–152.

1048. Nademanee K, Singh BN. Effects of sotalol on ventricular tachycardia and fibrillation produced by programmed electrical stimulation: comparison with other antiarrhythmic agents. Am J Cardiol 1990; 65:53A–57A.

1049. Kus T, Campa MA, Nadeau R, Dubuc M, Kaltenbrunner W, Shenasa M. Efficacy and electrophysiologic effects of oral sotalol in patients with sustained ventricular tachycardia caused by coronary artery disease. Am Heart J 1992; 123:82–89.

1050. Winters SL, Kukin M, Pe E, Stewart D, Deitchman D, Gomes JA. Effect of oral sotalol on systemic hemodynamics and programmed electrical stimulation in patients with ventricular arrhythmias and structural heart disease. Am J Cardiol 1993; 72:38A–43A.

1051. Lazzara R. Results of Holter ECG guided therapy for ventricular arrhythmias: the ESVEM trial. PACE 1994; 17:473–477.

1052. Young GD, Kerr CR, Mohama R, Boone J, Yeung-Lai-Wah JA. Efficacy of sotalol guided by programmed electrical stimulation for sustained ventricular arrhythmias secondary to coronary artery disease. Am J Cardiol 1994; 73:677–682.

1053. Reisinger J, Shenasa M, Lubinski A, et al. Clinical implications of pleomorphic ventricular tachycardias on oral sotalol therapy. Eur Heart J 1995; 16:377–382.

1054. Antz M, Cappato R, Kuck KH. Metoprolol versus sotalol in the treatment of sustained ventricular tachycardia. J Cardiovasc Pharmacol 1995; 26:627–635.

1055. Amiodarone Vs Sotalol Study Group. Multicentre randomized trial of sotalol vs amiodarone for chronic malignant ventricular tachyarrhythmias. Eur Heart J 1989; 10:685–694.

1056. Singh BN, Kehoe R, Woosley RL, Scheinman M, Quart B. Multicenter trial of sotalol compared with procainamide in the suppression of inducible ventricular tachycardia: a double-blind, randomized parallel evaluation: Sotalol Multicenter Study Group. Am Heart J 1995; 129:87–97.

1057. Kehoe RF, MacNeil DJ, Zheutlin TA, et al. Safety and efficacy of oral sotalol for sustained ventricular tachyarrhythmias refractory to other antiarrhythmic agents. Am J Cardiol 1993; 72:56A–66A.

1058. Klein RC. Comparative efficacy of sotalol and class I antiarrhythmic agents in patients with ventricular tachycardia or fibrillation: results of the Electrophysiology Study Versus Electrocardiographic Monitoring (ESVEM) Trial. Eur Heart J 1993; 14:78–84.

1059. Mason JW. A comparison of seven antiarrhythmic drugs in patients with ventricular tachyarrhythmias: electrophysiologic study versus electrocardiographic monitoring investigators. N Engl J Med 1993; 329:452–458.

1060. Biblo LA, Carlson MD, Waldo AL. Insights into the electrophysiology study versus electrocardiographic monitoring trial: its programmed stimulation protocol may introduce bias when assessing long-term antiarrhythmic drug therapy. J Am Coll Cardiol 1995; 25:1601–1604.

1061. Gill JS, Mehta D, Ward DE, Camm AJ. Efficacy of flecainide, sotalol, and verapamil in the treatment of right ventricular tachycardia in patients without overt cardiac abnormality. Br Heart J 1992; 68:392–397.

1062. Yli-Mayry S, Garcia-Alberola A, Haverkamp W, et al. Effect of sotalol on RR interval variability during induced ventricular tachycardia. Am J Cardiol 1996; 78:372–376.

1063. Dorian P, Newman D, Berman N, Hardy J, Mitchell J. Sotalol and type Ia drugs in combination prevent recurrence of sustained ventricular tachycardia. J Am Coll Cardiol 1993; 22:106–113.

1064. Lee SD, Newman D, Ham M, Dorian P. Electrophysiologic mechanisms of antiarrhythmic efficacy of a sotalol and class Ia drug combination: elimination of reverse use dependence. J Am Coll Cardiol 1997; 29:100–105.

1065. Horrigan MC, Davis MJ, May C, Smith P. Dual chamber rate responsive pacing to allow sotalol therapy for ventricular tachycardia. Pacing Clin Electrophysiol 1992; 15:2108–2110.

1066. Brachmann J, Schols W, Beyer T, Montero M, Enders B, Kubler W. Acute and chronic antiarrhythmic efficacy of d-sotalol in patients with sustained ventricular tachyarrhythmias. Eur Heart J 1993; 14:85–87.

1067. Cobbe SM. Class III antiarrhythmics: put to the sword? Heart 1996; 75:111–113.

1068. Waldo AL, Camm AJ, deRuyter H, et al. Effect of *d*-sotalol on mortality in patients with left ventricular dysfunction after recent and remote myocardial infarction. The SWORD Investigators: survival with oral *d*-sotalol. Lancet 1996; 348:7–12.

1069. Keefe DL, Williams S, Torres V, Flowers D, somberg JC. Prophylactic tocainide or lidocaine in acute myocardial infarction. Am J Cardiol 1986; 57:527–531.

1070. Ryden L, Arnman K, Conradson T-B, Hofvendahl S, Mortensen O, Smedgard P. Prophylaxis of ventricular tachyarrhythmias with intravenous and oral tocainide in patients with and recovering from acute myocardial infarction. Am Heart J 1980; 100:1006–1012.

1071. Belhassen B, Pines A, Laniado S. Failure of corticosteroid therapy to prevent induction of ventricular tachycardia in sarcoidosis. Chest 1989; 95:918–920.

1072. Stone N, Klein MD, Lown B. Diphenylhydantoin in the prevention of recurring ventricular tachycardia. Circulation 1971; 43:420–427.

1073. DeSilva RA, Graboys, TB, Podrid PJ, Lown B. Cardioversion and defibrillation. Am Heart J 1980; 100:881–895.

1074. Miller DI, Nachlas MM. Electrocardiographic patterns during resuscitation after experimentally induced ventricular fibrillation. Circ Res 1964; 15:199–207.

1075. DeSanctis RW. Electrical conversion of ventricular tachycardia. JAMA 1965; 191:632–636.

1076. Szekely P, Batson GA, stark DC. Direct current shock therapy of cardiac arrhythmias. Bri Heart J 1966; 28:366–373.

1077. Lown B, Shillingford JP. Symposium on coronary care units. Introduction. Coronary care unit: promise and challenge. Am J Cardiol 1967; 20:449–450.

1078. Resnekov L, McDonald L. Appraisal of electroconversion in treatment of cardiac dysrhythmias. Br Heart J 1968; 30:786–811.

1079. Diem SJ, Lantos JD, Tulsky JA. Cardiopulmonary resuscitation on television: miracles and misinformation. N Engl J Med 1996; 334:1578–1582.

1080. Waldecker B, Brugada P, Zehender M, Stevenson W, Wellens HJJ. Dysrhythmias after direct-current cardioversion. Am J Cardiol 1986; 57:120–123.

1081. Marchlinski FE, Gansler TS, Waxman HL, Josephson ME. Amiodarone pulmonary toxicity. Ann Intern Med 1982; 97:839–845.

1082. O'Neill PG, Faitelson L, Taylor A, Puleo P, Roberts R, Pacifico A. Time course of creatine kinase release after termination of sustained ventricular dysrhythmias. Am Heart J 1991; 122:709–714.

1083. Eysmann SB, Marchlinski FE, Buxton AE, Josephson ME. Electrocardiographic changes after cardioversion of ventricular arrhythmias. Circulation 1986; 73:73–81.

1084. Salerno DM, Katz A, Dunbar DN, Fjeldos-Sperbeck K. Serum electrolytes and catecholamines after cardioversion from ventricular tachycardia and atrial fibrillation. Pacing Clin Electrophysiol 1993; 16:1862–1871.

1085. Moss AJ. Therapeutic uses of permanent pervenous atrial pacemakers: a review. J Electrocardiol 1975; 8:373–380.

1086. Kastor JA, DeSanctis RW, Harthorne JW, Schwartz GH. Transvenous atrial pacing in the treatment of refractory ventricular irritability. Ann Intern Med 1967; 66:939–945.

1087. DeSanctis RW, Kastor JA. Rapid intracardiac pacing for treatment of recurrent ventricular tachyarrhythmias in the absence of heart block. Am Heart J 1968; 76:168–172.

1088. Zipes DP, Festoff B, Schaal SF, Cox C, Sealy WC, Wallace AG. Treatment of ventricular arrhythmia by permanent atrial pacemaker and cardiac sympathectomy. Ann Intern Med 1968; 68:591–597.

1089. Zipes DP, Wallace AG, Sealy WC, Floyd WL. Artificial atrial and ventricular pacing in the treatment of arrhythmias. Ann Intern Med 1969; 70:885–896.

1090. Lichstein E, Chadda K, Fenig S. Atrial pacing in the treatment of refractory ventricular tachycardia associated with hypokalemia. Am J Cardiol 1972; 30:550–553.

1091. Sowton E, Leatham A, Carson P. The suppression of arrhythmias by artificial pacemaking. Lancet 1964; 1098–1100.

1092. Swedberg J, Malm A. Pacemaker stimulation in ventricular paroxysmal tachycardia. Acta Chir Scand 1964; 128:610–615.

1093. Schoonmaker FW, Osteen RT, Greenfield JC. Thioridazine (Mellaril)-induced ventricular tachycardia controlled with an artificial pacemaker. Ann Intern Med 1966; 65:1076–1078.

1094. Heiman DF, Helwig J Jr. Suppression of ventricular arrhythmias by transvenous intracardiac pacing. JAMA 1966; 195:1150–1152.

1095. Bayley TJ, Lightwood R. Double and triple pulse pacemaking in treatment of ventricular tachycardia. Lancet 1966; 235–237.

1096. Lew HT, March HW. Control of recurrent ventricular fibrillation by transvenous pacing in the absence of heart block. Am Heart J 1967; 73:794–797.

1097. Cohen LS, Buccino RA, Morrow AG, Braunwald E. Recurrent ventricular tachycardia and fibrillation treated with a combination of beta-adrenergic blockade and electrical pacing. Ann Intern Med 1967; 66:945–949.

1098. Conrad JK, Mowry FM, Luan LL. Transvenous pacing in two patients with repetitive ventricular arrhythmias. Arch Intern Med 1968; 122:507–511.

1099. Kahn DR, Vathayanon S, Reynolds EW, Sloan H. Successful treatment of paroxysmal ventricular tachycardia with the cardiac pacemaker. Ann Thorac Surg 1968; 5:362–366.

1100. Beller BM, Kotler MN, Collens R. The use of ventricular pacing for suppression of ectopic ventricular activity. Am J Cardiol 1970; 25:467–473.

1101. Friedberg CK, Lyon LJ, Donoso E. Suppression of refractory recurrent ventricular tachycardia by transvenous rapid cardiac pacing and antiarrhythmic drugs. Am Heart J 1970; 79:44–50.

1102. Bennett MA, Pentecost BL. Reversion of ventricular tachycardia by pacemaker stimulation. Br Heart J 1971; 33:922–927.

1103. Fisher JD, Mehra R, Furman S. Termination of ventricular tachycardia with bursts of rapid ventricular pacing. Am J Cardiol 1978; 41:94–102.

1104. Haozhu C, Yuanzhu H, Yang JS, Leng J. Preliminary report on the termination of refractory tachyarrhythmias by cardiac pacing. PACE 1980; 3:302–310.

1105. McCallister BD, McGoon DC, Connolly DC. Paroxysmal ventricular tachycardia and fibrillation without complete heart block: report of a case treated with a permanent internal cardiac pacemaker. Am J Cardiol 1966; 18:898–903.

1106. DeFrancis NA, Giordano RP. Permanent epicardial atrial pacing in the treatment of refractory ventricular tachycardia. Am J Cardiol 1968; 22:742–745.

1107. Hornbaker JH, Humphries JO, Ross RS. Permanent pacing in the absence of heart block: an approach to the management of intractable arrhythmias. Circulation 1969; 39:189–195

1108. Kastor JA, DeSanctis RW, Leinbach RC, Harthorne JW, Wolfson IN. Long-term pervenous atrial pacing. Circulation 1969; 40:535–544.

1109. Feldman AE, Hellerstein HK, Driscol TE, Botti RE. Repetitive ventricular fibrillation in myocardial infarction refractory to bretylium tosylate subsequently controlled by ventricular pacing. Am J Cardiol 1971; 27:227–230.

1110. Johnson RA, Hutter AM, DeSanctis RW, Yurchak PM, Leinbach RC, Harthorne JW. Chronic overdrive pacing in the control of refractory ventricular arrhythmias. Ann Intern Med 1974; 80:380–383.

1111. Hartzler GO. Treatment of recurrent ventricular tachycardia by patient-activated radiofrequency ventricular stimulation. Mayo Clin Proc 1979; 54:75–82.

1112. Di Segni E, David D, Katzenstein M, Klein HO, Kaplinsky E, Levy MJ. Permanent overdrive pacing for the suppression of recurrent ventricular tachycardia in a newborn with long QT syndrome. J Electrocardiol 1980; 13:189–192.

1113. Ruskin JN, Garan H, Poulin F, Harthorne JW. Permanent radiofrequency ventricular pacing for management of drug-resistant ventricular tachycardia. Am J Cardiol 1980; 46:317–321.

1114. Griffin JC, Mason JW, Ross DL, Calfee RV. The treatment of ventricular tachycardia using an automatic tachycardia terminating pacemaker. PACE 1981; 4:582–588.

1115. Hartzler GO, Holmes DR, Osborn MJ. Patient-activated transvenous cardiac stimulation for the treatment of supraventricular and ventricular tachycardia. Am J Cardiol 1981; 47:903–909.

1116. Engler R, Curtis GP. Patient activated asynchronous ventricular pacing at normal rates for termination of ventricular tachycardia. J Electrocardiol 1981; 14:409–412.

1117. Greene HL, Gross BW, Preston TA, et al. Termination of ventricular tachycardia by programmed extrastimuli from an externally-activated permanent pacemaker. PACE 1982; 5:434–439.

1118. Fisher JD, Kim SG, Furman S, Matos JA. Role of implantable pacemakers in control of recurrent ventricular tachycardia. Am J Cardiol 1982; 49:194–206.

1119. Fisher JD, Kim SG, Matos JA, Ostrow E. Comparative effectiveness of pacing techniques for termination of well-tolerated sustained ventricular tachycardia. PACE 1983; 6:915–922.

1120. Fisher JD, Kim SG, Waspe LE, Matos JA. Mechanisms for the success and failure of pacing for termination of ventricular tachycardia: clinical and hypothetical considerations. PACE 1983; 6:1094–1105.

1121. Fisher JD, Ostrow E, Kim SG, Matos JA. Ultrarapid single-capture train stimulation for termination of ventricular tachycardia. Am J Cardiol 1983; 51:1334–1338.

1122. Fisher JD, Johnston DR, Furman S, Mercando AD, Kim SG. Long-term efficacy of antitachycardia pacing for supraventricular and ventricular tachycardias. Am J Cardiol 1987; 60:1311–1316.

1123. Newman DM, Lee MA, Herre JM, Langberg JJ, Scheinman MM, Griffin JC. Permanent antitachycardia pacemaker therapy for ventricular tachycardia. Pacing Clin Electrophysiol 1989; 12:1387–1395.

1124. Connelly DT, de Belder MA, Cunningham D, Lopes AN, Rickards AF, Rowland E. Long-term follow up of patients treated with a software based antitachycardia pacemaker. Br Heart J 1993; 69:250–254.

1125. Jentzer JH, Hoffmann RM. Acceleration of ventricular tachycardia by rapid overdrive pacing combined with extrastimuli. PACE 1984; 7:922–924.

1126. Fries R, Heisel A, Kalweit G, Jung J, Schieffer H. Antitachycardia pacing in patients with implantable cardioverter defibrillators: how many attempts are useful? Pacing Clin Electrophysiol 1997; 20:198–202.

1127. Wietholt D, Block M, Isbruch F, et al. Clinical experience with antitachycardia pacing and improved detection algorithms in a new implantable cardioverter-defibrillator. J Am Coll Cardiol 1993; 21:885–894.

1128. PCD Investigator Group. Clinical outcome of patients with malignant ventricular tachyarrhythmias and a multiprogrammable implantable cardioverter-defibrillator implanted with or without thoracotomy: an international multicenter study. PCD investigator group. J Am Coll Cardiol 1994; 23:1521–1530.

1129. Moss AJ, Hall WJ, Cannom DS, et al. Improved survival with an implanted defibrillator in patients with coronary disease at high risk for ventricular arrhythmia. N Engl J Med 1996; 335:1933–1940.

1130. Friedman PL, Stevenson WG. Unsustained ventricular tachycardia: to treat or not to treat? N Engl J Med 1996; 335:1984–1985.

1131. Josephson ME, Nisam S. The AVID trial: evidence based or randomized control trials: is the AVID study too late? Antiarrhythmics versus implantable defibrillators. Am J Cardiol 1997; 80:194–197.

1132. Ferguson TB Jr, Smith JM, Cox JL, Cain ME, Lindsay BD. Direct operation versus ICD therapy for ischemic ventricular tachycardia. Ann Thorac Surg 1994; 58:1291–1296.

1133. Belhassen B, Miller HI, Laniado S. Catheter ablation of incessant ventricular tachycardia refractory to external cardioversions. Am J Cardiol 1985; 55:1637–1639.

1134. Breithardt G, Borggrefe M, Podczeck A, Rohner D, Budde T.

Clinical experience with catheter ablation of ventricular tachycardia using defibrillator pulses. In Breithardt G, Borggrefe M, Zipes DP (eds.) Nonpharmacological Therapy of Tachyarrhythmias. Mount Kisco, NY: Futura Publishing Co., 1987, pp. 299–314.

1135. Fitzgerald DM, Friday KJ, Yeung Lai Wah JA, Lazzara R, Jackman WM. Electrogram patterns predicting successful catheter ablation of ventricular tachycardia. Circulation 1988; 77:806–814.

1136. Fisher JD, Kim SG, Mercando AD. Electrical devices for treatment of arrhythmias. Am J Cardiol 1988; 61:45A–57A.

1137. Aizawa Y, Chinushi M, Naitoh N, et al. Catheter ablation with radiofrequency current of ventricular tachycardia originating from the right ventricle. Am Heart J 1993; 125:1269–1275.

1138. Dubuc M, Nadeau R, Tremblay G, Kus T, Molin F, Savard P. Pace mapping using body surface potential maps to guide catheter ablation of accessory pathways in patients with Wolff-Parkinson-White syndrome. Circulation 1993; 87:135–143.

1139. Hindricks G. The Multicentre European Radiofrequency Survey (MERFS): complications of radiofrequency catheter ablation of arrhythmias. The Multicentre European Radiofrequency Survey (MERFS) investigators of the working group on arrhythmias of the European Society of Cardiology. Eur Heart J 1993; 14:1644–1653.

1140. Morady F, Calkins H, Langberg JJ, et al. A prospective randomized comparison of direct current and radiofrequency ablation of the atrioventricular junction. J Am Coll Cardiol 1993; 21:102–109.

1141. Wellens HJJ, Smeets JL. Idiopathic left ventricular tachycardia: cure by radiofrequency ablation. Circulation 1993; 88:2978–2979.

1142. American College of Cardiology Cardiovascular Technology Assessment Committee. Catheter ablation for cardiac arrhythmias: clinical applications, personnel and facilities: American College of Cardiology Cardiovascular Technology Assessment Committee. J Am Coll Cardiol 1994; 24:828–833.

1143. Bashir Y, Ward DE. Radiofrequency catheter ablation: a new frontier in interventional cardiology. Br Heart J 1994; 71:119–124.

1144. Blanck Z, Dhala A, Deshpande S, Sra J, Jazayeri M, Akhtar M. Catheter ablation of ventricular tachycardia. Am Heart J 1994; 127:1126–1133.

1145. Gonska B-D, Cao K, Schaumann A, Dorszewski A, von zur Muhlen F, Kreuzer H. Management of patients after catheter ablation of ventricular tachycardia. PACE 1994; 17:542–549.

1146. Manolis AS, Wang PJ, Estes NA III. Radiofrequency catheter ablation for cardiac tachyarrhythmias. Ann Intern Med 1994; 121:452–461.

1147. Scheinman MM. NASPE survey on catheter ablation. Pacing Clin Electrophysiol 1995; 18:1474–1478.

1148. Stevenson WG, Friedman PL, Ganz LI. Catheter ablation for ventricular tachycardia. American College of Cardiology Education Highlights. American College of Cardiology, 1996, pp. 10–14.

1149. Reek S, Klein HU, Ideker RE. Can catheter ablation in cardiac arrest survivors prevent ventricular fibrillation recurrence? Pacing Clin Electrophysiol 1997; 20:1840–1859.

1150. Stevenson WG, Friedman PL, Sweeney MO. Catheter ablation as an adjunct to ICD therapy. Circulation 1997; 96:1378–1380.

1151. Stevenson WG, Ellison KE, Lefroy DC, Friedman PL. Ablation therapy for cardiac arrhythmias. Am J Cardiol 1997; 80:56G–66G.

1152. Cohen TJ, Chien WW, Lurie KG, et al. Radiofrequency catheter ablation for treatment of bundle branch reentrant ventricular tachycardia: results and long-term follow-up. J Am Coll Cardiol 1991; 18:1767–1773.

1153. Aizawa Y, Chinushi M, Naitoh N, et al. Catheter ablation of ventricular tachycardia with radiofrequency currents, with special reference to the termination and minor morphologic change of reinduced ventricular tachycardia. Am J Cardiol 1995; 76:574–579.

1154. Cao K, Gonska BD. Catheter ablation of incessant

ventricular tachycardia: acute and long-term results. Eur Heart J 1996; 17:756–763.

1155. Rothman SA, Hsia HH, Cossu SF, Chmielewski L, Buxton AE, Miller JM. Radiofrequency catheter ablation of postinfarction ventricular tachycardia: long-term success and the significance of inducible nonclinical arrhythmias. Circulation 1997; 96:3499–3508.

1156. Nademanee K, Kosar EM. A nonfluoroscopic catheter-based mapping technique to ablate focal ventricular tachycardia. PACE 1998; 21:1442–1447.

1157. Morady F, Frank R, Kou WH, et al. Identification and catheter ablation of a zone of slow conduction in the reentrant circuit of ventricular tachycardia in humans. J Am Coll Cardiol 1988; 11:775–782.

1158. Borggrefe M, Breithardt G, Podczeck A, Rohner D, Budde T, Martinez-Rubio A. Catheter ablation of ventricular tachycardia using defibrillator pulses: electrophysiological findings and long-term results. Eur Heart J 1989; 10:591–601.

1159. Haissaguerre M, Warin JF, Lemetayer P, Guillem JP, Blanchot P. Fulguration of ventricular tachycardia using high cumulative energy: results in thirty-one patients with a mean follow-up of twenty-seven months. Pacing Clin Electrophysiol 1989; 12:245–251.

1160. Morady F, Scheinman MM, Griffin JC, Herre JM, Kou WH. Results of catheter ablation of ventricular tachycardia using direct current shocks. Pacing Clin Electrophysiol 1989; 12:252–257.

1161. Mukai J, Nakagawa H, Nagata K, et al. Long-term results of catheter ablation for idiopathic ventricular tachycardia originated from the right ventricular outflow. Jpn Circ J 1993; 57:960–968.

1162. Sreeram N, Smeets JL, Wellens HJJ. Radiofrequency catheter ablation of idiopathic left ventricular tachycardia in young adults. Int J Cardiol 1993; 42:288–291.

1163. Brugada P, de Swart H, Smeets JLRM, Wellens HJJ. Transcoronary chemical ablation of ventricular tachycardia. Circulation 1989; 79:475–482.

1164. Man KC, Daoud EG, Knight BP, et al. Accuracy of the unipolar electrogram for identification of the site of origin of ventricular activation. J Cardiovasc Electrophysiol 1997; 8:974–979.

1165. Willems S, Borggrefe M, Shenasa M, et al. Radiofrequency catheter ablation of ventricular tachycardia following implantation of an automatic cardioverter defibrillator. Pacing Clin Electrophysiol 1993; 16:1684–1692.

1166. Blanchard SM, Walcott GP, Wharton JM, Ideker RE. Why is catheter ablation less successful than surgery for treating ventricular tachycardia that results from coronary artery disease? Pacing Clin Electrophysiol 1994; 17:2315–2335.

1167. d'Avila A, Nellens P, Andries E, Brugada P. Catheter ablation of ventricular tachycardia occurring late after myocardial infarction: a point-of-view. Pacing Clin Electrophysiol 1994; 17:532–541.

1168. Hartzler GO. Electrode catheter ablation of refractory focal ventricular tachycardia. J Am Coll Cardiol 1983; 2:1107–1113.

1169. Belhassen B, Miller HI, Laniado S. Catheter ablation of incessant ventricular tachycardia refractory to external cardioversions. Am J Cardiol 1985; 55:1637–1639.

1170. Trappe HJ, Klein H, Auricchio A, Wenzlaff P, Lichtlen PR. Catheter ablation of ventricular tachycardia: role of the underlying etiology and the site of energy delivery. Pacing Clin Electrophysiol 1992; 15:411–424.

1171. Ometto R, Bedogni F, La Vecchia L, Finocchi G, Mosele GM, Vincenzi M. Radiofrequency catheter ablation of the slow reentrant pathway of sustained ventricular tachycardia. Pacing Clin Electrophysiol 1993; 16:1898–1905.

1172. Kim YH, Sosa-Suarez G, Trouton TG, et al. Treatment of ventricular tachycardia by transcatheter radiofrequency ablation in patients with ischemic heart disease. Circulation 1994; 89:1094–1102.

1173. Schwartzman D, Jadonath RL, Callans DJ, Gottlieb CD, Marchlinski FE. Radiofrequency catheter ablation for control of frequent ventricular tachycardia with healed myocardial infarction. Am J Cardiol 1995; 74:297–299.

1174. Wilber DJ, Kopp DE, Glascock DN, Kinder CA, Kall JG. Catheter ablation of the mitral isthmus for ventricular tachycardia associated with inferior infarction. Circulation 1995; 92:3481–3489.

1175. Strickberger SA, Man KC, Daoud EG, et al. A prospective evaluation of catheter ablation of ventricular tachycardia as adjuvant therapy in patients with coronary artery disease and an implantable cardioverter-defibrillator. Circulation 1997; 96:1525–1531.

1176. Stevenson WG, Khan H, Sager P, et al. Identification of reentry circuit sites during catheter mapping and radiofrequency ablation of ventricular tachycardia late after myocardial infarction. Circulation 1993; 88:1647–1670.

1177. Morady F, Harvey M, Kalbfleisch J, el-Atassi R, Calkins H, Langberg JJ. Radiofrequency catheter ablation of ventricular tachycardia in patients with coronary artery disease. Circulation 1993; 87:363–372.

1178. Gonska B-D, Cao K, Schaumann S, Dorszewski A, von zur Muhlen F, Kreuzer H. Catheter ablation of ventricular tachycardia in 136 patients with coronary artery disease: results and long-term follow-up. J Am Coll Cardiol 1994; 24:1506–1514.

1179. Stevenson WG, Friedman PL, Kocovic D, Sager PT, Saxon LA, Pavri B. Radiofrequency catheter ablation of ventricular tachycardia after myocardial infarction. Circulation 1998; 98:308–314.

1180. Menz V, Duthinh V, Callans DJ, Schwartzman D, Gottlieb CD, Marchlinski FE. Right ventricular radiofrequency ablation of ventricular tachycardia after myocardial infarction. Pacing Clin Electrophysiol 1997; 20:1727–1731.

1181. Blanck Z, Deshpande S, Jazayeri MR, Akhtar M. Catheter ablation of the left bundle branch for the treatment of sustained bundle branch reentrant ventricular tachycardia. J Cardiovasc Electrophysiol 1995; 6:40–43.

1182. Crijns HJGM, Smeets JLRM, Rodriguez LM, Meijer A, Wellens HJJ. Cure of interfasicular reentrant tachycardia by ablation of the anterior fascicle of the left bundle branch. J Cardiovasc Electrophysiol 1995; 6:486–492.

1183. Tchou P, Jazayeri M, Denker S, Dongas J, Caceres J, Akhtar M. Transcatheter electrical ablation of right bundle branch. A method of treating macroreentrant ventricular tachycardia attributed to bundle branch reentry. Circulation 1988; 78:246–257.

1184. Langberg JJ, Desai J, Dullet N, Scheinman MM. Treatment of macroreentrant ventricular tachycardia with radiofrequency ablation of the right bundle branch. Am J Cardiol 1989; 63:1010–1013.

1185. Kusniec J, Strasberg B, Birnbaum Y, Sclarovsky S. Bundle-branch reentry tachycardia. Clin Cardiol 1993; 16:892–894.

1186. Mehdirad AA, Keim S, Rist K, Tchou P. Long-term clinical outcome of right bundle branch radiofrequency catheter ablation for treatment of bundle branch reentrant ventricular tachycardia. Pacing Clin Electrophysiol 1995; 18:2135–2143.

1187. Wang CW, Sterba R, Tchou P. Bundle branch reentry ventricular tachycardia with two distinct left bundle branch block morphologies. J Cardiovasc Electrophysiol 1997; 8:688–693.

1188. Rodriguez LM, Smeets JL, Timmermans C, et al. Radiofrequency catheter ablation of sustained monomorphic ventricular tachycardia in hypertrophic cardiomyopathy. J Cardiovasc Electrophysiol 1997; 8:803–806.

1189. Stark SI, Arthur A, Lesh MD. Radiofrequency catheter ablation of ventricular tachycardia in right ventricular cardiomyopathy: use of concealed entrainment to identify the slow conduction isthmus bounded by an aneurysm and the tricuspid annulus. J Cardiovasc Electrophysiol 1996; 7:967–971.

1190. Kottkamp H, Hindricks G, Chen X, et al. Radiofrequency catheter ablation of sustained ventricular tachycardia in idiopathic dilated cardiomyopathy. Circulation 1995; 92:1159–1168.

1191. Burton ME, Leon AR. Radiofrequency catheter ablation of right ventricular outflow tract tachycardia late after complete repair of tetralogy of Fallot using the pace mapping technique. Pacing Clin Electrophysiol 1993; 16:2319–2325.

1192. Goldner BG, Cooper R, Blau W, Cohen TJ. Radiofrequency catheter ablation as a primary therapy for treatment of ventricular tachycardia in a patient after repair of tetralogy of Fallot. PACE 1994; 17:1441–1446.

1193. Biblo LA, Carlson MD. Transcatheter radiofrequency ablation of ventricular tachycardia following surgical correction of tetralogy of Fallot. Pacing Clin Electrophysiol 1994; 17:1556–1560.

1194. Chinushi M, Aizawa Y, Kitazawa H, Kusano Y, Washizuka T, Shibata A. Successful radiofrequency catheter ablation for macroreentrant ventricular tachycardias in a patient with tetralogy of Fallot after corrective surgery. Pacing Clin Electrophysiol 1995; 18:1713–1716.

1195. Horton RP, Canby RC, Kessler DJ, et al. Ablation of ventricular tachycardia associated with tetralogy of Fallot: demonstration of bidirectional block. J Cardiovasc Electrophysiol 1997; 8:432–435.

1196. Breithardt G, Borggrefe M, Wichter T. Catheter ablation of idiopathic right ventricular tachycardia. Circulation 1990; 82:2273–2276.

1197. Silka MJ, Kron J. Radiofrequency catheter ablation for idiopathic right ventricular tachycardia: first, last or only therapy—who decides? J Am Coll Cardiol 1996; 27:875–876.

1198. Varma N, Josephson ME. Therapy of "idiopathic" ventricular tachycardia. J Cardiovasc Electrophysiol 1997; 8:104–116.

1199. Hartzler GO. Electrode catheter ablation of refractory focal ventricular tachycardia. J Am Coll Cardiol 1983; 2:1107–1113.

1200. Morady F, Kadish AH, DiCarlo L, et al. Long-term results of catheter ablation of idiopathic right ventricular tachycardia. Circulation 1990; 82:2093–2099.

1201. Stevenson GW, Schuster J, Kross J, Hall SC. Transoesophageal pacing for perioperative control of neonatal paroxysmal supraventricular tachycardia. Can J Anaesth 1990; 37:672–674.

1202. Ashan AJ, Cunningham D, Rowland E. Low energy catheter ablation of right ventricular outflow tract tachycardia. Br Heart J 1991; 65:231–233.

1203. Klein LS, Shih HT, Hackett FK, Zipes DP, Miles WM. Radiofrequency catheter ablation of ventricular tachycardia in patients without structural heart disease. Circulation 1992; 85:1666–1674.

1204. Calkins H, Kalbfleisch SJ, el-Atassi R, Langberg JJ, Morady F. Relation between efficacy of radiofrequency catheter ablation and site of origin of idiopathic ventricular tachycardia. Am J Cardiol 1993; 71:827–833.

1205. O'Connor BK, Case CL, Sokoloski MC, Gementi A, Cooper K, Gillette PC. Radiofrequency catheter ablation of right ventricular outflow tachycardia in children and adolescents. J Am Coll Cardiol 1996; 27:869–874.

1206. Chinushi M, Aizawa Y, Takahashi K, et al. Morphological variation of nonreentrant idiopathic ventricular tachycardia originating from the right ventricular outflow tract and effect of radiofrequency lesion. Pacing Clin Electrophysiol 1997; 20:325–326.

1207. Chinushi M, Aizawa Y, Takahashi K, Kitazawa H, Shibata A. Radiofrequency catheter ablation for idiopathic right ventricular tachycardia with special reference to morphological variation and long-term outcome. Heart 1997; 78:255–261.

1208. Gumbrielle TP, Bourke JP, Doig JC, et al. Electrocardiographic features of septal location of right ventricular outflow tract tachycardia. Am J Cardiol 1997; 79:213–216.

1209. Rodriguez LM, Smeets JL, Timmermans C, Wellens HJJ. Predictors for successful ablation of right- and left-sided idiopathic ventricular tachycardia. Am J Cardiol 1997; 79:309–314.

1210. Smeets JL, Rodriguez LM, Timmermans C, Wellens HJJ. Radiofrequency catheter ablation of idiopathic ventricular tachycardias in children. Pacing Clin Electrophysiol 1997; 20:2068–2071.

1211. Breithardt G, Borggrefe M, Wichter T. Catheter ablation of idiopathic right ventricular tachycardia. Circulation 1990; 82:2273–2276.

1212. Page RL, Shenasa RA, Evans JJ, Sorrentino RA, Wharton JM, Prystowsky EN. Radiofrequency catheter ablation of idiopathic recurrent ventricular tachycardia with right bundle branch block, left axis morphology. PACE 1993; 16:327–336.

1213. Gaita F, Giustetto C, Leclercq JF, et al. Idiopathic verapamil-responsive left ventricular tachycardia: clinical characteristics and long-term follow-up of 33 patients. Eur Heart J 1994; 15:1252–1260.

1214. Wagshal AB, Mittleman RS, Schuger CD, Huang SKS. Coincident idiopathic left ventricular tachycardia and atrioventricular nodal reentrant tachycardia: control by radiofrequency catheter ablation of the slow atrioventricular nodal pathway. PACE 1994; 17:386–396.

1215. Wen MS, Yeh SJ, Wang CC, Lin FC, Chen IC, Wu D. Radiofrequency ablation therapy in idiopathic left ventricular tachycardia with no obvious structural heart disease. Circulation 1994; 89:1690–1696.

1216. Underwood RD, Deshpande SS, Biehl M, Cowan M, Akhtar M, Jazayeri MR. Radiofrequency catheter ablation of multiple morphologies of ventricular tachycardia by targeting a single region of the left ventricle. J Cardiovasc Electrophysiol 1995; 6:1015–1022.

1217. Washizuka T, Aizawa Y, Chinushi M, et al. Alternation of QRS morphology and effect of radiofrequency ablation in idiopathic ventricular tachycardia. Pacing Clin Electrophysiol 1995; 18:18–27.

1218. Zardini M, Thakur RK, Klein GJ, Yee R. Catheter ablation of idiopathic left ventricular tachycardia. Pacing Clin Electrophysiol 1995; 18:1255–1265.

1219. Katritsis D, Heald S, Ahsan A, et al. Catheter ablation for successful management of left posterior fascicular tachycardia: an approach guided by recording of fascicular potentials. Heart 1996; 75:384–388.

1220. Rodriguez LM, Smeets JL, Timmermans C, Trappe HJ, Wellens HJJ. Radiofrequency catheter ablation of idiopathic ventricular tachycardia originating in the anterior fascicle of the left bundle branch. J Cardiovasc Electrophysiol 1996; 7:1211–1216.

1221. Bennett DH. Experience with radiofrequency catheter ablation of fascicular tachycardia. Heart 1997; 77:104–107.

1222. Greenspon AJ, Hsu SS, Datorre S. Successful radiofrequency catheter ablation of sustained ventricular tachycardia postmyocardial infarction in man guided by a multielectrode "basket" catheter. J Cardiovasc Electrophysiol 1997; 8:565–570.

1223. Damle RS, Landers M, Kelly PA, Reiter MJ, Mann DE. Radiofrequency catheter ablation of idiopathic left ventricular tachycardia originating in the left anterior fascicle. PACE 1998; 21:1155–1158.

1224. Shimoike E, Ohba Y, Yanagi N, et al. Radiofrequency catheter ablation of left ventricular outflow tract tachycardia: report of two cases. J Cardiovasc Electrophysiol 1998; 9:196–202.

1225. Pons M, Beck L, Leclercq F, Ferriere M, Albat B, Davy JM. Chronic left main coronary artery occlusion: a complication of radiofrequency ablation of idiopathic left ventricular tachycardia. Pacing Clin Electrophysiol 1997; 20:1874–1876.

1226. Kottkamp H, Chen X, Hindricks G, et al. Induction of transient third degree atrioventricular block during radiofrequency catheter ablation in a patient with ventricular tachycardia and remote myocardial infarction. Eur Heart J 1995; 16:647–650.

1227. Hilton TC, Aguirre F, Greenwalt T, Janosik DL, Kern MJ. Successful treatment of complex ventricular arrhythmias with percutaneous transluminal coronary angioplasty. Am Heart J 1991; 122:230–231.

1228. Gallagher JJ. Surgical treatment of arrhythmias: current status and future directions. Am J Cardiol 1978; 41:1035–1044.

1229. Harrison DC, Buda AJ, Stinson EB. Surgery for ventricular arrhythmias. In Sandoe E, Julian DG, Bell JW (eds). Management of Ventricular Tachycardia. Role of Mexiletine. Amsterdam: Excerpta Medica, 1978, pp. 643–654.

1230. Fontaine G, Guiraudon G, Frank R, Vedel J, Grosgogeat Y,

Cabrol C. Modern concepts of ventricular tachycardia: the value of electrocardiological investigations and delayed potentials in ventricular tachycardia of ischemic and nonischemic etiology (31 operated cases). Eur J Cardiol 1978; 8:565–580.

1231. Gallagher JJ, Sealy WC, Kasell J. Intraoperative mapping studies in the Wolff-Parkinson-White syndrome. Pacing Clin Electrophysiol 1979; 2:523–537.

1232. Fontaine G, Guiraudon G, Frank R, Cabrol C, Grosgogeat Y. The surgical management of ventricular tachycardia. Herz 1979; 4:276–284.

1233. Sealy WC. The cause of the hemodynamic disturbances in Ebstein's anomaly based on observations at operation. Ann Thorac Surg 1979; 27:536–546.

1234. Anonymous. Surgery for ventricular tachycardia. Lancet 1980; 1:579.

1235. Collins JJ Jr. Surgery for intractable ventricular arrhythmias (editorial). N Engl J Med 1980; 302:627–628.

1236. Horowitz LN, Harken AH, Josephson ME, Kastor JA. Surgical treatment of ventricular arrhythmias in coronary artery disease. Ann Intern Med 1981; 95:88–97.

1237. Waldo AL, Arciniegas JG, Klein H. Surgical treatment of life-threatening ventricular arrhythmias: the role of intraoperative mapping and consideration of the presently available surgical techniques. Prog Cardiovasc Dis 1981; 23:247–264.

1238. Boineau JP, Cox JL. Rationale for a direct surgical approach to control ventricular arrhythmias: relation of specific intraoperative techniques to mechanism and location of arrhythmic circuit. Am J Cardiol 1982; 49:381–396.

1239. Wellens HJJ, Bar FWHM, Vanagt EJDM, Brugada P. Medical treatment of ventricular tachycardia: considerations in the selection of patients for surgical treatment. Am J Cardiol 1982; 49:186–193.

1240. Cox JL. Anatomic-electrophysiologic basis for the surgical treatment of refractory ischemic ventricular tachycardia. Ann Surg 1983; 198:119–129.

1241. Klein GJ, Guiraudon GM. Surgical therapy of cardiac arrhythmias. Cardiol Clin 1983; 1:323–340.

1242. Ferguson TB Jr. The future of arrhythmia surgery. J Cardiovasc Electrophysiol 1994; 5:621–634.

1243. Marchlinski FE, Buxton AE, Vassallo JA, et al. Comparative electrophysiologic effects of intravenous and oral procainamide in patients with sustained ventricular arrhythmias. J Am Coll Cardiol 1984; 4:1247–1254.

1244. Cox JL. Patient selection criteria and results of surgery for refractory ischemic ventricular tachycardia. Circulation 1989; 79:1163–1177.

1245. Hargrove WC, Miller JM. Risk stratification and management of patients with recurrent ventricular tachycardia and other malignant ventricular arrhythmias. Circulation 1989; 79(Suppl I):I-178–I-181.

1246. Fontaine G, Guiraudon G, Frank R, et al. Stimulation studies and epicardial mapping in ventricular tachycardia: study of mechanisms and selection for surgery. In Kulbertus HE (ed). Re-entrant Arrhythmias. Mechanisms and Treatment. Baltimore: University Park Press, 1976, pp. 334–350.

1247. Hargrove WC, 3rd, Addonizio VP, Miller JM. Surgical therapy of ventricular tachyarrhythmias in patients with coronary artery disease. J Cardiovasc Electrophysiol 1996; 7:469–480.

1248. DiMarco JP, Lerman BB, Kron IL, Sellers TD. Sustained ventricular tachyarrhythmias within 2 months of acute myocardial infarction: results of medical and surgical therapy in patients from the initial episode. J Am Coll Cardiol 1985; 6:759–768.

1249. Haines DE, Lerman BB, Kron IL, DiMarco JP. Surgical ablation of ventricular tachycardia with sequential map-guided subendocardial resection: electrophysiologic assessment and long-term follow-up. Circulation 1988; 77:131–141.

1250. Platia EV, Griffith LS, Watkins L Jr. et al. Treatment of malignant ventricular arrhythmias with endocardial resection and implantation of the automatic cardioverter-defibrillator. N Engl J Med 1986; 314:213–216.

1251. Wittig JH, Boineau JP. Surgical treatment of ventricular arrhythmias using epicardial, transmural, and endocardial mapping. Ann Thoracaa Surg 1975; 20:117–126.

1252. Moran JM, Talano JV, Euler D, Moran JF, Montoya A, Pifarre R. Refractory ventricular arrhythmia: the role of intraoperative electrophysiological study. Surgery 1977; 82:809–815.

1253. Harken AH, Josephson ME, Horowitz LN. Surgical endocardial resection for the treatment of malignant ventricular tachycardia. Ann Surg 1979; 190:456–460.

1254. Josephson ME, Harken AH, Horowitz LN. Endocardial excision: a new surgical technique for the treatment of recurrent ventricular tachycardia. Circulation 1979; 60:1430–1439.

1255. Harken AH, Horowitz LN, Josephson ME. Comparison of standard aneurysmectomy and aneurysmectomy with directed endocardial resection for the treatment of recurrent sustained ventricular tachycardia. J Thorac Cardiovasc Surg 1980; 80:527–534.

1256. Engel TR. Endocardial surgery for ventricular tachycardia: the inside story. Ann Intern Med 1981; 94:402–403.

1257. Cox JL, Gallagher JJ, Ungerleider RM. Encircling endocardial ventriculotomy for refractory ischemic ventricular tachycardia. IV. Clinical indication, surgical technique, mechanism of action, and results. J Thorac Cardiovasc Surg 1982; 83:865–872.

1258. Josephson ME, Harken AH, Horowitz LN. Long-term results of endocardial resection for sustained ventricular tachycardia in coronary disease patients. Am Heart J 1982; 104:51–57.

1259. Moran JM, Kehoe RF, Loeb JM, Lichtenthal PR, Sanders JH Jr, Michaelis LL. Extended endocardial resection for the treatment of ventricular tachycardia and ventricular fibrillation. Ann Thorac Surg 1982; 34:538–552.

1260. Moran JM, Kehoe RF, Loeb JM, Sanders JH Jr, Tommaso CL, Michaelis LL. Operative therapy of malignant ventricular rhythm disturbances. Ann Surg 1983; 198:479–486.

1261. Brodman R, Fisher JD, Johnston DR, et al. Results of electrophysiologically guided operations for drug-resistant recurrent ventricular tachycardia and ventricular fibrillation due to coronary artery disease. J Thorac Cardiovasc Surg 1984; 87:431–438.

1262. Miller JM, Kienzle MG, Harken AH, Josephson ME. Subendocardial resection for ventricular tachycardia: predictors of surgical success. Circulation 1984; 70:624–631.

1263. Bolooki H, Palatianos GM, Zaman L, Thurer RJ, Luceri RM, Myerburg RJ. Surgical management of post-myocardial infarction ventricular tachyarrhythmia by myocardial debulking, septal isolation, and myocardial revascularization. J Thorac Cardiovasc Surg 1986; 92:716–725.

1264. Garan H, Nguyen K, McGovern B, Buckley M, Ruskin JN. Perioperative and long-term results after electrophysiologically directed ventricular surgery for recurrent ventricular tachycardia. J Am Coll Cardiol 1986; 8:201–209.

1265. Hammon JW Jr, Echt DS, Merrill WH, et al. Indications for different modes of surgical therapy in medically refractory ventricular arrhythmias. Ann Surg 1986; 203:679–684.

1266. Hargrove WC 3d, Miller JM, Vassallo JA, Josephson ME. Improved results in the operative management of ventricular tachycardia related to inferior wall infarction: importance of the annular isthmus. J Thorac Cardiovasc Surg 1986; 92:726–732.

1267. Krafchek J, Lawrie GM, Roberts R, Magro SA, Wyndham CR. Surgical ablation of ventricular tachycardia: improved results with a map-directed regional approach. Circulation 1986; 73:1239–1247.

1268. Kron IL, DiMarco JP, Lerman BB, Nolan SP. Resection of scarred papillary muscles improves outcome after surgery for ventricular tachycardia. Ann Surg 1986; 203:685–690.

1269. Saksena S, Hussain SM, Wasty N, Gielchinsky I, Parsonnet V. Long-term efficacy of subendocardial resection in refractory ventricular tachycardia: relationship to site of arrhythmia origin. Ann Thorac Surg 1986; 42:685–689.

1270. Swerdlow CD, Mason JW, Stinson EB, Oyer PE, Winkle RA, Derby GC. Results of operations for ventricular tachycardia in 105 patients. J Thorac Cardiovasc Surg 1986; 92:105–113.

1271. Vigano M, Martinelli L, Salerno JA, et al. Ventricular tachycardia in post-myocardial infarction patients: results of surgical therapy. Eur Heart J 1986; 7 (Suppl A):165–8.

1272. Kron IL, Lerman BB, Nolan SP, Flanagan TL, Haines DE, DiMarco JP. Sequential endocardial resection for the surgical treatment of refractory ventricular tachycardia. J Thorac Cardiovasc Surg 1987; 94:843–847.

1273. McGiffin DC, Kirklin JK, Plumb VJ, et al. Relief of life-threatening ventricular tachycardia and survival after direct operations. Circulation 1987; 76:93–103.

1274. Ostermeyer J, Borggrefe M, Breithardt G, et al. Direct operations for the management of life-threatening ischemic ventricular tachycardia. J Thorac Cardiovasc Surg 1987; 94:848–865.

1275. Yee ES, Schienman MM, Griffin JC, Ebert PA. Surgical options for treating ventricular tachyarrhythmia and sudden death. J Thorac Cardiovasc Surg 1987; 94:866–873.

1276. Hargrove WC, 3d, Josephson ME, Marchlinski FE, Miller JM. Surgical decisions in the management of sudden cardiac death and malignant ventricular arrhythmias: subendocardial resection, the automatic internal defibrillator, or both. J Thorac Cardiovasc Surg 1989; 97:923–928.

1277. Landymore RW, Gardner MA, McIntyre AJ, Barker RA. Surgical intervention for drug-resistant ventricular tachycardia. J Am Coll Cardiol 1990; 16:37–41.

1278. Hobson CE, DiMarco JP, Haines DE, Flanagan TL, Kron IL. The influence of preoperative shock on outcome in sequential endocardial resection for ventricular tachycardia. J Thorac Cardiovasc Surg 1991; 102:348–353.

1279. Lawrie GM, Pacifico A, Kaushik R, Nahas C, Earle N. Factors predictive of results of direct ablative operations for drug-refractory ventricular tachycardia: analysis of 80 patients. J Thorac Cardiovasc Surg 1991; 101:44–55.

1280. Kron IL, Kern JA, Theodore P, et al. Does a posterior aneurysm increase the risk of endocardial resection? Ann Thorac Surg 1992; 54:617–620.

1281. Niebauer MJ, Kirsh M, Kadish A, Calkins H, Morady F. Outcome of endocardial resection in 33 patients with coronary artery disease: correlation with ventricular tachycardia morphology. Am Heart J 1992; 124:1500–1506.

1282. Trappe H-J, Klein H, Frank G, Wenzlaff P, Lichtlen PR. Role of mapping-guided surgery in patients with recurrent ventricular tachycardia. Am Heart J 1992; 124:636–644.

1283. Lee R, Mitchell JD, Garan H, et al. Operation for recurrent ventricular tachycardia: predictors of short- and long-term efficacy. J Thorac Cardiovasc Surg 1994; 107:732–742.

1284. Sarter BH, Finkle JK, Gerszten RE, Buxton AE. What is the risk of sudden cardiac death in patients presenting with hemodynamically stable sustained ventricular tachycardia after myocardial infarction? J Am Coll Cardiol 1996; 28:122–129.

1285. Sosa E, Jatene A, Kaeriyama JV, et al. Recurrent ventricular tachycardia associated with postinfarction aneurysm: results of left ventricular reconstruction. J Thorac Cardiovasc Surg 1992; 103:855–860.

1286. Gallagher JJ, Anderson RW, Kasell J, et al. Cryoablation of drug-resistant ventricular tachycardia in a patient with a variant of scleroderma. Circulation 1978; 57:190–197.

1287. Camm J, Ward DE, Cory-Pearce R, Rees GM, Spurrell RAJ. The successful cryosurgical treatment of paroxysmal ventricular tachycardia. Chest 1979; 75:621–624.

1288. Krafchek J, Lawrie GM, Wyndham CR. Cryoablation of arrhythmias from the interventricular septum: initial experience with a new biventricular approach. J Thorac Cardiovasc Surg 1986; 91:419–427.

1289. Ott DA, Garson A Jr, Cooley DA, Smith RT, Moak J. Cryoablative techniques in the treatment of cardiac tachyarrhythmias. Ann Thorac Surg 1987; 43:138–143.

1290. Caceres J, Werner P, Jazayeri M, Akhtar M, Tchou P. Efficacy of cryosurgery alone for refractory monomorphic sustained ventricular tachycardia due to inferior wall infarction. J Am Coll Cardiol 1988; 11:1254–1259.

1291. Page PL, Cardinal R, Shenasa M, Kaltenbrunner W, Cossette R, Nadeau R. Surgical treatment of ventricular tachycardia. Regional cryoablation guided by computerized epicardial and endocardial mapping. Circulation 1989; 80(Suppl I):I-124–I-134.

1292. Shumway SJ, Johnson EM, Svendsen CA, Kriett JM, Ring WS. Surgical management of ventricular tachycardia. Ann Thorac Surg 1997; 63:1589–1591.

1293. Selle JG, Svenson RH, Sealy WC, et al. Successful clinical laser ablation of ventricular tachycardia: a promising new therapeutic method. Ann Thorac Surg 1986; 42:380–384.

1294. Isner JM, Estes NA, Payne DD, Rastegar H, Clarke RJ, Cleveland RJ. Laser-assisted endocardiectomy for refractory ventricular tachyarrhythmias: preliminary intraoperative experience. Clin Cardiol 1987; 10:201–204.

1295. Svenson RH, Gallagher JJ, Selle JG, Zimmern SH, Fedor JM, Robicsek F. Neodymium: YAG laser photocoagulation: a successful new map-guided technique for the intraoperative ablation of ventricular tachycardia. Circulation 1987; 76:1319–1328.

1296. Saksena S, Gielchinsky I, Tullo NG. Argon laser ablation of malignant ventricular tachycardia associated with coronary artery disease. Am J Cardiol 1989; 64:1298–1304.

1297. Svenson RH, Littmann L, Gallagher JJ, et al. Termination of ventricular tachycardia with epicardial laser photocoagulation: a clinical comparison with patients undergoing successful endocardial photocoagulation alone. J Am Coll Cardiol 1990; 15:163–170.

1298. Moosdorf R, Pfeiffer D, Schneider C, Jung W. Intraoperative laser photocoagulation of ventricular tachycardia. Am Heart J 1994; 127:1133–1138.

1299. Miller JM, Kienzle MG, Harken AH, Josephson ME. Morphologically distinct sustained ventricular tachycardias in coronary artery disease: significance and surgical results. J Am Coll Cardiol 1984; 4:1073–1079.

1300. Kienzle MG, Doherty JU, Roy D, Waxman HL, Harken AH, Josephson ME. Subendocardial resection for refractory ventricular tachycardia: effects on ambulatory electrocardiogram, programmed stimulation and ejection fraction, and relation to outcome. J Am Coll Cardiol 1983; 2:853–858.

1301. Kienzle MG, Martin JL, Horowitz LN, Harken AH, Josephson ME. Electrocardiographic changes following endocardial resection for ventricular tachycardia. Am Heart J 1982; 104:753–761.

1302. Manolis AS, Rastegar H, Payne D, Cleveland R, Estes NA III. Surgical therapy for drug-refractory ventricular tachycardia: results with mapping-guided subendocardial resection. J Am Coll Cardiol 1989; 14:199–208.

1303. Moran JM, Kehoe RF, Loeb JM, et al. The role of papillary muscle resection and mitral valve replacement in the control of refractory ventricular arrhythmia. Circulation 1983; 68(Suppl II):II-154.

1304. Gallagher JJ, Oldham HN, Wallace WG, Peter RH, Kasell J. Ventricular aneurysm with ventricular tachycardia: report of a case with epicardial mapping and successful resection. Am J Cardiol 1975; 35:696–700.

1305. Spurrell RA, Yates AK, Thorburn CW, Sowton GE, Deuchar DC. Surgical treatment of ventricular tachycardia after epicardial mapping studies. Br Heart J 1975; 37:115–126.

1306. Guiraudon G, Fontaine G, Frank R, Escande G, Etievent P, Cabrol C. Encircling endocardial ventriculotomy: a new surgical treatment for life-threatening ventricular tachycardias resistant to medical treatment following myocardial infarction. Ann Thorac Surg 1978; 26:438–444.

1307. Ostermeyer J, Breithardt G, Borggrefe M, Godehardt E, Seipel L, Bircks W. Surgical treatment of ventricular tachycardias: complete versus partial encircling endocardial ventriculotomy. J Thorac Cardiovasc Surg 1984; 87:517–525.

1308. Zee-Cheng CS, Kouchoukos NT, Connors JP, Ruffy R. Treatment of life-threatening ventricular arrhythmias with nonguided surgery supported by electrophysiologic testing and drug therapy. J Am Coll Cardiol 1989; 13:153–162.

1309. Lehrman KL, Tilkian AG, Hultgren HN, Fowles RE. Effect of coronary arterial bypass surgery on exercise-induced ventricular arrhythmias: long-term follow-up of a prospective randomized study. Am J Cardiol 1979; 44:1056–1061.

1310. Leutenegger F, Giger G, Fuhr P, et al. Evaluation of

aortocoronary venous bypass grafting for prevention of cardiac arrhythmias. Am Heart J 1979; 98:15–19.

1311. Garan H, Ruskin JN, DiMarco JP, et al. Electrophysiologic studies before and after myocardial revascularization in patients with life-threatening ventricular arrhythmias. Am J Cardiol 1983; 51:519–524.

1312. Kelly P, Ruskin JN, Vlahakes GJ, Buckley MJ Jr, Freeman CS, Garan H. Surgical coronary revascularization in survivors of prehospital cardiac arrest: its effect on inducible ventricular arrhythmias and long-term survival. J Am Coll Cardiol 1990; 15:267–273.

1313. Ecker RR, Mullins CB, Grammer JC, Rea WJ, Atkins JM. Control of intractable ventricular tachycardia by coronary revascularization. Circulation 1971; 44:666–670.

1314. Nakhjavan FK, Morse DP, Nichols HT, Goldberg H. Emergency aortocoronary bypass: treatment of ventricular tachycardia due to ischemic heart disease. JAMA 1971; 216:2138–2140.

1315. Berntsen RF, Gunnes P, Lie M, Rasmussen K. Surgical revascularization in the treatment of ventricular tachycardia and fibrillation exposed by exercise-induced ischaemia. Eur Heart J 1993; 14:1297–1303.

1316. Pfeiffer D, Moosdorf R, Svenson RH, et al. Epicardial neodymium: YAG laser photocoagulation of ventricular tachycardia without ventriculotomy in patients after myocardial infarction. Circulation 1996; 94:3221–3225.

1317. Guiraudon G, Fontaine G, Frank R, Leandri R, Barra J, Cabrol C. Surgical treatment of ventricular tachycardia guided by ventricular mapping in 23 patients without coronary artery disease. Ann Thorac Surg 1981; 32:439–450.

1318. Fontaine G, Guiraudon G, Frank R, Fillette F, Cabrol C, Grosgogeat Y. Surgical management of ventricular tachycardia unrelated to myocardial ischemia or infarction. Am J Cardiol 1982; 49:397–410.

1319. Guiraudon GM, Klein GJ, Jones D, Kerr CR. Surgical treatment of Wolff-Parkinson-White syndrome. Can J Surg 1983; 26:147–149.

1320. Nimkhedkar K, Hilton CJ, Furniss SS, et al. Surgery for ventricular tachycardia associated with right ventricular dysplasia: disarticulation of right ventricle in 9 of 10 cases. J Am Coll Cardiol 1992; 19:1079–1084.

1321. Harken AH, Horowitz LN, Josephson ME. Surgical correction of recurrent sustained ventricular tachycardia following complete repair of tetralogy of Fallot. J Thorac Cardiovasc Surg 1980; 80:779–781.

1322. Horowitz LN, Vetter VL, Harken AH, Josephson ME. Electrophysiologic characteristics of sustained ventricular tachycardia occurring after repair of tetralogy of Fallot. Am J Cardiol 1980; 46:446–452.

1323. Mantica M, Della Bella P, Arena V. Hypertrophic cardiomyopathy with apical aneurysm: a case of catheter and surgical therapy of sustained monomorphic ventricular tachycardia. Heart 1997; 77:481–483.

1324. Ott DA, Cooley DA, Moak J, Friedman RA, Perry J, Garson A Jr. Computer-guided surgery for tachyarrhythmias in children: current results and expectations. J Am Coll Cardiol 1993; 21:1205–1210.

1325. Gillette PC, Garson A Jr, Hesslein PS, et al. Successful surgical treatment of atrial, junctional, and ventricular tachycardia unassociated with accessory connections in infants and children. Am Heart J 1981; 102:984–991.

1326. Bavaria JE, Miller JM, Josephson ME, Hargrove WC III. Endocardial resection in the treatment of ventricular tachycardia secondary to cardiac trauma. J Cardiovasc Surg 1991; 32:50–52.

1327. Bitar J, Lakier J, Goldstein S. General anesthesia for intractable ventricular tachycardia. Am J Cardiol 1988; 62:1318.

1328. Anderson MH. Risk Assessment of Ventricular Tachyarrhythmias. Armonk, NY: Futura Publishing Company, 1995.

1329. Kastor JA. Michel Mirowski and the automatic implantable defibrillator. Am J Cardiol 1989; 63:977–982.

1330. Kastor JA. Michel Mirowski and the automatic implantable defibrillator. Am J Cardiol 1989; 63:1121–1126.

1331. Lampert S, Lown B, Graboys TB, Podrid PJ, Blatt CM. Determinants of survival in patients with malignant ventricular arrhythmia associated with coronary artery disease. Am J Cardiol 1988; 61:791–797.

1332. Buxton AE, Marchlinski FE, Waxman HL, Flores BT, Cassidy DM, Josephson ME. Prognostic factors in nonsustained ventricular tachycardia. Am J Cardiol 1984; 53:1275–1279.

1333. Roy D, Marchlinski FE, Doherty JU, Buxton AE, Waxman HL, Josephson ME. Electrophysiologic testing of survivors of cardiac arrest. Cardiovasc Clin 1985; 15:171–177.

1334. Kowey PR, Waxman HL, Greenspon A, et al. Value of electrophysiologic testing in patients with previous myocardial infarction and nonsustained ventricular tachycardia. Am J Cardiol 1990; 65:594–598.

1335. Andresen D, Steinbeck G, Bruggemann T, Haberl R, Fink L, Schroder R. Prognosis of patients with sustained ventricular tachycardia and of survivors of cardiac arrest not inducible by programmed stimulation. Am J Cardiol 1992; 70:1250–1254.

1336. Swerdlow CD, Winkle RA, Mason JW. Determinants of survival in patients with ventricular tachyarrhythmias. N Engl J Med 1983; 308:1436–1442.

1337. Willems AR, Tijssen JG, van Capelle FJ, et al. Determinants of prognosis in symptomatic ventricular tachycardia or ventricular fibrillation late after myocardial infarction: the Dutch Ventricular Tachycardia Study Group of the Interuniversity Cardiology Institute of the Netherlands. J Am Coll Cardiol 1990; 16:521–530.

1338. Hamer A, Vohra J, Hunt D, Sloman G. Prediction of sudden death by electrophysiologic studies in high risk patients surviving acute myocardial infarction. Am J Cardiol 1982; 50:223–229.

1339. Richards DA, Cody DV, Denniss AR, Russell PA, Young AA, Uther JB. Ventricular electrical instability: a predictor of death after myocardial infarction. Am J Cardiol 1983; 51:75–80.

1340. Lindsay BD, Osborn JL, Schechtman KB, Kenzora JL, Ambos HD, Cain ME. Prospective detection of vulnerability to sustained ventricular tachycardia in patients awaiting cardiac transplantation. Am J Cardiol 1992; 69:619–624.

1341. Richards DA, Byth K, Ross DL, Uther JB. What is the best predictor of spontaneous ventricular tachycardia and sudden death after myocardial infarction? Circulation 1991; 83:756–763.

1342. Gomes JA, Hariman RI, Kang PS, el-Sherif N, Chowdhry I, Lyons J. Programmed electrical stimulation in patients with high-grade ventricular ectopy: electrophysiologic findings and prognosis for survival. Circulation 1984; 70:43–51.

1343. Wasilewski SJ, Ferrick KJ, Roth JA, Kim SG, Fisher JD. Evaluation of end points of serial drug testing in patients with sustained ventricular tachycardia after healing of acute myocardial infarction. Am J Cardiol 1995; 76:1247–1252.

1344. Freedman RA, Swerdlow CD, Soderholm-Difatte V, Mason JW. Prognostic significance of arrhythmia inducibility or noninducibility at initial electrophysiologic study in survivors of cardiac arrest. Am J Cardiol 1988; 61:578–582.

1345. Podrid PJ, Lown B. Tocainide for refractory symptomatic ventricular arrhythmias. Am J Cardiol 1982; 49:1279–1286.

1346. Vlay SC, Kallman CH, Reid PR. Prognostic assessment of survivors of ventricular tachycardia and ventricular fibrillation with ambulatory monitoring. Am J Cardiol 1984; 54:87–90.

1347. Hariman RJ, Hu D, Gallastegui JL, Beckman KJ, Bauman JL. Long-term follow-up in patients with incessant ventricular tachycardia. Am J Cardiol 1990; 66:831–836.

1348. DiMarco JP, Lerman BB. Role of invasive electrophysiologic studies in the evaluation and treatment of supraventricular tachycardia. Pacing Clin Electrophysiol 1985; 8:132–139.

1349. Hernandez M, Taylor J, Marinchak R, Rials S, Rubin A, Kowey P. Outcome of patients with nonsustained ventricular tachycardia and severely impaired ventricular function who have negative electrophysiologic studies. Am Heart J 1995; 129:492–496.

1350. Bigger JT Jr, Fleiss JL, Kleiger R, Miller JP, Rolnitzky LM, Multicenter Post-Infarction Research Group. The relationships among ventricular arrhythmias, left ventricular dysfunction, and mortality in the 2 years after myocardial infarction. Circulation 1984; 69:250–258.

1351. Kleiman RB, Miller JM, Buxton AE, Josephson ME, Marchlinski FE. Prognosis following sustained ventricular tachycardia occurring early after myocardial infarction. Am J Cardiol 1988; 62:528–533.

1352. Zoni-Berisso M, Molini D, Mela GS, Vecchio C. Value of programmed ventricular stimulation in predicting sudden death and sustained ventricular tachycardia in survivors of acute myocardial infarction. Am J Cardiol 1996; 77:673–680.

1353. Trappe H-J, Brugada P, Talajic M, et al. Prognosis of patients with ventricular tachycardia and ventricular fibrillation: role of the underlying etiology. J Am Coll Cardiol 1988; 12:166–174.

1354. Kowey PR, Taylor JE, Marinchak RA, Rials SJ. Does programmed stimulation really help in the evaluation of patients with nonsustained ventricular tachycardia? Results of a meta-analysis. Am Heart J 1992; 123:481–485.

1355. Mercando AD, Aronow WS, Epstein S, Fishbach M. Signal-averaged electrocardiography and ventricular tachycardia as predictors of mortality after acute myocardial infarction in elderly patients. Am J Cardiol 1995; 76:436–440.

1356. Kron J, Li CK, Murphy E, et al. Prognostic value of programmed electrical stimulation in patients with a recent episode of unstable angina. Am Heart J 1986; 112:1–8.

1357. Holmes J, Kubo SH, Cody RJ, Kligfield P. Arrhythmias in ischemic and nonischemic dilated cardiomyopathy: prediction of mortality by ambulatory electrocardiography. Am J Cardiol 1985; 55:146–151.

1358. Chakko S, De Marchena E, Kessler KM, Myerburg RJ. Ventricular arrhythmias in congestive heart failure. Clin Cardiol 1989; 12:525–530.

1359. Singh SN. Congestive heart failure and arrhythmias: therapeutic modalities. J Cardiovasc Electrophysiol 1997; 8:89–97.

1360. Stevenson WG, Stevenson LW, Weiss J, Tillisch JH. Inducible ventricular arrhythmias and sudden death during vasodilator therapy of severe heart failure. Am Heart J 1988; 116:1447–1454.

1361. Doval HC, Nul DR, Grancelli HO, et al. Nonsustained ventricular tachycardia in severe heart failure: independent marker of increased mortality due to sudden death. Circulation 1996; 94:3198–3203.

1362. Reese DB, Silverman ME, Gold MR, Gottlieb SS. Prognostic importance of the length of ventricular tachycardia in patients with nonischemic congestive heart failure. Am Heart J 1995; 130:489–493.

1363. Galinier M, Balanescu S, Fourcade J, et al. Prognostic value of arrhythmogenic markers in systemic hypertension. Eur Heart J 1997; 18:1484–1491.

1364. Tanabe T, Goto Y. Long-term prognostic assessment of ventricular tachycardia with respect to sudden death in patients with and without overt heart disease. Jpn Circ J 1989; 53:1557–1564.

1365. Tsuji A, Nagashima M, Hasegawa S, et al. Long-term follow-up of idiopathic ventricular arrhythmias in otherwise normal children. Jpn Circ J 1995; 59:654–662.

1366. Hinkle LE Jr, Carver ST, Stevens M. The frequency of asymptomatic disturbances of cardiac rhythm and conduction in middle-aged men. Am J Cardiol 1969; 24:629–650.

1367. Malik M, Odemuyiwa O, Poloniecki J, et al. Late potentials after acute myocardial infarction: performance of different criteria for the prediction of arrhythmic complications. Eur Heart J 1992; 13:599–607.

1368. Kinoshita O, Kamakura S, Ohe T, et al. Frequency analysis of signal-averaged electrocardiogram in patients with right ventricular tachycardia. J Am Coll Cardiol 1992; 20:1230–1237.

1369. Klein GJ, Yee R, Sharma AD. Longitudinal electrophysiologic assessment of asymptomatic patients with the Wolff-Parkinson-White electrocardiographic pattern. N Engl J Med 1989; 320:1229–1233.

1370. Morady F, Sledge C, Shen E, Sung RJ, Gonzales R, Scheinman MM. Electrophysiologic testing in the management of patients with the Wolff-Parkinson-White syndrome and atrial fibrillation. Am J Cardiol 1983; 51:1623–1628.

1371. Morady F, Scheinman MM. Transvenous catheter ablation of a posteroseptal accessory pathway in a patient with the Wolff-Parkinson-White syndrome. N Engl J Med 1984; 310:705–707.

1372. Mitchell LB, Wyse DG, Duff HJ. Electropharmacology of sotalol in patients with Wolff-Parkinson-White syndrome. Circulation 1987; 76:810–818.

1373. Selzer A, Walter RM. Adequacy of preoperative digitalis therapy in controlling ventricular rate in postoperative atrial fibrillation. Circulation 1966; 34:119–122.

1374. Lemery R, Brugada P, Della Bella P, Dugernier T, van den Dool A, Wellens HJJ. Nonischemic ventricular tachycardia: clinical course and long-term follow-up in patients without clinically overt heart disease. Circulation 1989; 79:990–999.

Polymorphic Ventricular Tachycardia, Including Torsades de Pointes, Long QT Syndrome, and Bidirectional Tachycardia[1–42a]

Polymorphic ventricular tachycardia, a tachyarrhythmia with wide QRS complexes having several forms, has, in its time, had many names[43–60] (Table 13.1). For several clinical, electrocardiographic, and electrophysiological reasons, the arrhythmia deserves separate consideration from monomorphic ventricular tachycardia.

---

[a]This chapter includes material from Chapter 16, "Polymorphic Ventricular Tachycardia, Including Torsades de Pointes,"[1] by Dr. Leonard N. Horowitz[2] in the first edition of this book.

Table 13.1	OTHER NAMES FOR POLYMORPHIC VENTRICULAR TACHYCARDIA AND TORSADES DE POINTES[a]

Atypical ventricular tachycardia[5]
Cardiac ballet[55]
Multiform ventricular tachycardia[68]
Paroxysmal ventricular fibrillation[51, 54]
Polymorphous ventricular tachycardia[57–59]
Recurrent ventricular fibrillation[52, 53]
Repetitive paroxysmal tachycardia[45]
Pseudoventricular fibrillation[43]
Transient ventricular fibrillation[44, 46–50]
Transient recurrent ventricular fibrillation[53]
Ventricular fibrilloflutter[56]

---

[a]Although a reference by John Parkinson and Cornelio Papp[45] is often cited, the ventricular arrhythmias they described were examples of repetitive monomorphic ventricular tachycardia; none were polymorphic.

In 1966, F. Dessertenne introduced the phrase "les torsades de pointes" (Fig. 13.1),[30, 61–63b] literally, "the twists (or twistings) of points," to describe a peculiar form of ventricular tachycardia in an 80-year-old woman with syncope and atrioventricular block.[63] It was the tachyarrhythmia that appeared when her heart rate was particularly slow and not the heart block that caused her to faint.[61] Dessertenne described her electrocardiogram as follows:[62]

At the initiation of the arrhythmia, polymorphous systolic activity was observed. This was followed by unidirectional and then bidirectional ventricular tachycardia, a pattern of "bulging" with variations in the bulge amplitude, and finally monomorphic systolic activity.

Most cardiologists,[6, 15, 18, 23, 24, 33, 36, 58, 64–67] although not all,[68–70] now use the phrase only for those patients whose electrocardiograms have long QT intervals dur-

---

[b]"Torsades" is also the term used for a military braid, the twisting appearance of which looks like the tachycardia.[30] Should the nouns in "torsades de pointes" be spelled in the singular or the plural as first used by Dessertenne who, incidentally, did not discuss prolonged QT intervals in his initial report?[6, 61, 62] I have insufficient knowledge and inadequate courage to debate such a point with my French colleagues[25] and refer interested readers to Dr. Guy Fontaine's paragraphs on "The Correct Spelling of Torsade(s) de Pointe(s)" at the end of an article published in 1992.[24]

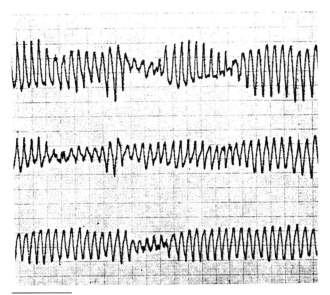

FIGURE 13.1   First illustration of torsades de pointes. An electrocardiogram of torsades de pointes from the 1966 publication in which Dessertenne introduced the phrase. (Adapted from Dessertenne F. La tachycardie ventriculaire a deux foyers opposés variables. Arch Mal Coeur 1966; 59:263–272, with permission.)[61]

ing sinus rhythm in addition to the changing QRS complexes during the arrhythmia.[c] Polymorphic ventricular tachycardia, considered apart from torsades de pointes, can arise in patients with normal as well as long QT intervals.

Torsades de pointes, strictly defined as that form of polymorphic ventricular tachycardia with the appearance first described by Dessertenne in patients with prolonged QT intervals, may be conveniently classified into two types:

- *Pause-dependent,* in which the arrhythmia begins after an asystolic interval resulting from bradycardia or premature beats. The most frequent cause is "proarrhythmia," the ability of antiarrhythmic drugs under some circumstances to produce dangerous ventricular arrhythmias.
- *Adrenergic-dependent,* arising during tachycardia from catecholamine excess produced by physical or emotional stress. The best known examples of adrenergic-dependent torsades de pointes are the relatively few, usually young, patients with the long QT syndrome, an idiopathic disease of genetic origin.

In 1957, Anton Jervell and Fred Lange-Nielsen from Norway first described the features of what came to be called the long QT syndrome in four siblings, three of whom died suddenly (Fig. 13.2):[71, 72d]

---

[c]Much ink has been spilled debating what should, and what should not, be called torsades de pointes.[15, 19, 58, 64, 65] In the most extreme case, one group has argued that "the term torsade de pointes has now become a chimera and should be abandoned."[22] Concerned and neighborly Italian authorities have countered with the warning that such action would upset "every man and woman in France."[33]

[d]Dr. Arthur J. Moss remembers that, in 1957, when he was an intern, Dr. Samuel A. Levine showed him the electrocardiogram of a patient with what would later be called the long QT syndrome just before Jervell and Lange-Nielsen published their cases. Dr. Levine reported his patients a year later.[72]

A combination of deaf-mutism and a peculiar heart disease has been observed in four children in a family of six. The parents were not related, and were, as the other two children, quite healthy and had normal hearing.

The deaf-mute children, who otherwise seemed quite healthy, suffered from "fainting attacks" occurring from the age of 3 to 5 years. By clinical and roentgen examination . . . no signs of heart disease could be discovered. The electrocardiograms, however, revealed a pronounced prolongation of the QT interval in all cases.[71]

In describing the last events in the life of the first case, a boy named Tormod J. who died at the age of 9 years, the foregoing authors wrote:

On Nov. 19, 1953 . . . he had another attack. He suddenly became pale and fell unconscious. On the doctor's arrival the patient was pulseless with cold skin and with marked cyanosis. He was taken to the hospital as soon as possible, but on arrival he presented definite signs of death with marked hypostasis.[71]

Patients with the long QT syndrome and normal hearing were first described by C. Romano and associates[73] from Italy in 1963 and O. Connor Ward from Dublin a year later.[74] Ward's cases were a brother and a sister, each with prolonged QT intervals on their electrocardiograms. "Ventricular fibrillation" was recorded in the girl who died after being given thioridazine for "a phase of marked irritability."[74] Ward was probably the first to connect the sympathetic nervous system to the long QT syndrome:[74]

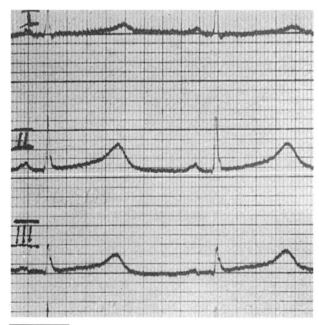

FIGURE 13.2   Electrocardiogram from first report of long QT syndrome. The prolonged QT intervals (0.50 sec) in the electrocardiogram of Tormod J., the first patient described by Jervell and Lange-Neilsen in their 1957 report of patients with "congenital deaf-mutism, functional heart disease with prolongation of the QT interval, and sudden death." (Adapted from Jervell A, Lange-Neilsen F. Congenital deaf-mutism, functional heart disease with prolongation of the QT interval and sudden death. Am Heart J 1957; 54:59–68, with permission.)[71]

Undue sensitivity of the myocardium to sympathetic stimulation is proposed. Excessive sympathetic stimulation may prolong QT interval and may also contribute to ventricular fibrillation . . . . The only evidence of excessive sympathetic tone was the unusual dilatation of the pupils. This was not a constant finding, but the parents come to recognize that the children were particularly at risk when the pupils were dilated.[74]

An international register of patients with the long QT syndrome assists in the study of their characteristics and progress.[75–81]

Bidirectional tachycardia, another form of polymorphic ventricular tachycardia, produces alternation in the direction of the QRS complexes, which are predominantly upward in one beat and downward in the next. It is often caused by digitalis intoxication in patients with severe heart disease.

SOME ADVANCES SINCE THE FIRST EDITION OF THIS BOOK

- Progress in understanding the clinical and molecular genetics of the long QT syndrome.
- Myocardial infarction or residual ischemia suggested when polymorphic ventricular tachycardia develops after coronary artery bypass graft surgery.
- Catecholamine-dependent polymorphic ventricular tachycardia documented in a few children with normal QT intervals and structurally normal hearts.
- Prolonged QT intervals in children with sudden infant death syndrome, suggesting that they may have died from polymorphic ventricular tachycardia.
- Assistance of QT interval dispersion in evaluating patients with possible polymorphic ventricular tachycardia.
- Removal of *d*-sotalol from use because some patients taking it die suddenly, possibly from torsades de pointes produced by the drug.

PREVALENCE

The risk that antiarrhythmic drugs will induce torsades de pointes and polymorphic ventricular tachycardia was estimated by three studies to be 1.5% to 6.6% per year.[82–84] In a fourth study, arrhythmias, including polymorphic ventricular tachycardia, developed in 8.4% of 782 patients with coronary heart disease who were taking a variety of antiarrhythmic drugs.[85e] Five cases (0.4%) of the Jervell–Lange-Nielsen syndrome[71]—torsades de pointes, long QT intervals, and deafness—appeared among 1,336 deaf-mute pupils in two epidemiological studies from Japan.[86]

AGE AND GENDER[87, 88]

Although men and women are similarly affected by acquired polymorphic ventricular tachycardia,[89]

Table 13.2	INCIDENCE OF HISTORICAL DATA, SYMPTOMS, AND FINDINGS IN PATIENTS WITH LONG QT SYNDROME[a]
History, Symptoms, and Findings	**Incidence**
Age	21 ± 15 years
Female	69%
Syncope or resuscitated cardiac arrest as reason for presentation	80%
Congenital deafness	7%
History of ventricular tachyarrhythmia	47%
Resting heart rate less than 60 beats per minute	31%
Corrected QT interval 0.50 second or more	50%

[a]When these patients first present to physicians specializing in the syndrome.[77] In each case, the probands exhibit the symptoms and findings sooner or more often than do their affected or unaffected relatives.[77]

women seem more prone to develop torsades de pointes from cardiovascular drugs than do men.[90f] The mean age of 287 children less than 21 years of age with long QT syndrome was 6.8 years. Patients with the condition may have no symptoms until middle age.[91]

Females predominate among those with the Romano-Ward syndrome—long QT intervals, torsades de pointes, and normal hearing.[86] Although QT intervals are more prolonged in females than males with the Romano-Ward syndrome,[86] males with the syndrome develop syncope earlier than females, usually before the age of 15 years, whereas more than half of females faint from the arrhythmia on or after the age of 15 years[86] (Table 13.2). Thus, in patients with the congenital long QT syndrome, cardiac events occur more often in males until puberty and in females during adult life.[92] A few children with normal QT intervals and structurally normal hearts develop a catecholamine-dependent polymorphic ventricular tachycardia.[93]

GENETICS[39, 94–100]

Most cases of the idiopathic long QT syndrome are inherited. The Jervell–Lange-Nielsen syndrome is transmitted in a recessive pattern,[86, 101–103] and the more frequently encountered Romano-Ward syndrome is transmitted as an autosomal dominant trait[86, 104–108] and occasionally in a recessive mode.[109] The genetic basis for the long QT syndrome, which is heterogeneous,[110g] has been mapped to loci on several chromosomes, and features of the molecular genetics of these patients explain many of their clinical characteristics.[110–134] Most cases of polymorphic ventricular tachycardia and torsades de pointes, however, are not, according to current knowledge, genetically determined. A few patients with bidirectional ventricular tachycardia[135, 136] and monomorphic ventricular tachycardia with normal QT intervals inherit their arrhythmia.[137]

---

[e]Proarrhythmia was defined in this study to include a more than 4-fold increase in ventricular premature beats, a more than 10-fold increase in repetitive forms, and the new occurrence of ventricular tachycardia or ventricular fibrillation.[85]

[f]From a review of 93 articles describing at least one case of torsades de pointes among 332 patients taking amiodarone, disopyramide, procainamide, or quinidine.[90]

[g]Heterogeneity of genetic loci means that two or more genes account for clinically similar or identical diseases in different families.[110]

CLINICAL SETTING

Most cases of polymorphic ventricular tachycardia are produced by drugs given to patients with organic heart disease.[89]

Drugs[138–153] (Table 13.3)[h]

Many drugs, including those prescribed specifically to suppress supraventricular and ventricular arrhythmias, produce monomorphic and polymorphic ventricular tachycardia and ventricular fibrillation. This unwanted property, called "proarrhythmia,"[154, 155] occurs in children[156] as well as adults.

The incidence of proarrhythmia is about 10% of patients given antiarrhythmic drugs.[157] Electrophysiological studies reveal a higher incidence, but this is expected because such patients are studied specifically for arrhythmias.

When the ventricular tachycardia induced is polymorphic, the arrhythmia may often be called torsades de pointes because many of these drugs prolong the QT interval. In North American clinical practice, antiarrhythmic drugs are the most frequent cause of torsades de pointes.[30]

Drug-induced arrhythmias are usually idiosyncratic. Most episodes occur in the first 4 days after the drug is started[89, 158, 159] and when patients are taking usual doses[51] or have subtherapeutic or therapeutic levels in the blood.[51, 84, 89, 160–162] Occasionally, polymorphic ventricular tachycardia can appear for the first time in patients who have taken the offending drug for months.[84, 89, 163]

Factors that increase the likelihood that a drug will induce an arrhythmia:

• Structural heart disease. Proarrhythmia is much more likely to develop in patients with, than in those without, organic heart disease.[57, 83, 89, 156, 164, 165] The more severe the myocardial disease, the more likely is the arrhythmia.[57, 157, 159, 162, 166, 167]
• Adding another drug that can produce arrhythmias.[158, 160, 163, 168, 169]
• Arrhythmia requiring antiarrhythmic treatment. Drug-induced arrhythmias more likely develop in patients receiving treatment for recurrent sustained ventricular tachycardia[157, 166, 167] or ventricular fibrillation[83, 166, 170] than for transient (nonsustained or unsustained) ventricular tachycardia[157, 167] or ventricular premature beats.[83, 157, 170i]
• Digitalis toxicity.[163]

---

[h]This is the section of the book in which I discuss proarrhythmia, the arrhythmias produced by drugs, particularly antiarrhythmic drugs. Although this chapter features polymorphic ventricular tachycardia and torsades de pointes, I include information about drug-induced monomorphic ventricular tachycardia and ventricular fibrillation. See Chapter 8 for information about the drugs that produce ventricular tachyarrhythmias by accelerating conduction in accessory pathways.

[i]According to one study of 1,330 patients taking flecainide, serious nonlethal proarrhythmic events occurred in 6.6% of patients being treated for sustained ventricular tachycardia, in 0.9% of those with transient ventricular tachycardia, and in none with ventricular premature beats.[83]

Table 13.3	**DRUGS THAT PRODUCE ARRHYTHMIAS (PROARRHYTHMIC EFFECT)**

Antiarrhythmic drugs that prolong the QT interval
  Almokalant[183]
  Aprindine[208, 209]
  Amiodarone[89, 90, 158, 179, 181, 184–186, 189–104, 207]
  Disopyramide[13, 89, 90, 158, 159, 168, 177, 210–217]
  Ibutilide[218–220]
  N-Acetyl procainamide[226–230]
  Procainamide[57, 89, 90, 159, 177, 221–225]
  Quinidine[13, 51, 52, 57, 59, 82, 84, 90, 156, 158, 159, 161, 163–165, 174, 177, 178, 180, 192, 222, 224, 231–245]
  Sotalol (d,l)[89, 169, 189, 246, 248–263]
  Sotalol (d)[189, 265]
Antiarrhythmic drugs that do not prolong the QT interval
  Encainide[167, 170, 182, 267]
  Flecainide[83, 182, 268–276]
  Lidocaine[209]
  Mexiletine[277]
  Moricizine[162]
  Propafenone[278]
  Tocainide[279, 280]
Other drugs used to treat cardiovascular disease
  Bepridil[281]
  Digitalis[282–285, 287]
  Indoramin[288]
  Prenylamine[191, 289–292]
  Probucol[293, 294]
  Verapamil[295]
Tranquilizers, tricyclic antidepressant drugs, and antipsychotic drugs
  Amitriptyline[303]
  Doxepin[307]
  Imipramine[302]
  Haloperidol[310–312]
  Maprotilene[306, 308]
  Thioridazine and other phenothiazine drugs[56, 57, 191, 296–301, 304–306, 309]
Antibiotics
  Erythromycin[313, 314]
  Pentamidine[315–318]
  Trimethoprim-sulfamethoxazole[319]
Histamine H₁-receptor antagonists[320]
  Astemizole (Hismanal)[3223–326, 328]
  Terfenadine (Seldane)[321, 322, 327]
Miscellaneous drugs and agents
  Aconites[329]
  Amantadine[330]
  Chloral hydrate[331]
  Chinese herbal remedy[332]
  Indoramin[288]
  Ioxaglate[333]
  Ketanserin[334]
  Terodiline[335]
Poisons
  Arsenic[336, 337]
  Organophosphorous insecticides[338, 339]

• Hypokalemia.[53, 56, 171–174]
• Hypomagnesemia.[54, 89, 175, 176]
• Previous episode of proarrhythmia.[162]
• Substituting a similar drug for the one that produced the arrhythmia, for example, changing quinidine to procainamide.[160]

Factors that do *not* predict who will develop proarrhythmia:

• Age.[157, 162, 167]
• Ambulatory electrocardiographic characteristics.[177]
• Cardiac diagnosis.[157, 162, 167, 177]

- Clinical status.[170]
- Electrocardiographic intervals both before[157] and after[157] the drug is given, including the amount that the drug increases the width of the QRS complexes.[170, 178]
- Gender.[157, 167]
- Level of drug in the blood.[156, 166, 179]
- Location of prior myocardial infarction.[167]
- Presence, absence, or amount of QT interval prolongation.[156, 179-181]
- Severity of heart failure (New York Heart Association functional classification).[167]

Antiarrhythmic drugs that prolong the QT interval. These drugs produce polymorphic ventricular tachycardia, including torsades de pointes, more frequently than any other cause. Most affected patients have organic heart disease that has caused the ventricular arrhythmias for which the antiarrhythmic drugs have been prescribed. However, proarrhythmia can also occur in patients without obvious structural heart disease who require antiarrhythmic drugs for arrhythmias such as supraventricular tachycardia.[182]

Almokalant. This new type III antiarrhythmic drug produces torsades de pointes when it is infused intravenously.[183]

Amiodarone.[184-189] This drug produces torsades de pointes[89, 90, 158, 179, 181, 184-186, 190-204] at all ages, including infancy.[179] However, amiodarone seems to be associated infrequently with proarrhythmia,[205j] less often than are type I agents,[201] and rarely during intravenous[198, 203, 206] or oral[198] loading.[k] However, once torsades de pointes occurs, the affected patient may soon have additional episodes, one of which may be fatal.[202]

Because the drug takes so long to be metabolized and excreted, patients with polymorphic ventricular tachycardia thought to be caused by amiodarone should be observed for up to 2 weeks after the drug is stopped.[179, 196, 207] Amiodarone can be safely given to some patients who develop torsades de pointes from other antiarrhythmic drugs.[89, 181, 201]

Aprindine. This type I antiarrhythmic drug investigated in the 1980s but seldom used now, can produce torsades de pointes.[208, 209]

Disopyramide. This drug, which has electrophysiological properties similar to those of quinidine and procainamide, produces torsades de pointes.[13, 89, 90, 158, 159, 168, 177, 210-217]

Ibutilide.[218] This recently released type III antiarrhythmic drug, for intravenous use primarily to convert atrial fibrillation and atrial flutter of recent onset to sinus rhythm, produces torsades de pointes and, if so, quite soon after it is administered.[219, 220]

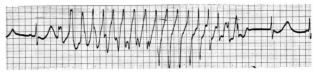

FIGURE 13.3 **Torsades de pointes in a patient taking quinidine.** This is the electrocardiogram of the first patient, a 54-year-old woman, described by Selzer and Wray in their influential article on ``quinidine syncope,'' which was published in 1964, 2 years before Dessertenne introduced the name ``torsades de pointes.'' Selzer and Wray called the arrhythmia ``paroxysmal ventricular fibrillation.'' (Adapted from Selzer A, Wray HW. Quinidine syncope: paroxysmal ventricular fibrillation occurring during treatment of chronic atrial arrhythmias. Circulation 1964; 30:17–26, by permission of the American Heart Association, Inc.)[51]

Procainamide. Because of its widespread use, procainamide is among the most frequently reported causes of drug-induced torsades de pointes.[57, 89, 90, 159, 177, 221-225] N-acetyl procainamide, a metabolite of procainamide that has itself been used as an antiarrhythmic drug, can also produce torsades de pointes.[226-230]

Quinidine.[231-233] This drug is an important cause of polymorphic ventricular tachycardia.[13, 51, 52, 57, 59, 82, 84, 90, 156, 158, 159, 161, 163-165, 174, 177, 178, 180, 192, 222, 224, 231, 232, 234-245l] As the principal antiarrhythmic drug in use at the time (1964), quinidine was the first to be shown to produce what we would now call torsades de pointes[51] (Fig. 13.3).[m]

Torsades de pointes produced by quinidine is usually an idiosyncratic reaction. The amount of drug given is low and seldom in toxic amounts,[51, 84, 166, 178] supratherapeutic blood levels are absent,[84, 222] and most patients who develop the arrhythmia are not suffering from the usual side effects of the drug.[51] Although most cases of torsades de pointes due to quinidine develop soon after starting treatment with the drug,[164] the arrhythmia can also appear for the first time 3 months or more after treatment has begun.[84, 163]

Quinidine rarely induces an arrhythmia when given for treatment of ventricular premature beats to patients whose clinical condition is stable and who do not have digitalis toxicity, hypokalemia, atrial fibrillation, or a prolonged QT interval.[82] However, the QT intervals are often prolonged in patients who develop quinidine-induced arrhythmias before or after taking the drug.[165n]

---

[j]In less than 1% of 2,878 patients, according to a comprehensive review.[205]

[k]Among 205 patients with advanced congestive heart failure, amiodarone induced torsades de pointes in only 4%.[202]

[l]One group has estimated that the risk of quinidine's producing an arrhythmia is 1.5% to 2% per year.[84]

[m]The potential for quinidine to produce ventricular arrhythmias and sudden death has been known since the earliest days of its use. "Quinidine Syncope," the title of an article that brought the problem to particular attention, was published by Arthur Selzer and H. Wesley Wray[51] in 1964, 2 years before Dessertenne's description of torsades de pointes.[61] Selzer and Wray described 36 syncopal episodes due to a ventricular tachyarrhythmia in eight patients taking quinidine for atrial arrhythmias. They called the arrhythmia "paroxysmal ventricular fibrillation."

[n]The corrected QT intervals were prolonged in 17 of 24 patients with torsades de pointes due to quinidine while these patients were not taking the drug.[165]

Sotalol (d,l).[189, 246–248] Sotalol produces torsades de pointes[89, 169, 249–261o] in adults as well as in children[262, 263] and probably more often than amiodarone, its fellow class III antiarrhythmic drug. Sotalol exhibits this tendency even in therapeutic concentrations,[259] in low doses in the presence of hypokalemia, or when given with other drugs that prolong the QT interval.[169] However, the incidence of the arrhythmia may increase when larger doses of sotalol are given.[187, 258] Whether or not sotalol will produce proarrhythmia does not depend on the length of the corrected QT interval before the drug is given.[187]

Sotalol (d). No episodes of torsades de pointes were reported in a study of 233 patients who were given this class III antiarrhythmic drug, which, unlike the racemic agent *d,l*-sotalol, has no beta-adrenergic–blocking properties.[264] However, the higher death rate of patients taking *d*-sotalol, compared with similar patients receiving placebo, who have had recent or remote myocardial infarction and left ventricular dysfunction suggests that the drug may produce fatal torsades de pointes in some such patients.[189, 265] Consequently, *d*-sotalol is no longer available for use.[265, 266p]

Antiarrhythmic drugs that have little effect on the QT interval

Encainide.[267q] This drug appears to be among the most potent producers of polymorphic ventricular tachycardia and consequently is no longer available in the United States. Of 110 patients receiving the drug in one series, 11.8% developed the arrhythmia.[167] Polymorphic ventricular tachycardia leading to cardiac arrest was the most frequent arrhythmia exacerbating the course of 11 of 90 patients receiving encainide for recurrent sustained ventricular tachycardia or ventricular fibrillation.[170]

Encainide-induced arrhythmias occur, according to one series, 17 to 48 hours after starting treatment or increasing chronic oral maintenance doses or 1 to 2 hours after single large doses.[170] The size of the dose, however, does not appear to influence the appearance of proarrhythmia.[170]

Youth does not protect patients. Proarrhythmia developed in 7.5% of young patients receiving encainide for ventricular and supraventricular arrhythmias.[182]

Flecainide.[268] This drug induced proarrhythmic events[83, 182, 268–275] in 6.8% of 1,330 patients receiving the drug as treatment for ventricular arrhythmias.[83] Drug-induced arrhythmias developed in 7.4% of young patients receiving flecainide for ventricular and supraventricular arrhythmias.[182] The drug may have also

produced monomorphic ventricular tachycardia in three patients with atrial fibrillation.[274] Exercise can produce ventricular tachycardia in patients taking flecainide.[271] Investigators, however, find the drug relatively safe in suppressing atrial tachyarrhythmias in patients with normal ventricular function.[276]

Lidocaine. This drug induced torsades de pointes in a patient with prolonged QT intervals.[209] An association between polymorphic ventricular tachycardia and administration of lidocaine, however, has seldom been otherwise reported despite its widespread use.

Mexiletine. This lidocaine-like drug, which can be taken orally, has been reported to produce polymorphic ventricular tachycardia.[277]

Moricizine. Although Moricizine is little used in the United States, it can cause polymorphic ventricular tachycardia.[162]

Propafenone. This type IC antiarrhythmic drug is seldom said to produce proarrhythmia, apparently less often than encainide or flecainide.[278]

Tocainide. This drug can produce polymorphic ventricular tachycardia.[279, 280]

Other drugs used to treat cardiovascular disease

Bepridil. This calcium-channel–blocking drug, which prolongs the QT interval, can produce torsades de pointes.[281]

Digitalis. Digitalis overdosage is a prominent cause of bidirectional ventricular tachycardia.[282–287] The patients who develop this arrhythmia almost always have severe organic heart disease.

Indoramin. This post-synaptic alpha-blocking agent, which has type III antiarrhythmic properties when given in large doses, produced polymorphic ventricular tachycardia.[288]

Prenylamine. This vasodilator, which inhibits uptake of catecholamines and is used in Europe principally for treatment of angina, can prolong the QT interval and produce torsades de pointes.[191, 242, 289–292] The drug produces the arrhythmia more often in women than in men.

Probucol.[293] A preview of the published literature and adverse reactions filed with the United States Food and Drug Administration uncovered 16 patients with tachyarrhythmias associated with this cholesterol-lowering agent, which prolongs the QT interval and is now being investigated and prescribed for its antioxidant properties.[294] Eleven of the patients had torsades de pointes, and each was a woman.[294]

Verapamil. Given intravenously, verapamil produced polymorphic ventricular tachycardia in a young woman with supraventricular tachycardia.[295]

---

*o*In 4.3% of 3,257 patients and 6.5% of those treated for ventricular tachycardia or ventricular fibrillation.[258]

*p*Mostly because of the results of the Survival with Oral *d*-Sotalol (SWORD) study.[265]

*q*Encainide and flecainide and probably moricizine increased mortality in the Cardiac Arrhythmia Suppression Trial (CAST), a study of the effects of three antiarrhythmic drugs that reduce the frequency of ventricular premature beats occurring in patients with previous myocardial infarction.[267] Proarrhythmia is assumed to have been a major reason that these patients died.[533]

Tranquilizers, tricyclic antidepressant drugs, and antipsychotic drugs. Several drugs used in the treatment of psychiatric disturbances can produce polymorphic ventricular tachycardia, including torsades de pointes.[56, 57, 191, 296–312]

Antibiotics. Erythromycin,[313, 314] pentamidine,[315–318] and trimethoprim-sulfamethoxazole[319] can produce polymorphic ventricular tachycardia and, in many cases, may prolong the QT interval.

Histamine H₁-receptor antagonists.[320] Usually prescribed for allergic conditions, these drugs can produce torsades de pointes.[321–328r]

Miscellaneous drugs and agents

Aconites. Present in a Chinese herbal concoction, aconites produced bidirectional tachycardia in a previously healthy woman.[329]

Amantadine. This tricyclic amine, used to treat viral infections and Parkinson disease, produced torsades de pointes in a woman who ingested a large amount in a suicide attempt.[330]

Chloral hydrate. This agent seemed to be the cause of prolonged QT intervals and torsades de pointes in a woman who took a large overdose of about 15 g.[331]

Glycyrrhizic acid. Thought to be the active agent in *chui-feng-su-ho-wan*, a Chinese herbal remedy,[332] this substance prolonged the QT intervals and produced polymorphic ventricular tachycardia in a 69-year-old Cambodian woman.

Ioxaglate. This low-osmolar contrast medium produced torsades de pointes when it was injected into a coronary artery in a patient with prolonged QT intervals.[333]

Indoramin. This alpha-blocking agent has some type III antiarrhythmic properties.[288]

Ketanserin. This competitive antagonist of 5-hydroxytryptamine₂–serotonergic receptors, used to treat hypertension, prolonged the QT interval and produced torsades de pointes in a patient.[334]

Terodiline. This drug, with anticholinergic and calcium-blocking effects used for management of bladder instability, produced torsades de pointes in five patients.[335]

Poisons

Arsenic. Arsenic intoxication can prolong the QT interval and can produce torsades de pointes.[336, 337]

Organophosphorous insecticides. These agents can prolong the QT interval and may produce torsades de pointes in patients who ingest or inhale these substances accidentally or in attempting suicide.[338, 339]

Coronary Heart Disease

Myocardial infarction.[340] Polymorphic ventricular tachycardia, which occasionally complicates acute myocardial infarction,[69, 89, 341–344s] often develops during recurrent myocardial ischemia.[343] The QT intervals in these patients are normal[69, 342–344] or only slightly prolonged,[341] and the appearance of the arrhythmia does not depend on sinus bradycardia, sinus pauses, or electrolyte abnormalities.[343]

Polymorphic ventricular tachycardia, monomorphic ventricular tachycardia, and ventricular fibrillation appear as reperfusion arrhythmias after successful thrombolytic treatment.[344, 345] The arrhythmias seem to occur most often in patients with particularly large elevations of ST segments that resolve soon after reperfusion.[344]

Angina. Occasionally,[t] polymorphic ventricular tachycardia appears during unstable angina.[68] Patients with Prinzmetal's variant angina develop ventricular arrhythmias including polymorphic ventricular tachycardia that has been recorded during episodes of vasospastic angina[346, 347] and during silent myocardial ischemia due to coronary vasospasm.[348] Polymorphic ventricular tachycardia can also be induced in the electrophysiology laboratory more readily in such patients than in healthy persons.[349]

Coronary artery bypass graft surgery. Ventricular tachycardia, both monomorphic and polymorphic, occasionally develops after coronary artery bypass graft surgery.[350, 351u] Transient perioperative abnormalities such as myocardial infarction and residual ischemia should be considered when polymorphic ventricular tachycardia occurs in this setting.[350, 351]

Cardiomyopathy and Myocarditis

Polymorphic ventricular tachycardia has been observed in some patients with idiopathic cardiomyopathy and normal QT intervals in the absence of other inciting factors such as antiarrhythmic drugs.[89] A patient with varicella-induced myocarditis sustained repeated paroxysms of polymorphic ventricular tachycardia.[352]

No Structural Heart Disease—Normal QT Intervals[353–355]

Polymorphic ventricular tachycardia occasionally develops in patients with normal QT intervals, no organic

---

[r]Torsades de pointes developed in a patient on astemizole after taking a single dose of quinine.[328]

[s]Sixteen (0.93%) of 1,725 patients from two series from Israeli hospitals.[341, 344] In one series, the tachycardia was polymorphic in 12.5% of all who developed ventricular tachycardia during the infarction.[341]

[t]But infrequently, judging by the paucity of reports on the subject.

[u]In one series of 21 patients, the ventricular tachycardia that appeared was polymorphic in 16 patients and monomorphic in five.[351] Polymorphic ventricular tachycardia tended to occur sooner after operation than monomorphic tachycardia, and the ejection fraction was higher in those with polymorphic tachycardia.[351]

heart disease, and no drugs known to produce the arrhythmia.[70, 93, 223, 356–358]v Bidirectional tachycardia has been reported in patients without structural heart disease who were taking no cardiac medications.[93, 359, 360]

Other Arrhythmias

Atrioventricular block. Polymorphic ventricular tachycardia and torsades de pointes occasionally develop in patients with atrioventricular block whether due to coronary heart disease or to idiopathic disease of the conduction system.[48, 68, 158, 174, 361–370] Patients with heart block who develop these tachyarrhythmias have more ventricular premature beats than those who do not.[364]

Two-to-one atrioventricular block occurs more often in children with long QT syndrome than in those without the syndrome.[370] Congenital complete atrioventricular block and abnormally prolonged QT intervals can provide the substrate for torsades de pointes.[371–374]

Sick sinus syndrome. The bradycardia of sick sinus syndrome can also give rise to polymorphic ventricular tachycardia and torsades de pointes.[362]

Metabolic Disturbances

Anorexia nervosa. A few patients with anorexia nervosa die suddenly, and prolonged QT intervals and torsades de pointes have been recorded in some of them.[375]

Hyperparathyroidism. This condition has presented as torsades de pointes.[376]

Hypothyroidism. This disorder, which may be associated with prolonged QT intervals, can occasionally provide the substrate for polymorphic ventricular tachycardia, which disappears when the endocrinopathy is treated.[377–379]

Liquid-protein diets.[380] Sudden death has occurred in a few dieters using these very-low-calorie programs. Prolonged QT intervals and ventricular tachycardia including torsades de pointes have been recorded in some of these patients.[381–384]

Periodic paralysis. Bidirectional ventricular tachycardia appears in a few patients with hyperkalemic[385, 386] and hypokalemic[387] periodic paralysis.

Neurological Disease

Acute severe damage of the central nervous system, such as subarachnoid hemorrhage, can be associated with QT interval prolongation and, in some cases, torsades de pointes.[56, 158, 388–395]w

Long QT Syndrome[1, 3, 4, 8, 10, 11, 17, 19, 26–28, 32, 33, 37–39, 355, 396–402]

Torsades de pointes is the characteristic arrhythmia that develops in patients with the idiopathic long QT syndrome (see Table 13.2). Adrenergic stimuli[401] such as excitement,[403, 404] vigorous physical activity,[104, 107] stress,[405] sinus tachycardia,[105] and adrenergic agonists prompt polymorphic ventricular tachycardia in these patients.

The long QT syndrome appears as the genetically determined Jervell–Lange-Nielsen syndrome[72, 101, 103, 406–415]x or the Romano-Ward syndrome.[86, 104–108, 397, 416–424] The long QT syndrome and its associated arrhythmias and symptoms also develop sporadically in a few patients without evidence of inheritance.[424]

In a variant of the long QT syndrome, polymorphic ventricular tachycardia appears when the sinus rate increases despite the patients' having normal QT intervals at rest.[425] In one such patient with no structural heart disease, the QT intervals did not appropriately shorten when the heart rate increased, giving prolonged corrected QT intervals when the arrhythmia started.[425]

Children with the long QT syndrome can also have atrioventricular block.[366, 423] The slow heart rates contribute to the occurrence of torsades de pointes.[366]

No structural heart disease has yet been described in patients with the long QT syndrome.

Miscellaneous Conditions

Auditory stimuli.[426] A 14-year-old girl fainted repeatedly from what we would now call polymorphic ventricular tachycardia on being awakened from sleep by the sound produced by thunder or an alarm clock[403] (Fig. 13.4).

Mitral valve prolapse. This has been the only cardiac diagnosis in a few patients with polymorphic ventricular tachycardia whose QT intervals are normal.[89]

Sudden infant death syndrome.[427–429] The QT intervals of infants with this syndrome are longer than normal children and those who die of other diseases, a finding suggesting that fatal ventricular arrhythmias, including polymorphic ventricular tachycardia, may account for the death of these children.[430]y However, earlier studies demonstrated that the QT intervals of resuscitated infants are not significantly different from

---

vOne group identifies as torsades de pointes the polymorphic ventricular tachycardia recorded from some patients with no structural heart disease and *normal* QT intervals.[70]

wIn one series of 70 patients with subarachnoid hemorrhage and no clinical evidence of heart disease, torsades de pointes was observed by 24-hour Holter recordings in three.[395] Occurrence of the arrhythmia does not correlate with the neurological condition, the site and extent of intracranial blood on computed tomography scan, or the location of the ruptured malformation.[395]

xAlso called the "surdo-cardiac syndrome" ("surdo," from the Latin *surdus,* meaning deaf).

yAccording to the 1-year follow-up of 33,034 infants.[430]

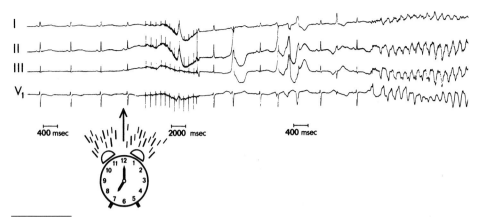

FIGURE 13.4 Auditory stimulus starting torsades de pointes. The electrocardiogram shows that a paroxysm of a multiform ventricular tachyarrhythmia was the cause of recurrent syncope in a 14-year-old girl.[403] The episodes occurred when she was awakened from sleep by a loud noise such as a thunderclap or the ringing of an alarm clock. Her QT intervals were normal at rest, but they became prolonged just before the onset of the tachycardia. The authors called the arrhythmia "ventricular fibrillation" when this well-known case was published in 1972.[a] (Adapted from Wellens HJJ, Vermeulen A, Durrer D. Ventricular fibrillation occurring on arousal from sleep by auditory stimuli. Circulation 1972; 46:661–665, by permission of the American Heart Association, Inc.)[403]

those of similarly aged healthy children,[431] nor are the QT intervals prolonged among most of the first-degree relatives of affected children.[432] A few cases of sudden infant death syndrome have been ascribed to inherited QT interval prolongation.[433, 434]

Epiglottitis. This condition produced cardiac syncope caused by an acquired adrenergic-dependent long QT syndrome and torsades de pointes.[435]

SYMPTOMS

Syncope during childhood or in the teenage years is the symptom that most frequently brings patients with familial idiopathic long QT syndrome to medical attention[77, 113, 370, 436] (see Table 13.2).[z] Sudden physical, emotional, or auditory stimuli often precede syncope resulting from an arrhythmia such as torsades de pointes in these patients.[77] Because seizures may be associated with syncope produced by a ventricular arrhythmia,[370, 437] patients with the long QT syndrome can be misdiagnosed as having idiopathic epilepsy.[77, 356, 417, 418, 437–439] Children who faint from quinidine-induced ventricular arrhythmias more often have structural heart disease than those with the syndrome who do not faint.[156]

---

[a]"I would now consider the arrhythmia polymorphic ventricular tachycardia or torsades de pointes," writes Dr. Hein J. J. Wellens, the senior author.[534] "Now she would be classified as a long-QT syndrome in view of the QT segment behavior. She probably falls in category LQT-2. . . . an abnormality on chromosome 7. The girl died approximately a year after the case report. She had met a boyfriend and he told her to stop all medication because he did not believe in using medication. She was found dead in bed 1 week after she had stopped propranolol."

[z]Of 23 children and young adults, 13 (69%) had syncope and 5 (26%) had aborted sudden death.[436]

ELECTROCARDIOGRAPHY

Rate and Rhythm

The average ventricular rate during polymorphic ventricular tachycardia in 32 patients was 227 beats per minute.[222] The range was 150 to 300 beats per minute in 88 patients.[84, 158, 165, 222]

Careful observation of the electrocardiogram reveals that the rhythm is irregularly irregular, but the rate is so rapid that detecting the irregularity by physical examination is very difficult. The RR intervals may become regular for short periods of time. The rate in most cases of bidirectional ventricular tachycardia is 140 to 180 beats per minute.[440]

P Waves

P waves are seldom seen during polymorphic ventricular tachycardia and torsades de pointes. They are usually buried within the rapid wide QRS complexes.

QRS Complexes

The morphology and axis of the QRS complexes change from beat to beat or within groups of beats. The width of these complexes is abnormally wide, and their duration varies. This appearance led many earlier observers to conclude that the arrhythmia was ventricular fibrillation.

When monitored in a single electrocardiographic lead, the tachycardia may appear to be monomorphic. Longer recordings with several leads reveal its polymorphic character.

Bidirectional tachycardia is a rapid, regular polymorphic ventricular tachycardia in which the morphology of the QRS complexes alternates (Figs. 13.5 and 13.6). The duration of the complexes usually, but not always,[283, 441] exceeds 120 milliseconds, and the form in

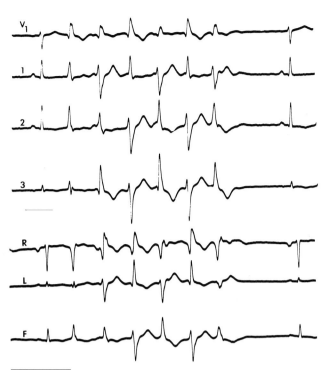

FIGURE 13.5 Bidirectional ventricular tachycardia at a rate of about 130 beats per minute (leads V₁, I, II, III, aVR, aVL, and aVF). A sinus beat starts and ends the sequence. Notice that all the beats of the tachycardia have the appearance of right bundle branch block in lead V₁ and that the axis in the frontal plane of the two types of ventricular beats is −75 degrees and +110 degrees. (Adapted from Kastor JA, Goldreyer BN. Ventricular origin of bidirectional tachycardia: case report of a patient not toxic from digitalis. Circulation 1973; 48:897–903, by permission of the American Heart Association, Inc.)[386]

lead V₁ is that of right bundle branch block.[440] The axis in the frontal plane of the QRS complexes is usually −60 to −80 degrees in one form and +120 degrees in the other.[440]

Onset and Termination of Polymorphic Ventricular Tachycardia[19, 58]

Bradycardia- or pause-dependent torsades de pointes. This arrhythmia, which is usually due to conditions such as atrioventricular block that slow the heart rate or to drugs that prolong the QT interval,[11, 19, 84, 165] characteristically begins after a "long-short" series of RR intervals.[84, 222, 442] This sequence starts with a ventricular premature beat, which is followed by a pause. The last sinus[aa] beat then appears and terminates the pause (the "long" cycle).[84] Soon afterward comes the ventricular beat, which initiates the arrhythmia (the "short" cycle). Although premature, this ventricular beat appears after a relatively long coupling interval[158] on or after the peak of the T wave of the last sinus beat[164, 222] (Figs. 13.7 and 13.8).[bb]

[aa] Or other supraventricular beat (in the case of atrial fibrillation, for example).

[bb] This sequence is also called "short-long-short" by adding the short interval preceding the first ventricular premature beat.[1, 38]

Other electrocardiographic findings when the tachycardias begin in these patients include

- Slowing[158, 443] or, occasionally, speeding[442] of the ventricular rate.
- Abnormalities of the QT intervals of the sinus beats just before the paroxysm begins, such as marked prolongation of the QT interval, corrected QT interval, or QU intervals[84, 158, 222, 443, 444] or striking changes in the morphology of the T waves.[222]
- Widening of the QRS complexes.[158]

Adrenergic-dependent torsades de pointes. This condition, of which the congenital long QT syndrome is a primary example,[445] demonstrates the following electrocardiographic changes:

- Speeding of the heart rate without shortening of the QT interval just before the arrhythmia begins.[17, 19]
- When the tachycardia ends, marked prolongation of the QT interval in the sinus complex.

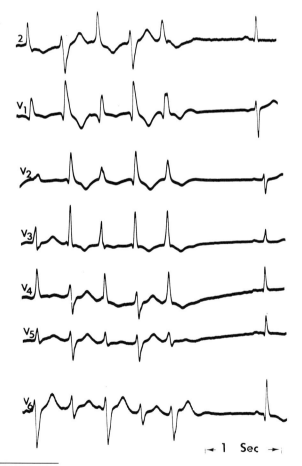

FIGURE 13.6 Bidirectional ventricular tachycardia (lead II and the precordial leads from the same patient as in Fig. 13.5). Notice the characteristic appearance of ventricular tachycardia with the morphology of right bundle branch block suggesting that both types of abnormal beats originate in the left ventricle. (Adapted from Kastor JA, Goldreyer BN. Ventricular origin of bidirectional tachycardia: case report of a patient not toxic from digitalis. Circulation 1973; 48:897–903, by permission of the American Heart Association, Inc.)[386]

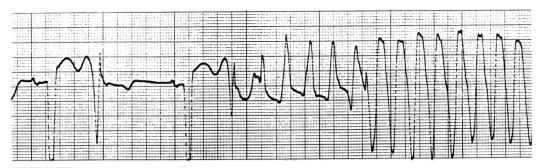

FIGURE 13.7 **Onset of torsades de pointes.** Note the characteristic *short* (beat 1 (sinus) to beat 2 (ventricular))–*long* (beat 2 to beat 3 (sinus))–*short* (beat 3 to beat 4 (ventricular)) sequence that initiates the paroxysm of torsades de pointes. The postextrasystolic pause produced by beat 2 contributes to the particularly abnormal QT interval in the next sinus complex (beat 3). Premature beat 4 occurs after the peak of the abnormal T wave of beat 3 and initiates torsades de pointes. (Adapted from Horowitz LN. Polymorphic ventricular tachycardia, including torsades de points. In Kastor JA (ed). Arrhythmias. Philadelphia: WB Saunders, 1994, pp. 376–394, with permission.)[1]

Polymorphic ventricular tachycardia without QT interval prolongation during sinus rhythm (and, hence, not torsades de pointes). Here are some of its electrocardiographic features:[341, 446]

- The paroxysm usually starts with a premature ventricular beat occurring soon after the last sinus beat. No "long-short" sequence occurs. Early coupling of the first beat of the tachycardia to the last sinus beat characterizes a few patients with polymorphic ventricular tachycardia, no structural heart disease, and normal QT intervals.[70, 356cc]
- R-on-T ventricular premature beats do not necessarily initiate polymorphic ventricular tachycardia associated with encainide.[170]
- The T and U waves during sinus rhythm are not prominent and do not alternate.

[cc]Which the authors called "torsades de pointes" in a few patients without structural heart disease and polymorphic ventricular tachycardia[70] despite the convention that prolonged QT intervals are considered by most to be one of the features of the diagnosis.

- The QT interval following the paroxysm has a normal duration and shortens appropriately with increasing rate.
- There may be associated ST- and T-wave abnormalities suggestive of ischemia.[346]

ELECTROCARDIOGRAM OF PATIENTS WHO DEVELOP POLYMORPHIC VENTRICULAR TACHYCARDIA AND TORSADES DE POINTES (Table 13.4)

Rate

Bradycardia is characteristic of the resting electrocardiograms of patients about to develop bradycardia- or pause-dependent torsades de pointes.[89, 447] The resting heart rate is more likely to be less than 60 beats per minute in the first member of a family with long QT syndrome to come to medical attention than in affected or unaffected relatives.[77]

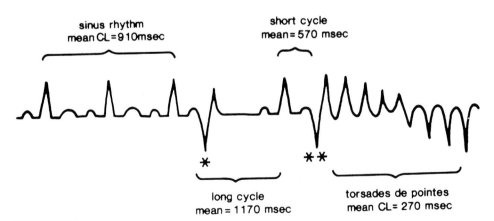

FIGURE 13.8 **Long-short sequence at the onset of pause-dependent torsades de pointes** caused by administration of quinidine (**diagram**). The first ventricular premature beat (*) is followed by a pause that is terminated by a sinus beat, followed by another ventricular beat (**) that initiates the tachyarrhythmia. Those workers who favor the phrase ``short-long-short'' would include the interval preceding the first ventricular beat (*). (Adapted from Bauman JL, Bauernfeind RA, Hoff JV, Strasberg B, Swiryn S, Rosen KM. Torsades de pointes due to quinidine: observations in 31 patients. Am Heart J 1984; 107:425–430, with permission.)[165]

Table 13.4			

Table 13.4 ELECTROCARDIOGRAPHIC CHARACTERISTICS OF PATIENTS WITH POLYMORPHIC VENTRICULAR TACHYCARDIA

Finding	Bradycardia- or Pause-Dependent PMVT (Torsades de Pointes)	Adrenergic-Dependent PMVT (Torsades de Pointes)	PMVT with Normal Repolarization
QT interval	Usually prolonged; when normal at rest, usually does not shorten or lengthen after premature complexes or tachycardias	Usually prolonged; when normal at rest, does not shorten or lengthen after premature complexes or tachycardias	Normal; shortens with increased rates
Abnormal U waves	Prominent	Prominent	No
T-wave abnormalities	Usually only slightly	Marked—biphasic or notched	No characteristic abnormalities
T- and/or U-wave alternans	Frequently	Frequently	No
Short-long-short initiation sequence	Typical	Infrequently	No
Initiation follows "long" or "short" coupled premature complex	Long	Long	Short
QT interval in complex following end of paroxysm	Prolonged	Prolonged	Normal or short

PMVT, polymorphic ventricular tachycardia.
   (Adapted from Horowitz LN: Polymorphic ventricular tachycardia, including torsades de pointes. In Kastor JA [ed]. Arrhythmias. Philadelphia: WB Saunders, 1994, p. 383.)

The resting heart rate of children up to the age of 3 years with the Romano-Ward syndrome is slower than in healthy persons of the same age.[448] Similarly, the heart rate of otherwise normal fetuses with the long QT syndrome appears to be slower than normal.[449]

QT Intervals and T Waves

Pause-dependent torsades de pointes. The QT and corrected QT (QTc) intervals are characteristically prolonged during sinus rhythm in patients who develop bradycardia- or pause-dependent torsades de pointes.[dd] Long QT intervals may be caused by the antiarrhythmic drugs such patients receive, by intrinsic myocardial disease, or both. The QT intervals of some patients taking antiarrhythmic drugs may remain prolonged even after the drug is discontinued.[165]

The QT interval is longer in patients with atrioventricular block who develop polymorphic ventricular tachycardia than in those with block who do not.[364, 450] This feature is clearly a function of the slow ventricular rate because the difference only applies when the paced heart rate is 60 beats per minute or less.[450]

Long QT syndrome (see Table 13.2). Prolonged corrected QT intervals, generally accepted as greater than 0.44 second,[370] are fundamental to the diagnosis of the idiopathic long QT syndrome.[86, 103–105, 107, 108, 407, 416, 451] The abnormal QT intervals take several forms,[27, 118] some of which are associated with specific chromosome abnormalities[118] (Fig. 13.9). One of them, notched T waves, predicts more syncope and cardiac arrest in patients with long QT syndrome.[452]

Among subjects with familial long QT syndrome linked to either chromosome 7q or 11p, the QTc intervals are longer in women and children than in men.[453]

In families affected by the Romano-Ward syndrome, the corrected QT interval is not always diagnostic in identifying patients who carry the abnormal genes for the condition.[113]

Compared with healthy persons, the QT interval in patients with the long QT syndrome is significantly longer during the following:

- Cold pressor test.[454]
- Exercise testing,[454] when one may only detect prolonged QT intervals despite the presence of the other characteristics of the syndrome.[417]
- Minimal and maximal heart rate on 24-hour ambulatory recordings.[454]
- Standard electrocardiogram recordings.[454]
- Valsalva maneuver,[454] which excessively lengthens the corrected QT interval in these patients and may produce T-wave alternans and ventricular arrhythmias.[455]

Propranolol, which suppresses the arrhythmias in patients with the long QT interval syndrome,[456] can shorten[424, 456] the QT interval in patients with long QT syndrome. In those patients, when propranolol has no effect, left cervicothoracic sympathetic ganglionectomy[313] and left stellate ganglion block[424] do not normalize the QT interval.

QT interval dispersion. This is the difference between the shortest and longest QT intervals measured either in the 12 electrocardiographic leads or in the precordial leads alone. Increasing QT interval dispersion while taking type Ia antiarrhythmic drugs, such as disopyramide, procainamide, and quinidine, identifies patients more likely to develop torsades de pointes.[201] Amiodarone, which produces less torsades de pointes, does not increase QT interval dispersion.[201ee]

[dd]The QTc is the QT interval corrected for rate; the QT interval normally shortens as the rate increases.

[ee]A case has been reported of increased QT interval dispersion and torsades de pointes produced by amiodarone in a patient also taking quinidine.[204]

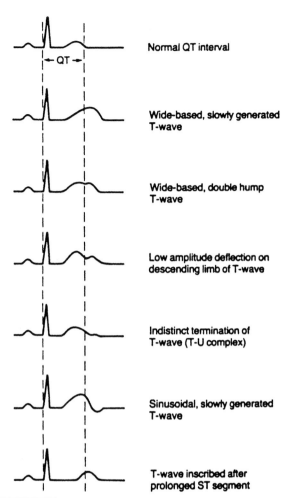

Normal QT interval

Wide-based, slowly generated T-wave

Wide-based, double hump T-wave

Low amplitude deflection on descending limb of T-wave

Indistinct termination of T-wave (T-U complex)

Sinusoidal, slowly generated T-wave

T-wave inscribed after prolonged ST segment

FIGURE 13.9 The different abnormal forms of the QT interval in patients with the long QT syndrome (lead II). (From Moss AJ, Robinson J. Clinical features of the idiopathic long QT syndrome. Circulation 1992; 85:140–144, by permission of the American Heart Association, Inc.)[27]

QT interval dispersion is greater in patients with long QT syndrome than in healthy persons[457–460] and in those with monomorphic ventricular tachycardia.[461] Greater QT interval dispersion characterizes Romano-Ward patients who fail to respond to antiadrenergic treatment.[459] Patients with QT interval dispersion[462] of 55 milliseconds or more[460] identify those most likely to sustain dangerous ventricular arrhythmias.[ff]

Epinephrine, because of its beta-adrenergic properties, but not phenylephrine, the alpha-adrenergic agonist, increases QT interval dispersion in patients with congenital long QT syndrome.[463] Propranolol decreases the dispersion of ventricular repolarization in newborns with long QT syndrome.[464]

T-wave alternans. This condition, in which the form of the T wave varies in an alternating sequence, can be detected in patients with the long QT syndrome,[79,]

180, 313, 423, 436, 465–467gg and emotional or physical stress can prompt the appearance of this finding in these patients.[465] However, T-wave alternans does not predict, apart from its association with prolonged QT intervals, which patients will have cardiac events.[79]

U-waves

About half the patients who develop quinidine-induced torsades de pointes have large U waves following the abnormal QT intervals.[165] However, prominent U waves do not persist, as long QT intervals may, when such patients stop taking quinidine.[165] "Diastolic waves" larger than the preceding T waves (possibly what other observers would call U waves) appear just before ventricular premature beats in patients with quinidine-induced torsades de pointes[180] and seem to predict that torsades de pointes will develop soon thereafter.[180]

Other Findings

Children with long QT syndrome have more 2:1 atrioventricular block and multiform ventricular premature beats than children without the syndrome.[370] Prominent J waves of unknown cause were present during sinus rhythm in a patient with idiopathic recurrent, self-terminating polymorphic ventricular tachycardia.[357] An index of complexity of repolarization developed from 12-lead Holter recordings assists in recognizing patients with long QT syndrome.[129]

OTHER ELECTROCARDIOGRAPHIC STUDIES

Exercise

Exercise shortens the QT interval less than normal in patients with the long QT syndrome[468] and may prolong the interval further.[103, 436] Moreover, shortening of the QT interval in patients with long QT syndrome persists longer after exercise than in healthy persons.[469] The QT interval decreases less during exercising in patients with procainamide- and quinidine-induced polymorphic ventricular tachycardia than in patients without the arrhythmia.[225]

The resting and maximal heart rates achieved during exercise are lower in patients with long QT syndrome than in healthy persons.[468] Similarly, the heart rate on exercise increases less in those with the long QT syndrome than in healthy persons after receiving propranolol.[422]

Ambulatory Monitoring

Holter recordings reveal much useful information about the incidence and characteristics of polymorphic ventricular tachycardia and torsades de pointes.[85, 164, 345, 357, 395, 442, 454]

---

ffAlthough not all have found that the degree of dispersion relates to the severity of symptoms.[458]

ggTwenty-nine (2.5%) of 1,171 patients in the International Long-QT syndrome Registry.[79]

ECHOCARDIOGRAPHY

Echocardiographic measurements show that acquired torsades de pointes and polymorphic ventricular tachycardia more frequently occur in hearts whose ventricular contractile function is low.[159] According to one study, increased number of ventricular arrhythmias produced by antiarrhythmic drugs correlates better with decreased systolic function when measured at the base of the left ventricle than from the global left ventricular ejection fraction.[167] Echocardiograms show that many patients with long QT syndrome have an as yet unexplained abnormal thickening of the left ventricular posterior wall.[470, 471]

PATHOLOGY[472]

The single consistent abnormality in the hearts of eight patients with long QT syndrome, three of whom were born deaf, was focal neuritis and neural degeneration within the sinus node, atrioventricular node, bundle of His, and ventricular myocardium.[473] The hearts of patients with acquired polymorphic ventricular tachycardia and torsades de pointes demonstrate the expected findings from their intrinsic heart disease, if they have any, but nothing with special connection to the arrhythmia. The heart of Tormod J., the index case of Jervell and Lange-Nielsen, showed no specific pathological changes.[71]

ELECTROPHYSIOLOGY[474-479]

Recognition

Polymorphic ventricular tachycardia is recognized during electrophysiological study by the same characteristics observed during monomorphic ventricular tachycardia.[hh] Electrophysiological techniques confirm that most[125, 283, 284, 386, 480–482] (Fig. 13.10), although not all,[483–486] cases of bidirectional tachycardia[487] originate in the ventricles, in some cases near the bundle of His[486] or within the bundle branches or their fascicles.[283ii]

Induction

Bradycardia- or pause-dependent torsades de pointes. Programmed stimulation rarely induces a sustained ventricular arrhythmia in patients whose torsades de pointes is associated with drugs that prolong the QT interval or is due to bradycardias such as atrioventricular block.[488] Programmed stimulation induced torsades de pointes in a patient with spontaneous episodes produced by the tricyclic antidepressant doxepin.[307]

Adrenergic-dependent torsades de pointes. Standard ventricular stimulation techniques can seldom in-

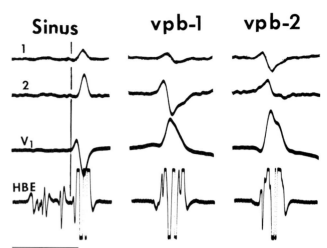

FIGURE 13.10 **Beats from both forms of bidirectional tachycardia** in surface leads I, II, and V$_1$ and a His bundle electrogram. Notice the presence of an H wave (from activation of the bundle of His) preceding the V wave in the sinus beat and its absence before the V waves in the ventricular beats (vpb). This finding establishes the ventricular origin of the tachycardia. (Adapted from Kastor JA, Goldreyer BN. Ventricular origin of bidirectional tachycardia: case report of a patient not toxic from digitalis. Circulation 1973; 48:897–903, by permission of the American Heart Association, Inc.)[386]

duce sustained arrhythmias in patients with long QT syndrome and spontaneous arrhythmias.[488–490]

Polymorphic ventricular tachycardia without QT interval prolongation during sinus rhythm. Polymorphic ventricular tachycardia with electrocardiographic form closely resembling spontaneous episodes can be induced in most patients[140, 446jj] with a history of the arrhythmia and no electrolyte disturbances, antiarrhythmic drug therapy, or ischemia[446] (Fig. 13.11). The induced polymorphic ventricular tachycardia may progress to monomorphic ventricular tachycardia or ventricular fibrillation.[446]

Procainamide and quinidine, in these patients, often convert the arrhythmia to monomorphic reentrant ventricular tachycardia[446] (Fig. 13.12). However, when given to patients without a clinical history of the arrhythmia in whom polymorphic ventricular tachycardia can be induced, procainamide more likely converts to monomorphic ventricular tachycardia those with coronary heart disease, previous myocardial infarction, decreased left ventricular function, and more abnormalities of left ventricular endocardial activation.[66] These findings suggest that polymorphic ventricular tachycardia may be a rapid reentrant ventricular tachycardia closely related to recurrent sustained monomorphic ventricular tachycardia and a precursor to ventricular fibrillation and cardiac arrest.[446]

Ventricular tachycardia of any form is seldom in-

[hh] See the electrophysiology section of Chapter 12.

[ii] Until electrophysiological work settled the issue, a favorite theory for the origin of bidirectional tachycardia postulated that the arrhythmia started in the bundle of His and was conducted to the ventricles by passing in sequence through the anterior or posterior fascicles of the left bundle branch and was blocked in the right bundle branch.[440]

[jj] Nineteen of 21 patients in one series.[446] Among 160 patients with ventricular tachycardia or ventricular fibrillation studied for their responses to antiarrhythmic drugs, proarrhythmic responses were elicited in 16%.[140] In another series of 248 electrophysiological tests, antiarrhythmic drugs aggravated the arrhythmia in 45 (18%) patients.[157]

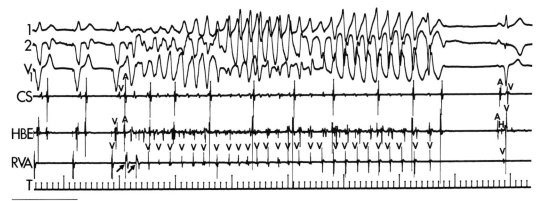

FIGURE 13.11 **Induction of polymorphic ventricular tachycardia** in the electrophysiology laboratory. After the first three paced ventricular beats, two premature ventricular extrastimuli are delivered (*arrows*) that induce a paroxysm of polymorphic ventricular tachycardia that terminates spontaneously. **Top** to **bottom**: Electrocardiographic leads I, II, and V₁, electrograms from the coronary sinus (CS), His bundle (HBE), and right ventricular apex (RVA). (From Horowitz LN. Polymorphic ventricular tachycardia, including torsades de points. In Kastor JA (ed). Arrhythmias. Philadelphia: WB Saunders, 1994, pp. 376–394, with permission.)[1]

duced in patients with spontaneous polymorphic ventricular tachycardia, no structural heart disease, normal QT intervals, and short coupling of the first beat of the tachycardia to the last sinus beat.[70] However, the arrhythmia was induced in a young woman with these findings,[356] and the same arrhythmia could be induced in her mother, who had similar symptoms and electrocardiogram features, except the spontaneous arrhythmia had not been recorded.[356] Polymorphic ventricular tachycardia can be induced more readily in asymptomatic patients with a history of vasospastic angina than in patients without Prinzmetal's angina.[349] Programmed stimulation did not induce a ventricular arrhythmia in any of 10 patients who developed polymorphic ventricular tachycardia after coronary artery bypass graft surgery.[351] Polymorphic ventricular tachycardia of uncertain significance can be induced in some patients who have had no spontaneous episodes.[491]

Ventricular Refractoriness and Repolarization

Ventricular refractoriness, as the characteristic electrocardiographic findings indicate, is prolonged in patients with the long QT syndrome.[489, 492–495kk] Epinephrine[494, 496] and isoproterenol[493] increase and verapamil[494] and propranolol[494] decrease the duration of ventricular refractoriness in patients with long QT syndrome more than in healthy persons. Exercise decreases and epinephrine increases differences in the duration of ventricular repolarization between those with the long QT syndrome and patients with normal QT intervals and no structural heart disease.[495]

The differences in refractoriness measured at separate locations within the left or right ventricles (dispersion of refractoriness) are greater in patients with long QT syndrome than in patients with normal QT intervals.[490, 493–495, 497] Thus, wide dispersion of local refractory periods appears to account for the prolonged electrical recovery of the left ventricle in patients with long QT syndrome.[490]

Left cardiac sympathetic denervation decreases the QT and corrected QT intervals, but they remain ab-

---

kkRefractoriness in the human heart can be measured directly by the use of monophasic action potentials, which are recorded with contact electrodes directly from the atrial or ventricular endocardium.[492, 495, 497]

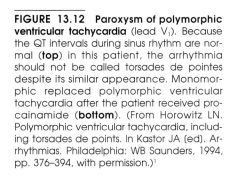

FIGURE 13.12 **Paroxysm of polymorphic ventricular tachycardia** (lead V₁). Because the QT intervals during sinus rhythm are normal (**top**) in this patient, the arrhythmia should not be called torsades de pointes despite its similar appearance. Monomorphic replaced polymorphic ventricular tachycardia after the patient received procainamide (**bottom**). (From Horowitz LN. Polymorphic ventricular tachycardia, including torsades de points. In Kastor JA (ed). Arrhythmias. Philadelphia: WB Saunders, 1994, pp. 376–394, with permission.)[1]

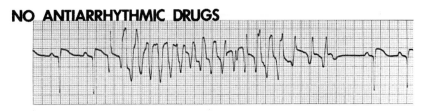

NO ANTIARRHYTHMIC DRUGS

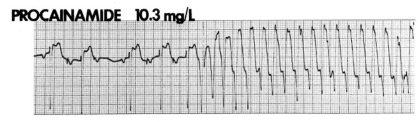

PROCAINAMIDE 10.3 mg/L

normally long.[459, 498] The dispersion of repolarization, however, is significantly reduced.[459] Blocking the left stellate ganglion and stimulating the right stellate ganglion in patients with the long QT syndrome shorten the QT interval.[499] Stimulating on the left and blocking on the right has the opposite effect.[499]

Other Advances

Other studies, beyond the scope of this book to discuss, on patients with long QT syndrome have added to cardiologists' knowledge of the scientific basis of this syndrome.[500]

TREATMENT[99, 355, 501–503] (Table 13.5)

Acute treatment of torsades de pointes and polymorphic ventricular tachycardia is seldom necessary because the arrhythmias are characteristically transient. However, when they persist or endanger the patient, cardioversion will usually produce sinus rhythm, at least temporarily. Temporary pacing is the most reliable method for suppressing recurrent episodes. Isoproterenol and magnesium are also often effective.

When the problem is due to proarrhythmia, stopping the drug that is causing the arrhythmia is essential. Further treatment for torsades de pointes is seldom required, although one may then need to decide how to treat the arrhythmia for which the drug causing torsades was given.

Beta-adrenergic–blocking drugs and/or left cardiac sympathetic denervation are the preferred methods of preventing torsades de pointes, syncope, and sudden death in patients with the inherited long QT syndrome. Occasionally, implantable cardioverter-defibrillators may be needed.

Drugs[504]

Amiodarone.[188] Given intravenously, amiodarone suppresses polymorphic as well as monomorphic ventricular tachycardia.[505] The drug can be administered safely both acutely[255] and on a long-term basis to many patients who develop torsades de pointes when they are taking other antiarrhythmic drugs.[89, 506]

Beta-adrenergic–blocking drugs. These drugs suppress torsades de pointes in many,[313, 419] but not all,[507] patients with the long QT syndrome and in some others with adrenergic-dependent polymorphic ventricular tachycardia and normal QT intervals.[403] Effective treatment with these drugs reduces the incidence of syncope and death.[76] Propranolol is as effective in treating long QT syndrome in children as other beta-adrenergic–blocking drugs.[370, 464, 508] Beta-blocking drugs can also suppress polymorphic ventricular tachycardia produced by antiarrhythmic drugs.[275]

Bretylium tosylate. Although infrequently used today, bretylium controls torsades de pointes in some patients.[238, 438]

Digoxin-specific Fab antibody fragments. These fragments reverse bidirectional tachycardia due to digitalis intoxication.[286]

Isoproterenol. Given by intravenous infusion, isoproterenol temporarily suppresses torsades de pointes in many cases.[57, 196, 446] It works like pacing by increasing the heart rate. The risk of isoproterenol's worsening myocardial ischemia must be considered before using the drug. Isoproterenol, taken orally, provided long-term suppression of torsades de pointes in the few patients with the long QT syndrome in whom its use has been reported.[356]

Lidocaine. Occasionally, but not frequently, lidocaine suppresses polymorphic ventricular tachycardia or acquired torsades de pointes.[56, 57, 89, 344, 446, 509, 510] The drug effectively treats bidirectional ventricular tachycardia.[285]

Table 13.5   TREATMENT OF POLYMORPHIC VENTRICULAR TACHYCARDIA

Treatment	Bradycardia- or Pause-Dependent PMVT (Torsades de Pointes)	Adrenergic-Dependent PMVT (Torsades de Pointes)	PMVT with Normal Repolarization
Eliminate the cause	Drugs or electrolyte abnormalities	—	—
Antiarrhythmic drugs	Only those that do not prolong the QT interval	Only those that do not prolong the QT interval	All drugs including types I and III
Beta-adrenergic–blocking drugs	—	Most effective	Effective if needed for ischemia
Magnesium sulfate	Can be effective	—	—
Isoproterenol to raise heart rate	Yes	—	—
Pacing	Yes	Yes	—
Cardioversion	Only for prolonged episodes or ventricular fibrillation	Only for prolonged episodes or ventricular fibrillation	Only for prolonged episodes or ventricular fibrillation
Implantable cardioverter-defibrillator	In refractory cases	In refractory cases	In refractory cases
Thoracic sympathectomy	—	Effective in many cases	—
Anti-ischemic treatment	—	—	Yes if indicated: avoid treatment that may worsen ischemia

PMVT, polymorphic ventricular tachycardia.
(Adapted from Horowitz LN: Polymorphic ventricular tachycardia, including torsades de pointes. In Kastor JA [ed]. Arrhythmias. Philadelphia: WB Saunders, 1994.

Magnesium.[511] Magnesium suppresses torsades de pointes quite effectively in many cases.[257, 368, 512, 513] Although bolus injections are acutely effective,[513] administering the agent by slow intravenous infusion reduces the incidence of cardiac and extracardiac side effects.[512] Despite suppressing the arrhythmia, magnesium does not usually shorten the QT intervals.[368, 512, 513]

Mexiletine and tocainide. These drugs suppressed polymorphic ventricular tachycardia in some of the few reported cases in which they were given.[509, 510]

Phenytoin. This drug has occasionally been administered successfully to control the ventricular arrhythmias of the long QT syndrome.[405]

Potassium. This substance corrects abnormalities of repolarization duration, T-wave morphology, QT/RR slope, and QT interval dispersion in patients with chromosome 7–linked long QT syndrome.[514] Potassium also normalizes long QT intervals in patients taking quinidine.[515]

Primidone. This anticonvulsant successfully suppressed dangerous ventricular arrhythmias in the members of a family with long QT syndrome.[516]

Quinidine, procainamide, or disopyramide. The most familiar type I agents, they seldom suppress and may aggravate polymorphic ventricular tachycardia when the arrhythmia is due to administration of another type I drug.[89]

Verapamil. This drug terminated three of four acute episodes of polymorphic ventricular tachycardia during myocardial infarction.[341] The drug also abolishes the abnormality of left ventricular wall motion found in patients with long QT syndrome.[473]

Pacing[517]

Temporarily pacing the atria[244] (Fig. 13.13)[ll] or ventricles (Figs. 13.14 and 13.15) is the most reliable method of acutely suppressing acquired or congenital polymorphic ventricular tachycardia and torsades de pointes in patients with prolonged QT intervals.[13, 57, 89, 91, 158, 191, 222, 240, 242, 313, 363, 371, 447, 507, 518] The technique can also be applied permanently.[191, 507, 519] The rate need seldom exceed 110 beats per minute to be effective.[89, 158, 222, 242, 507]

Pacing shortens the prolonged QT intervals, but it does not reduce the corrected QT intervals[242, 507] until the cause, such as a QT interval–prolonging drug, has disappeared.[191] In cases of acquired polymorphic ventricular tachycardia due to proarrhythmia, temporary pacing may be required for up to 10 days until all effects of the drugs have worn off.[191, 196] Temporary overdrive pacing did not suppress polymorphic ventricular tachycardia developing in three patients during myocardial infarction.[341]

Cardioversion

Prolonged paroxysms of polymorphic ventricular tachycardia and torsades de pointes, as well as the monomorphic ventricular tachycardia or ventricular fibrillation into which they may progress, usually re-

---

[ll]Which can be conducted in the esophagus.[244]

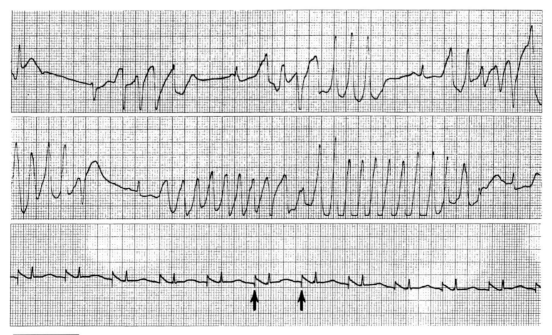

FIGURE 13.13 Atrial pacing at 80 beats per minute (*arrows,* **bottom**) suppressing quinidine-induced, pause-dependent torsades de pointes (**top** and **middle**). (From Horowitz LN. Polymorphic ventricular tachycardia, including torsades de points. In Kastor JA (ed). Arrhythmias. Philadelphia: WB Saunders, 1994, pp. 376–394, with permission.)[1]

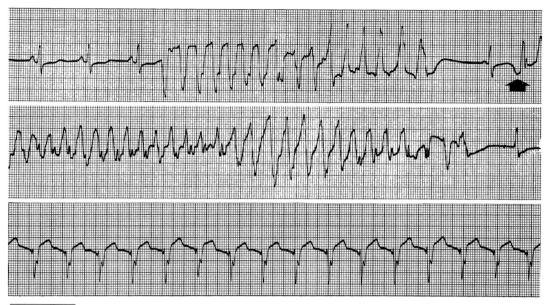

FIGURE 13.14 **Ventricular pacing** at a rate of 100 beats per minute (**bottom**) suppressing procainamide-induced torsades de pointes (**top** and **middle**). Notice the markedly prolonged and abnormally formed QT interval in the sinus complex after the termination of the paroxysm of torsades de pointes (*arrow*, **top**). (From Horowitz LN. Polymorphic ventricular tachycardia, including torsades de points. In Kastor JA (ed). Arrhythmias. Philadelphia: WB Saunders, 1994, pp. 376–394, with permission.)[1]

spond transiently to synchronized electric shock.[57, 222, 341, 344, 446, 510, 520] However, the arrhythmia often recurs because cardioversion does not remove the cause of the problem.

Left Cardiac Sympathetic Denervation[521, 522]

First described in 1971 as left stellate ganglionectomy, this procedure is based on the presumption that the idiopathic long QT syndrome is caused by an imbalance of the autonomic supply to the heart that prolongs repolarization and provides the substrate for torsades de pointes.[523]

Surgically interrupting the output from the left sympathetic system,[370, 498, 507, 524–526] although not universally effective,[414] reduces the incidence of syncope resulting from torsades de pointes and sudden death in patients with long QT syndrome.[76mm] Left stellate ganglion

---

[mm]Temporary block of the left stellate ganglion with lidocaine suppressed torsades de pointes caused by subarachnoid hemorrhage.[390]

blockade can abolish T-wave alternans,[527] but it does not appear to affect cardiac function at rest or during exercise.[528] The procedure can be performed with transthoracic video-assisted endoscopic coagulation.[529]

Implantable Cardioverter-Defibrillators[nn]

When other treatment does not prevent polymorphic ventricular tachycardia or torsades de pointes and the danger of cardiac arrest persists, a cardioverter-defibrillator should be implanted.[354, 370, 530]

PROGNOSIS

The presence of proarrhythmia predicts death from a cardiac event independent of a history of myocardial infarction, ventricular tachycardia, ventricular fibrillation, left ventricular ejection fraction less than 40%, or corrected QT interval longer than 440 milliseconds.[85]

[nn]See Chapter 14 for the discussion about the use of implantable cardioverter-defibrillators.

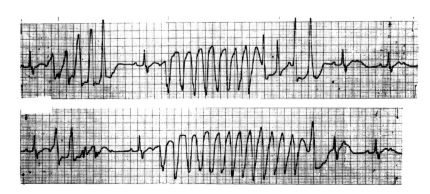

FIGURE 13.15 Bradycardia-dependent torsades de pointes in a patient with second-degree atrioventricular block. Notice the prolonged QT intervals after the sinus beats. The arrhythmia was successfully suppressed with ventricular pacing. Dessertenne's index case was also bradycardia-dependent; his patient had complete atrioventricular block. (Adapted from Keren A, Tzivoni D, Gavish D, et al. Etiology, warning signs and therapy of torsades de pointes: a study of 10 patients. Circulation 1981; 64:1167–1174, by permission of the American Heart Association, Inc.)[158]

Administering amiodarone to patients with congestive heart failure markedly increases the mortality if the patients had previously developed torsades de pointes from taking other antiarrhythmic drugs or amiodarone.[202] Quinidine is associated with a higher mortality, presumably from proarrhythmia, than flecainide, mexiletine, or tocainide.[531][oo] The prognosis does not significantly differ whether the tachycardia induced in the electrophysiological study is polymorphic or monomorphic.[532]

Long QT Syndrome

Syncope recurs in 5.0% per year, and death occurs in 0.9% per year in patients with the long QT syndrome.[77] The risk of these events in affected and unaffected family members is considerably lower.[77] The corrected QT interval, history of a cardiac event, and the heart rate independently contribute to the likelihood of subsequent syncope or death before the age of 50 years.[77] The risk of sudden death in children is particularly high when the QT interval is more than 0.60 second.[370]

SUMMARY

Polymorphic ventricular tachycardia is an uncommon tachyarrhythmia distinguished by the changing morphology of its QRS complexes. Most patients have organic heart disease and are taking drugs, often antiarrhythmic drugs, many of which prolong the QT intervals during sinus rhythm.

The polymorphic ventricular tachycardia that develops in patients with long QT intervals is known as torsades de pointes and also occurs in patients with the long QT syndrome, a genetically determined, uncommon condition. Patients with the Jervell–Lange-Nielsen syndrome, which is transmitted in an autosomal recessive pattern, are deaf in addition to having the long QT syndrome. Those with the Romano-Ward syndrome, which is more frequent, are not deaf and inherit their condition as an autosomal dominant trait.

Polymorphic ventricular tachycardia also develops in patients whose QT intervals are normal during sinus rhythm. Most of these patients have coronary heart disease or cardiomyopathy, but a few have no structural heart disease. The bradycardia produced by atrioventricular block or sick sinus syndrome can give rise to polymorphic ventricular tachycardia. Syncope is the most dramatic symptom that brings patients with polymorphic ventricular tachycardia to medical attention.

The most characteristic feature of polymorphic ventricular tachycardia is the changing form of the QRS complexes. Their morphology and axis change from beat to beat or within groups of beats, their width is abnormally wide, and their duration varies.

A special variety of polymorphic ventricular tachycardia is known as bidirectional tachycardia. In this arrhythmia, which is rapid and regular, the morphology of the abnormally wide QRS complexes alternates. The form in lead V_1 is that of right bundle branch block, and the axes in the frontal plane alternate between left and right.

Abnormally prolonged corrected QT intervals during sinus rhythm are the fundamental feature of the long QT syndrome. The dispersion of the QT intervals is greater than normal in patients with the long QT syndrome and those prone to developing torsades de pointes while they are taking antiarrhythmic drugs. Exercise shortens the QT intervals less than normal in patients with drug-induced torsades de pointes or the long QT syndrome. Echocardiograms confirm the clinical observation that torsades de pointes occurs more often in patients whose left ventricular function is poor.

Polymorphic ventricular tachycardia usually begins in one of two patterns. A ventricular premature beat starts bradycardia- or pause-dependent torsades de pointes after supraventricular beats with particularly long or abnormally formed QT intervals. A pause follows the premature beat before the final supraventricular beat ("long-short" interval) that precedes the first beat of the tachycardia. The QT intervals during sinus rhythm are normal in patients with the second pattern. In them, the arrhythmia begins immediately after a ventricular premature beat that occurs relatively soon after the last supraventricular beat.

Programmed stimulation in the electrophysiology laboratory seldom starts torsades de pointes or another sustained ventricular arrhythmia in patients with long QT intervals, even when these patients have had spontaneous episodes of polymorphic ventricular tachycardia. However, the arrhythmia can be induced, with electrocardiographic form closely resembling spontaneous episodes in most patients with a history of the arrhythmia and no electrolyte disturbances, antiarrhythmic drug therapy, or ischemia. Induced polymorphic ventricular tachycardia may progress to monomorphic ventricular tachycardia or ventricular fibrillation.

Ventricular refractoriness is prolonged in patients with the long QT syndrome, and the dispersion of refractoriness measured at different sites in the ventricles is greater in patients with long QT syndrome than in patients with normal QT intervals. Blocking the left and stimulating the right stellate ganglion in patients with the long QT syndrome shorten the QT interval. Stimulating on the left and blocking on the right have the opposite effect.

Acute treatment of torsades de pointes and polymorphic ventricular tachycardia is seldom necessary. On the occasions when the arrhythmia persists and acutely endangers the patient, cardioversion usually produces sinus rhythm, at least temporarily. Temporary pacing is the most reliable method for suppressing recurrent episodes. Isoproterenol and magnesium are also often effective. When the problem is due to proarrhythmia, the drug causing the arrhythmia must be discontinued.

[oo]According to a meta-analysis of four randomized double-blind studies.[531]

Beta-adrenergic–blocking drugs and left cardiac sympathetic denervation are the preferred methods of preventing torsades de pointes, syncope, and sudden death in patients with the inherited long QT syndrome. Occasionally, implantable cardioverter-defibrillators may be needed.

The likelihood of death from a cardiac event is greater in those with proarrhythmia than in patients without this complication. Syncope recurs in 5.0% per year, and death occurs in 0.9% per year in patients with the long QT syndrome. Children whose QT intervals are greater than 0.60 second have a high risk of sudden death.[370]

REFERENCES

1. Horowitz LN. Polymorphic ventricular tachycardia, including torsades de pointes. In Kastor JA (ed). Arrhythmias. Philadelphia: WB Saunders, 1994, pp. 376–394.
2. Kastor JA. Leonard Norman Horowitz, M.D., 1947–1992. In Kastor JA (ed). Arrhythmias. Philadelphia: WB Saunders, 1994, pp. xi–xii.
3. Jervell A. Surdocardiac and related syndromes in children. Adv Intern Med 1971; 17:425–438.
4. Schwartz PJ, Periti M, Malliani A. The long Q-T syndrome. Am Heart J 1975; 89:378 390.
5. Krikler DM, Curry PV. Torsade de pointes, an atypical ventricular tachycardia. Br Heart J 1976; 38:117–120.
6. Smith WM, Gallagher JJ. "Les torsades de pointes": an unusual ventricular arrhythmia. Ann Intern Med 1980; 93:578–584.
7. Fontaine G, Frank R, Grosgogeat Y. Torsades de pointes: definition and management. Mod Concepts Cardiovasc Dis 1982; 51:103–108.
8. Moss AJ, Schwartz PJ. Delayed repolarization (QT or QTU prolongation) and malignant ventricular arrhythmias. Mod Concepts Cardiovasc Dis 1982; 51:85–90.
9. Soffer J, Dreifus LS, Michelson EL. Polymorphous ventricular tachycardia associated with normal and long Q-T intervals. Am J Cardiol 1982; 49:2021–2029.
10. Schwartz PJ. The idiopathic long Q-T syndrome. Ann Intern Med 1983; 99:561–562.
11. Jackman WM, Clark M, Friday KJ, Aliot EM, Anderson J, Lazzara R. Ventricular tachyarrhythmias in the long QT syndromes. Med Clin North Am 1984; 68:1079–1109.
12. Motte G, Davy JM, Slama M, Laine JF. Specific aspects of ventricular arrhythmias: torsades de pointes, bidirectional tachycardias. In Levy S, Scheinman MM (eds). Cardiac Arrhythmias. From Diagnosis to Therapy. Mount Kisco, NY: Futura Publishing Co., 1984, pp. 371–389.
13. Stern S, Keren A, Tzivoni D. Torsade de pointes: definitions, causative factors, and therapy: experience with sixteen patients. Ann NY Acad Sci 1984; 427:234–240.
14. Surawicz B, Knoebel SB. Long QT: good, bad or indifferent? J Am Coll Cardiol 1984; 4:398–413.
15. Levy S. Torsades de pointes: a clearly defined syndrome or an electrocardiographic curiosity? Int J Cardiol 1985; 7:421–427.
16. Schwartz PJ, Locati E. The idiopathic long QT syndrome: pathogenetic mechanisms and therapy. Eur Heart J 1985; 6:103–114.
17. Schwartz PJ. Idiopathic long QT syndrome: progress and questions. Am Heart J 1985; 109:399–411.
18. Brugada P. "Torsade de pointes." Pacing Clin Electrophysiol 1988; 11:2246–2249.
19. Jackman WM, Friday KJ, Anderson JL, Aliot EM, Clark M, Lazzara R. The long QT syndromes: a critical review, new clinical observations and a unifying hypothesis. Prog Cardiovasc Dis 1988; 31:115–172.
20. Kastor JA. Ventricular tachycardia. Clin Cardiol 1989; 12:586–599.
21. Dessertenne F, Coumel P, Fabiato A. Ventricular fibrillation

and torsades de pointes. Cardiovasc Drugs Ther 1990; 4:1177–1182.
22. Curtis MJ. Torsades de pointes: arrhythmia, syndrome, or chimera? A perspective in the light of the Lambeth conventions. Cardiovasc Drugs Ther 1991; 5:191–200.
23. Cleland JG, Krikler DM. Torsade de pointes: chaos, sixteen years on? Br Heart J 1992; 67:1–3.
24. Fontaine G. A new look at torsades de pointes. Ann NY Acad Sci 1992; 644:157–177.
25. Leenhardt A, Coumel P, Slama R. Torsades de pointes. J Cardiovasc Electrophysiol 1992; 3:281–291.
26. Moss AJ, Robinson JL. Clinical aspects of the idiopathic long QT syndrome. Ann NY Acad Sci 1992; 644:103–111.
27. Moss AJ, Robinson J. Clinical features of the idiopathic long QT syndrome. Circulation 1992; 85:140–144.
28. Schwartz PJ, Bonazzi O, Locati E, Napolitano C, Sala S. Pathogenesis and therapy of the idiopathic long QT syndrome. Ann NY Acad Sci 1992; 644:112–141.
29. Grogin HR, Scheinman M. Evaluation and management of patients with polymorphic ventricular tachycardia. Cardiol Clinics 1993; 11:39–54.
30. Roden DM. Torsade de pointes. Clin Cardiol 1993; 16:683–686.
31. Roden DM. Polymorphic ventricular tachycardia: mechanisms and therapeutic implications. In Josephson ME, Wellens HJJ (eds). Tachycardias. Mechanisms and Management. Mount Kisco, NY: Futura Publishing Co., 1993, pp. 273–282.
32. Schwartz PJ, Moss AJ, Vincent GM, Crampton RS. Diagnostic criteria for the long QT syndrome: an update. Circulation 1993; 88:782–784.
33. Priori SG, Diehl L, Schwartz PJ. Torsade de pointes. In Podrid PJ, Kowey PR (eds). Cardiac Arrhythmia. Mechanisms, Diagnosis and Management. Baltimore: Williams & Wilkins, 1995, pp. 951–963.
34. el-Sherif N. Polymorphic ventricular tachycardia. In Podrid PJ, Kowey PR (eds). Cardiac Arrhythmia. Mechanisms, Diagnosis and Management. Baltimore: Williams & Wilkins, 1995, pp. 936–950.
35. Grimm W, Marchlinski FE. Accelerated idioventricular rhythm, bidirectional ventricular tachycardia. In Zipes DP, Jalife J (eds). Cardiac Electrophysiology. From Cell to Bedside. 2nd ed. Philadelphia: WB Saunders, 1995, pp. 920–926.
36. Haverkamp W, Shenasa M, Borggrefe M, Breithardt G. Torsades de pointes. In Zipes DP, Jalife J (eds). Cardiac Electrophysiology. From Cell to Bedside. 2nd ed. Philadelphia: WB Saunders, 1995, pp. 885–899.
37. Moss AJ. Long QT syndrome. In Podrid PJ, Kowey PR (eds). Cardiac Arrhythmia. Mechanisms, Diagnosis and Management. Baltimore: Williams & Wilkins, 1995: 1110–1120.
38. Schwartz PJ, Locati EH, Napolitano C, Priori SG. The long QT syndrome. In Zipes DP, Jalife J (eds). Cardiac Electrophysiology. From Cell to Bedside. 2nd ed. Philadelphia: WB Saunders, 1995, pp. 788–811.
39. Roden DM, Lazzara R, Rosen M, Schwartz PJ, Towbin J, Vincent GM. Multiple mechanisms in the long-QT syndrome: Current knowledge, gaps, and future directions. The SADS foundation task force on LQTS. Circulation 1996; 94:1996–2012.
40. Lazzara R. Twisting of the points. J Am Coll Cardiol 1997; 29:843–845.
41. Moss AJ. The long QT syndrome revisited: current understanding and implications for treatment. PACE 1997; 20:2879–2881.
42. Roden DM. Taking the "idio" out of "idiosyncratic": predicting torsades de pointes. PACE 1998; 21:1029–1034.
43. MacWilliam JA. Some applications of physiology to medicine. II. Ventricular fibrillation and sudden death. BMJ 1923; 2:215–219.
44. Schwartz SP. Transient ventricular fibrillation: a study of the fibrillatory process in man. J Mt Sinai Hosp 1942; 8:1005–1014.
45. Parkinson J, Papp C. Repetitive paroxysmal tachycardia. Br Heart J 1947; 9:241–262.

46. Schwartz SP, Orloff J, Fox C. Transient ventricular fibrillation. I. The prefibrillary period during established auriculo-ventricular dissociation with a note on the phonocardiograms obtained at such times. Am Heart J 1949; 37:21–35.

47. Schwartz SP, De Sola Pool N. Transient ventricular fibrillation. III. The effects of bodily rest, atropine sulfate, and exercise on patients with transient ventricular fibrillation during established atrioventricular dissociation: a study of the influence of the extrinsic nerves on the idioventricular pacemaker of the heart. Am Heart J 1950; 39:361–386.

48. Schwartz SP, Hallinger L, Imperialli A. Transient ventricular fibrillation. IV. The effects of procainamide on patients with transient ventricular fibrillation during established auriculo-ventricular dissociation. Circulation 1952; 6:193–200.

49. Schwartz SP, Margolies MP, Firenze A. Transient ventricular fibrillation. V. The effects of the oral administration of quinidine sulfate on patients with transient ventricular fibrillation during established atrioventricular dissociation. Am Heart J 1953; 45:404–415.

50. Schwartz SP, Hallinger LN. Transient ventricular fibrillation. VI. Observations on the peripheral arterial pulse pressures in the course of transient ventricular fibrillation during established auriculoventricular dissociation. Am Heart J 1954; 48:390–404.

51. Selzer A, Wray HW. Quinidine syncope-paroxysmal ventricular fibrillation occurring during treatment of chronic atrial arrhythmias. Circulation 1964; 30:17–26.

52. Oravetz J, Slodki SJ. Recurrent ventricular fibrillation precipitated by quinidine: report of a patient with recovery after 28 paroxysms. Arch Intern Med 1968; 122:63–65.

53. Tamura K, Tamura T, Yoshida S, Inui M, Fukuhara N. Transient recurrent ventricular fibrillation due to hypopotassemia with a special note on the U wave. Jpn Heart J 1967; 8:652–660.

54. Loeb HS, Pietras RJ, Gunnar RM, Tobin JR Jr. Paroxysmal ventricular fibrillation in two patients with hypomagnesemia: treatment by transvenous pacing. Circulation 1968; 37:210–215.

55. Smirk FH, Ng J. Cardiac ballet: repetitions of complex electrocardiographic patterns. Br Heart J 1969; 31:426–434.

56. Ranquin R, Parizel G. Ventricular fibrillo-flutter ("torsade de pointe"): an established electrocardiographic and clinical entity. Angiology 1977; 28:115–118.

57. Sclarovsky S, Strasberg B, Lewin RF, Agmon J. Polymorphous ventricular tachycardia: clinical features and treatment. Am J Cardiol 1979; 44:339–344.

58. Tzivoni D, Keren A, Stern S. Torsades de pointes versus polymorphous ventricular tachycardia. Am J Cardiol 1983; 52:639–640.

59. Della Bella P, Tondo C, Marenzi G, Grazi S. Polymorphous ventricular tachycardia as undesirable effect of the association of quinidine treatment with hysteresis ventricular inhibited pacing. Eur Heart J 1990; 11:1124–1126.

60. Clayton RH, Murray A, Higham PD, Campbell RW. Self-terminating ventricular tachyarrhythmias: a diagnostic dilemma? Lancet 1993; 341:93–95.

61. Dessertenne F. La tachycardie ventriculaire a deux foyers opposés variables. Arch Mal Coeur 1966; 59:263–272.

62. Dessertenne F. Ventricular tachycardia with two variable foci. Cardiovasc Drugs Ther 1990; 4:1171–1176.

63. Fabiato A, Coumel P. Torsades de pointes, a quarter of a century later: a tribute to Dr. F. Dessertenne. Cardiovasc Drugs Ther 1991; 5:167–169.

64. Kossmann CE. Torsade de pointes: an addition to the nosography of ventricular tachycardia. Am J Cardiol 1978; 42:1054–1056.

65. Horowitz LN. Torsades de pointes: twisting of the points or confusion of the points? Int J Cardiol 1985; 7:427–430.

66. Buxton AE, Josephson ME, Marchlinski FE, Miller JM. Polymorphic ventricular tachycardia induced by programmed stimulation: response to procainamide. J Am Coll Cardiol 1993; 21:90–98.

67. el-Sherif N. Clinical significance of polymorphic ventricular tachycardia induced by programmed stimulation. J Am Coll Cardiol 1993; 21:99–101.

68. Zilcher H, Glogar D, Kaindl F. Torsades de pointes: occurrence in myocardial ischaemia as a separate entity: multiform ventricular tachycardia or not? Eur Heart J 1980; 1:63–71.

69. Bashour TT, Lehrman K, Edgett J. Torsade de pointes: a maximal vulnerability arrhythmia. Am Heart J 1985; 109:167–169.

70. Leenhardt A, Glaser E, Burguera M, Nurnberg M, Maison-Blanche P, Coumel P. Short-coupled variant of torsade de pointes: a new electrocardiographic entity in the spectrum of idiopathic ventricular tachyarrhythmias. Circulation 1994; 89:206–215.

71. Jervell A, Lange-Nielson F. Congenital deaf-mutism, functional heart disease with prolongation of the QT interval and sudden death. Am Heart J 1957; 54:59–68.

72. Levine SA, Woodworth CR. Congenital deaf-mutism, prolonged QT interval, syncopal attacks and sudden death. N Engl J Med 1958; 259:412–417.

73. Romano C, Gemme G, Pongiglione R. Aritmie cardiache rare in etá pediatrica. Clin Pediatr 1963; 45:656–683.

74. Ward OC. New familial cardiac syndrome in children. J Irish Med Assoc 1964; 54:103–106.

75. Schwartz PJ. The idiopathic long QT syndrome: the need for a prospective registry. Eur Heart J 1983; 4:529–531.

76. Moss AJ, Schwartz PJ, Crampton RS, Locati E, Carleen E. The long QT syndrome: a prospective international study. Circulation 1985; 71:17–21.

77. Moss AJ, Schwartz PJ, Crampton RS, et al. The long QT syndrome: prospective longitudinal study of 328 families. Circulation 1991; 84:1136–1144.

78. Moss AJ. Measurement of the QT interval and the risk associated with QTc interval prolongation: a review. Am J Cardiol 1993; 72:23B–25B.

79. Zareba W, Moss AJ, le Cessie S, Hall WJ. T wave alternans in idiopathic long QT syndrome. J Am Coll Cardiol 1994; 23:1541–1546.

80. Zareba W, Moss AJ, le Cessie S, et al. Risk of cardiac events in family members of patients with long QT syndrome. J Am Coll Cardiol 1995; 26:1685–1691.

81. Zareba W, Moss AJ. Dispersion of repolarization: relation to heart rate and repolarization duration. J Electrocardiol 1995; 28:202–206.

82. Morganroth J, Horowitz LN. Incidence of proarrhythmic effects from quinidine in the outpatient treatment of benign or potentially lethal ventricular arrhythmias. Am J Cardiol 1985; 56:585–587.

83. Morganroth J, Anderson JL, Gentzkow GD. Classification by type of ventricular arrhythmia predicts frequency of adverse cardiac events from flecainide. J Am Coll Cardiol 1986; 8:607–615.

84. Roden DM, Woosley RL, Primm RK. Incidence and clinical features of the quinidine-associated long QT syndrome: implications for patient care. Am Heart J 1986; 111:1088–1093.

85. Trusz-Gluza M, Giec L, Dabrowski A, et al. Proarrhythmic response to antiarrhythmic drug as a risk factor for sudden cardiac death in patients with ischemic heart disease. Pacing Clin Electrophysiol 1991; 14:1947–1950.

86. Hashiba K. Hereditary QT prolongation syndrome in Japan: genetic analysis and pathological findings of the conducting system. Jpn Circ J 1978; 42:1133–1150.

87. Larsen JA, Kadish AH. Effects of gender on cardiac arrhythmias. J Cardiovasc Electrophysiol 1998; 9:655–664.

88. Rubart M, von der Lohe E. Sex steroids and cardiac arrhythmias: more questions than answers. J Cardiovasc Electrophysiol 1998; 9:665–667.

89. Nguyen PT, Scheinman MM, Seger J. Polymorphous ventricular tachycardia: clinical characterization, therapy, and the QT interval. Circulation 1986; 74:340–349.

90. Makkar RR, Fromm BS, Steinman RT, Meissner MD, Lehmann MH. Female gender as a risk factor for torsades de pointes associated with cardiovascular drugs. JAMA 1993; 270:2590–2597.

91. Schneider RR, Bahler A, Pincus J, Stimmel B. Asymptomatic idiopathic syndrome of prolonged Q-T interval in a 45-year-

old woman: ventricular tachyarrhythmias precipitated by hypokalemia and therapy with amitriptyline and perphenazine. Chest 1977; 71:210–213.

92. Locati EH, Zareba W, Moss AJ, et al. Age- and sex-related differences in clinical manifestations in patients with congenital long-QT syndrome: findings from the International LQTS Registry. Circulation 1998; 97:2237–2244.

93. Leenhardt A, Lucet V, Denjoy I, Grau F, Ngoc DD, Coumel P. Catecholaminergic polymorphic ventricular tachycardia in children: a 7-year follow-up of 21 patients. Circulation 1995; 91:1512–1519.

94. Keating M. Linkage analysis and long QT syndrome: using genetics to study cardiovascular disease. Circulation 1992; 85:1973–1986.

95. Moss AJ. Molecular genetics and ventricular arrhythmias. N Engl J Med 1992; 327:885–887.

96. Eggeling T, Hoher M, Osterhues HH, Kochs M, Weismuller P, Hombach V. The arrhythmogenic substrate of the long QT syndrome: genetic basis, pathology, and pathophysiologic mechanisms. Eur Heart J 1993; 14:73–79.

97. Ackerman MJ, Clapham DE. Ion channels: basic science and clinical disease. N Engl J Med 1997; 336:1575–1586.

98. Priori SG. Is long QT syndrome entering the era of molecular diagnosis? Heart 1997; 77:5–6.

99. Priori SG, Napolitano C, Paganini V, Cantu F, Schwartz PJ. Molecular biology of the long QT syndrome: impact on management. Pacing Clin Electrophysiol 1997; 20:2052–2057.

100. Wilde AA, Veldkamp MW. Ion channels, the QT interval, and arrhythmias. Pacing Clin Electrophysiol 1997; 20:2048–2051.

101. Fraser GR, Froggatt P, Murphy T. Genetical aspects of the cardio-auditory syndrome of Jervell and Lange-Nielsen (congenital deafness and electrocardiographic abnormalities). Ann Hum Genet 1964; 28:133–157.

102. Fraser GR, Froggatt P, James TN. Congenital deafness associated with electrocardiographic abnormalities, fainting attacks and sudden death. Q J Med 1964; 33:361–385.

103. Jervell A, Thingstad R, Endsjo TO. The surdo-cardiac syndrome: three new cases of congenital deafness with syncopal attacks and Q-T prolongation in the electrocardiogram. Am Heart J 1966; 72:582–593.

104. Gale GE, Bosman CK, Tucker RB, Barlow JB. Hereditary prolongation of QT interval: study of two families. Br Heart J 1970; 32:505–509.

105. Garza LA, Vick RL, Nora JJ, McNamara DG. Heritable Q-T prolongation without deafness. Circulation 1970; 41:39–48.

106. Hanazono N, Ando Y, Onishi M, Oda H, Yuhara N. Heritable Q-T prolongation without deafness: the Romano-Ward syndrome. Jpn Heart J 1973; 14:479–493.

107. Chaudron JM, Heller F, Van den Berghe HB, LeBacq EG. Attacks of ventricular fibrillation and unconsciousness in a patient with prolonged QT interval: a family study. Am Heart J 1976; 91:783–791.

108. Roy PR, Emanuel R, Ismail SA, El Tayib MH. Hereditary prolongation of the Q-T interval: genetic observations and management in three families with twelve affected members. Am J Cardiol 1976; 37:237–243.

109. Priori SG, Schwartz PJ, Napolitano C, et al. A recessive variant of the Romano-Ward long-QT syndrome? Circulation 1998; 97:2420–2425.

110. Towbin JA, Li H, Taggart RT, et al. Evidence of genetic heterogeneity in Romano-Ward long QT syndrome: analysis of 23 families. Circulation 1994; 90:2635–2644.

111. Keating M, Atkinson D, Dunn C, Timothy K, Vincent GM, Leppert M. Linkage of a cardiac arrhythmia, the long QT syndrome, and the Harvey ras-1 gene. Science 1991; 252:704–706.

112. Keating M, Dunn C, Atkinson D, Timothy K, Vincent GM, Leppert M. Consistent linkage of the long-QT syndrome to the Harvey ras-1 locus on chromosome 11. Am J Hum Genet 1991; 49:1335–1339.

113. Vincent GM, Timothy KW, Leppert M, Keating M. The spectrum of symptoms and QT intervals in carriers of the gene for the long-QT syndrome. N Engl J Med 1992; 327:846–852.

114. Curran M, Atkinson D, Timothy K, et al. Locus heterogeneity

of autosomal dominant long QT syndrome. J Clin Invest 1993; 92:799–803.

115. Jiang C, Atkinson D, Towbin JA, et al. Two long QT syndrome loci map to chromosomes 3 and 7 with evidence for further heterogeneity. Nat Genet 1994; 8:141–147.

116. Bennett PB, Yazawa K, Makita N, George AL Jr. Molecular mechanism for an inherited cardiac arrhythmia. Nature 1995; 376:683–685.

117. Curran ME, Splawski I, Timothy KW, Vincent GM, Green ED, Keating MT. A molecular basis for cardiac arrhythmia: herg mutations cause long QT syndrome. Cell 1995; 80:795–803.

118. Moss AJ, Zareba W, Benhorin J, et al. ECG T-wave patterns in genetically distinct forms of the hereditary long QT syndrome. Circulation 1995; 92:2929–2934.

119. Sanguinetti MC, Jiang C, Curran ME, Keating MT. A mechanistic link between an inherited and an acquired cardiac arrhythmia: herg encodes the IKR potassium channel. Cell 1995; 81:299–307.

120. Schott JJ, Charpentier F, Peltier S, et al. Mapping of a gene for long QT syndrome to chromosome 4q25-27. Am J Hum Genet 1995; 57:1114–1122.

121. Wang Q, Shen J, Splawski I, et al. Scn5a mutations associated with an inherited cardiac arrhythmia, long QT syndrome. Cell 1995; 80:805–811.

122. Schwartz PJ, Priori SG, Locati EH, et al. Long QT syndrome patients with mutations of the scn5a and herg genes have differential responses to Na⁺ channel blockade and to increases in heart rate: implications for gene-specific therapy. Circulation 1995; 92:3381–3386.

123. Wang Q, Shen J, Li Z, et al. Cardiac sodium channel mutations in patients with long QT syndrome, an inherited cardiac arrhythmia. Hum Mol Genet 1995; 4:1603–1607.

124. Dumaine R, Wang Q, Keating MT, et al. Multiple mechanisms of Na⁺ channel–linked long-QT syndrome. Circ Res 1996; 78:916–924.

125. Tesson F, Donger C, Denjoy I, et al. Exclusion of kcne 1 (isk) as a candidate gene for Jervell and Lange-Nielsen syndrome. J Mol Cell Cardiol 1996; 28:2051–2055.

126. Wang Q, Curran ME, Splawski I, et al. Positional cloning of a novel potassium channel gene: kvlqt1 mutations cause cardiac arrhythmias. Nat Genet 1996; 12:17–23.

127. Donger C, Denjoy I, Berthet M, et al. KVLQT1 C-terminal missense mutation causes a forme fruste long-QT syndrome. Circulation 1997; 96:2778–2781.

128. Neyroud N, Tesson F, Denjoy I, et al. A novel mutation in the potassium channel gene kvlqt1 causes the Jervell and Lange-Nielsen cardioauditory syndrome. Nat Genet 1997; 15:186–189.

129. Priori SG, Mortara DW, Napolitano C, et al. Evaluation of the spatial aspects of T-wave complexity in the long-QT syndrome. Circulation 1997; 96:3006–3012.

130. Splawski I, Timothy KW, Vincent GM, Atkinson DL, Keating MT. Molecular basis of the long-QT syndrome associated with deafness. N Engl J Med 1997; 336:1562–1567.

131. Splawski I, Timothy KW, Vincent GM, Atkinson DL, Keating MT. Molecular basis of the long-QT syndrome associated with deafness. Proc Assoc Am Physicians 1997; 109:504–511.

132. Duggal P, Vesely MR, Wattanasirichaigoon D, Villafane J, Kaushik V, Beggs AH. Mutation of the gene for IsK associated with both Jervell and Lange-Nielsen and Romano-Ward forms of long-QT syndrome. Circulation 1998; 97:142–146.

133. Kanters JK, Larsen LA, Orholm M, et al. Novel donor splice site mutation in the KVLQT1 gene is associated with long QT syndrome. J Cardiovasc Electrophysiol 1998; 9:620–624.

134. Li H, Chen Q, Moss AJ, et al. New mutations in the KVLQT1 potassium channel that cause long-QT syndrome. Circulation 1998; 97:1264–1269.

135. Gault JH, Cantwell J, Lev M, Braunwald E. Fatal familial cardiac arrhythmias: histologic observations on the cardiac conduction system. Am J Cardiol 1972; 29:548–553.

136. Cohen TJ, Liem LB, Hancock EW. Association of bidirectional ventricular tachycardia with familial sudden death syndrome. Am J Cardiol 1989; 64:1078–1079.

137. Sacks HS, Matisson R, Kennelly BM. Familial paroxysmal ventricular tachycardia in two sisters. Am Heart J 1974; 87:217–222.

138. Bigger JT Jr, Sahar DI. Clinical types of proarrhythmic response to antiarrhythmic drugs. Am J Cardiol 1987; 59:2E–9E.

139. Cowan JC, Bourke J, Campbell RW. Arrhythmogenic effects of antiarrhythmic drugs. Eur Heart J 1987; 8:133–136.

140. Horowitz LN, Zipes DP, Bigger JT Jr, et al. Proarrhythmia, arrhythmogenesis or aggravation of arrhythmia: a status report, 1987. Am J Cardiol 1987; 59:54E–56E.

141. Stratmann HG, Kennedy HL. Torsades de pointes associated with drugs and toxins: recognition and management. Am Heart J 1987; 113:1470–1482.

142. Zipes DP. Proarrhythmic effects of antiarrhythmic drugs. Am J Cardiol 1987; 59:26E–31E.

143. Levine JH, Morganroth J, Kadish AH. Mechanisms and risk factors for proarrhythmia with type Ia compared with Ic antiarrhythmic drug therapy. Circulation 1989; 80:1063–1069.

144. Podrid PJ. Aggravation of arrhythmia: a complication of antiarrhythmic drug therapy. Eur Heart J 1989; 10:66–72.

145. Singh BN. When is QT prolongation antiarrhythmic and when is it proarrhythmic? Am J Cardiol 1989; 63:867–869.

146. Fauchier JP, Cosnay P, Babuty RD. Drug-induced atrial arrhythmias. In Touboul P, Waldo AL (eds). Atrial Arrhythmias. Current Concepts and Management. St. Louis: Mosby–Year Book, 1990, pp. 288–310.

147. Benditt DG, Bailin S, Remole S, Milstein S. Proarrhythmia: recognition of patients at risk. J Cardiovasc Electrophysiol 1991; 2:S221–S232.

148. Zehender M, Hohnloser S, Just H. QT-interval prolonging drugs: mechanisms and clinical relevance of their arrhythmogenic hazards. Cardiovasc Drugs Ther 1991; 5:515–530.

149. Falk RH. Proarrhythmia in patients treated for atrial fibrillation or flutter. Ann Intern Med 1992; 117:141–150.

150. Ben-David J, Zipes DP. Torsades de pointes and proarrhythmia. Lancet 1993; 341:1578–1582.

151. Lazzara R. Antiarrhythmic drugs and torsade de pointes. Eur Heart J 1993; 14:88–92.

152. Crijns HJ. Torsade de pointes: the Achilles' heel of arrhythmia therapy with drugs that prolong the cardiac action potential. Eur Heart J 1995; 16:580–581.

153. Capucci A, Villani GQ, Aschieri D. Risk of complications of atrial fibrillation. PACE 1997; 20:2684–2691.

154. Martyn R, Somberg JC, Kerin NZ. Proarrhythmia of nonantiarrhythmic drugs. Am Heart J 1993; 126:201–205.

155. Kerin NZ, Somberg J. Proarrhythmia: definition, risk factors, causes, treatment, and controversies. Am Heart J 1994; 128:575–585.

156. Webb CL, Dick M II, Rocchini AP, et al. Quinidine syncope in children. J Am Coll Cardiol 1987; 9:1031–1037.

157. Podrid PJ, Lampert S, Graboys TB, Blatt CM, Lown B. Aggravation of arrhythmia by antiarrhythmic drugs: incidence and predictors. Am J Cardiol 1987; 59:38E–44E.

158. Keren A, Tzivoni D, Gavish D, et al. Etiology, warning signs and therapy of torsade de pointes: a study of 10 patients. Circulation 1981; 64:1167–1174.

159. Minardo JD, Heger JJ, Miles WM, Zipes DP, Prystowsky EN. Clinical characteristics of patients with ventricular fibrillation during antiarrhythmic drug therapy. N Engl J Med 1988; 319:257–262.

160. Velebit V, Podrid P, Lown B, Cohen BH, Graboys TB. Aggravation and provocation of ventricular arrhythmias by antiarrhythmic drugs. Circulation 1982; 65:886–894.

161. Thompson KA, Murray JJ, Blair IA, Woosley RL, Roden DM. Plasma concentrations of quinidine, its major metabolites, and dihydroquinidine in patients with torsades de pointes. Clin Pharmacol Ther 1988; 43:636–642.

162. Tschaidse O, Graboys TB, Lown B, Lampert S, Ravid S. The prevalence of proarrhythmic events during moricizine therapy and their relationship to ventricular function. Am Heart J 1992; 124:912–916.

163. Oberg KC, O'Toole MF, Gallastegui JL, Bauman JL. "Late" proarrhythmia due to quinidine. Am J Cardiol 1994; 74:192–194.

164. Denes P, Gabster A, Huang SK. Clinical, electrocardiographic and follow-up observations in patients having ventricular fibrillation during Holter monitoring. Am J Cardiol 1981; 48:9–16.

165. Bauman JL, Bauernfeind RA, Hoff JV, Strasberg B, Swiryn S, Rosen KM. Torsade de pointes due to quinidine: observations in 31 patients. Am Heart J 1984; 107:425–430.

166. Slater W, Lampert S, Podrid PJ, Lown B. Clinical predictors of arrhythmia worsening by antiarrhythmic drugs. Am J Cardiol 1988; 61:349–353.

167. Stanton MS, Prystowsky EN, Fineberg NS, Miles WM, Zipes DP, Heger JJ. Arrhythmogenic effects of antiarrhythmic drugs: a study of 506 patients for ventricular tachycardia or fibrillation. J Am Coll Cardiol 1989; 14:209–215.

168. Tzivoni D, Keren A, Stern S, Gottlieb S. Disopyramide-induced torsade de pointes. Arch Intern Med 1981; 141:946–947.

169. McKibbin JK, Pocock WA, Barlow JB, Millar RN, Obel IW. Sotalol, hypokalaemia, syncope, and torsade de pointes. Br Heart J 1984; 51:157–162.

170. Winkle RA, Mason JW, Griffin JC, Ross D. Malignant ventricular tachyarrhythmias associated with the use of encainide. Am Heart J 1981; 102:857–864.

171. Scherf D, Cohen J, Shafiiha H. Ectopic ventricular tachycardia, hypokalemia and convulsions in alcoholics. Cardiology 1967; 50:129–139.

172. Redleaf PD, Lerner IJ. Thiazide-induced hypokalemia with associated major ventricular arrhythmias: report of a case and comment on therapeutic use of bretylium. JAMA 1968; 206:1302–1304.

173. Curry P, Fitchett D, Stubbs W, Krikler D. Ventricular arrhythmias and hypokalaemia. Lancet 1976; 2:231–233.

174. Cokkinos DV, Mallios C, Philias N, Vorides EM. "Torsades de pointe": a distinct entity of ventricular arrhythmia? Acta Cardiol 1978; 33:167–184.

175. Topol EJ, Lerman BB. Hypomagnesemic torsades de pointes. Am J Cardiol 1983; 52:1367–1368.

176. Ramee SR, White CJ, Svinarich JT, Watson TD, Fox RF. Torsade de pointes and magnesium deficiency. Am Heart J 1985; 109:164–167.

177. Au PK, Bhandari AK, Bream R, Schreck D, Siddiqi R, Rahimtoola SH. Proarrhythmic effects of antiarrhythmic drugs during programmed ventricular stimulation in patients without ventricular tachycardia. J Am Coll Cardiol 1987; 9:389–397.

178. Koster RW, Wellens HJJ. Quinidine-induced ventricular flutter and fibrillation without digitalis therapy. Am J Cardiol 1976; 38:519–523.

179. Pohlgeers A, Villafane J. Ventricular fibrillation in two infants treated with amiodarone hydrochloride. Pediatr Cardiol 1995; 16:82–84.

180. Ejvinsson G, Orinius E. Prodromal ventricular premature beats preceded by a diastolic wave. Acta Med Scand 1980; 208:445–450.

181. Mattioni TA, Zheutlin TA, Sarmiento JJ, Parker M, Lesch M, Kehoe RF. Amiodarone in patients with previous drug-mediated torsade de pointes: long-term safety and efficacy. Ann Intern Med 1989; 111:574–580.

182. Fish FA, Gillette PC, Benson DW. Proarrhythmia, cardiac arrest and death in young patients receiving encainide and flecainide: the Pediatric Electrophysiology Group. J Am Coll Cardiol 1991; 18:356–365.

183. Houltz B, Darpo B, Edvardsson N, et al. Electrocardiographic and clinical predictors of torsades de pointes induced by almokalant infusion in patients with chronic atrial fibrillation or flutter: a prospective study. PACE 1998; 21:1044–1057.

184. Jorens PG, Van Den Heuvel PA, Van Cauwelaert PA, Parizel GA. Myxoma with a left-to-left shunt and fistula. Chest 1989; 96:945–946.

185. Lazzara R. Amiodarone and torsade de pointes. Ann Intern Med 1989; 111:549–551.

186. Mattioni TA, Zheutlin TA, Dunnington C, Kehoe RF. The proarrhythmic effects of amiodarone. Prog Cardiovasc Dis 1989; 31:439–446.

187. Hohnloser SH, Singh BN. Proarrhythmia with class III antiarrhythmic drugs: definition, electrophysiologic

mechanisms, incidence, predisposing factors, and clinical implications. J Cardiovasc Electrophysiol 1995; 6:920–936.

188. Desai AD, Chun S, Sung RJ. The role of intravenous amiodarone in the management of cardiac arrhythmias. Ann Intern Med 1997; 127:294–303.

189. Hohnloser SH. Proarrhythmia with class III antiarrhythmic drugs: types, risks, and management. Am J Cardiol 1997; 80:82G–89G.

190. McComb JM, Logan KR, Khan MM, Geddes JS, Adgey AA. Amiodarone-induced ventricular fibrillation. Eur J Cardiol 1980; 11:381–385.

191. Khan MM, Logan KR, McComb JM, Adgey AA. Management of recurrent ventricular tachyarrhythmias associated with Q-T prolongation. Am J Cardiol 1981; 47:1301–1308.

192. Tartini R, Kappenberger L, Steinbrunn W, Meyer UA. Dangerous interaction between amiodarone and quinidine. Lancet 1982; 1:1327–1329.

193. Westveer DC, Gadowski GA, Gordon S, Timmis GC. Amiodarone-induced ventricular tachycardia. Ann Intern Med 1982; 97:561–562.

194. Cui G, Huang W, Urthaler F. Ventricular flutter during treatment with amiodarone. Am J Cardiol 1983; 51:609–610.

195. Fogoros RN, Anderson KP, Winkle RA, Swerdlow CD, Mason JW. Amiodarone: clinical efficacy and toxicity in 96 patients with recurrent, drug-refractory arrhythmias. Circulation 1983; 68:88–94.

196. Sclarovsky S, Lewin RF, Kracoff O, Strasberg B, Arditti A, Agmon J. Amiodarone-induced polymorphous ventricular tachycardia. Am Heart J 1983; 105:6–12.

197. Brown MA, Smith WM, Lubbe WF, Norris RM. Amiodarone-induced torsades de pointes. Eur Heart J 1986; 7:234–239.

198. Leroy G, Haiat R, Barthelemy M, Lionnet F. Torsade de pointes during loading with amiodarone. Eur Heart J 1987; 8:541–543.

199. Bajaj BP, Baig MW, Perrins EJ. Amiodarone-induced torsades de pointes: the possible facilitatory role of digoxin. Int J Cardiol 1991; 33:335–337.

200. Morgan JM, Lopes A, Rowland E. Sudden cardiac death while taking amiodarone therapy: the role of abnormal repolarization. Eur Heart J 1991; 12:1144–1147.

201. Hii JT, Wyse DG, Gillis AM, Duff HJ, Solylo MA, Mitchell LB. Precordial QT interval dispersion as a marker of torsade de pointes: disparate effects of class Ia antiarrhythmic drugs and amiodarone. Circulation 1992; 86:1376–1382.

202. Middlekauff HR, Stevenson WG, Saxon LA, Stevenson LW. Amiodarone and torsades de pointes in patients with advanced heart failure. Am J Cardiol 1995; 76:499–502.

203. Levine JH, Massumi A, Scheinman MM, et al. Intravenous amiodarone for recurrent sustained hypotensive ventricular tachyarrhythmias: intravenous amiodarone multicenter trial group. J Am Coll Cardiol 1996; 27:67–75.

204. Tran HT, Chow MS, Kluger J. Amiodarone induced torsades de pointes with excessive QT dispersion following quinidine induced polymorphic ventricular tachycardia. Pacing Clin Electrophysiol 1997; 20:2275–2278.

205. Hohnloser SH, Klingenheben T, Singh BN. Amiodarone-associated proarrhythmic effects: a review with special reference to torsade de pointes tachycardia. Ann Intern Med 1994; 121:529–535.

206. Scheinman MM, Levine JH, Cannom DS, et al. Dose-ranging study of intravenous amiodarone in patients with life-threatening ventricular tachyarrhythmias. Circulation 1995; 92:3264–3272.

207. Forfar JC, Gribbin B. Torsade de pointes after amiodarone withdrawal: effects of mild hypokalaemia on repolarization. Eur Heart J 1984; 5:510–512.

208. Scagliotti D, Strasberg B, Hai HA, Kehoe R, Rosen K. Aprindine-induced polymorphous ventricular tachycardia. Am J Cardiol 1982; 49:1297–1300.

209. Burket MW, Fraker TD Jr, Temesy-Armos PN. Polymorphous ventricular tachycardia provoked by lidocaine. Am J Cardiol 1985; 55:592–593.

210. Meltzer RS, Robert EW, McMorrow M, Martin RP. Atypical ventricular tachycardia as a manifestation of disopyramide toxicity. Am J Cardiol 1978; 42:1049–1053.

211. Nicholson WJ, Martin CE, Gracey JG, Knoch HR. Disopyramide-induced ventricular fibrillation. Am J Cardiol 1979; 43:1053–1055.

212. Commerford PJ, Beck W. Ventricular tachycardia with torsade de pointes morphology induced by oral disopyramide. S Afr Med J 1980; 58:447–448.

213. Wald RW, Waxman MB, Colman JM. Torsade de pointes ventricular tachycardia: a complication of disopyramide shared with quinidine. J Electrocardiol 1981; 14:301–307.

214. Ko PT, Gulamhusein S, Kostuk WJ, Klein GJ. Torsades de pointes, a common arrhythmia, induced by medication. Can Med Assoc J 1982; 127:368–372.

215. Schweitzer P, Mark H. Torsade de pointes caused by disopyramide and hypokalemia. Mt Sinai J Med 1982; 49:110–114.

216. Schattner A, Gindin J, Geltner D. Fatal torsade de pointes following jaundice in a patient treated with disopyramide. Postgrad Med J 1989; 65:333–334.

217. Kasanuki H, Ohnishi S, Tamura K, Nirei T, Shoda M, Hosoda S. Acquired long QT syndrome due to antiarrhythmic drugs and bradyarrhythmias. Ann NY Acad Sci 1992; 644:57–73.

218. Murray KT. Ibutilide. Circulation 1998; 97:493–497.

219. Ellenbogen KA, Stambler BS, Wood MA, et al. Efficacy of intravenous ibutilide for rapid termination of atrial fibrillation and atrial flutter: a dose-response study. J Am Coll Cardiol 1996; 28:130–136.

220. Volgman AS, Carberry PA, Stambler B, et al. Conversion efficacy and safety of intravenous ibutilide compared with intravenous procainamide in patients with atrial flutter or fibrillation. J Am Coll Cardiol 1998; 31:1414–1419.

221. Strasberg B, Sclarovsky S, Erdberg A, Duffy CE, Lam W, Swiryn S, et al. Procainamide-induced polymorphous ventricular tachycardia. Am J Cardiol 1981; 47:1309–1314.

222. Kay GN, Plumb VJ, Arciniegas JG, Henthorn RW, Waldo AL. Torsade de pointes: the long-short initiating sequence and other clinical features: observations in 32 patients. J Am Coll Cardiol 1983; 2:806–817.

223. Schweitzer P, Mark H. Delayed repolarization syndrome. Am J Med 1983; 75:393–401.

224. Sarmiento JJ, Shea PM, Goldberger AL. Unusual ventricular depolarizations associated with torsade de pointes. Am Heart J 1985; 109:377–379.

225. Kadish AH, Weisman HF, Veltri EP, Epstein AE, Slepian MJ, Levine JH. Paradoxical effects of exercise on the QT interval in patients with polymorphic ventricular tachycardia receiving type Ia antiarrhythmic agents. Circulation 1990; 81:14–19.

226. Olshansky B, Martins J, Hunt S. N-acetyl procainamide causing torsades de pointes. Am J Cardiol 1982; 50:1439–1441.

227. Chow MJ, Piergies AA, Bowsher DJ, et al. Torsade de pointes induced by N-acetylprocainamide. J Am Coll Cardiol 1984; 4:621–624.

228. Herre JM, Thompson JA. Polymorphic ventricular tachycardia and ventricular fibrillation due to N-acetyl procainamide. Am J Cardiol 1985; 55:227–228.

229. Stevenson W.G., Weiss J. Torsades de pointes due to N-acetylprocainamide. Pacing Clin Electrophysiol 1985; 8:528–531.

230. Stratmann HG, Walter KE, Kennedy HL. Torsade de pointes associated with elevated N-acetylprocainamide levels. Am Heart J 1985; 109:375–377.

231. Roden DM, Thompson KA, Hoffman BF, Woosley RL. Clinical features and basic mechanisms of quinidine-induced arrhythmias. J Am Coll Cardiol 1986; 8:83A–78A.

232. Salerno DM. Quinidine: worse than adverse? Circulation 1991; 84:2196–2198.

233. Grace AA, Camm AJ. Quinidine. N Engl J Med 1998; 338:35–45.

234. Rainier-Pope CR, Schrire V, Beck W, Barnard CN. The treatment of quinidine-induced ventricular fibrillation by closed-chest resuscitation and external defibrillation. Am Heart J 1962; 63:582–590.

235. Davies P, Leak D, Oram S. Quinidine-induced syncope. BMJ 1965; 2:517–520.

236. Seaton A. Quinidine-induced paroxysmal ventricular

fibrillation treated with propranolol. BMJ 1966;
5502:1522–1523.

237. Kaplinsky E, Yahini JH, Barzilai J, Neufeld HN. Quinidine syncope: report of a case successfully treated with lidocaine. Chest 1972; 62:764–766.

238. VanderArk CR, Reynolds EW, Kahn DR, Tullett G. Quinidine syncope: a report of successful treatment with bretylium tosylate. J Thorac Cardiovasc Surg 1976; 72:464–467.

239. Cohen IS, Jick H, Cohen SI. Adverse reactions to quinidine in hospitalized patients: findings based on data from the Boston Collaborative Drug Surveillance Program. Prog Cardiovasc Dis 1977; 20:151–163.

240. Anderson KP, DeCamilla J, Moss AJ. Clinical significance of ventricular tachycardia (3 beats or longer) detected during ambulatory monitoring after myocardial infarction. Circulation 1978; 57:890–897.

241. Anderson JL, Mason JW. Successful treatment by overdrive pacing of recurrent quinidine syncope due to ventricular tachycardia. Am J Med 1978; 64:715–718.

242. DiSegni E, Klein HO, David D, Libhaber C, Kaplinsky E. Overdrive pacing in quinidine syncope and other long QT-interval syndromes. Arch Intern Med 1980; 140:1036–1040.

243. Koenig W, Schinz AM. Spontaneous ventricular flutter and fibrillation during quinidine medication. Am Heart J 1983; 105:863–865.

244. Smith MS, Lindsay WC, Flowers NC. Treatment of torsades de pointes with esophageal atrial pacing. Am J Med 1987; 83:971–972.

245. el-Sherif N, Bekheit SS, Henkin R. Quinidine-induced long QTU interval and torsade de pointes: role of bradycardia-dependent early afterdepolarizations. J Am Coll Cardiol 1989; 14:252–257.

246. Soyka LF, Wirtz C, Spangenberg RB. Clinical safety profile of sotalol in patients with arrhythmias. Am J Cardiol 1990; 65:74A–81A.

247. Hohnloser SH, Woosley RL. Sotalol. N Engl J Med 1994; 331:31–38.

248. MacNeil DJ. The side effect profile of class III antiarrhythmic drugs: focus on d,l-sotalol. Am J Cardiol 1997; 80:90G–98G.

249. Elonen E, Neuvonen PJ, Tarssanen L, Kala R. Sotalol intoxication with prolonged Q-T interval and severe tachyarrhythmias. BMJ 1979; 1:1184.

250. Kontopoulos A, Filindris A, Manoudis F, Metaxas P. Sotalol-induced torsade de pointes. Postgrad Med J 1981; 57:321–323.

251. Neuvonen PJ, Elonen E, Vuorenmaa T, Laakso M. Prolonged Q-T interval and severe tachyarrhythmias, common features of sotalol intoxication. Eur J Clin Pharmacol 1981; 20:85–89.

252. Kuck KH, Kunze KP, Roewer N, Bleifeld W. Sotalol-induced torsade de pointes. Am Heart J 1984; 107:179–180.

253. Gonzalez R, Scheinman MM, Herre JM, Griffin JC, Sauve MJ, Sharkey H. Usefulness of sotalol for drug-refractory malignant ventricular arrhythmias. J Am Coll Cardiol 1988; 12:1568–1572.

254. Jordaens LJ, Palmer A, Clement DL. Low-dose oral sotalol for monomorphic ventricular tachycardia: effects during programmed electrical stimulation and follow-up. Eur Heart J 1989; 10:218–226.

255. Rankin AC, Pringle SD, Cobbe SM. Acute treatment of torsades de pointes with amiodarone: proarrhythmic and antiarrhythmic association of QT prolongation. Am Heart J 1990; 119:185–186.

256. Anastasiou-Nana MI, Gilbert EM, Miller RH, et al. Usefulness of d,l sotalol for suppression of chronic ventricular arrhythmias. Am J Cardiol 1991; 67:511–516.

257. Arstall MA, Hii JT, Lehman RG, Horowitz JD. Sotalol-induced torsade de pointes: management with magnesium infusion. Postgrad Med J 1992; 68:289–290.

258. MacNeil DJ, Davies RO, Deitchman D. Clinical safety profile of sotalol in the treatment of arrhythmias. Am J Cardiol 1993; 72:44A–50A.

259. Krapf R, Gertsch M. Torsade de pointes induced by sotalol despite therapeutic plasma sotalol concentrations. BMJ 1994; 1985:1784–1785.

260. Haverkamp W, Martinez-Rubio A, Hief C, et al. Efficacy and safety of d,l-sotalol in patients with ventricular tachycardia and

in survivors of cardiac arrest. J Am Coll Cardiol 1997; 30:487–495.

261. Krishnan SC, Galvin J, McGovern B, Garan H, Ruskin JN. Reproducible induction of "atypical" torsades de pointes by programmed electrical stimulation: a novel form of sotalol-induced proarrhythmia? J Cardiovasc Electrophysiol 1997; 8:1055–1061.

262. Pfammatter JP, Paul T, Lehmann C, Kallfelz HC. Efficacy and proarrhythmia of oral sotalol in pediatric patients. J Am Coll Cardiol 1995; 26:1002–1007.

263. Sasse M, Paul T, Bergmann P, Kallfelz HC. Sotalol associated torsades de pointes tachycardia in a 15-month-old child: successful therapy with magnesium aspartate. PACE 1998; 21:1164–1166.

264. Hohnloser SH, Meinertz T, Stubbs P, et al. Efficacy and safety of d-sotalol, a pure class III antiarrhythmic compound, in patients with symptomatic complex ventricular ectopy: results of a multicenter, randomized, double-blind, placebo-controlled dose-finding study. Circulation 1995; 92:1517–1525.

265. Waldo AL, Camm AJ, deRuyter H, et al. Effect of d-sotalol on mortality in patients with left ventricular dysfunction after recent and remote myocardial infarction. The SWORD Investigators: survival with oral d-sotalol. Lancet 1996; 348:7–12.

266. Cobbe SM. Class III antiarrhythmics: put to the sword? Heart 1996; 75:111–113.

267. Echt DS, Liebson PR, Mitchell LB, et al. Mortality and morbidity in patients receiving encainide, flecainide, or placebo: the Cardiac Arrhythmia Suppression Trial. N Engl J Med 1991; 324:781–788.

268. Lui HK, Lee G, Dietrich P, Low RI, Mason DT. Flecainide-induced QT prolongation and ventricular tachycardia. Am Heart J 1982; 103:567–569.

269. Oetgen WJ, Tibbits PA, Abt ME, Goldstein RE. Clinical and electrophysiologic assessment of oral flecainide acetate for recurrent ventricular tachycardia: evidence for exacerbation of electrical instability. Am J Cardiol 1983; 52:746–750.

270. Nathan AW, Hellestrand KJ, Bexton RS, Banim SO, Spurrell RA, Camm AJ. Proarrhythmic effects of the new antiarrhythmic agent flecainide acetate. Am Heart J 1984; 107:222–228.

271. Anastasiou-Nana MI, Anderson JL, Stewart JR, et al. Occurrence of exercise-induced and spontaneous wide complex tachycardia during therapy with flecainide for complex ventricular arrhythmias: a probable proarrhythmic effect. Am Heart J 1987; 113:1071–1077.

272. Bauman JL, Gallastegui JL, Tanenbaum SR, Hariman RJ. Flecainide-induced sustained ventricular tachycardia successfully treated with lidocaine. Chest 1987; 92:573–575.

273. Morganroth J. Risk factors for the development of proarrhythmic events. Am J Cardiol 1987; 59:32E–37E.

274. Falk RH. Flecainide-induced ventricular tachycardia and fibrillation in patients treated for atrial fibrillation. Ann Intern Med 1989; 111:107–111.

275. Myerburg RJ, Kessler KM, Cox MM, et al. Reversal of proarrhythmic effects of flecainide acetate and encainide hydrochloride by propranolol. Circulation 1989; 80:1571–1579.

276. Chimienti M, Cullen Mt Jr, Casadei G. Safety of flecainide versus propafenone for the long-term management of symptomatic paroxysmal supraventricular tachyarrhythmias: report from the Flecainide and Propafenone Italian Study (FAPIS) group. Eur Heart J 1995; 16:1943–1951.

277. Cocco G, Strozzi C, Chu D, Pansini R. Torsades de pointes as a manifestation of mexiletine toxicity. Am Heart J 1980; 100:878–880.

278. Janousek J, Paul T. Safety of oral propafenone in the treatment of arrhythmias in infants and children (European Retrospective Multicenter Study). Am J Cardiol 1998; 81:1121–1124.

279. Engler RL, LeWinter M. Tocainide-induced ventricular fibrillation. Am Heart J 1981; 101:494–496.

280. Cheesman M, Ward DE. Exacerbation of ventricular tachycardia by tocainide. Clin Cardiol 1985; 8:47–50.

281. Manouvrier J, Sagot M, Caron C, et al. Nine cases of torsade

de pointes with bepridil administration. Am Heart J 1986; 111:1005–1007.

282. Dolara A, Manetti A, Pozzi L, Tordini G. Bidirectional tachycardia. Cardiology 1971; 55:302–309.

283. Cohen HC, Gozo EG Jr, Pick A. Ventricular tachycardia with narrow QRS complexes (left posterior fascicular tachycardia). Circulation 1972; 45:1035–1043.

284. Morris SN, Zipes DP. His bundle electrocardiography during bidirectional tachycardia. Circulation 1973; 48:32–36.

285. Castellanos A, Ferreiro J, Pefkaros K, Rozanski JJ, Moleiro F, Myerburg RJ. Effects of lignocaine on bidirectional tachycardia and on digitalis-induced atrial tachycardia with block. Br Heart J 1982; 48:27–32.

286. Chan T, Vilke GM, Williams S. Bidirectional tachycardia associated with digoxin toxicity. J Emerg Med 1995; 13:89.

287. Valent S, Kelly P. Images in clinical medicine. Digoxin-induced bidirectional ventricular tachycardia. N Eng J Med 1997; 336:550.

288. James MA, Culling W, Vann Jones J. Polymorphous ventricular tachycardia due to alpha-blockade. Int J Cardiol 1987; 14:225–227.

289. Puritz R, Henderson MA, Baker SN, Chamberlain DA. Ventricular arrhythmias caused by prenylamine. BMJ 1977; 2:608–609.

290. Grenadier E, Keidar S, Alpan G, Marmor A, Palant A. Prenylamine-induced ventricular tachycardia and syncope controlled by ventricular pacing. Br Heart J 1980; 44:330–334.

291. Meanock CI, Noble MI. A case of prenylamine toxicity showing the torsade de pointes phenomenon in sinus rhythm. Postgrad Med J 1981; 57:381–384.

292. Abinader EG, Shahar J. Possible female preponderance in prenylamine-induced "torsade de pointes" tachycardia. Cardiology 1983; 70:37–40.

293. Matsuhashi H, Onodera S, Kawamura Y, et al. Probucol-induced QT prolongation and torsades de pointes. Jpn J Med 1989; 28:612–615.

294. Reinoehl J, Frankovich D, Machado C, et al. Probucol-associated tachyarrhythmic events and QT prolongation: importance of gender. Am Heart J 1996; 131:1184–1191.

295. Winters SL, Schweitzer P, Kupersmith J, Gomes JA. Verapamil-induced polymorphous ventricular tachycardia. J Am Coll Cardiol 1985; 6:257–259.

296. Kelly HG, Fay JE, Laverty SG. Thioridizine hyrochloride (Mellaril): its effect on the electrocardiogram and a report of two fatalities with electrocardiographic abnormalities. Can Med Asso J 1963; 89:546–554.

297. Desautels S, Filteau C, St-Jean A. Ventricular tachycardia associated with administration of thioridazine hydrochloride (Mellaril). Can Med Asso J 1964; 90:1030–1031.

298. Schoonmaker FW, Osteen RT, Greenfield JC. Thioridazine (Mellaril)-induced ventricular tachycardia controlled with an artificial pacemaker. Ann Intern Med 1966; 65:1076–1078.

299. Giles TD, Modlin RK. Death associated with ventricular arrhythmia and thioridazine hydrochloride. JAMA 1968; 205:108–110.

300. Leestma JE, Koenig KL. Sudden death and phenothiazines. Arch Gen Psychiatry 1968; 18:137–148.

301. Moore MT, Book MH. Sudden death in phenothiazine therapy: a clinicopathologic study of 12 cases. Psychiatr Q 1970; 44:389–402.

302. Fouron JC, Chicoine R. ECG changes in fatal imipramine (tofranil) intoxication. Pediatrics 1971; 48:777–781.

303. Moir DC, Cornwell WB, Dingwall-Fordyce I, et al. Cardiotoxicity of amitriptyline. Lancet 1972; 2:561–564.

304. Fowler NO, McCall D, Chou TC, Holmes JC, Hanenson IB. Electrocardiographic changes and cardiac arrhythmias in patients receiving psychotropic drugs. Am J Cardiol 1976; 37:223–230.

305. Kounis NG. Iatrogenic "torsade de pointes" ventricular tachycardia. Postgrad Med J 1979; 55:832–835.

306. Magorien RD, Jewell GM, Schaal SF, Leier CV. Electrophysiologic studies of perphenazine and protriptyline in a patient with psychotropic drug-induced ventricular fibrillation. Am J Med 1979; 67:353–357.

307. Strasberg B, Coelho A, Welch W, Swiryn S, Bauernfeind R,

Rosen K. Doxepin induced torsade de pointes. Pacing Clin Electrophysiol 1982; 5:873–877.

308. Herrmann HC, Kaplan LM, Bierer BE. Q-T prolongation and torsades de pointes ventricular tachycardia produced by the tetracyclic antidepressant agent maprotiline. Am J Cardiol 1983; 51:904–906.

309. Kemper AJ, Dunlap R, Pietro DA. Thioridazine-induced torsade de pointes: successful therapy with isoproterenol. JAMA 1983; 249:2931–2934.

310. Kriwisky M, Perry GY, Tarchitsky D, Gutman Y, Kishon Y. Haloperidol-induced torsades de pointes. Chest 1990; 98:482–484.

311. Wilt JL, Minnema AM, Johnson RF, Rosenblum AM. Torsade de pointes associated with the use of intravenous haloperidol. Ann Intern Med 1993; 119:391–394.

312. Sharma ND, Rosman HS, Padhi D, Tisdale JE. Torsades de pointes associated with intravenous haloperidol in critically ill patients. Am J Cardiol 1998; 81:238–240.

313. Freedman RA, Anderson KP, Green LS, Mason JW. Effect of erythromycin on ventricular arrhythmias and ventricular repolarization in idiopathic long QT syndrome. Am J Cardiol 1987; 59:168–169.

314. Schoenenberger RA, Haefeli WE, Weiss P, Ritz RF. Association of intravenous erythromycin and potentially fatal ventricular tachycardia with Q-T prolongation (torsades de pointes). BMJ 1990; 300:1375–1376.

315. Wharton JM, Demopulos PA, Goldschlager N. Torsade de pointes during administration of pentamidine isethionate. Am J Med 1987; 83:571–576.

316. Bibler MR, Chou TC, Toltzis RJ, Wade PA. Recurrent ventricular tachycardia due to pentamidine-induced cardiotoxicity. Chest 1988; 94:1303–1306.

317. Mitchell P, Dodek P, Lawson L, Kiess M, Russell J. Torsades de pointes during intravenous pentamidine isethionate therapy. Can Med Assoc J 1989; 140:173–174.

318. Stein KM, Haronian H, Mensah GA, Acosta A, Jacobs J, Kligfield P. Ventricular tachycardia and torsades de pointes complicating pentamidine therapy of *Pneumocystis carinii* pneumonia in the acquired immunodeficiency syndrome. Am J Cardiol 1990; 66:888–889.

319. Lopez JA, Harold JG, Rosenthal MC, Oseran DS, Schapira JN, Peter T. QT prolongation and torsades de pointes after administration of trimethoprim-sulfamethoxazole. Am J Cardiol 1987; 59:376–377.

320. Woosley RL, Chen Y, Freiman JP, Gillis RA. Mechanism of the cardiotoxic actions of terfenadine. JAMA 1993; 269:1532–1536.

321. Monahan BP, Ferguson CL, Killeavy ES, Lloyd BK, Troy J, Cantilena LR Jr. Torsades de pointes occurring in association with terfenadine use. JAMA 1990; 264:2788–2790.

322. Zimmermann M, Duruz H, Guinand O, et al. Torsades de pointes after treatment with terfenadine and ketoconazole. Eur Heart J 1992; 13:1002–1003.

323. Broadhurst P, Nathan AW. Cardiac arrest in a young woman with the long QT syndrome and concomitant astemizole ingestion. Br Heart J 1993; 70:469–470.

324. Sakemi H, VanNatta B. Torsade de pointes induced by astemizole in a patient with prolongation of the QT interval. Am Heart J 1993; 125:1436–1438.

325. Craft TM. Torsade de pointes after astemizole overdose. BMJ 1994; 1986:660.

326. Rao KA, Adlakha A, Verma-Ansil B, Meloy TD, Stanton MS. Torsades de pointes ventricular tachycardia associated with overdose of astemizole. Mayo Clin Proc 1994; 69:589–593.

327. Feroze H, Suri R, Silverman DI. Torsades de pointes from terfenadine and sotalol given in combination. Pacing Clin Electrophysiol 1996; 19:1519–1521.

328. Martin ES, Rogalski K, Black JN. Quinine may trigger torsades de pointes during astemizole therapy. Pacing Clin Electrophysiol 1997; 20:2024–2025.

329. Tai YT, Lau CP, But PP, Fong PC, Li JP. Bidirectional tachycardia induced by herbal aconite poisoning. Pacing Clin Electrophysiol 1992; 15:831–839.

330. Sartori M, Pratt CM, Young JB. Torsade de pointe: malignant cardiac arrhythmia induced by amantadine poisoning. Am J Med 1984; 77:388–391.

331. Young JB, Vandermolen LA, Pratt CM. Torsade de pointes: an unusual manifestation of chloral hydrate poisoning. Am Heart J 1986; 112:181–184.

332. Bryer-Ash M, Zehnder J, Angelchik P, Maisel A. Torsades de pointes precipitated by a Chinese herbal remedy. Am J Cardiol 1987; 60:1186–1187.

333. Emori T, Fujieda H, Ohe T. Polymorphic ventricular tachycardia induced by intracoronary injection of ioxaglate in a patient with borderline QT prolongation. J Cardiovasc Electrophysiol 1996; 7:962–966.

334. Aldariz AE, Romero H, Baroni M, Baglivo H, Esper RJ. QT prolongation and torsade de pointes ventricular tachycardia produced by ketanserin. Pacing Clin Electrophysiol 1986; 9:836–841.

335. Connolly MJ, Astridge PS, White EG, Morley CA, Cowan JC. Torsades de pointes ventricular tachycardia and terodiline. Lancet 1991; 338:344–345.

336. Goldsmith S, From AH. Arsenic-induced atypical ventricular tachycardia. N Engl J Med 1980; 303:1096–1098.

337. Little RE, Kay GN, Cavender JB, Epstein AE, Plumb VJ. Torsade de pointes and T-U Wave alternans associated with arsenic poisoning. Pacing Clin Electrophysiol 1990; 13:164–170.

338. Kiss Z, Fazekas T. Arrhythmias in organophosphate poisonings. Acta Cardiol 1979; 34:323–330.

339. Ludomirsky A, Klein HO, Sarelli P, et al. Q-T prolongation and polymorphous ("torsade de pointes") ventricular arrhythmias associated with organophosphorus insecticide poisoning. Am J Cardiol 1982; 49:1654–1658.

340. Dalle XS, Meltzer E, Kravitz B. A new look at ventricular tachycardia. Acta Cardiol 1967; 22:519–535.

341. Grenadier E, Alpan G, Maor N, et al. Polymorphous ventricular tachycardia in acute myocardial infarction. Am J Cardiol 1984; 53:1280–1283.

342. Griffin J, Most AS. Torsade de pointes complicating acute myocardial infarction. Am Heart J 1984; 107:169–170.

343. Wolfe CL, Nibley C, Bhandari A, Chatterjee K, Scheinman M. Polymorphous ventricular tachycardia associated with acute myocardial infarction. Circulation 1991; 84:1543–1551.

344. Birnbaum Y, Sclarovsky S, Ben-Ami R, et al. Polymorphous ventricular tachycardia early after acute myocardial infarction. Am J Cardiol 1993; 71:745–749.

345. Gressin V, Louvard Y, Pezzano M, Lardoux H. Holter recording of ventricular arrhythmias during intravenous thrombolysis for acute myocardial infarction. Am J Cardiol 1992; 69:152–159.

346. Kerin NZ, Rubenfire M, Naini M, Wajszczuk WJ, Pamatmat A, Cascade PN. Arrhythmias in variant angina pectoris: relationship of arrhythmias to ST-segment elevation and R-wave changes. Circulation 1979; 60:1343–1350.

347. Sawaya JI, Rubeiz GA. Prinzmetal's angina with torsade de pointes ventricular tachycardia. Acta Cardiol 1980; 35:47–54.

348. Myerburg RJ, Kessler KM, Mallon SM, et al. Life-threatening ventricular arrhythmias in patients with silent myocardial ischemia due to coronary artery spasm. N Engl J Med 1992; 326:1451–1455.

349. Nishizaki M, Arita M, Sakurada H, et al. Induction of polymorphic ventricular tachycardia by programmed ventricular stimulation in vasospastic angina pectoris. Am J Cardiol 1996; 77:355–360.

350. Saxon LA, Wiener I, Natterson PD, Laks H, Drinkwater D, Stevenson WG. Monomorphic versus polymorphic ventricular tachycardia after coronary artery bypass grafting. Am J Cardiol 1995; 75:403–405.

351. Azar RR, Berns E, Seecharran B, Veronneau J, Lippman N, Kluger J. De novo monomorphic and polymorphic ventricular tachycardia following coronary artery bypass grafting. Am J Cardiol 1997; 80:76–78.

352. Fiddler GI, Campbell RW, Pottage A, Godman MJ. Varicella myocarditis presenting with unusual ventricular arrhythmias. Br Heart J 1997; 39:1150–1153.

353. Coumel P. Polymorphous ventricular tachyarrhythmias in the absence of structural heart disease. PACE 1995; 18:633–636.

354. Coumel P. Polymorphous ventricular tachyarrhythmias in the absence of structural heart disease. Pacing Clin Electrophysiol 1997; 20:2065–2067.

355. Bourke JP, Doig JC. Ventricular Tachyarrhythmias in the Normal Heart. Armonk, NY: Futura Publishing Co., 1998.

356. Strasberg B, Welch W, Palileo E, Swiryn S, Bauernfeind R, Rosen KM. Familial inducible torsade de pointes with normal QT interval. Eur Heart J 1983; 4:383–390.

357. Bjerregaard P, Gussak I, Kotar SL, Gessler JE, Janosik D. Recurrent syncope in a patient with prominent J wave. Am Heart J 1994; 127:1426–1430.

358. Masrani K, Cowley C, Bekheit S, el-Sherif N. Recurrent syncope for over a decade due to idiopathic ventricular fibrillation. Chest 1994; 106:1601–1603.

359. Dyk T, Janukowicz C. Bidirectional tachycardia in a case of recurrent paroxysmal tachycardia with ventricular fibrillation. Cardiology 1968; 52:132–137.

360. Martini B, Buja GF, Canciani B, Nava A. Bidirectional tachycardia: a sustained form, not related to digitalis intoxication, in an adult without apparent cardiac disease. Jpn Heart J 1988; 29:381–387.

361. Chiche P, Haiat R, Steff P. Angina pectoris with syncope due to paroxysmal atrioventricular block: role of ischaemia: report of two cases. Br Heart J 1974; 36:577–581.

362. Jensen G, Sigurd B, Sandoe E. Adams-Stokes seizures due to ventricular tachydysrhythmias in patients with heart block: prevalence and problems of management. Chest 1975; 67:43–48.

363. Steinbrecher UP, Fitchett DH. Torsade de pointes: a cause of syncope with atrioventricular block. Arch Intern Med 1980; 140:1223–1226.

364. Strasberg B, Kusniec J, Erdman S, et al. Polymorphous ventricular tachycardia and atrioventricular block. Pacing Clin Electrophysiol 1986; 9:522–526.

365. Maor N, Weiss D, Lorber A. Torsade de pointe complicating atrioventricular block: report of two cases. Int J Cardiol 1987; 14:235–238.

366. Scott WA, Dick M II. Two:one atrioventricular block in infants with congenital long QT syndrome. Am J Cardiol 1987; 60:1409–1410.

367. Cosio FG, Goicolea A, Lopez Gil M, Kallmeyer C, Barroso JL. Suppression of torsades de pointes with verapamil in patients with atrio-ventricular block. Eur Heart J 1991; 12:635–638.

368. Kurita T, Ohe T, Shimizu W, Hotta D, Shimomura K. Early afterdepolarization in a patient with complete atrioventricular block and torsades de pointes. Pacing Clin Electrophysiol 1993; 16:33–38.

369. de Meester A, Djian D, Jacques JM, Luwaert R, Chaudron JM. Torsades de pointes and aborted sudden death after implantation of a cardioverter defibrillator. Acta Cardiol 1994; 49:543–548.

370. Garson A Jr, Dick M II, Fournier A, et al. The long QT syndrome in children: an international study of 287 patients. Circulation 1993; 87:1866–1872.

371. Gascho JA, Schieken R. Congenital complete heart block and long Q-T syndrome requiring ventricular pacing for control of refractory ventricular tachycardia and fibrillation. J Electrocardiol 1979; 12:331–335.

372. Scott JS, Maddison PJ, Taylor PV, Esscher E, Scott O, Skinner RP. Connective-tissue disease, antibodies to ribonucleoprotein, and congenital heart block. N Engl J Med 1983; 309:209–212.

373. Case CL, Gillette PC. Conduction system disease in a child with long QT syndrome. Am Heart J 1990; 120:984–986.

374. Solti F, Szatmary L, Vecsey T, Renyi-Vamos F Jr, Bodor E. Congenital complete heart block associated with QT prolongation. Eur Heart J 1992; 13:1080–1083.

375. Isner JM, Roberts WC, Heymsfield SB, Yager J. Anorexia nervosa and sudden death. Ann Intern Med 1985; 102:49–52.

376. Kearney P, Reardon M, O'Hare J. Primary hyperparathyroidism presenting as torsades de pointes. Br Heart J 1993; 70:473.

377. Fredlund BO, Olsson SB. Long QT interval and ventricular tachycardia of "torsade de pointe" type in hypothyroidism. Acta Med Scand 1983; 213:231–235.

378. Kumar A, Bhandari AK, Rahimtoola SH. Torsade de pointes and marked QT prolongation in association with hypothyroidism. Ann Intern Med 1987; 106:712–713.

379. Nesher G, Zion MM. Recurrent ventricular tachycardia in

hypothyroidism: report of a case and review of the literature. Cardiology 1988; 75:301–306.

380. Moss AJ. Caution: very-low-calorie diets can be deadly. Ann Intern Med 1985; 102:121–123.

381. Brown JM, Yetter JF, Spicer MJ, Jones JD. Cardiac complications of protein-sparing modified fasting. JAMA 1978; 240:120–122.

382. Singh BN, Gaarder TD, Kanegae T, Goldstein M, Montgomerie JZ, Mills H. Liquid protein diets and torsade de pointes. JAMA 1978; 240:115–119.

383. Isner JM, Sours HE, Paris AL, Ferrans VJ, Roberts WC. Sudden, unexpected death in avid dieters using the liquid-protein-modified-fast diet: observations in 17 patients and the role of the prolonged QT interval. Circulation 1979; 60:1401–1412.

384. Siegel RJ, Cabeen WR Jr, Roberts WC. Prolonged QT interval–ventricular tachycardia syndrome from massive rapid weight loss utilizing the liquid-protein-modified-fast diet: sudden death with sinus node ganglionitis and neuritis. Am Heart J 1981; 102:121–122.

385. Lisak RP, Lebeau J, Tucker SH, Rowland LP. Hyperkalemic periodic paralysis and cardiac arrhythmia. Neurology 1972; 22:810–815.

386. Kastor JA, Goldreyer BN. Ventricular origin of bidirectional tachycardia: case report of a patient not toxic from digitalis. Circulation 1973; 48:897–903.

387. Fukuda K, Ogawa S, Yokozuka H, Handa S, Nakamura Y. Long-standing bidirectional tachycardia in a patient with hypokalemic periodic paralysis. J Electrocardiol 1988; 21:71–75.

388. Parizel G. Life-threatening arrhythmias in subarachnoid hemorrhage. Angiology 1973; 24:17–21.

389. Estanol BV, Marin OS. Cardiac arrhythmias and sudden death in subarachnoid hemorrhage. Stroke 1975; 6:382–386.

390. Grossman MA. Cardiac arrhythmias in acute central nervous system disease: successful management with stellate ganglion block. Arch Intern Med 1976; 136:203–207.

391. Estanol Vidal B, Badui Dergal E, Cesarman E, et al. Cardiac arrhythmias associated with subarachnoid hemorrhage: prospective study. Neurosurgery 1979; 5:675–680.

392. Carruth JE, Silverman ME. Torsade de pointe atypical ventricular tachycardia complicating subarachnoid hemorrhage. Chest 1980; 78:886–888.

393. Hust MH, Nitsche K, Hohnloser S, Bohm B, Just H. Q-T prolongation and torsades de pointes in a patient with subarachnoid hemorrhage. Clin Cardiol 1984; 7:44–48.

394. Sen S, Stober T, Burger L, Anstatt T, Rettig G. Recurrent torsade de pointes type ventricular tachycardia in intracranial hemorrhage. Intensive Care Med 1984; 10:263–264.

395. Andreoli A, Di Pasquale G, Pinelli G, Grazi P, Tognetti F, Testa A. Subarachnoid hemorrhage: frequency and severity of cardiac arrhythmias: a survey of 70 cases studied in the acute phase. Stroke 1987; 18:558–564.

396. Vincent GM, Abildskov JA, Burgess MJ. Q-T interval syndromes. Prog Cardiovasc Dis 1974; 16:523–530.

397. Ovsyshcher IA, Gueron M. Congenital QT interval prolongation: a review with a survey of three families. Isr J Med Sci 1978; 14:833–840.

398. Moss AJ, Schwartz PJ. Sudden death and the idiopathic long Q-T syndrome. Am J Med 1979; 66:6–7.

399. Jervell A. The surdo-cardiac syndrome. Eur Heart J 1985; 6:97–102.

400. Moss AJ. Prolonged QT-interval syndromes. JAMA 1986; 256:2985–2987.

401. Schwartz PJ, Zaza A, Locati E, Moss AJ. Stress and sudden death: the case of the long QT syndrome. Circulation 1991; 83(Suppl I):I-171–I-180.

402. Zipes DP. The long QT interval syndrome: a rosetta stone for sympathetic related ventricular tachyarrhythmias. Circulation 1991; 84:1414–1419.

403. Wellens HJJ, Vermeulen A, Durrer D. Ventricular fibrillation occurring on arousal from sleep by auditory stimuli. Circulation 1972; 46:661–665.

404. Wennevold A, Kringelbach J. Prolonged Q-interval and cardiac syncopes. Acta Paediatr Scand 1971; 60:239–242.

405. Ratshin RA, Hunt D, Russell RO Jr, Rackley CE. QT-interval prolongation, paroxysmal ventricular arrhythmias, and convulsive syncope. Ann Intern Med 1971; 75:919–924.

406. Lisker SA, Finkelstein D. The cardio-auditory syndrome of Jervell and Lange-Nielsen: report of an additional case with radioelectrocardiographic monitoring during exercise. Am J Med Sci 1966; 252:458–464.

407. James TN. Congenital deafness and cardiac arrhythmias. Am J Cardiol 1967; 19:627–643.

408. van Bruggen HW, Sebus J, van Heyst AN. Convulsive syncope resulting from arrhythmia in a case of congenital deafness with ECG abnormalities. Am Heart J 1969; 78:81–86.

409. Sanchez Cascos A, Sanchez-Harguindey L, De Rabago P. Cardio-auditory syndromes: cardiac and genetic study of 511 deaf-mute children. Br Heart J 1969; 31:26–33.

410. Olley PM, Fowler RS. The surdo-cardiac syndrome and therapeutic observations. Br Heart J 1970; 32:467–471.

411. Furlanello F, Macca F, Dal Palu C. Observation on a case of Jervell and Lange-Neilsen syndrome in an adult. Br Heart J 1972; 34:648–652.

412. Mathews EC, Blount AW, Townsend JI. Q-T prolongation and ventricular arrhythmias, with and without deafness, in the same family. Am J Cardiol 1972; 29:702–711.

413. Behera M. Jervell and Lange-Nielsen syndrome in a middle aged patient. Postgrad Med J 1987; 63:395–396.

414. Till JA, Shinebourne EA, Pepper J, Camm AJ, Ward DE. Complete denervation of the heart in a child with congenital long QT and deafness. Am J Cardiol 1988; 62:1319–1321.

415. Holland JJ. Cardiac arrest under anaesthesia in a child with previously undiagnosed Jervell and Lange-Nielsen syndrome. Anaesthesia 1993; 48:149–151.

416. Karhunen P, Luomanmaki K, Heikkila J, Eisalo A. Syncope and Q-T prolongation without deafness: the Romano-Ward syndrome. Am Heart J 1970; 80:820–823.

417. Phillips J, Ichinose H. Clinical and pathologic studies in the hereditary syndrome of a long QT interval, syncopal spells and sudden death. Chest 1970; 58:236–243.

418. Johansson BW, Jorming B. Hereditary prolongation of QT interval. Br Heart J 1972; 34:744–751.

419. Csanady M, Kiss Z. Heritable Q-T prolongation without congenital deafness (Romano-Ward syndrome). Chest 1973; 64:359–362.

420. Kernohan RJ, Froggatt P. Atrioventricular dissociation with prolonged QT interval and syncopal attacks in a 10-year-old boy. Br Heart J 1974; 36:516–519.

421. Moothart RW, Pryor R, Hawley RL, Clifford NJ, Blount SG Jr. The heritable syndrome of prolonged Q-T interval, syncope, and sudden death: electron microscopic observation. Chest 1976; 70:263–266.

422. Curtiss EI, Heibel RH, Shaver JA. Autonomic maneuvers in hereditary Q-T interval prolongation (Romano-Ward syndrome). Am Heart J 1978; 95:420–428.

423. Sharma S, Nair KG, Gadekar HA. Romano-Ward prolonged QT syndrome with intermittent T wave alternans and atrioventricular block. Am Heart J 1981; 101:500–501.

424. Milne JR, Ward De, Spurrell RA, Camm AJ. The long QT syndrome; effects of drugs and left stellate ganglion block. Am Heart J 1982; 104:194–198.

425. Santinelli V, Chiariello M. Heart rate acceleration without changes in the QT interval and severe ventricular tachyarrhythmias: a variant of the long QT syndrome? Int J Cardiol 1983; 4:69–71.

426. Topaz O, Castellanos A, Grobman LR, Myerburg RJ. The role of arrhythmogenic auditory stimuli in sudden cardiac death. Am Heart J 1988; 116:222–226.

427. Schwartz PJ. Cardiac sympathetic innervation and the sudden infant death syndrome: a possible pathogenetic link. Am J Med 1976; 60:167–172.

428. Schwartz PJ, Segantini A. Cardiac innervation, neonatal electrocardiography, and SIDS: a key for a novel preventive strategy? Ann N Y Acad Sci 1988; 533:210–220.

429. Towbin JA, Friedman RA. Prolongation of the QT interval and the sudden infant death syndrome. N Engl J Med 1998; 338: 1760–1761.

430. Schwartz PJ, Stramba-Badiale M, Segantini A, et al.

Prolongation of the QT interval and the sudden infant death syndrome. N Engl J Med 1998; 338:1709–1714.

431. Kelly DH, Shannon DC, Liberthson RR. The role of the QT interval in the sudden infant death syndrome. Circulation 1977; 55:633–635.

432. Kukolich MK, Telsey A, Ott J, Motulsky AG. Sudden infant death syndrome: normal QT interval on ECGs of relatives. Pediatrics 1977; 60:51–54.

433. Maron BJ, Clark CE, Goldstein RE, Epstein SE. Potential role of QT interval prolongation in sudden infant death syndrome. Circulation 1976; 54:423–430.

434. Southall DP, Arrowsmith WA, Oakley JR, McEnery G, Anderson RH, Shinebourne EA. Prolonged QT interval and cardiac arrhythmias in two neonates: sudden infant death syndrome in one case. Arch Dis Child 1979; 54:776–779.

435. Pripp CM, Blomstrom P. Epiglottitis and torsade de pointes tachycardia. Br Heart J 1994; 72:205–208.

436. Weintraub RG, Gow RM, Wilkinson JL. The congenital long QT syndromes in childhood. J Am Coll Cardiol 1990; 16:674–680.

437. Bricker JT, Garson A Jr, Gillette PC. A family history of seizures associated with sudden cardiac deaths. Am J Dis Child 1984; 138:866–868.

438. Singer PA, Crampton RS, Bass NH. Familial Q-T prolongation syndrome: convulsive seizures and paroxysmal ventricular fibrillation. Arch Neurol 1974; 31:64–66.

439. Gospe SM Jr, Choy M. Hereditary long Q-T syndrome presenting as epilepsy: electroencephalography laboratory diagnosis. Ann Neurol 1989; 25:514–516.

440. Rosenbaum MB, Elizari MV, Lazzari JO. The mechanism of bidirectional tachycardia. Am Heart J 1969; 78:4–12.

441. Rothfeld EL. Bidirectional tachycardia with normal QRS duration. Am Heart J 1976; 92:231–233.

442. Locati EH, Maison-Blanche P, Dejode P, Cauchemez B, Coumel P. Spontaneous sequences of onset of torsade de pointes in patients with acquired prolonged repolarization: quantitative analysis of Holter recordings. J Am Coll Cardiol 1995; 25:1564–1575.

443. Gilmour RF Jr, Riccio ML, Locati EH, Maison-Blanche P, Coumel P, Schwartz PJ. Time- and rate-dependent alterations of the QT interval precede the onset of torsade de pointes in patients with acquired QT prolongation. J Am Coll Cardiol 1997; 30:209–217.

444. Lewis BH, Antman EM, Graboys TB. Detailed analysis of 24 hour ambulatory electrocardiographic recordings during ventricular fibrillation or torsade de pointes. J Am Coll Cardiol 1983; 2:426–436.

445. Abildskov JA, Lux RL. Mechanisms in adrenergic dependent onset of torsades de pointes. Pacing Clin Electrophysiol 1997; 20:88–94.

446. Horowitz LN, Greenspan AM, Spielman SR, Josephson ME. Torsades de pointes: electrophysiologic studies in patients without transient pharmacologic or metabolic abnormalities. Circulation 1981; 63:1120–1128.

447. Keren A, Tzivoni D, Golhman JM, Corcos P, Benhorin J, Stern S. Ventricular pacing in atypical ventricular tachycardia. J Electrocardiol 1981; 14:201–206.

448. Vincent GM. The heart rate of Romano-Ward syndrome patients. Am Heart J 1986; 112:61–64.

449. Hofbeck M, Ulmer H, Beinder E, Sieber E, Singer H. Prenatal findings in patients with prolonged QT interval in the neonatal period. Heart 1997; 77:198–204.

450. Kurita T, Ohe T, Marui N, et al. Bradycardia-induced abnormal QT prolongation in patients with complete atrioventricular block with torsades de pointes. Am J Cardiol 1992; 69:628–633.

451. Benhorin J, Merri M, Alberti M, et al. Long QT syndrome: new electrocardiographic characteristics. Circulation 1990; 82:521–527.

452. Malfatto G, Beria G, Sala S, Bonazzi O, Schwartz PJ. Quantitative analysis of T wave abnormalities and their prognostic implications in the idiopathic long QT syndrome. J Am Coll Cardiol 1994; 23:296–301.

453. Lehmann MH, Timothy KW, Frankovich D, et al. Age-gender influence on the rate-corrected QT interval and the QT-heart rate relation in families with genotypically characterized long QT syndrome. J Am Coll Cardiol 1997; 29:93–99.

454. Eggeling T, Hoeher M, Osterhues HH, Weismueller P, Hombach V. Significance of noninvasive diagnostic techniques in patients with long QT syndrome. Am J Cardiol 1992; 70:1421–1426.

455. Mitsutake A, Takeshita A, Kuroiwa A, Nakamura M. Usefulness of the Valsalva maneuver in management of the long QT syndrome. Circulation 1981; 63:1029–1035.

456. Schechter E, Freeman CC, Lazzara R. Afterdepolarizations as a mechanism for the long QT syndrome: electrophysiologic studies of a case. J Am Coll Cardiol 1984; 3:1556–1561.

457. De Ambroggi L, Negroni MS, Monza E, Bertoni T, Schwartz PJ. Dispersion of ventricular repolarization in the long QT syndrome. Am J Cardiol 1991; 68:614–620.

458. Linker NJ, Colonna P, Kekwick CA, Till J, Camm AJ, Ward DE. Assessment of QT dispersion in symptomatic patients with congenital long QT syndromes. Am J Cardiol 1992; 69:634–638.

459. Priori SG, Napolitano C, Diehl L, Schwartz PJ. Dispersion of the QT interval: a marker of therapeutic efficacy in the idiopathic long QT syndrome. Circulation 1994; 89:1681–1689.

460. Shah MJ, Wieand TS, Rhodes LA, Berul CI, Vetter VL. QT and JT dispersion in children with long QT syndrome. J Cardiovasc Electrophysiol 1997; 8:642–648.

461. Yuan S, Blomstrom-Lundqvist C, Pehrson S, Pripp CM, Wohlfart B, Olsson SB. Dispersion of repolarization following double and triple programmed stimulation: a clinical study using the monophasic action potential recording technique. Eur Heart J 1996; 17:1080–1091.

462. Day CP, McComb JM, Campbell RW. QT dispersion: an indication of arrhythmia risk in patients with long QT intervals. Br Heart J 1990; 63:342–344.

463. Sun ZH, Swan H, Viitasalo M, Toivonen L. Effects of epinephrine and phenylephrine on QT interval dispersion in congenital long QT syndrome. J Am Coll Cardiol 1998; 31:1400–1405.

464. Stramba-Badiale M, Goulene K, Schwartz PJ. Effects of beta-adrenergic blockade on dispersion of ventricular repolarization in newborn infants with prolonged QT interval. Am Heart J 1997; 134:406–410.

465. Schwartz PJ, Malliani A. Electrical alternation of the T-wave: clinical and experimental evidence of its relationship with the sympathetic nervous system and with the long Q-T syndrome. Am Heart J 1975; 89:45–50.

466. Hiejima K, Sano T. Electrical alternans of TU wave in Romano-Ward syndrome. Br Heart J 1976; 38:767–770.

467. Habbab MA, el-Sherif N. TU alternans, long QTU, and torsade de pointes: clinical and experimental observations. Pacing Clin Electrophysiol 1992; 15:916–931.

468. Vincent GM, Jaiswal D, Timothy KW. Effects of exercise on heart rate, QT, QTC and QT/QS2 in the Romano-Ward inherited long QT syndrome. Am J Cardiol 1991; 68:498–503.

469. Krahn AD, Klein GJ, Yee R. Hysteresis of the RT interval with exercise: a new marker for the long-QT syndrome? Circulation 1997; 96:1551–1556.

470. Nador F, Beria G, De Ferrari GM, et al. Unsuspected echocardiographic abnormality in the long QT syndrome: diagnostic, prognostic, and pathogenetic implications. Circulation 1991; 84:1530–1542.

471. De Ferrari GM, Nador F, Beria G, Sala S, Lotto A, Schwartz PJ. Effect of calcium channel block on the wall motion abnormality of the idiopathic long QT syndrome. Circulation 1994; 89:2126–2132.

472. Rossi L, Thiene G. Recent advances in clinicohistopathologic correlates of sudden cardiac death. Am Heart J 1981; 102:478–484.

473. James TN, Froggatt P, Atkinson WJ Jr, et al. De subitaneis mortibus. XXX. Observations on the pathophysiology of the long QT syndromes with special reference to the neuropathology of the heart. Circulation 1978; 57:1221–1231.

474. Coumel P, Leclercq JF, Lucet V. Possible mechanisms of the arrhythmias in the long QT syndrome. Eur Heart J 1985; 6:115–129.

475. Surawicz B. Electrophysiologic substrate of torsade de pointes: dispersion of repolarization or early afterdepolarizations? J Am Coll Cardiol 1989; 14:172–184.

476. Attwell D, Lee JA. A cellular basis for the primary long Q-T syndromes. Lancet 1988; 1:1136–1139.

477. Cranefield PF, Aronson RS. Torsade de pointes and other pause-induced ventricular tachycardias: the short-long-short sequence and early afterdepolarizations. Pacing Clin Electrophysiol 1988; 11:670–678.

478. Vincent GM. Hypothesis for the molecular physiology of the Romano-Ward long QT syndrome. J Am Coll Cardiol 1992; 20:500–503.

479. Surawicz B. Long QT interval, torsade de pointes, and early after depolarizations. In Surawicz B (ed). Electrophysiologic Basis of ECG and Cardiac Arrhythmias. Baltimore: Williams & Wilkins, 1995, pp. 191–229.

480. Cohen SI, Deisseroth A, Hecht HS. Infra-His bundle origin of bidirectional tachycardia. Circulation 1973; 47:1260–1266.

481. Reid DS, Tynan M, Braidwood L, Fitzgerald GR. Bidirectional tachycardia in a child: a study using His bundle electrography. Br Heart J 1975; 37:339–344.

482. Stubbs WA. Bidirectional ventricular tachycardia in familial hypokalaemic periodic paralysis. Proc R So Med 1976; 69:223–224.

483. Cohen SI, Voukydis P. Supraventricular origin of bidirectional tachycardia: report of a case. Circulation 1974; 50:634–638.

484. Gavrilescu S, Luca C. His bundle electrogram during bidirectional tachycardia. Br Heart J 1975; 37:1198–1201.

485. Gavrilescu S, Luca C, Streian C, Cristodorescu R. Bidirectional tachycardia: a study of five cases. Acta Cardiol 1976; 31:147–160.

486. Levy S, Hilaire J, Clementy J, et al. Bidirectional tachycardia: mechanism derived from intracardiac recordings and programmed electrical stimulation. Pacing Clin Electrophysiol 1982; 5:633–638.

487. Levy S, Aliot E. Bidirectional tachycardia: a new look on the mechanism. Pacing Clin Electrophysiol 1989; 12:827–834.

488. Bhandari AK, Shapiro WA, Morady F, Shen EN, Mason J, Scheinman MM. Electrophysiologic testing in patients with the long QT syndrome. Circulation 1985; 71:63–71.

489. Hartzler GO, Osborn MJ. Invasive electrophysiological study in the Jervell and Lange-Nielsen syndrome. Bri Heart J 1981; 45:225–229.

490. Vassallo JA, Cassidy DM, Kindwall E, Marchlinski FE, Josephson ME. Nonuniform recovery of excitability in the left ventricle. Circulation 1988; 78:1365–1372.

491. Evans TR, Curry PV, Fitchett DH, Krikler DM. "Torsade de pointes" initiated by electrical ventricular stimulation. J Electrocardiol 1976; 9:255–258.

492. Gavrilescu S, Luca C. Right ventricular monophasic action potentials in patients with long QT syndrome. Br Heart J 1978; 40:1014–1018.

493. Shimizu W, Ohe T, Kurita T, et al. Early after depolarizations induced by isoproterenol in patients with congenital long QT syndrome. Circulation 1991; 84:1915–1923.

494. Shimizu W, Ohe T, Kurita T, et al. Effects of verapamil and propranolol on early after depolarizations and ventricular arrhythmias induced by epinephrine in congenital long QT syndrome. J Am Coll Cardiol 1995; 26:1299–1309.

495. Hirao H, Shimizu W, Kurita T, et al. Frequency-dependent electrophysiologic properties of ventricular repolarization in patients with congenital long QT syndrome. J Am Coll Cardiol 1996; 28:1269–1277.

496. Shimizu W, Kamakura S, Kurita T, Suyama K, Aihara N, Shimomura K. Influence of epinephrine, propranolol, and atrial pacing on spatial distribution of recovery time measured by body surface mapping in congenital long QT syndrome. J Cardiovasc Electrophysiol 1997; 8:1102–1114.

497. Bonatti V, Rolli A, Botti G. Recording of monophasic action potentials of the right ventricle in long QT syndromes complicated by severe ventricular arrhythmias. Eur Heart J 1983; 4:168–179.

498. Bhandari AK, Scheinman MM, Morady F, Svinarich J, Mason J, Winkle R. Efficacy of left cardiac sympathectomy in the treatment of patients with the long QT syndrome. Circulation 1984; 70:1018–1023.

499. Crampton R. Preeminence of the left stellate ganglion in the long Q-T syndrome. Circulation 1979; 59:769–778.

500. Shimizu W, Kurita T, Matsuo K, Suyama K, Aihara N, Kamakura S, et al. Improvement of repolarization abnormalities by a K+ channel opener in the LQT1 form of congenital long-QT syndrome. Circulation 1998; 97:1581–1588.

501. Locati EH, Schwartz PJ. The idiopathic long QT syndrome: therapeutic management. Pacing Clin Electrophysiol 1992; 15:1374–1379.

502. Moss AJ. Clinical management of patients with the long QT syndrome: drugs, devices, and gene-specific therapy. Pacing Clin Electrophysiol 1997; 20:2058–2060.

503. Moss AJ. Management of patients with the hereditary long QT syndrome. J Cardiovasc Electrophysiol 1998; 9:668–674.

504. Banai S, Tzivoni D. Drug therapy for torsade de pointes. J Cardiovasc Electrophysiol 1993; 4:206–210.

505. Kowey PR, Marinchak RA, Rials SJ, Rubin AM, Smith L. Electrophysiologic testing in patients who respond acutely to intravenous amiodarone for incessant ventricular tachyarrhythmias. Am Heart J 1993; 125:1628–1632.

506. Bashour T, Jokhadar M, Cheng TO. Effective management of the long Q-T syndrome with amiodarone. Chest 1981; 79:704–706.

507. Eldar M, Griffin JC, Abbott JA, et al. Permanent cardiac pacing in patients with the long QT syndrome. J Am Coll Cardiol 1987; 10:600–607.

508. Noh CI, Song JY, Kim HS, Choi JY, Yun YS. Ventricular tachycardia and exercise related syncope in children with structurally normal hearts: emphasis on repolarisation abnormality. Br Heart J 1995; 73:544–547.

509. Shah A, Schwartz H. Mexiletine for treatment of torsade de pointes. Am Heart J 1984; 107:589–591.

510. Bansal AM, Kugler JD, Pinsky WW, Norberg WJ, Frank WE. Torsade de pointes: successful acute control by lidocaine and chronic control by tocainide in two patients—one each with acquired long QT and the congenital long QT syndrome. Am Heart J 1986; 112:618–621.

511. Keren A, Tzivoni D. Magnesium therapy in ventricular arrhythmias. Pacing Clin Electrophysiol 1990; 13:937–945.

512. Perticone F, Adinolfi L, Bonaduce D. Efficacy of magnesium sulfate in the treatment of torsade de pointes. Am Heart J 1986; 112:847–849.

513. Tzivoni D, Banai S, Schuger C, Benhorin J, Keren A, Gottlieb S, et al. Treatment of torsade de pointes with magnesium sulfate. Circulation 1988; 77:392–397.

514. Compton SJ, Lux RL, Ramsey MR, et al. Genetically defined therapy of inherited long-QT syndrome: correction of abnormal repolarization by potassium. Circulation 1996; 94:1018–1022.

515. Choy AM, Lang CC, Chomsky DM, Rayos GH, Wilson JR, Roden DM. Normalization of acquired QT prolongation in humans by intravenous potassium. Circulation 1997; 96:2149–2154.

516. DeSilvey DL, Moss AJ. Primidone in the treatment of the long QT syndrome: QT shortening and ventricular arrhythmia suppression. Ann Intern Med 1980; 93:53–54.

517. Glikson M, Hayes DL, Nishimura RA. Newer clinical applications of pacing. J Cardiovasc Electrophysiol 1997; 8:1190–1203.

518. Lyon LJ, Donoso E, Friedberg CK. Temporary control of ventricular arrhythmias by drug-induced sinus tachycardia. Arch Intern Med 1969; 123:436–438.

519. Moss AJ, Liu JE, Gottlieb S, Locati EH, Schwartz PJ, Robinson JL. Efficacy of permanent pacing in the management of high-risk patients with long QT syndrome. Circulation 1991; 84:1524–1529.

520. Rubeiz GA, El-Hajj M, Touma A. Successful use of external electrical cardioversion in the treatment of ventricular fibrillation caused by quinidine. Am J Cardiol 1965; 16:118–121.

521. Schwartz PJ. The rationale and the role of left stellectomy for the prevention of malignant arrhythmias. Ann N Y Acad Sci 1984; 427:199–221.

522. Schwartz PJ, Zaza A. The rational basis and the clinical value

of selective cardiac sympathetic denervation in the prevention of malignant arrhythmias. Eur Heart J 1986; 7:107–118.

523. Moss AJ, McDonald J. Unilateral cervicothoracic sympathetic ganglionectomy for the treatment of long QT interval syndrome. N Engl J Med 1971; 285:903–904.

524. Packer DL, Coltorti F, Smith MS, et al. Sudden death after left stellectomy in the long QT syndrome. Am J Cardiol 1984; 54:1365–1366.

525. Malfatto G, Rosen MR, Foresti A, Schwartz PJ. Idiopathic long QT syndrome exacerbated by beta-adrenergic blockade and responsive to left cardiac sympathetic denervation: implications regarding electrophysiologic substrate and adrenergic modulation. J Cardiovasc Electrophysiol 1992; 3:295–305.

526. Ouriel K, Moss AJ. Long QT syndrome: an indication for cervicothoracic sympathectomy. Cardiovasc Surg 1995; 3:475–478.

527. Crampton RS. Another link between the left stellate ganglion and the long Q-T syndrome. Am Heart J 1978; 96:130–132.

528. Gardner MJ, Kimber S, Johnstone DE, et al. The effects of unilateral stellate ganglion blockade on human cardiac function during rest and exercise. J Cardiovasc Electrophysiol 1993; 4:2–8.

529. Wong CW, Wang CH, Wen MS, Yeh SJ, Wu D. Effective therapy with transthoracic video-assisted endoscopic coagulation of the left stellate ganglion and upper sympathetic trunk in congenital long-QT syndrome. Am Heart J 1996; 132:1060–1063.

530. Platia EV, Griffith LS, Watkins L, Mirowski M, Mower MM, Reid PR. Management of the prolonged QT syndrome and recurrent ventricular fibrillation with an implantable automatic cardioverter-defibrillator. Clin Cardiol 1985; 8:490–493.

531. Morganroth J, Goin JE. Quinidine-related mortality in the short-to-medium-term treatment of ventricular arrhythmias: a meta-analysis. Circulation 1991; 84:1977–1983.

532. Torres V, Flowers D, Somberg J. The clinical significance of polymorphic ventricular tachycardia provoked at electrophysiologic testing. Am Heart J 1985; 110:17–24.

533. Wyse DG, Morganroth J, Ledingham R, et al. New insights into the definition and meaning of proarrhythmia during initiation of antiarrhythmic drug therapy from the Cardiac Arrhythmia Suppression Trial and its pilot study: the CAST and CAPS investigators. J Am Coll Cardiol 1994; 23:1130–1140.

534. Wellens HJJ. Personal communication, 1997.

14

Ventricular Fibrillation[1-25a]

The treatment of few arrhythmias has been so affected by the computer and by miniaturization, that great spin-off from the space program, than that of ventricular fibrillation. Almost always fatal until the introduction of the external defibrillator and now preventable with the implantable cardioverter-defibrillator, ventricular fibrillation can finally take its place among the treatable and preventable arrhythmias. Only unawareness of how to treat and limited financial resources prevent application of proper therapy to those patients whose risk of ventricular fibrillation is known to be high.

The contemporary story of ventricular fibrillation begins with the development of a practical method of external defibrillation in the mid 1950s.[26, 27] Then came the cardiac or coronary care unit,[28, 29] effective techniques of cardiac resuscitation,[30-32] and efficient electrocardiographic monitoring,[33] allowing the arrhythmia to be recognized early and its precursors to be identified and suppressed.[34] Other developments increasing the chances of survival from ventricular fibrillation include special ambulances,[35] staffed by trained medical and paramedical personnel equipped with devices such as automated external defibrillator-pacemakers,[36-55] and cardiac resuscitation performed by members of the public who witness cardiac arrest.[36, 43, 44, 47-49, 56-63]

One is only certain that ventricular fibrillation has produced cardiac arrest if the event occurs when the patient is being monitored electrocardiographically in a hospital unit, is wearing an ambulatory recorder, or has an implantable cardioverter-defibrillator with memory capability, circumstances that are seldom present. Consequently, much of our understanding of the prevalence of ventricular fibrillation and the likelihood of its occurring are based on other data from patients who die suddenly.[9, 10, 64, 65b] The records we do have, however, suggest that most, although not all, cardiac arrests in adults are due to tachyarrhythmias, and the terminal arrhythmia is usually ventricular fibrillation.[66-89] The cause of the infrequent instances of cardiac arrest recorded in children, however, is more frequently asystole.[90]

Our hope that antiarrhythmic drugs would prevent ventricular fibrillation in susceptible patients was dashed in 1989, by the Cardiac Arrhythmia Suppression Trial (CAST),[91-95c] but, most fortunately, the implantable cardioverter-defibrillator was then available and has become the definitive method of preventing cardiac arrest due to ventricular fibrillation.

SOME ADVANCES SINCE THE FIRST EDITION OF THIS BOOK

- Definition of patients at risk of sudden unexplained death, including those with Brugada's syndrome.
- Better understanding of the circadian pattern of ventricular fibrillation, thanks to study of the memory capabilities of implantable cardioverter-defibrillators.
- Data suggesting that sudden death following trauma to the chest in healthy young people may be due to ventricular fibrillation started when the ventricles are struck during their vulnerable period of repolarization.
- QT dispersion helps to select who may develop cardiac arrest due to ventricular fibrillation.
- Increasing information that hearts are not

---

[a]This chapter contains material from Chapter 17, "Ventricular Fibrillation," by Robert J. Myerburg and Kenneth M. Kessler,[1] in the first edition of this book.

[b]Data collected from implantable cardioverter-defibrillators in patients who die suddenly of cardiac disease, however, reveal that mechanisms other than ventricular tachyarrhythmia may be the cause.[65] The correct diagnosis often hinges on the definition of sudden death,[9, 10] which ranges from instantaneous to within 1 hour after the onset of symptoms.[64]

[c]CAST established that suppressing ventricular premature beats with antiarrhythmic drugs in asymptomatic or mildly symptomatic patients with mild or moderate ventricular dysfunction after myocardial infarction does not prolong, and may reduce, survival.[91-95]

"normal" in patients with ventricular fibrillation who have no structural heart disease (idiopathic ventricular fibrillation).

- Value of portable automatic defibrillators for use by lay workers who encounter patients with cardiac arrest.
- Greater understanding of which patients at risk of ventricular fibrillation should receive implantable cardioverter-defibrillators.

PREVALENCE[3, 7, 16, 17, 96–102]

When patients die of heart disease, more than half die outside the hospital,[103] and at least 80% die suddenly.[64, 65, 104, 105] Patients succumbing to atherosclerotic coronary heart disease die suddenly three times more often than from acute myocardial infarction.[106] However, study of risk factors does not distinguish who will die suddenly from who will die more slowly.[107]

Although the proximate event is undocumented in most cases, records from ambulatory electrocardiographic monitors or electrogram-storing implantable cardioverter-defibrillators in patients with cardiac arrest reveal that ventricular fibrillation, often preceded by ventricular tachycardia, is the most frequent cause.[78, 82, 84, 101, 108–114] However, by the time rescue squads reach such patients and take electrocardiograms, cardiac standstill has often replaced ventricular fibrillation.[115, 116d]

In hospitalized patients, ventricular fibrillation is less frequently the final cardiac rhythm. Adults and children with poor hemodynamic function and noncardiac terminal illnesses such as pulmonary disease, sepsis, and cancer die more often of bradyarrhythmias, asystole, or electromechanical dissociation.[100, 117–119]

AGE

Sudden death is rare among children and adolescents,[120e] only occasionally resulting from cardiac disease,[121] and uncommon in healthy, young subjects[122] under the age of 45 years.[112] The incidence subsequently doubles with each decade.[100] The *proportion* of deaths that are sudden, however, decreases with age.[112f] The younger the patient, the more likely it is ventricular fibrillation rather than electromechanical dissociation will be the mechanism of cardiac arrest.[123g]

GENDER[124–126]

Sudden death due to coronary heart disease is predominantly a male affliction.[98, 112, 127–131] In the fourth

and fifth decades of life, the male-to-female ratio is 5 to 7:1, in the sixth decade 2:1.[98] Women must be 20 years older before their incidence approaches that of men.[100] Women who suffer cardiac arrest are less likely than men to have coronary heart disease and more likely to have other forms of, or no, structural heart disease.[132]

RACE[133, 134]

Black men and women are more likely than white men and women to die out of hospital of myocardial infarction,[135] often, presumably, with ventricular fibrillation.[h]

SOCIAL AND ECONOMIC FACTORS

Most patients who die suddenly are awake (88%), many are active (42%), and few are asleep (8.5%).[72i] Most are at home.[128, 136] Cardiac arrest occurs in about three-fourths of survivors of out-of-hospital cardiac arrest while performing low-level activity and in one-fourth during exertion.[137]

Certain socioeconomic factors, many of which also increase the risk of coronary heart disease, raise the likelihood of dying suddenly:[100]

- Cigarette smokers[98, 104, 128, 129, 138] with coronary heart disease, aged 39 to 59 years, who are two to three times more likely to die suddenly than nonsmokers. The risk of dying increases from 19% to 37% in patients who survive out-of-hospital ventricular fibrillation and continue to smoke.
- High levels of physical activity.[98, 139–141]
- Lower educational accomplishments,[142, 143] the risk of sudden cardiac death being three times greater in men with complex ventricular premature beats who have had 8 or less years of schooling than in those with similar arrhythmias who are better educated.[144]
- Obesity.[98, 104, 145, 146j]
- Recent "life-change events."[147]
- Type A personality, possibly.[148]
- Women who are single,[129, 149] have fewer children,[149] an educational discrepancy with their spouse,[149] a history of psychiatric treatment,[149] increased alcohol consumption,[149] and greater cigarette smoking.[129, 149]

CLINICAL SETTING[125, 150, 151]

Primary versus Secondary Ventricular Fibrillation

Primary ventricular fibrillation develops from specific electrophysiological abnormalities in the absence of

---

[d]Thirty-two percent in one study;[116] 72% in another.[115]

[e]1.3 per 100,000 patient-years in subjects aged 3 to 10 years (median, 13 years).[120] Of 12 children and adolescents who died suddenly in Olmsted County, Minnesota, the cause in 7 was definitely or probably cardiac.[120]

[f]Ranging from 75% in 35- to 44-year-old black men to 47% in 65- to 74-year-old white women in a study in 40 states from 1980 to 1985 in which sudden cardiac death was defined as occurring out of hospital or in emergency departments.[112]

[g]Ventricular fibrillation caused cardiac arrest in 83% of 102 patients less than 70 years of age but in only 71% in those more than 70 years of age in one study.[123]

---

[h]Death is sudden among patients aged 55 to 65 years in[112]
- Sixty-six percent of black men.
- Sixty-one percent of white men.
- Fifty-six percent of black women.
- Half of white women.

[i]From a study of 142 deaths in 1,020 men aged 40 to 65 years who were observed for 5 years with frequent examinations and 24-hour electrocardiographic recordings.[72]

[j]Hippocrates is reputed to have observed: "Sudden death is more common in those who are naturally fat than in the lean."[145]

hemodynamic factors of sufficient severity to initiate the arrhythmia. *Secondary* or *complicating* ventricular fibrillation results from myocardial damage sufficient to produce congestive heart failure.[152–154k]

More than half of patients dying of cardiac disease suffer an arrhythmic death—sudden collapse with the pulse stopping without prior circulatory failure. Fewer die in circulatory failure—the pulse ceasing after the circulation has failed.[105l]

Patients with Out-of-Hospital Ventricular Fibrillation

Ventricular fibrillation or ventricular tachycardia recurs in about half of patients admitted to the hospital after out-of-hospital ventricular fibrillation.[155] Congestive heart failure, cardiogenic shock, and pulmonary problems are frequent complications.[155]

Coronary Heart Disease[98, 104]

Coronary heart disease due to atherosclerosis is the underlying pathological process in most people with cardiac arrest.[104, 115, 131, 156–166] Many have had previous myocardial infarctions, even though some have no symptoms of heart disease[72, 104, 167–169] (Table 14.1), and many have not previously sought medical attention for heart disease.[170] About half of survivors of cardiac arrest, according to one angiographic study, have acute coronary occlusion.[166]

Characteristic of patients with coronary heart disease who die of, rather than survive, cardiac arrest are[171]

- Three-vessel disease.
- Left bundle branch block.
- Moderate or severe mitral regurgitation.

---

[k]Most investigators include, but some do not[154] include, its occurrence during cardiogenic shock[153] or as a terminal arrhythmia within their definition of secondary ventricular fibrillation.

[l]Of 142 deaths, 58% were primarily arrhythmic, and 42% were primarily circulatory.[105]

- Previous myocardial infarctions.
- Reduced left ventricular function as shown by abnormal ventricular contraction, cardiac index less than 2.5 liters/minute/meter,[2] and left ventricular end-diastolic pressure greater than 18 millimeters of mercury.

Angina.[172] Although some survivors of cardiac arrest have angina,[173] only occasionally does the episode occur during an anginal attack.[174, 175] However, patients with coronary heart disease who die suddenly have more angina than those without cardiac arrest.[171] The ischemia of survivors of ventricular fibrillation who have coronary heart disease is frequently silent.[86, 176–180m]

Ventricular fibrillation and cardiac arrest sometimes complicate paroxysms of Prinzmetal's angina variant due to coronary vasospasm.[181–199] Although it usually occurs during chest pain, ventricular fibrillation may develop in the absence of pain[200] and occasionally after relief of pain (Fig. 14.1), during the period of early reperfusion.[190, 198, 201]

Myocardial infarction (Fig. 14.2).[202–214] Ventricular fibrillation was documented in as many as 19% of patients with acute myocardial infarction in the late 1960s and early 1970s.[215, 216n] Its incidence, however, decreased throughout the 1970s,[217] from 1980 to 1985,[112] and thereafter with such advances in the treatment of acute myocardial infarction as coronary care units and then aspirin, beta-adrenergic–blocking drugs, intravenous nitrates, acute angioplasty, and

---

[m]Only 1 (6%) of 16 patients with coronary heart disease, ventricular fibrillation, and a positive treadmill stress test or radionuclide ventriculogram had painful ischemia.[179]

[n]Nineteen percent includes episodes of ventricular fibrillation occurring in mobile coronary care unit ambulances.[215] Eight percent of patients with myocardial infarction who were transported by helicopters sustained ventricular fibrillation before takeoff in one study.[216]

Table 14.1 CLINICAL FEATURES OF 142 PATIENTS WITH CORONARY HEART DISEASE WHO WERE SUCCESSFULLY RESUSCITATED FROM CARDIAC ARREST[167]

Patients and Clinical Features	Acute Myocardial Infarction	Ischemic Event	Primary Arrhythmia
How Defined	*New Q Waves*	*ST Segment and T-wave Changes, Diagnostic Enzyme Elevations*	*Insignificant ST Segment or T-wave Changes, No Diagnostic Enzyme Elevations*
142 patients	62 (44%)	49 (34%)	31 (22%)
Cardiac arrest as the first cardiac event	35%	16%	6%
Previous myocardial infarction	27%	55%	71%
Taking digitalis	10%	31%	55%
Prodromal symptoms	78%	57%	73%
Chest pain	56%	22%	40%
Dyspnea	34%	27%	37%
Indigestion	30%	13%	0
Syncope	12%	7%	25%

(From Goldstein S, Landis JR, Leighton R, et al. Characteristics of the resuscitated out-of-hospital cardiac arrest victim with coronary heart disease. Circulation 1981; 64:977–984. By permission of the American Heart Association, Inc.)

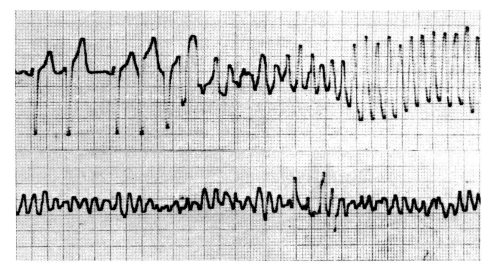

FIGURE 14.1 Ventricular fibrillation developing after relief of Prinzmetal's angina. (Adapted from Tzivoni D, Keren A, Granot H, Gottlieb S, Benhorin J, Stern S. Ventricular fibrillation caused by myocardial reperfusion in Prinzmetal's angina. Am Heart J 1983; 105:323–325, with permission.)[201]

thrombolysis (Fig. 14.3).[218–225][o] About half of survivors of cardiac arrest sustain myocardial infarction.[178, 226]

Occurrence. Ventricular fibrillation occurs most often during the first hour after the onset of symptoms.[215] For example, among 284 patients with confirmed myocardial infarction treated in a mobile coronary care unit,[215] ventricular fibrillation developed in:

• Twenty-eight (10%) during the first hour.
• Twelve (4%) during the second hour.
• Two (1%) during the third and fourth hours.

In the hospital, the incidence of ventricular fibrillation is highest soon after admission,[227, 228] specifically

• Three percent during the first day.[229]
• From 3% to 4% while in the coronary care unit.[230]
• All instances of primary ventricular fibrillation within the first 3 days.[231][p]

---

[o]Although not all agree.[225]

[p]Some episodes of *secondary* ventricular fibrillation occurred later,[231] according to one series of 74 patients with ventricular fibrillation (68 patients) or ventricular tachycardia (six patients) requiring resuscitation.[231]

• Between 5% and 6% during the course of the hospitalization.[152, 215, 232–238][q]

Secondary ventricular fibrillation develops in 2% to 3% of patients with myocardial infarction.[154][r]

Factors affecting incidence. Ventricular fibrillation and cardiac arrest more often occur during myocardial infarction in younger patients,[232] particularly those less than 65 years of age,[239] and in those who have the following:

• History or presence of left ventricular failure.[221, 240–243]
• Anterior[152, 237, 240, 242, 244–246][s] or right ventricular infarctions.[247]
• Atrial fibrillation.[222]
• Atrioventricular block.[222]
• Bundle branch block.[245, 248]

---

[q]This incidence is not much different from 4.5% (range, 2% to 10%) among 2,651 hospitalized patients from nine series reported in the 1960s and early 1970s when coronary care units and continuous electrocardiographic monitoring were being developed.[152, 232–238, 251]

[r]One hundred forty-two (2.4%) of 5,839 patients with myocardial infarction.[154]

[s]Some reports disagree on this point.[152, 237, 246]

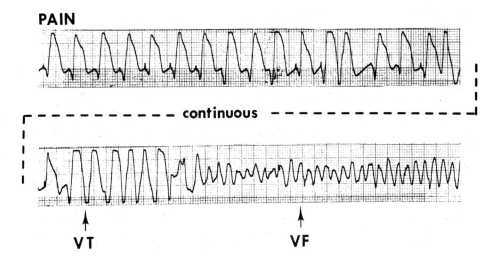

FIGURE 14.2 Ventricular fibrillation produced by myocardial infarction. The ST segments are greatly elevated during chest pain (**top**) in this patient with an acute myocardial infarction. Ventricular tachycardia (VT) develops (**bottom,** *left*) and is followed by ventricular fibrillation (VF) (**bottom,** *right*).

PAIN

continuous

V T   VF

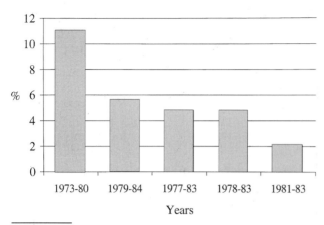

FIGURE 14.3 The incidence of primary ventricular fibrillation during myocardial infarction in hospitalized patients (%) decreased from 1973 to 1983. Meta-analysis indicates that in patients not given prophylactic lidocaine the incidence of primary ventricular fibrillation during myocardial infarction may be even lower—4.51% in 1970 and 0.35% in 1990. (Adapted from Antman EM, Berlin JA. Declining incidence of ventricular fibrillation in myocardial infarction: implications for the prophylactic use of lidocaine. Circulation 1992; 86:764–773, by permission of the American Heart Association, Inc.)[223]

- Higher levels of serum aspartic transaminase,[249] creatinine phosphokinase,[221] alpha-hydroxybutyrate dehydrogenase,[250] glutamic oxaloacetic transaminase,[222, 251] or lactic dehydrogenase.[222, 252]
- More diseased coronary arteries seen in coronary arteriography.[253]
- Persistent sinus tachycardia.[240]

Reports differ on whether ventricular fibrillation develops more often in men or in women with acute myocardial infarction.[254, 255]

The younger the patients, the more frequently will they sustain primary ventricular fibrillation during myocardial infarction[152, 232, 244, 256] or will myocardial infarction be the cause of cardiac arrest from which they have been resuscitated.[167] The infarction that develops in those patients successfully resuscitated from cardiac arrest is more often anterior than inferior.[115]

Thrombolytic treatment does not remove[239] or affect the risk of[229] sustaining ventricular fibrillation during the first hours of a myocardial infarction, but it does reduce the occurrence of the arrhythmia throughout the hospital course.[229t] Furthermore, successful reperfusion in normotensive patients without heart failure during myocardial infarction does not produce ventricular fibrillation or ventricular tachycardia ("reperfusion arrhythmias").[257]

Recurrence. Ventricular fibrillation recurs more frequently in patients with

- Acute ischemic episodes rather than myocardial infarction.
- Reduced left ventricular ejection fraction.[162, 258, 259]

- Secondary, rather than primary, ventricular fibrillation.[260, 261]
- Severe abnormalities of left ventricular contraction.[162, 262u]
- Severe triple-vessel disease.[162]

Ventricular fibrillation during the acute phase of myocardial infarction does not predict its recurrence during early convalescence.[263] Furthermore, recurrence of ventricular fibrillation during myocardial infarction is *not* related to[260, 261]

- Adequacy of initial resuscitation.
- Age.
- Delay before initial attempted defibrillation.
- Place of cardiac arrest.
- Previous myocardial infarction.
- Sex.
- Site of infarction.
- Time from onset of symptoms to initial cardiac arrest.

Coronary disease not due to atherosclerosis. Ischemia and myocardial damage from coronary disease other than atherosclerosis can produce cardiac arrest and ventricular fibrillation in patients with such lesions as

- Coronary emboli.[264]
- Coronary ostial stenosis.[265, 266]
- Dissection of the coronary arteries with or without aortic dissection in Marfan syndrome[267] or after delivery.[268]
- Inflammation from Kawasaki disease (mucocutaneous lymph node syndrome),[269–271] polyarteritis nodosa, and other vascular syndromes.[272]
- Intussusception of a coronary artery.[273]

Congenital anomalies of the coronary arteries.[274–276] These anomalies are associated with an increased risk of cardiac arrest, presumably because of ventricular fibrillation.[266, 267, 270, 277–282v]

Hypertension[98, 283–289]

Hypertension increases the risk of dying suddenly.[138, 283] The annual rate of sudden death rises progressively with the blood pressure. Men with systolic blood pressure of 160 millimeters of mercury or more have three times the incidence of sudden death than men with blood pressure lower than 140 millimeters of mercury.[104] Even in patients whose hypertension has been treated, electrocardiographic evidence of left ventricular hypertrophy,[290] myocardial injury,[290] or QT prolongation[290] predicts a higher risk of cardiac arrest.

---

[t]From a meta-analysis, published in 1993, of more than 20,000 patients collected from 15 series.[229]

[u]Patients with two separate areas of infarction are more likely to have cardiac arrest than ventricular tachycardia.[262]
[v]Thirty-two percent of deaths among 242 patients with isolated congenital coronary artery anomalies were sudden.[281] In 96 children with myocardial infarction, many of whom had anomalies of the coronary arteries, ventricular fibrillation developed in eight.[288]

Valvular Heart Disease

Patients with severe, uncorrected valvular aortic stenosis frequently die suddenly.[291–294w] Although aortic valve replacement has diminished the risk of sudden death, cardiac arrest—after cardiac failure, the second most common mode of death[295]—still accounts for about one-fifth of deaths after aortic or mitral valve replacement.[295]

Mitral valve prolapse.[296–298] Although mitral valve prolapse is frequently associated with ventricular arrhythmias, patients with this common condition seldom die suddenly.[299–307] Furthermore, despite the absence of another obvious cause, one should not assume that when a patient dies suddenly, mitral valve prolapse is the culprit.[298, 308] The few who die without other recognized conditions are usually young,[309] female, and without mitral regurgitation or ruptured chordae tendineae.[310] ST segment and T-wave abnormalities in the electrocardiogram[305] and mitral valve redundancy in the echocardiogram[311] may predict higher risk.

Congenital Heart Disease[276, 312]

Congenital heart disease accounts for about half of the cases of fatal cardiac arrest due to cardiac disease in young soldiers.[313] The principal congenital lesions producing cardiac arrest in young patients are

- Aortic stenosis.[314–317]
- Anomalous origin of the coronary arteries.[316, 317]
- Ebstein's disease.[316–318x]
- Eisenmenger syndrome (intra- or extracardiac shunt with pulmonary hypertension).[315–317, 319]
- Sinus of Valsalva aneurysm.[315–317]
- Tetralogy of Fallot.[316, 317, 320]
- Vena caval–left atrial communication.[316, 317]

After surgical correction of congenital lesions, cardiac arrest, either from ventricular fibrillation or a bradyarrhythmia, occurs in a few patients, particularly those with[312, 316]

- Atrioventricular canal and ventricular septal defect.
- Complete transposition of the great vessels.
- Tetralogy of Fallot.

---

[w]An autopsy study published in 1968 reported that 44 (73%) of 60 patients with unrepaired aortic stenosis had died suddenly.[292]

T. Bonet wrote in 1679: "A Parisian tailor . . . full-blooded and inclined to obesity and not yet old, having dined and left his house had walked hardly 40 paces when he suddenly fell to the ground and expired. Carried back to his house, his body was opened, and no disease was found anywhere except that the 3 semilunar cusps, situated at the entrance to the aorta from the left ventricle were discovered to be bony; I received 1 of these as a gift and found it of whitish color and so hard that it could hardly be incised with a knife" (translated by Paul D. White).[291]

[x]Physical stimulation of the atrialized ventricle in patients with Ebstein's disease may induce ventricular tachycardia and ventricular fibrillation. Before these arrhythmias could be effectively treated, cardiac catheterization could be fatal. In the third edition of his cardiology text (1968), Paul Wood warned: "I have catheterized eight cases of Ebstein's disease, but do not propose to catheterize another wittingly."[318]

Patients with congenital complete atrioventricular block also sustain cardiac arrest, and the mechanism may, in some cases, be ventricular fibrillation.

Cardiomyopathy[276, 321–325] **and Myocarditis**

Death is sudden in 28% of patients with dilated cardiomyopathy.[323y] However, cardiac arrest is unusual in children with dilated cardiomyopathy,[326] except in those with the familial variety.[327]

Hypertrophic cardiomyopathy.[328–334] From 2% to 3% of adults with hypertrophic cardiomyopathy die suddenly each year.[335] In the young,[271, 315] the annual mortality from sudden death is approximately 6%.[335] Most fatalities among patients with hypertrophic cardiomyopathy occur suddenly and unexpectedly[336, 337] (Table 14.2).[z]

Most patients with hypertrophic cardiomyopathy who die suddenly or who are resuscitated from cardiac arrest have had no functional limitations.[338] Those who die suddenly during or immediately after strenuous activity—a common setting for sudden death among patients with hypertrophic cardiomyopathy[336, 339]—tend to be younger than 30 years of age, whereas older patients more likely have cardiac arrest during mild activities or while resting or asleep.[337] Abnormal genetic mutations identify patients with familial hypertrophic cardiomyopathy who are at particularly high risk of sudden death.[340, 341]

A few patients with hypertrophic cardiomyopathy also have accessory pathways and the Wolff-Parkinson-White syndrome. Ventricular fibrillation in these patients may be due to rapid conduction in the accessory

---

[y]From an analysis of the data on 1,432 patients with idiopathic dilated cardiomyopathy collected in 14 studies.[323]

[z]Sixty-eight percent of cardiac deaths among 314 patients with hypertrophic cardiomyopathy.[337]

Table 14.2 RISK OF SUDDEN DEATH IN PATIENTS WITH HYPERTROPHIC CARDIOMYOPATHY

Characteristics	High	Low
Family history of hypertrophic cardiomyopathy	Yes	No
Age	<30 years	≥30 years
Previous episode of cardiac arrest	Yes	No
Onset of symptoms	In childhood	Later
Symptoms	Moderate or severe	None or slight
Left atrium	Marked enlargement	—
Left ventricular hypertrophy	Severe	—
Left ventricular outflow tract gradient	Large	—
Response to exercise test	Hypotension	Normal

(Data from references 122, 334, 337, 376, and 803.)

pathway from atrial fibrillation or atrial flutter rather than from the cardiomyopathy itself.[342, 343]

Myocarditis.[131, 165, 266, 344–347] This condition is a leading cardiac diagnosis in children and adolescents who die suddenly.[282, 348] Myocarditis was the second most common cardiac cause of fatal cardiac arrest, exceeded only by congenital heart disease, among a group of Israeli soldiers.[313]

The etiologic factors associated with myocarditis and ventricular fibrillation include

- Chagas disease.[349]
- Coxsackie viral infection.[350]
- Diphtheria.[351]
- Human immunodeficiency virus.[352]
- Lymphocytic infiltration.[353]

Miscellaneous conditions. Other less common types of cardiomyopathy that can also produce cardiac arrest, presumably, from ventricular fibrillation include

- Amyloid heart disease.[354, 355]
- Arrhythmogenic right ventricular dysplasia.[356–364aa]
- Morbid obesity, the cardiomyopathy of which is the most frequent cause of sudden death in patients with this affliction.[146]
- Sarcoid heart disease.[365]

Congestive Heart Failure[366–369]

The death of 40% to 50% of patients with congestive heart failure is sudden.[370bb] Congestive heart failure increases the risk of dying suddenly[371] five fold[370bb] over that of the general population. In the presence of coronary heart disease, the likelihood is doubled further.[370] The risk of sudden death remains high in those with severe congestive heart failure even when they are well treated with vasodilators and diuretics.[372]

More men than women with congestive heart failure die suddenly.[370] Patients older than 70 years who have cardiac arrest are more likely than younger subjects to have a history of congestive heart failure.[116]

Left Ventricular Hypertrophy[98, 286, 287, 373–375]

Left ventricular hypertrophy is an independent risk factor for sudden death.[373] Marked left ventricular hypertrophy increases the likelihood of cardiac arrest in patients with hypertrophic cardiomyopathy.[376]

Cardiac Surgery

Ventricular fibrillation or polymorphic ventricular tachycardia occasionally develops for the first time in patients who have had recent coronary artery bypass graft surgery.[377–382] Many have had an acute myocardial infarction within 2 weeks before the operation.[383]

Supraventricular Tachyarrhythmias and Wolff-Parkinson-White Syndrome[384, 385]

About 2% of patients with Wolff-Parkinson-White syndrome referred to a center specializing in arrhythmias and clinical electrophysiology have been resuscitated from cardiac arrest.[386cc] Characteristically,

- Most are men.
- Two-thirds are exercising or under emotional stress when cardiac arrest occurs.
- In half, ventricular fibrillation is the first manifestation of Wolff-Parkinson-White syndrome.[386]

Supraventricular tachyarrhythmias, including a rapid response to atrial fibrillation[387] with and without the Wolff-Parkinson-White syndrome, was the cause of cardiac arrest from ventricular fibrillation in 5% of 290 patients evaluated for "aborted sudden death" at one center.[388] The incidence of sudden death is higher when patients have had atrial fibrillation.[389dd]

Whether a child with Wolff-Parkinson-White syndrome will have cardiac arrest does not depend on age, duration of symptoms, incidence of congenital heart disease, presence of multiple pathways, or the location of the accessory pathway.[390]

Neuropsychiatric Influences[391–395]

Severe environmental stress can trigger cardiac arrest.[396–398ee] Sudden death also occurs more often in patients who have recently sustained stressful changes in health, work, home, or family[147, 391, 394, 399–403ff] and in male survivors of myocardial infarction with high levels of stress and social isolation.[143]

Auditory stimuli.[404] A 14-year-old girl fainted repeatedly from what was then (1972) called "spontaneously reversible ventricular fibrillation"[405gg] on being awakened from sleep by the sound produced by thunder or an alarm clock. One young patient with cardiac arrest was "listening to extremely loud music at the time of his collapse."[406]

[aa]An uncommon cause of sudden death. Three cases of arrhythmogenic right ventricular dysplasia were found among 547 cardiac deaths.[360]

[bb]From the Framingham study of 232 men and 229 women with congestive heart failure and followed for 30 years.[370]

[cc]Fifteen of 690 patients with Wolff-Parkinson-White syndrome.[386] The incidence of ventricular fibrillation in all patients with Wolff-Parkinson-White syndrome is lower.

[dd]Eight percent in one study of 26 patients.[389]

[ee]The number of sudden deaths in patients with atherosclerotic cardiovascular disease in Los Angeles County rose from a daily average of 4.6 to 24 on January 17, 1994, the day of the Northridge, California earthquake.[397] Most of the deaths occurred within 1 hour of the beginning of the earthquake at 4:31 a.m.[397] Only three victims were engaging in unusual physical exertion when they collapsed. During the 6 days after the earthquake, the number of patients who died suddenly decreased to an average of 2.7 per day.[397]

The incidence of sudden death, which rose in Israel during the Iraqi missile attacks of the Gulf War of 1991,[396, 398] returned to normal levels after the first days of the war despite the continued threat of attack.[396]

[ff]The stress of the first day in medical school may have contributed to the cardiac arrest of a 22-year-old woman with Marfan syndrome.[403] Dr. Samuel A. Levine, one of the founders of American cardiology, reported the sudden death in 1961 of a 63-year-old man with chronic atrial fibrillation and little coronary disease on autopsy who had been greatly distressed by the illegal shooting of a fawn.[399]

[gg]The arrhythmia would now be considered polymorphic ventricular tachycardia[1327] (see Chapter 13).

Exercise, Athletes, and Sports[140, 276, 359, 407–414]

Athletes and physical activity. Competitive athletes who die suddenly may also have[415]

- Aortic valve stenosis.
- Congenital coronary anomalies.
- Idiopathic left ventricular hypertrophy.
- Mitral valve prolapse.
- Myocarditis.
- Ruptured aorta from cystic medial necrosis.
- Sarcoidosis.

Sudden death in apparently healthy children[271] and young adults[416] usually occurs during strenuous physical activity.[417, 418hh] However, only 5% of patients, age 14 to 40 years, who die suddenly are engaged in sports-related activities.[419ii]

The risk of dying suddenly rises in subjects who avoid physical activity and decreases in habitually well-conditioned people.[139] For example, the risk of sudden death among habitually vigorous men is 40% that of sedentary men.[139]

Hypertrophic cardiomyopathy is the most common cause of sudden death in athletes younger than 35 years of age, according to reports from the United States,[415, 419–421jj] whereas coronary heart disease is usually the cause among older athletes.[141, 415, 422, 423kk] Screening athletes for hypertrophic cardiomyopathy and then disqualifying those with the disease from competitive sports may prevent their dying suddenly.[424] Arrhythmogenic right ventricular dysplasia is an important cause of cardiac arrest and sudden death in young Italian athletes.[358, 359, 424–426ll]

Miscellaneous diseases and activities. Daily physical activities or sports are not important factors in producing sudden death in the general population.[427] The cardiovascular disease that causes sudden death in those patients is usually severe.[427, 428]

Sudden death, presumably from ventricular fibrillation, occurs more often in patients with coronary heart disease if they develop frequent ventricular premature beats during exercise.[429] Recruits with sickle cell trait have a substantially increased, age-dependent risk of exercise-related sudden death unexplained by any known preexisting cause.[430] Exercise has occasionally produced ventricular fibrillation during swimming[89] and through anaphylaxis.[199]

Exercise testing. Cardiac arrest[431, 432] and ventricular fibrillation occur occasionally, but infrequently,[433–435] during properly supervised exercise testing:

- Six (0.1%) of 7,500 patients during maximal exercise testing.[436]
- Nine (3%) of 283 patients who were referred for treatment of malignant ventricular arrhythmias during maximal exercise testing.[437]
- One patient per 6,000 man-hours of supervised exercise training.[438]

Exercise decreases or limits to no more than 10 millimeters of mercury the increase in blood pressure in the patients most likely to sustain ventricular fibrillation during exercise testing.[439] These patients frequently have severe coronary disease,[440] particularly of the left main or proximal left anterior descending coronary artery.[441] Exercise testing, however, does not usually provoke the arrhythmia in survivors of ventricular fibrillation.[442]

Commotio cordis (concussion of the heart)[412, 443–445] occasionally and most dramatically suddenly kills young patients[446] during contact sports or when struck by a baseball,[447, 448] hockey puck,[449] or other similar object. Experimental studies suggest that the mechanism is ventricular fibrillation produced by stimulation of the heart during the "vulnerable phase" of ventricular repolarization.[450]

No Structural Heart Disease[451–461mm]

Rarely,[456, 462nn] cardiac arrest due to ventricular fibrillation occurs in patients without structural heart disease who are said to have "idiopathic ventricular fibrillation" or "primary electrical disease."[463, 464] By definition, none of these patients has the long QT interval or Wolff-Parkinson-White syndrome. Studies are beginning to reveal that the hearts of many patients with no obvious structural heart disease are not entirely normal.[465–469]

Among patients with idiopathic ventricular fibrillation,[451oo]

- Males predominate.[pp]
- The average age is younger than among all who sustain cardiac arrest.
- A family history of sudden death is uncommon.
- Ventricular fibrillation occurs almost invariably during the daytime and when the patients are awake; about 15% of patients are engaged in physical exertion.

[hh]Such was the case among 1,606,167 United States Air Force male recruits, 19 of whom died suddenly during a 42-day basic training period between 1965 and 1985.[122]

[ii]Thirty-four of 690 cases examined in the Maryland Medical Examiner's office.[419]

[jj]Fourteen (48%) of 29 highly conditioned, competitive athletes who died suddenly during or soon after severe exertion on the athletic field had hypertrophic cardiomyopathy.[420]

[kk]For example, significant coronary heart disease was found in 23 (77%) of 29 men and one woman (average age, 46.7 years) who died suddenly while playing squash.[423]

[ll]In a report from Trento in northern Italy, arrhythmogenic right ventricular dysplasia was present in 23% to 25% of athletes with sports-related cardiac arrest or sudden cardiac death.[426] In Italy, this cardiomyopathy is responsible for more sudden deaths in athletes than hypertrophic cardiomyopathy.[424]

[mm]Investigators interested in studying patients with cardiac arrest and no apparent structural heart disease have organized registries in the United States and Europe.[455, 460]

[nn]For example, in one series of 104 patients who sustained out-of-hospital cardiac arrest, heart disease was absent in only four men and two women.[462] In another, only nine patients without structural heart disease who survived arrhythmic sudden death presented to one of the most renowned centers for the study of arrhythmias in Europe during the 10-year period from 1979 to 1989.[456]

[oo]From a review of 54 patients reported in 18 series.[451]

[pp]Seventy-three percent were male among 45 patients with idiopathic ventricular fibrillation.[451] Males predominate by a similar ratio (79%) among patients with lone (idiopathic) atrial fibrillation.

- Although a history of syncope is present in about one-fourth of these patients when they come to medical attention, many have no symptoms suggesting cardiovascular disease.
- Psychological stress precedes ventricular fibrillation in 22%.

The combination of right bundle branch block, ST segment elevation in leads V_1 to V_3, and cardiac arrest due to ventricular fibrillation appears to constitute a syndrome among patients without structural heart disease ("Brugada's syndrome").[470–479] The electrocardiographic features of Brugada's syndrome also identify patients at risk of cardiac arrest.[477] The same electrocardiographic pattern is also found among residents and immigrants from Southeast Asia[480–482] who die suddenly with what has been called "sudden unexplained death syndrome."[483qq] "Pokkuri disease," sudden death at night in young, otherwise healthy Japanese men,[484rr] may be the same entity.[483]

Although follow-up of Brugada's own series revealed no progression to cardiomyopathy,[474] other investigators[466, 468, 469] have found that some patients with the syndrome have cardiomyopathy, including right ventricular dysplasia, acute ischemia of the right ventricle, or tricyclic drug overdose. Despite careful evaluation, the hearts of some, and perhaps many, patients with cardiac arrest and no apparent structural heart disease have cardiac abnormalities, not yet discernible with the methods currently available to us.[460]

Sudden death occurs in a few children and adolescents with normal hearts and without discoverable cause.[485ss]

Pulmonary Disease

Cardiac arrest[486] may be the initial manifestation of primary pulmonary hypertension.[487]

Cardiac Catheterization

Ventricular fibrillation occasionally complicates cardiac catheterization, coronary angioplasty, and angiography, but the rate of occurrence depends on the procedure and the illness of the patients, for example:

- Five percent among 20,142 patients undergoing coronary angiography.[488]
- Five episodes in 300 patients having outpatient cardiac catheterization.[489]
- Eleven percent of 708 patients treated with thrombolysis and angioplasty during acute myocardial infarction.[490]

Electricity

Several electrical events can produce ventricular fibrillation.

- *Cardioversion.* Ventricular fibrillation, often brief and self-reverting, occasionally appears after elective cardioversion.[491–497tt]
- *Catheter ablation* of cardiac structures.[498–501]
- *Electrocution,* including that produced by inadequate grounding of an injector used in cardioangiography[502] and from a faulty switch in an operating table.[503] The arrhythmia may not appear until several hours after the shock.[504]
- *Electrophysiological study.* Programmed stimulation during electrophysiological evaluation of ventricular arrhythmias frequently induces ventricular fibrillation.[505]
- *Low-energy shocks* from implantable cardioverter-defibrillators in patients with coronary heart disease.[506] In testing defibrillators, operators frequently induce ventricular fibrillation with this technique during the T waves.
- *Pacing* from the right ventricle in patients with right ventricular infarction[507] or from esophageal stimulation of the left atrium in a patient with hypertrophic cardiomyopathy.[508]

Drugs

Many antiarrhythmic drugs can produce potentially fatal arrhythmias, including ventricular fibrillation ("proarrhythmic" effect).[uu]

Other drugs that can occasionally induce ventricular fibrillation include:

- Atropine.[509–516]
- Catecholamines such as dobutamine given during stress echocardiographic study.[517]
- Cocaine[131, 518–521vv] and other substance abuse,[522] such as inhalation of freon.[523]
- Digitalis.[524–527]
- Lidocaine.[509]
- Nitroglycerin.[81] Non–potassium-sparing diuretics given to hypertensive patients.[528]
- Verapamil in patients with Wolff-Parkinson-White syndrome and atrial fibrillation.[529, 530]

Miscellaneous Conditions

Ventricular fibrillation has been occasionally associated with

- Alcohol.[387]
- Carotid sinus pressure.[531–535]
- Hypokalemia.[536, 537]

---

qqCalled *Lai Tai* ("died during sleep") in northeast Thailand and *Bangungut* ("moaning and dying during sleep") in the Philippines.[483]
rrFrom the colloquial Japanese word *pokkuri,* which means "a sudden and an unexpected occurrence."[484]
ssA study from the University of Lund, Sweden found sudden, natural death occurring in four children and adolescents, none of whom were infants. This equals 0.007 deaths per 1,000 live births, very low compared with the incidence of sudden infant death syndrome.[485]

---

ttWhat was called ventricular fibrillation during the early days of cardioversion in the 1960s could now be considered polymorphic ventricular tachycardia.
uuThis topic is discussed in Chapter 13.
vvThe increasing importance of cocaine in producing cardiac arrest is shown by the experience of Olmsted County, Minnesota during 1980 to 1989 where, among 54 subjects aged 20 to 40 years with cardiac arrest, 27 (33%) had a history of cocaine abuse.[131]

- Hypomagnesemia.[538]
- Thyroid hormone abuse.[539]
- Thyrotoxic periodic paralysis.[540]

Heart Rate

Cardiac arrest occurs five times more often in men whose heart rates are at least 90 beats per minute than in those with heart rates of less than 60 beats per minute, irrespective of age, systolic blood pressure, blood cholesterol, smoking, social class, heavy drinking, or physical activity.[541][ww]

Circadian Effects[542, 543]

Cardiac arrest occurs most often in the daytime,[544, 545] particularly in the morning,[546–560][xx] and least often in the middle of the night.[557] The incidence seems to peak from 8 a.m. to 11 a.m. and 4 p.m. to 7 p.m., the evening peak particularly due to ventricular fibrillation.[560] The time of rearrest is random and is unrelated to when the previous cardiac arrest occurred.[560]

The time of the event is unaffected by age,[554] ejection fraction,[554] frequency of cardiac arrests,[554] use of amiodarone,[559] or presence of congestive heart failure.[555]

Implantable cardioverter-defibrillators shock life-threatening ventricular arrhythmias most frequently in the late[561] morning[558, 562] and to a lesser degree from 4 p.m. to 8 p.m.,[558] on Mondays and to a lesser extent on Fridays.[563] Weekends are particularly free of the arrhythmias that produce defibrillator shocks.[563] Antiarrhythmic[545] and beta-adrenergic–blocking[563, 564] drugs eliminate the hourly[545, 564] and day-to-day[563] circadian pattern. Among travelers to Hawaii, the incidence of sudden death rises steadily throughout the day rather than peaking in the morning, a difference postulated to be caused by "stress related to travel and time zone changes."[565]

The highest rate of sudden death among patients with hypertrophic cardiomyopathy also occurs early in the daytime, from 7 a.m. to 1 p.m., but a second peak appears from 8 p.m. to 10 p.m.[339] Age, gender, severity of symptoms, subaortic gradient, and left ventricular wall thickness do not affect this pattern.[339] In the hospital, resuscitation from ventricular fibrillation is more likely to be successful when the episodes occur during the day rather than during the evening or at night.[566]

OTHER ARRHYTHMIAS IN PATIENTS WITH VENTRICULAR FIBRILLATION

Ventricular Premature Beats[567]

Ventricular premature beats, often frequent and complex, are frequently recorded in patients who will have or have had ventricular fibrillation.[74, 568–586] However, the beats are less likely to be complex when cardiac arrest occurs during exertion.[137]

[ww]In 7,735 men aged 40 to 59 years seen in general practices in 24 British towns.[541]

[xx]Or in the afternoon, according to one report.[545]

Ventricular Tachycardia

At the onset of the arrhythmia, fibrillation is usually the ventricular arrhythmia of acute ischemia, whereas tachycardia is the ventricular arrhythmia of chronic coronary disease. Patients presenting with cardiac arrest are three times more likely to suffer cardiac rearrest than those presenting with ventricular tachycardia.[587] Certain characteristics distinguish patients presenting with sustained ventricular tachycardia from those resuscitated from ventricular fibrillation[262, 588–593] (Table 14.3):

- Sustained ventricular tachycardia appears more often in patients presenting with monomorphic sustained ventricular tachycardia than in those whose cardiac arrest is due solely to ventricular fibrillation.
- The rate of induced monomorphic sustained ventricular tachycardia in patients who have survived primary ventricular fibrillation is faster than in those who present with ventricular tachycardia.

Ventricular tachycardia,[79, 82, 84, 87, 110, 594] frequently sustained, rapid or polymorphic,[78][yy] often precedes ventricular fibrillation.[78, 82] The R-on-T phenomenon, however, seldom introduces the ventricular tachycardia that precedes ventricular fibrillation.[82]

Ventricular tachycardia that changes into ventricular fibrillation is more likely to be:[595]

- Faster than 180 beats per minute.
- Initiated by an R-on-T beat.
- Polymorphic.
- Present for more than 100 beats.[zz]

[yy]Ventricular tachycardia preceded ventricular fibrillation in each of 27 ambulatory patients whose electrocardiogram was monitored when cardiac arrest occurred.[78, 82] In 15 of these patients, the average length of the runs of ventricular tachycardia was 560 beats and the average rate was 241 beats per minute.[78]

[zz]Ventricular fibrillation is then 20 times more likely.[595]

Table 14.3	CHARACTERISTICS OF PATIENTS PRESENTING WITH SUSTAINED VENTRICULAR TACHYCARDIA VERSUS VENTRICULAR FIBRILLATION[588]	
Characteristics of Patients	Presenting with Ventricular Tachycardia	Resuscitated from Ventricular Fibrillation
Coronary disease[592]	Less severe	More severe
Myocardial infarctions[590]	More	Fewer
Left ventricular aneurysms	More	Fewer
Left ventricular ejection fraction[591]	Lower	Higher

(From Adhar GC, Larson LW, Bardy GH, Greene HL. Sustained ventricular arrhythmias: differences between survivors of cardiac arrest and patients with recurrent sustained ventricular tachycardia. J Am Coll Cardiol 1988; 12:159–165. Reprinted with permission from the American College of Cardiology.)

The heart rate may vary just before ventricular fibrillation develops.[74]

Miscellaneous Conditions

Such nonventricular arrhythmias as complete heart block, reentrant supraventricular tachycardia, and sinus arrest may precede the ventricular fibrillation.[596]

SYMPTOMS

Many,[108] probably between one-third[597] and one-half,[115, 170] of cardiac arrests occur without warning. On close questioning, however, many patients successfully resuscitated from cardiac arrest will recall prodromal symptoms[165] such as chest pain, dyspnea, indigestion, or ringing in the ears[598] during the hour before the event[167] (see Table 14.1). Even young patients, previously thought to have few symptoms, often report, on careful questioning, palpitations, chest pain, or previous episodes of syncope or cardiac arrest.[406] Relatives can sometimes recall symptoms that the victim complained of before the cardiac arrest even though survivors may not remember such events.[597]

Older patients more often complain of dyspnea and younger patients complain of chest pain.[116] Although two-thirds of patients have chest pain or dyspnea during the 4 weeks before dying suddenly, in only one-fourths are the symptoms new or different.[115] Few[aaa] consult physicians for new or changing chest pain or dyspnea shortly before death.[115]

The severity of the symptoms correlates more or less with the arrhythmia. Syncope or dizziness that prevents the patient's ability to stand or walk is usually associated with ventricular fibrillation or sustained ventricular tachycardia, whereas mild symptoms, such as palpitations or slight dizziness, tend to occur with transient ventricular tachycardia or nonventricular arrhythmias.[599]

Syncope[600]

The preeminent symptom of ventricular fibrillation is syncope. Having had syncope predicts that cardiac arrest is likely to occur in patients with congestive heart failure, independent of age, presence of atrial fibrillation, cardiac index, serum sodium, or angiotensin-converting enzyme inhibition.[601] Left ventricular function is better preserved in patients with sustained ventricular tachyarrhythmias, including ventricular fibrillation, who present with syncope rather than with cardiac arrest.[602]

Although fatal cardiac arrest is unpredictable in most young people, syncope often precedes such events, as was the case in 23 of 44 soldiers in one report.[313] Syncope occurs in about one-fourth of young patients but seldom in adults with arrhythmogenic right ventricular dysplasia.[603]

PHYSICAL EXAMINATION

The physical examination during ventricular fibrillation reveals an unconscious patient without a palpable pulse or audible heart sounds. These patients frequently have seizures and breathe poorly with inspiratory snoring.

ELECTROCARDIOGRAPHY

The electrocardiographic tracing of ventricular fibrillation presents a continuous undulating pattern without discrete P waves, QRS complexes, or T waves. The atria can sustain organized activity soon after the onset of ventricular fibrillation, but one usually cannot identify the P waves.

The appearance of the fibrillatory waves has given rise to the terms *fine* and *coarse* to describe their size (Fig. 14.4). The electrocardiographic amplitude of the waveforms of fine fibrillation is defined as less than 0.2 millivolts.[604] When ventricular fibrillation begins, the waveforms tend to be large; their amplitude subsequently diminishes.[604]

The distinction between coarse and fine fibrillation has more than descriptive importance. Coarse fibrillation usually identifies patients who can be more easily defibrillated and have a better prognosis.[604]

Ventricular fibrillation can be transient.[605] Spontaneous conversion occurred in 53% of episodes in one series documented from the memory of implantable cardioverter-defibrillators.[606]

Electrocardiogram during Sinus Rhythm

WARNING OR PREMONITORY ARRHYTHMIAS[607]

"Warning arrhythmias."[211, 608] These arrhythmias are those ventricular beats that predict that patients may develop ventricular tachycardia and ventricular fibrillation. Their characteristics include

- Frequency; more than 5 per minute is a commonly used figure.
- Multiform appearance.
- Coupling (two in a row).
- Appearance in the "vulnerable phase" of the preceding T wave ("R-on-T phenomenon").

During myocardial infarction. Warning arrhythmias appear before many, but not all, episodes of ventricular fibrillation that develop during myocardial infarction.[152, 237, 256, 569, 595, 609bbb] R-on-T ventricular premature beats precede about half the paroxysms of ventricular fibrillation;[244, 256, 610, 611] their presence as a harbinger of ventricular fibrillation is probably highest soon after the infarction begins.[228]

HARBINGERS OF VENTRICULAR FIBRILLATION DURING DAILY ACTIVITIES[612]

Ventricular fibrillation recorded during daily activities is often preceded by

---

[aaa]Seventeen percent in one series.[115]

[bbb]Warning arrhythmias appeared in only half of 18 patients with ventricular fibrillation during myocardial infarction in one study.[256]

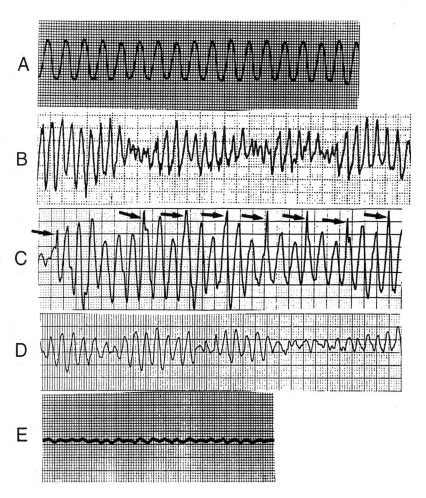

FIGURE 14.4 Electrocardiographic patterns related to ventricular fibrillation. A, Ventricular flutter (*panel A*), a sinusoidal regular tachycardia at cycle lengths in the range of 200 to 240 milliseconds. The rhythm is regular, and mechanical function may be preserved, although patients may be hypotensive or unconscious. This rhythm commonly precedes ventricular fibrillation. **B,** Torsades de pointes (*panel B*), a rapid polymorphic ventricular tachycardia associated with a long QT interval during sinus rhythm (see Chapter 13). **C,** "Pseudoventricular fibrillation" (*panel C*) produced by an electrocardiographic artifact caused by a loose electrode. The *arrows* indicate subtle but identifiable QRS complexes from the patient's sinus rhythm. **D,** Coarse ventricular fibrillation (*panel D*). **E,** Fine ventricular fibrillation (*panel E*). (From Myerburg RJ, Kessler KM. Ventricular fibrillation. In Kastor JA (ed). Arrhythmias. Philadelphia: WB Saunders, 1994, pp. 395–420, with permission.)

- Changing,[613] usually increasing,[82, 87, 614ccc] heart rate particularly during the hour preceding the cardiac arrest.[87]
- Complex ventricular premature beats[74, 77, 78, 594] whose frequency rises during the pre-arrest hour.[87]
- Repolarization abnormalities, including ST segment elevations,[87] which may last for several hours before the cardiac arrest,[77] and QT prolongation, occasionally,[614] but seldom.[78ddd]

PRINZMETAL'S ANGINA

Coronary vasospasm that produces ischemia in the absence of pain or flow-limiting coronary lesions may induce life-threatening ventricular arrhythmias including ventricular fibrillation.[200] Ventricular premature beats instituting ventricular tachycardia and ventricular fibrillation occur earlier in the T wave of the preceding QRS complex during vasospasm than during reperfusion.[198] Electrical alternation of the ST segments and T waves predicts that ventricular arrhythmias, including ventricular fibrillation, may appear while the ST segments are maximally elevated.[188]

IDIOPATHIC VENTRICULAR FIBRILLATION

Ventricular fibrillation in patients without structural heart disease spontaneously begins after a burst of rapid polymorphic ventricular tachycardia initiated by ventricular premature beats with very short coupling intervals.[615eee]

ST SEGMENTS

The ST segments are characteristically elevated in patients with "Brugada's syndrome," survivors of cardiac arrest with no structural heart disease whose electrocardiograms show right bundle branch block and elevated ST segments in leads V_1, V_2, and V_3 (Fig. 14.5).

QT INTERVALS, PROLONGATION, AND DISPERSION[616–618]

Sudden death, presumably from ventricular fibrillation, more likely occurs in patients after myocardial infarction whose corrected QT intervals are persistently longer than normal[619–621] and in subjects aged 55 years or more with increased dispersion of ventricular electrophysiological recovery, measured as QT disper-

---

ccc In 11 (55%) of 20 patients, the heart rate increased by an average of 20% during the hour before cardiac arrest.[82]

ddd In only three (20%) of 15 patients; the mean QT interval for all 15 patients was 0.42 seconds.[78]

eee As found in a study of 22 episodes of ventricular fibrillation in nine patients without identifiable structural heart disease.[615]

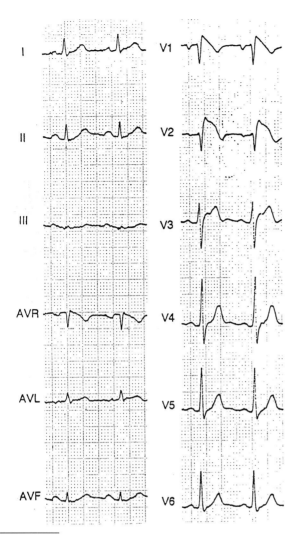

FIGURE 14.5 Brugada's syndrome. Notice the pattern of right bundle branch block and the elevated ST segments in the left precordial leads in this patient with no structural heart disease who was resuscitated from cardiac arrest. (Adapted from Brugada J, Brugada P. What to do in patients with no structural heart disease and sudden arrhythmic death? Am J Cardiol 1996; 78:69–75, with permission.)[457]

sion.[622]*fff* The circadian variation of the QT interval found in healthy people is almost undetectable in patients who have had myocardial infarction and who die suddenly.[621]

QT dispersion, differences in the QT interval among electrocardiographic leads, is greater in patients who have had ventricular fibrillation during myocardial infarction than in those without the arrhythmia at this time.[623] QT interval dispersion has been thought to predict which patients,[624–626] after myocardial infarction,[627–630] will die or will develop sustained ventricular arrhythmias. A 1998 report, however, suggests that this is not the case and that QT interval dispersion does not predict these events in patients who have had myocardial infarction.[631] QT interval dispersion may predict potentially fatal events in patients with hyper-

trophic cardiomyopathy[632] or congestive heart failure,[633, 634] but the test does not discriminate in this respect among patients with dilated cardiomyopathy,[635, 636] nor does it identify patients with idiopathic ventricular fibrillation.[637] QT interval dispersion tends to be greater in patients with ventricular fibrillation or polymorphic ventricular tachycardia than with monomorphic ventricular tachycardia.[638]

T-WAVE ALTERNANS[639, 640]

Some patients susceptible to ventricular arrhythmias have slight alternating changes in the amplitude of the T waves.[641–643]

OTHER ELECTROCARDIOGRAPHIC FINDINGS

Patients with bundle branch block are more likely to develop ventricular fibrillation than those without this finding,[644] but whether bundle branch block is an independent risk factor is not known. Electrocardiographic evidence of left ventricular hypertrophy, myocardial injury, or QT prolongation predicts a higher risk of cardiac arrest in patients with treated hypertension.[290] ST segment and T-wave abnormalities persist in about half of patients without overt cardiac disease who have been resuscitated from cardiac arrest.[425] A spontaneous supraventricular beat occasionally induces ventricular fibrillation,[645] particularly during acute myocardial infarction.[646] Late sudden death occurs more frequently in children with tetralogy of Fallot whose QRS complexes and JT intervals are abnormally prolonged.[647]*ggg*

Compared with other patients with coronary heart disease, survivors of ventricular fibrillation more commonly have more[648]

- QTc prolongation.
- ST segment depression.
- T-wave flattening.
- Ventricular premature beats.

OTHER ELECTROCARDIOGRAPHIC STUDIES

Ambulatory Monitoring[649, 650]

With respect to ventricular fibrillation, continuous electrocardiographic (Holter) monitoring reveals the following:

- Electrocardiographic examples of the arrhythmia in adults (Fig. 14.6)[66–70, 72–89, 614] and children[119] during cardiac arrest.
- The influence of changes in heart rate.[82, 613]
- The relation of the arrhythmia to transient myocardial ischemia[86, 198] and to Prinzmetal's angina.[188]
- The significance of supraventricular[646] and ventricular arrhythmias in patients during and after myocardial infarction,[228, 244, 569, 595, 610, 611, 613, 651–656] with

---

*fff*From a study of 2,358 men and 3,454 women in Rotterdam, the Netherlands.

*ggg*The JT interval is measured from the J point at the end of the QRS complex to the end of the T wave.[647]

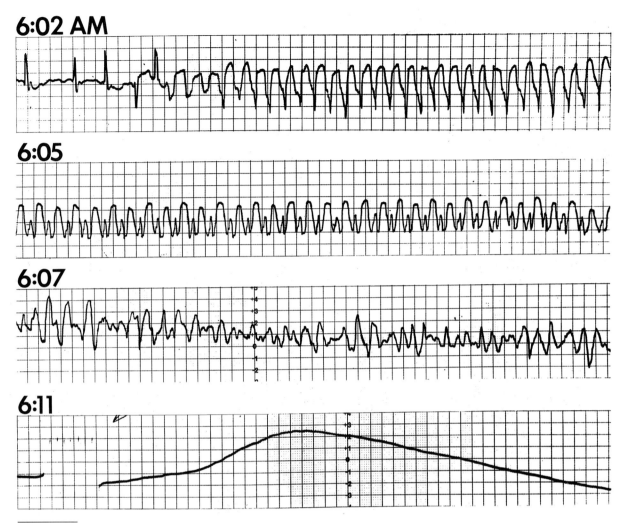

FIGURE 14.6 Cardiac arrest recorded on a Holter monitor. Uniform ventricular tachycardia at a rate of 215 beats per minute interrupts sinus rhythm (**top** *6:02 a.m.*). Approximately 5 minutes later, (**third panel,** *6:07*), the rhythm degenerates into polymorphic ventricular tachycardia and then cardiac arrest and asystole (**bottom,** *6:11*). (From Josephson ME, Callans DJ. Sustained ventricular tachycardia. In Kastor JA (ed). Arrhythmias. Philadelphia: WB Saunders, 1994, pp. 336–362, with permission.)

dilated[584, 654] and hypertrophic cardiomyopathy[657, 658] or if resuscitated from cardiac arrest.[75]

Implantable Cardioverter-Defibrillator Memory[659]

The memory built into contemporary implantable cardioverter-defibrillators reveals that spontaneous conversion occurs in 95% of patients with ventricular tachyarrhythmias (monomorphic or polymorphic ventricular tachycardia or ventricular fibrillation).[606] Of the *episodes* of ventricular tachyarrhythmias detected,[606]

• Three-quarters revert spontaneously.
• Twenty-two percent require antitachycardia pacing.
• Shock is required in 1.7%.

In survivors of cardiac arrest without inducible arrhythmias at electrophysiological study, ventricular fibrillation is usually present at the beginning and throughout recurrences of cardiac arrest.[660]

Signal-averaged Electrocardiogram[661, 662]

Most patients with documented ventricular fibrillation have abnormal late potentials.[589, 663–665hhh] The risk of developing malignant ventricular arrhythmias is higher in persons with abnormal signal-averaged electrocardiograms,[355, 655, 666–670] but not in elderly patients with ejection fraction of 40% or more.[671] Moreover, the presence of late potentials in elderly patients without clinical evidence of heart disease does not increase their incidence of sudden death, total cardiac death, or total death.[672]

Late potentials do not predict whether ventricular fibrillation can be induced at electrophysiological study.[590] The signal-averaged electrocardiogram has a limited role in deciding whether to implant a defibrillator in patients with life-threatening arrhythmias because the test does not predict which patients with

---

[hhh]The signal-averaged electrocardiograms of patients with ventricular fibrillation or ventricular tachycardia differ in some details[589, 663] (see Table 14.4).

implantable cardioverter-defibrillators will receive the most discharges.[673] Abnormal late potentials predict life-threatening arrhythmias slightly more reliably than do 24-hour ambulatory electrocardiograms or left ventricular ejection fraction.[674]

Myocardial infarction and dilated cardiomyopathy.[675, 676] In patients with old myocardial infarctions, the presence of either abnormal late potentials[655, 656, 677, 678] or increased width of the filtered QRS complexes[677, 679] raises the risk of dying suddenly. Abnormal signal-averaged electrocardiograms[680] or, according to one report,[681] both abnormal late potentials and increased width of the QRS complexes predict a higher likelihood of sudden death in patients with dilated cardiomyopathy.[iii] Signal-averaged electrocardiography does not predict which patients with advanced congestive heart failure due to ischemic or idiopathic cardiomyopathy will have cardiac arrest.[682]

Hypertrophic cardiomyopathy. Although some patients with hypertrophic cardiomyopathy who survive cardiac arrest have abnormal signal-averaged electrocardiograms,[683] the test will not identify which young patients with hypertrophic cardiomyopathy will die suddenly.[684] Furthermore, there is no association, among subjects with hypertrophic cardiomyopathy, between an abnormal signal-averaged electrocardiogram and a history of syncope or a family history of premature sudden cardiac death.[683]

Ventricular tachycardia. Survivors of cardiac arrest due to ventricular fibrillation are less likely to have late potentials than those with a history of sustained ventricular tachycardia.[590, 591]

Familial sudden death syndromes. Abnormal signal-averaged electrocardiograms may select those at highest risk among members of families with an inherited tendency to develop cardiac arrest.[685]

Heart Rate Variability[543, 686–688]

The variability of the heart rate among survivors of cardiac arrest is lower than normal,[594] particularly in the morning after awakening, when the incidence of sudden death is the greatest.[689] The heart rate varies less in patients who die after being resuscitated from cardiac arrest than in those who recover after resuscitation and go home to resume the activities of daily living.[690] Healthy persons have more rate variability than both groups.[690]

The risk of cardiac arrest rises in patients with old myocardial infarction whose heart rate varies less than normal.[655, 677, 678, 691–697][jjj] The normal variability in heart rate decreases during the 5 minutes preceding the ST segment changes precipitated by ischemic cardiac arrest.[698] Heart rate variability tends to be abnormal in those patients with idiopathic dilated cardiomyopathy who are prone to having major ventricular arrhythmias including ventricular fibrillation.[699]

Heart rate variability predicts sudden death better than does left ventricular ejection fraction.[700] However, in patients with comparable left ventricular ejection fractions, the variation of the heart rate is not different between those who are about to have ventricular fibrillation—as documented on ambulatory electrocardiograms—and others who will not suffer ventricular fibrillation.[701]

Exercise Testing[650]

About half of patients with ventricular fibrillation and coronary heart disease have positive exercise tests.[179kkk] However, exercise testing produces angina in few survivors of out-of-hospital cardiac arrest, although ST changes of ischemia develop in about half.[702] The failure of systolic blood pressure to rise 10 millimeters of mercury or more predicts a worse prognosis.[702] Exercise testing selects with high sensitivity but low specificity which patients with the Wolff-Parkinson-White syndrome have had or will develop ventricular fibrillation.[703, 704]

Body-surface QRST Mapping

This technique reveals abnormalities in patients with ventricular arrhythmias including ventricular fibrillation.[705]

HEMODYNAMICS

When ventricular fibrillation ensues, pulsatile arterial waveforms quickly disappear. The mean arterial pressure decreases rapidly at first and then more gradually[706] (Fig. 14.7). The systolic pressure returns to its prefibrillatory level about 10 seconds after conversion. The longer the fibrillation persists, the lower the aortic systolic and diastolic pressures become,[707] and the longer the time before the blood pressure achieves pre-arrhythmic levels.[706]

Hemodynamic studies show that as left ventricular function decreases, the likelihood of dying suddenly rises.[78, 259, 579, 584, 656, 679, 700, 708–710] Thus, in survivors of cardiac arrest,

- Cardiac index is decreased.[711]
- Ejection fraction is decreased,[711] and when less than 35%, it predicts that cardiac arrest is likely to recur within the next 6 months.[655, 712]
- Left ventricular end-diastolic pressure is raised.[711]

The ejection fraction is lower in survivors of primary ventricular fibrillation during myocardial infarction who have[258]

[iii]None of 154 patients with old myocardial infarction or dilated cardiomyopathy and normal signal-averaged electrocardiograms died suddenly during follow-up of about 2 years.[681]

[jjj]However, according to one study[697] in patients with ventricular tachycardia or ventricular fibrillation who have had myocardial infarction at least 1 year previously, heart rate variability is not abnormal, whereas vagal reflexes, measured in the baroreflex sensitivity test, are depressed.

[kkk]Thirteen (54%) of 24 patients with 1 millimeter or more of downsloping ST segment depression.[179]

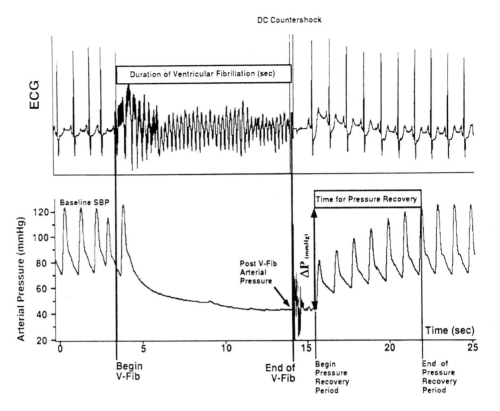

FIGURE 14.7 Hemodynamic effect of ventricular fibrillation. The blood pressure (SBP), recorded from the brachial artery (**bottom**), decreases continuously during ventricular fibrillation (V = Fib) (**top**) and returns toward normal after countercheck reestablishes sinus rhythm (*right portion of figure*). (The horizontal axis records time in seconds.) (Adapted from Park WM, Amirhamzeh MM, Jia CX, et al. Systolic arterial pressure recovery after ventricular fibrillation/flutter in humans. Pacing Clin Electrophysiol 1994; 17:1100–1106, with permission.)[706]

- Myocardial infarction and no ventricular fibrillation.
- Anterior rather than inferior infarction.
- Recurrences of ventricular fibrillation.

ECHOCARDIOGRAPHY AND NUCLEAR CARDIOLOGY

The lower the left ventricular ejection fraction, whether measured with echocardiography[78, 584, 679, 713] or with nuclear techniques,[78, 259, 580, 582, 583, 656, 700, 708, 714–717] the greater is the likelihood that a patient will die suddenly.

The incidence of sudden death, presumably from ventricular fibrillation, rises in patients with coronary heart disease who have echocardiographically determined left ventricular hypertrophy.[718] Some patients without structural heart disease who have been resuscitated from cardiac arrest will have mild to moderate left ventricular dilatation or hypertrophy.[425]

Sudden cardiac death is uncommon in asymptomatic or mildly symptomatic patients with hypertrophic cardiomyopathy and mild left ventricular hypertrophy. The likelihood of cardiac arrest rises in such patients if they have echocardiographically determined severe, diffuse left ventricular hypertrophy.[376]

At the onset of ventricular fibrillation, transesophageal echocardiography[719]*III* reveals chaotic motion of the myocardium and valves and abrupt decrease of left ventricular end-diastolic volume and area, ejection fraction, and fractional area change. About 10 seconds later, the oscillatory movements of the heart walls increase and become regular, the mitral and aortic valves show cyclical closure and opening with forward flow, and spontaneous contrast in the echocardiogram appears within the atria and ventricles.

Exercise radionuclide ventriculography is superior to exercise thallium scintigraphy in predicting which patients after myocardial infarction will have nonfatal ventricular fibrillation, will have another myocardial infarction, or will die of their heart disease.[717] Discharge of implantable cardioverter-defibrillators does not affect echocardiographically determined atrial mechanical function.[720]

PATHOLOGY[265, 721–725]

Coronary Heart Disease

Most patients who die suddenly of ventricular fibrillation have coronary heart disease.[726, 727]

Ventricular myocardium. Pathologists observe *healed* myocardial infarctions in 40% to 70% of patients with coronary heart disease who die suddenly.[727–731] However, pathological evidence of *acute* myocardial infarction appears in only about 20%.

The myocardium of victims of sudden cardiac death also shows many effects of chronic coronary heart disease including interstitial, diffuse fibrosis of minimal, moderate, marked, or multicentric severity and ventricular aneurysms. Eyelets of retained muscle may persist within the scar and around the aneurysms and infarctions.[732]

---

*III*Performed in men with poor left ventricular function during installation of implantable cardioverter-defibrillator.[719] Repeated episodes of ventricular fibrillation and defibrillation did not seem to worsen left ventricular dynamics in these patients.

Cardiomegaly (heart weight more than 400 grams) is frequently present in patients who die suddenly.[115, 727, 733, 734] The hearts of those who die suddenly weigh slightly more than the hearts of cardiac patients who die more gradually despite a similar prevalence of hypertension.[732]

Coronary arteries. Severe, chronic multivessel coronary stenosis is present in most victims of sudden cardiac death.[115, 726] However, 15% have major involvement of only one vessel, most commonly the left anterior descending or left main coronary artery.[115]

The coronary lesions are usually ruptured or fissured atherosclerotic plaques, platelet aggregation, acute or organized thrombus, or spasm.[115, 727, 734–736]mmm "Type II" coronary lesions (irregular rather than smooth obstructions), which are taken to represent ruptured plaques, are more prevalent among survivors of cardiac arrest without the electrophysiological substrate for reentrant ventricular tachycardia than those with it.[737]

The prevalence and extent of coronary heart disease in patients who die suddenly exceed that seen in patients whose death is not sudden.[265, 734, 738] Eighty-one percent of patients who die suddenly with coronary heart disease have obstruction of 75% or more in at least one coronary artery.[727]nnn However, the distribution of stenosis among the different coronary arteries is no different among patients who die suddenly or who succumb more gradually.[734, 738]

Recent coronary thrombosis occurs in about half of patients who die suddenly.[115, 727, 732, 739–743]ooo However, among patients who die within 6 hours after the beginning of symptoms, fewer than 40% have evidence of recent coronary thrombosis.[744]ppp Chronic organized thrombus, frequently associated with significant lesions, is seen in about one-third of victims of sudden cardiac death.[745] This finding could lead one to conclude that an asymptomatic myocardial infarction may precede the arrhythmias producing cardiac arrest by about 1 week.

Necropsy may reveal fixed narrowing of the coronary arteries, not demonstrated with coronary angiography, in patients dying with Prinzmetal's angina variant.[267] Systolic constriction of mural left anterior descending coronary arteries may occasionally produce cardiac arrest during strenuous exercise.[746]

Valvular and Myocardial Disease

Pathological studies reveal that aortic valvular stenosis, hypertrophic cardiomyopathy,[747] and mitral valve prolapse are present in most of the 10% to 20% of victims

of sudden death whose structural heart disease is other than coronary.[165, 265]qqq The hearts of black men, who die suddenly more frequently than white men, weigh over 500 grams.[129]

Mitral valve prolapse. Pathological study of the hearts of patients who die suddenly with,[282] but not necessarily of, mitral valve prolapse reveals the following:

- Endocardial plaques[309] and friction lesions[748] consisting of thickening of the mural endocardium[305] of the left ventricle beneath the posterior leaflet.
- Greater circumference of the mitral valve annulus,[301] length of the leaflets, and thickness of the posterior leaflet.[309]
- Mitral regurgitation, but infrequently.[310]
- Thrombotic lesions containing fibrin and platelets in the angle between the posterior leaflet and the left atrial wall.[748]

Cardiomyopathy of morbid obesity. This most common cause of sudden death in such patients is characterized by cardiomegaly, left ventricular dilatation, and myocyte hypertrophy without interstitial fibrosis.[146]

Disease of the Conducting System[749]

Sudden death is occasionally caused by, or associated with, injury to the conduction system.[345, 610, 750–756] Ischemic damage of the conduction system occurs with equal frequency in patients with myocardial infarctions and in those who die suddenly.[256, 610] Such injury may predispose patients to bradyarrhythmias as well as to ventricular fibrillation.

Sclerosis of the left side of the intraventricular septum with involvement of the conduction system was found in three teenagers who died suddenly.[757] Young athletes[758] and young, apparently healthy Japanese men dying suddenly of Pokkuri disease have fibrosis and other pathological abnormalities of the sinus node and surrounding tissues with minor anomalies of the artery to the sinus node.[754]

Cardiac neural involvement may also have a role in sudden cardiac death.[759, 760] Accessory pathways found in patients who die suddenly may contribute to their deaths despite the absence of electrocardiographic evidence during life.[761]

Young Patients

The pathological causes of sudden, unexpected, nontraumatic death in young adults are cardiac in most cases[131]rrr and coronary in about one-third.[131] Coronary artery anomalies are found in one-fourth of those

---

mmmThe hearts of 51 (57%) of 90 victims of sudden coronary death revealed "active" coronary lesions, defined as demonstrating a disrupted plaque, luminal fibrin/platelet thrombus, or both.[736]

nnnFrom autopsies of 220 victims of sudden cardiac death.[727]

oooThe range was 15% to 64% in eight studies.[115, 727, 732, 738–741, 743] One series reported six victims of sudden death each with only nonobstructive coronary disease.[742]

pppPathologists cannot always ascertain the effects of post-mortem thrombus formation and pre-mortem clot lysis on these data.

qqqNo relationship between mitral valve prolapse and sudden cardiac death resulting from ventricular fibrillation has been firmly established.

rrrThirty-one (57%) of 54 subjects aged 20 to 40 years from a study in Olmsted County, Minnesota from 1960 to 1989; the remainder died of noncardiac causes.[131]

under the age of 21 years who die suddenly.[266] Congenital cardiac abnormalities, particularly of the aortic origin of the coronary arteries, appear in the majority of infants who die suddenly.[266] Autopsy may also reveal unexpected pathological lesions of the conducting system.[345]

Trauma. Injury to the chest as occurs during such contact sports as professional football may lead to coronary blockage, myocardial infarction, and cardiac arrest in patients with premature coronary atherosclerosis.[762]

No Structural Heart Disease[454]

Examination of the hearts at autopsy or of tissue from hearts during myocardial biopsy of patients with idiopathic ventricular fibrillation usually reveals no pathological process.[sss] However, some patients with cardiac arrest from idiopathic ventricular fibrillation have

- Active myocarditis,[763] hypertrophic cardiomyopathy, right ventricular dysplasia, or nonspecific cardiomyopathic changes in biventricular biopsies.[425ttt]
- Multifocal Purkinje cell tumors in an infant aged 9 months.[764]
- Myocardial cellular hypertrophy, interstitial fibrosis, endocardial fibrosis, myocardial degenerative changes, and increased interstitial cellularity.[765uuu]
- Right ventricular dysplasia.[469, 766vvv]

Pathological lesions were found in the conducting system of half of a series of patients with Pokkuri disease, sudden nocturnal death in young Japanese men in apparent good health, even though these patients are thought to have no structural heart disease.[767]

CLINICAL ELECTROPHYSIOLOGY[768–771]

Induction of Ventricular Fibrillation and Sustained Ventricular Arrhythmias
(Fig. 14.8)[www]

Ventricular fibrillation can be induced in the following circumstances:

- Infrequently, when using unaggressive stimulation protocols, in patients without clinical ventricular tachyarrhythmias.[772]
- In about 4%[773xxx] of patients with suspected or documented ventricular arrhythmias and no recent

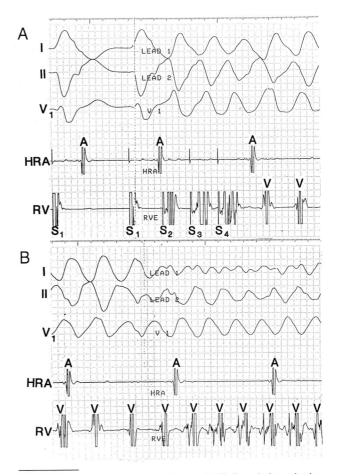

FIGURE 14.8 Induction of ventricular fibrillation during electrophysiologic testing. A paced ventricular beat S₁ (*vertical line*, **A**) induces ventricular tachycardia, which soon changes into ventricular fibrillation (**B**). The lack of relationship between atrial (A) and ventricular (V) activation establishes the presence of atrioventricular dissociation. Parts **A** and **B** of the tracing are continuous. Electrode recordings are from the high right atrium (HRA) and right ventricle (RVE); S indicates pacing stimuli. (From Myerburg RJ, Kessler KM. Ventricular fibrillation. In Kastor JA (ed). Arrhythmias. Philadelphia: WB Saunders, 1994, pp. 395–420, with permission.)[1]

myocardial infarction; about one-third will have had out-of-hospital ventricular fibrillation.[773]
- In about 11% of patients with transient (nonsustained) ventricular tachycardia.[774yyy]
- In more than one-third of patients with valvular heart disease presenting with either ventricular fibrillation or syncope.[775zzz]
- Less frequently in patients treated with amiodarone who have had clinical episodes of ventricular fibrillation than can ventricular tachycardia be induced in similarly treated patients with sustained ventricular tachycardia.[776]

Survivors of cardiac arrest. Sustained ventricular arrhythmias can be induced in the majority of patients who have been resuscitated from cardiac arrest[262, 711,

---

sssIncluding an immigrant from Southeast Asia who had been resuscitated from ventricular fibrillation.[482]

tttOf 8 of 17 young patients without overt heart disease resuscitated from cardiac arrest.[425]

uuuAmong 12 patients with life-threatening ventricular arrhythmias and normal coronary anatomy and mechanical function.[765]

vvvIn six of nine patients with presumed idiopathic ventricular fibrillation[766] and in five of six Japanese men with "Brugada's syndrome" (right bundle branch block, ST segment elevation and sudden death).[469]

wwwSee also the section on electrophysiology in Chapter 12.

xxxTwenty-eight (3.9%) of 718 patients.[773]

yyyTen (11%) of 90 patients each of whom had coronary heart disease or idiopathic cardiomyopathy.[774]

zzzSeven (39%) of 18 patients.[775]

[712, 777–783] and in one-half to two-thirds of those with documented ventricular fibrillation.[590, 784, 785] Patients with coronary heart disease most likely to be inducible have prior myocardial infarction, ventricular aneurysms, or decreased ejection fraction.[786]

Programmed stimulation induces ventricular arrhythmias in patients with cardiac arrest less often than in those with stable sustained ventricular tachycardia.[591, 787] In patients who have had cardiac arrest, programmed stimulation often induces fast[788] polymorphic ventricular tachycardia,[789] whereas in those evaluated for ventricular tachycardia, the procedure is more likely to produce a sustained,[789] slower,[788] monomorphic and hemodynamically well-tolerated ventricular tachycardia.[790]

Depending on the number of premature stimuli employed, ventricular fibrillation itself can be directly induced in only a few[262, 711, 712, 777, 780–782] survivors of cardiac arrest, despite the likelihood or certainty, according to some reports, that ventricular fibrillation occurred during the cardiac arrest, for example:

- Four percent (5 of 142) of patients each of whom had coronary heart disease.[712]
- Eight percent (15 of 196) of patients with two premature stimuli, 27 (19%) of 140 patients with three premature stimuli.[781]
- Eight percent (4 of 52) of patients directly into ventricular fibrillation; 13% (7 of 52) into ventricular fibrillation which followed induction into ventricular tachycardia.[711]
- Eleven percent (9 of 84) of patients with documented ventricular fibrillation as the cause of cardiac arrest.[780]
- Fifteen percent (23 of 150) of patients.[782]

Ventricular tachycardia and ventricular fibrillation can be induced in more men than women who are survivors of cardiac arrest and have coronary heart disease[791] and in more survivors who have coronary heart disease than in those with no structural heart disease.[792aaaa]

Coronary heart disease and myocardial infarction. Ventricular fibrillation is more likely to be induced in patients presenting with ventricular fibrillation who have anterior wall motion abnormalities or significant obstructions of the left anterior descending coronary artery proximal to or involving the first septal perforator branch than in those without these lesions.[793]

Sustained ventricular arrhythmias, including ventricular fibrillation can be induced in

- About one-fourth of patients who have had myocardial infarction.[794bbbb]
- Half of those with ventricular fibrillation during myocardial infarction.[246cccc]

- Fewer patients with coronary heart disease who present with ventricular fibrillation than with sustained ventricular tachycardia.[793dddd]
- Patients receiving amiodarone for ventricular arrhythmias after myocardial infarction in whom ventricular fibrillation can be induced have a high risk of sudden death.[795]

Cardiomyopathy.[325, 334] Ventricular fibrillation can be induced in about 15% of patients with dilated cardiomyopathy.[796, 797eeee] The rate of inducibility of ventricular fibrillation is similar even in patients with dilated cardiomyopathy who have had clinically documented ventricular fibrillation or sustained ventricular tachycardia.[798ffff] In most patients with idiopathic dilated cardiomyopathy, however, extrastimulation with up to two beats fails to produce an electrophysiological correlation to clinical ventricular arrhythmias.[799]

Ventricular fibrillation or sustained polymorphic ventricular tachycardia that deteriorates into ventricular fibrillation can be induced in about one-third of patients with hypertrophic cardiomyopathy and no history of sudden death[800] and in at least half of such patients who have sustained cardiac arrest.[801–803gggg] The ventricular electrogram is more fragmented in patients with hypertrophic cardiomyopathy who have ventricular fibrillation than in those without the arrhythmia.[804–806] The value of electrophysiological testing to identify patients with hypertrophic cardiomyopathy at high risk for sudden death remains controversial.

No structural heart disease.[451] Sustained ventricular arrhythmias can be induced in one-third[462, 807] to over half[454, 808–810] of patients with clinical ventricular fibrillation and no overt cardiac disease. Polymorphic ventricular tachycardia[807] or ventricular fibrillation is produced in about one-third,[425, 462, 464, 811hhhh] but sustained ventricular tachycardia occurs infrequently.[454, 807] Data obtained from electrophysiological studies predict poorly whether the arrhythmia will recur.[462] The duration of the fragmented electrograms recorded from patients with primary ventricular fibrillation is greater than in patients without this arrhythmia.[812]

No inducible ventricular tachyarrhythmias. Ventricular fibrillation, not ventricular tachycardia, is usually present from the beginning of the arrhythmia in those survivors of cardiac arrest in whom no sustained ventricular tachyarrhythmias can be induced at electrophysiological study.[660]

Selection of drugs.[813–818] Administering antiarrhythmic drugs may decrease the ability to induce ventricular fibrillation in the electrophysiology laboratory.[819] Although early studies promised useful results,[814] fur-

---

aaaaSixty-nine percent with coronary heart disease and 40% with no structural heart disease.[792]

bbbbThirty-eight of 165 (23%) of patients with acute myocardial infarction.[794]

ccccIn 17 such patients, five were induced into sustained ventricular tachycardia—which in four of whom degenerated into ventricular fibrillation—and four more into transient ventricular tachycardia. No ventricular arrhythmias were induced in eight.[246]

ddddForty-three percent versus 95% according to one study.[793]

eeeeIn 9 of 62 patients from two series.[796, 797]

ffffSeven of 39 (18%) who have had ventricular fibrillation and 9 of 63 (14%) with sustained ventricular tachycardia.[798]

ggggTwenty-two of 38 (58%) of patients with hypertrophic cardiomyopathy and cardiac arrest.[801, 803]

hhhhIn 8 (35%) of 23 patients from two studies.[425, 811]

ther work demonstrated a poor correlation between the drugs' effect on inducibility of ventricular fibrillation and their prevention of future arrhythmic events and cardiac arrest.[463, 773, 775, 780, 797, 798, 820–823]

Technical considerations.[iiii] To induce ventricular fibrillation, at least two extrastimuli are usually required,[824] and the coupling intervals must be shorter than is needed to start ventricular tachycardia.[825] Ventricular fibrillation induced in the electrophysiology laboratory in patients without previous clinical episodes of ventricular fibrillation or ventricular tachycardia may be a nonspecific response unrelated to clinical disease, particularly in patients

- Without previous clinical episodes of ventricular tachycardia or ventricular fibrillation.[826]
- Subjected to aggressive stimulation protocols such as three or four premature stimuli that produce nonclinical arrhythmias more than single or double premature stimuli.[827–830]

Wolff-Parkinson-White Syndrome[iiii]

Ventricular fibrillation can develop in patients with the Wolff-Parkinson-White syndrome when impulses transmitted from the atria in flutter or fibrillation conduct over rapidly conducting accessory pathways. Those with ventricular preexcitation at particular risk of this potentially fatal complication can be identified at electrophysiological study by measuring the shortest RR interval produced by atrial fibrillation induced by rapid atrial stimulation.[524, 529, 703, 704, 778, 831–853] Those who have multiple accessory pathways seem to be at especially high risk.[850]

Miscellaneous Electrophysiological Findings

Coupling interval, latency, local activation, and left ventricular activation time differ among patients who can, or cannot, be induced into sustained ventricular tachycardia or ventricular fibrillation[854, 855] (Table 14.4). Refractory periods are more dispersed distantly from regions of infarcted myocardium in patients with

---

[iiii]See the section on electrophysiology in Chapter 12 for further details about technical features of inducing ventricular arrhythmias.
[iiii]See the paragraphs on the electrophysiology of Wolff-Parkinson-White syndrome in Chapter 8.

post-infarction ventricular fibrillation than in those with ventricular tachycardia.[856]

Studies in the operating room show that

- Patients who have had clinical ventricular tachycardia are more likely to develop ventricular fibrillation.[857]
- The ventricular fibrillation threshold is lower in patients with coronary heart disease than in those with other forms of heart disease.[858]

TREATMENT[859]

CONVERSION AND RESUSCITATION[203, 860–871]

Successful treatment of ventricular fibrillation requires that a hemodynamically effective cardiac rhythm be reestablished as quickly as possible.

Thumpversion[872, 873]

The operator should forcefully strike the precordium once or twice of all patients who are pulseless, apneic, and unconscious. Because thumpversion is more effective in converting ventricular tachycardia than ventricular fibrillation,[873] the treatment should be used even if a faint, rapid pulse is present.[860kkkk]

Airway

A functioning airway must be quickly established. The operator tilts the patient's head backward, lifts the chin, and removes foreign bodies, including dentures, from the patient's mouth and oropharynx. Then the operator inserts a plastic oral airway and begins respiratory resuscitation by mouth-to-mouth breathing or with an AMBU bag. The lungs should be inflated once every 5 seconds when a full staff is available or twice every 15 seconds if one person is performing the resuscitation. The operator should not intubate the trachea unless he or she is experienced in the procedure.

[kkkk]Because precordial thumps may occasionally change ventricular tachycardia to ventricular fibrillation, some recommend not performing precordial thump when ventricular tachycardia is suspected.[860] I do not agree.

Table 14.4 **ELECTROPHYSIOLOGIC FINDINGS AMONG PATIENTS WITH VENTRICULAR FIBRILLATION, VENTRICULAR TACHYCARDIA, OR NO INDUCIBLE ARRHYTHMIA**

Inducible Arrhythmia	Ventricular Fibrillation	Ventricular Tachycardia	None
Number of patients	40	51	45
Last coupling interval	≤190 milliseconds[854]	Longest	—
Latency	Higher	Lower	Highest
Local activation of last stimulated beat	Shortest	—	—
Left ventricular ejection fraction	45 ± 13%	32 ± 15%	51 ± 17%

(From Avitall B, McKinnie J, Jazayeri M, Akhtar M, Anderson AJ, Tchou P. Induction of ventricular fibrillation versus monomorphic ventricular tachycardia during programmed stimulation: role of premature beat conduction delay. Circulation 1992; 85:1271–1278. By permission of the American Heart Association, Inc.)[855]

Chest Compression[874]

The operator should reestablish cardiovascular circulation by compressing the chest with the palm of one hand placed over the lower sternum and the heel of the other hand resting on the dorsum of the lower hand. The arm of the person performing the resuscitation should be straight at the elbow to provide a less tiring and more forceful effect. Sternal pressure should be applied about 80 to 100 times per minute, with depression of 3 to 5 centimeters, followed by abrupt relaxation.[860, 875]*llll*

Defibrillation[50, 876–880]

If ventricular fibrillation is likely to be the arrhythmia, one should administer a nonsynchronized shock of at least 300 joules (watt-seconds)[215, 860, 881, 882] because 200 joules converts only half of cases (Fig. 14.9).[883] A few patients require more than 300 joules.[882]*mmmm* The longer ventricular fibrillation persists, the greater is the amount of energy required for successful conversion.[707] Two joules per kilogram (1 joule per pound) is usually adequate to defibrillate most children weighing less than 50 kilograms.[884]

The patients most likely to recover are defibrillated soon after the arrhythmia begins.[40, 46, 50, 170, 566, 885] Consequently, one should apply defibrillation even when ventricular fibrillation is suspected rather than proven electrocardiographically. Survival is enhanced when trained ambulance attendants and bystanders begin resuscitation as soon as the patient collapses.[36, 43, 44, 47, 48, 56–63] Lay workers should use automatic external defibrillators rather than manual defibrillators to decrease the duration of ventricular fibrillation.[38, 39, 41, 50–55] These devices enable the first-responding worker to deliver an appropriate shock quickly. Cardiopulmonary resuscitation alone without defibrillation when indicated leads to further cardiac deterioration and a poor prognosis.[886] Unfortunately, either no one is present when many fatal events occur or relatively few people who witness a person collapsing with what may be ventricular fibrillation apply resuscitation.[887, 888]*nnnn*

Efficacy (Table 14.5). Transthoracic shock converts ventricular fibrillation in 90% of victims weighing up to 90 kilograms.[876, 889–891] The arrhythmia reverts more easily in patients with coronary heart disease or primary ventricular fibrillation than in those without cor-

---

*llll*Because no gradient of pressure across the heart can be measured during successful cardiopulmonary resuscitation, investigators have concluded that changes in pressure are transmitted within the entire thoracic cavity rather than only to the cardiac chambers.[874] The active compression-decompression device that decompresses the patient's chest between downward compressions does not improve survival or neurological outcome.[875] (See elsewhere for original sources and reviews on cardiopulmonary resuscitation.[860])

*mmmm*Six of 13 episodes of ventricular fibrillation induced in an electrophysiology laboratory.[883] Whether high-energy shocks are deleterious has never been settled.[877, 881]

*nnnn*For example, in a study from Glasgow, the deaths of 40% of those who died outside the hospital were not witnessed, and in over half the cases, a witness to the collapse, including a spouse or other close relative, did not apply resuscitation.[887]

MONITOR LEAD II   (CONTINUOUS)

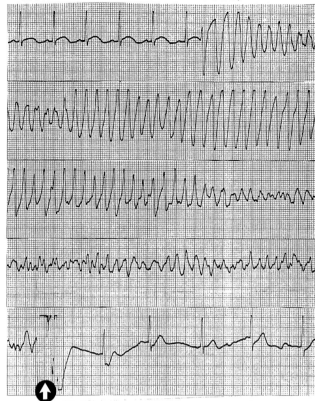

FIGURE 14.9 Ventricular fibrillation following polymorphic ventricular tachycardia. A ventricular premature beat interrupts the downslope of the T wave of the previous sinus beat (**top**) and initiates polymorphic ventricular tachycardia, which degenerates into ventricular fibrillation (*middle* of **middle**). A 200-joule DC shock (*arrow*) converts ventricular fibrillation into an organized, probably junctional, rhythm. (From Myerburg RJ, Kessler KM. Ventricular fibrillation. In Kastor JA (ed). Arrhythmias. Philadelphia: WB Saunders, 1994, pp. 395–420, with permission.)[1]

onary heart disease or with secondary ventricular fibrillation during myocardial infarction.[881] The first shock is more likely to succeed in patients taking antiarrhythmic drugs and in those treated in the hospital compared with those treated out of hospital.[892] One can predict from their clinical characteristics which

Table 14.5 LIKELIHOOD OF SUCCESSFUL DEFIBRILLATION

Unlikely to Be Defibrillated		**No Effect on Defibrillation**
All Patients	**Patients with Myocardial Infarction**[900]	**All Patients**
Acidosis[891]	Cardiogenic shock[900]	Age[881]
Lengthy cardiopulmonary resuscitation before first shock[891]	Congestive heart failure[900]	Body weight[881, 890]
One or two shocks did not convert[892, 893]	Hypotension[900]	Duration of the pulse wave[881]
Systemic hypoxia[891]	—	Heart weight[890]

patients can be successfully defibrillated (see Table 14.1).[893]*oooo*

When standard transthoracic shocks do not defibrillate, the following techniques occasionally succeed:[894–897]

- Intracardiac defibrillation from electrode catheters temporarily in the right ventricle, a technique particularly applicable in the electrophysiology laboratory.
- Simultaneous transthoracic and epicardial defibrillation in the operating room.
- Transesophageal defibrillation.

Although 10 to 20 joules[898] applied through paddles directly on the heart can reliably convert most patients in ventricular fibrillation induced during cardiac surgery, as little as 1 joule can be effective in some cases.[899] The cause of cardiac arrest in some patients who cannot be defibrillated is asystole,[900] severe bradycardia, or electromechanical dissociation. In these patients, ventricular fibrillation develops as a late, secondary arrhythmia.[891]

Survival. Factors that independently predict survival to discharge in descending order are

- Age less than or equal to 70 years.[892]
- Defibrillation requiring no more than two shocks.[892]
- Electrocardiographic amplitude of ventricular fibrillation[604] of at least 0.5 millivolts;[892] few patients survive resuscitation who have asystole or arrhythmias other than ventricular fibrillation or ventricular tachycardia when first treated.[71, 226, 901]

Out-of-hospital resuscitation and defibrillation.[36, 49, 62, 205, 902–904] Survival to discharge from the hospital decreases as the time from the onset of the cardiac arrest to the beginning of resuscitation increases:[905]*pppp*

- Twelve percent when less than 5 minutes.
- Two percent when 5 to 10 minutes.
- None when greater than 10 minutes.
- Twelve percent when resuscitated in a public space.
- Five percent when resuscitated at home.

Antiarrhythmic Drugs[906, 907]

All drugs should be administered intravenously.

Lidocaine. Lidocaine, 1 milligram per kilogram repeated in 2 minutes and followed with an infusion of 1 to 4 milligrams per minute is the first drug usually chosen to suppress ventricular fibrillation during or after resuscitation.

Procainamide. Procainamide hydrochloride, a 100-milligram bolus every 5 minutes to a total dose of 500

to 1,000 milligrams followed by an infusion of 2 to 4 milligrams per minute, can suppress recurrent ventricular tachycardia and ventricular fibrillation when lidocaine fails.

Amiodarone.[908, 909] A 5 milligram per kilogram bolus over 30 minutes followed by 1 gram per 24 hours often suppresses recurrent ventricular tachycardia and occasionally persistent ventricular fibrillation.[910, 911] Many physicians now choose amiodarone over procainamide for this purpose.[778, 912–916]

Bretylium Tosylate.[917–922] This drug, at 5 milligrams per kilogram repeated if defibrillation is unsuccessful with additional doses every 15 minutes to a maximum of 25 milligrams per kilogram, can suppress recurrent ventricular tachycardia and ventricular fibrillation, but it is no more effective than lidocaine.[923]

Other Drugs

Epinephrine. Epinephrine, 0.5 to 1.0 milligrams or 5 to 10 milliliters of a 1:10,000 solution repeated every 5 minutes if necessary, given to patients who do not respond to defibrillation shocks is seldom useful[893] in making the next defibrillation successful. Epinephrine is sometimes administered by the endotracheal route but no longer by direct injection into the heart.[860]

Calcium. Calcium, 5 to 10 milliliters of a 10% solution of calcium gluconate at a rate of 2 to 4 milliliters per minute, may be useful for treating hyperkalemia, hypocalcemia, or toxicity from the effects of calcium entry–blocking drugs.

TREATMENT

PREVENTION[457, 567, 924–929]

Every patient resuscitated from cardiac arrest or with documented ventricular fibrillation occurring in the absence of acute myocardial infarction should be evaluated by a cardiologist with expertise in clinical electrophysiology and access to an electrophysiology laboratory. Only by this means can a successful program be developed to prevent a potentially fatal recurrence.

Drugs[930–937]

As implantable cardioverter-defibrillators have improved and their efficacy has been established, cardiologists less frequently prescribe drugs alone to treat patients with, or at risk of developing, ventricular fibrillation. When drugs are chosen to prevent recurrent episodes, only type III and occasionally beta-adrenergic–blocking agents should be used.

Amiodarone.[938–942] This leading type III antiarrhythmic drug suppresses recurrent drug-refractory ventricular tachycardia and ventricular fibrillation[819, 912, 943–955] in most patients more effectively for ventricular fibrillation than for ventricular tachycardia.[956] However, in

---

*oooo*Nevertheless, several defibrillations should be attempted. The possibility of success with repeated defibrillations significantly outweighs the benefit of drug therapy even with lidocaine and epinephrine.[893]

*pppp*In the experience of ambulance rescue squads in Denmark.[905]

patients with congestive heart failure, amiodarone suppresses ventricular tachycardia more effectively than ventricular fibrillation.[957] Sudden death in patients taking amiodarone occurs most often in those who are older, have reduced ventricular function, or have had a previous cardiac arrest.[587] Amiodarone does not protect all patients with Brugada's syndrome against recurrent cardiac arrest.[477] When given intravenously[778, 912–915, 942, 958] or by rapid oral dosing,[959] amiodarone suppresses incessant ventricular fibrillation even when lidocaine, procainamide, or bretylium fails.[916qqqq]

Orally administered amiodarone reduces total mortality by 10% to 19% in patients at risk of cardiac arrest.[960rrrr] In individual trials, amiodarone

- Reduced the recurrence of out-of-hospital cardiac arrest[780, 961–964] unassociated with myocardial infarction.[783]
- Reduced the incidence of arrhythmic events and death better than "conventional" drugs[783, 965] in those relatively low-risk patients whose left ventricular ejection fractions are more than 39%;[966] amiodarone also reduced the incidence of sudden death in patients with severe congestive heart failure in one trial, in which the patients took 300 milligrams per day after loading,[967ssss] but, it did not prolong survival or reduce the incidence of sudden death in patients with congestive heart failure and asymptomatic ventricular arrhythmias in another.[968]
- Reduced the incidence of sudden death after recovery from myocardial infarction[940, 969–971] in patients with preserved left ventricular function (ejection fraction greater than or equal to 40%),[972] but not in those with diminished left ventricular function (ejection fraction less than or equal to 40%).[973, 974tttt]
- Reduced the incidence of ventricular fibrillation or arrhythmic death among survivors of myocardial infarction who have frequent or repetitive ventricular premature beats.[975uuuu]

Amiodarone probably reduces the incidence of sudden death in patients with hypertrophic cardiomyopathy.[970, 976]

Atropine. By increasing the sinus rate, atropine temporarily suppresses recurrent ventricular fibrillation in some patients.[977] The drug is seldom used for this purpose now.

Beta-adrenergic–blocking drugs.[111, 978–983] These drugs reduce the incidence of ventricular fibrillation

- During acute myocardial infarction,[984–987vvvv] although not, apparently, in patients treated with thrombolytic agents.
- When induced by programmed stimulation during electrophysiological study.[821]
- In some children with stress- and exercise-induced ventricular fibrillation;[988, 989] in those who do arrest, the presence of beta-blocking drugs leads to more successful resuscitation.

Patients who take beta-blocking drugs after myocardial infarction have fewer cardiac arrests[990–993] and are resuscitated more successfully than those not taking the drugs.[992] This advantage applies even in those with reduced left ventricular ejection fractions.[710] Beta-blocker drugs reduce the number of shocks from implantable cardioverter-defibrillators required by patients with life-threatening arrhythmias.[994]

Beta-adrenergic–blocking drugs do not protect each patient with Brugada's syndrome against recurrent cardiac arrest.[477, 478] Beta-adrenergic–blocking drugs reported in the treatment or prevention of ventricular fibrillation include atenolol,[250, 985, 994] metoprolol,[984] nadolol,[994] and propranolol.[821, 986, 988]

Bretylium tosylate. Bretylium tosylate suppresses further ventricular arrhythmias after resuscitation from cardiac arrest no better or worse than lidocaine.[923]

Digoxin specific antibodies. Fab fragments of digoxin specific antibodies can suppress ventricular fibrillation produced by digoxin intoxication.[525]

Isoproterenol. Like atropine, isoproterenol may help to temporarily suppress ventricular fibrillation by increasing the sinus rate.[977]

Lidocaine.[111, 879, 995–998] In adequate doses, lidocaine reduces the incidence of primary ventricular fibrillation in patients with acute myocardial infarction,[210, 211, 214, 245, 999–1010wwww] and it is the first drug usually administered to suppress complex ventricular beating and ven-

---

qqqqIn one study, amiodarone and bretylium were similarly effective, but the use of bretylium was limited by its hypotensive effects.[914]

rrrrAccording to a meta-analysis of 15 randomized trials.[960]

ssssAccording to the Grupo de Estudio de la Sobrevida en la Insuficiencia Cardiaca en Argentina (GESICA) trial.[967]

ttttAccording to the European Myocardial Infarct Amiodarone Trial (EMIAT) of 1,486 patients.[973, 974, 1217] The authors suggest: "Our findings do not support the systematic prophylactic use of amiodarone in all patients with depressed left-ventricular function after myocardial infarction."[974]

uuuuAccording to the Canadian Amiodarone Myocardial Infarction Arrhythmia Trial (CAMIAT) of 1,202 patients.[975, 1217] This favorable result with amiodarone conflicts with the neutral or negative results of the Cardiac Arrhythmia Suppression Trial (CAST) with encainide, flecainide, and moricizine.

---

vvvvThe MIAMI Trial Research Group observed that metoprolol reduces the number of episodes of ventricular fibrillation from the onset through the 15 days after myocardial infarction, but the difference compared with a placebo group did not reach significance.[987]

wwwwAlthough *intramuscular* administration of lidocaine before admission to the hospital has been proposed to reduce early mortality from myocardial infarction,[1002, 1004] studies have shown that the drug is ineffective in preventing ventricular fibrillation during myocardial infarction when given as:

- Three hundred milligrams intramuscularly,[245] although 400 milligrams administered by paramedics with an autoinjector may work.[1005, 1006]
- One hundred milligrams intravenous bolus followed by 300 milligrams intramuscularly in Norway where the majority of patients must be transported for more than 1 hour in ambulances without defibrillators or personnel trained in cardiopulmonary resuscitation.[1009]

tricular tachycardia that arise during acute myocardial infarction and may progress to ventricular fibrillation.[1011, 1012]

When given prophylactically,[1013] however, lidocaine must be administered to about 400 patients with presumed or confirmed myocardial infarction to prevent one episode of ventricular fibrillation,[223] and the drug can produce serious side effects.[1014–1018] In some hospitalized patients with myocardial infarction, lidocaine

- Decreases the blood pressure.[1019]
- Increases congestive heart failure.[1020]
- Produces asystole when repeated defibrillations are required.[893]
- Produces petit and grand mal seizures.[1021]
- Raises the mortality.[1019, 1022]

In view of these facts, lidocaine should not be administered routinely to each patient admitted with an established or suspected myocardial infarction.[223, 998, 1012, 1014, 1018, 1022, 1023]*xxxx*

In the operating room, surgeons and anesthesiologists use lidocaine to reduce the incidence of

- Ventricular tachyarrhythmias, including ventricular fibrillation, for 24 hours after coronary artery bypass graft surgery.[1024]
- Ventricular fibrillation during reperfusion after cardiopulmonary bypass when given immediately after unclamping the aorta.[1025]

Magnesium. A patient with digitalis intoxication producing repetitive ventricular fibrillation responded "dramatically" to magnesium sulfate.[526]

Sotalol *(d,l)*.[1026–1032] This drug, which has some beta-adrenergic–blocking properties, exerts most of its antiarrhythmic properties through type III activity. The racemic *(d,l)* form decreases

- The number of arrhythmic events in patients with sustained ventricular tachyarrhythmias,[1033–1039] and more effectively with ventricular fibrillation than with ventricular tachycardia.[1040]
- The inducibility of ventricular tachycardia and fibrillation in the electrophysiology laboratory in many patients with these arrhythmias.[1033, 1039, 1041–1043]

Sotalol improves survival in patients with ventricular fibrillation and ventricular tachycardia.[1043] However, the drug produces more of what are presumed to be arrhythmic deaths in patients with left ventricular dysfunction and recent myocardial infarctions or congestive heart failure.[1044]*yyyy* Implantable cardioverter-defibrillators prevent sudden death more effectively than sotalol.[1039]

Ineffective drugs. No data conclusively support the value of the following drugs in suppressing ventricular fibrillation or reducing the incidence of cardiac arrest:

- Calcium-channel antagonists, although in one report, verapamil was thought to suppress recurrent ventricular fibrillation during cardiac surgery in four patients with ventricular hypertrophy.[1045]
- Class I antiarrhythmic drugs such as disopyramide, flecainide, procainamide, propafenone, and quinidine.[822, 992, 1046–1049]*zzzz*
- Isoproterenol.[1050]*aaaaa*

Surgery[1051]

Ischemia occasionally produces cardiac arrest from ventricular fibrillation. Such patients have severe stenoses of their coronary arteries, and imaging studies show marked ischemia at low workloads or at rest. Successful coronary revascularization can relieve the ischemia and prevent recurrence of the arrhythmia.[176, 387, 435, 440, 592, 785, 1052–1062]

Surgical revascularization, however, does not reduce the likelihood that most survivors of cardiac arrest whose arrhythmias cannot be induced at electrophysiological study will require fewer shocks from implantable cardioverter-defibrillators.[1063] These data suggest that relief of ischemia seldom removes all the factors that lead to arrest in such patients. Moreover, coronary artery bypass graft surgery does not prevent induction of sustained ventricular arrhythmias or spontaneous ventricular fibrillation in all patients with coronary heart disease who have been resuscitated from cardiac arrest.[1064, 1065]

Pacing

Pacing seldom *converts* ventricular fibrillation, but it can *suppress* recurrent ventricular fibrillation[1066] and ventricular tachycardia. The technique is seldom used by itself, however, in the management of the arrhythmia. Ventricular pacing at 90 beats per minute, rather than at 70 beats per minute or less, seems to prevent episodes of ventricular fibrillation after atrioventricular junctional ablation for rapid supraventricular tachycardias.[501]

Implantable Cardioverter-Defibrillator[932, 934, 1067–1112]*bbbbb*

The implantable cardioverter-defibrillator, in its latest models a highly versatile instrument[596, 599, 1112–1122] (Table 14.6), is the most effective means of preventing cardiac arrest in patients of all ages at risk of ventricular tachycardia and ventricular fibrillation (Fig.

---

*xxxx*Many will remember when lidocaine was given prophylactically to most patients admitted with a documented or suspected myocardial infarction to prevent development of ventricular fibrillation.[210, 211, 1000, 1001, 1008]

*yyyy*According to the Survival with Oral *d*-Sotalol (SWORD) trial.[1044] The left ventricular ejection fraction the patients was 40% or less.[1044]

---

*zzzz*Which are implicated in increasing cardiac arrest. (See the discussion of proarrhythmia in Chapter 13.)

*aaaaa*Isoproterenol was employed before pacemakers were developed to suppress ventricular fibrillation produced by complete atrioventricular block.[1050]

*bbbbb*The implantable cardioverter-defibrillator was developed by Michel Mirowski (1924–1990) and associates in Baltimore during the 1970s[1067, 1068, 1079, 1080] (see Chapter 2).

Table 14.6	**FEATURES OF IMPLANTABLE CARDIOVERTER-DEFIBRILLATORS THAT CAN BE PROGRAMMED NONINVASIVELY**

Defibrillate ventricular fibrillation
Convert ventricular tachycardia by rapid pacing or low energy shock[596, 1119]
Prevent bradycardia-induced asystole by pacing, with ability to pace atria as well as ventricles in the latest models[1120, 1122a]
Reveal the presence of arrhythmias through memory[599, 1113, 1115]
Induce arrhythmias on instruction during electrophysiological evaluation[1118]

---

*a*Experience with installing both implantable cardioverter-defibrillators and dual-chamber pacers support the value of defibrillators that incorporate this feature.[1121]

14.10).[114, 596, 1123–1160][ccccc] Neither age[1140, 1161–1163] nor pregnancy[1164] limits use of the devices. However, survival in patients with implantable cardioverter-defibrillators is lower in those older than 74 years of age compared with younger patients in the same functional class and with similar left ventricular ejection fractions.[1162]

Patients now selected for implantable cardioverter-defibrillators are older[ddddd] and have better left ventricular function[eeeee] than those who received the device during the 1980s, the first decade of its use.[1154] However, implanting cardioverter-defibrillators may be indicated even when left ventricular function is severely reduced.[1165]

[ccccc]The Antiarrhythmics versus Implantable Defibrillators (AVID) trial demonstrated that, among survivors of sustained ventricular tachycardia or ventricular fibrillation, implantable cardioverter-defibrillators increase overall survival better than do antiarrhythmic drugs.[1110, 1159, 1160]

[ddddd]60.9 years for patients receiving implantable cardioverter-defibrillators during the 1980s versus 63 years for patients receiving them recently.[1154]

[eeeee]Left ventricular ejection fraction of 29.7% during the 1980s versus 32.7% recently.[1154]

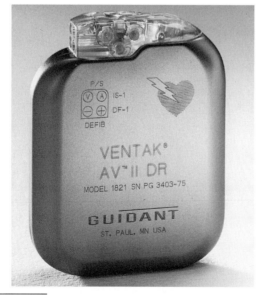

FIGURE 14.10 Implantable cardioverter defibrillator. Model VENTAK AV II. (Courtesy of Guidant/CPI, St. Paul, MN.)

The development of models which can be installed without thoracotomy[1119, 1166–1171] has eliminated most of the mortality from the procedure,[1154, 1172] which was troublingly high,[1173, 1174] particularly in patients with poor ventricular function,[1175] and has reduced the morbidity, length of hospitalization, and expense of implanting the devices.[1149, 1176–1182] An external wearable transthoracic defibrillator is under study for use by patients awaiting implantation.[1183]

Syncope. However, syncope still occurs in patients with implantable cardioverter-defibrillators,[1184][fffff] most frequently in those with low left ventricular ejection fractions, chronic atrial fibrillation, and fast ventricular tachycardia induced at electrophysiological study.[1185] The absence of syncope during one shock does not preclude patients fainting during subsequent shocks.[1184] None of the following predict which patients with implantable cardioverter-defibrillators will faint:[1184]

- Age.
- Antiarrhythmic drugs.
- Electrophysiological findings.
- Gender.
- Heart disease.
- History of syncope.
- Left ventricular function.
- Pulse generator.
- Ventricular tachycardia rate.

Indications[1186–1188] (Table 14.7).[ggggg] Implantation of cardioverter-defibrillators should be considered for all patients presenting with ventricular fibrillation, regardless of the etiologic diagnosis,[1189] except when the arrhythmia is due to[591]

- Acute myocardial infarction.
- Myocardial ischemia which can be treated with revascularization.[387]
- Proarrhythmia from a drug that can be discontinued.[387]
- Sepsis, hemorrhage, or another treatable cause.

Compared with men who require implantable cardioverter-defibrillators, women tend to be younger and more likely have[1190]

- Greater left ventricular ejection fraction.
- No structural heart disease.
- Spontaneous ventricular fibrillation.

Reduced ventricular function identifies best the patients in whom implantable cardioverter-defibrillators will discharge[1133, 1191–1195] and, presumably, prevent fatal ventricular arrhythmias.[1139, 1142, 1145, 1150, 1192] The devices

---

[fffff]Loss of consciousness occurred in 16 (9%) of 180 patients with implantable cardioverter-defibrillators during a follow-up period averaging 16 months.[1184]

[ggggg]The American College of Cardiology/American Heart Association Task Force on Practice Guidelines (Committee on Pacemaker Implantation) has published (1998) guidelines for the use of implantable cardioverter-defibrillators that I have summarized in Table 14.8.[1188]

Table 14.7 USE OF IMPLANTABLE CARDIOVERTER-DEFIBRILLATORS[1188]

Indicated (class I)
1. Cardiac arrest due to ventricular fibrillation or ventricular tachycardia not due to a transient or reversible cause
2. Spontaneous sustained ventricular tachycardia
3. Syncope of undetermined origin with clinically relevant, hemodynamically significant sustained ventricular tachycardia or ventricular fibrillation induced at electrophysiological study when drug therapy is ineffective, not tolerated, or not preferred
4. Transient ventricular tachycardia with coronary disease, prior myocardial infarction, left ventricular dysfunction, and inducible ventricular fibrillation or sustained ventricular tachycardia at electrophysiological study that is not suppressible by a class I antiarrhythmic drug

Possible indicated (class IIb)
1. Cardiac arrest presumed to be due to ventricular fibrillation when other medical conditions prevent an electrophysiological study
2. Severe symptoms attributable to sustained ventricular tachyarrhythmias while awaiting cardiac transplantation
3. Familial or inherited conditions with a high risk of life-threatening ventricular tachyarrhythmias such as long QT syndrome or hypertrophic cardiomyopathy
4. Transient ventricular tachycardia with coronary heart disease, prior myocardial infarction, and left ventricular dysfunction, and inducible sustained ventricular tachycardia or ventricular fibrillation at electrophysiological study
5. Recurrent syncope of undetermined origin in the presence of ventricular dysfunction and inducible ventricular arrhythmias at electrophysiological study when other causes of syncope have been excluded

Not indicated and possibly harmful (class III)
1. Syncope of undetermined cause in a patient without inducible tachyarrhythmias
2. Incessant ventricular tachycardia or ventricular fibrillation
3. Ventricular tachycardia or ventricular tachycardia from arrhythmias treatable with surgical or catheter ablation (such as atrial arrhythmias associated with Wolff-Parkinson-White syndrome, ventricular tachycardia from the right ventricular outflow track, idiopathic left ventricular tachycardia, or fascicular ventricular tachycardia)
4. Ventricular tachyarrhythmias due to a transient or reversible cause (such as myocardial infarction, electrolyte imbalance, drugs, or trauma)
5. Psychiatric illnesses that may be aggravated by implantation of a device or that may prevent systematic follow-up
6. Terminal illnesses with projected life expectancy of no more than 6 months
7. Patients with coronary heart disease, left ventricular dysfunction, and prolonged duration of the QRS complexes in the absence of spontaneous sustained or transient ventricular tachycardia who are undergoing coronary artery bypass graft surgery
8. Patients who are not candidates for cardiac transplantation and who have congestive heart failure with New York Heart Association classification class IV

(Adapted from Gregoratos G, Cheitlin MD, Conill A, et al. ACC/AHA Guidelines for Implantation of Cardiac Pacemakers and Antiarrhythmia Devices (Committee on Pacemaker Implantation). Circulation 1998; 97:1325–1335. By permission of the American Heart Association, Inc.)

discharge more frequently in those patients in whom ventricular tachycardia rather than polymorphic ventricular tachycardia or ventricular fibrillation is induced during electrophysiological study.[1195] Whether cardioverter-defibrillators should be implanted prophylactically without electrophysiological study in patients at high risk of cardiac arrest is a topic of continuing debate,[1077, 1196–1205] as is the prophylactic use of defibrillators to treat dangerous arrhythmias that could arise in patients awaiting cardiac transplantation.[1206]

Survivors of cardiac arrest. Implantable cardioverter-defibrillators, rather than drugs, are becoming the leading therapeutic choice for those who survive cardiac arrest and who have had previous myocardial infarction.[1207] Nevertheless, some survivors of cardiac arrest with implantable cardioverter-defibrillators die suddenly, presumably from irreversible ventricular arrhythmias; the device does not provide eternal relief from cardiac arrest due to advanced heart disease.[1208]

Coronary heart disease. Most patients with coronary heart disease who have ventricular fibrillation or cardiac arrest presumed due to ventricular fibrillation have inducible sustained ventricular tachycardia. They should be evaluated and treated like patients being evaluated for sustained ventricular tachycardia and may require an implantable cardioverter-defibrillator.

When the arrhythmia that causes cardiac arrest in patients with coronary heart disease is ventricular fibrillation alone, an implantable cardioverter-defibrillator is the appropriate treatment. Of course, ischemia, susceptible to treatment with angioplasty or coronary artery bypass graft surgery, must be excluded. Furthermore, when ventricular fibrillation complicates the first days of acute myocardial infarction, specific treatment after recovery is not required unless the later course is complicated by additional ventricular arrhythmias.

Implantable cardioverter-defibrillators reduce mortality, including that due to cardiac arrest, by as much as 50% in patients with prior Q-wave myocardial infarction, documented transient ventricular tachycardia not producing syncope, and[1209–1217hhhhh]

- Left ventricular ejection fraction less than 35%.
- New York Heart Association classification I, II, or III.
- No indications for coronary revascularization.
- Ventricular arrhythmias inducible during electrophysiological study and unsuppressible with procainamide.

---

hhhhhAccording to MADIT (Multicenter Automatic Defibrillator Implantation Trial).[1209, 1211–1217] The results of MUSTT (Multicenter Unsustained Tachycardia Trial) should further help physicians to decide what form of therapy will best prevent sudden death in patients with transient ventricular tachycardia resulting from coronary heart disease.[1210]

Radiofrequency current ablation of ventricular tachycardia reduces the number of discharges from implantable cardioverter-defibrillators in patients with coronary heart disease.[1218] The survival of patients undergoing coronary artery bypass graft surgery who receive cardioverter-defibrillators implanted prophylactically and without specific indications is not superior when compared with that in similar, operated patients without the devices.[1219–1222][iiiii]

Cardiomyopathy. Although type III antiarrhythmic drugs, particularly amiodarone, are sometimes employed, most clinical electrophysiologists advise that a cardioverter-defibrillator be implanted in all patients with dilated cardiomyopathy who have cardiac arrest in ventricular fibrillation. Electrophysiological study of such patients is often unhelpful,[796] except when bundle branch reentry susceptible to ablation can be demonstrated.

Compared with patients with coronary heart disease, those with idiopathic cardiomyopathy who need implantable cardioverter-defibrillators for ventricular fibrillation are younger and are more likely to be female.[1223] However, implantable cardioverter-defibrillators discharge with similar frequency in patients with idiopathic dilated cardiomyopathy as in patients with coronary heart disease.[1223]

No studies have yet established the value of the implantable cardioverter-defibrillator in hypertrophic cardiomyopathy, although it seems reasonable that this treatment could be lifesaving in patients at high risk of cardiac arrest.[800, 1224] These devices, when implanted in patients with hypertrophic cardiomyopathy who have survived cardiac arrest or who have sustained ventricular tachycardia, seldom discharge, confirming the favorable short-term prognosis in many of these patients.[1225] In deciding whether to advise the use of the device, one should also remember that most patients with hypertrophic cardiomyopathy do not die suddenly.[334]

No structural heart disease.[452, 457, 461] Predicting which patients with no demonstrable structural heart disease who have been resuscitated from cardiac arrest will have cardiac arrest again is very difficult. The electrophysiological study of those with ventricular fibrillation, rather than sustained ventricular tachycardia, seldom supplies therapeutic information[462, 807] because programmed stimulation infrequently induces reproducible arrhythmias in these patients.[jjjjj] Although the number of such patients saved from recurrent cardiac arrest by implantable cardioverter-defibrillators is relatively low,[807] selecting those at risk is not possible at this time. Consequently, several authorities advise implanting cardioverter-defibrillators in most patients with idiopathic ventricular fibrillation[462, 807, 1226] including all with Brugada's syndrome.[475, 477, 478]

Cost.[1227, 1228] Implantable cardioverter-defibrillators are costly, and investigators debate whether their expense is justified.[933, 1229–1237] At this writing, it appears that early implantation of cardioverter-defibrillators may be more cost-effective for patients with recurrent ventricular tachyarrhythmias than drug therapy guided by electrophysiological study,[1238–1242] including patients who fulfill the criteria for the Multicenter Automatic Defibrillator Implantation Trial.[1243][kkkkk] The procedure reduces the frequency and duration of readmissions to hospitals, often to the more expensive intensive care monitoring units.[1244]

Catheter Ablation[593]

Ablating accessory pathways in patients with Wolff-Parkinson-White syndrome can prevent their having ventricular fibrillation caused by rapid antegrade conduction from fibrillating or fluttering atria.[lllll] Ablating the sites where ventricular tachycardia originates can, by suppressing that arrhythmia, prevent the ventricular fibrillation that may follow.[mmmmm] Ablation of arrhythmogenic foci producing ventricular fibrillation has been attempted,[1245] but the efficacy of the procedure for this purpose has not been established.

Acute Angioplasty

Opening obstructed coronary vessels soon after the admission of survivors of out-of-hospital cardiac arrest may improve survival.[166, 1246, 1247] The usual clinical and electrocardiographic clues to the presence of ischemia or injury are often absent in these patients.[166] Angioplasty can also prevent further exercise-induced ventricular fibrillation in patients with obstructing coronary lesions.[434]

Activity

Survivors of cardiac arrest that appears to be provoked by physical activities, such as competitive athletics, must stop these activities unless the cause of the arrhythmia is removed or the patient has received treatment certain to prevent a recurrence, such as an implantable cardioverter-defibrillator.[426]

Driving. Syncope still occurs in patients with implantable cardioverter-defibrillators,[1184] so even though accidents follow only about 11% of discharges from implantable cardioverter-defibrillators in patients while driving,[1248] most physicians, at least those surveyed in the midwestern United States,[1249] advise their patients not to drive after receiving these devices. Not every patient follows this advice.[1250–1252][nnnnn]

[kkkkk]See the earlier paragraphs on implantable cardioverter-defibrillators in patients with coronary heart disease.

[lllll]See Chapter 8 for a discussion of the ablation of accessory pathways.

[mmmmm]See Chapter 12 for a discussion of the ablation of ventricular sites of origin.

[nnnnn]According to a paper published in 1991, only eight states of the United States have specific laws about driving by patients with arrhythmias and none distinguish between patients being treated with drugs or implantable cardioverter-defibrillators.[1250]

[iiiii]According to the CABG Patch Trial.[1219–1222]

[jjjjj]Ventricular fibrillation in the absence of structural heart disease is often lethal, whereas sustained ventricular tachycardia in the absence of structural heart disease carries a more favorable prognosis.

The hazard of recurrent ventricular fibrillation, hemodynamically unstable ventricular tachycardia, syncope, cardiac arrest, or discharge of an implantable cardioverter-defibrillator continues after discharge from the hospital and is[1253]

- Highest in the first month.[ooooo]
- Intermediate from months 2 through 7.[ppppp]
- Lowest after 8 to 12 months.[qqqqq]

Accordingly, it seems reasonable that survivors of ventricular fibrillation not drive during the first month after discharge and seriously consider abstaining through the eighth month. Furthermore, patients and their physicians should bear in mind that in those for whom electrophysiological study finds no satisfactory conventional antiarrhythmic agent, the risk remains higher than average even after 7 months.[1253]

PROGNOSIS[859, 1254, 1255]

Predictors of Potentially Fatal Cardiac Arrest[1256]

Before reviewing how we can predict which patients are most likely to suffer cardiac arrest, one should realize, as Hein J. J. Wellens has written: "The majority of sudden death victims cannot be identified before the event."[63] As for what is known, the following predict a greater likelihood of cardiac arrest regardless of the cause of the heart disease:

- Reduced ventricular function.[78, 114, 162, 259, 579, 580, 582–584, 587, 656, 664, 679, 700, 708–710, 713–717, 795, 822, 963, 966, 1193, 1195, 1207, 1257–1270] Left ventricular ejection fraction of less than 40% predicts more strongly than any other factor the cardiac and total mortality of men who survive cardiac arrest.[132]
- Complex ventricular premature beats and ventricular tachycardia,[74, 568–573, 576–586, 651, 654, 713, 714, 716, 1257, 1259, 1260, 1267, 1271–1278] which, when hemodynamically unstable, predict higher mortality even in patients with implantable cardioverter-defibrillators.[114]

[ooooo]4.22% per month.[1253]
[ppppp]1.81% per month.[1253]
[qqqqq]0.63% per month.[1253]

- Abnormal signal-averaged electrocardiogram.[655, 656, 664, 665, 667, 674, 677–681, 685, 693, 1260, 1279, 1280]
- Decreased heart rate variability.[543, 594, 655, 677, 686, 688–692, 696, 698, 700]
- Increased dispersion of recovery time (QT dispersion) in patients 55 years of age or older.[622]
- Induction of at least five ventricular beats[1281] or of ventricular fibrillation rather than monomorphic ventricular tachycardia[rrrrr] at electrophysiological study after myocardial infarction.[795]

Rehospitalization

Fifty percent of survivors of cardiac arrest and 65% of those whose left ventricular ejection fraction is less than 30% are rehospitalized within the first year after sustaining arrest.[1282] The rate is lower in those taking amiodarone or in those with implantable cardioverter-defibrillators.[1282]

Out-of-Hospital Ventricular Fibrillation and Cardiac Arrest

About one-third of patients who sustain out-of-hospital ventricular fibrillation reach a hospital alive, and about 50% of those hospitalized are discharged alive.[155, 178] Fatal rearrest occurs in about 17% in 1 year,[1283, 1284sssss] and about one-third of those who are discharged die within 3 years[1285, 1286] (Fig. 14.11). The incidence of recurrent cardiac arrest is highest during the first month after discharge in patients admitted for cardiac arrest or for sustained ventricular tachycardia.[587ttttt]

Factors associated with increased mortality in survivors of out-of-hospital ventricular fibrillation include

- Older age,[1287] particularly more than 59 years.[1288]
- Digitalis taken before the arrest or after discharge.[1288]
- Diuretic taken before the arrest.[1288]
- Hypertension.[1288]

[rrrrr]In patients taking amiodarone.[795]
[sssss]According to a study reported in 1991;[1284] 10% according to an earlier study (1984).[1283]
[ttttt]The median time to recurrent cardiac arrest in 234 survivors in the Seattle experience was 20 weeks.[108]

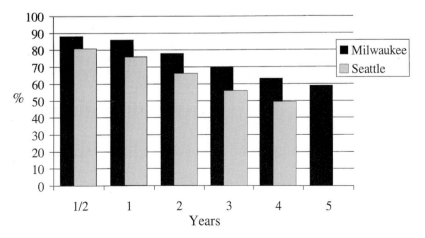

FIGURE 14.11 Prognosis of patients resuscitated from cardiac arrest by paramedics and discharged from the hospital alive (%), according to two series: Milwaukee (*black columns*), 139 patients presenting from December 1973 to March 1992; Seattle (*stippled columns*), 302 patients from April 1, 1976 to June 1, 1981. None of the patients had electrophysiological studies or received cardioverter-defibrillators. (Adapted from Tresch DD, Keelan MH Jr, Siegel R, et al. Long-term survival after prehospital sudden cardiac death. Am Heart J 1984; 108:1–5; and Eisenberg MS, Hallstrom A, Bergner L. Long-term survival after out-of-hospital cardiac arrest. N Engl J Med 1982; 306:1340–1343, with permission.)[1285, 1286]

- Longer interval between collapse and defibrillation.[1287]
- Myocardial infarction in the past.[1288]
- No bystander-initiated cardiopulmonary resuscitation.[1287]
- Smoking after discharge in patients who smoked before the cardiac arrest.[1288]
- Ventricular fibrillation occurring *without* myocardial infarction.[1288]*uuuuu*

Recurrent cardiac arrest occurs more often in patients without myocardial infarction who have

- Impaired contraction of many left ventricular segments.[1289]
- Persistent inducible ventricular fibrillation despite treatment with antiarrhythmic drugs.[1290]
- Reduced left ventricular ejection fraction.[1289, 1290]
- Triple-vessel congenital heart disease.[1289]
- Unstable blood levels of antiarrhythmic drugs.[1291]

Coronary Heart Disease

Impaired ventricular function predicts more strongly than any other factor the cardiac and total mortality of women who survive cardiac arrest.[132]

Myocardial infarction. As one would expect, patients who have survived myocardial infarction die suddenly more often than persons of similar age who have not had myocardial infarction.[1292] Furthermore, those who have had myocardial infarction, develop symptomatic sustained ventricular tachycardia and ventricular fibrillation, and are treated with standard antiarrhythmic drugs have a poor prognosis, particularly when they also have[1293]

- Cardiac arrest during the first arrhythmia episode.
- Killip class III or IV symptoms.
- Multiple previous infarctions.
- Q-wave infarction.

The in-hospital mortality rate is higher when primary ventricular fibrillation complicates the early course of myocardial infarction.[154, 222, 231, 239, 243, 1023, 1294, 1295]*vvvvv* However, primary ventricular fibrillation early during myocardial infarction, although it slows rehabilitation,[1296] does not worsen the prognosis after discharge[153, 221, 222, 231, 651, 1294, 1295, 1297–1300]*wwwww* or affect

- Driving.[1296]
- Resumption of normal sexual activity.[1296]
- Return to work.[1296]

Patients with ventricular fibrillation or sustained ventricular tachycardia after the acute period have a poor prognosis.[1301] Moreover, as expected, the worse the ventricular function, the worse is their prognosis.[709, 1207, 1262, 1264]

Other factors that increase the likelihood that patients with previous myocardial infarction and ventricular tachycardia or fibrillation will die suddenly or otherwise from coronary heart disease include[1302]

- Cardiac arrest at the time of the first spontaneous episode of the arrhythmia.[1302]
- New York Heart Association functional class III for dyspnea.[1302]
- Ventricular tachycardia or fibrillation occurring between 4 days and 2 months after myocardial infarction.[1302]
- Multiple myocardial infarctions before the first episode of ventricular tachyarrhythmia.[1302]

A potentially fatal ventricular arrhythmia occurs more often after recovery from myocardial infarction in patients with a closed, rather than open, infarct-related artery.[1280]

Inducing ventricular tachycardia in the electrophysiology laboratory after myocardial infarction predicts better than any other factor whether a patient will sustain ventricular tachycardia or cardiac arrest afterward.[1303] However, the prognosis is not adversely affected when electrophysiological study induces ventricular fibrillation in patients whose recent myocardial infarction was uncomplicated by *spontaneous* ventricular tachycardia or ventricular fibrillation.[1304] When ventricular tachycardia or fibrillation complicates the course of myocardial infarction in children, the mortality rises from 59% to 80%.[288]

Ischemia. Successful revascularization improves the prognosis for survivors of ventricular fibrillation who have severe, operable coronary heart disease,[592, 1058] particularly those with ventricular fibrillation inducible at electrophysiological study preoperatively and not postoperatively.[1057] The rate of sudden death is lower in patients with coronary heart disease treated surgically than medically.[1305] *xxxxx*

Cardiomyopathy

Idiopathic dilated cardiomyopathy. Neither the electrophysiological study[796, 798, 1306] nor the arrhythmia on presentation[1307] predicts which patients with dilated cardiomyopathy will have cardiac arrest, nor does empiric antiarrhythmic treatment reliably prevent fatal cardiac arrest in such patients.[820, 1306] Although an antiarrhythmic drug may reduce its incidence, cardiac arrest still occurs unpredictably.[798]

---

*uuuuu*Patients die three times more often within 2 years if they have *not* had a myocardial infarction than if they have had one.[1328] Of 146 patients resuscitated from out-of-hospital ventricular fibrillation, 14% who had a myocardial infarction died during the next 2 years, whereas 47% died whose cardiac arrest was unassociated with myocardial infarction.[226]

*vvvvv*In one large series of patients with myocardial infarction,[1295] 94% of 6,781 patients without ventricular fibrillation were discharged alive compared with 89% of 332 patients with ventricular fibrillation.[1295] Although revealing a higher in-hospital mortality for *all* patients with ventricular fibrillation, the authors of a smaller series of 849 patients found that those with *primary* ventricular fibrillation did not suffer a higher in-hospital mortality.[231]

*wwwww*One study found that ventricular fibrillation associated with myocardial infarction worsened the prognosis for the first 60 days after the infarction but not thereafter.[1329]

---

*xxxxx*4.9% of 5,258 patients treated medically and 1.6% of 6,250 patients treated surgically died suddenly according to the Coronary Artery Surgery Study (CASS) (1986) of 13,476 patients.[1305]

Patients with idiopathic cardiomyopathy more likely to die suddenly have

- Abnormal signal-averaged electrocardiograms.[680]
- Atrial fibrillation.[585]
- Complex ventricular arrhythmias.[585, 1307, 1308]
- Decreased left ventricular function.[1308, 1309]
- Left bundle branch block.

Absence of high-risk ventricular arrhythmias (Lown grades III to V) on Holter monitoring, however, selects those at low risk of cardiac arrest.[1307] Fatal cardiac arrest is uncommon in children with dilated cardiomyopathy, and their arrhythmias detected on monitoring do not predict outcome.[326] However, the risk of fatal cardiac arrest is greater in older children—age is an independent risk factor—if their echocardiographic dimensions remain abnormal.[1310]

Hypertrophic cardiomyopathy.[333, 334] Fatal cardiac arrest occurs more often in patients with hypertrophic cardiomyopathy who are 14 years of age or less[122] or who have

- Family history of hypertrophic cardiomyopathy and fatal cardiac arrest.[122]
- Reduced left ventricular ejection fraction.[1311]
- Severe dyspnea when last examined.[122]
- Syncope as the presenting symptom when the diagnosis is made.[122, 1311]

The rate of fatal cardiac arrest in adults with hypertrophic cardiomyopathy increases if Holter monitoring reveals transient ventricular tachycardia. In children, however, the absence of ventricular arrhythmias does not necessarily indicate a low risk of subsequent cardiac arrest.[335, 1312] The prognosis is poor in some, but not in all, survivors of cardiac arrest who have hypertrophic cardiomyopathy.[1313]

Chagas disease. Ventricular tachycardia on exercise testing is significantly associated with sudden cardiac death in patients with chronic chagasic cardiomyopathy and ventricular arrhythmias.[1314]

No Major Structural Heart Disease[452, 454]

The prognosis of most patients with idiopathic ventricular fibrillation is good,[454, 1315, 1316] but we do not yet know how to select in advance the many who will survive from the few who will rearrest.[807] However, cardiac arrest recurs in many survivors of cardiac arrest with no major structural heart disease[462] and most often in those who have wall motion or electrocardiographic abnormalities and are, surprisingly, younger.[465] The risk is greater in patients who present specifically with ventricular fibrillation; a major arrhythmic event occurred in 37% of such patients in one series.[464]yyyyy Sufficiently long refractoriness of accessory pathways and RR intervals during atrial fibrillation in patients

---

yyyyyDuring follow-up of 43 months (range 5 to 85 months).[464]

with Wolff-Parkinson-White syndrome predict that sudden death is unlikely but still possible.[845]

No Inducible Ventricular Fibrillation during Electrophysiological Study

Cardiac arrest, often fatal,[1285, 1317zzzzz] most likely recurs in those survivors of cardiac arrest in whom ventricular tachyarrhythmias cannot be induced at electrophysiological study and who have[1317]

- Dilated cardiomyopathy.
- Ventricular premature beats or transient ventricular tachycardia.
- Left ventricular ejection fractions of less than 40%.

Few survivors of ventricular fibrillation with good ventricular function in whom sustained ventricular arrhythmias cannot be induced, however, die suddenly.[808, 1318] The prognosis, moreover, can be excellent for such patients when ischemia that can be relieved with coronary artery bypass graft surgery causes the cardiac arrest.[1319] The prognosis of survivors of cardiac arrest who do not have coronary heart disease is much superior to that in those who have coronary disease.[792] Implantation of cardioverter-defibrillators reduces the likelihood of cardiac rearrest better than other treatments for survivors in whom ventricular arrhythmias cannot be induced at electrophysiological study.[1320]

Syncope

The incidence of fatal cardiac arrest is low in patients with unexplained syncope and a nondiagnostic electrophysiological study.[1321] Syncope, however, frequently recurs.[1321] Women have a better short-term survival than men after admission for syncope.[1322]

Effect of the Implantable Cardioverter-Defibrillator

The implantable cardioverter-defibrillator has significantly reduced mortality in victims of ventricular fibril-

---

zzzzzEleven of 26 (42%) in one series.[1317]

| Table 14.8 | EFFECT OF THE IMPLANTABLE CARDIOVERTER-DEFIBRILLATOR ON THE PROBABILITY OF NOT DYING OF HEART DISEASE AMONG 331 SURVIVORS OF OUT-OF-HOSPITAL CARDIAC ARREST UNASSOCIATED WITH MYOCARDIAL INFARCTION[1150] |

Left ventricular ejection fraction	>0.39%		<0.40%	
Implantable cardioverter-defibrillator	Yes	No	Yes	No
1-year survival	97.7%	95.4%	94.3%	82.1%
5-year survival	94.5%	86.9%	69.6%	43.5%
Number of patients	150	181	150	181

(From Powell AC, Fuchs T, Finkelstein DM, et al. Influence of implantable cardioverter-defibrillators on the long-term prognosis of survivors of out-of-hospital cardiac arrest. Circulation 1993; 88:1083–1092. By permission of the American Heart Association, Inc.)

lation,[1127, 1135, 1323] particularly those with reduced ventricular function[1150] (Table 14.8). The lower the left ventricular ejection fraction[1324] and the greater the extent of regional malfunction of the ventricular walls[1324] and of myocardial scarring,[1325] the worse the prognosis.[1324] In preventing them from dying suddenly from arrhythmias, implantable cardioverter-defibrillators allow the sickest patients to succumb eventually to progressive congestive heart failure[1324] and electromechanical dissociation[1326] and not to a treatable arrhythmia.[1326] The mortality is three times greater in patients who receive implantable cardioverter-defibrillators when they are older than 74 years of age compared with younger patients with the same functional classes and left ventricular ejection fractions.[1162]

SUMMARY

Patients who die suddenly in cardiac arrest usually succumb to ventricular fibrillation, the arrhythmia that most frequently causes cardiac arrest and the setting for at least 80% of those who die suddenly outside the hospital. Men die suddenly much more often than women, and blacks die slightly more frequently than whites. Few who are young die suddenly, the incidence rising rapidly over the age of 45 years. Cardiac arrest occurs more frequently in patients who are awake, active or highly active, cigarette smokers, obese, less educated, or have survived previous cardiac arrests. Cardiac arrest occurs more often on Monday than on other days of the week and in the morning rather than at other times of the day or night.

Primary ventricular fibrillation develops from specific electrophysiological abnormalities in the absence of hemodynamic factors of sufficient severity to initiate the arrhythmia. Secondary or complicating ventricular fibrillation results from myocardial damage sufficient to produce congestive failure.

Patients with cardiac arrest who are more than 30 years of age most frequently have coronary heart disease, often involving three vessels, previous myocardial infarction, and reduced ventricular function. About half of survivors of out-of-hospital cardiac arrest have a myocardial infarction. However, ventricular fibrillation develops in relatively few patients with myocardial infarction once they come under medical care. The incidence is highest early after the onset of the infarction and occurs most often in those with anterior or large infarctions, congestive heart failure, more diseased coronary arteries, atrial fibrillation, atrioventricular block, or bundle branch block. Ventricular fibrillation recurs most often in those with ischemia rather than infarction, secondary rather than primary ventricular fibrillation, or reduced ventricular function. Thrombolytic therapy reduces the probability that ventricular fibrillation will develop during hospitalization. Complex ventricular premature beats and ventricular tachycardia during and after myocardial infarction identify those patients most likely to sustain cardiac arrest after discharge.

About one-fourth of patients with dilated cardiomyopathy die suddenly, and cardiac arrest accounts for the majority of deaths in patients with hypertrophic cardiomyopathy. Valvular heart disease produces fewer cardiac arrests in developed countries than in former years; mitral valve prolapse seldom kills suddenly. The death of up to half of patients with congestive heart failure is sudden. Aortic stenosis, congenital anomalies of the coronary arteries, congenital complete atrioventricular block, Ebstein's disease, Eisenmenger syndrome, and tetralogy of Fallot are the principal congenital lesions producing cardiac arrest and ventricular fibrillation. Certain drugs, including some used to treat arrhythmias, Wolff-Parkinson-White syndrome, strenuous physical activity in healthy-appearing athletes and other young people, exercise testing, and pulmonary disease have been associated with sudden death. Finally, some subjects without any objective evidence for cardiac disease have cardiac arrest ("idiopathic ventricular fibrillation").

About half of patients resuscitated from cardiac arrest recall no prodromal symptoms. When severe symptoms such as syncope or marked dizziness and weakness are remembered, the arrhythmia is more likely to be ventricular fibrillation; when palpitations or slight dizziness can be perceived, it is more likely to be ventricular tachycardia. The physical examination reveals an unconscious patient without palpable pulse or audible heart sounds.

A continuous undulating pattern characterizes the electrocardiographic pattern of ventricular fibrillation. The warning arrhythmias that may predict ventricular fibrillation are ventricular premature beats, which are multiform or coupled or occur more frequently than 5 per minute or in the early portion of the preceding T wave ("vulnerable phase"). Ventricular tachycardia during myocardial infarction more frequently changes into ventricular fibrillation when it persists for more than 100 beats or is faster than 180 beats per minute, polymorphic, or initiated by an R-on-T beat. Most patients with ventricular fibrillation have abnormal signal-averaged electrocardiograms and heart rate variability. About half of patients with ventricular fibrillation and coronary heart disease have positive exercise tests. Spontaneous conversion occurs in many episodes of ventricular tachyarrhythmias including ventricular fibrillation.

When ventricular fibrillation ensues, pulsatile arterial waveforms quickly disappear. The longer the fibrillation persists, the lower the aortic systolic and diastolic pressures and the longer before the blood pressure achieves pre-arrhythmic levels.

In the electrophysiology laboratory, sustained ventricular tachyarrhythmias, but infrequently ventricular fibrillation, can be induced in the majority of patients successfully resuscitated from cardiac arrest but less often than in those with stable sustained ventricular tachycardia and more often in those with organic heart disease compared with patients who have idiopathic ventricular fibrillation. Ventricular fibrillation can seldom be induced in survivors of cardiac arrest with dilated cardiomyopathy.

Ventricular fibrillation must be converted quickly if the patient is to recover. The operator should apply thumpversion, and if a pulse does not immediately return, chest compression and artificial respiration. Early electrical defibrillation and electrocardiographic monitoring are vital. If the arrhythmia recurs, intravenous lidocaine, procainamide, or amiodarone should be given.

Each patient resuscitated from cardiac arrest should have an electrophysiological evaluation. If the history or the study suggests that ventricular fibrillation was the cause of the cardiac arrest and no reversible cause, such as acute ischemia or taking a pro-arrhythmic drug can be found, a cardioverter-defibrillator should be implanted. Survivors of out-of-hospital cardiac arrest with idiopathic ventricular fibrillation should receive implantable cardioverter-defibrillators even if no arrhythmia can be induced at electrophysiological study.

If a pharmacological approach is chosen, beta-blocking drugs and amiodarone are the most useful drugs to prevent a recurrence of ventricular fibrillation. Prophylactic administration of lidocaine to prevent ventricular fibrillation in the absence of specific arrhythmic complications to patients with acute myocardial infarction is no longer recommended. Whether drugs can prevent induction of a ventricular arrhythmia correlates poorly with the prevention of spontaneous ventricular arrhythmias. Patients who have had ventricular fibrillation should not drive for up to 8 months after discharge from the hospital because the hazard of another dangerous cardiac event is highest during that period.

About 30% of patients who sustain out-of-hospital cardiac arrest survive the initial event. Half of the survivors die in the hospital, and about one-third of those who are discharged die within 3 years. The implantable carioverter-defibrillator dramatically reduces mortality in discharged survivors.

Cardiac arrest most likely occurs in patients whose heart disease has reduced ventricular function, has aroused complex ventricular premature beats or ventricular tachycardia, or is associated with an abnormal signal-averaged electrocardiogram or decreased heart rate variability. Ventricular fibrillation in myocardial infarction worsens the prognosis for survivors during the acute infarction but not after discharge. The prognosis is excellent for patients resuscitated from out-of-hospital cardiac arrest due to acute ischemia who can be successfully revascularized.

REFERENCES

1. Myerburg RJ, Kessler KM. Ventricular fibrillation. In Kastor JA (ed). Arrhythmias. Philadelphia: WB Saunders, 1994, pp. 395–420.
2. Vaughan Williams EM. Fibrillation. Am Heart J 1963; 66:569–572.
3. Kuller L. Sudden and unexpected non-traumatic deaths in adults: a review of epidemiological and clinical studies. J Chronic Dis 1966; 19:1165–1192.
4. Paul O, Schatz M. On sudden death. Circulation 1971; 43:7–10.
5. Biorck G. "Sudden death": what are we talking about? Circulation 1972; 45:256–258.
6. Vedin JA, Wilhelmsson C, Elmfeldt D, Tibblin G, Wilhelmsen L, Werko L. Sudden death: identification of high risk groups. Am Heart J 1973; 86:124–132.
7. Kuller L H. Sudden death: definition and epidemiologic considerations. Prog Cardiovasc Dis 1980; 23:1–12.
8. Zipes DP, Heger JJ, Prystowsky EN. Sudden cardiac death. Am J Med 1981; 70:1151–1153.
9. Myerburg RJ. Sudden death. I. Risk factors and epidemiology, pathology and pathophysiology. Circulation 1981; 64:1070–1074.
10. Myerburg RJ. Sudden death. II. Clinical interventions, survival, neurophysiologic and psychophysiologic factors, and miscellaneous. Circulation 1981; 64:1291–1296.
11. Surawicz B. Ventricular fibrillation. J Am Coll Cardiol 1985; 5:43B–54B.
12. Roberts WC. Sudden cardiac death: definitions and causes. Am J Cardiol 1986; 57:1410–1413.
13. Garson A Jr. Ventricular arrhythmias. In Gillette PC, Garson A Jr (eds). Pediatric Arrhythmias. Electrophysiology and Pacing. Philadelphia: WB Saunders, 1990, pp. 427–500.
14. Meissner MD, Akhtar M, Lehmann MH. Nonischemic sudden tachyarrhythmic death in atherosclerotic heart disease. Circulation 1991; 84:905–912.
15. Hurwitz JL, Josephson ME. Sudden cardiac death in patients with chronic coronary heart disease. Circulation 1992; 85 (Suppl I): I-43–I-49.
16. Myerburg RJ, Kessler KM, Castellanos A. Sudden cardiac death: structure, function, and time-dependence of risk. Circulation 1992; 85 (Suppl I): I-2–I-10.
17. Myerburg RJ, Kessler KM, Castellanos A. Sudden cardiac death: epidemiology, transient risk, and intervention assessment. Ann Intern Med 1993; 119:1187–1197.
18. Prystowsky EN, Klein GJ. Cardiac arrest. In Prystowsky EN, Klein GJ (eds). Cardiac Arrhythmias. An Integrated Approach for the Clinician. New York: McGraw-Hill, 1994, pp. 272–286.
19. Wellens HJJ. Key references on sudden death: 1980–1994. Circulation 1994; 90:2547–2553.
20. Epstein AE, Ideker RE. Ventricular fibrillation. In Zipes DP, Jalife J (eds). Cardiac Electrophysiology. From Cell to Bedside. 2nd ed. Philadelphia: WB Saunders, 1995, pp. 927–933.
21. Kowey PR, Podrid PJ. Sudden cardiac death: evaluation and management. In Podrid PJ, Kowey PR (eds). Cardiac Arrhythmia. Mechanisms, Diagnosis and Management. Baltimore: Williams & Wilkins, 1995, pp. 974–1003.
22. Myerburg RJ, Demirovic J. Epidemiologic considerations in cardiac arrest and sudden cardiac death: etiology and prehospital and posthospital outcomes. In Podrid PJ, Kowey PR (eds). Cardiac Arrhythmia. Mechanisms, Diagnosis and Management. Baltimore: Williams & Wilkins, 1995, pp. 964–974.
23. Poole JE, Bardy GH. Sudden cardiac death. In Zipes DP, Jalife J (eds). Cardiac Electrophysiology. From Cell to Bedside. 2nd ed. Philadelphia: WB Saunders, 1995, pp. 812–832.
24. Jordaens LJ, 'T Kindt H. Primary ventricular fibrillation: a reason to be cautious. Eur Heart J 1997; 18:890–892.
25. Myerburg RJ, Interian A Jr, Mitrani RM, Kessler KM, Castellanos A. Frequency of sudden cardiac death and profiles of risk. Am J Cardiol 1997; 80:10F–19F.
26. Zoll PM, Linenthal AJ, Gibson W, Paul MH, Norman LR. Termination of ventricular fibrillation in man by externally applied electric countershock. N Engl J Med 1956; 254:727–732.
27. Kouwenhoven WB. The development of the defibrillator. Ann Intern Med 1969; 71:449–458.
28. Brown KWG, MacMillan RL, Norbath N, Mel'Grano F, Scott JW. Coronary unit: an intensive care centre for acute myocardial infarction. Lancet 1963; 2:349–352.
29. Day HW. Effectiveness of an intensive coronary care area. Am J Cardiol 1965; 15:51–54.
30. Kouwenhoven WB, Jude JR, Knickerbocker GG. Closed-chest cardiac massage. JAMA 1960; 173:94–97.

31. Baringer JR, Salzman EW, Jones WA, Friedlich AL. External cardiac massage. N Engl J Med 1961; 265:62–65.
32. Jude JR, Kouwenhoven WB, Knickerbocker GG. Cardiac arrest: report of application of external cardiac massage on 118 patients. JAMA 1961; 178:85–92.
33. Spann JF, Moellering RC. Haber E, Wheeler EO. Arrhythmias in acute myocardial infarction: a study utilizing an electrocardiographic monitor for automatic detection and recording of arrhythmias. N Engl J Med 1964; 271:427–431.
34. Lown B, Fakhro AM, Hood WB Jr, Thorn GW. The coronary care unit: new perspectives and directions. JAMA 1967; 199:188–198.
35. Pantridge JF, Geddes JS. Cardiac arrest after myocardial infarction. Lancet 1966; 1:807–808.
36. Thompson RG, Hallstrom AP, Cobb LA. Bystander-initiated cardiopulmonary resuscitation in the management of ventricular fibrillation. Ann Intern Med 1979; 90:737–740.
37. Jaggarao NS, Heber M, Grainger R, et al. Use of an automated external defibrillator-pacemaker by ambulance staff. Lancet 1982; 2:73–75.
38. Heber M. Out-of-hospital resuscitation using the "heart-aid," an automated external defibrillator-pacemaker. Int J Cardiol 1983; 3:456–458.
39. Cummins RO, Eisenberg M, Bergner L, Murray JA. Sensitivity, accuracy, and safety of an automatic external defibrillator. Lancet 1984; 2:318–320.
40. Eisenberg MS, Hallstrom AP, Copass MK, Bergner L, Short F, Pierce J. Treatment of ventricular fibrillation: emergency medical technician defibrillation and paramedic services. JAMA 1984; 251:1723–1726.
41. Weaver WD, Copass MK, Hill DL, Fahrenbruch C, Hallstrom AP, Cobb LA. Cardiac arrest treated with a new automatic external defibrillator by out-of-hospital first responders. Am J Cardiol 1986; 57:1017–1021.
42. Chadda KD, Kammerer R. Early experiences with the portable automatic external defibrillator in the home and public places. Am J Cardiol 1987; 60:732–733.
43. Cummins RO, Eisenberg MS, Litwin PE, Graves JR, Hearne TR, Hallstrom AP. Automatic external defibrillators used by emergency medical technicians: a controlled clinical trial. JAMA 1987; 257:1605–1610.
44. Weaver WD, Hill D, Fahrenbruch CE, et al. Use of the automatic external defibrillator in the management of out-of-hospital cardiac arrest. N Engl J Med 1988; 319:661–666.
45. Eisenberg MS, Moore J, Cummins RO, et al. Use of the automatic external defibrillator in homes of survivors of out-of-hospital ventricular fibrillation. Am J Cardiol 1989; 63:443–446.
46. Haynes BE, Mendoza A, McNeil M, Schroeder J, Smiley DR. A statewide early defibrillation initiative including laypersons and outcome reporting. JAMA 1991; 266:545–547.
47. Kellermann AL, Hackman BB, Somes G. Predicting the outcome of unsuccessful prehospital advanced cardiac life support. JAMA 1993; 270:1433–1436.
48. Kellermann AL, Hackman BB, Somes G, Kreth TK, Nail L, Dobyns P. Impact of first-responder defibrillation in an urban emergency medical services system. JAMA 1993; 270:1708–1713.
49. Weisfeldt ML, Kerber RE, McGoldrick RP, et al. Public access defibrillation: a statement for healthcare professionals from the American Heart Association Task Force on Automatic External Defibrillation. Circulation 1995; 92:2763.
50. Kloeck W, Cummins RO, Chamberlain D, et al. Early defibrillation: an advisory statement from the Advanced Life Support Working Group of the International Liaison Committee on Resuscitation. Circulation 1997; 95:2183–2184.
51. American Heart Association Task Force on Automatic External Defibrillation. Automatic external defibrillators for public access defibrillation: recommendations for specifying and reporting arrhythmia analysis algorithm performance, incorporating new waveforms, and enhancing safety. Biomed Instrum Technol 1997; 31:238–244.
52. Becker L, Eisenberg M, Fahrenbruch C, Cobb L. Public locations of cardiac arrest: implications for public access defibrillation. Circulation 1998; 97:2106–2109.
53. Nichol G, Hallstrom AP, Kerber R, et al. American Heart Association report on the Second Public Access Defibrillation conference, April 17–19, 1997. Circulation 1998; 97:1309–1314.
54. Nichol G, Hallstrom AP, Ornato JP, et al. Potential cost-effectiveness of public access defibrillation in the United States. Circulation 1998; 97:1315–1320.
55. Smith SC, Hamburg RS. Automated external defibrillators: time for federal and state advocacy and broader utilization. Circulation 1998; 97:1321–1324.
56. Rose LB, Press E. Cardiac defibrillation by ambulance attendants. JAMA 1972; 219:63–68.
57. Eisenberg MS, Copass MK, Hallstrom A, Cobb LA, Bergner L. Management of out-of-hospital cardiac arrest: failure of basic emergency medical technician services. JAMA 1980; 243:1049–1051.
58. Ornato JP, McNeill SE, Craren EJ, Nelson NM. Limitation on effectiveness of rapid defibrillation by emergency medical technicians in a rural setting. Ann Emerg Med 1984; 13:1096–1099.
59. Stults KR, Brown DD, Schug VL, Bean JA. Prehospital defibrillation performed by emergency medical technicians in rural communities. N Engl J Med 1984; 310:219–223.
60. Cummins RO, Eisenberg MS, Hallstrom AP, Litwin PE. Survival of out-of-hospital cardiac arrest with early initiation of cardiopulmonary resuscitation. Am J Emerg Med 1985; 3:114–119.
61. Herlitz J, Ekstrom L, Wennerblom B, Axelsson A, Bang A, Holmberg S. Effect of bystander initiated cardiopulmonary resuscitation on ventricular fibrillation and survival after witnessed cardiac arrest outside hospital. Br Heart J 1994; 72:408–412.
62. Weisfeldt ML, Kerber RE, McGoldrick RP, et al. American Heart Association report on the public access defibrillation conference December 8–10, 1994: Automatic External Defibrillation Task Force. Circulation 1995; 92:2740–2747.
63. Wellens HJ, de Vreede J, Gorgels AP. Sudden cardiac death: how to reduce the number of victims? Eur Heart J 1995; 16:G7–G9.
64. Greene HL, Richardson DW, Barker AH, et al. Classification of deaths after myocardial infarction as arrhythmic or nonarrhythmic (the Cardiac Arrhythmia Pilot Study). Am J Cardiol 1989; 63:1–6.
65. Pratt CM, Greenway PS, Schoenfeld MH, Hibben ML, Reiffel JA. Exploration of the precision of classifying sudden cardiac death: implications for the interpretation of clinical trials. Circulation 1996; 93:519–524.
66. Gradman AH, Bell PA, DeBusk RF. Sudden death during ambulatory monitoring: clinical and electrocardiographic correlations: report of a case. Circulation 1977; 55:210–211.
67. Hinkle J, LE Jr, Argyros DC, Hayes JC, et al. Pathogenesis of an unexpected sudden death: role of early cycle ventricular premature contractions. Am J Cardiol 1977; 39:873–879.
68. Pool J, Kunst K, van Wermeskerken JL. Two monitored cases of sudden death outside hospital. Br Heart J 1978; 40:627–629.
69. Lahiri A, Balasubramanian V, Raftery EB. Sudden death during ambulatory monitoring. BMJ 1979; 1:1676–1678.
70. Bissett JK, Watson JW, Scovil JA, deSoyza N, Ohrt DW. Sudden death in cardiomyopathy: role of bradycardia-dependent repolarization changes. Am Heart J 1980; 99:625–629.
71. Myerburg RJ, Conde CA, Sung RJ, et al. Clinical, electrophysiologic and hemodynamic profile of patients resuscitated from prehospital cardiac arrest: Am J Med 1980; 68:568–576.
72. Hinkle LE Jr. The immediate antecedents of sudden death. Acta Med Scand 1981; 210:207–217.
73. Denes P, Gabster A, Huang SK. Clinical, electro-cardiographic and follow-up observations in patients having ventricular fibrillation during Holter monitoring: role of quinidine therapy. Am J Cardiol 1981; 48:9–16.
74. Nikolic G, Bishop RL, Singh JB. Sudden death recorded during Holter monitoring. Circulation 1982; 66:218–225.

75. Weaver WD, Cobb LA, Hallstrom AP. Ambulatory arrhythmias in resuscitated victims of cardiac arrest. Circulation 1982; 66:212–218.

76. Clark MB, Dwyer EM Jr, Greenberg H. Sudden death during ambulatory monitoring: analysis of six cases. Am J Med 1983; 75:801–806.

77. Lewis BH, Antman EM, Graboys TB. Detailed analysis of 24 hour ambulatory electrocardiographic recordings during ventricular fibrillation or torsade de pointes. J Am Coll Cardiol 1983; 2:426–436.

78. Pratt CM, Francis MJ, Luck JC, Wyndham CR, Miller RR, Quinones MA. Analysis of ambulatory electrocardiograms in 15 patients during spontaneous ventricular fibrillation with special reference to preceding arrhythmic events. J Am Coll Cardiol 1983; 2:789–797.

79. Panidis IP, Morganroth J. Sudden death in hospitalized patients: cardiac rhythm disturbances detected by ambulatory electrocardiographic monitoring. J Am Coll Cardiol 1983; 2:798–805.

80. Savage DD, Castelli WP, Anderson SJ, Kannel WB. Sudden unexpected death during ambulatory electrocardiographic monitoring: the Framingham study. Am J Med 1983; 74:148–152.

81. Berisso MZ, Cavallini A, Iannetti M. Sudden death during continuous Holter monitoring out of hospital after nitroglycerin consumption. Am J Cardiol 1984; 54:677–679.

82. Kempf FC, Josephson ME. Cardiac arrest recorded on ambulatory electrocardiograms. Am J Cardiol 1984; 53:1577–1582.

83. Roelandt J, Klootwijk P, Lubsen J, Janse MJ. Sudden death during longterm ambulatory monitoring. Eur Heart J 1984; 5:7–20.

84. Milner PG, Platia EV, Reid PR, Griffith LS. Ambulatory electrocardiographic recordings at the time of fatal cardiac arrest. Am J Cardiol 1985; 56:588–592.

85. Nicod P, Polikar R, Peterson KL. Hypertrophic cardiomyopathy and sudden death. N Engl J Med 1988; 318:1255–1257.

86. Hohnloser SH, Kasper W, Zehender M, Geibel A, Meinertz T, Just H. Silent myocardial ischemia as a predisposing factor for ventricular fibrillation. Am J Cardiol 1988; 61:461–463.

87. Olshausen KV, Witt T, Pop T, Treese N, Bethge KP, Meyer J. Sudden cardiac death while wearing a Holter monitor. Am J Cardiol 1991; 67:381–386.

88. Pepine CJ, Morganroth J, McDonald JT, Gottlieb SO. Sudden death during ambulatory electrocardiographic monitoring. Am J Cardiol 1991; 68:785–788.

89. Niebauer J, Hambrecht R, Hauer K, et al. Identification of patients at risk during swimming by Holter monitoring. Am J Cardiol 1994; 74:651–656.

90. Eisenberg M, Bergner L, Hallstrom A. Epidemiology of cardiac arrest and resuscitation in children. Ann Emerg Med 1983; 12:672–674.

91. Cardiac Arrhythmia Suppression Trial (CAST) investigators. Preliminary report: effect of encainide and flecainide on mortality in a randomized trial of arrhythmia suppression after myocardial infarction. N Engl J Med 1989; 321:406–412.

92. Akhtar M, Breithardt G, Camm AJ, et al. CAST and beyond: implications of the Cardiac Arrhythmia Suppression Trial. Circulation 1990; 81:1123–1127.

93. Morganroth J, Bigger JT Jr. Pharmacologic management of ventricular arrhythmias after the Cardiac Arrhythmia Suppression Trial. Am J Cardiol 1990; 65:1497–1503.

94. Echt DS, Liebson PR, Mitchell LB, et al. Mortality and morbidity in patients receiving encainide, flecainide, or placebo: the Cardiac Arrhythmia Suppression Trial. N Engl J Med 1991; 324:781–788.

95. Cardiac Arrhythmia Suppression Trial II Investigators. Effect of the antiarrhythmic agent moricizine on survival after myocardial infarction. N Engl J Med 1992; 327:227–233.

96. Kuller L, Lilienfeld A, Fisher R. An epidemiological study of sudden and unexpected deaths in adults. Medicine 1967; 46:341–361.

97. Kuller L. Sudden death in arteriosclerotic heart disease: the case for preventive medicine. Am J Cardiol 1969; 24:617–628.

98. Kannel WB, Thomas HE Jr. Sudden coronary death: the Framingham study. I. Epidemiology and pathology of sudden coronary death. Ann N Y Acad Sci 1982; 382:3–21.

99. Gillum RF, Folsom AR, Blackburn H. Decline in coronary heart disease mortality: old questions and new facts. Am J Med 1984; 76:1055–1065.

100. Kannel WB, Schatzkin A. Sudden death: lessons from subsets in population studies. J Am Coll Cardiol 1985; 5:141B–149B.

101. Bayes de Luna A, Coumel P, Leclercq JF. Ambulatory sudden cardiac death: mechanisms of production of fatal arrhythmia on the basis of data from 157 cases. Am Heart J 1989; 117:151–159.

102. Akhtar M, Jazayeri MR, Sra JS, Blanck Z, Deshpande S, Dhala A. Sudden cardiac death: prevalence, causes, underlying substrates, and triggers. In Kroll MW, Lehmann MH (eds). Implantable Cardioverter Defibrillator Therapy. The Engineering-Clinical Interface. Norwell, MA: Kluwer Academic Publishers, 1996, pp. 1–15.

103. McNeilly RH, Pemberton J. Duration of last attack in 998 fatal cases of coronary artery disease and its relation to possible cardiac resuscitation. BMJ 1968; 3:139–142.

104. Kannel WB, Doyle JT, McNamara PM, Quickenton P, Gordon T. Precursors of sudden coronary death: factors related to the incidence of sudden death. Circulation 1975; 51:606–613.

105. Hinkle LE Jr, Thaler HT. Clinical classification of cardiac deaths. Circulation 1982; 65:457–464.

106. Waller BF, Catellier MJ, Clark MA, Hawley DA, Pless JE. Cardiac pathology in 2,007 consecutive forensic autopsies. Clin Cardiol 1992; 15:760–765.

107. Doyle JT, Kannel WB, McNamara PM, Quickenton P, Gordon T. Factors related to suddenness of death from coronary disease: combined Albany-Framingham studies. Am J Cardiol 1976; 37:1073–1078.

108. Schaffer WA, Cobb LA. Recurrent ventricular fibrillation and modes of death in survivors of out-of-hospital ventricular fibrillation. N Engl J Med 1975; 293:259–262.

109. Goldstein S. The necessity of a uniform definition of sudden coronary death: witnessed death within 1 hour at the onset of acute symptoms. Am Heart J 1982; 103:156–159.

110. Geuze RH, Koster RW. Ventricular fibrillation and transient arrhythmias after defibrillation in patients with acute myocardial infarction. J Electrocardiol 1984; 17:353–360.

111. Chamberlain DA. Overview of completed sudden death trials: European experience. Cardiology 1987; 74:10–23.

112. Gillum RF. Sudden coronary death in the United States. 1980-1985. Circulation 1989; 79:756–765.

113. Zaim BR, Zaim SH, Rankin AC, McGovern BA, Garan H, Ruskin JN. Comparison of cycle lengths between induced and spontaneous sustained ventricular tachycardia during concordant antiarrhythmic therapy associated with healed myocardial infarction. Am J Cardiol 1996; 77:202–204.

114. Li YG, Gronefeld G, Hohnloser SH. Radiofrequency catheter ablation of atrial flutter after orthotopic heart transplantation. J Cardiovasc Electrophysiol 1996; 7:1086–1090.

115. Liberthson RR, Nagel EL, Hirschman JC, Nussenfeld SR, Blackbourne BD, Davis JH. Pathophysiologic observations in prehospital ventricular fibrillation and sudden cardiac death. Circulation 1974; 49:790–798.

116. Tresch DD, Thakur RK, Hoffmann RG, Aufderheide TP, Brooks HL. Comparison of outcome of paramedic-witnessed cardiac arrest in patients younger and older than 70 years. Am J Cardiol 1990; 65:453–457.

117. Camarata SJ, Weil MH, Hanashiro PK, Shubin H. Cardiac arrest in the critically ill. I. A study of predisposing causes in 132 patients. Circulation 1971; 44:688–695.

118. Luu M, Stevenson, WG, Stevenson LW, Baron K, Walden J. Diverse mechanisms of unexpected cardiac arrest in advanced heart failure. Circulation 1989; 80:1675–1680.

119. Walsh CK, Krongrad E. Terminal cardiac electrical activity in pediatric patients. Am J Cardiol 1983; 51:557–561.

120. Driscoll DJ, Edwards WD. Sudden unexpected death in

children and adolescents. J Am Coll Cardiol 1985; 5:118B–121B.

121. Vetter VL. Sudden death in infants, children, and adolescents. Cardiovasc Clin 1985; 15:301–313.

122. McKenna W, Deanfield J, Faruqui A, England D, Oakley C, Goodwin J. Prognosis in hypertrophic cardiomyopathy: role of age and clinical, electrocardiographic and hemodynamic features. Am J Cardiol 1981; 47:532–538.

123. Tresch DD, Thakur RK, Hoffmann RG, Olson D, Brooks HL. Should the elderly be resuscitated following out-of-hospital cardiac arrest? Am J Med 1989; 86:145–150.

124. Larsen JA, Kadish AH. Effects of gender on cardiac arrhythmias. J Cardiovasc Electrophysiol 1998; 9:655–664.

125. Oparil S. Pathophysiology of sudden coronary death in women: implications for prevention. Circulation 1998; 97:2103–2105.

126. Rubart M, von der Lohe E. Sex steroids and cardiac arrhythmias: more questions than answers. J Cardiovasc Electrophysiol 1998; 9:665–667.

127. Chiang BN, Perlman LV, Fulton M, Ostrander LD Jr, Epstein FH. Predisposing factors in sudden cardiac death in Tecumseh, Michigan: a prospective study. Circulation 1970; 41:31–37.

128. Romo M. Factors related to sudden death in acute ischaemic heart disease: a community study in Helsinki. Acta Med Scand Suppl 1972; 547:1–92.

129. Kuller L, Perper J, Cooper M. Demographic characteristics and trends in arteriosclerotic heart disease mortality: sudden death and myocardial infarction. Circulation 1975; 52(Suppl III):III-1–III-15.

130. Zehender M, Buchner C, Meinertz T, Just H. Prevalence, circumstances, mechanisms, and risk stratification of sudden cardiac death in unipolar single-chamber ventricular pacing. Circulation 1992; 85:596–605.

131. Shen WK, Edwards WD, Hammill SC, Bailey KR, Ballard DJ, Gersh BJ. Sudden unexpected nontraumatic death in 54 young adults: a 30-year population-based study. Am J Cardiol 1995; 76:148–152.

132. Albert CM, McGovern BA, Newell JB, Ruskin JN. Sex differences in cardiac arrest survivors. Circulation 1996; 93:1170–1176.

133. Gillum RF. Coronary heart disease in black populations. I. Mortality and morbidity. Am Heart J 1982; 104:839–851.

134. Gillum RF, Grant CT. Coronary heart disease in black populations. II. Risk factors. Am Heart J 1982; 104:852–864.

135. Keil JE, Saunders DE Jr, Lackland DT, et al. Acute myocardial infarction: period prevalence, case fatality, and comparison of black and white cases in urban and rural areas of South Carolina. Am Heart J 1985; 109:776–784.

136. de Vreede-Swagemakers JJM, Gorgels APM, Dubois-Arbouw WI, et al. Out-of-hospital cardiac arrest in the 1990s: a population-based study in the Maastricht area on incidence, characteristics and survival. J Am Coll Cardiol 1997; 30:1500–1505.

137. Weaver WD, Cobb LA, Hallstrom AP. Characteristics of survivors of exertion- and nonexertion-related cardiac arrest: value of subsequent exercise testing. Am J Cardiol 1982; 50:671–676.

138. Schatzkin A, Cupples LA, Heeren T, Morelock S, Mucatel M, Kannel WB. The epidemiology of sudden unexpected death: risk factors for men and women in the Framingham heart study. Am Heart J 1984; 107:1300–1306.

139. Siscovick DS, Weiss NS, Fletcher RH, Lasky T. The incidence of primary cardiac arrest during vigorous exercise. N Engl J Med 1984; 311:874–877.

140. Coplan NL, Gleim GW, Nicholas JA. Exercise and sudden cardiac death. Am Heart J 1988; 115:207–212.

141. Sadaniantz A, Clayton MA, Sturner WQ, Thompson PD. Sudden death immediately after a record-setting athletic performance. Am J Cardiol 1989; 63:375.

142. Jenkins CD. Low education: a risk factor for death. N Engl J Med 1978; 299:95–97.

143. Ruberman W, Weinblatt E, Goldberg JD, Chaudhary BS. Psychosocial influences on mortality after myocardial infarction. N Engl J Med 1984; 311:552–559.

144. Weinblatt E, Ruberman W, Goldberg JD, Frank CW, Shapiro S, Chaudhary BS. Relation of education to sudden death after myocardial infarction. N Engl J Med 1978; 299:60–65.

145. Messerli FH, Nunez BD, Ventura HO, Snyder DW. Overweight and sudden death: increased ventricular ectopy in cardiomyopathy of obesity. Arch Intern Med 1987; 147:1725–1728.

146. Duflou J, Virmani R, Rabin I, Burke A, Farb A, Smialek J. Sudden death as a result of heart disease in morbid obesity. Am Heart J 1995; 130:306–313.

147. Rahe RH, Romo M, Bennett L, Siltman P. Recent life changes, myocardial infarction, and abrupt coronary death. Arch Intern Med 1974; 133:221–228.

148. Friedman M, Rosenman RH. Association of specific overt behavior pattern with blood and cardiovascular findings. JAMA 1959; 169:1286–1296.

149. Talbott E, Kuller LH, Detre K, Perper J. Biologic and psychological risk factors of sudden death from coronary disease in white women. Am J Cardiol 1977; 39:858–864.

150. Doyle JT. Profile of risk of sudden death in apparently healthy people. Circulation 1975; 52(Suppl III):III-176–III-179.

151. Killip T. Time, place, event of sudden death. Circulation 1975; 52(Suppl III):III-160–III-163.

152. Lawrie DM, Higgins MR, Godman MG, Oliver MF, Julian DG, Donald KW. Ventricular fibrillation complicating acute myocardial infarction. Lancet 1968; 2:523–528.

153. Thygesen K, Haghfelt T, Steinmetz E, Nielsen BL. Long-term survival after myocardial infarction as related to early complications. Eur J Cardiol 1977; 6:41–51.

154. Behar S, Reicher-Reiss H, Shechter M, et al. Frequency and prognostic significance of secondary ventricular fibrillation complicating acute myocardial infarction. Am J Cardiol 1993; 71:152–156.

155. Liberthson RR, Nagel EL, Hirschman JC, Nussenfeld SR. Prehospital ventricular defibrillation: prognosis and follow-up course. N Engl J Med 1974; 291:317–321.

156. Moritz AR, Zamcheck N. Sudden and unexpected deaths of young soldiers. Arch Pathol 1947; 42:459–494.

157. Kuller L, Lilienfeld A, Fisher R. Sudden and unexpected deaths in young adults: an epidemiological study. JAMA 1966; 198:248–252.

158. Kuller L, Lilienfeld A, Fisher R. Epidemiological study of sudden and unexpected deaths due to arteriosclerotic heart disease. Circulation 1966; 34:1056–1068.

159. Luke JL, Helpern M. Sudden unexpected death from natural causes in young adults: a review of 275 consecutive autopsied cases. Arch Pathol 1968; 85:10–17.

160. Koskenvuo K. Sudden deaths among Finnish conscripts. BMJ 1976; 2:1413–1415.

161. Tresch DD, Grove JR, Keelan MH Jr, et al. Long-term follow-up of survivors of prehospital sudden coronary death. Circulation 1981; 64(Suppl II):II-1–II-6.

162. Weaver WD, Lorch GS, Alvarez HA, Cobb LA. Angiographic findings and prognostic indicators in patients resuscitated from sudden cardiac death. Circulation 1976; 54:895–900.

163. Lundberg GD, Voigt GE. Reliability of a presumptive diagnosis in sudden unexpected death in adults: the case for the autopsy. JAMA 1979; 242:2328–2330.

164. Raymond JR, van den Berg EK Jr, Knapp MJ. Nontraumatic prehospital sudden death in young adults. Arch Intern Med 1988; 148:303–308.

165. Drory Y, Turetz Y, Hiss Y, et al. Sudden unexpected death in persons less than 40 years of age. Am J Cardiol 1991; 68:1388–1392.

166. Spaulding CM, Joly LM, Rosenberg A, et al. Immediate coronary angiography in survivors of out-of-hospital cardiac arrest. N Engl J Med 1997; 336:1629–1633.

167. Goldstein S, Landis JR, Leighton R, et al. Characteristics of the resuscitated out-of-hospital cardiac arrest victim with coronary heart disease. Circulation 1981; 64:977–984.

168. Stevenson WG, Linssen GCM, Havenith MG, Brugada P, Wellens HJJ. Late death after myocardial infarction: mechanisms, etiologies, and implications for prevention of sudden death. In Brugada P, Wellens HJJ (eds). Cardiac

Arrhythmias. Where To Go From Here? Mount Kisco, NY: Futura Publishing Co. 1987, pp. 377–389.

169. Hwang S, Stevenson WG, Wiener I. Hearts too good to die: ventricular fibrillation due to small infarctions or ischemia. Am Heart J 1991; 121:938–939.

170. Dickey W, Adgey AA. Out-of-hospital ventricular fibrillation in patients under the age of 40 years and the long-term prognosis. Q J Med 1991; 81:821–827.

171. Margolis JF, Hirshfeld JW Jr, McNeer JF, et al. Sudden death due to coronary artery disease: a clinical, hemodynamic, and angiographic profile. Circulation 1975; 51 and 52(Suppl III):III-180–III-183.

172. Amsterdam EA. Relation of silent myocardial ischemia to ventricular arrhythmias and sudden death. Am J Cardiol 1988; 62:24II–27II.

173. Stevenson WG, Wiener I, Yeatman L, Wohlgelernter D, Weiss JN. Complicated atherosclerotic lesions: a potential cause of ischemic ventricular arrhythmias in cardiac arrest survivors who do not have inducible ventricular tachycardia? Am Heart J 1988; 116:1–6.

174. Schwartz LS, Schwedel JB, Schwartz SP. Adams-Stokes syndrome during angina pectoris associated with coronary artery disease. Am J Cardiol 1966; 17:426–432.

175. Takayanagi K, Fujito T, Morooka S, Takabatake Y, Nakamura Y. Headache angina with fatal outcome. Jpn Heart J 1990; 31:503–507.

176. Hong RA, Bhandari AK, McKay CR, Au PK, Rahimtoola SH. Life-threatening ventricular tachycardia and fibrillation induced by painless myocardial ischemia during exercise testing. JAMA 1987; 257:1937–1940.

177. Sharma B, Asinger R, Francis GS, Hodges M, Wyeth RP. Demonstration of exercise-induced painless myocardial ischemia in survivors of out-of-hospital ventricular fibrillation. Am J Cardiol 1987; 59:740–745.

178. Sharma B, Wyeth RP. Six-year survival of patients with and without painless myocardial ischemia and out-of-hospital ventricular fibrillation. Am J Cardiol 1988; 61:9F–15F.

179. Whitaker MP, Sheps DS. Prevalence of silent myocardial ischemia in survivors of cardiac arrest. Am J Cardiol 1989; 64:591–593.

180. Sheps DS, Heiss G. Sudden death and silent myocardial ischemia. Am Heart J 1989; 117:177–184.

181. Gorfinkel HJ, Inglesby TV, Lansing AM, Goodin RR. ST-segment elevation, transient left-posterior hemiblock, and recurrent ventricular arrhythmias unassociated with pain. Ann Intern Med 1973; 79:795–799.

182. Levi GF, Proto C. Ventricular fibrillation in the course of Prinzmetal's angina pectoris: report of two cases. Br Heart J 1973; 35:601–603.

183. Kerin NZ, Rubenfire M, Naini M, Wajszczuk WJ, Pamatmat A, Cascade PN. Arrhythmias in variant angina pectoris: relationship of arrhythmias to ST-segment elevation and R-wave changes. Circulation 1979; 60:1343–1350.

184. Rozanski JJ, Kleinfeld M. TQ segment (baseline) alternans during Prinzmetal's variant angina. Pacing Clin Electrophysiol 1980; 3:724–729.

185. Kerin NZ, Rubenfire M, Naini M, Wajszczuk WJ, Rao P. Prinzmetal's variant angina: electrocardiographic and angiographic correlations. J Electrocardiol 1982; 15:365–380.

186. Maseri A, Severi S, Marzullo P. Role of coronary arterial spasm in sudden coronary ischemic death. Ann N Y Acad Sci 1982; 382:204–217.

187. Miller DD, Waters DD, Szlachcic J, Theroux P. Clinical characteristics associated with sudden death in patients with variant angina. Circulation 1982; 66:588–592.

188. Rozanski JJ, Kleinfeld M. Alternans of the ST segment of T wave: a sign of electrical instability in Prinzmetal's angina. Pacing Clin Electrophysiol 1982; 5:359–365.

189. Conti CR, Feldman RL, Pepine CJ. Coronary artery spasm: prevalence, clinical significance, and provocative testing. Am Heart J 1982; 103:584–588.

190. Kerin NZ, Rubenfire M, Willens HJ, Rao P, Cascade PN. The mechanism of dysrhythmias in variant angina pectoris: occlusive versus reperfusion. Am Heart J 1983; 106:1332–1340.

191. Previtali M, Klersy C, Salerno JA, et al. Ventricular tachyarrhythmias in Prinzmetal's variant angina: clinical significance and relation to the degree and time course of S-T segment elevation. Am J Cardiol 1983; 52:19–25.

192. Puddu PE, Bourassa MG, Waters DD, Lesperance J. Sudden death in two patients with variant angina and apparently minimal fixed coronary stenoses. J Electrocardiol 1983; 16:213–220.

193. Bashour T. Cardiac rhythm disorders complicating coronary arterial spasm. Clin Cardiol 1984; 7:510–512.

194. Szlachcic J, Waters DD, Miller D, Theroux P. Ventricular arrhythmias during ergonovine-induced episodes of variant angina. Am Heart J 1984; 107:20–24.

195. Simpson IA, Hutton I. An unusual presentation of variant angina. Scot Med J 1986; 31:37–38.

196. Nakamura M, Takeshita A, Nose Y. Clinical characteristics associated with myocardial infarction, arrhythmias, and sudden death in patients with vasospastic angina. Circulation 1987; 75:1110–1116.

197. Nakaya Y, Hiasa Y, Fujino K, Aihara T, Mori H. The nature of ventricular arrhythmias during ergonovine-induced vasospastic angina pectoris. Clin Cardiol 1987; 10:497–502.

198. Turitto G, Dini P, Prati PL. The R on T phenomenon during transient myocardial ischemia. Am J Cardiol 1989; 63:1520–1522.

199. Attenhofer C, Speich R, Salomon F, Burkhard R, Amann FW. Ventricular fibrillation in a patient with exercise-induced anaphylaxis, normal coronary arteries, and a positive ergonovine test. Chest 1994; 105:620–622.

200. Myerburg RJ, Kessler KM, Mallon SM, et al. Life-threatening ventricular arrhythmias in patients with silent myocardial ischemia due to coronary artery spasm. N Engl J Med 1992; 326:1451–1455.

201. Tzivoni D, Keren A, Granot H, Gottlieb S, Benhorin J, Stern S. Ventricular fibrillation caused by myocardial reperfusion in Prinzmetal's angina. Am Heart J 1983; 105:323–325.

202. Meltzer LE, Kitchell JB. The incidence of arrhythmias associated with acute myocardial infarction. Prog Cardiovasc Dis 1966; 9:50–63.

203. Lown B, Klein MD, Hershberg PI. Coronary and precoronary care. Am J Med 1969; 46:705–724.

204. Fulton M, Julian DG, Oliver MF. Sudden death and myocardial infarction. Circulation 1969; 39 and 40(Suppl IV):IV-182–IV-193.

205. Adgey AAJ, Scott ME, Allen JD, et al. Management of ventricular fibrillation outside hospital. Lancet 1969; 1:1169–1171.

206. Pantridge JF, Adgey AAJ. Pre-hospital coronary care: the mobile coronary care unit. Am J Cardiol 1969; 24:666–673.

207. James TN. Sudden death related to myocardial infarction. Circulation 1972; 45:205–214.

208. DeSanctis RW, Block P, Hutter, AM Jr. Tachyarrhythmias in myocardial infarction. Circulation 1972; 45:681–702.

209. Lie KI, Wellens HJJ, Liem KL, Durrer D. Treatment and prevention of primary ventricular fibrillation complicating acute myocardial infarction. Acta Cardiol Suppl 1977; 22:107–120.

210. Noneman JW, Rogers JF. Lidocaine prophylaxis in acute myocardial infarction. Medicine 1978; 57:501–515.

211. Ribner HS, Isaacs ES, Frishman WH. Lidocaine prophylaxis against ventricular fibrillation in acute myocardial infarction. Prog Cardiovasc Dis 1979; 21:287–313.

212. Richards D, Taylor A, Fahey P, Irwig L, Koo CC, Ross D, Identification of patients at risk of sudden death after myocardial infarction: the continued Australian experience. In Brugada P. Wellens HJJ (eds). Cardiac Arrhythmias. Where To Go From Here? Mount Kisco, NY: Futura Publishing Co., 1987, pp. 329–341.

213. Roy D, Arenal A, Godin D, Marchand E, Cassidy D, Theroux P. The Canadian experience on the identification of candidates for sudden cardiac death after myocardial infarction. In Brugada P, Wellens HJJ eds. Cardiac Arrhythmias. Where To Go From Here? Mount Kisco, NY: Futura Publishing Co., 1987, pp. 343–351.

214. Tisdale JE. Lidocaine prophylaxis in acute myocardial infarction. Henry Ford Hosp Med J 1991; 39:217–225.

215. Adgey AAJ, Geddes JS, Webb SW, et al. Acute phase of myocardial infarction. Lancet 1971; 2:501–504.

216. Bellinger RL, Califf RM, Mark DB, et al. Helicopter transport of patients during acute myocardial infarction. Am J Cardiol 1988; 61:718–722.

217. Gillum RF, Folsom A, Luepker RV, et al. Sudden death and acute myocardial infarction in a metropolitan area. 1970–1980: the Minnesota heart survey. N Engl J Med 1983; 309:1353–1358.

218. O'Doherty M, Tayler DI, Quinn E, Vincent R, Chamberlain DA. Five hundred patients with myocardial infarction monitored within one hour of symptoms. BMJ 1994; 1983:1405–1408.

219. Dubois C, Smeets JP, Demoulin JC, et al. Incidence, clinical significance and prognosis of ventricular fibrillation in the early phase of myocardial infarction. Eur Heart J 1986; 7:945–951.

220. Miles WM, Klein LS, Minardo JD, Zipes DP. Two retrograde atrial responses from one ventricular complex in the permanent form of junctional reciprocating tachycardia. Am J Cardiol 1987; 59:1004–1006.

221. Nicod P, Gilpin E, Dittrich H, et al. Late clinical outcome in patients with early ventricular fibrillation after myocardial infarction. J Am Coll Cardiol 1988; 11:464–470.

222. Behar S, Goldbourt U, Reicher-Reiss H, Kaplinsky E. Prognosis of acute myocardial infarction complicated by primary ventricular fibrillation. Am J Cardiol 1990; 66:1208–1211.

223. Antman EM, Berlin JA. Declining incidence of ventricular fibrillation in myocardial infarction: implications for the prophylactic use of lidocaine. Circulation 1992; 86:764–773.

224. Antman EM, Berlin JA. Reply. Circulation 1993; 87:2068–2069.

225. Wyman MG. Declining incidence of ventricular fibrillation in myocardial infarction. Circulation 1993; 87:2067–2068.

226. Baum RS, Alvarez H III, Cobb LA. Survival after resuscitation from out-of-hospital ventricular fibrillation. Circulation 1974; 50:1231–1235.

227. Ruosteenoja R, Inkovaara J, Koskinen PJ. Long-term prognosis after ventricular fibrillation in acute myocardial infarction. Acta Med Scand 1972; 191:229–232.

228. Campbell RWF, Murray A, Julian DG. Ventricular arrhythmias in first 12 hours of acute myocardial infarction: natural history study. Br Heart J 1981; 46:351–357.

229. Solomon SD, Ridker PM, Antman EM. Ventricular arrhythmias in trials of thrombolytic therapy for acute myocardial infarction: a meta-analysis. Circulation 1993; 88:2575–2581.

230. Gheorghiade M, Anderson J, Rosman H, et al. Risk identification at the time of admission to coronary care unit in patients with suspected myocardial infarction. Am Heart J 1988; 116:1212–1217.

231. Tofler GH, Stone PH, Muller JE, et al. Prognosis after cardiac arrest due to ventricular tachycardia or ventricular fibrillation associated with acute myocardial infarction (the MILIS study): Multicenter Investigation of the Limitation of Infarct Size. Am J Cardiol 1987; 60:755–761.

232. Julian DG, Valentine PA, Miller GG. Disturbances of rate, rhythm and conduction in acute myocardial infarction: a prospective study of 100 consecutive unselected patients with the aid of electrocardiographic monitoring. Am J Med 1964; 37:915–927.

233. Killip T III, Kimball JT. Treatment of myocardial infarction in a coronary care unit: a two year experience with 250 patients. Am J Cardiol 1967; 20:457–464.

234. Stock E, Goble A, Sloman G. Assessment of arrhythmias in myocardial infarction. BMJ 1967; 2:719–723.

235. Langhorne WH. The coronary care unit: a year's experience in a community hospital. JAMA 1967; 201:92–95.

236. Wyman MG, Hammersmith L. Coronary care in the small community hospital. Dis Chest 1968; 53:584–591.

237. Dhurandhar RW, MacMillan RL, Brown KWG. Primary ventricular fibrillation complicating acute myocardial infarction. Am J Cardiol 1971; 27:347–351.

238. Scheinman MM, Abbott JA. Clinical significance of transmural versus nontransmural electrocardiographic changes in patients with acute myocardial infarction. Am J Med 1973; 55:602–607.

239. Volpi A, Maggioni A, Franzosi G, Pampallona S, Mauri F, Tognoni G. In-hospital prognosis of patients with acute myocardial infarction complicated by primary ventricular fibrillation. N Engl J Med 1987; 317:257–309.

240. Thompson P, Sloman G. Sudden death in hospital after discharge from coronary care unit. BMJ 1971; 4:136–139.

241. Wilson C, Adgey AA. Survival of patients with late ventricular fibrillation after acute myocardial infarction. Lancet 1974; 2:124–126.

242. Bornheimer J, de Guzman M, Haywood LJ. Analysis of in-hospital deaths from myocardial infarction after coronary care unit discharge. Arch Intern Med 1975; 135:1035–1038.

243. Conley MJ, McNeer JF, Lee KL, Wagner GS, Rosati RA. Cardiac arrest complicating acute myocardial infarction: predictability and prognosis. Am J Cardiol 1977; 39:7–12.

244. el-Sherif N, Myerburg RJ, Scherlag BJ, et al. Electrocardiographic antecedents of primary ventricular fibrillation: value of the R-on-T phenomenon in myocardial infarction. Br Heart J 1976; 38:415–422.

245. Lie KI, Liem KL, Louridtz WJ, Janse MJ, Willebrands AF, Durrer D. Efficacy of lidocaine in preventing primary ventricular fibrillation within 1 hour after a 300 mg intramuscular injection: a double-blind, randomized study of 300 hospitalized patients with acute myocardial infarction. Am J Cardiol 1978; 42:486–488.

246. Kowey PR, Friehling T, Meister SG, Engel TR. Late induction of tachycardia in patients with ventricular fibrillation associated with acute myocardial infarction. J Am Coll Cardiol 1984; 3:690–695.

247. Zehender M, Kasper W, Kauder E, et al. Right ventricular infarction as an independent predictor of prognosis after acute inferior myocardial infarction. N Engl J Med 1993; 328:981–988.

248. Hauer RNW, Lie KI, Liem KL, Durrer D. Long-term prognosis in patients with bundle branch block complicating acute anteroseptal infarction. Am J Cardiol 1982; 49:1581–1585.

249. Chapman BL. Relation of cardiac complications to SGOT level in acute myocardial infarction. Br Heart J 1972; 34:890–896.

250. Heidbuchel H, Tack J, Vanneste L, Ballet A, Ector H, Van de Werf F. Significance of arrhythmias during the first 24 hours of acute myocardial infarction treated with alteplase and effect of early administration of a beta-blocker or a bradycardiac agent on their incidence. Circulation 1994; 89:1051–1059.

251. Restieaux N, Bray C, Bullard H, et al. 150 patients with cardiac infarction treated in a coronary unit. Lancet 1967; 1:1285–1289.

252. Herlitz J, Hjalmarson A, Swedberg K, Waagstein F, Holmberg S, Waldenstrom J. Relationship between infarct size and incidence of severe ventricular arrhythmias in a double-blind trial with metoprolol in acute myocardial infarction. Int J Cardiol 1984; 6:47–60.

253. Kyriakidis M, Petropoulakis P, Antonopoulos A, et al. Early ventricular fibrillation in patients with acute myocardial infarction: correlation with coronary angiographic findings. Eur Heart J 1993; 14:364–368.

254. Lie KI, Wellens HJJ, Durrer D. Characteristics and predictability of primary ventricular fibrillation. Eur J Cardiol 1974; 1:379–384.

255. Greenland P, Reicher-Reiss H, Goldbourt U, Behar S, Israeli SPRINT investigators. In-hospital and 1-year mortality in 1,524 women after myocardial infarction: comparison with 4,315 men. Circulation 1991; 83:484–491.

256. Lie JT, Hunt D. The cardiac conduction system in acute myocardial infarction: a clinicopathological correlation. Aust N Z J Med 1974; 4:331–338.

257. Berger PB, Ruocco NA, Ryan TJ, Frederick MM, Podrid PJ. Incidence and significance of ventricular tachycardia and fibrillation in the absence of hypotension or heart failure in acute myocardial infarction treated with recombinant tissue-

type plasminogen activator: results from the thrombolysis in myocardial infarction (TIMI) phase II trial. J Am Coll Cardiol 1993; 22:1773–1779.

258. Dewhurst NG, Hannan WJ, Muir AL. Ventricular performance and prognosis after primary ventricular fibrillation complicating acute myocardial infarction. Eur Heart J 1984; 5:275–281.

259. Kelly MJ, Thompson PL, Quinlan MF. Prognostic significance of left ventricular ejection fraction after acute myocardial infarction: a bedside radionuclide study. Br Heart J 1985; 53:16–24.

260. Logan KR, McIlwaine WJ, Adgey AA, Pantridge JF. Ventricular fibrillation and its recurrence in early acute myocardial infarction. Lancet 1981; 1:242–244.

261. Logan KR, McIlwaine WJ, Adgey AAJ, Pantridge JF. Recurrence of ventricular fibrillation in acute ischemic heart disease. Circulation 1981; 64:1163–1167.

262. Stevenson WG, Brugada P, Waldecker B, Zehender M, Wellens HJJ. Clinical, angiographic, and electrophysiologic findings in patients with aborted sudden death as compared with patients with sustained ventricular tachycardia after myocardial infarction. Circulation 1985; 76:1146–1152.

263. Morrison GW, Kumar EB, Portal RW, Aber CP. Cardiac arrhythmias 48 hours before, during, and 48 hours after discharge from hospital following acute myocardial infarction. Br Heart J 1981; 45:500–511.

264. El-Maraghi N, Genton E. The relevance of platelet and fibrin thromboembolism of the coronary microcirculation, with special reference to sudden cardiac death. Circulation 1980; 62:936–944.

265. Davies MJ. Pathological view of sudden cardiac death. Br Heart J 1981; 45:88–96.

266. Steinberger J, Lucas RV Jr, Edwards JE, Titus JL. Causes of sudden unexpected cardiac death in the first two decades of life. Am J Cardiol 1996; 77:992–995.

267. Roberts WC, Siegel RJ, Zipes DP. Origin of the right coronary artery from the left sinus of Valsalva and its functional consequences: analysis of 10 necropsy patients. Am J Cardiol 1982; 49:863–868.

268. Shaver PJ, Carrig TF, Baker WP. Postpartum coronary artery dissection. Br Heart J 1978; 40:83–86.

269. Kegel SM, Dorsey TJ, Rowen M, Taylor WF. Cardiac death in mucocutaneous lymph node syndrome. Am J Cardiol 1977; 40:282–286.

270. Okuni M, Sumitomo N. Sudden death of school children in Japan. Jpn Circ J 1987; 51:1397–1399.

271. Niimura I, Maki T. Sudden cardiac death in childhood. Jpn Circ J 1989; 53:1571–1580.

272. Thiene G, Valente M, Rossi L. Involvement of the cardiac conducting system in panarteritis nodosa. Am Heart J 1978; 95:716–724.

273. Roberts WC, Silver MA, Sapala JC. Intussusception of a coronary artery associated with sudden death in a college football player. Am J Cardiol 1986; 57:179–180.

274. Perloff JK. The Clinical Recognition of Congenital Heart Disease. 4th ed. Philadelphia: WB Saunders, 1994, pp. 546–561.

275. Perloff JK. The Clinical Recognition of Congenital Heart Disease. 4th ed. Philadelphia: WB Saunders, 1994, pp. 738–755.

276. Liberthson RR. Sudden death from cardiac causes in children and young adults. N Engl J Med 1996; 334:1039–1044.

277. Harthorne JW, Scannell JG, Dinsmore RE. Anomalous origin of the left coronary artery: remediable cause of sudden death in adults. N Engl J Med 1966; 275:660–663.

278. Wesselhoeft H, Fawcett JS, Johnson AL. Anomalous origin of the left coronary artery from the pulmonary trunk: its clinical spectrum, pathology, and pathophysiology, based on a review of 140 cases with seven further cases. Circulation 1968; 38:403–425.

279. Cheitlin MD, De Castro CM, McAllister HA. Sudden death as a complication of anomalous left coronary origin from the anterior sinus of Valsalva, a not-so-minor congenital anomaly. Circulation 1974; 50:780–787.

280. Corrado D, Thiene G, Cocco P, Frescura C. Non-atherosclerotic coronary artery disease and sudden death in the young. Br Heart J 1992; 68:601–607.

281. Taylor AJ, Rogan KM, Virmani R. Sudden cardiac death associated with isolated congenital coronary artery anomalies. J Am Coll Cardiol 1992; 20:640–647.

282. Topaz O, Edwards JE. Pathologic features of sudden death in children, adolescents, and young adults. Chest 1985; 87:476–482.

283. Heuzey JL. Cardiac prognosis in hypertensive patients: incidence of sudden death and ventricular arrhythmias. Am J Med 1988; 84:65–68.

284. Kannel WB. Hypertension, hypertrophy, and the occurrence of cardiovascular disease. Am J Med Sci 1991; 302:199–204.

285. Messerli FH, Grodzicki T. Hypertension, left ventricular hypertrophy, ventricular arrhythmias and sudden death. Eur Heart J 1992; 13:D66–D69.

286. Almendral J, Villacastin JP, Arenal A, Tercedor L, Merino JL, Delcan JL. Evidence favoring the hypothesis that ventricular arrhythmias have prognostic significance in left ventricular hypertrophy secondary to systemic hypertension. Am J Cardiol 1995; 76:60D–63D.

287. Bayes-Genis A, Guindo J, Tomas L, Elosua R, Duran I, Bayes de Luna A. Cardiac arrhythmias and left ventricular hypertrophy in systemic hypertension and their influences on prognosis. Am J Cardiol 1995; 76:54D–59D.

288. Johnsrude CL, Towbin JA, Cecchin F, Perry JC. Postinfarction ventricular arrhythmias in children. Am Heart J 1995; 129:1171–1177.

289. Zehender, M, Faber T, Koscheck U, Meinertz T, Just H. Ventricular tachyarrhythmias, myocardial ischemia, and sudden cardiac death in patients with hypertensive heart disease. Clin Cardiol 1995; 18:377–383.

290. Siscovick DS, Raghunathan TE, Rautaharju P, Psaty BM, Cobb LA, Wagner EH. Clinically silent electrocardiographic abnormalities and risk of primary cardiac arrest among hypertensive patients Circulation 1996; 94:1329–1333.

291. White PD. Heart Disease. 4th ed. New York: Macmillan, 1951, p. 692.

292. Campbell M. Calcific aortic stenosis and congenital bicuspid aortic valves. Br Heart J 1968; 30:606–616.

293. Iskandrian AS, Segal BL, Wasserman L, Kimbiris D, Bemis CE. Sudden death in severe aortic stenosis following cardiac catheterization. Cathet Cardiovasc Diagn 1978; 4:419–425.

294. Siostrzonek P, Gossinger H, Prischl F, et al. Electrophysiologic testing after aortic valve replacement in two patients with aortic stenosis and preoperative ventricular fibrillation. Eur Heart J 1990; 11:372–376.

295. Blackstone EH, Kirklin JW. Death and other time-related events after valve replacement. Circulation 1985; 72:753–767.

296. Jeresaty RM. Sudden death in the mitral valve prolapse-click syndrome. Am J Cardiol 1976; 37:317–318.

297. Oakley CM. Mitral valve prolapse: harbinger of death or variant of normal? BMJ 1984; 288:1853–1854.

298. Kligfield P, Levy D, Devereux RB, Savage DD. Arrhythmias and sudden death in mitral valve prolapse. Am Heart J 1987; 113:1298–1307.

299. Campbell RWF, Godman MG, Fiddler GI, Marquis RM, Julian DG. Ventricular arrhythmias in syndrome of balloon deformity of mitral valve: definition of possible high risk group. Br Heart J 1976; 38:1053–1057.

300. Winkle RA, Lopes MG, Popp RL, Hancock, EW. Life-threatening arrhythmias in the mitral valve prolapse syndrome. Am J Med 1976; 60:961–967.

301. Davies MJ, Moore BP, Braimbridge MV. The floppy mitral valve. Study of incidence, pathology, and complications in surgical, necropsy, and forensic material. Br Heart J 1978; 40:468–481.

302. Wei JY, Bulkley BH, Schaeffer AH, Greene, HL, Reid PR. Mitral-valve prolapse syndrome and recurrent ventricular tachyarrhythmias: a malignant variant refractory to conventional drug therapy. Ann Intern Med 1978; 89:6–9.

303. Salmela PI, Ikaheimo M, Juustila H. Fatal ventricular fibrillation after treatment with digoxin in a 27-year-old man with mitral leaflet prolapse syndrome. Br Heart J 1981; 46:338–341.

304. Kolibash AJ, Bush CA, Fontana MB, Ryan JM, Kilman J, Wooley CF. Mitral valve prolapse syndrome: analysis of 62 patients aged 60 years and older. Am J Cardiol 1983; 52:534–539.

305. Pocock WA, Bosman CK, Chesler E, Barlow JB, Edwards JE. Sudden death in primary mitral valve prolapse. Am Heart J 1984; 107:378–382.

306. Duren DR, Becker AE, Dunning AJ. Long-term follow-up of idiopathic mitral valve prolapse in 300 patients: a prospective study. J Am Coll Cardiol 1988; 11:42–47.

307. Boudoulas H, Schaal SF, Stang JM, Fontana ME, Kolibash AJ, Wooley CF. Mitral valve prolapse: cardiac arrest with long-term survival. Int J Cardiol 1990; 26:37–44.

308. Martini, B, Basso C, Thiene G. Sudden death in mitral valve prolapse with Holter monitoring–documented ventricular fibrillation: evidence of coexisting arrhythmogenic right ventricular cardiomyopathy. Int J Cardiol 1995; 49:274–278.

309. Farb A, Tang AL, Atkinson JB, McCarthy WF, Virmani R. Comparison of cardiac findings in patients with mitral valve prolapse who die suddenly to those who have congestive heart failure from mitral regurgitation and to those with fatal noncardiac conditions. Am J Cardiol 1992; 70:234–239.

310. Dollar AL, Roberts WC. Morphologic comparison of patients with mitral valve prolapse who died suddenly with patients who died from severe valvular dysfunction or other conditions. J Am Coll Cardiol 1991; 17:921–931.

311. Nishimura RA, McGoon MD, Shub, C, Miller FA Jr, Ilstrup DM, Tajik, AJ. Echocardiographically documented mitral-valve prolapse: long-term follow-up of 237 patients. N Engl J Med 1985; 313:1305–1309.

312. Natterson PD, Perloff JK. Klitzner TS, Stevenson WG. Electrophysiologic abnormalities: unoperated occurrence and postoperative residua and sequelae. In: Perloff JK, Child JS (eds). Congenital Heart Disease in Adults. 2nd ed. Philadelphia: WB Saunders, 1998, pp. 316–345.

313. Kramer MR, Drori Y, Lev B. Sudden death in young soldiers: high incidence of syncope prior to death. Chest 1988; 93:345–347.

314. Glew RH, Varghese PJ, Krovetz LJ, Dorst JP, Rowe RD. Sudden death in congenital aortic stenosis: a review of eight cases with an evaluation of premonitory clinical features. Am Heart J 1969; 78:615–625.

315. Lambert EC, Menon VA, Wagner HR, Vlad P. Sudden unexpected death from cardiovascular disease in children: a cooperative international study. Am J Cardiol 1974; 34:89–96.

316. Garson A Jr, McNamara DG. Sudden death in a pediatric cardiology population, 1958 to 1983: relation to prior arrhythmias. J Am Coll Cardiol 1985; 5:134B–137B.

317. Perloff JK. The Clinical Recognition of Congenital Heart Disease. 4th ed. Philadelphia: WB Saunders, 1994.

318. Anonymous. Paul Wood's Diseases of the Heart and Circulation. 3rd ed. Philadelphia: JB Lippincott, 1968, pp. 415–416.

319. Young D, Mark H. Fate of the patient with the Eisenmenger syndrome. Am J Cardiol 1971; 28:658–669.

320. Kugler JD. Predicting sudden death in patients who have undergone tetralogy of Fallot repair: is it really as simple as measuring ECG intervals? J Cardiovasc Electrophysiol 1998; 9:103–106.

321. Brandenburg, R.O. Cardiomyopathies and their role in sudden death. J Am Coll Cardiol 1985; 5:185B–189B.

322. Anderson KP, Freedman RA, Mason JW. Sudden death in idiopathic dilated cardiomyopathy. Ann Intern Med 1987; 107:104–106.

323. Tamburro P, Wilber D. Sudden death in idiopathic dilated cardiomyopathy. Am Heart J 1992; 124:1035–1045.

324. Larsen L, Markham J, Haffajee CI. Sudden death in idiopathic dilated cardiomyopathy: role of ventricular arrhythmias. PACE 1993; 16:1051–1059.

325. Brachmann J. Hilbel T, Grunig E, Benz A, Haass M, Kubler W. Ventricular arrhythmias in dilated cardiomyopathy. PACE 1997; 20:2714–2718.

326. Friedman RA, Moak JP, Garson A. Clinical course of idiopathic dilated cardiomyopathy in children. J Am Coll Cardiol 1991; 18:152–156.

327. Mestroni L, Miani D, Di Lenarda A, et al. Clinical and pathologic study of familial dilated cardiomyopathy. Am J Cardiol 1990; 65:1449–1453.

328. Goodwin JF, Krikler DM. Arrhythmia as a cause of sudden death in hypertrophic cardiomyopathy. Lancet 1976; 2:937–940.

329. McKenna WJ. Sudden death in hypertrophic cardio-myopathy: identification of the "high risk" patient. In Brugada P, Wellens HJJ (eds). Cardiac Arrhythmias. Where To Go From Here? Mount Kisco, NY: Futura Publishing Co., 1987, pp. 353–365.

330. Maron BJ, Bonow RO. Cannon, RO. Leon MB, Epstein SE. Hypertrophic cardiomyopathy: interrelations of clinical manifestations, pathophysiology, and therapy. N Engl J Med 1987; 316:780–789.

331. Maron BJ, Bonow RO, Cannon RO, Leon MB, Epstein SE. Hypertrophic cardiomyopathy: interrelations of clinical manifestations, pathophysiology, and therapy. N Engl J Med 1987; 316:844–852.

332. Maron BJ. Right ventricular cardiomyopathy: another cause of sudden death in the young. N Engl J Med 1988; 318:178–180.

333. Kuck KH. Arrhythmias in hypertrophic cardiomyopathy. PACE 1997; 20:2706–2713.

334. Spirito P, Seidman CE, McKenna WJ, Maron BJ. The management of hypertrophic cardiomyopathy. N Engl J Med 1997; 336:775–785.

335. McKenna WJ, Franklin RC, Nihoyannopoulos P, Robinson KC, Deanfield JE. Arrhythmia and prognosis in infants, children and adolescents with hypertrophic cardiomyopathy. J Am Coll Cardiol 1988; 11:147–153.

336. Maron BJ, Lipson LC, Roberts WC Savage DD, Epstein SE. "Malignant" hypertrophic cardiomyopathy: identification of a subgroup of families with unusually frequent premature death. Am J Cardiol 1978; 41:1133–1140.

337. Koga Y, Ogata M, Kihara K, Tsubaki K, Toshima H. Sudden death in hypertrophic and dilated cardiomyopathy. Jpn Cir J 1989; 53:1546–1556.

338. Maron BJ, Roberts WC, Epstein SE. Sudden death in hypertrophic cardiomyopathy: a profile of 78 patients. Circulation 1982; 65:1388–1394.

339. Maron BJ, Kogan J, Proschan MA, Hecht GM, Roberts WC. Circadian variability in the occurrence of sudden cardiac death in patients with hypertrophic cardiomyopathy. J Am Coll Cardiol 1994; 23:1405–1409.

340. Marian AJ. Sudden cardiac death in patients with hypertrophic cardiomyopathy: from bench to bedside with an emphasis on genetic markers. Clin Cardiol 1995; 18:189–198.

341. Moolman JC, Corfield VA, Posen B, et al. Sudden death due to troponin T mutations. J Am Coll Cardiol 1997; 29:549–555.

342. Krikler DM, Davies MJ, Rowland E, Goodwin JF, Evans RC, Shaw DB. Sudden death in hypertrophic cardiomyopathy: associated accessory atrioventricular pathways. B Heart J 1980; 43:245–251.

343. Wiedermann CJ, Becker AE, Hopferwieser T, Muhlberger V, Knapp E. Sudden death in a young competitive athlete with Wolff-Parkinson-White syndrome. Eur Heart J 1987; 8:651–655.

344. James TN, Armstrong RS, Silverman J, Marshall TK. De subitaneis mortibus. VI. Two young soldiers. Circulation 1974; 49:1239–1246.

345. Bharati S, Lev M. Congenital abnormalities of the conduction system in sudden death in young adults. J Am Coll Cardiol 1986; 8:1096–1104.

346. Fukuda K, Arakawa K. Pathological substratum for clinical features of fatal myocarditis. Jpn Cir J 1987; 51:1379–1384.

347. See DM, Tilles JG. Viral myocarditis. Rev Infect Dis 1991; 13:951–956.

348. Neuspiel DR, Kuller LH. Sudden and unexpected natural death in childhood and adolescence. JAMA 1985; 254:1321–1325.

349. Elizari MV, Chiale PA. Cardiac arrhythmias in Chagas' heart disease. J Cardiovasc Electrophysiol 1993; 4:596–608.

350. Levi G, Scalvini S, Volterrani M, Marangoni S, Arosio G, Quadri A. Coxsackie virus heart disease: 15 years after. Eur Heart J 1988; 9:1303–1307.

351. Stockins BA. Lanas FT, Saavedra JG, Opazo JA. Prognosis in patients with diphtheric myocarditis and bradyarrhythmias: assessment of results of ventricular pacing. Br Heart J 1994; 72:190–191.

352. Turnicky RP, Goodin J, Smialek JE, Herskowitz A, Beschorner WE. Incidental myocarditis with intravenous drug abuse: the pathology, immunopathology, and potential implications for human immunodeficiency virus-associated myocarditis. Hum Pathol 1992; 23:138–143.

353. Vignola PA, Aonuma K, Swaye PS, et al. Lymphocytic myocarditis presenting as unexplained ventricular arrhythmias: diagnosis with endomyocardial biopsy and response to immunosuppression. J Am Coll Cardiol 1984; 4:812–819.

354. Roberts WC, Waller BF. Cardiac amyloidosis causing cardiac dysfunction: analysis of 54 necropsy patients. Am J Cardiol 1983; 52:137–146.

355. Dubrey SW, Bilazarian S, Lavalley M, Reisinger J, Skinner M, Falk, RH. Signal-averaged electrocardiography in patients with AL (primary) amyloidosis. Am Heart J 1997; 134:994–1001.

356. Blomstrom-Lundqvist C, Sabel KG, Olsson SB. A long term follow up of 15 patients with arrhythmogenic right ventricular dysplasia. B Heart J 1987; 58:477–488.

357. Nava A, Thiene G, Canciani B, et al. Familial occurrence of right ventricular dysplasia: a study involving nine families. J Am Coll Cardiol 1988; 12:1222–1228.

358. Thiene G, Nava A, Corrado D, Rossi L, Pennelli N. Right ventricular cardiomyopathy and sudden death in young people. N Engl J Med 1988; 318:129–133.

359. Corrado D, Thiene G, Nava A, Rossi L, Pennelli N. Sudden death in young competitive athletes: clinicopathologic correlations in 22 cases. Am J Med 1990; 89:588–596.

360. Goodin JC, Farb A, Smialek JE, Field F, Virmani R. Right ventricular dysplasia associated with sudden death in young adults. Mod Pathol 1991: 4:702–706.

361. Dalal P, Fujisic K, Hupart P, Schwietzer P. Arrhythmogenic right ventricular dysplasia: a review. Cardiology 1994; 85:361–369.

362. Kullo IJ, Edwards WD, Seward JB. Right ventricular dysplasia: the Mayo Clinic experience. Mayo Clinic Proc 1995; 70:541–548.

363. Peters S, Reil GH. Risk factors of cardiac arrest in arrhythmogenic right ventricular dysplasia. Eur Heart J 1995; 16:77–80.

364. Marcus FI, Fontaine G. Arrhythmogenic right ventricular dysplasia/cardiomyopathy: a review. Pacing Clin Electrophysiol 1995; 18:1298–1314.

365. Silverman KJ, Hutchins GM, Bulkley BH. Cardiac sarcoid: a clinicopathologic study of 84 unselected patients with systemic sarcoidosis. Circulation 1978; 58:1204–1211.

366. Packer M. Sudden unexpected death in patients with congestive heart failure: a second frontier. Circulation 1985; 72:681–685.

367. Chakko S, De Marchena E, Kessler KM, Myerburg RJ. Ventricular arrhythmias in congestive heart failure. Clin Cardiol 1989; 12:525–530.

368. Singh SN. Congestive heart failure and arrhythmias: therapeutic modalities. J Cardiovasc Electrophysiol 1997; 8:89–97.

369. Uretsky BF, Sheahan RG. Primary prevention of sudden cardiac death in heart failure: will the solution be shocking? J Am Coll Cardiol 1997; 30:1589–1597.

370. Kannel WB, Plehn JF, Cupples A. Cardiac failure and sudden death in the Framingham study. Am Heart J 1988; 115:869–875.

371. Wilson JR, Schwartz JS, St. John Sutton M, et al. Prognosis in severe heart failure: relation to hemodynamic measurements and ventricular ectopic activity. J Am Coll Cardiol 1983; 2:403–410.

372. Stevenson WG, Stevenson LW, Weiss J, Tillisch JH. Inducible ventricular arrhythmias and sudden death during vasodilator

373. Borhani NO. Left ventricular hypertrophy, arrhythmias and sudden death in systemic hypertension. Am J Cardiol 1987; 60:13I–18I.

374. Kannel WB. Left ventricular hypertrophy as a risk factor: the Framingham experience. J Hypertens 1991; 9:S3–S8.

375. Messerli FH, Grodzicki T. Hypertension, left ventricular hypertrophy, ventricular arrhythmias and sudden death. Eur Heart J 1992; 13:D66–D69.

376. Spirito P, Maron BJ. Relation between extent of left ventricular hypertrophy and occurrence of sudden cardiac death in hypertrophic cardiomyopathy. J Am Coll Cardiol 1990; 15:1521–1526.

377. Salerno TA, Stefaniszyn HJ. Spontaneous ventricular fibrillation occurring immediately after institution of cardiopulmonary bypass: possible clinical implications. J Thorac Cardiovasc Surg 1983; 86:306–309.

378. Topol EJ, Lerman BB, Baughman KL, Platia EV, Griffith LSC. De novo refractory ventricular tachyarrhythmias after coronary revascularization. Am J Cardiol 1986; 57:57–59.

379. Kron IL, DiMarco JP, Harman PK, et al. Unanticipated postoperative ventricular tachyarrhythmias. Ann Thorac Surg 1984; 38:317–322.

380. Sapin PM, Woelfel AK, Foster JR. Unexpected ventricular tachyarrhythmias soon after cardiac surgery. Am J Cardiol 1991; 68:1099–1100.

381. Costeas XF, Schoenfeld MH. Usefulness of electrophysiologic studies for new-onset sustained ventricular tachyarrhythmias shortly after coronary artery bypass grafting. Am J Cardiol 1993; 72:1291–1294.

382. Pires LA, Wagshal AB, Lancey R, Huang SK. Arrhythmias and conduction disturbances after coronary artery bypass graft surgery: epidemiology, management, and prognosis. Am Heart J 1995; 129:799–808.

383. Saxon LA, Wiener I, Natterson PD, Laks H, Drinkwater D, Stevenson WG. Monomorphic versus polymorphic ventricular tachycardia after coronary artery bypass grafting. Am J Cardiol 1995; 75:403–405.

384. Dreifus LS, Haiat R, Watanabe Y, Arriaga J, Reitman N. Ventricular fibrillation: a possible mechanism of sudden death in patients and Wolff-Parkinson-White syndrome. Circulation 1971; 43:520–527.

385. Dreifus LS, Wellens HJJ, Watanabe Y, Kimbiris D, Truex R. Sinus bradycardia and atrial fibrillation associated with the Wolff-Parkinson-White syndrome. Am J Cardiol 1976; 38:149–156.

386. Timmermans, C, Smeets JL, Rodriguez LM, Vrouchos G, van den Dool A, Wellens HJJ. Aborted sudden death in the Wolff-Parkinson-White syndrome. Am J Cardiol 1995; 76:492–494.

387. Zheutlin TA, Steinman RT. Mattioni TA, Kehoe RF. Long-term arrhythmic outcome in survivors of ventricular fibrillation with absence of inducible ventricular tachycardia. Am J Cardiol 1988; 62:1213–1217.

388. Wang YS, Scheinman MM, Chien WW, Cohen TJ, Lesh MD, Griffin JC. Patients with supraventricular tachycardia presenting with aborted sudden death: incidence, mechanism and long-term follow-up. J Am Coll Cardiol 1991; 18:1711–1719.

389. Pietersen AH, Andersen ED, Sandoe E. Atrial fibrillation in the Wolff-Parkinson-White syndrome. Am J Cardiol 1992; 70:38A–43A.

390. Bromberg BI, Lindsay BD, Cain ME, Cox JL. Impact of clinical history and electrophysiologic characterization of accessory pathways on management strategies to reduce sudden death among children with Wolff-Parkinson-White syndrome. J Am Coll Cardiol 1996; 27:690–695.

391. Engel GL. Sudden and rapid death during psychological stress: folklore or folk wisdom? Ann Intern Med 1971; 74:771–782.

392. Lynch JJ, Paskewitz DA, Gimbel KS, Thomas SA. Psychological aspects of cardiac arrhythmia. Am Heart J 1977; 93:645–657.

393. Engel GL. Psychologic stress, vasodepressor (vasovagal)

syncope, and sudden death. Ann Intern Medicine 1978; 89:403–412.

394. Lown B, Verrier RL. Neural activity and ventricular fibrillation. N Engl J Med 1976; 294:1165–1170.

395. Lown B. Mental stress, arrhythmias and sudden death. Am J Med 1982; 72:177–180.

396. Meisel SR, Kutz I, Dayan KI, et al. Effect of Iraqi missile war on incidence of acute myocardial infarction and sudden death in Israeli civilians. Lancet 1991; 338:660–661.

397. Leor J, Poole WK, Kloner RA. Sudden cardiac death triggered by an earthquake. N Engl J Med 1996; 334:413–419.

398. Weisenberg D, Meisel SR, David D. Sudden death among the Israeli civilian population during the Gulf War: incidence and mechanisms. Isr J Med Sci 1996; 32:95–99.

399. Levine, SA. Benign atrial fibrillation of forty years' duration with sudden death from emotion. Ann Intern Med 1963; 58:681–684.

400. Greene WA, Goldstein S, Moss AJ. Psychosocial aspects of sudden death: a preliminary report. Arch Intern Med 1972; 129:725–731.

401. Reich P, DeSilva RA, Lown B, Murawski BJ. Acute psychological disturbances preceding life-threatening ventricular arrhythmias. JAMA 1981; 246:233–235.

402. Eliot RS, Buell JC. Role of emotions and stress in the genesis of sudden death. J Am Coll Cardiol 1985; 5:95B–98B.

403. Vlay, SC. Ventricular tachycardia/fibrillation on the first day of medical school. Am J Cardiol 1986; 57:483.

404. Topaz O, Castellanos A, Grobman LR, Myerburg RJ. The role of arrhythmogenic auditory stimuli in sudden cardiac death. Am Heart J 1988; 116:222–226.

405. Wellens HJJ, Schuilenburg RM, Durrer, D. Electrical stimulation of the heart in patients with ventricular tachycardia. Circulation 1972; 46:216–226.

406. Topaz O, Perin E, Cox M, Mallon SM, Castellanos A, Myerburg, RJ. Young adult survivors of sudden cardiac arrest: analysis of invasive evaluation of 22 subjects. Am Heart J 1989; 118:281–287.

407. Opie LH. Sudden death and sport. Lancet 1975; February 1:263–266.

408. Cobb LA, Weaver WD. Exercise: a risk for sudden death in patients with coronary heart disease. J Am Coll Cardiol 1986; 7:215–219.

409. Amsterdam EA. Sudden death during exercise. Cardiology 1990; 77:441–417.

410. Friedewald VE Jr, Spence DW. Sudden cardiac death associated with exercise: the risk-benefit issue. Am J Cardiol 1990; 66:183–188.

411. Zehender M, Meinertz T, Keul J, Just H. ECG variants and cardiac arrhythmias in athletes: clinical relevance and prognostic importance. Am Heart J 1990: 119:1378–1391.

412. Estes NA, III. Sudden death in young athletes. N Engl J Med 1995; 333:380–381.

413. Wight JN Jr, Salem D. Sudden cardiac death and the "athlete's heart." Arch Intern Med 1995; 155:1473–1480.

414. Josephson ME, Schibgilla VH. Athletes and arrhythmias: clinical considerations and perspectives. Eur Heart J 1996; 17:498–505.

415. Maron BJ, Epstein SE, Roberts WC. Causes of sudden death in competitive athletes. J Am Coll Cardiol 1986; 7:204–214.

416. Green LH, Cohen SI, Kurland G. Fatal myocardial infarction in marathon racing. Ann Intern Med 1976; 84:704–706.

417. Thompson PD, Funk EJ, Carleton RA, Sturner WQ. Incidence of death during jogging in Rhode Island from 1975 through 1980. JAMA 1982; 247:2535–2538.

418. Phillips M, Robinowitz M, Higgins JR, Boran KJ, Reed T, Virmani R. Sudden cardiac death in Air Force recruits: a 20-year review. JAMA 1986; 256:2696–2699.

419. Burke AP, Farb A, Virmani R, Goodin J, Smialek JE. Sports-related and non-sports-related sudden cardiac death in young adults. Am Heart J 1991; 121:568–575.

420. Maron BJ, Roberts WC, McAllister, HA, Rosing DR, Epstein SE. Sudden death in young athletes. Circulation 1980; 62:218–229.

421. Maron BJ, Epstein SE, Roberts WC. Hypertrophic cardiomyopathy: a common cause of sudden death in the young competitive athlete. Eur Heart J 1983; 4:135–144.

422. Waller BF, Roberts WC. Sudden death while running in conditioned runners aged 40 years or over. Am J Cardiol 1980; 45:1292–1300.

423. Northcote RJ, Evans AD, Ballantyne D. Sudden death in squash players. Lancet 1984; 1:148–150.

424. Corrado D, Basso C, Schiavon M, Thiene G. Screening for hypertrophic cardiomyopathy in young athletes. N Engl J Med 1998; 339:364–369.

425. Frustaci A, Bellocci F, Olsen EG. Results of biventricular endomyocardial biopsy in survivors of cardiac arrest with apparently normal hearts. Am J Cardiol 1994; 74:890–895.

426. Furlanello F, Bertoldi A, Dallago M, et al. Cardiac arrest and sudden death in competitive athletes with arrhythmogenic right ventricular dysplasia. PACE 1998; 21:331–335.

427. Vuori I, Makarainen M, Jaskelainen A. Sudden death and physical activity. Cardiology 1978; 63:287–304.

428. Lynch P. Soldiers, sport, and sudden death. Lancet 1980; 1:1235–1237.

429. Murayama M, Shimomura K. Exercise and arrhythmia. Jpn Circ J 1979; 43:247–256.

430. Kark JA, Posey DM, Schumacher HR, Ruehle CJ. Sickle-cell trait as a risk factor for sudden death in physical training. N Engl J Med 1987; 317:781–787.

431. Pyfer HR, Doane BL. Cardiac arrest during exercise training: report of a successfully treated case attributed to preparedness. JAMA 1969; 210:101–102.

432. Rochmis P, Blackburn H. Exercise tests: a survey of procedures, safety, and litigation experience in approximately 170,000 tests. JAMA 1971; 217:1061–1066.

433. Bruce RA, Kluge W. Defibrillatory treatment of exertional cardiac arrest in coronary disease. JAMA 1971; 216:653–658.

434. Molajo AO, Summers GD, Bennett DH. Effect of percutaneous transluminal coronary angioplasty on arrhythmias complicating angina. Br Heart J 1985; 54:375–377.

435. Berntsen RF, Gunnes P, Lie M, Rasmussen K. Surgical revascularization in the treatment of ventricular tachycardia and fibrillation exposed by exercise-induced ischaemia. Eur Heart J 1993; 14:1297–1303.

436. Detry JM, Abouantoun S, Wyns W. Incidence and prognostic implications of severe ventricular arrhythmias during maximal exercise testing. Cardiology 1981; 68:35–43.

437. Young DZ, Lampert S, Graboys TB, Lown B. Safety of maximal exercise testing in patients at high risk for ventricular arrhythmia. Circulation 1984; 70:184–191.

438. Mead WF, Pyfer HR, Thrombold JC, Frederick RC. Successful resuscitation of two near simultaneous cases of cardiac arrest with a review of fifteen cases occurring during supervised exercise. Circulation 1976; 53:187–189.

439. Irving JB, Bruce RA. Exertional hypotension and postexertional ventricular fibrillation in stress testing. Am J Cardiol 1977; 39:849–851.

440. Fletcher GF, Cantwell JD. Ventricular fibrillation in a medically supervised cardiac exercise program: clinical, angiographic, and surgical correlations. JAMA 1977; 238:2627–2629.

441. Berntsen RF, Gunnes P, Rasmussen K. Pattern of coronary artery disease in patients with ventricular tachycardia and fibrillation exposed by exercise-induced ischemia. Am Heart J 1995; 129:733–738.

442. Allen BJ, Casey TP, Brodsky MA, Luckett CR, Henry WL. Exercise testing in patients with life-threatening ventricular tachyarrhythmias: results and correlation with clinical and arrhythmia factors. Am Heart J 1988; 116:997–1002.

443. Frazer M, Mirchandani H. Commotio cordis, revisited. Am J Forensic Med Pathol 1984; 5:249–251.

444. American Academy of Pediatrics Committee on Sports Medicine. Risk of injury from baseball and softball in children 5 to 14 years of age. Pediatrics 1994; 93:690–692.

445. Curfman GD. Fatal impact: concussion of the heart. N Engl J Med 1998; 338:1841–1843.

446. Maron BJ, Poliac LC, Kaplan JA, Mueller FO. Blunt impact to the chest leading to sudden death from cardiac arrest during sports activities. N Engl J Med 1995; 333:337–342.

447. Abrunzo TJ. Commotio cordis: the single, most common cause of traumatic death in youth baseball. Am J Dis Child 1991; 145:1279–1282.

448. van Amerongen R, Rosen M, Winnik G, Horwitz J. Ventricular fibrillation following blunt chest trauma from a baseball. Pediatr Emerg Care 1997; 13:107–110.

449. Kaplan JA, Karofsky PS, Volturo GA. Commotio cordis in two amateur ice hockey players despite the use of commercial chest protectors: case reports. J Trauma 1993; 34:151–153.

450. Link MS, Wang PJ, Pandian NG. An experimental model of sudden death due to low-energy chest-wall impact (commotio cordis). N Engl J Med 1998; 338:1805–1811.

451. Viskin S, Belhassen B. Acute management of paroxysmal atrioventricular junctional reentrant supraventricular tachycardia: pharmacologic strategies. Am Heart J 1990; 120:180–188.

452. Almendral J, Ormaetxe J, Delcan JL. Idiopathic ventricular tachycardia and fibrillation: incidence, prognosis, and therapy. PACE 1992; 15:627–630.

453. Campbell RW. Ventricular rhythm disturbances in the normal heart. Eur Heart J 1992; 13:139–143.

454. Belhassen B, Viskin S. Idiopathic ventricular tachycardia and fibrillation. J Cardiovasc Electrophysiol 1993; 4:356–368.

455. Priori SG, Borggrefe M, Camm AJ, et al. Unexplained cardiac arrest: the need for a prospective registry. Eur Heart J 1992; 13:1445–1446.

456. Wellens HJJ, Lemery R, Smeets JL, et al. Sudden arrhythmic death without overt heart disease. Circulation 1992; 85(Suppl I):I-92–I-97.

457. Brugada J, Brugada P. What to do in patients with no structural heart disease and sudden arrhythmic death? Am J Cardiol 1996; 78:69–75.

458. Jordaens L, Tavernier R, Kazmierczak J, Dimmer C. Ventricular arrhythmias in apparently healthy subjects. Pacing Clin Electrophysiol 1997; 20:2692–2698.

459. Marcus FI. Idiopathic ventricular fibrillation. J Cardiovasc Electrophysiol 1997; 8:1075–1083.

460. Joint Steering Committees of the Unexplained Cardiac Arrest Registry of Europe and of the Idiopathic Ventricular Fibrillation Registry of the United States. Survivors of out-of-hospital cardiac arrest with apparently normal heart: need for definition and standardized clinical evaluation. Circulation 1997; 95:265–272.

461. Bourke JP, Doig JC. Ventricular Tachyarrhythmias in the Normal Heart. Armonk, NY: Futura Publishing Co., 1998.

462. Tung RT, Shen W-K, Hammill SC, Gersh BJ. Idiopathic ventricular fibrillation in out-of-hospital cardiac arrest survivors. PACE 1994; 17:1405–1412.

463. Belhassen B, Pelleg A, Miller HI, Laniado S. Serial electrophysiological studies in a young patient with recurrent ventricular fibrillation. PACE 1981; 4:92–99.

464. Wever EF, Hauer RN, Oomen A, Peters RH, Bakker PF, Robles de Medina EO. Unfavorable outcome in patients with primary electrical disease who survived an episode of ventricular fibrillation. Circulation 1993; 88:1021–1029.

465. Kudenchuk PJ, Cobb LA, Greene HL, Fahrenbruch CE, Sheehan FH. Late outcome of survivors of out-of-hospital cardiac arrest with left ventricular ejection fractions greater than or equal to 50% and without significant coronary arterial narrowing. Am J Cardiol 1991; 67:704–708.

466. Corrado D, Nava A, Buja G, et al. Familial cardiomyopathy underlies syndrome of right bundle branch block, ST segment elevation and sudden death. J Am Coll Cardiol 1996; 27:443–448.

467. American Heart Association Task Force on Automatic External Defibrillation. Automatic external defibrillators for public access defibrillation: recommendations for specifying and reporting arrhythmia analysis algorithm performance, incorporating new waveforms, and enhancing safety. Biomed Instrum Technol 1997; 31:238–244.

468. Scheinman MM. Is the Brugada syndrome a distinct clinical entity? J Cardiovasc Electrophysiol 1997; 8:332–336.

469. Tada H, Aihara N, Ohe T, et al. Arrhythmogenic right ventricular cardiomyopathy underlies syndrome of right bundle branch block, ST-segment elevation, and sudden death. Am J Cardiol 1998; 81:519–522.

470. Brugada P, Brugada J. Right bundle branch block, persistent ST segment elevation and sudden cardiac death: a distinct clinical and electrocardiographic syndrome: a multicenter report. J Am Coll Cardiol 1992; 20:1391–1396.

471. Viskin S, Belhassen B. When you only live twice. N Engl J Med 1995; 332:1221–1225.

472. Atarashi H, Ogawa S, Harumi K, et al. Characteristics of patients with right bundle branch block and ST-segment elevation in right precordial leads: idiopathic ventricular fibrillation investigators. Am J Cardiol 1996; 78:581–583.

473. Miyazaki T, Mitamura H, Miyoshi S, Soejima K, Aizawa Y, Ogawa S. Autonomic and antiarrhythmic drug modulation of ST segment elevation in patients with Brugada syndrome. J Am Coll Cardiol 1996; 27:1061–1070.

474. Brugada J, Brugada P. Further characterization of the syndrome of right bundle branch block, ST segment elevation, and sudden cardiac death. J Cardiovasc Electrophysiol 1997; 8:325–331.

475. Kasanuki H, Ohnishi S, Ohtuka M, et al. Idiopathic ventricular fibrillation induced with vagal activity in patients without obvious heart disease. Circulation 1997; 95:2277–2285.

476. Antzelevitch C. The Brugada syndrome. J Cardiovasc Electrophysiol 1998; 9:513–516.

477. Brugada J, Brugada R, Brugada P. Right bundle-branch block and ST-segment elevation in leads V$_1$ through V$_3$: a marker for sudden death in patients without demonstrable structural heart disease. Circulation 1998; 97:457–460.

478. Garg A, Finneran W, Feld GK. Familial sudden cardiac death associated with a terminal QRS abnormality on surface 12-lead electrocardiogram in the index case. J Cardiovasc Electrophysiol 1998; 9:642–647.

479. Matsuo K, Shimizu W, Kurita T, Inagaki M, Aihara N, Kamakura S. Dynamic changes of 12-lead electrocardiograms in a patient with Brugada syndrome. J Cardiovasc Electrophysiol 1998; 9:508–512.

480. Baron RC, Thacker SB, Gorelkin L, Vernon AA, Taylor WR, Choi K. Sudden death among southeast Asian refugees: an unexplained nocturnal phenomenon. JAMA 1983; 250:2947–2951.

481. Otto CM, Tauxe RV, Cobb LA, et al. Ventricular fibrillation causes sudden death in southeast Asian immigrants. Ann Intern Med 1984; 100:45–47.

482. Gilbert J, Gold RL, Haffajee CI, Alpert JS. Sudden cardiac death in a southeast Asian immigrant: clinical, electrophysiologic, and biopsy characteristics. PACE 1986; 9:912–914.

483. Nademanee K, Veerakul G, Nimmannit S, et al. Arrhythmogenic marker for the sudden unexplained death syndrome in Thai men. Circulation 1997; 96:2595–2600.

484. Hayashi M, Murata M, Satoh M, et al. Sudden nocturnal death in young males from ventricular flutter. Jpn Heart J 1985; 26:585–591.

485. Molander N. Sudden natural death in later childhood and adolescence. Arch Dis Child 1982; 57:572–576.

486. D'Alonzo GE, Barst RJ, Ayres SM, et al. Survival in patients with primary pulmonary hypertension: results from a national prospective registry. Ann Intern Med 1991; 115:343–349.

487. Ackermann DM, Edwards WD. Sudden death as the initial manifestation of primary pulmonary hypertension: report of four cases. Am J Forensic Med Pathol 1987; 8:97–102.

488. Epstein AE, Davis KB, Kay GN, Plumb VJ, Rogers WJ. Significance of ventricular tachyarrhythmias complicating cardiac catheterization: a CASS registry study. Am Heart J 1990; 119:494–502.

489. Clements SD Jr, Gatlin S. Outpatient cardiac catheterization: a report of 3,000 cases. Clin Cardiol 1991; 14:477–480.

490. Mark DB, Sigmon K, Topol EJ, et al. Identification of acute myocardial infarction patients suitable for early hospital discharge after aggressive interventional therapy: results from the thrombolysis and angioplasty in acute myocardial infarction registry. Circulation 1991; 83:1186–1193.

491. Oram S, Davies JPH. Further experience of electrical conversion of atrial fibrillation to sinus rhythm: analysis of 100 patients. Lancet 1964; 1:1294–1298.

492. Turner JRB, Towers JRH. Complications of cardioversion. Lancet 1965; 2:612–614.

493. Castellanos A, Lemberg L, Fonseca EJ. Significance of ventricular and pseudoventricular arrhythmias appearing after DC countershock. Am Heart J 1965; 70:583–594.

494. Robinson JS, Sloman G, Hogan J, McConchie IH. Ventricular tachycardia and fibrillation with implanted electrical pacemakers. Br Heart J 1965; 27:937–941.

495. Morris JJ, Peter RH, McIntosh HD. Electrical conversion of atrial fibrillation. Ann Intern Med 1966; 65:216–231.

496. Resnekov L, McDonald L. Complications in 220 patients with cardiac dysrhythmias treated by phased direct current shock, and indications for electroconversion. Br Heart J 1967; 29:926–936.

497. Bjerkelund C, Orning OM. An evaluation of DC shock treatment of atrial arrhythmias. Acta Med Scand 1968; 184:481–491.

498. Bharati S, Scheinmann MM, Morady F, Hess DS, Lev M. Sudden death after catheter-induced atrioventricular junctional ablation. Chest 1985; 88:883–889.

499. Perry JC, Kearney DL, Friedman RA, Moak JP, Garson A Jr. Late ventricular arrhythmia and sudden death following direct-current catheter ablation of the atrioventricular junction. Am J Cardiol 1992; 70:765–768.

500. Lacroix D, Kacet S, Lekieffre J. Ventricular fibrillation after successful radiofrequency catheter ablation of idiopathic right ventricular tachycardia. Am Heart J 1994; 128: 1044–1045.

501. Geelen P, Brugada J, Andries E, Brugada P. Ventricular fibrillation and sudden death radiofrequency catheter ablation of the atrioventricular junction. PACE 1997; 20:343–348.

502. Rowe GG, Zarnstorff WC. Ventricular fibrillation during selective angiocardiography. JAMA 1965; 192:947–950.

503. Chambers JJ, Saha AK. Electrocution during anaesthesia. Anaesthesia 1979; 34:173–175.

504. Jensen PJ, Thomsen PEB, Bagger JP, Norgaard A, Baandrup U. Electrical injury causing ventricular arrhythmias. Br Heart J 1987; 57:279–283.

505. Marchlinski FE, Waxman HL, Shaw LM, Ezri MD, Josephson ME. Electrophysiologic study for ventricular arrhythmia: effect on total and myocardial-specific creatine kinase activity. Am J Cardiol 1982; 50:1061–1065.

506. Lauer MR, Young C, Liem B, et al. Ventricular fibrillation induced by low-energy shocks from programmable implantable cardioverter-defibrillators in patients with coronary artery disease. Am J Cardiol 1994; 73:559–563.

507. Sclarovsky S, Zafrir N, Strasberg B, et al. Ventricular fibrillation complicating temporary ventricular pacing in acute myocardial infarction: significance of right ventricular infarction. Am J Cardiol 1981; 48:1160–1166.

508. Favale S, Di Biase M, Rizzo U, Minafra F, Rizzon P. Ventricular fibrillation induced by transesophageal atrial pacing in hypertrophic cardiomyopathy. Eur Heart J 1987; 8:912–916.

509. Massumi RA, Mason DT, Amsterdam EA, et al. Ventricular fibrillation and tachycardia after intravenous atropine for treatment of bradycardias. N Engl J Med 1972; 287:336–338.

510. Scheinman MM, Thorburn D, Abbott JA. Use of atropine in patients with acute myocardial infarction and sinus bradycardia. Circulation 1975; 52:627–633.

511. Lunde P. Ventricular fibrillation after intravenous atropine for treatment of sinus bradycardia. Acta Med Scand 1976: 199:369–371.

512. Warren JV, Lewis RP. Beneficial effects of atropine in the pre-hospital phase of coronary care. Am J Cardiol 1976; 37:68–72.

513. Cooper MJ, Abinader EG. Atropine-induced ventricular fibrillation: case report and review of the literature. Am Heart J 1979; 97:225–228.

514. Schweitzer P, Mark H. The effect of atropine on cardiac arrhythmias and conduction. Am Heart J 1980; 100:255–261.

515. Lazzari JO, Benchuga EG, Elizari MV, Rosenbaum MB. Ventricular fibrillation after intravenous atropine in a patient with atrioventricular block. Pacing Clin Electrophysiol 1982; 5:196–200.

516. Santinelli V, Chiariello M, Condorelli M. Rapid increase of intraventricular conduction delay in the genesis of ventricular fibrillation after atropine. Int J Cardiol 1983; 3:109–111.

517. Shaheen J, Mendzelevski B, Tzivoni D. Dobutamine-induced ST segment elevation and ventricular fibrillation with nonsignificant coronary artery disease. Am Heart J 1996; 132:1058–1060.

518. Nanji AA, Filipenko JD. Asystole and ventricular fibrillation associated with cocaine intoxication. Chest 1984; 85:132–133.

519. Isner JM, Estes NA. III, Thompson PD, et al. Acute cardiac events temporally related to cocaine abuse. N Engl J Med 1986; 315:1438–1443.

520. Kloner RA, Hale S, Alker K, Rezkalla S. The effects of acute and chronic cocaine use on the heart. Circulation 1992; 85:407–419.

521. Warner EA. Cocaine abuse. Ann Intern Med 1993; 119:226–235.

522. Adgey AA, Johnston PW, McMechan S. Sudden cardiac death and substance abuse. Resuscitation 1995; 29:219–221.

523. Brady WJ Jr, Stremski E, Eljaiek L, Aufderheide TP. Freon inhalational abuse presenting with ventricular fibrillation. Am J Emerg Med 1994; 12:533–536.

524. Byrum CJ, Wahl RA, Behrendt DM, Dick M. Ventricular fibrillation associated with use of digitalis in a newborn infant with Wolff-Parkinson-White syndrome. J Pediatr 1982; 101:400–403.

525. Zucker AR, Lacina SJ, DasGupta DS, et al. Fab fragments of digoxin-specific antibodies used to reverse ventricular fibrillation induced by digoxin ingestion in a child. Pediatrics 1982; 70:468–471.

526. French JH, Thomas RG, Siskind AP, Brodsky M, Iseri LT. Magnesium therapy in massive digoxin intoxication. Ann Emerg Med 1984; 13:562–566.

527. Clarke W, Ramoska EA. Acute digoxin overdose: use of digoxin-specific antibody fragments. Am J Emerg Med 1988; 6:465–470.

528. Hoes AW, Grobbee DE, Lubsen J, Man in't Veld AJ, van der Does E, Hofman A. Diuretics, beta-blockers, and the risk for sudden cardiac death in hypertensive patients. Ann Intern Med 1995; 123:481–487.

529. Gulamhusein S, Ko P, Klein GJ. Ventricular fibrillation following verapamil in the Wolff-Parkinson-White syndrome. Am Heart J 1983; 106:145–147.

530. McGovern B, Garan H, Ruskin JN. Precipitation of cardiac arrest by verapamil in patients with Wolff-Parkinson-White syndrome. Ann Intern Med 1986; 104:791–794.

531. Greenwood RJ, Dupler DA. Death following carotid sinus pressure. JAMA 1962; 181:605–609.

532. Porus RL, Marcus FI. Ventricular fibrillation during carotid-sinus stimulation. N Engl J Med 1963; 268:1338–1342.

533. Hilal H, Massumi R. Fatal ventricular fibrillation after carotid-sinus stimulation. N Engl J Med 1966; 275:157–158.

534. Alexander S, Ping WC. Fatal ventricular fibrillation during carotid sinus stimulation. Am J Cardiol 1966; 18:289–291.

535. Cohen MV. Ventricular fibrillation precipitated by carotid sinus pressure: case report and review of the literature. Am Heart J 1972; 84:681–686.

536. Nordrehaug JE, von der Lippe G. Hypokalaemia and ventricular fibrillation in acute myocardial infarction. Br Heart J 1983; 50:525–529.

537. Podrid PJ. Potassium and ventricular arrhythmias. Am J Cardiol 1990; 65:33E–44E.

538. Loeb HS, Pietras RJ, Gunnar RM, Tobin JR Jr. Paroxysmal ventricular fibrillation in two patients with hypomagnesemia: treatment by transvenous pacing. Circulation 1968; 37:210–215.

539. Bhasin S, Wallace W, Lawrence JB, Lesch M. Sudden death associated with thyroid hormone abuse. Am J Med 1981; 71:887–890.

540. Fisher J. Thyrotoxic periodic paralysis with ventricular fibrillation. Arch Intern Med 1982; 142:1362–1364.

541. Shaper AG, Wannamethee G, Macfarlane PW, Walker M. Heart rate, ischaemic heart disease, and sudden cardiac death in middle-aged British men. Br Heart J 1993; 70:49–55.

542. Willich SN, Maclure M, Mittleman M, Arntz H-R, Muller JE. Sudden cardiac death: support for a role of triggering in causation. Circulation 1993; 87:1442–1450.

543. Hohnloser SH, Klingenheben T. Insights into the pathogenesis of sudden cardiac death from analysis of circadian fluctuations of potential triggering factors. Pacing Clin Electrophysiol 1994; 17:428–433.

544. Mifune J, Takeda Y. Sudden cardiac arrest: clinical characteristics and predictors of survival. Jpn Circ J 1989; 53:1536–1540.

545. Wood MA, Simpson PM, London WB, et al. Circadian pattern of ventricular tachyarrhythmias in patients with implantable cardioverter-defibrillators. J Am Coll Cardiol 1995; 25:901–907.

546. Muller JE, Ludmer PL, Willich SN, et al. Circadian variation in the frequency of sudden cardiac death. Circulation 1987; 75:131–138.

547. Tofler GH, Brezinski D, Schafer AI, et al. Concurrent morning increase in platelet aggregability and the risk of myocardial infarction and sudden cardiac death. N Engl J Med 1987; 316:1514–1518.

548. Willich SN, Levy D, Rocco MB, Tofler GH, Stone PH, Muller JE. Circadian variation in the incidence of sudden cardiac death in the Framingham heart study population. Am J Cardiol 1987; 60:801–806.

549. Willich SN. Epidemiologic studies demonstrating increased morning incidence of sudden cardiac death. Am J Cardiol 1990; 66:15G–17G.

550. Willich SN, Goldberg RJ, Maclure M, Perriello L, Muller JE. Increased onset of sudden cardiac death in the first three hours after awakening. Am J Cardiol 1992; 70:65–68.

551. Levine RL, Pepe PE, Fromm RE Jr, Curka PA, Clark PA. Prospective evidence of a circadian rhythm for out-of-hospital cardiac arrests. JAMA 1992; 267:2935–2937.

552. Arntz HR, Willich SN, Oeff M, et al. Circadian variation of sudden cardiac death reflects age-related variability in ventricular fibrillation. Circulation 1993; 88:2284–2289.

553. Aronow WS, Ahn C. Circadian variation of primary cardiac arrest or sudden cardiac death in patients aged 62 to 100 years (mean 82). Am J Cardiol 1993; 71:1455–1456.

554. Lampert R, Rosenfeld L, Batsford W, Lee F, McPherson C. Circadian variation of sustained ventricular tachycardia in patients with coronary artery disease and implantable cardioverter-defibrillators. Circulation 1994; 90:241–247.

555. Moser DK, Stevenson WG, Woo MA, Stevenson LW. Timing of sudden death in patients with heart failure. J Am Coll Cardiol 1994; 24:963–967.

556. Peters RW, Mitchell B, Brooks MM, et al. Circadian pattern of arrhythmic death in patients receiving encainide, flecainide or moricizine in the Cardiac Arrhythmia Suppression Trial (CAST). J Am Coll Cardiol 1994; 23:283–289.

557. Mallavarapu C. Pancholy S, Schwartzman D, et al. Circadian variation of ventricular arrhythmia recurrences after cardioverter-defibrillator implantation in patients with healed myocardial infarcts. Am J Cardiol 1995; 75:1140–1144.

558. Behrens S, Galecka M, Bruggemann T, et al. Circadian variation of sustained ventricular tachyarrhythmias terminated by appropriate shocks in patients with an implantable cardioverter defibrillator. Am Heart J 1995; 130:79–84.

559. Behrens S, Ney G, Fisher SG, Fletcher RD, Franz MR, Singh SN. Effects of amiodarone on the circadian pattern of sudden cardiac death (Department of Veterans Affairs Congestive Heart Failure–Survival Trial of Antiarrhythmic Therapy). Am J Cardiol 1997; 80:45–48.

560. Peckova M, Fahrenbruch CE, Cobb LA, Hallstrom AP. Circadian variations in the occurrence of cardiac arrests: initial and repeat episodes. Circulation 1998; 98:31–39.

561. Tofler GH, Gebara OC, Mittleman MA, et al. Morning peak in ventricular tachyarrhythmias detected by time of implantable cardioverter/defibrillator therapy: the CPI investigators. Circulation 1995; 92:1203–1208.

562. d'Avila A, Wellens F, Andries E, Brugada P. At what time are implantable defibrillator shocks delivered? Evidence for individual circadian variance in sudden cardiac death. Eur Heart J 1995; 16:1231–1233.

563. Peters RW, McQuillan S, Resnick SK, Gold M. Increased Monday incidence of life-threatening ventricular arrhythmias: experience with a third-generation implantable defibrillator. Circulation 1996; 94:1346–1349.

564. Behrens S, Ehlers C, Bruggemann T, et al. Modification of the circadian pattern of ventricular tachyarrhythmias by beta-blocker therapy. Clin Cardiol 1997; 20:253–257.

565. Couch RD. Travel, time zones, and sudden cardiac death: emporiatric pathology. Am J Forensic Med Pathol 1990; 11:106–111.

566. Wright D, Bannister J, Mackintosh, AF. Automatic recording and timing of defibrillation on general wards by day and night. Eur Heart J 1994; 15:631–636.

567. Lown B, Wolf M. Approaches to sudden death from coronary heart disease. Circulation 1971; 44:130–142.

568. Chiang BN, Perlman LV, Ostrander LD Jr, Epstein FH. Relationship of premature systoles to coronary heart disease and sudden death in the Tecumseh epidemiologic study. Ann Intern Med 1969; 70:1159–1166.

569. Bennett MA, Pentecost BL. Warning of cardiac arrest due to ventricular fibrillation and tachycardia. Lancet 1972; 2:1351–1352.

570. Coronary Drug Project Research Group. Prognostic importance of premature beats following myocardial infarction: experience in the Coronary Drug Project. JAMA 1973; 223:1116–1124.

571. Kotler MN, Tabatznik B, Mower MM, Tominaga S. Prognostic significance of ventricular ectopic beats with respect to sudden death in the late postinfarction period. Circulation 1973; 47:959–966.

572. Hinkle LE, Carver ST, Argyros DC, Stevens M, Horvath J. The prognostic significance of ventricular premature contractions in healthy people and in people with coronary heart disease. Acta Cardiol 1974; 18:5–32.

573. Ruberman W, Weinblatt E, Goldberg JD, Frank CW, Shapiro S. Ventricular premature beats and mortality after myocardial infarction. N Engl J Med 1977; 297:750–757.

574. Schulze RA Jr, Strauss HW, Pitt B. Sudden death in the year following myocardial infarction: relation to ventricular premature contractions in the late hospital phase and left ventricular ejection fraction. Am J Med 1977; 62:192–199.

575. Boudoulas H, Dervenagas S, Schaal SF, Lewis RP, Dalamangas G. Malignant premature ventricular beats in ambulatory patients. Ann Intern Med 1979; 91:723–726.

576. Moss AJ, Davis HT, DeCamilla J, Bayer LW. Ventricular ectopic beats and their relation to sudden and nonsudden cardiac death after myocardial infarction. Circulation 1979; 60:998–1003.

577. Ruberman W, Weinblatt E, Goldberg JD, Frank CW, Chaudhary BS, Shapiro S. Ventricular premature complexes and sudden death after myocardial infarction. Circulation 1981; 64:297–305.

578. Bigger JT Jr, Weld FM. Analysis of prognostic significance of ventricular arrhythmias after myocardial infarction: shortcomings of Lown grading system. Br Heart J 1981; 45:717–724.

579. Califf RM, McKinnis RA, Burks J, et al. Prognostic implications of ventricular arrhythmias during 24 hour ambulatory monitoring in patients undergoing cardiac catheterization for coronary artery disease. Am J Cardiol 1982; 50:23–31.

580. Multicenter Post-Infarction Research Group. Risk stratification and survival after myocardial infarction. N Engl J Med 1983; 309:331–336.

581. Olson HG, Lyons KP, Troop P, Butman SM, Piters KM. Prognostic implications of complicated ventricular arrhythmias early after hospital discharge in acute myocardial infarction: a serial ambulatory electrocardiography study. Am Heart J 1984; 108:1221–1228.

582. Gomes JAC, Hariman RI, Kang PS, el-Sherif N, Chowdhry I, Lyons J. Programmed electrical stimulation in patients with high-grade ventricular ectopy: electrophysiologic findings and prognosis for survival. Circulation 1984; 70:43–51.

583. Mukharji J, Rude RE, Poole K, et al. Risk factors for sudden death after acute myocardial infarction: two-year follow-up. Am J Cardiol 1984; 54:31–36.

584. Meinertz T, Hofmann T, Kasper W, et al. Significance of ventricular arrhythmias in idiopathic dilated cardiomyopathy. Am J Cardiol 1984; 53:902–907.

585. Romeo F, Pelliccia F, Cianfrocca C, Cristofani R, Reale A. Predictors of sudden death in idiopathic dilated cardiomyopathy. Am J Cardiol 1989; 63:138–140.

586. Maggioni AP, Zuanetti G, Franzosi MG, et al. Prevalence and prognostic significance of ventricular arrhythmias after acute myocardial infarction in the fibrinolytic era: GISSI-2 results. Circulation 1993; 87:312–322.

587. Herre JM, Sauve MJ, Malone P, et al. Long-term results of amiodarone therapy in patients with recurrent sustained ventricular tachycardia or ventricular fibrillation. J Am Coll Cardiol 1989; 13:442–449.

588. Adhar GC, Larson LW, Bardy GH, Greene HL. Sustained ventricular arrhythmias: differences between survivors of cardiac arrest and patients with recurrent sustained ventricular tachycardia. J Am Coll Cardiol 1988; 12:159–165.

589. Denniss AR, Ross DL, Richards DA, et al. Differences between patients with ventricular tachycardia and ventricular fibrillation as assessed by signal-averaged electrocardiogram, radionuclide ventriculography and cardiac mapping. J Am Coll Cardiol 1988; 11:276–283.

590. Dolack GL, Callahan DB, Bardy GH, Greene HL. Signal-averaged electrocardiographic late potentials in resuscitated survivors of out-of-hospital ventricular fibrillation. Am J Cardiol 1990; 65:1102–1104.

591. Raitt MH, Dolack GL, Kudenchuk PJ, Poole JE, Bardy GH. Ventricular arrhythmias detected after transvenous defibrillator implantation in patients with a clinical history of only ventricular fibrillation: implications for use of implantable defibrillator. Circulation 1995; 91:1996–2001.

592. Wiesfeld AC, Crijns HJ, Hillege HL, Tuininga YS, Lie KL. The clinical significance of coronary anatomy in post-infarct patients with late sustained ventricular tachycardia or ventricular fibrillation. Eur Heart J 1995; 16:818–824.

593. Reek S, Klein HU, Ideker RE. Can catheter ablation in cardiac arrest survivors prevent ventricular fibrillation recurrence? Pacing Clin Electrophysiol 1997; 20:1840–1859.

594. Martin GJ, Magid NM, Myers G, et al. Heart rate variability and sudden death secondary to coronary artery disease during ambulatory electrocardiographic monitoring. Am J Cardiol 1987; 60:86–89.

595. Bluzhas J, Lukshiene D, Shalpikiene B, Ragaishis J. Relation between ventricular arrhythmia and sudden cardiac death in patients with acute myocardial infarction: the predictors of ventricular fibrillation. J Am Coll Cardiol 1986; 8:69A–72A.

596. Leitch JW, Gillis AM, Wyse DG, et al. Reduction in defibrillator shocks with an implantable device combining antitachycardia pacing and shock therapy. J Am Coll Cardiol 1991; 18:145–151.

597. Hunt D, Baker G, Hamer A, Penington C, Duffield A, Sloman G. Predictors of reinfarction and sudden death in a high-risk group of acute myocardial infarction survivors. Lancet 1979;13:233–236.

598. Sheps DS, Conde CA, Mayorga-Cortes A, et al. Primary ventricular fibrillation: some unusual features. Chest 1977; 72:235–238.

599. Grimm W, Flores BF, Marchlinski FE. Symptoms and electrocardiographically documented rhythm preceding spontaneous shocks in patients with implantable cardioverter-defibrillator. Am J Cardiol 1993; 71:1415–1418.

600. Olshansky B. Is syncope the same thing as sudden death except that you wake up? J Cardiovasc Electrophysiol 1997; 8:1098–1101.

601. Middlekauff HR, Stevenson WG, Stevenson LW, Saxon LA. Syncope in advanced heart failure: high risk of sudden death regardless of origin of syncope. J Am Coll Cardiol 1993; 21:110–116.

602. Saxon LA, Uretz EF, Denes P. Significance of the clinical presentation in ventricular tachycardia/fibrillation. Am Heart J 1989; 118:695–701.

603. Daliento L, Turrini P, Nava A, et al. Arrhythmogenic right ventricular cardiomyopathy in young versus adult patients: similarities and differences. J Am Coll Cardiol 1995; 25:655–664.

604. Weaver WD, Cobb LA, Dennis D, Ray R, Hallstrom AP, Copass MK. Amplitude of ventricular fibrillation waveform and outcome after cardiac arrest. Ann Intern Med 1985; 102:53–55.

605. Goble AJ. Paroxysmal ventricular fibrillation with spontaneous reversion to sinus rhythm. Br Heart J 1965; 27:62–68.

606. Wood MA, Stambler BS, Damiano RJ, Greenway, P Ellenbogen KA. Lessons learned from data logging in a multicenter clinical trial using a late-generation implantable cardioverter-defibrillator: the Guardian ATP 4210 Multicenter Investigators Group. J Am Coll Cardiol 1994; 24:1692–1699.

607. Rozanski JJ, Castellanos A, Myerburg RJ. Ventricular ectopy and sudden death. Cardiovasc Clin 1980; 11:127–142.

608. Engel TR, Meister SG, Frankl WS. The "R-on-T" phenomenon: an update and critical review. Ann Intern Med 1978; 88:221–225.

609. Talbot S. Prognostic importance of ventricular extrasystoles in acute myocardial infarction. Postgrad Med J 1977; 53:69–74.

610. Lie JT. Histopathology of the conduction system in sudden death from coronary heart disease. Circulation 1975; 51:446–452.

611. Tye KH, Samant A, Desser DB, Benchimol A. R on T or R on P phenomenon? Relation to the genesis of ventricular tachycardia. Am J Cardiol 1979; 44:632–637.

612. Cobb LA, Werner JA. Antiarrhythmic therapy, ventricular premature depolarizations and sudden cardiac death: the tip of the iceberg. Circulation 1979; 59:864–865.

613. Yusuf S, Lopez R, Sleight P. Heart rate and ectopic prematurity in relation to sustained ventricular arrhythmias. Br Heart J 1980; 44:233–239.

614. Singh JP, Sleight P, Kardos A, Hart G. QT interval dynamics and heart rate variability preceding a case of cardiac arrest. Heart 1997; 77:375–377.

615. Viskin S, Lesh MD, Eldar M, et al. Mode of onset of malignant ventricular arrhythmias in idiopathic ventricular fibrillation. J Cardiovasc Electrophysiol 1997; 8:1115–1120.

616. Higham PD, Campbell RW. QT dispersion. Br Heart J 1994; 71:508–510.

617. Amlie JP. QT dispersion and sudden cardiac death. Eur Heart J 1997; 18:189–190.

618. Coumel P, Maison-Blanche P, Badilini F. Dispersion of ventricular repolarization. Reality? Illusion? Significance? Circulation 1998; 97:2491–2493.

619. Schwartz PJ, Wolf S. QT interval prolongation as predictor of sudden death in patients with myocardial infarction. Circulation 1978; 57:1074–1077.

620. Mobitz W. Uber den partiellen Herzblock. Z Klin Med 1928; 107:450.

621. Yi G, Guo XH, Reardon M, et al. Circadian variation of the QT interval in patients with sudden cardiac death after myocardial infarction. Am J Cardiol 1998; 81:950–956.

622. de Bruyne MC, Hoes AW, Kors JA, Hofman A, van Bemmel JH, Grobbee DE. QTc dispersion predicts cardiac mortality in the elderly: the Rotterdam study. Circulation 1998; 97:467–472.

623. Higham PD, Furniss SS, Campbell RW. QT dispersion and components of the QT interval in ischaemia and infarction. Br Heart J 1995; 73:32–36.

624. Pye M, Quinn AC, Cobbe SM. QT interval dispersion: a non-invasive marker of susceptibility to arrhythmia in patients with sustained ventricular arrhythmias? Br Heart J 1994; 71:511–514.

625. Manttari M, Oikarinen L, Manninen V, Viitasalo M. QT dispersion as a risk factor for sudden cardiac death and fatal myocardial infarction in a coronary risk population. Heart 1997; 78:268–272.

626. Tavernier R, Jordaens L, Haerynck F, Derycke E, Clement DL. Changes in the QT interval and its adaptation to rate,

assessed with continuous electrocardiographic recordings in
patients with ventricular fibrillation, as compared to normal
individuals without arrhythmias. Eur Heart J 1997;
18:994–999.

627. Nakagawa M, Saikawa T, Ito M. Progressive reduction of
heart rate variability with eventual sudden death in two
patients. Br Heart J 1994; 71:87–88.

628. Glancy JM, Garratt CJ, Woods KL, de Bono DP. QT
dispersion and mortality after myocardial infarction. Lancet
1995; 345:945–948.

629. Perkiomaki JS, Koistinen MJ, Yli-Mayry S, Huikuri HV.
Dispersion of QT interval in patients with and without
susceptibility to ventricular tachyarrhythmias after previous
myocardial infarction. J Am Coll Cardiol 1995; 26:174–179.

630. Perkiomaki JS, Huikuri HV, Koistinen JM, Makikallio T,
Castellanos A, Myerburg RJ. Heart rate variability and
dispersion of QT interval in patients with vulnerability to
ventricular tachycardia and ventricular fibrillation after
previous myocardial infarction. J Am Coll Cardiol 1997;
30:1331–1338.

631. Zabel M, Klingenheben T, Franz MR, Hohnloser SH.
Assessment of QT dispersion for prediction of mortality or
arrhythmic events after myocardial infarction: results of a
prospective, long-term follow-up study. Circulation 1998;
97:2543–2550.

632. Buja G, Miorelli M, Turrini P, Melacini P, Nava A.
Comparison of QT dispersion in hypertrophic
cardiomyopathy between patients with and without
ventricular arrhythmias and sudden death. Am J Cardiol
1993; 72:973–976.

633. Barr CS, Naas A, Freeman M, Lang CC, Struthers AD. QT
dispersion and sudden unexpected death in chronic heart
failure. Lancet 1994; 343:327–329.

634. Fu GS, Meissner A, Simon R. Repolarization dispersion and
sudden cardiac death in patients with impaired left
ventricular function. Eur Heart J 1997; 18:281–289.

635. Fei L, Goldman JH, Prasad K, et al. QT dispersion and RR
variations on 12-lead ECGS in patients with congestive heart
failure secondary to idiopathic dilated cardiomyopathy. Eur
Heart J 1996; 17:258–263.

636. Grimm W, Steder U, Menz V, Hoffman J, Maisch B. QT
dispersion and arrhythmic events in idiopathic dilated
cardiomyopathy. Am J Cardiol 1996; 78:458–461.

637. Peeters HAP, SippensGroenewegen A, Wever EFD, et al.
Electrocardiographic identification of abnormal ventricular
depolarization and repolarization in patients with idiopathic
ventricular fibrillation. J Am Coll Cardiol 1998;
31:1406–1413.

638. Yuan S, Blomstrom-Lundqvist C, Pehrson S, Pripp CM,
Wohlfart B, Olsson SB. Dispersion of repolarization
following double and triple programmed stimulation: a
clinical study using the monophasic action potential
recording technique. Eur Heart J 1996; 17:1080–1091.

639. Surawicz B, Fisch C. Cardiac alternans: diverse mechanisms
and clinical manifestations. J Am Coll Cardiol 1992;
20:483–499.

640. Rosenbaum DS, Albrecht P, Cohen RJ. Predicting sudden
cardiac death from T wave alternans of the surface
electrocardiogram: promise and pitfalls. J Cardiovasc
Electrophysiol 1996; 7:1095–1111.

641. Rosenbaum DS, Jackson LE, Smith JM, Garan H, Ruskin JN,
Cohen RJ. Electrical alternans and vulnerability to
ventricular arrhythmias. N Engl J Med 1994; 330:235–241.

642. Hohnloser SH, Klingenheben T, Zabel M, Li YG, Albrecht P,
Cohen RJ. T wave alternans during exercise and atrial
pacing in humans. J Cardiovasc Electrophysiol 1997;
8:987–993.

643. Verrier RL, Stone PH. Exercise stress testing for T wave
alternans to expose latent electrical instability. J Cardiovasc
Electrophysiol 1997; 8:994–997.

644. Fisch GR, Zipes DP, Fisch C. Bundle branch block and
sudden death. Prog Cardiovasc Dis 1980; 23:187–222.

645. Sakamoto T, Yamada T, Hiejima K. Ventricular fibrillation
induced by conducted sinus or supraventricular beat.
Circulation 1973; 48:438–442.

646. Bekheit S, Turitto G, Fontaine J, el-Sherif N. Initiation of
ventricular fibrillation by supraventricular beats in patients
with acute myocardial infarction. Br Heart J 1988;
59:190–195.

647. Berul CI, Hill SL, Geggel RL, et al. Electrocardiographic
markers of late sudden death risk in postoperative tetralogy
of Fallot children. J Cardiovasc Electrophysiol 1997;
8:1349–1356.

648. Haynes RE, Hallstrom AP, Cobb LA. Repolarization
abnormalities in survivors of out-of-hospital ventricular
fibrillation. Circulation 1978;57:654–658.

649. Armstrong WF, McHenry PL. Ambulatory
electrocardiographic monitoring: can we predict sudden
death? J Am Coll Cardiol 1985; 5:13B–16B.

650. Zehender M, Geibel A, Hohnloser S, Meinertz T, Just H.
Standardization of noninvasive and invasive studies in the
assessment of patients with ventricular arrhythmias. In
Brugada P, Wellens HJJ (eds). Cardiac Arrhythmias. Where
To Go From Here? Mount Kisco, NY: Futura Publishing Co.
1987, pp. 435–455.

651. Vismara LA, Amsterdam EA, Mason DT. Relation of
ventricular arrhythmias in the late hospital phase of acute
myocardial infarction to sudden death after hospital
discharge. Am J Med 1975; 59:6–12.

652. Campbell RWF, Julian DG. Incidence, prevalence and
significance of ventricular ectopic activity in acute
myocardial infarction. In Sandoe E, Julian DG, Bell JW
(eds). Management of Ventricular Tachycardia. Role of
Mexiletine. Amsterdam: Excerpta Medica, 1978, pp.
457–464.

653. Moller M. Reliability of serial 24 h ambulatory
electrocardiography in predicting cardiac death after
myocardial infarction. Eur Heart J 1982; 3:67–74.

654. Holmes J, Kubo SH, Cody RJ, Kligfield P. Arrhythmias in
ischemic and nonischemic dilated cardiomyopathy:
prediction of mortality by ambulatory electrocardiography.
Am J Cardiol 1985; 55:146–151.

655. Farrell TG, Bashir Y, Cripps T, et al. Risk stratification for
arrhythmic events in postinfarction patients based on heart
rate variability, ambulatory electrocardiographic variables
and the signal-averaged electrocardiogram. J Am Coll
Cardiol 1991; 18:687–697.

656. Steinberg JS, Regan A, Sciacca RR, Bigger JT Jr, Fleiss JL.
Predicting arrhythmic events after acute myocardial
infarction using the signal-averaged electrocardiogram. Am J
Cardiol 1992; 69:13–21.

657. McKenna WJ, England D, Doi YL, Deanfield JE, Oakley C,
Goodwin JF. Arrhythmia in hypertrophic cardiomyopathy. I.
Influence on prognosis. Br Heart J 1981; 46:168–172.

658. von Olshausen K, Schafer A, Mehmel HC, Schwarz F, Senges
J, Kubler W. Ventricular arrhythmias in idiopathic dilated
cardiomyopathy. Br Heart J 1984; 51:195–201.

659. Bach SM Jr, Lehmann MH, Kroll MW. Tachyarrhythmia
detection. In Kroll MW, Lehmann MH (eds). Implantable
Cardioverter-Defibrillator Therapy. The Engineering-Clinical
Interface. Norwell, MA: Kluwer Academic Publishers, 1996,
pp. 303–323.

660. Zaim S, Zaim B, Rottman J, Mendoza I, Nasir N Jr, Pacifico
A. Characterization of spontaneous recurrent ventricular
arrhythmias detected by electrogram-storing defibrillators in
sudden cardiac death survivors with no inducible ventricular
arrhythmias at baseline electrophysiologic testing. Am Heart
J 1996; 132:274–279.

661. Gomes JA, Winters SL, Ip J. Signal averaging of the surface
QRS complex: practical applications. J Cardiovasc
Electrophysiol 1991; 2:316–330.

662. Steinberg JS, Berbari EJ. The signal-averaged
electrocardiogram: update on clinical applications. J
Cardiovasc Electrophysiol 1996; 7:972–988.

663. Freedman RA, Gillis AM, Keren A, Soderholm-Difatte V,
Mason JW. Signal-averaged electrocardiographic late
potentials in patients with ventricular fibrillation or
ventricular tachycardia: correlation with clinical arrhythmia
and electrophysiologic study. Am J Cardiol 1985;
55:1350–1353.

664. Gomes JA, Winters SL, Stewart D, Horowitz S, Milner M, Barreca P. A new noninvasive index to predict sustained ventricular tachycardia and sudden death in the first year after myocardial infarction: based on signal-averaged electrocardiogram, radionuclide ejection fraction and Holter monitoring. J Am Coll Cardiol 1987; 10:349–357.

665. Lindsay BD, Ambos HD, Schechtman KB, Arthur RM, Cain ME. Noninvasive detection of patients with ischemic and nonischemic heart disease prone to ventricular fibrillation. J Am Coll Cardiol 1990; 16:1656–1664.

666. Malik M, Farrell T, Cripps T, Camm AJ. Heart rate variability in relation to prognosis after myocardial infarction: selection of optimal processing techniques. Eur Heart J 1989; 10:1060–1074.

667. Nalos PC, Pappas JM, Nyitray W, Ishimori T, DonMichael TA. Prospective community evaluation of the signal-averaged electrocardiogram in predicting malignant ventricular arrhythmias: beneficial outcome with electrophysiology guided therapy. Clin Cardiol 1991; 14:963–970.

668. Rosenthal ME, Hamer A, Gang ES, Oseran DS, Mandel WJ, Peter T. The yield of programmed ventricular stimulation in mitral valve prolapse patients with ventricular arrhythmias. Am Heart J 1985; 110:970–976.

669. Tobe TJ, de Langen CD, Crijns HJ, et al. Late potentials, QTc prolongation, and prediction of arrhythmic events after myocardial infarction. Int J Cardiol 1994; 46:121–128.

670. Lander P, Gomis P, Goyal R, et al. Analysis of abnormal intra-QRS potentials: improved predictive value for arrhythmic events with the signal-averaged electrocardiogram. Circulation 1997; 95:1386–1393.

671. Mercando AD, Aronow WS, Epstein S, Fishbach M. Signal-averaged electrocardiography and ventricular tachycardia as predictors of mortality after acute myocardial infarction in elderly patients. Am J Cardiol 1995; 76:436–440.

672. Aronow WS, Mercando AD, Epstein S. Usefulness of an abnormal signal-averaged electrocardiogram for predicting cardiac death in elderly persons without heart disease. Am J Cardiol 1995; 75:1273–1274.

673. Epstein AE, Dailey SM, Shepard RB, Kirk KA, Kay GN, Plumb VJ. Inability of the signal-averaged electrocardiogram to determine risk of arrhythmia recurrence in patients with implantable cardioverter defibrillators. PACE 1991; 14:1169–1178.

674. Zhang YZ, Wang SW, Hu DY, Zhu GY. Prediction of life-threatening arrhythmia in patients after myocardial infarction by late potentials, ejection fraction and Holter monitoring. Jpn Heart J 1992; 33:15–23.

675. Winters SL, Ip J, Deshmukh P, et al. Determinants of induction of ventricular tachycardia in nonsustained ventricular tachycardia after myocardial infarction and the usefulness of the signal-averaged electrocardiogram. Am J Cardiol 1993; 72:1281–1285.

676. Borggrefe M, Fetsch T, Martinez-Rubio A, Makijarvi M, Breithardt G. Prediction of arrhythmia risk based on signal-averaged ECG in postinfarction patients. PACE 1997; 20:2566–2576.

677. Hartikainen JEK, Malik M, Staunton A, Poloniecki J, Camm AJ. Distinction between arrhythmic and nonarrhythmic death after acute infarction based on heart rate variability, signal-averaged electrocardiogram, ventricular arrhythmias and left ventricular ejection fraction. J Am Coll Cardiol 1996; 28:296–304.

678. Faber TS, Staunton A, Hnatkova K, Camm AJ, Malik M. Stepwise strategy of using short- and long-term heart rate variability for risk stratification after myocardial infarction. Pacing Clin Electrophysiol 1996; 19:1845–1851.

679. Rodriguez LM, Krijne R, van den Dool A, Brugada P, Smeets J, Wellens HJJ. Time course and prognostic significance of serial signal-averaged electrocardiograms after a first acute myocardial infarction. Am J Cardiol 1990; 66:1199–1202.

680. Mancini DM, Wong KL, Simson MB. Prognostic value of an abnormal signal-averaged electrocardiogram in patients with nonischemic congestive cardiomyopathy. Circulation 1993; 87:1083–1092.

681. Ohnishi Y, Inoue T, Fukuzaki H. Value of the signal-averaged electrocardiogram as a predictor of sudden death in myocardial infarction and dilated cardiomyopathy. Jpn Circ J 1990; 54:127–136.

682. Middlekauff HR, Stevenson WG, Woo MA, Moser DK, Stevenson LW. Comparison of frequency of late potentials in idiopathic dilated cardiomyopathy and ischemic cardiomyopathy with advanced congestive heart failure and their usefulness in predicting sudden death. Am J Cardiol 1990; 66:1113–1117.

683. Cripps TR, Counihan PJ, Frenneaux MP, Ward DE, Camm AJ, McKenna WJ. Signal-averaged electrocardiography in hypertrophic cardiomyopathy. J Am Coll Cardiol 1990; 15:956–961.

684. Kulakowski P, Counihan PJ, Camm AJ, McKenna WJ. The value of time and frequency domain, and spectral temporal mapping analysis of the signal-averaged electrocardiogram in identification of patients with hypertrophic cardiomyopathy at increased risk of sudden death. Eur Heart J 1993; 14:941–950.

685. Chambers JW, Denes P, Dahl W, et al. Familial sudden death syndrome with an abnormal signal-averaged electrocardiogram as a potential marker. Am Heart J 1995; 130:318–323.

686. Singer DH, Martin GJ, Magid N, et al. Low heart rate variability and sudden cardiac death. J Electrocardiol 1988; 21:S46–S55.

687. van Ravenswaaij-Arts CMA, Kollee LAA, Hopman JCW, Stoelinga GBA, Geijn HP. Heart rate variability. Ann Intern Med 1993; 118:436–447.

688. Bigger JT Jr. Spectral analysis of R-R variability to evaluate autonomic physiology and pharmacology and to predict cardiovascular outcomes in humans. In Zipes DP, Jalife J (eds). Cardiac Electrophysiology. From Cell to Bedside. 2nd ed. Philadelphia: WB Saunders, 1995, pp. 1151–1170.

689. Huikuri HV, Linnaluoto MK, Seppanen T, et al. Circadian rhythm of heart rate variability in survivors of cardiac arrest. Am J Cardiol 1992; 70:610–615.

690. Dougherty AH, Jackman WM, Naccarelli GV, Friday KJ, Dias VC. Acute conversion of paroxysmal supraventricular tachycardia with intravenous diltiazem. IV. Diltiazem study group. Am J Cardiol 1992; 70:587–592.

691. Kleiger RE, Miller JP, Bigger JT Jr, Moss AJ. Decreased heart rate variability and its association with increased mortality after acute myocardial infarction. Am J Cardiol 1987; 59:256–262.

692. Cripps TR, Malik M, Farrell TG, Camm AJ. Prognostic value of reduced heart rate variability after myocardial infarction: clinical evaluation of a new analysis method. Br Heart J 1991; 65:14–19.

693. Odemuyiwa O, Malik M, Farrell T, et al. Multifactorial prediction of arrhythmic events after myocardial infarction: combination of heart rate variability and left ventricular ejection fraction with other variables. Pacing Clin Electrophysiol 1991; 14:1986–1991.

694. Bigger JT Jr, Fleiss JL, Steinman RC, Rolnitzky LM, Kleiger RE, Rottman JN. Frequency domain measures of heart period variability and mortality after myocardial infarction. Circulation 1992; 85:164–171.

695. Bigger JT Jr, Fleiss JL, Rolnitzky LM, Steinman RC. The ability of several short-term measures of RR variability to predict mortality after myocardial infarction. Circulation 1993; 88:927–934.

696. Hohnloser SH, Klingenheben T, van de Loo A, Hablawetz E, Just H, Schwartz PJ. Reflex versus tonic vagal activity as a prognostic parameter in patients with sustained ventricular tachycardia or ventricular fibrillation. Circulation 1994; 89:1068–1073.

697. De Ferrari GM, Landolina M, Mantica Mr, Manfredini R, Schwartz PJ, Lotto A. Baroreflex sensitivity, but not heart rate variability, is reduced in patients with life-threatening ventricular arrhythmias long after myocardial infarction. Am Heart J 1995; 130:473–480.

698. Pozzati A, Pancaldi LG, DiPasquale G, Pinelli G, Bugiardini R. Transient sympathovagal imbalance triggers "ischemic" sudden death in patients undergoing electrocardiographic Holter monitoring. J Am Coll Cardiol 1996; 27:847–852.

699. Hoffmann J, Grimm W, Menz V, Knop U, Maisch B. Heart rate variability and major arrhythmic events in patients with idiopathic dilated cardiomyopathy. PACE 1996; 19:1841–1844.

700. Odemuyiwa O, Malik M, Farrell T, Bashir Y, Poloniecki J, Camm J. Comparison of the predictive characteristics of heart rate variability index and left ventricular ejection fraction for all-cause mortality, arrhythmic events and sudden death after acute myocardial infarction. Am J Cardiol 1991; 68:434–439.

701. Vybiral T, Glaeser DH, Goldberger AL, et al. Conventional heart rate variability analysis of ambulatory electrocardiographic recordings fails to predict imminent ventricular fibrillation. J Am Coll Cardiol 1993; 22:557–565.

702. Weaver WD, Cobb LA, Hallstrom AP. Characteristics of survivors of exertion- and nonexertion-related cardiac arrest: value of subsequent exercise testing. Am J Cardiol 1982; 50:671–676.

703. Sharma AD, Yee R, Guiraudon G, Klein GJ. Sensitivity and specificity of invasive and noninvasive testing for risk of sudden death in Wolff-Parkinson-White syndrome. J Am Coll Cardiol 1987; 10:373–381.

704. Gaita F, Giustetto C, Riccardi R, Mangiardi L, Brusca A. Stress and pharmacologic tests as methods to identify patients with Wolff-Parkinson-White syndrome at risk of sudden death. Am J Cardiol 1989; 64:487–490.

705. Gardner MJ, Montague TJ, Armstrong CS, Horacek BM, Smith ER. Vulnerability to ventricular arrhythmia: assessment by mapping of body surface potential. Circulation 1986; 73:684–692.

706. Park WM, Amirhamzeh MM, Jia CX, et al. Systolic arterial pressure recovery after ventricular fibrillation/flutter in humans. Pacing Clin Electrophysiol 1994; 17:1100–1106.

707. Winkle RA, Mead RH, Ruder MA, Smith NA, Buch WS, Gaudiani VA. Effect of duration of ventricular fibrillation on defibrillation efficacy in humans. Circulation 1990; 81:1477–1481.

708. Ritchie JL, Hallstrom AP, Troubaugh GB, Caldwell JH, Cobb LA. Out-of-hospital sudden coronary death: rest and exercise radionuclide left ventricular function in survivors. Am J Cardiol 1985; 55:645–651.

709. Trappe HJ, Brugada P, Talajic M, et al. Prognosis of patients with ventricular tachycardia and ventricular fibrillation: role of the underlying etiology. J Am Coll Cardiol 1988; 12:166–174.

710. Szabo BM, Crijns HJGM, Wiesfeld ACP, van Veldhuisen DJ, Hillege HL, Lie KI. Predictors of mortality in patients with sustained ventricular tachycardias or ventricular fibrillation and depressed left ventricular function: importance of B-blockade. Am Heart J 1995; 130:281–286.

711. Josephson ME, Horowitz LN, Spielman SR, Greenspan AM. Electrophysiologic and hemodynamic studies in patients resuscitated from cardiac arrest. Am J Cardiol 1980; 46:948–955.

712. Furukawa T, Rozanski JJ, Nogami A, Moroe K, Gosselin AJ, Lister JW. Time-dependent risk of and predictors for cardiac arrest recurrence in survivors of out-of-hospital cardiac arrest with chronic coronary artery disease. Circulation 1989; 80:599–608.

713. De Maria R, Gavazzi A, Caroli A, Ometto R, Biagini A, Camerini F. Ventricular arrhythmias in dilated cardiomyopathy as an independent prognostic hallmark: Italian Multicenter Cardiomyopathy Study (SPIC) Group. Am J Cardiol 1992; 69:1451–1457.

714. Schulze RA, Jr, Strauss HW, Pitt B. Sudden death in the year following myocardial infarction: relation to ventricular premature contractions in the late hospital phase and left ventricular ejection fraction. Am J Med 1977; 62:192–199.

715. Ritchie JL, Hamilton GW, Trobaugh GB, Weaver WD, Williams DL, Cobb LA. Myocardial imaging and radionuclide angiography in survivors of sudden cardiac death due to ventricular fibrillation: preliminary report. Am J Cardiol 1977; 39:852–857.

716. Bigger JT Jr, Fleiss JL, Kleiger R, Miller JP, Rolnitzky LM, Multicenter Post-Infarction Research Group. The relationships among ventricular arrhythmias, left ventricular dysfunction, and mortality in the 2 years after myocardial infarction. Circulation 1984; 69:250–258.

717. Hung JS, Yeh SJ, Lin FC, Fu M, Lee YS, Wu D. Usefulness of intravenous diltiazem in predicting subsequent electrophysiologic and clinical responses to oral diltiazem. Am J Cardiol 1984; 54:1259–1262.

718. Levy D, Garrison RJ, Savage DD, Kannel WB, Castelli WP. Prognostic implications of echocardiographically determined left ventricular mass in the Framingham heart study. N Engl J Med 1990; 322:1561–1566.

719. De Piccoli B, Rigo F, Raviele A, et al. Transesophageal echocardiographic evaluation of the morphologic and hemodynamic cardiac changes during ventricular fibrillation. J Am Soc Echocardiogr 1996; 9:71–78.

720. Perera R, Steinberg JS, Ehlert F, Mogtader A, Hillel Z. Left atrial function is unchanged by implantable defibrillator shocks on hearts in sinus rhythm. Am J Cardiol 1998; 81:787–789.

721. Schwartz CJ, Walsh WJ. The pathologic basis of sudden death. Prog Cardiovasc Dis 1971; 13:465–481.

722. Davies MJ, Popple A. Sudden unexpected cardiac death: a practical approach to the forensic problem. Histopathology 1979; 3:255–277.

723. Rossi L, Thiene G. Recent advances in clinicohistopathologic correlates of sudden cardiac death. Am Heart J 1981; 102:478–484.

724. Davies MJ, Thomas AC. Plaque fissuring: the cause of acute myocardial infarction, sudden ischaemic death, and crescendo angina. Br Heart J 1985; 53:363–373.

725. Bharati S, Lev M. The conduction system findings in sudden cardiac death. J Cardiovasc Electrophysiol 1994; 5:356–366.

726. Rissanen V, Romo M, Siltanen P. Prehospital sudden death from ischaemic heart disease: a postmortem study. Br Heart J 1978; 40:1025–1033.

727. Baroldi G, Falzi G, Mariani F. Sudden coronary death: a postmortem study in 208 selected cases compared to 97 "control" subjects. Am Heart J 1979; 98:20–31.

728. Bashe WJ Jr, Baba N, Keller MD, Geer JC, Anthony JR. Pathology of atherosclerotic heart disease in sudden death. II. The significance of myocardial infarction. Circulation 1975; 52(Suppl III):III-63–III-77.

729. Schwartz CJ, Gerrity RG. Anatomical pathology of sudden unexpected cardiac death. Circulation 1975; 52(Suppl III):III-18–III-26.

730. Reichenbach DD, Moss NS, Meyer E. Pathology of the heart in sudden cardiac death. Am J Cardiol 1977; 39:865–872.

731. Newman WP III, Tracy RE, Strong JP, Johnson WD, Oalmann MC. Pathology on sudden coronary death. Ann N Y Acad Sci 1982; 382:39–49.

732. Friedman M, Manwaring JH, Rosenman RH, Donlon G, Ortego P, Grube SM. Instantaneous and sudden deaths: clinical and pathological differentiation in coronary artery disease. JAMA 1973; 225:1319–1328.

733. Kuller L, Cooper M, Perper J. Epidemiology of sudden death. Arch Intern Med 1972; 129:714–719.

734. Warnes CA, Roberts WC. Sudden coronary death: relation of amount and distribution of coronary narrowing at necropsy to previous symptoms of myocardial ischemia, left ventricular scarring and heart weight. Am J Cardiol 1984; 54:67–73.

735. Kragel AH, Gertz SD, Roberts WC. Morphologic comparison of frequency and types of acute lesions in the major epicardial coronary arteries in unstable angina pectoris, sudden coronary death and acute myocardial infarction. J Am Coll Cardiol 1991; 18:801–808.

736. Farb A, Tang AL, Burke AP, Sessums L, Liang Y, Virmani R. Sudden coronary death: frequency of active coronary lesions, inactive coronary lesions, and myocardial infarction. Circulation 1995; 92:1701–1709.

737. Lo YS, Cutler JE, Blake K, Wright AM, Kron J, Swerdlow CD. Angiographic coronary morphology in survivors of cardiac arrest. Am Heart J 1988; 115:781–785.

738. Roberts WC, Jones AA. Quantitation of coronary arterial narrowing at necropsy in sudden coronary death. Am J Cardiol 1979; 44:39–45.

739. Roberts WC, Buja LM. The frequency and significance of coronary arterial thrombi and other observations in fatal acute myocardial infarction: a study of 107 necropsy patients. Am J Med 1972; 52:425–443.

740. Haerem JW. Mural platelet microthrombi and major acute lesions of main epicardial arteries in sudden coronary death. Atherosclerosis 1974; 19:529–541.

741. Myers A, Dewar HA. Circumstances attending 100 sudden deaths from coronary artery disease with coroner's necropsies. Br Heart J 1975; 37:1133–1143.

742. Frink RJ, Trowbridge JO, Rooney PA Jr. Nonobstructive coronary thrombosis in sudden cardiac death. Am J Cardiol 1978; 42:48–51.

743. Davies MJ, Thomas A. Thrombosis and acute coronary-artery lesions in sudden cardiac ischemic death. N Engl J Med 1984; 310:1137–1140.

744. Crawford T, Dexter D, Teare RD. Coronary artery pathology in sudden death from myocardial ischaemia. Lancet 1961; 1:181–185.

745. Baba N, Bashe WJ Jr, Keller MD, Geer JC, Anthony JR. Pathology of atherosclerotic heart disease in sudden death. I. Organizing thrombosis and acute coronary vessel lesions. Circulation 1975; 52(Suppl III):III-53–III-59.

746. Morales AR, Romanelli R, Boucek RJ. The mural left anterior descending coronary artery, strenuous exercise and sudden death. Circulation 1980; 62:230–237.

747. James TN, Marshall TK. De subitaneis mortibus. XII. Asymmetrical hypertrophy of the heart. Circulation 1975; 51:1149–1166.

748. Chesler E, King RA, Edwards JE. The myxomatous mitral valve and sudden death. Circulation 1983; 67:632–639.

749. Bharati S, Lev M. Sudden death in athletes—conduction system: practical approach to dissection and pertinent pathology. Cardiovasc Pathol 1994; 3:117–127.

750. Green JR Jr, Korovetz MJ, Shanklin DR, DeVito JJ, Taylor WJ. Sudden unexpected death in three generations. Arch Intern Med 1969; 124:359–363.

751. James TN, Puech P. De subitaneis mortibus. IX. Type A Wolff-Parkinson-White syndrome. Circulation 1974;50:1264–1280.

752. James TN, Marilley RJ Jr, Marriott HJ. De subitaneis mortibus. XI. Young girl with palpitations. Circulation 1975; 51:743–748.

753. Bharati S, Granston AS, Liebson PR, Loeb HS, Rosen KM, Lev M. The conduction system in mitral valve prolapse syndrome with sudden death. Am Heart J 1981; 101:667–670.

754. Okada R, Kawai S. Histopathology of the conduction system in sudden cardiac death. Jpn Circ J 1983; 47:573–580.

755. Bharati S, Dreifus LS, Chopskie E, Lev M. Conduction system in a trained jogger with sudden death. Chest 1988; 93:348–351.

756. Bharati S, Lev M. Conduction system in sudden unexpected death a considerable time after repair of atrial septal defect. Chest 1988; 94:142–148.

757. Bharati S, Bauernfeind R, Miller LB, Strasberg B, Lev M. Sudden death in three teenagers: conduction system studies. J Am Coll Cardiol 1983; 1:879–886.

758. James TN, Froggatt P, Marshall TK. Sudden death in young athletes. Ann Intern Med 1967; 67:1013–1021.

759. Rossi L. Pathologic changes in the cardiac conduction and nervous system in sudden coronary death. Ann N Y Acad Sci 1982; 382:50–68.

760. James TN. Primary and secondary cardioneuropathies and their functional significance. J Am Coll Cardiol 1983; 2:983–1002.

761. Thiene G, Pennelli N, Rossi L. Cardiac conduction system abnormalities as a possible cause of sudden death in young athletes. Hum Pathol 1983; 14:704–709.

762. Roberts WC, Maron BJ. Sudden death while playing professional football. Am Heart J 1981; 102:1061–1066.

763. Bharati S, Olshansky B, Lev M. Pathological study of an explanted heart due to intractable ventricular fibrillation. J Cardiovasc Electrophysiol 1992; 3:437–441.

764. James TN, Beeson CW, II, Sherman EB, Mowry RW. Clinical conference: de subitaneis mortibus. XIII. Multifocal Purkinje cell tumors of the heart. Circulation 1975; 52:333–344.

765. Sugrue DD, Holmes DR, Gersh BJ, et al. Cardiac histologic findings in patients with life-threatening ventricular arrhythmias of unknown origin. J Am Coll Cardiol 1984; 4:952–957.

766. Wiesfeld ACP, Crijns HJGM, Van Dijk RB, et al. Potential role for endomyocardial biopsy in the clinical characterization of patients with idiopathic ventricular fibrillation: arrhythmogenic right ventricular dysplasia—an undervalued cause. Am Heart J 1994; 127:1421–1424.

767. Gotoh, K. A histopathological study on the conduction system of the so-called "Pokkuri disease" (sudden unexpected cardiac death of unknown origin in Japan). Jpn Circ 1976; 40:753–768.

768. Horowitz LN, Spielman SR, Greenspan SR, Josephson ME. Role of programmed stimulation in assessing vulnerability to ventricular arrhythmias. Am Heart J 1982; 103:604–610.

769. Horowitz LN, Spielman SR, Greenspan AM, Josephson ME. Mechanisms in the genesis of recurrent ventricular tachyarrhythmias as revealed by clinical electrophysiologic studies. Ann N Y Acad Sci 1982; 382:116–135.

770. Gottlieb C, Josephson ME. The preference of programmed stimulation-guided therapy for sustained ventricular arrhythmias. In Brugada P, Wellens IJJ (eds). Cardiac Arrhythmias. Where To Go From Here? Mount Kisco, NY: Futura Publishing Co., 1987, pp. 421–434.

771. Wellens HJJ, Brugada P, Stevenson WG. Programmed electrical stimulation of the heart in patients with life-threatening ventricular arrhythmias: what is the significance of induced arrhythmias and what is the correct stimulation protocol? Circulation 1985; 72:1–7.

772. Morady F, Shapiro W, Shen E, Sung RJ, Scheinman MM. Programmed ventricular stimulation in patients without spontaneous ventricular tachycardia. Am Heart J 1984; 107:875–882.

773. Mahmud R, Denker S, Lehmann MH, Tchou P, Dongas J, Akhtar M. Incidence and clinical significance of ventricular fibrillation induced with single and double ventricular extrastimuli. Am J Cardiol 1986; 58:75–79.

774. Turitto G, Fontaine JM, Ursell S, Caref EB, Bekheit S, el-Sherif N. Risk stratification and management of patients with organic heart disease and nonsustained ventricular tachycardia: role of programmed stimulation, left ventricular ejection fraction, and the signal-averaged electrocardiogram. Am J Med 1990; 88:35N–41N.

775. Martinez-Rubio A, Schwammenthal Y, Schwammenthal E, et al. Patients with valvular heart disease presenting with sustained ventricular tachyarrhythmias or syncope: results of programmed ventricular stimulation and long-term follow-up. Circulation 1997; 96:500–508.

776. Strasberg B, Kusniec J, Zlotikamien B, Mager A, Sclarovsky S. Long-term follow-up of postmyocardial infarction patients with ventricular tachycardia or ventricular fibrillation treated with amiodarone. Am J Cardiol 1990; 66:673–678.

777. Ruskin JN, DiMarco JP, Garan H. Out-of-hospital cardiac arrest: electrophysiologic observations and selection of long-term antiarrhythmic therapy. N Engl J Med 1980; 303:607–613.

778. Morady F, Sledge C, Shen E, Sung RJ, Gonzales R, Scheinman MM. Electrophysiologic testing in the management of patients with the Wolff-Parkinson-White syndrome and atrial fibrillation. Am J Cardiol 1983; 51:1623–1628.

779. Skale BT, Miles WM, Heger JJ, Zipes DP, Prystowsky EN. Survivors of cardiac arrest: prevention of recurrence by drug therapy as predicted by electrophysiologic testing or electrocardiographic monitoring. Am J Cardiol 1986; 57:113–119.

780. Eldar M, Sauve MJ, Scheinman MM. Electrophysiologic testing and follow-up of patients with aborted sudden death. J Am Coll Cardiol 1987; 10:291–298.

781. Swerdlow CD, Bardy GH, McAnulty J, et al. Determinants of induced sustained arrhythmias in survivors of out-of-hospital ventricular fibrillation. Circulation 1987; 76:1053–1060.

782. Freedman RA, Swerdlow CD, Soderholm-Difatte V, Mason JW. Prognostic significance of arrhythmia inducibility or noninducibility at initial electrophysiologic study in survivors of cardiac arrest. Am J Cardiol 1988; 61:578–582.

783. CASCADE investigators. Randomized antiarrhythmic drug therapy in survivors of cardiac arrest (the CASCADE study). Am J Cardiol 1993; 72:280–287.

784. Schoenfeld MH, McGovern B, Garan H, Kelly E, Grant G, Ruskin JN. Determinants of the outcome of electrophysiologic study in patients with ventricular tachyarrhythmias. J Am Coll Cardiol 1985; 6:298–306.

785. Kehoe R, Tommaso C, Zheutlin T, et al. Factors determining programmed stimulation responses and long-term arrhythmic outcome in survivors of ventricular fibrillation with ischemic heart disease. Am Heart J 1988; 116:355–363.

786. Roy D, Waxman HL, Kienzle MG, Buxton AE, Marchlinski FE, Josephson ME. Clinical characteristics and long-term follow-up in 119 survivors of cardiac arrest: relation to inducibility at electrophysiologic testing. Am J Cardiol 1983; 52:969–974.

787. Buxton AE, Waxman HL, Marchlinski FE, Untereker WJ, Waspe LE, Josephson ME. Role of triple extrastimuli during electrophysiologic study of patients with documented sustained ventricular tachyarrhythmias. Circulation 1984; 69:532–540.

788. Stevenson WG, Brugada P, Kersschot I, et al. Electrophysiologic characteristics of ventricular tachycardia or fibrillation in relation to age of myocardial infarction. Am J Cardiol 1986; 57:387–391.

789. Li HG, Klein GJ, Yee R, Thakur RK. Fatigue phenomenon in accessory pathways. J Cardiovasc Electrophysiol 1994; 5:818–823.

790. Adhar GC, Larson LW, Bardy GH, Greene HL. Sustained ventricular arrhythmias: differences between survivors of cardiac arrest and patients with recurrent sustained ventricular tachycardia. J Am Coll Cardiol 1988; 12:159–165.

791. Vaitkus PT, Kindwall KE, Miller JM, Marchlinski FE, Buxton AE, Josephson ME. Influence of gender on inducibility of ventricular arrhythmias in survivors of cardiac arrest with coronary artery disease. Am J Cardiol 1991; 67:537–539.

792. McLaran CJ, Gersh BJ, Sugrue DD, et al. Out-of-hospital cardiac arrest in patients without clinically significant coronary artery disease: comparison of clinical, electrophysiological, and survival characteristics with those in similar patients who have clinically significant coronary artery disease. Br Heart J 1987; 58:583–591.

793. Vorperian VR, Gittelsohn AM, Veltri EP. Predictors of inducible sustained ventricular tachyarrhythmias in patients with coronary artery disease. J Am Coll Cardiol 1989; 13:637–645.

794. Richards DA, Cody DV, Denniss AR, Russell PA, Young AA, Uther JB. Ventricular electrical instability: a predictor of death after myocardial infarction. Am J Cardiol 1983; 51:75–80.

795. Rodriguez LM, Sternick EB, Smeets JL, et al. Induction of ventricular fibrillation predicts sudden death in patients treated with amiodarone because of ventricular tachyarrhythmias after a myocardial infarction. Heart 1996; 75:23–28.

796. Das SK, Morady F, Dicarlo J LA Jr, Baerman J, DeBuitleir M, Crevey B. Prognostic usefulness of programmed ventricular stimulation in idiopathic dilated cardiomyopathy without symptomatic ventricular arrhythmias. Am J Cardiol 1986; 58:998–1000.

797. Rae AP, Spielman SR, Kutalek SP, Kay HR, Horowitz LN. Electrophysiologic assessment of antiarrhythmic drug efficacy for ventricular tachyarrhythmias associated with dilated cardiomyopathy. Am J Cardiol 1987; 59:291–295.

798. Chen X, Shenasa M, Borggrefe M, et al. Role of programmed ventricular stimulation in patients with idiopathic dilated cardiomyopathy and documented sustained ventricular tachyarrhythmias: inducibility and prognostic value in 102 patients. Eur Heart J 1994; 15:76–82.

799. Meinertz T, Treese N, Kasper W, et al. Determinants of prognosis in idiopathic dilated cardiomyopathy as determined by programmed electrical stimulation. Am J Cardiol 1985; 56:337–341.

800. Zhu DWX, Sun H, Hill R, Roberts R. The value of electrophysiology study and prophylactic implantation of cardioverter defibrillator in patients with hypertrophic cardiomyopathy. PACE 1998; 21:299–302.

801. Watson RM, Schwartz JL, Maron BJ, Tucker E, Rosing DR, Josephson ME. Inducible polymorphic ventricular tachycardia and ventricular fibrillation in a subgroup of patients with hypertrophic cardiomyopathy at high risk for sudden death. J Am Coll Cardiol 1987; 10:761–764.

802. Jansson K, Dahlstrom U, Karlsson E, Nylander E, Walfridsson H, Sonnhag C. The value of exercise test, Holter monitoring, and programmed electrical stimulation in detection of ventricular arrhythmias in patients with hypertrophic cardiomyopathy. Pacing Clin Electrophysiol 1990; 13:1261–1267.

803. Fananapazir L, Epstein SE. Hemodynamic and electrophysiologic evaluation of patients with hypertrophic cardiomyopathy surviving cardiac arrest. Am J Cardiol 1991; 67:280–287.

804. Saumarez RC, Camm AJ, Panagos A, et al. Ventricular fibrillation in hypertrophic cardiomyopathy is associated with increased fractionation of paced right ventricular electrograms. Circulation 1992; 86:467–474.

805. Saumarez RC. Electrophysiological investigation of patients with hypertrophic cardiomyopathy: evidence that slowed intraventricular conduction is associated with an increased risk of sudden death. Br Heart J 1994; 72:S19–S23.

806. Saumarez RC, Slade AK, Grace AA, Sadoul N, Camm AJ, McKenna WJ. The significance of paced electrogram fractionation in hypertrophic cardiomyopathy: a prospective study. Circulation 1995; 91:2762–2768.

807. Meissner MD, Lehmann MH, Steinman RT, et al. Ventricular fibrillation in patients without significant structural heart disease: a multicenter experience with implantable cardioverter-defibrillator therapy. J Am Coll Cardiol 1993; 21:1406–1412.

808. Kron J, Kudenchuk PJ, Murphy ES, et al. Ventricular fibrillation survivors in whom tachyarrhythmia cannot be induced: outcome related to selected therapy. Pacing Clin Electrophysiol 1987; 10:1291–1300.

809. Benson DW Jr, Dunnigan A, Benditt DG, Pritzker MR, Thompson TR. Transesophageal study of infant supraventricular tachycardia: electrophysiologic characteristics. Am J Cardiol 1983; 52:1002–1006.

810. Aizawa Y, Naitoh N, Washizuka T, et al. Electrophysiological findings in idiopathic recurrent ventricular fibrillation: special reference to mode of induction, drug testing, and long-term outcomes. Pacing Clin Electrophysiol 1996; 19:929–939.

811. Lemery R, Brugada P, Janssen J, Cheriex E, Dugernier T, Wellens HJJ. Nonischemic sustained ventricular tachycardia: clinical outcome in 12 patients with arrhythmogenic right ventricular dysplasia. J Am Coll Cardiol 1989; 14:96–105.

812. Saumarez RC, Heald S, Gill J, et al. Primary ventricular fibrillation is associated with increased paced right ventricular electrogram fractionation. Circulation 1995; 92:2565–2571.

813. Horowitz LN, Josephson ME, Kastor JA. Intracardiac electrophysiologic studies as a method for the optimization of drug therapy in chronic ventricular arrhythmia. Prog Cardiovasc Dis 1980; 23:81–98.

814. Benditt DG, Benson DW Jr, Klein GJ, Pritzker MR, Kriett JM, Anderson RW. Prevention of recurrent sudden cardiac arrest: role of provocative electropharmacologic testing. J Am Coll Cardiol 1983; 2:418–425.

815. Hamer A, Vohra J, Sloman G, Hunt D. Electrophysiologic studies in survivors of late cardiac arrest after myocardial infarction. Am Heart J 1983; 105:921–927.

816. Breithardt G, Borggrefe M, Seipel L. Selection of optimal drug treatment of ventricular tachycardia by programmed electrical stimulation of the heart. Ann N Y Acad Sci 1984; 427:49–66.

817. Anderson JL, Mason JW. Testing the efficacy of antiarrhythmic drugs. N Engl J Med 1986; 315:391–393.

818. Singh BN. Choice and chance in drug therapy of cardiac arrhythmias: technique versus drug-specific responses in evaluation of efficacy. Am J Cardiol 1993; 72:114F–124F.

819. Kuchar DL, Garan H, Venditti FJ, et al. Usefulness of sotalol in suppressing ventricular tachycardia or ventricular fibrillation in patients with healed myocardial infarcts. Am J Cardiol 1989; 64:33–36.

820. Poll DS, Marchlinski FE, Buxton AE, Josephson ME. Usefulness of programmed stimulation in idiopathic dilated cardiomyopathy. Am J Cardiol 1986; 58:992–997.

821. Huikuri HV, Cox M, Interian A, et al. Efficacy of intravenous propranolol for suppression of inducibility of ventricular tachyarrhythmias with different electrophysiologic characteristics in coronary artery disease. Am J Cardiol 1989; 64:1305–1309.

822. Poole JE, Mathisen TL, Kudenchuk PJ, et al. Long-term outcome in patients who survive out of hospital ventricular fibrillation and undergo electrophysiologic studies: evaluation by electrophysiologic subgroups. J Am Coll Cardiol 1990; 16:657–665.

823. Foster MT, Peters RW, Froman D, Shorofsky SR, Gold MR. Electrophysiologic effects and predictors of success of combination therapy with class Ia and Ib antiarrhythmic drugs for sustained ventricular arrhythmias. Am J Cardiol 1996; 78:47–50.

824. Spielman SR, Farshidi A, Horowitz LN, Josephson ME. Ventricular fibrillation during programmed ventricular stimulation: incidence and clinical implications. Am J Cardiol 1978; 42:913–918.

825. Martinez-Rubio A, Shenasa M, Borggrefe M, Chen X, Benning F, Breithardt G. Electrophysiologic variables characterizing the induction of ventricular tachycardia versus ventricular fibrillation after myocardial infarction: relation between ventricular late potentials and coupling intervals for the induction of sustained ventricular tachyarrhythmias. J Am Coll Cardiol 1993; 21:1624–1631.

826. DiCarlo LA Jr, Morady F, Schwartz AB, et al. Clinical significance of ventricular fibrillation-flutter induced by ventricular programmed stimulation. Am Heart J 1985; 109:959–963.

827. Brugada P, Abdollah H, Heddle B, Wellens HJJ. Results of a ventricular stimulation protocol using a maximum of 4 premature stimuli in patients without documented or suspected ventricular arrhythmias. Am J Cardiol 1983; 52:1214–1218.

828. Morady F, Scheinman MM. The role and limitations of electrophysiologic testing in patients with unexplained syncope. Int J Cardiol 1983; 4:229–234.

829. Brugada P, Green M, Abdollah H, Wellens HJJ. Significance of ventricular arrhythmias initiated by programmed ventricular stimulation: the importance of the type of ventricular arrhythmia induced and the number of premature stimuli required. Circulation 1984; 69:87–92.

830. Estes NAM III, Garan H, McGovern B, Ruskin JN. Influence of drive cycle length during programmed stimulation on induction of ventricular arrhythmias: analysis of 403 patients. Am J Cardiol 1986; 57:108–112.

831. Tonkin AM, Miller HC, Svenson RH, Wallace AG, Gallagher JJ. Refractory periods of the accessory pathway in the Wolff-Parkinson-White syndrome. Circulation 1975; 52:563–569.

832. Sellers TD Jr, Bashore TM, Gallagher JJ. Digitalis in the pre-excitation syndrome: analysis during atrial fibrillation. Circulation 1977; 56:260–267.

833. Klein GJ, Bashore TM, Sellers TD, Pritchett EL, Smith WM, Gallagher JJ. Ventricular fibrillation in the Wolff-Parkinson-White syndrome. N Engl J Med 1979; 301:1080–1085.

834. Gulamhusein S, Ko P, Carruthers SG, Klein GJ. Acceleration of the ventricular response during atrial fibrillation in the Wolff-Parkinson-White syndrome after verapamil. Circulation 1982; 65:348–354.

835. Critelli G, Grassi G, Perticone F, Coltorti F, Monda V, Condorelli M. Transesophageal pacing for prognostic evaluation of preexcitation syndrome and assessment of protective therapy. Am J Cardiol 1983; 51:513–518.

836. Critelli G, Gallagher JJ, Perticone F, Coltorti F, Monda V, Condorelli M. Evaluation of noninvasive tests for identifying patients with preexcitation syndrome at risk of rapid ventricular response. Am Heart J 1984; 108:905–909.

837. Meijler FL, van der Tweel I, Herbschleb JN, Hauer RN, Robles de Medina EO. Role of atrial fibrillation and atrioventricular conduction (including Wolff-Parkinson-White syndrome) in sudden death. J Am Coll Cardiol 1985; 5:17B–22B.

838. Waspe LE, Brodman R, Kim SG, Fisher JD. Susceptibility to atrial fibrillation and ventricular tachyarrhythmia in the Wolff-Parkinson-White syndrome: role of the accessory pathway. Am Heart J 1986; 112:1141–1152.

839. Stafford WJ, Trohman RG, Bilsker M, Zaman L, Castellanos A, Myerburg RJ. Cardiac arrest in an adolescent with atrial fibrillation and hypertrophic cardiomyopathy. J Am Coll Cardiol 1986; 7:701–704.

840. Milstein S, Sharma AD, Klein GJ. Electrophysiologic profile of asymptomatic Wolff-Parkinson-White pattern. Am J Cardiol 1986; 57:1097–1100.

841. Szabo TS, Klein GJ, Guiraudon GM, Yee R, Sharma AD. Localization of accessory pathways in the Wolff-Parkinson-White syndrome. Pacing Clin Electrophysiol 1989; 12:1691–1705.

842. Leitch JW, Klein GJ, Yee R, Murdock C. Prognostic value of electrophysiology testing in asymptomatic patients with Wolff-Parkinson-White pattern. Circulation 1990; 82:1718–1723.

843. Paul T, Guccione P, Garson A Jr. Relation of syncope in young patients with Wolff-Parkinson-White syndrome to rapid ventricular response during atrial fibrillation. Am J Cardiol 1990; 65:318–321.

844. Fukatani M, Tanigawa M, Mori M, et al. Prediction of a fatal atrial fibrillation in patients with asymptomatic Wolff-Parkinson-White pattern. Jpn Circ J 1990; 54:1331–1339.

845. Beckman KJ, Gallastegui JL, Bauman JL, Hariman RJ. The predictive value of electrophysiologic studies in untreated patients with Wolff-Parkinson-White syndrome. J Am Coll Cardiol 1990; 15:640–647.

846. Boahene KA, Klein GJ, Sharma AD, Yee, R, Fujimura O. Value of a revised procainamide test in the Wolff-Parkinson-White syndrome. Am J Cardiol 1990; 65:195–200.

847. Crosby LH, Pifalo WB, Woll KR, Burkholder JA. Risk factors for atrial fibrillation after coronary artery bypass grafting. Am J Cardiol 1990; 66:1520–1522.

848. Della Bella P, Brugada P, Talajic M, et al. Atrial fibrillation in patients with an accessory pathway: importance of the conduction properties of the accessory pathway. J Am Coll Cardiol 1991; 17:1352–1356.

849. Montoya PT, Brugada P, Smeets J, et al. Ventricular fibrillation in the Wolff-Parkinson-White syndrome. Eur Heart J 1991; 12:144–150.

850. Teo WS, Klein GJ, Guiraudon GM, Yee R, Leitch JW. Predictive accuracy of electrophysiologic localization of accessory pathways. J Am Coll Cardiol 1991; 18:527–531.

851. Vignati G, Mauri L, Lunati M, Gasparini M, Figini A. Transesophageal electrophysiological evaluation of paediatric patients with Wolff-Parkinson-White syndrome. Eur Heart J 1992; 13:220–222.

852. Brembilla-Perrot B, Dechaux JP. Ventricular fibrillation induced by transesophageal atrial pacing in asymptomatic Wolff-Parkinson-White syndrome. Am Heart J 1992; 123:536–537.

853. Brembilla-Perrot B, Ghawi R. Electrophysiological characteristics of asymptomatic Wolff-Parkinson-White syndrome. Eur Heart J 1993; 14:511–515.

854. Silka MJ, Kron J, Cutler JE, McAnulty JH. Analysis of programmed stimulation methods in the evaluation of ventricular arrhythmias in patients 20 years old and younger. Am J Cardiol 1990; 66:826–830.

855. Avitall B, McKinnie J. Jazayeri M, Akhtar M, Anderson AJ, Tchou P. Induction of ventricular fibrillation versus monomorphic ventricular tachycardia during programmed stimulation: role of premature beat conduction delay. Circulation 1992; 85:1271–1278.

856. Misier ARR, Opthof T, van Hemel NM, et al. Dispersion of

"refractoriness" in noninfarcted myocardium of patients with ventricular tachycardia or ventricular fibrillation after myocardial infarction. Circulation 1995; 91:2566–2572.

857. Kowey PR, Khuri S, Josa M, et al. Vulnerability to ventricular fibrillation in patients with clinically manifest ventricular tachycardia. Am Heart J 1984; 108:884–889.

858. Horowitz LN, Spear JF, Josephson ME, Kastor JA, Moore EN. The effects of coronary artery disease on the ventricular fibrillation threshold in man. Circulation 1979; 60:792–797.

859. Myerburg RJ, Kessler KM, Zaman L, Conde CA, Castellanos A. Survivors of prehospital cardiac arrest. JAMA 1982; 247:1485–1490.

860. Montgomery WH. The 1985 conference on standards and guidelines for cardiopulmonary resuscitation and emergency cardiac care. JAMA 1986; 255:2990–2991.

861. Brugada P, Lemery R, Talajic M, Della Bella P, Wellens HJJ. Treatment of patients with ventricular tachycardia or ventricular fibrillation: first lessons from the "parallel study." In Brugada P, Wellens HJJ (eds). Cardiac Arrhythmias. Where To Go From Here? Mount Kisco, NY: Futura Publishing Co., 1987, pp. 457–470.

862. Fisher JD, Mercando AD, Kim SG. Prospective criteria for the selection of therapy for ventricular tachycardia and ventricular fibrillation. In Brugada P, Wellens HJJ (eds). Cardiac Arrhythmias. Where To Go From Here? Mount Kisco, NY: Futura Publishing Co., 1987, pp. 471–482.

863. Fisher JD, Brodman RF, Kim SG, Ferrick KJ, Roth JA. VT/VF: 60/60 protection. PACE 1990; 13:218–222.

864. Cummins RO, Chamberlain DA, Abramson NS, et al. Recommended guidelines for uniform reporting of data from out-of-hospital cardiac arrest. Circulation 1991; 84:960–975.

865. Cummins RO, Ornato JP, Thies WH, Pepe PE. Improving survival from sudden cardiac arrest: the "chain of survival" concept. Circulation 1991; 83:1832.

866. Cobb LA, Weaver WD, Fahrenbruch CE, Hallstrom AP, Copass MK. Community-based interventions for sudden cardiac death: impact, limitations, and changes. Circulation 1992; 85(Suppl I):I-98–I-102.

867. Bocker D, Breithardt G, Block M, Borggrefe M. Management of patients with ventricular tachyarrhythmias: does an optimal therapy exist? PACE 1994; 17:559–570.

868. Eisenberg MS, Pantridge JF, Cobb LA, Geddes JS. The revolution and evolution of prehospital cardiac care. Arch Intern Med 1996; 156:1611–1619.

869. Johnston PW, Adgey AAJ. Out-of-hospital resuscitation: room for improvement. Heart 1996; 75:431–432.

870. Cummins RO, Sanders A, Mancini E, Hazinski MF. In-hospital resuscitation: a statement for healthcare professionals from the American Heart Association Emergency Cardiac Care Committee and the Advanced Cardiac Life Support, Basic Life Support, Pediatric Resuscitation, and Program Administration Subcommittees. Circulation 1997; 95:2211–2212.

871. Lurie KG, Lindner KH. Recent advances in cardiopulmonary resuscitation. J Cardiovasc Electrophysiol 1997; 8:584–600.

872. Lown B, Taylor J. "Thump-version." N Engl J Med 1970; 283:1223–1224.

873. Caldwell G, Millar G, Quinn E, Vincent R, Chamberlain DA. Simple mechanical methods for cardioversion: defence of the precordial thump and cough version. BMJ 1985; 291:627–630.

874. Weisfeldt ML, Chandra N. Physiology of cardiopulmonary resuscitation. Annu Rev Med 1981; 32:435–442.

875. Stiell IG, Hebert PC, Wells GA, et al. The Ontario trial of active compression-decompression cardiopulmonary resuscitation for in-hospital and prehospital cardiac arrest. JAMA 1996; 275:1417–1423.

876. Lown B, Crampton RS, DeSilva RA, Gascho J. Health-manpower needs. N Engl J Med 1978; 298:1252–1253.

877. Adgey AA, Patton JN, Campbell NP, Webb SW. Ventricular defibrillation: appropriate energy levels. Circulation 1979; 60:219–223.

878. DeSilva RA, Graboys TB, Podrid PJ, Lown B. Cardioversion and defibrillation. Am Heart J 1980; 100:881–895.

879. American College of Cardiology, American Heart Association Task Force on Assessment of Diagnostic and Therapeutic Cardiovascular Procedures. ACC/AHA guidelines for the early management of patients with acute myocardial infarction. Circulation 1990; 82:664, 671–672.

880. Kerber RE. External direct current cardioversion-defibrillation. In Zipes DP, Jalife J (eds). Cardiac Electrophysiology. From Cell to Bedside. 2nd ed. Philadelphia: WB Saunders, 1995, pp. 1360–1365.

881. Gascho JA, Crampton RS, Cherwek ML, Sipes JN, Hunter FP, O'Brien WM. Determinants of ventricular defibrillation in adults. Circulation 1979; 60:231–240.

882. Tacker WA Jr, Ewy GA. Emergency defibrillation dose: recommendations and rationale. Circulation 1979; 60:223–225.

883. Eysmann SB, Marchlinski FE, Buxton AE, Josephson ME. Electrocardiographic changes after cardioversion of ventricular arrhythmias. Circulation 1986; 73:73–81.

884. Gutgesell HP, Tacker WA, Geddes LA, Davis S, Lie JT, McNamara DG. Energy dose for ventricular defibrillation of children. Pediatrics 1976; 58:898–901.

885. Kuisma M, Maatta T. Out-of-hospital cardiac arrests in Helsinki: Utstein style reporting. Heart 1996; 76:18–23.

886. Enns J, Tweed WA, Donen N. Prehospital cardiac rhythm deterioration in a system providing only basic life support. Ann Emerg Med 1983; 12:478–481.

887. Fitzpatrick B, Watt GC, Tunstall-Pedoe H. Potential impact of emergency intervention on sudden deaths from coronary heart disease in Glasgow. Br Heart J 1992; 67:250–254.

888. Leslie WS, Fitzpatrick B, Morrison CE, Watt GC, Tunstall-Pedoe H. Out-of-hospital cardiac arrest due to coronary heart disease: a comparison of survival before and after the introduction of defibrillators in ambulances. Heart 1996; 75:195–199.

889. Pantridge JF, Adgey AA, Webb SW, Anderson J. Electrical requirements for ventricular defibrillation. BMJ 1975; 2:313–315.

890. Kerber RE, Sarnat W. Factors influencing the success of ventricular defibrillation in man. Circulation 1979; 60:226–230.

891. Kerber RE, Jensen SR, Gascho JA, Grayzel J, Hoyt R, Kennedy J. Determinants of defibrillation: prospective analysis of 183 patients. Am J Cardiol 1983; 52:739–745.

892. Dalzell GW, Adgey AA. Determinants of successful transthoracic defibrillation and outcome in ventricular fibrillation. Br Heart J 1991; 65:311–316.

893. Weaver WD, Fahrenbruch CE, Johnson DD, Hallstrom AP, Cobb LA, Copass MK. Effect of epinephrine and lidocaine therapy on outcome after cardiac arrest due to ventricular fibrillation. Circulation 1990; 82:2027–2034.

894. Cohen TJ, Scheinman MM, Pullen BT, et al. Emergency intracardiac defibrillation for refractory ventricular fibrillation during routine electrophysiologic study. J Am Coll Cardiol 1991; 18:1280–1284.

895. Cohen TJ. Innovative emergency defibrillation methods for refractory ventricular fibrillation in a variety of hospital settings. Am Heart J 1993; 126:962–968.

896. Cohen TJ, Chin MC, Oliver DG, Scheinman MM, Griffin JC. Transesophageal defibrillation: animal studies and preliminary clinical observations. PACE 1993; 16:1285–1292.

897. Cohen TJ, Scheinman MM, Pullen BT, et al. Emergency simultaneous transthoracic and epicardial defibrillation for refractory ventricular fibrillation during routine implantable cardioverter-defibrillator testing in the operating room. Am J Cardiol 1993; 71:619–622.

898. Kerber RE, Carter J, Klein S, Grayzel J, Kennedy J. Open chest defibrillation during cardiac surgery: energy and current requirements. Am J Cardiol 1980; 46:393–396.

899. Lake CL, Sellers TD, Nolan SP, Crosby IK, Wellons HA, Crampton RS. Low-energy defibrillation: safe and effective. Am J Emerg Med 1985; 3:104–107.

900. Robinson JS, Sloman G, Mathew TH, Goble AJ. Survival after resuscitation from cardiac arrest in acute myocardial infarction. Am Heart J 1965; 69:740–747.

901. Roth R, Stewart RD, Rogers K, Cannon GM. Out-of-hospital

cardiac arrest: factors associated with survival. Ann Emerg Med 1984; 13:237–243.

902. Lund I, Skulberg A. Cardiopulmonary resuscitation by lay people. Lancet 1976; 2:702–704.

903. Ventricular fibrillation outside hospital (editorial). Lancet 1979; 2:508–509.

904. Eisenberg MS, Copass MK, Hallstrom AP, et al. Treatment of out-of-hospital cardiac arrests with rapid defibrillation by emergency medical technicians. N Engl J Med 1980; 302:1379–1383.

905. Torp-Pedersen C, Birk Madsen E, Pedersen A. Sudden cardiac arrest outside the hospital: value of defibrillators in ambulances. Resuscitation 1991; 21:283–288.

906. Kowey PR. An overview of antiarrhythmic drug management of electrical storm. Can J Cardiol 1996; 12:3B–8B.

907. Ryan TJ, Anderson JL, Antman EM, et al. ACC/AHA guidelines for the management of patients with acute myocardial infarction. Circulation 1996; 94:2341–2350.

908. Koch-Weser J. Drug therapy. Bretylium. N Engl J Med 1979; 300:473–477.

909. Desai AD, Chun S, Sung RJ. The role of intravenous amiodarone in the management of cardiac arrhythmias. Ann Intern Med 1997; 127:294–303.

910. Schmidt A Konig W, Binner L, Mayer U, Stauch M. Efficacy and safety of intravenous amiodarone in acute refractory arrhythmias. Clin Cardiol 1988; 11:481–485.

911. Williams ML, Woelfel A, Cascio WE, Simpson RJ Jr, Gettes LS, Foster JR. Intravenous amiodarone during prolonged resuscitation from cardiac arrest. Ann Intern Med 1989; 110:839–842.

912. Helmy I, Herre JM, Gee G, et al. Use of intravenous amiodarone for emergency treatment of life-threatening ventricular arrhythmias. J Am Coll Cardiol 1988; 12:1015–1022.

913. Weinberg BA, Miles WM, Klein LS, et al. Five-year follow-up of 589 patients treated with amiodarone. Am Heart J 1993; 125:109–120.

914. Kowey PR, Levine JH, Herre JM, et al. Randomized, double-blind comparison of intravenous amiodarone and bretylium in the treatment of patients with recurrent, hemo-dynamically destabilizing ventricular tachycardia or fibrillation. Circulation 1995; 92:3255–3263.

915. Scheinman MM, Levine JH, Cannom DS, et al. Dose-ranging study of intravenous amiodarone in patients with life-threatening ventricular tachyarrhythmias. Circulation 1995; 92:3264–3272.

916. Levine JH, Massumi A, Scheinman MM, et al. Intravenous amiodarone for recurrent sustained hypotensive ventricular tachyarrhythmias. J Am Coll Cardiol 1996; 27:67–75.

917. Bacaner MB. Treatment of ventricular fibrillation and other acute arrhythmias with bretylium tosylate. Am J Cardiol 1968; 21:530–543.

918. Terry G, Vellani CW, Higgins MR, Doig A. Bretylium tosylate in treatment of refractory ventricular arrhythmias complicating myocardial infarction. Br Heart J 1970; 32:21–25.

919. Dhurandhar RW, Teasdale SJ, Mahon WA. Bretylium tosylate in the management of refractory ventricular fibrillation. Can Med Assoc J 1971; 105:161–166.

920. Bernstein JG, Koch-Weser J. Effectiveness of bretylium tosylate against refractory ventricular arrhythmias. Circulation 1972; 45:1024–1034.

921. Holder DA, Sniderman AD, Fraser G, Fallen EL. Experience with bretylium tosylate by a hospital cardiac arrest team. Circulation 1977; 55:541–544.

922. Heissenbuttel RH, Bigger JT Jr. Bretylium tosylate: a newly available antiarrhythmic drug for ventricular arrhythmias. Ann Intern Med 1979; 91:229–238.

923. Haynes RE, Chinn TL, Copass MK, Cobb LA. Comparison of bretylium tosylate and lidocaine in management of out of hospital ventricular fibrillation: a randomized clinical trial. Am J Cardiol 1981; 48:353–356.

924. Horowitz LN, Morganroth J. Can we prevent sudden cardiac death? Am J Cardiol 1982; 50:535–538.

925. Campbell RWF. Treatment and prophylaxis of ventricular arrhythmias in acute myocardial infarction. Am J Cardiol 1983; 52:55C–59C.

926. Cobb LA, Hallstrom AP, Weaver WD, Trobaugh GB, Greene HL. Considerations in the long-term management of survivors of cardiac arrest. Ann N Y Acad Sci 1984; 432:247–257.

927. Middlekauff HR, Stevenson WG, Tillisch JH. Prevention of sudden death in survivors of myocardial infarction: a decision analysis approach. Am Heart J 1992; 123:475–480.

928. Gilman JK, Jalal S, Naccarelli GV. Predicting and preventing sudden death from cardiac causes. Circulation 1994; 90:1083–1092.

929. Domanski MJ, Zipes DP, Schron E. Treatment of sudden cardiac death: current understandings from randomized trials and future research directions. Circulation 1997; 95:2694–2699.

930. Singh BN. Advantages of beta blockers versus antiarrhythmic agents and calcium antagonists in secondary prevention after myocardial infarction. Am J Cardiol 1990; 66:9C–20C.

931. Andresen D, Bruggemann T, Ehlers C, Behrens S. Management and prophylaxis of life-threatening arrhythmias: recent achievements. Eur Heart J 1995; 16:20–23.

932. Kim SG. Evolution of the management of malignant ventricular tachyarrhythmias: the roles of drug therapy and implantable defibrillators. Am Heart J 1995; 130:1144–1150.

933. Anderson J. Implantable defibrillators are preferable to pharmacologic therapy for patients with ventricular tachyarrhythmias: an antagonist's viewpoint. Prog Cardiovasc Dis 1996; 38:393–400.

934. Haverkamp W, Eckardt L, Borggrefe M, Breithardt G. Drugs versus devices in controlling ventricular tachycardia, ventricular fibrillation, and recurrent cardiac arrest. Am J Cardiol 1997; 80:67G–73G.

935. Landers MD, Reiter MJ. General principles of antiarrhythmic therapy for ventricular tachyarrhythmias. Am J Cardiol 1997; 80:31G–44G.

936. Reiffel JA. Prolonging survival by reducing arrhythmic death: pharmacologic therapy of ventricular tachycardia and fibrillation. Am J Cardiol 1997; 80:45G–55G.

937. Singh BN. Controlling cardiac arrhythmias: an overview with a historical perspective. Am J Cardiol 1997; 80:4G–15G.

938. Fisher JD, Kim SG, Waspe LE, Johnston DR. Amiodarone: value of programmed electrical stimulation and Holter monitoring. Pacing Clin Electrophysiol 1986; 9:422–435.

939. Mason JW. Amiodarone. N Engl J Med 1987; 316:455–466.

940. Nademanee K, Singh BN, Stevenson WG, Weiss JN. Amiodarone and post-MI patients. Circulation 1993; 88:764–774.

941. Julian DG. The amiodarone trials. Eur Heart J 1997; 18:1361–1362.

942. Kowey PR, Marinchak RA, Rials SJ, Filart RA. Intravenous amiodarone. J Am Coll Cardiol 1997; 29:1190–1198.

943. Heger JJ, Prystowsky EN, Jackman WM, et al. Clinical efficacy and electrophysiology during long-term therapy for recurrent ventricular tachycardia or ventricular fibrillation. N Engl J Med 1981; 305:539–544.

944. Nademanee K, Hendrickson J, Kannan R, Singh BN. Antiarrhythmic efficacy and electrophysiologic actions of amiodarone in patients with life-threatening ventricular arrhythmias: potent suppression of spontaneously occurring tachyarrhythmias versus inconsistent abolition of induced ventricular tachycardia. Am Heart J 1982; 103:950–959.

945. Greene HL, Graham EL, Werner JA, et al. Toxic and therapeutic effects of amiodarone in the treatment of cardiac arrhythmias. J Am Coll Cardiol 1983; 2:1114–1128.

946. Morady F, Scheinman MM, Hess DS. Amiodarone in the management of patients with ventricular tachycardia and ventricular fibrillation. Pacing Clin Electrophysiol 1983; 6:609–615.

947. Heger JJ, Prystowsky EN, Zipes DP. Clinical efficacy of amiodarone in treatment of recurrent ventricular tachycardia and ventricular fibrillation. Am Heart J 1983; 106:887–894.

948. Fogoros RN, Anderson KP, Winkle RA, Swerdlow CD, Mason

ventricular fibrillation during acute myocardial infarction by intravenous propranolol. Lancet 1984; 2:883–886.

987. Miami Trial Research Group. Metoprolol in acute myocardial infarction (MIAMI): a randomised placebo-controlled international trial. Eur Heart J 1985; 6:199–226.

988. Wennevold A, Sandoe E. Paroxysmal ventricular fibrillation in children: long-term follow-up of three cases treated with β-blocking agents. Acta Med Scand 1977; 202:425–427.

989. von Bernuth G, Bernsau U, Gutheil H, et al. Tachyarrhythmic syncopes in children with structurally normal hearts with and without QT-prolongation in the electrocardiogram. Eur J Pediatr 1982; 138:206–210.

990. Hansteen V. Beta blockade after myocardial infarction: the Norwegian propranolol study in high-risk patients. Circulation 1983; 67(Suppl I):I-57–I-60.

991. Olsson G, Ryden L. Prevention of sudden death using beta-blockers: review of possible contributory actions. Circulation 1991; 84(Suppl V):V-133–V-137.

992. Hallstrom AP, Cobb LA, Yu BH, Weaver WD, Fahrenbruch CE. An antiarrhythmic drug experience in 941 patients resuscitated from an initial cardiac arrest between 1970 and 1985. Am J Cardiol 1991; 68:1025–1031.

993. Kennedy HL, Brooks MM, Barker AH, et al. Beta-blocker therapy in the Cardiac Arrhythmia Suppression Trial: CAST investigators. Am J Cardiol 1994; 74:674–680.

994. Leclercq JF, Leenhardt A, Coumel P, Slama R. Efficacy of beta-blocking agents in reducing the number of shocks in patients implanted with first-generation automatic defibrillators. Eur Heart J 1992; 13:1180–1184.

995. Mogensen L. Ventricular tachyarrhythmias and lignocaine prophylaxis in acute myocardial infarction. Acta Med Scand 1970; 513:1–89.

996. Borak J, Veilleux S. Prophylactic lidocaine: uncertain benefits in emergency settings. Ann Emerg Med 1982; 11:493–496.

997. Singh BN. Routine prophylactic lidocaine administration in acute myocardial infarction: an idea whose time is all but gone? Circulation 1992; 86:1033–1035.

998. Hennekens CH, Albert CM, Godfried SL, Gaziano JM, Buring JE. Adjunctive drug therapy of acute myocardial infarction: evidence from clinical trials. N Engl J Med 1996; 335:1660–1667.

999. Pitt A, Lipp H, Anderson ST. Lignocaine given prophylactically to patients with acute myocardial infarction. Lancet 1971; 1:612–616.

1000. Lie KI, Wellens, HJJ, van Capelle FJ, Durrer D. Lidocaine in the prevention of primary ventricular fibrillation: a double-blind, randomized study of 212 consecutive patients. N Engl J Med 1974; 291:1324–1326.

1001. Wyman MG, Hammersmith L. Comprehensive treatment plan for the prevention of primary ventricular fibrillation in acute myocardial infarction. Am J Cardiol 1974; 33:661–667.

1002. Valentine PA, Frew JL, Mashford ML, Sloman JG. Lidocaine in the prevention of sudden death in the pre-hospital phase of acute infarction: a double-blind study. N Engl J Med 1974; 291:1327–1331.

1003. Wennerblom B, Holmberg S, Wedel H. The effect of a mobile coronary care unit on mortality in patients with acute myocardial infarction or cardiac arrest outside hospital. Eur Heart J 1982; 3:504–515.

1004. Wennerblom B, Holmberg S, Ryden L, Wedel H. Antiarrhythmic efficacy and side-effects of lidocaine given in the prehospital phase of acute myocardial infarction. Eur Heart J 1982; 3:516–524.

1005. Lie KI. Pre- and in-hospital antiarrhythmic prevention of ventricular fibrillation complicating acute myocardial infarction. Eur Heart J 1984; 5:B95–B97.

1006. Koster RW, Dunning AJ. Intramuscular lidocaine for prevention of lethal arrhythmias in the prehospitalization phase of acute myocardial infarction. N Engl J Med 1985; 313:1105–1110.

1007. MacMahon S, Collins R, Peto R, Koster RW, Yusuf S. Effects of prophylactic lidocaine in suspected acute myocardial infarction: an overview of results from the randomized, controlled trials. JAMA 1988; 260:1910–1916.

1008. Harrison DC. Arrhythmia prophylaxis after acute myocardial infarction: a decade of controversy. Cardiovasc Drugs Ther 1989; 2:783–789.

1009. Berntsen RF, Rasmussen K. Lidocaine to prevent ventricular fibrillation in the prehospital phase of suspected acute myocardial infarction: the north-Norwegian lidocaine intervention trial. Am Heart J 1992; 124:1478–1483.

1010. Bertini G, Giglioli C, Rostagno C, et al. Early out-of-hospital lidocaine administration decreases the incidence of primary ventricular fibrillation in acute myocardial infarction. J Emerg Med 1993; 11:667–672.

1011. Lofmark R, Orinius E. Restricted lignocaine prophylaxis in acute myocardial infarction. Acta Med Scand 1977; 201:89–91.

1012. Zehender M, Kasper W, Just H. Lidocaine in the early phase of acute myocardial infarction: the controversy over prophylactic or selective use. Clinical Cardiol 1990; 13:534–539.

1013. Harrison DC. Should lidocaine be administered routinely to all patients after acute myocardial infarction? Circulation 1978; 58:581–584.

1014. Bleifeld W, Merx KW, Heinrich KW, Effert S. Controlled trial of prophylactic treatment with lidocaine in acute myocardial infarction. Eur J Clin Pharmacol 1973; 6:119–126.

1015. Pfeifer HJ, Greenblatt DJ, Koch-Weser J. Clinical use and toxicity of intravenous lidocaine: a report from the Boston Collaborative Drug Surveillance Program. Am Heart J 1976; 92:168–173.

1016. Lown B. Lidocaine to prevent ventricular fibrillation: easy does it. N Engl J Med 1985; 313:1154–1156.

1017. Rademaker AW, Kellen J, Tam YK, Wyse DG. Character of adverse effects of prophylactic lidocaine in the coronary care unit. Clin Pharmacol Ther 1986; 40:71–80.

1018. Wyse DG, Kellen J, Rademaker AW. Prophylactic versus selective lidocaine for early ventricular arrhythmias of myocardial infarction. J Am Coll Cardiol 1988; 12:507–513.

1019. Dunn HM, McComb JM, Kinney CD, et al. Prophylactic lidocaine in the early phase of suspected myocardial infarction. Am Heart J 1985; 110:353–362.

1020. Pharand C, Kluger J, O'Rangers E, Ujhelyi M, Fisher J, Chow M. Lidocaine prophylaxis for fatal ventricular arrhythmias after acute myocardial infarction. Clin Pharmacol Ther 1995; 57:471–478.

1021. Crampton RS, Oriscello RG. Petit and grand mal convulsions during lidocaine hydrochloride treatment of ventricular tachycardia. JAMA 1968; 204:201–204.

1022. Hine LK, Laird N, Hewitt P, Chalmers TC. Meta-analytic evidence against prophylactic use of lidocaine in acute myocardial infarction. Arch Intern Med 1989: 149:2694–2698.

1023. Carruth JE, Silverman ME. Ventricular fibrillation complicating acute myocardial infarction: reasons against the routine use of lidocaine. Am Heart J 1982; 104:545–550.

1024. King FG, Addetia AM, Peters SD, Peachey GO. Prophylactic lidocaine for postoperative coronary artery bypass patients, a double-blind, randomized trial. Can J Anaesth 1990; 37:363–368.

1025. Fall SM, Burton NA, Graeber GM, et al. Prevention of ventricular fibrillation after myocardial revascularization. Ann Thorac Surg 1987; 43:182–184.

1026. Gonzalez R, Scheinman MM, Herre JM, Griffin JC, Sauve MJ, Sharkey H. Usefulness of sotalol for drug-refractory malignant ventricular arrhythmias. J Am Coll Cardiol 1988; 12:1568–1572.

1027. Aliot E, Sadoul N, de Chillou C. Effects of sotalol and *d*-sotalol on ventricular tachycardia and fibrillation induced by programmed electrical stimulation. Eur Heart J 1993; 14:H74–H77.

1028. Campbell RW, Furniss SS. Practical considerations in the use of sotalol for ventricular tachycardia and ventricular fibrillation. Am J Cardiol 1993; 72:80A–85A.

1029. Ruffy R. Sotalol. J Cardiovasc Electrophysiol 1993; 4:89–98.

1030. Hohnloser SH, Woosley RL. Sotalol. N Engl J Med 1994; 331:31–38.

JW. Amiodarone: clinical efficacy and toxicity in 96 patients with recurrent, drug-refractory arrhythmias. Circulation 1983; 68:88–94.

949. Raviele A, Di Pede F, Delise P, Piccolo E. Value of serial electropharmacological testing in managing patients resuscitated from cardiac arrest. Pacing Clin Electrophysiol 1984; 7:850–860.

950. Leak D. Intravenous amiodarone in the treatment of refractory life-threatening cardiac arrhythmias in the critically ill patient. Am Heart J 1986; 111:456–462.

951. Lavery D, Saksena S. Management of refractory sustained ventricular tachycardia with amiodarone: a reappraisal. Am Heart J 1987; 113:49–56.

952. Schmitt C, Brachmann J, Waldecker B, Rizos I, Senges J, Kubler W. Amiodarone in patients with recurrent sustained ventricular tachyarrhythmias: results of programmed electrical stimulation and long-term clinical outcome in chronic treatment. Am Heart J 1987; 114:279–283.

953. Ochi RP, Goldenberg IF, Almquist A, et al. Intravenous amiodarone for the rapid treatment of life-threatening ventricular arrhythmias in critically ill patients with coronary artery disease. Am J Cardiol 1989; 64:599–603.

954. Myers M, Peter T, Weiss D, et al. Benefit and risks of long-term amiodarone therapy for sustained ventricular tachycardia/fibrillation: minimum of three-year follow-up in 145 patients. Am Heart J 1990; 119:8–14.

955. Kowey PR, Marinchak RA, Rials SJ, Rubin AM, Smith L. Electrophysiologic testing in patients who respond acutely to intravenous amiodarone for incessant ventricular tachyarrhythmias. Am Heart J 1993; 125:1628–1632.

956. Young GD, Kerr CR, Mohama R, Boone J, Yeung-Lai-Wah JA. Efficacy of sotalol guided by programmed electrical stimulation for sustained ventricular arrhythmias secondary to coronary artery disease. Am J Cardiol 1994; 73:677–682.

957. Schmitt C, Miller JM, Josephson ME. Atrioventricular nodal supraventricular tachycardia with 2:1 block above the bundle of His. Pacing Clin Electrophysiol 1988; 11:1018–1023.

958. Schutzenberger W, Leisch F, Kerschner K, Harringer W, Herbinger W. Clinical efficacy of intravenous amiodarone in the short term treatment of recurrent sustained ventricular tachycardia and ventricular fibrillation. Br Heart J 1989; 62:367–371.

959. Russo AM, Beauregard LM, Waxman HL. Oral amiodarone loading for the rapid treatment of frequent, refractory, sustained ventricular arrhythmias associated with coronary artery disease. Am J Cardiol 1993; 72:1395–1399.

960. Sim I, McDonald KM, Lavori PW, Norbutas CM, Hlatky MA. Quantitative overview of randomized trials of amiodarone to prevent sudden cardiac death. Circulation 1997; 96:2823–2829.

961. Morady F, Scheinman MM, Hess DS, Sung RJ, Shen E, Shapiro W. Electrophysiologic testing in the management of survivors of out-of-hospital cardiac arrest. Am J Cardiol 1983; 51:85–89.

962. Peter T, Hamer A, Weiss D, Mandel WJ. Prognosis after sudden cardiac death without associated myocardial infarction: one year follow-up of empiric therapy with amiodarone. Am Heart J 1984; 107:209–213.

963. McGovern B, Garan H, Malacoff RF, et al. Long-term clinical outcome of ventricular tachycardia of fibrillation treated with amiodarone. Am J Cardiol 1984; 53:1558–1563.

964. Steinbeck G, Greene HL. Management of patients with life-threatening sustained ventricular tachyarrhythmias: the role of guided antiarrhythmic drug therapy. Prog Cardiovasc Dis 1996; 38:419–428.

965. Greene HL. The CASCADE study: randomized antiarrhythmic drug therapy in survivors of cardiac arrest in Seattle: CASCADE investigators. Am J Cardiol 1993; 72:70F–74F.

966. Olson PJ, Woelfel A, Simpson RJ Jr, Foster JR. Stratification of sudden death risk in patients receiving long-term amiodarone treatment for sustained ventricular tachycardia or ventricular fibrillation. Am J Cardiol 1993; 71:823–826.

967. Doval HC, Nul DR, Grancelli HO, Perrone SV, Bortman GR, Curiel R. Randomised trial of low-dose amiodarone in severe congestive heart failure: Grupo de Estudio de la Sobre[v] en la Insuficiencia Cardiaca en Argentina (GESICA). L[ ] 1994; 344:493–498.

968. Singh SN, Fletcher RD, Fisher SG, et al. Amiodarone i[n] patients with congestive heart failure and asymptomatic ventricular arrhythmia: survival trial of antiarrhythmic therapy in congestive heart failure. N Engl J Med 1995; 333:77–82.

969. Burkart F, Pfisterer M, Kiowski W, Follath F, Burckhard[t] Effect of antiarrhythmic therapy on mortality in survivo[r] myocardial infarction with asymptomatic complex ventr[ ] arrhythmias: Basel Antiarrhythmic Study of Infarct Surv[ ] (BASIS). J Am Coll Cardiol 1990; 16:1711–1718.

970. Ceremuzynski L, Kleczar E, Krzeminska-Pakula M, et al. Effect of amiodarone on mortality after myocardial infarction: a double-blind, placebo-controlled, pilot stud[y] Am Coll Cardiol 1992; 20:1056–1062.

971. Pfisterer ME, Kiowski W, Brunner H, Burckhardt D, Bu[ ] F. Long-term benefit of 1-year amiodarone treatment fo[r] persistent complex ventricular arrhythmias after myocar[ ] infarction. Circulation 1993; 87:309–311.

972. Pfisterer M, Kiowski W, Burckhardt D, Follath F, Burkar[t] Beneficial effect of amiodarone on cardiac mortality in patients with asymptomatic complex ventricular arrhyth[ ] after acute myocardial infarction and preserved but not impaired left ventricular function. Am J Cardiol 1992; 69:1399–1402.

973. Schwartz PJ, Camm AJ, Frangin G, Janse MJ, Julian DG, Simon P. Does amiodarone reduce sudden death and cardiac mortality after myocardial infarction? The Europ[ ] Myocardial Infarct Amiodarone Trial (EMIAT). Eur Hea[ ] 1994; 15:620–624.

974. Julian DG, Camm AJ Frangin G, et al. Randomised trial effect of amiodarone on mortality in patients with left-ventricular dysfunction after recent myocardial infarctio[n] EMIAT: European Myocardial Infarct Amiodarone Trial Investigators. Lancet 1997; 349:667–674.

975. Cairns JA, Connolly SJ, Roberts R, Gent M. Randomise[d] of outcome after myocardial infarction in patients with frequent or repetitive ventricular premature depolarisati[ ] CAMIAT: Canadian Amiodarone Myocardial Infarction Arrhythmia Trial Investigators. Lancet 1997; 349:675–68[ ]

976. Anonymous. Randomized antiarrhythmic drug therapy i[n] survivors of cardiac arrest (the CASCADE study): the CASCADE investigators. Am J Cardiol 1993; 72:280–287.

977. Lyon LJ, Donoso E, Friedberg CK. Temporary control of ventricular arrhythmias by drug-induced sinus tachycardi[a] Arch Intern Med 1969; 123:436–438.

978. Depelchin P, Sobolski J, Jottrand M, Flament C. Seconda[ry] prevention after myocardial infarction: effects of beta blocking agents and calcium antagonists. Cardiovasc Dru[g] Ther 1988; 2:139–148.

979. Held PH, Yusuf S. Effects of beta-blockers and calcium channel blockers in acute myocardial infarction. Eur Hea[ ] 1993; 14:18–25.

980. Coumel P, Escoubet B, Attuel P. Beta-blocking therapy in atrial and ventricular tachyarrhythmias: experience with nadolol. Am Heart J 1984; 108:1098–1108.

981. Hjalmarson A. Empiric therapy with beta-blockers. Pacing Clin Electrophysiol 1994; 17:460–466.

982. Kendall MJ, Lynch KP, Hjalmarson A, Kjekshus J. β-blocke[r] and sudden cardiac death. Ann Intern Med 1995; 123:358–367.

983. Wiesfeld ACP, Crijns JGM, Tuininga YS, Lie KI. Beta adrenergic blockade in the treatment of sustained ventricular tachycardia or ventricular fibrillation. PACE 19[ ] 19:1026–1035.

984. Ryden L, Ariniego R, Arnman K, et al. A double-blind tria[l] of metoprolol in acute myocardial infarction. N Engl J Me[d] 1983; 308:614–618.

985. Rossi PRF, Yusuf S, Ramsdale D, Furze L, Sleight P. Reduction of ventricular arrhythmias by early intravenous atenolol in suspected acute myocardial infarction. BMJ 198[ ] 286:506–510.

986. Norris RM, Barnaby PF, Brown MA, et al. Prevention of

1031. Winters SL, Curwin JH. Sotalol and the management of ventricular arrhythmias: implications of ESVEM. PACE 1995; 18:377–378.

1032. Claudel JP, Touboul P. Sotalol: from "Just another beta blocker" to "the prototype of class III antidysrhythmic compound." PACE 1995; 18:451–467.

1033. Steinbeck G, Bach P, Haberl R. Electrophysiologic and antiarrhythmic efficacy of oral sotalol for sustained ventricular tachyarrhythmias: evaluation by programmed stimulation and ambulatory electrocardiogram. J Am Coll Cardiol 1986; 8:949–958.

1034. Amiodarone vs Sotalol Study Group. Multicentre randomized trial of sotalol vs amiodarone for chronic malignant ventricular tachyarrhythmias. Eur Heart J 1989; 10:685–694.

1035. Klein RC. Comparative efficacy of sotalol and class I antiarrhythmic agents in patients with ventricular tachycardia or fibrillation: results of the Electrophysiology Study Versus Electrocardiographic Monitoring (ESVEM) Trial. Eur Heart J 1993; 14:78–84.

1036. Mason JW. Implications of the ESVEM trial for use of antiarrhythmic drugs that prolong cardiac repolarization. Am J Cardiol 1993; 72:59F–61F.

1037. Mason JW. A comparison of seven antiarrhythmic drugs in patients with ventricular tachyarrhythmias: electrophysiologic study versus electrocardiographic monitoring investigators. N Engl J Med 1993; 329:452–458.

1038. Lazzara R. Results of Holter ECG guided therapy for ventricular arrhythmias: the ESVEM trial. PACE 1994; 17:473–477.

1039. Bocker D, Haverkamp W, Block M, Borggrefe M, Hammel D, Breithardt G. Comparison of d,l-sotalol and implantable defibrillators for treatment of sustained ventricular tachycardia or fibrillation in patients with coronary artery disease. Circulation 1996; 94:151–157.

1040. Young GD, Kerr CR, Mohama R, Boone J, Yeung-Lai-Wah JA. Efficacy of sotalol guided by programmed electrical stimulation for sustained ventricular arrhythmias secondary to coronary artery disease. Am J Cardiol 1994; 73:677–682.

1041. Nademanee K, Singh BN. Effects of sotalol on ventricular tachycardia and fibrillation produced by programmed electrical stimulation: comparison with other antiarrhythmic agents. Am J Cardiol 1990; 65:53A–57A.

1042. Singh BN, Kehoe R, Woosley RL, Scheinman M, Quart B. Multicenter trial of sotalol compared with procainamide in the suppression of inducible ventricular tachycardia: a double-blind, randomized parallel evaluation. Sotalol Multicenter Study Group. Am Heart J 1995; 129:87–97.

1043. Haverkamp W, Martinez-Rubio A, Hief C, et al. Efficacy and safety of d,l-sotalol in patients with ventricular tachycardia and in survivors of cardiac arrest. J Am Coll Cardiol 1997; 30:487–495.

1044. Waldo AL, Camm AJ, deRuyter H, et al. Effect of d-sotalol on mortality in patients with left ventricular dysfunction after recent and remote myocardial infarction. The SWORD Investigators: survival with oral d-sotalol. Lancet 1996; 348:7–12.

1045. Fyke FE III, Vlietstra RE, Danielson GK, Beynen FM. Verapamil for refractory ventricular fibrillation during cardiac operations in patients with cardiac hypertrophy. J Thorac Cardiovasc Surg 1983; 86:108–111.

1046. Wellens HJJ, Atie J, Smeets JL, Cruz FE, Gorgels AP, Brugada P. The electrocardiogram in patients with multiple accessory atrioventricular pathways. J Am Coll Cardiol 1990; 16:745–751.

1047. Moosvi AR, Goldstein S, VanderBrug Medendorp S, et al. Effect of empiric antiarrhythmic therapy in resuscitated out-of-hospital cardiac arrest victims with coronary artery disease. Am J Cardiol 1990; 65:1192–1197.

1048. Siebels J, Cappato R, Ruppel R, Schneider MAE, Kuck KH, CASH Investigators. ICD versus drugs in cardiac arrest survivors: preliminary results of the Cardiac Arrest Study Hamburg. PACE 1993; 16:552–558.

1049. Singh BN. Acute management of ventricular arrhythmias: role of antiarrhythmic agents. Pharmacotherapy 1997; 17:56S–64S.

1050. Linenthal, AJ, Zoll PM. Prevention of ventricular tachycardia and fibrillation by intravenous isoproterenol and epinephrine. Circulation 1963; 27:5–11.

1051. Hargrove WC III, Addonizio VP, Miller JM. Surgical therapy of ventricular tachyarrhythmias in patients with coronary artery disease. J Cardiovasc Electrophysiol 1996; 7:469–480.

1052. Bryson AL, Parisi AF, Schechter E, Wolfson S. Life-threatening ventricular arrhythmias induced by exercise: cessation after coronary bypass surgery. Am J Cardiol 1973; 32:995–999.

1053. Kaiser GA, Ghahramani A, Bolooki H, et al. Role of coronary artery surgery in patients surviving unexpected cardiac arrest. Surgery 1975; 78:749–754.

1054. Myerburg RJ, Ghahramani A, Mallon SM, Castellanos A Jr, Kaiser G. Coronary revascularization in patients surviving unexpected ventricular fibrillation. Circulation 1975; 52(Suppl III):III-219–III-222.

1055. Bonchek LI, Olinger GN, Keelan MH Jr, Tresch DD, Siegel R. Management of sudden coronary death. Ann Thorac Surg 1977; 24:337–345.

1056. Morady F, Higgins J, Peters RW, et al. Electrophysiologic testing in bundle branch block and unexplained syncope. Am J Cardiol 1984; 54:587–591.

1057. Kelly P, Ruskin JN, Vlahakes GJ, Buckley MJ, Freeman CS, Garan H. Surgical coronary revascularization in survivors of prehospital cardiac arrest: its effect on inducible ventricular arrhythmias and long-term survival. J Am Coll Cardiol 1990; 15:267–273.

1058. Every NR, Fahrenbruch CE, Hallstrom AP, Weaver WD, Cobb LA. Influence of coronary bypass surgery on subsequent outcome of patients resuscitated from out of hospital cardiac arrest. J Am Coll Cardiol 1992; 19:1435–1439.

1059. O'Rourke RA. Role of myocardial revascularization in sudden cardiac death. Circulation 1992; 85(Suppl I):I-112–I-117.

1060. Amarasena NL, Pillai RP, Forfar JC. Atypical ventricular tachycardia and syncope with left coronary artery origin from the right coronary sinus. Br Heart J 1993; 70:391–392.

1061. Manolis AS, Rastegar H, Estes NAM III. Effects of coronary artery bypass grafting on ventricular arrhythmias: results with electrophysiological testing and long-term follow-up. PACE 1993; 16:984–991.

1062. Autschbach R, Falk V, Gonska BD, Dalichau H. The effect of coronary bypass graft surgery for the prevention of sudden cardiac death: recurrent episodes after ICD implantation and review of literature. PACE 1994; 17:552–558.

1063. Daoud EG, Niebauer M, Kou WH, et al. Incidence of implantable defibrillator discharges after coronary revascularization in survivors of ischemic sudden cardiac death. Am Heart J 1995; 130:277–280.

1064. Garan H, Ruskin JN, DiMarco JP, et al. Electrophysiologic studies before and after myocardial revascularization in patients with life-threatening ventricular arrhythmias. Am J Cardiol 1983; 51:519–524.

1065. Kron IL, Lerman BB, Haines DE, Flanagan TL, DiMarco JP. Coronary artery bypass grafting in patients with ventricular fibrillation. Ann Thorac Surg 1989; 48:85–89.

1066. Feldman AE, Hellerstein HK, Driscol TE, Botti RE. Repetitive ventricular fibrillation in myocardial infarction refractory to bretylium tosylate subsequently controlled by ventricular pacing. Am J Cardiol 1971; 27:227–230.

1067. Mirowski M, Mower MM, Staewen WS, Tabatznik B, Mendeloff AI. Standby automatic defibrillator: an approach to prevention of sudden coronary death. Arch Intern Med 1970; 126:158–161.

1068. Mirowski M, Mower MM, Staewen WS, Denniston RH, Mendeloff AI. The development of the transvenous automatic defibrillator. Arch Intern Med 1972; 129:773–779.

1069. Mirowski M, Mower MM, Reid PR. The automatic implantable defibrillator. Am Heart J 1980; 100:1089–1092.

1070. Mirowski M, Reid PR, Mower MM, Watkins L, Gott VL, Schauble JF, and others. Termination of malignant ventricular arrhythmias with an implanted automatic defibrillator in human beings. N Engl J Med 1980; 303:322–324.

1071. Mirowski M, Reid PR, Watkins L, Weisfeldt ML, Mower MM. Clinical treatment of life-threatening ventricular tachyarrhythmias with the automatic implantable defibrillator. Am Heart J 1981; 102:265–270.

1072. Mirowski M. Prevention of sudden arrhythmic death with implanted automatic defibrillators. Ann Intern Med 1982; 97:606–608.

1073. Mirowski M, Mower MM, Reid PR, Watkins L, Langer A. The automatic implantable defibrillator: new modality for treatment of life-threatening ventricular arrhythmias. Pacing Clin Electrophysiol 1982; 5:384–401.

1074. Winkle RA, Stinson EB, Echt DS, Mead RH, Schmidt P. Practical aspects of automatic cardioverter/defibrillator implantation. Am Heart J 1984; 108:1335–1346.

1075. Mirowski M. The automatic implantable cardioverter-defibrillator: an overview. J Am Coll Cardiol 1985; 6:461–466.

1076. Guarnieri T, Levine JH, Griffith LC, Veltri EP. When "sudden cardiac death" is not so sudden: lessons learned from the automatic implantable defibrillator. Am Heart J 1988; 115:205–207.

1077. Lehmann MH, Steinman RT, Schuger CD, Jackson K. The automatic implantable cardioverter defibrillator as antiarrhythmic treatment modality of choice for survivors of cardiac arrest unrelated to acute myocardial infarction. Am J Cardiol 1988; 62:803–805.

1078. Mirowski M, Mower MM. Transvenous catheter defibrillation for prevention of sudden cardiac death. J Am Coll Cardiol 1988; 11:371–372.

1079. Kastor JA. Michel Mirowski and the automatic implantable defibrillator. Am J Cardiol 1989; 63:977–982.

1080. Kastor JA. Michel Mirowski and the automatic implantable defibrillator. Am J Cardiol 1989; 63:1121–1126.

1081. Kay GN, Plumb VJ, Dailey SM, Epstein AE. Current role of the automatic implantable cardioverter-defibrillator in the treatment of life-threatening ventricular arrhythmias. Am J Med 1990; 88:25N–34N.

1082. Fogoros RN. The implantable defibrillator backlash. Am J Cardiol 1991; 67:1424–1427.

1083. Lehmann MH, Saksena S. Implantable cardioverter defibrillators in cardiovascular practice: report of the policy conference of the North American Society of Pacing and Electrophysiology: NASPE policy conference committee. Pacing Clin Electrophysiol 1991; 14:969–979.

1084. Akhtar M, Avitall B, Jazayeri M, et al. Role of implantable cardioverter defibrillator therapy in the management of high-risk patients. Circulation 1992; 85(Suppl I):I-131–I-139.

1085. Connolly SJ, Yusuf S. Evaluation of the implantable cardioverter defibrillator in survivors of cardiac arrest: the need for randomized trials. Am J Cardiol 1992; 69:959–962.

1086. Saksena S. Survival of implantable cardioverter-defibrillator recipients: can the iceberg remain submerged? Circulation 1992; 85:1616–1618.

1087. Adler SW, Remole S, Benditt DG. Impact of implantable cardioverter-defibrillators on prognosis of cardiac arrest survivors: a continuing controversy. Circulation 1993; 88:1348–1350.

1088. Epstein AE. Avid necessity. Pacing Clin Electrophysiol 1993; 16:1773–1775.

1089. Kim SG. Implantable defibrillator therapy: does it really prolong life? How can we prove it? Am J Cardiol 1993; 71:1213–1218.

1090. Moss AJ. One randomized defibrillator trial is worth 1,000 descriptive reports. Pacing Clin Electrophysiol 1993; 16:247–250.

1091. Singh BN. Implantable cardioverter-defibrillators: not the ultimate gold standard for gauging therapy of VT/fibrillation. Am J Cardiol 1994; 73:1211–1213.

1092. Sweeney MO, Ruskin JN. Mortality benefits and the implantable cardioverter-defibrillator. Circulation 1994; 89:1851–1858.

1093. Trappe HJ, Pfitzner P, Figuth HG, Wenzlaff P, Kielblock B, Klein H. Nonpharmacological therapy of ventricular tachyarrhythmias: observations in 554 patients. Pacing Clin Electrophysiol 1994; 17:2172–2177.

1094. Zipes DP. The implantable cardioverter defibrillator revolution continues. Mayo Clin Proc 1994; 69:395–396.

1095. Zipes DP. Implantable cardioverter-defibrillator: lifesaver or a device looking for a disease? Circulation 1994; 89:2934–2936.

1096. Block M, Breithardt G. Long-term follow-up and clinical results of implantable cardioverter-defibrillators. In Zipes DP, Jalife J (eds). Cardiac Electrophysiology. From Cell to Bedside. 2nd ed. Philadelphia: WB Saunders, 1995, pp. 1412–1425.

1097. Mitrani RD, Klein LS, Rardon DP, Zipes DP, Miles WM. Current trends in the implantable cardioverter-defibrillator. In Zipes DP, Jalife J (eds). Cardiac Electrophysiology. From Cell to Bedside. 2nd ed. Philadelphia: WB Saunders, 1995, pp. 1393–1403.

1098. Schlepper M, Neuzner J, Pitschner HF. Implantable cardioverter defibrillator: effect on survival. Pacing Clin Electrophysiol 1995; 18:569–578.

1099. Fogoros RN. Impact of the implantable defibrillator on mortality: the axiom of overall implantable cardioverter-defibrillator survival. Am J Cardiol 1996; 78:57–61.

1100. Kuck KH, Cappato R, Siebels J. Clinical Approaches to Tachyarrhythmias. Armonk NY: Futura Publishing Co., 1996, pp. 1–63.

1101. Josephson M, Nisam S. Prospective trials of implantable cardioverter defibrillators versus drugs: are they addressing the right question? Am J Cardiol 1996; 77:859–863.

1102. Kroll MW, Lehmann MH. Implantable Cardioverter Defibrillator Therapy. The Engineering-Clinical Interface. Norwell MA: Kluwer Academic Publishers, 1996.

1103. Raviele A. Implantable cardioverter-defibrillator (ICD) indications in 1996: have they changed? Am J Cardiol 1996; 78:21–25.

1104. Staewen WS, Mower MM. History of the ICD. In Kroll MW, Lehmann MH (eds). Implantable Cardioverter-Defibrillator Therapy. The Engineering-Clinical Interface. Norwell MA: Kluwer Academic Publishers, 1996, pp. 17–30.

1105. Fogoros RN. Clinical results. In Kroll MW, Lehmann MH (eds). Implantable Cardioverter Defibrillator Therapy. The Engineering-Clinical Interface. Norwell MA: Kluwer Academic Publishers, 1996, pp. 477–500.

1106. Kuck KH, Cappato R, Siebels J. ICD Therapy. Armonk NY: Futura Publishing Co. 1996.

1107. Lehmann MH, Pires LA, Olson WH, Ivan V, Steinman RT, Baga JJ. Sudden death despite ICD therapy: why does it happen? In Kroll MW, Lehmann MH (eds). Implantable Cardioverter-Defibrillator Therapy. The Engineering-Clinical Interface. Norwell MA: Kluwer Academic Publishers, 1996, pp. 501–523.

1108. Bocker D, Block M, Borggrefe M, Breithardt G. Defibrillators are superior to antiarrhythmic drugs in the treatment of ventricular tachyarrhythmias. Eur Heart J 1997; 18:26–30.

1109. Nisam S, Breithardt G. Mortality trials with implantable defibrillators. Am J Cardiol 1997; 79:468–471.

1110. Josephson ME, Nisam S. The AVID trial: evidence based or randomized control trials—is the AVID study too late? Antiarrhythmics versus implantable defibrillators. Am J Cardiol 1997; 80:194–197.

1111. Nisam S, Mower M. ICD trials: an extraordinary means of determining patient risk? PACE 1998; 21:1341–1346.

1112. Sarter BH, Callans DJ, Gottlieb CD, Schwartzman DS, Marchlinski FE. Implantable defibrillator diagnostic storage capabilities: evolution, current status, and future utilization. PACE 1998; 21:1287–1298.

1113. Hook BG, Callans DJ, Kleiman RB, Flores BT, Marchlinski FE. Implantable cardioverter-defibrillator therapy in the absence of significant symptoms: rhythm diagnosis and management aided by stored electrogram analysis. Circulation 1993; 87:1897–1906.

1114. Hurwitz JL, Hook BG, Flores BT, Marchlinski FE. Importance of abortive shock capability with electrogram storage in cardioverter-defibrillator devices. J Am Coll Cardiol 1993; 21:895–900.

1115. Marchlinski FE, Gottlieb CD, Sarter B, et al. ICD data storage: value in arrhythmia management. Pacing Clin Electrophysiol 1993; 16:527–534.

1116. Rankin AC, Zaim S, Powell A, et al. Efficacy of a tiered therapy defibrillator system used to treat recurrent ventricular arrhythmias refractory to drugs. Br Heart J 1993; 70:61–69.

1117. Wietholt D, Block M, Isbruch F, et al. Clinical experience with antitachycardia pacing and improved detection algorithms in a new implantable cardioverter-defibrillator. J Am Coll Cardiol 1993; 21:885–894.

1118. Kleiman RB, Callans DJ, Hook BG, Marchlinski FE. Effectiveness of noninvasive programmed stimulation for initiating ventricular tachyarrhythmias in patients with third-generation implantable cardioverter defibrillators. Pacing Clin Electrophysiol 1994; 17:1462–1468.

1119. PCD Investigator Group. Clinical outcome of patients with malignant ventricular tachyarrhythmias and a multiprogrammable implantable cardioverter-defibrillator implanted with or without thoracotomy: an international multicenter study. PCD Investigator Group. J Am Coll Cardiol 1994; 23:1521–1530.

1120. Geelen P, Lorga Filho A, Chauvin M, Wellens F, Brugada P. The value of DDD pacing in patients with an implantable cardioverter defibrillator. Pacing Clin Electrophysiol 1997; 20:177–181.

1121. Iskos D, Shultz JJ, Benditt DG. Recurrent supine syncope: an unusual manifestation of the neurally mediated faint. J Cardiovasc Electrophysiol 1998; 9:441–444.

1122. Higgins SL, Williams SK, Pak JP, Meyer DB. Indications for implantation of a dual-chamber pacemaker combined with an implantable cardioverter-defibrillator. Am J Cardiol 1998; 81:1360–1362.

1123. Mirowski M, Reid PR, Winkle RA, et al. Mortality in patients with implanted automatic defibrillators. Ann Intern Med 1983; 98:585–588.

1124. Mirowski M, Reid PR, Mower MM, et al. Clinical performance of the implantable cardioverter-defibrillator. Pacing Clin Electrophysiol 1984; 7:1345–1350.

1125. Mirowski M, Reid PR, Mower MM, et al. The automatic implantable cardioverter-defibrillator. Pacing Clin Electrophysiol 1984; 7:534–540.

1126. Mirowski M, Reid PR, Mower MM, et al. Clinical experience with the implantable cardioverter-defibrillator. Ann N Y Acad Sci 1984; 427:297–306.

1127. Echt DS, Armstrong K, Schmidt P, Oyer PE, Stinson EB, Winkle RA. Clinical experience, complications, and survival in 70 patients with the automatic implantable cardioverter/defibrillator. Circulation 1985; 71:289–296.

1128. Stults KR, Brown DD, Kerber RE. Efficacy of an automated external defibrillator in the management of out-of-hospital cardiac arrest: validation of the diagnostic algorithm and initial clinical experience in a rural environment. Circulation 1986; 73:701–709.

1129. Fogoros RN, Fiedler SB, Elson JJ. The automatic implantable cardioverter-defibrillator in drug-refractory ventricular tachyarrhythmias. Ann Intern Med 1987; 107:635–641.

1130. Gabry MD, Brodman R, Johnston D, et al. Automatic implantable cardioverter-defibrillator: patient survival, battery longevity and shock delivery analysis. J Am Coll Cardiol 1987; 9:1349–1356.

1131. Lehmann MH, Steinman RT. Preventing sudden cardiac death. Postgrad Med 1987; 82:36–39.

1132. Yee ES, Scheinman MM, Griffin JC, Ebert PA. Surgical options for treating ventricular tachyarrhythmia and sudden death. J Thorac Cardiovasc Surg 1987; 94:866–873.

1133. Kelly PA, Cannom DS, Garan H, et al. The automatic implantable cardioverter-defibrillator: efficacy, complications and survival in patients with malignant ventricular arrhythmias. J Am Coll Cardiol 1988; 11:1278–1286.

1134. Fonger JD, Guarnieri T, Griffith LS, et al. Impending sudden cardiac death: treatment with myocardial revascularization and the automatic implantable cardioverter defibrillator. Ann Thorac Surg 1988; 46:13–19.

1135. Tchou PJ, Kadri N, Anderson J, Caceres JA, Jazayeri M, Akhtar M. Automatic implantable cardioverter defibrillators and survival of patients with left ventricular dysfunction and malignant ventricular arrhythmias. Ann Intern Med 1988; 109:529–534.

1136. Thomas AC, Moser SA, Smutka ML, Wilson PA. Implantable defibrillation: eight years clinical experience. Pacing Clin Electrophysiol 1988; 11:2053–2058.

1137. Hargrove WC III, Josephson ME, Marchlinski FE, Miller JM. Surgical decisions in the management of sudden cardiac death and malignant ventricular arrhythmias: subendocardial resection, the automatic internal defibrillator, or both. J Thorac Cardiovasc Surg 1989; 97:923–928.

1138. Winkle RA, Mead RH, Ruder MA, et al. Long-term outcome with the automatic implantable cardioverter-defibrillator. J Am Coll Cardiol 1989; 13:1353–1361.

1139. Fogoros RN, Elson JJ, Bonnet CA, Fiedler SB, Burkholder JA. Efficacy of the automatic implantable cardioverter-defibrillator in prolonging survival in patients with severe underlying cardiac disease. J Am Coll Cardiol 1990; 16:381–386.

1140. Kron J, Oliver RP, Norsted S, Silka MJ. The automatic implantable cardioverter-defibrillator in young patients. J Am Coll Cardiol 1990; 16:896–902.

1141. Ropella KM, Baerman JM, Sahakian AV, Swiryn S. Differentiation of ventricular tachyarrhythmias. Circulation 1990; 82:2035–2043.

1142. De Marchena E, Chakko S, Fernandez P, et al. Usefulness of the automatic implantable cardioverter defibrillator in improving survival of patients with severely depressed left ventricular function associated with coronary artery disease. Am J Cardiol 1991; 67:812–816.

1143. Kim SG, Fisher JD, Furman S, et al. Benefits of implantable defibrillators are overestimated by sudden death rates and better represented by the total arrhythmic death rate. J Am Coll Cardiol 1991; 17:1587–1592.

1144. Palatianos GM, Thurer RJ, Cooper DK, et al. The implantable cardioverter-defibrillator: clinical results. Pacing Clin Electrophysiol 1991; 14:297–301.

1145. Axtell K, Tchou P, Akhtar M. Survival in patients with depressed left ventricular function treated by implantable cardioverter defibrillator. Pacing Clin Electrophysiol 1991; 14:291–296.

1146. Nisam S, Mower M, Moser S. ICD clinical update: first decade, initial 10,000 patients. Pacing Clin Electrophysiol 1991; 14:255–262.

1147. Newman D, Sauve MJ, Herre J, et al. Survival after implantation of the cardioverter defibrillator. Am J Cardiol 1992; 69:899–903.

1148. Saksena S, Poczobutt-Johanos M, Castle LW, et al. Long-term multicenter experience with a second-generation implantable pacemaker-defibrillator in patients with malignant ventricular tachyarrhythmias: the Guardian Multicenter Investigators Group. J Am Coll Cardiol 1992; 19:490–499.

1149. Bardy GH, Hofer B, Johnson G, et al. Implantable transvenous cardioverter-defibrillators. Circulation 1993; 87:1152–1168.

1150. Powell AC, Fuchs T, Finkelstein DM, et al. Influence of implantable cardioverter-defibrillators on the long-term prognosis of survivors of out-of-hospital cardiac arrest. Circulation 1993; 88:1083–1092.

1151. Bocker D, Block M, Isbruch F, et al. Do patients with an implantable defibrillator live longer? J Am Coll Cardiol 1993; 21:1638–1644.

1152. Nisam S, Mower MM, Thomas A, Hauser R. Patient survival comparison in three generations of automatic implantable cardioverter defibrillators: review of 12 years, 25,000 patients. Pacing Clin Electrophysiol 1993; 16:174–178.

1153. Choue CW, Kim SG, Fisher JD, et al. Comparison of defibrillator therapy and other therapeutic modalities for sustained ventricular tachycardia or ventricular fibrillation associated with coronary artery disease. Am J Cardiol 1994; 73:1075–1079.

1154. Nisam S, Kaye SA, Mower MM, Hull M. AICD automatic cardioverter defibrillator clinical update: 14 years experience in over 34,000 patients. Pacing Clin Electrophysiol 1995; 18:142–147.

1155. Fogoros RN. Why the Antiarrhythmics versus Implantable Defibrillator (AVID) Trial sets the wrong precedent. Am J Cardiol 1997; 80:762–765.

1156. Kim SG, Hallstrom A, Love JC, et al. Comparison of clinical characteristics and frequency of implantable defibrillator use between randomized patients in the Antiarrhythmics vs Implantable Defibrillators (AVID) Trial and nonrandomized registry patients. Am J Cardiol 1997; 80:454–457.

1157. Raviele A, Gasparini G. Italian multicenter clinical experience with endocardial defibrillation: acute and long-term results in 307 patients. The Italian Endotak Investigator Group. Pacing Clin Electrophysiol 1995; 18:599–608.

1158. Singer I, Nisam S. There should never be another Antiarrhythmics versus Implantable Defibrillator (AVID) Trial. Am J Cardiol 1997; 80:766–768.

1159. Antiarrhythmics versus Implantable Defibrillators (AVID) Investigators. A comparison of antiarrhythmic-drug therapy with implantable defibrillators in patients resuscitated from near-fatal ventricular arrhythmias: the Antiarrhythmics versus Implantable Defibrillators (AVID) Investigators. N Engl J Med 1997; 337:1576–1583.

1160. Antiarrhythmics versus Implantable Defibrillators (AVID) Trial Executive Committee. Are implantable cardioverter-defibrillators or drugs more effective in prolonging life? Am J Cardiol 1997; 79:661–663.

1161. Geelen P, Lorga Filho A, Primo J, Wellens F, Brugada P. Experience with implantable cardioverter defibrillator therapy in elderly patients. Eur Heart J 1997; 18:1339–1342.

1162. Panotopoulos PT, Axtell K, Anderson AJ, et al. Efficacy of the implantable cardioverter-defibrillator in the elderly. J Am Coll Cardiol 1997; 29:556–560.

1163. Trappe HJ, Pfitzner P, Achtelik M, Fieguth HG, Age dependent efficacy of implantable cardioverter-defibrillator treatment: observations in 450 patients over an 11 year period. Heart 1997; 78:364–370.

1164. Natale A, Davidson T, Geiger MJ, Newby K. Implantable cardioverter-defibrillators and pregnancy: a safe combination? Circulation 1997; 96:2808–2812.

1165. Narasimhan C, Dhala A, Axtell K, et al. Comparison of outcome of implantable cardioverter defibrillator implantation in patients with severe versus moderately severe left ventricular dysfunction secondary to atherosclerotic coronary artery disease. Am J Cardiol 1997; 80:1305–1308.

1166. Saksena S, Parsonnet V. Implantation of a cardioverter/ defibrillator without thoracotomy using a triple electrode system. JAMA 1988; 259:69–72.

1167. Brooks R, Garan H, Torchiana D, et al. Determinants of successful nonthoracotomy cardioverter-defibrillator implantation: experience in 101 patients using two different lead systems. J Am Coll Cardiol 1993; 22:1835–1842.

1168. Jordaens L, Trouerbach JW, Vertongen P, Herregods L, Poelaert J, Van Nooten G. Experience of cardioverter-defibrillators inserted without thoracotomy: evaluation of transvenously inserted intracardiac leads alone or with a subcutaneous axillary patch. Br Heart J 1993; 69:14–19.

1169. Schmitt C, Alt E, Plewan A, Schomig A. Initial experience with implantation of internal cardioverter/defibrillators under local anaesthesia by electrophysiologists. Eur Heart J 1996; 17:1710–1716.

1170. Stix G, Anvari A, Grabenwoger M, et al. Implantation of a unipolar cardioverter/defibrillator system under local anaesthesia. Eur Heart J 1996; 17:764–768.

1171. van Rugge FP, Savalle LH, Schalij MJ. Subcutaneous single-incision implantation of cardioverter-defibrillators under local anesthesia by electrophysiologists in the electrophysiology laboratory. Am J Cardiol 1998; 81:302–305.

1172. Zipes DP, Roberts D. Results of the international study of the implantable pacemaker cardioverter-defibrillator: a comparison of epicardial and endocardial lead systems. The Pacemaker-Cardioverter-Defibrillator Investigators. Circulation 1995; 92:59–65.

1173. Gartman DM, Bardy GH, Allen MD, Misbach GA, Ivey TD. Short-term morbidity and mortality of implantation of automatic implantable cardioverter-defibrillator. J Thorac Cardiovasc Surg 1990; 100:353–357.

1174. Mosteller RD, Lehmann MH, Thomas AC, Jackson K. Operative mortality with implantation of the automatic cardioverter-defibrillator. Am J Cardiol 1991; 68:1340–1345.

1175. Kim SG, Fisher JD, Choue CW, et al. Influence of left ventricular function on outcome of patients treated with implantable defibrillators. Circulation 1992; 85:1304–1310.

1176. Bardy GH, Johnson G, Poole JE, et al. A simplified, single-lead unipolar transvenous cardioversion-defibrillation system. Circulation 1993; 88:543–547.

1177. Marchlinski FE. Nonthoracotomy defibrillator lead systems: a welcomed addition but still a lot to learn. Circulation 1993; 87:1410–1411.

1178. Kleman JM, Castle LW, Kidwell GA, et al. Nonthoracotomy-versus thoracotomy-implantable defibrillators: intention-to-treat comparison of clinical outcomes. Circulation 1994; 90:2833–2842.

1179. Williamson BD, Man KC, Niebauer M, et al. The economic impact of transvenous defibrillation lead systems. Pacing Clin Electrophysiol 1994; 17:2297–2303.

1180. Ong JJ, Hsu PC, Lin L, et al. Arrhythmias after cardioverter-defibrillator implantation: comparison of epicardial and transvenous systems. Am J Cardiol 1995; 75:137–140.

1181. Venditti FJ, Jr, O'Connell M, Martin DT, Shahian DM. Transvenous cardioverter defibrillators: cost implications of a less invasive approach. Pacing Clin Electrophysiol 1995; 18:711–715.

1182. Pacifico A, Wheelan KR, Nasir, N, et al. Long-term follow-up of cardioverter-defibrillator implanted under conscious sedation in prepectoral subfascial position. Circulation 1997; 95:946–950.

1183. Auricchio A, Klein H, Geller CJ, Reek S, Heilman MS, Szymkiewicz SJ. Clinical efficacy of the wearable cardioverter-defibrillator in acutely terminating episodes of ventricular fibrillation. Am J Cardiol 1998; 81:1253–1256.

1184. Kou WH, Calkins H, Lewis RR, et al. Incidence of loss of consciousness during automatic implantable cardioverter-defibrillator shocks. Ann Intern Med 1991; 115:942–945.

1185. Bansch D, Brunn J, Castrucci M, et al. Syncope in patients with an implantable cardioverter-defibrillator: incidence, prediction and implications for driving restrictions. J Am Coll Cardiol 1998; 31:608–615.

1186. Henthorn RW, Waller TJ, Hiratzka LF. Are the benefits of the automatic implantable cardioverter-defibrillator (AICD) overestimated by sudden death rate? J Am Coll Cardiol 1991; 17:1593–1594.

1187. Zipes DP. Are implantable cardioverter-defibrillators better than conventional antiarrhythmic drugs for survivors of cardiac arrest? Circulation 1995; 91:2115–2117.

1188. Gregoratos G, Cheitlin MD, Conill A, et al. ACC/AHA Guidelines for Implantation of Cardiac Pacemakers and Antiarrhythmia Devices (Committee on Pacemaker Implantation). Circulation 1998; 97:1325–1335.

1189. Muratore C, Rabinovich R, Iglesias R, Gonzalez M Daru, V, Liprandi AS. Implantable cardioverter defibrillators in patients with Chagas' disease: are they different from patients with coronary disease? Pacing Clin Electrophysiol 1997; 20:194–197.

1190. Kudenchuk PJ, Bardy GH, Poole JE, et al. Malignant sustained ventricular tachyarrhythmias in women: characteristics and outcome of treatment with an implantable cardioverter defibrillator. J Cardiovasc Electrophysiol 1997; 8:2–10.

1191. Myerburg RJ, Luceri RM, Thurer R, et al. Time to first shock and clinical outcome in patients receiving an automatic implantable cardioverter-defibrillator. J Am Coll Cardiol 1989; 14:508–514.

1192. Levine JH, Mellits ED, Baumgardner RA, et al. Predictors of first discharge and subsequent survival in patients with automatic implantable cardioverter-defibrillators. Circulation 1991; 84:558–566.

1193. Mehta D, Saksena S, Krol RB. Survival of implantable cardioverter-defibrillator recipients: role of left ventricular function and its relationship to device use. Am Heart J 1992; 124:1608–1614.

1194. Grimm W, Flores BT, Marchlinski FE. Shock occurrence and survival in 241 patients with implantable cardioverter-defibrillator therapy. Circulation 1993; 87:1880–1888.

1195. Tebbenjohanns J, Schumacher B, Jung W, et al. Predictors of outcome in patients with implantable transvenous cardioverter defibrillators. Am Heart J 1994; 127:1086–1089.

1196. Kim SG. Management of survivors of cardiac arrest: is electrophysiologic testing obsolete in the era of implantable defibrillators? J Am Coll Cardiol 1990; 16:756–762.

1197. Bigger JT Jr. Prophylactic use of implantable cardioverter defibrillators: medical, technical, economic considerations. Pacing Clin Electrophysiol 1991; 14:376–380.

1198. Nisam S, Thomas A, Mower M, Hauser R. Identifying patients for prophylactic automatic implantable cardioverter defibrillator therapy: status of prospective studies. Am Heart J 1991; 122:607–612.

1199. Brugada P, Andries E. The rationale for prophylactic implantation of a defibrillator in "high risk" patients. PACE 1993; 16:547–551.

1200. Li HG, Thakur RK, Yee R, Klein GJ. The value of electrophysiologic testing in patients resuscitated from documented ventricular fibrillation. J Cardiovasc Electrophysiol 1994; 5:805–809.

1201. Dolack GL, Poole JE, Kudenchuk PJ, et al. Management of ventricular fibrillation with transvenous defibrillators without baseline electrophysiologic testing or antiarrhythmic drugs. J Cardiovasc Electrophysiol 1996; 7:197–202.

1202. Josephson ME. ICD implantation: cost conscious or patient conscious. J Cardiovasc Electrophysiol 1996; 7:203–205.

1203. Andresen D, Bruggemann T, Behrens S, Ehlers C. Risk of ventricular arrhythmias in survivors of myocardial infarction. Pacing Clin Electrophysiol 1997; 20:2699–2705.

1204. Bocker D, Block M, Borggrefe M, Breithardt G. Are electrophysiological studies needed before implantable cardioverter defibrillator surgery? Eur Heart J 1997; 18:548–551.

1205. Wilber DJ, Kall JG, Kopp DE. What can we expect from prophylactic implantable defibrillators? Am J Cardiol 1997; 80:20F–27F.

1206. Haverich A, Troster J, Wahlers T, Fieguth HG, Klein H. The automatic implantable cardioverter defibrillator (AICD) as a bridge to heart transplantation. Pacing Clin Electrophysiol 1992; 15:701–707.

1207. Wever EFD, Hauer RNW, Van Capelle FJL, et al. randomized study of implantable defibrillator as first-choice therapy versus conventional strategy in postinfarct sudden death survivors. Circulation 1995; 91:2195–2203.

1208. Gross JN, Song SL, Buckingham T, Furman S. Influence of clinical characteristics and shock occurrence on ICD patient outcome: a multicenter report. The BILITCH Registry Group. Pacing Clin Electrophysiol 1991; 14:1881–1886.

1209. MADIT Executive Committee. Multicenter Automatic Defibrillator Implantation Trial (MADIT): design and clinical protocol. MADIT Executive Committee. Pacing Clin Electrophysiol 1991; 14:920–927.

1210. Buxton AE, Fisher JD, Josephson ME, et al. Prevention of sudden death in patients with coronary artery disease: the Multicenter Unsustained Tachycardia Trial (MUSTT). Prog Cardiovasc Dis 1993; 36:215–226.

1211. Moss AJ, Hall WJ, Cannom DS, et al. Improved survival with an implanted defibrillator in patients with coronary disease at high risk for ventricular arrhythmia. N Eng J Med 1996; 335:1933–1940.

1212. Friedman PL, Stevenson WG. Unsustained ventricular tachycardia: to treat or not to treat? N Engl J Med 1996; 335:1984–1985.

1213. Higgins SL, Klein H, Nisam S. Which device should "MADIT protocol" patients receive? Multicenter Automatic Defibrillator Implantation Trial. Am J Cardiol 1997; 79:31–35.

1214. Moss AJ. Background, outcome, and clinical implications of the Multicenter Automatic Defibrillator Implantation Trial (MADIT). Am J Cardiol 1997; 80:28F–32F.

1215. Mushlin AI, Zwanziger J, Gajary E, Andrews M, Marron R. Approach to cost-effectiveness assessment in the MADIT trial: Multicenter Automatic Defibrillator Implantation Trial. Am J Cardiol 1997; 80:33F–41F.

1216. Nisam S. Do MADIT results apply only to "MADIT patients"? Multicenter Automatic Defibrillator Implantation Trial. Am J Cardiol 1997; 79:27–30.

1217. Myerburg RJ, Mitrani R, Interian A, Castellanos A. Interpretation of outcomes of antiarrhythmic clinical trials: design features and population impact. Circulation 1998; 97:1514–1521.

1218. Strickberger SA, Man KC, Daoud EG, et al. A prospective evaluation of catheter ablation of ventricular tachycardia as adjuvant therapy in patients with coronary artery disease and an implantable cardioverter-defibrillator. Circulation 1997; 96:1525–1531.

1219. CABG Patch Trial Investigators and Coordinators. The Coronary Artery Bypass Graft (CABG) Patch Trial. Pro Cardiovasc Dis 1993; 36:97–114.

1220. Spotnitz HM, Herre JM, Baker LD Jr, Fitzgerald DM, Kron IL, Bigger JT Jr. Surgical aspects of a randomized trial of defibrillator implantation during coronary artery bypass surgery: the CABG Patch Trial. Circulation 1996; 94 (Suppl I):I-1248–I-1253.

1221. Bigger JT. Prophylactic use of implanted cardiac defibrillators in patients at high risk for ventricular arrhythmias after coronary-artery bypass graft surgery. N Eng J Med 1997; 337:1569–1575.

1222. Curtis AB, Cannom DS, Bigger JT, et al. Baseline characteristics of patients in the Coronary Artery Bypass Graft (CABG) Patch Trial. Am Heart J 1997; 133:787–798.

1223. Lessmeier TJ, Lehmann MH, Steinman RT, et al. Outcome with implantable cardioverter-defibrillator therapy for survivors of ventricular fibrillation secondary to idiopathic dilated cardiomyopathy or coronary artery disease without myocardial infarction. Am J Cardiol 1993; 72:911–915.

1224. Borggrefe M, Breithardt G. Is the implantable defibrillator indicated in patients with hypertrophic cardiomyopathy and aborted sudden death? J Am Coll Cardiol 1998; 31:1086–1088.

1225. Primo J, Geelen P, Brugada J, et al. Hypertrophic cardiomyopathy: role of the implantable cardioverter-defibrillator. J Am Coll Cardiol 1998; 31:1081–1085.

1226. Fan W, Peter CT. Survival and incidence of appropriate shocks in implantable cardioverter defibrillator recipients who have no detectable structural heart disease: Cedars investigators. Am J Cardiol 1994; 74:687–690.

1227. Levy S. Is the implantable cardioverter-defibrillator cost-effective? Eur Heart J 1996; 17:1458–1459.

1228. Hlatky MA, Owens DK. Cost-effectiveness of tests to assess the risk of sudden death after acute myocardial infarction. J Am Coll Cardiol 1998; 31:1490–1492.

1229. Kuppermann M, Luce BR, McGovern B, Podrid PJ, Bigger JT Jr, Ruskin JN. An analysis of the cost effectiveness of the implantable defibrillator. Circulation 1990; 81:91–100.

1230. Winkle RA. Early automatic implantable cardioverter-defibrillator implantation: medical and economic considerations and inequities in health care reimbursement. J Am Coll Cardiol 1990; 16:1264–1266.

1231. O'Brien BJ, Buxton MJ, Rushby JA. Cost effectiveness of the implantable cardioverter defibrillator: a preliminary analysis. Br Heart J 1992; 68:241–245.

1232. Larsen GC, Manolis AS, Sonnenberg FA, Beshansky JR, Estes NA, Pauker SG. Cost-effectiveness of the implantable cardioverter-defibrillator: effect of improved battery life and comparison with amiodarone therapy. J Am Coll Cardiol 1992; 19:1323–1334.

1233. Saksena S, Camm AJ. Implantable defibrillators for prevention of sudden death: technology at a medical and economic crossroad. Circulation 1992; 85:2316–2321.

1234. Anderson MH, Camm AJ. Implications for present and future applications of the implantable cardioverter-defibrillator resulting from the use of a simple model of cost efficacy. Br Heart J 1993; 69:83–92.

1235. Saksena S, Madan N, Lewis C. Implanted cardioverter-defibrillators are preferable to drugs as primary therapy in sustained ventricular tachyarrhythmias. Prog Cardiovasc Dis 1996; 38:445–454.

1236. Brugada P, Wellens F, Andries E. A prophylactic implantable cardioverter-defibrillator? Am J Cardiol 1996; 78:128–133.

1237. Owens DK, Sanders GD, Harris RA, et al. Cost-effectiveness of implantable cardioverter defibrillators relative to amiodarone for prevention of sudden cardiac death. Ann Intern Med 1997; 126:1–12.

1238. O'Donoghue S, Platia EV, Brooks-Robinson S, Mispireta L. Automatic implantable cardioverter-defibrillator: is early implantation cost-effective? J Am Coll Cardiol 1990; 16:1258–1263.

1239. Akhtar M, Jazayeri M, Sra J, et al. Implantable cardioverter defibrillator for prevention of sudden cardiac death in patients with ventricular tachycardia and ventricular fibrillation: ICD therapy in sudden cardiac death. Pacing Clin Electrophysiol 1993; 16:511–518.

1240. Kupersmith J, Hogan A, Guerrero P, et al. Evaluating and improving the cost-effectiveness of the implantable cardioverter-defibrillator. Am Heart J 1995; 130:507–515.

1241. Wever EFD, Hauer RNW, Schrijvers G, et al. Cost-effectiveness of implantable defibrillator as first-choice therapy versus electrophysiologically guided, tiered strategy in postinfarct sudden death survivors: a randomized study. Circulation 1996; 93:489–496.

1242. Hauer RN, Derksen R, Wever EF. Can implantable cardioverter-defibrillator therapy reduce healthcare costs? Am J Cardiol 1996; 78:134–139.

1243. Mushlin AI, Hall J, Zwanziger J, et al. The cost-effectiveness of automatic implantable cardiac defibrillators: results from MADIT. Circulation 1998; 97:2129–2135.

1244. Valenti R, Schlapfer J, Fromer M, Fischer A, Kappenberger L. Impact of the implantable cardioverter-defibrillator on rehospitalizations. Eur Heart J 1996; 17:1565–1571.

1245. Aizawa Y, Tamura M, Chinushi M, et al. An attempt at electrical catheter ablation of the arrhythmogenic area in idiopathic ventricular fibrillation. Am Heart J 1992; 123:257–260.

1246. Fitzpatrick AP, Dawkins K, Conway N. Emergency percutaneous transluminal coronary angioplasty for intractable ventricular arrhythmias associated with acute anterior myocardial infarction. Br Heart J 1993; 69:453–454.

1247. Kahn JK, Glazier S, Swor R, Savas V, O'Neill WW. Primary coronary angioplasty for acute myocardial infarction complicated by out-of-hospital cardiac arrest. Am J Cardiol 1995; 75:1069–1070.

1248. Curtis AB, Conti JB, Tucker KJ, Kubilis PS, Reilly RE, Woodard DA. Motor vehicle accidents in patients with an implantable cardioverter-defibrillator. J Am Coll Cardiol 1995; 26:180–184.

1249. DiCarlo LA, Winston SA, Honoway S, Reed P. Driving restrictions advised by midwestern cardiologists implanting cardioverter defibrillators: present practices, criteria utilized, and compatibility with existing state laws. Pacing Clin Electrophysiol 1992; 15:1131–1136.

1250. Strickberger SA, Cantillon CO, Friedman PL. When should patients with lethal ventricular arrhythmia resume driving? An analysis of state regulations and physician practices. Ann Intern Med 1991; 115:560–563.

1251. Finch NJ, Leman RB, Kratz JM, Gillette PC. Driving safety among patients with automatic implantable cardioverter defibrillators. JAMA 1993; 270:1587–1588.

1252. Conti JB, Woodard DA, Tucker KJ, Bryant B, King LC, Curtis AB. Modification of patient driving behavior after implantation of a cardioverter defibrillator. Pacing Clin Electrophysiol 1997; 20:2200–2204.

1253. Larsen GC, Stupey MR, Walance CG, et al. Recurrent cardiac events in survivors of ventricular fibrillation or tachycardia: implications for driving restrictions. JAMA 1994; 271:1335–1339.

1254. Surawicz B. Prognosis of ventricular arrhythmias in relation to sudden cardiac death: therapeutic implications. J Am Coll Cardiol 1987; 10:435–447.

1255. Anderson MH. Risk Assessment of Ventricular Tachyarrhythmias. Armonk, NY: Futura Publishing Co., 1995.

1256. Breithardt G, Borggrefe M, Fetsch T, Bocker D, Makijarvi M, Reinhardt L. Prognosis and risk stratification after myocardial infarction. Eur Heart J 1995; 16:G10–G19.

1257. Rehnqvist N, Lundman T, Sjogren A. Prognostic implications of ventricular arrhythmias registered before discharge and one year after acute myocardial infarction. Acta Med Scand 1978; 204:203–209.

1258. Norris RM, Barnaby PF, Brandt PW, et al. Prognosis after recovery from first acute myocardial infarction: determinants of reinfarction and sudden death. Am J Cardiol 1984; 53:408–413.

1259. DiCarlo LA, Jr, Morady F, Sauve MJ, et al. Cardiac arrest and sudden death in patients treated with amiodarone for sustained ventricular tachycardia or ventricular fibrillation: risk stratification based on clinical variables. Am J Cardiol 1985; 55:372–374.

1260. Kuchar DL, Thorburn CW, Sammel, NL. Prediction of serious arrhythmic events after myocardial infarction: signal-averaged electrocardiogram, Holter monitoring and radionuclide ventriculography. J Am Coll Cardiol 1987; 9:531–538.

1261. Lampert S, Lown B, Graboys TB, Podrid, PJ, Blatt CM. Determinants of survival in patients with malignant ventricular arrhythmia associated with coronary artery disease. Am J Cardiol 1988; 61:791–797.

1262. Marcus FI, Cobb LA, Edwards JE, et al. Mechanism of death and prevalence of myocardial ischemic symptoms in the terminal event after acute myocardial infarction. Am J Cardiol 1988; 61:8–15.

1263. Andresen D, Steinbeck G, Bruggemann T, Haberl, R, Fink L, Schroder R. Prognosis of patients with sustained ventricular tachycardia and of survivors of cardiac arrest not inducible by programmed stimulation. Am J Cardiol 1992; 70:1250–1254.

1264. Rodriguez LM, Oyarzun R, Smeets, J, et al. Identification of patients at high risk for recurrence of sustained ventricular tachycardia after healing of acute myocardial infarction. Am J Cardiol 1992; 69:462–464.

1265. Rodriguez LM, Smeets J, O'Hara, GE, et al. Incidence and timing of recurrences of sudden death and ventricular tachycardia during antiarrhythmic drug treatment after myocardial infarction. Am J Cardiol 1992; 69:1403–1406.

1266. Kim SG, Maloney JD, Pinski SL, et al. Influence of left ventricular function on survival and mode of death after implantable defibrillator therapy (Cleveland Clinic Foundation and Montefiore Medical Center experience). Am J Cardiol 1993; 72:1263–1267.

1267. Szabo BM, van Veldhuisen DJ, Crijns HJ, Wiesfeld AC, Hillege HL, Lie K.I. Value of ambulatory electrocardiographic monitoring to identify increased risk of sudden death in patients with left ventricular dysfunction and heart failure. Eur Heart J 1994; 15:928–933.

1268. Caruso AC, Marcus FI, Hahn EA, Hartz VL, Mason JW. Predictors of arrhythmic death and cardiac arrest in the ESVEM Trial: Electrophysiologic Study Versus Electromagnetic Monitoring. Circulation 1997; 96:1888–1892.

1269. Giorgberidze I. Saksena S, Krol RB, et al. Risk stratification and clinical outcome of minimally symptomatic and asymptomatic patients with nonsustained ventricular tachycardia and coronary disease: a prospective single-center study. Am J Cardiol 1997; 80:3F–9F.

1270. Gomes JA, Mehta D, Ip J, et al. Predictors of long-term survival in patients with malignant ventricular arrhythmias. Am J Cardiol 1997; 79:1054–1060.

1271. Bigger JT Jr, Dresdale FJ, Heissenbuttel RH, Weld FM, Wit AL. Ventricular arrhythmias in ischemic heart disease: mechanism, prevalence, significance, and management. Prog Cardiovasc Dis 1977; 19:255–300.

1272. Ruberman W, Weinblatt E, Frank, CW, Goldberg JD, Shapiro S. Repeated 1 hour electrocardiographic monitoring of survivors of myocardial infarction at 6 month intervals: arrhythmia detection and relation to prognosis. Am J Cardiol 1981; 47:1197–1204.

1273. Bigger JT Jr, Weld FM, Rolnitzky LM. Prevalence, characteristics and significance of ventricular tachycardia (three or more complexes) detected with ambulatory electrocardiographic recording in the late hospital phase of acute myocardial infarction. Am J Cardiol 1981; 48:815–823.

1274. Bigger JT Jr, Weld FM, Rolnitzky LM. Which postinfarction ventricular arrhythmias should be treated? Am Heart J 1982; 103:660–666.

1275. Bigger JT Jr. Identification of patients at high risk for sudden cardiac death. Am J Cardiol 1984; 54:3D–8D.

1276. Bigger JT Jr, Coromilas J, Weld, FM, Reiffel, JA, Rolnitzky LM. Prognosis after recovery from acute myocardial infarction. Annu Rev Med 1984; 35:127–147.

1277. Bigger JT Jr, Coromilas J. Identification of patients at risk for arrhythmic death: role of Holter ECG recording. Cardiovasc Clin 1985; 15:131–143.

1278. Gradman A, Deedwania P, Cody R, et al. Predictors of total mortality and sudden death in mild to moderate heart failure: Captopril-Digoxin Study Group. J Am Coll Cardiol 1989; 14:564–570.

1279. Lindsay BD, Osborn JL, Schechtman KB, Kenzora JL, Ambos HD, Cain, ME. Prospective detection of vulnerability to sustained ventricular tachycardia in patients awaiting cardiac transplantation. Am J Cardiol 1992; 69:619–624.

1280. Zimmerman M, Sentici A, Adamec R, Metzger J, Mermillod B, Rutishauser W. Long-term prognostic significance of ventricular late potentials after a first acute myocardial infarction. Am Heart J 1997; 134:1019–1028.

1281. Hamer, A, Vohra J, Hunt D, Sloman G. Prediction of sudden death by electrophysiologic studies in high risk patients surviving acute myocardial infarction. Am J Cardiol 1982; 50:223–229.

1282. Maynard C. Rehospitalization in surviving patients of out-of-hospital ventricular fibrillation (the CASCADE Study). Am J Cardiol 1993; 72:1295–1300.

1283. Myerburg RJ, Kessler KM, Estes D, et al. Long-term survival after prehospital cardiac arrest: analysis of outcome during an 8 year study. Circulation 1984; 70:538–546.

1284. CASCADE Investigators. Cardiac arrest in Seattle: Conventional versus Amiodarone Drug Evaluation (the CASCADE Study). Am J Cardiol 1991; 67:578–584.

1285. Eisenberg MS, Hallstrom A, Bergner L. Long-term survival after out-of-hospital cardiac arrest. N Engl J Med 1982; 306:1340–1343.

1286. Tresch DD, Keelan MH Jr, Siegel R, et al. Long-term survival after prehospital sudden cardiac death. Am Heart J 1984; 108:1–5.

1287. Herlitz J, Ekstrom L, Wennerblom B, Axelsson A, Bang A, Holmberg S. Survival in patients found to have ventricular fibrillation after cardiac arrest witnessed outside hospital. Eur Heart J 1994; 15:1628–1633.

1288. Dickey W, MacKenzie G, Adgey AA. Long-term survival after resuscitation from ventricular fibrillation occurring before hospital admission. Q J Med 1991; 80:729–737.

1289. Weaver WD. Calcium-channel blockers and advanced cardiac life support. Circulation 1986; 74(Suppl IV):IV-94–IV-97.

1290. Wilber DJ, Garan H, Finkelstein D, et al. Out-of-hospital cardiac arrest: use of electrophysiologic testing in the prediction of long-term outcome. N Engl J Med 1988; 318:19–24.

1291. Myerburg RJ, Conde C, Sheps DS, et al. Antiarrhythmic drug therapy in survivors of prehospital cardiac arrest: comparison of effects on chronic ventricular arrhythmias and recurrent cardiac arrest. Circulation 1979; 59:855–863.

1292. Hagstrom RM, Billings FT Jr, Ball COT, Meneely GR. The risk of sudden death following myocardial infarction. Arch Environ Health 1967; 15:450–454.

1293. Willems AR, Tijssen JG, van Capelle FJ, et al. Determinants of prognosis in symptomatic ventricular tachycardia or ventricular fibrillation late after myocardial infarction: the Dutch Ventricular Tachycardia Study Group of the Interuniversity Cardiology Institute of the Netherlands. J Am Coll Cardiol 1990; 16:521–530.

1294. Goldberg R, Szklo M, Tonascia JA, Kennedy HL. Acute myocardial infarction: Prognosis complicated by ventricular fibrillation or cardiac arrest. JAMA 1979; 241:2024–2027.

1295. Volpi A, Cavalli A, Franzosi MG, et al. One-year prognosis of primary ventricular fibrillation complicating acute myocardial infarction. Am J Cardiol 1989; 63:1174–1178.

1296. Kushnir B, Fox KM, Tomlinson IW, Portal RW, Aber CP. Primary ventricular fibrillation and resumption of work, sexual activity, and driving after first acute myocardial infarction. BMJ 1975; 4:609–611.

1297. Geddes JS, Adgey AA, Pantridge JF. Prognosis after recovery from ventricular fibrillation complicating ischaemic heart-disease. Lancet 1967; 2:273–275.

1298. Lawrie DM. Long-term survival after ventricular fibrillation complicating acute myocardial infarction. Lancet 1969; 2:1085–1087.

1299. Stannard M, Sloman G. Ventricular fibrillation in acute myocardial infarction: prognosis following successful resuscitation. Am Heart J 1969; 77:573.

1300. Fabricius-Bjerre N, Astvad K, Kjaerulff J. Cardiac arrest following acute myocardial infarction: a study of 285 cases from three medical departments using a joint acute admission section containing a coronary care unit. Acta Med Scand 1974; 195:261–265.

1301. DiMarco JP, Lerman BB, Kron IL, Sellers TD. Sustained ventricular tachyarrhythmias within 2 months of acute myocardial infarction: results of medical and surgical therapy in patients from the initial episode. J Am Coll Cardiol 1985; 6:759–768.

1302. Brugada P, Talajic M, Smeets J, Mulleneers R, Wellens, HJJ. The value of the clinical history to assess prognosis of patients with ventricular tachycardia or ventricular fibrillation after myocardial infarction. Eur Heart J 1989; 10:747–752.

1303. Richards DA, Byth K, Ross DL, Uther JB. What is the best predictor of spontaneous ventricular tachycardia and sudden death after myocardial infarction? Circulation 1991; 83:756–763.

1304. Denniss AR, Richards DA, Cody DV, et al. Prognostic significance of ventricular tachycardia and fibrillation induced at programmed stimulation and delayed potentials detected on the signal-averaged electrocardiograms of survivors of acute myocardial infarction. Circulation 1986; 74:731–745.

1305. Holmes DR Jr, Davis KB, Mock MB, et al. The effect of medical and surgical treatment on subsequent sudden cardiac death in patients with coronary artery disease: a report from the Coronary Artery Surgery Study. Circulation 1986; 73:1254–1263.

1306. Poll DS, Marchlinski FE, Buxton AE, Doherty JU, Waxman HL, Josephson ME. Sustained ventricular tachycardia in patients with idiopathic dilated cardiomyopathy: electrophysiologic testing and lack of response to antiarrhythmic drug therapy. Circulation 1984; 70:451–456.

1307. Kron J, Hart M, Schual-Berke S, Niles NR, Hosenpud JD, McAnulty JH. Idiopathic dilated cardiomyopathy: role of programmed electrical stimulation and Holter monitoring in predicting those at risk of sudden death. Chest 1988; 93:85–90.

1308. Hofmann T, Meinertz T, Kasper W, et al. Mode of death in idiopathic dilated cardiomyopathy: a multivariate analysis of prognostic determinants. Am Heart J 1988; 116:1455–1463.

1309. Olshausen KV, Stienen U, Math D, Schwarz F, Kubler W, Meyer J. Long-term prognostic significance of ventricular arrhythmias in idiopathic dilated cardiomyopathy. Am J Cardiol 1988; 61:146–151.

1310. Burch M, Siddiqi SA, Celermajer DS, Scott C, Bull C, Deanfield JE. Dilated cardiomyopathy in children: determinant of outcome. Br Heart J 1994; 72:246–250.

1311. Romeo F, Cianfrocca C, Pelliccia F, Colloridi V, Cristofani R, Reale A. Long-term prognosis in children with hypertrophic cardiomyopathy: an analysis of 37 patients aged less than or equal to 14 years at diagnosis. Clin Cardiol 1990; 13:101–107.

1312. McKenna WJ, Deanfield JE. Hypertrophic cardiomyopathy: an important cause of sudden death. Arch Dis Child 1984; 59:971–975.

1313. Cecchi F, Maron BJ, Epstein SE. Long-term outcome of patients with hypertrophic cardiomyopathy successfully resuscitated after cardiac arrest. J Am Coll Cardiol 1989; 13:1283–1288.

1314. de Paola AA, Gomes JA, Terzian AB, Miyamoto MH, Martinez Fo EE. Ventricular tachycardia during exercise testing as a predictor of sudden death in patients with chronic chagasic cardiomyopathy and ventricular arrhythmias. Br Heart J 1995; 74:293–295.

1315. Goy JJ, Tauxe F, Fromer M, Schlapfer J, Vogt P, Kappenberger L. Ten-years follow-up of 20 patients with idiopathic ventricular tachycardia. Pacing Clin Electrophysiol 1990; 13:1142–1147.

1316. Mewis C, Kuhlkamp V, Spyridopoulos S, Bosch RF, Seipel L. Late outcome of survivors of idiopathic ventricular fibrillation. Am J Cardiol 1998; 81:999–1003.

1317. Sager PT, Choudhary R, Leon C, Rahimtoola SH, Bhandari AK. The long-term prognosis of patients with out-of-hospital cardiac arrest but no inducible ventricular tachycardia. Am Heart J 1990; 120:1334–1342.

1318. Kim YN, Sousa J, el-Atassi R, Calkins H, Langberg JJ, Morady F. Magnitude of ST segment depression during paroxysmal supraventricular tachycardia. Am Heart J 1991; 122:1486–1487.

1319. Morady F, DiCarlo L, Winston S, Davis JC, Scheinman MM. Clinical features and prognosis of patients with out of hospital cardiac arrest and a normal electrophysiologic study. J Am Coll Cardiol 1984; 4:39–44.

1320. Crandall B, Morris CD, Cutler JE, et al. Implantable cardioverter-defibrillator therapy in survivors of out-of-hospital sudden cardiac death without inducible arrhythmias. J Am Coll Cardiol 1993; 21:1186–1192.

1321. Sharma AD, Klein GJ, Milstein S. Diagnostic assessment of recurrent syncope. PACE 1984; 7:749–759.

1322. Freed LA, Eagle KA, Mahjoub ZA, et al. Gender differences in presentation, management, and cardiac event-free survival in patients with syncope. Am J Cardiol 1997; 80:1183–1187.

1323. Lessmeier TJ, Lehmann MH, Steinman RT, et al. Implantable cardioverter-defibrillator therapy in 300 patients with coronary artery disease presenting exclusively with ventricular fibrillation. Am Heart J 1994; 128:211–218.

1324. Nath S, DeLacey WA, Haines DE, et al. Use of a regional wall motion score to enhance risk stratification of patients receiving an implantable cardioverter-defibrillator. J Am Coll Cardiol 1993; 22:1093–1099.

1325. Gioia G, Bagheri B, Gottlieb CD, et al. Prediction of outcome of patients with life-threatening ventricular arrhythmias treated with automatic implantable cardioverter-defibrillators using SPECT perfusion imaging. Circulation 1997; 95:390–395.

1326. Luceri RM, Habal SM, Castellanos A, Thurer RJ, Waters RS, Brownstein SL. Mechanism of death in patients with the automatic implantable cardioverter defibrillator. Pacing Clin Electrophysiol 1988; 11:2015–2022.

1327. Wellens HJJ. Personal communication, 1997

1328. Cobb LA, Baum RS, Alvarez H III, Schaffer WA. Resuscitation from out-of-hospital ventricular fibrillation: 4 years follow-up. Circulation 1975; 52(Suppl III):III-223–III-235.

1329. Jensen GV, Torp-Pedersen C, Hildebrandt P, et al. Does in-hospital ventricular fibrillation affect prognosis after myocardial infarction? Eur Heart J 1997; 18:919–924.

Atrioventricular
Block[1-5]

Intracardiac electrocardiography, continuous recording of the electrocardiogram, the concept of hemiblocks, and, of course, cardiac pacing significantly advanced our understanding and methods of treating heart block during the second half of the twentieth century. Atrioventricular block was one of the first cardiac arrhythmias studied when His bundle electrocardiography was developed in the late 1960s.[6, 7] We quickly learned to localize block to the atrioventricular node, bundle of His, or bundle branch–fascicular system, and these electrophysiological findings correlated well with clinical and pathological[8] observations. Clinical electrophysiologists then defined more precisely the characteristics of atrioventricular nodal and infranodal conduction with programmed atrial stimulation.[9, 10] Continuous electrocardiographic recording in hospitalized and ambulatory patients revealed more precisely the frequency and characteristics of atrioventricular block, which complicates acute myocardial infarction and occurs during daily life.[11a]

The diseases responsible for atrioventricular block changed as the incidence of rheumatic fever in Western countries decreased. Newly described infections such as Lyme disease and procedures such as cardiac surgery and catheter ablation became occasional causes of temporary or permanent block. Cardiac pathologists found that most acquired atrioventricular block was due to idiopathic fibrosis of the conduction system rather than to coronary heart disease, as was previously assumed.[12] Hemiblocks that may progress to trifascicular block provided electrocardiographic representation of this process.[13, 14]

Few practitioners can now remember when effective pacing was unavailable for the treatment of heart block.[15–20] In 1952, external stimulation was first reported to produce ventricular systole in patients with complete block.[21] Although this method was lifesaving, conscious patients could not tolerate the discomfort of continuous electrical stimulation indefinitely. Within 5 years, stainless steel sutures inserted into the myocardium at surgery and passed through the skin to an external pacemaker provided the means for painlessly activating the heart.[22] This development was followed soon afterward by pacing with transvenously introduced catheters.[23] An implanted system activated by an external radiofrequency generator appeared in 1959,[24] and a totally implanted system was developed 2 years later.[25] Chronic transvenous ventricular pacing followed in the mid-1960s.[26–28]

The early pacers discharged continuously and did not sense intrinsic cardiac activity. Demand ventricular pacing, in which the pacemaker was suppressed when the ventricles beat spontaneously, became available by the late 1960s.[29] Although atrial synchronous pacing was also developed during this decade,[30] its widespread application awaited the development of reliable transvenous atrial leads and the refinement of pacemaker units in the 1970s and 1980s. Pacemakers that respond to physiological needs whatever the atrial rhythm and implantable cardioverter-defibrillators with pacemaking capabilities have found increasing use during the past decade.

Because of improvement in batteries and other elements of the circuits, pacemakers may now work for more than a decade. Only veteran pacerologists remember the problems of broken electrodes and malfunctioning impulse generators and when the lifespan of pacemakers was measured in months. The applications for pacemakers have broadened; although these devices were initially used for treatment of atrioventricular block, more are now inserted—at least in the United States—for abnormalities of sinus node function.[31]

---

[a]The name of Norman J. Holter, D.Sc., has been associated with ambulatory electrocardiography for more than 40 years.[11]

SOME ADVANCES SINCE THE FIRST EDITION OF THIS BOOK

- Atrioventricular block as a complication of nodal ablation for supraventricular tachycardia.
- Factors influencing the relation of atrioventricular block to right ventricular infarction.
- Symptoms suggesting whether atrioventricular block or neurocardiogenic factors produce syncope.
- Indications for pacing in children and adults with congenital complete heart block.

PREVALENCE

First-Degree Atrioventricular Block

The PR interval, which is seldom prolonged beyond normal in young, healthy adults, lengthens beyond 0.20 to 0.24 second as people age, even in those without heart disease:

- In 0.52% of 72,375 asymptomatic, young men in the United States Air Force and the Canadian Air Force.[32, 33]
- In 2% of 4,678 adults older than 20 years in Tecumseh, Michigan.[34]
- In 2.3% of 4,264 patients examined at a general hospital in Atlanta.[35]
- In 3% of 50,000 consecutive patients at a general hospital in Chicago.[36]
- In 5.3% of 1,832 men without obvious heart disease aged 40 to 59 years.[37]
- In 5% of 300 men over the age of 60.[38]
- In 7.2% of 559 persons 85 years of age or older in Tempere, Finland.[39]

When intrinsic heart disease is present, the frequency of first-degree atrioventricular block rises.[40–45b] First-degree atrioventricular block occurs more frequently in healthy children than in adults.[46–48c]

Second-Degree Atrioventricular Block

Second-degree atrioventricular block occasionally occurs in normal healthy subjects.[49] Among the Air Force personnel studied, the arrhythmia was rarely observed,[32, 33] but Wenckebach periods were recorded in 3% to 11% of 335 children studied by ambulatory electrocardiography.[46–48]

Second-degree block was also found

- In 2.7% of 10,000 patients with heart disease.[43]
- In 0.7% of 50,000 patients at a general hospital.[36]
- In 0.7% of 559 subjects aged 85 years or more.[50]

Third-Degree Atrioventricular Block

Complete atrioventricular block occurs rarely in healthy people. It was observed in one of the Air Force personnel,[32, 33] none of the children,[46–48] and 0.4% of the older subjects.[50] Among 100,000 people in Devon, England, the prevalence of third-degree block was 15.6 (0.016%).[51]

The incidence rises in patients with heart disease:

- In 428 patients (0.18%) of 234,286 electrocardiograms taken in adults with and without heart disease.[52–54]
- In 0.5% of 50,000 patients in a general hospital.[36]
- In 8% of 10,000 patients with heart disease.[43]

Congenital complete heart block occurs in 1 of 20,000 to 25,000 live births.[55] The incidence *in utero* is higher.[56d] Of patients evaluated for congenital heart disease at two large children's hospitals, 0.5% had congenital complete heart block.[57, 58e]

Complete atrioventricular block accounts for only a small fraction of cardiac arrests as recorded by emergency rescue squads.[59] Second- or third-degree atrioventricular block caused pauses of 3 or more seconds in 5 (0.2%) of 2,350 consecutive Holter recordings.[60]

AGE

The prevalence of high-degree atrioventricular block increases with age.[51] Acquired complete block appears most frequently in patients during the seventh decade of life (age 60 to 69 years) and somewhat less often in the sixth and eighth decades.[52, 53, 61, 62f] Seventy-eight percent of cases develop in patients who are older than age 50 years.[52, 53, 61, 62]

GENDER

Males develop acquired complete heart block more often than females.[52–54, 61, 62g] Conversely, congenital complete atrioventricular block occurs more often in females.[58, 63–65h]

GENETICS

Atrioventricular block that develops after birth and in adults can be transmitted in a familial manner.[66–73] Atrial septal defect is the most common structural lesion with which familial heart block has been associated.[74–80] Atrioventricular block appeared in two brothers with hypertrophic cardiomyopathy.[81] Familial congenital atrioventricular block, sometimes complete but

---

[b]In 1,359 older patients taken from five series of subjects who were mostly older than the age of 70 years and many of whom had heart disease, the PR interval was long in 10% (range, 3% to 29%).[40–42, 44, 45] In electrocardiograms taken between 1916 and 1930 on 10,000 patients with symptoms or signs of cardiac disease, 3% had prolonged PR intervals.[43]

[c]It was found in 8% to 12% of children aged 7 to 16 years old.[46–48]

[d]Thirty-seven (0.6%) of 6,000 fetuses examined by echocardiography had congenital complete heart block.[56]

[e]One hundred fifty-five cases of congenital complete heart block from 31,786 patients at the Toronto Children's Hospital[57] and the Texas Children's Hospital.[58] Sixty-nine percent had isolated congenital complete heart block, which means that no other structural heart disease was present.

[f]In one series, complete heart block was observed slightly more commonly in patients in their seventies than in those in their sixties.[52]

[g]Of 725 patients in five series, 457 (63%) were male.[52–54, 61, 62] The male-to-female ratio was 1.7:1, with a range of 1.3:1 to 3.9:1.[52–54, 61, 62] In the Devon series, the male-to-female ratio was 1.4:1.

[h]Of 213 patients in four series, 127 (60%) were female.[58, 63–65] The female-to-male ratio was 1.5:1.[58, 63–65]

also of lesser degrees, appears in patients without associated structural heart disease.[66, 73, 82–89] Bifascicular block, which may progress to atrioventricular block, occurs with a familial tendency that becomes more pronounced in older patients.[90]

CLINICAL SETTING (Table 15.1)
Healthy People[91]

Transient atrioventricular block develops, presumably from autonomic imbalance, in some otherwise healthy subjects,[92] in the supine position and resolves when they stand[93–97] or exercise.[94] Conversely, 10.5 seconds of ventricular asystole resulting from paroxysmal high-grade atrioventricular block developed during head-up tilting in a healthy young man who had volunteered for the test.[98]

Coughing,[99–101] hiccups,[102] and swallowing[103–110i] occasionally produce transient atrioventricular block. Even the sight of food has induced heart block.[109] The Valsalva maneuver may produce block, particularly when the sinus rate does not appropriately decrease.[111] Sinus tachycardia may rarely induce atrioventricular block.[112]

First- and second-degree atrioventricular block frequently may appear in well-trained athletes, particularly when they are resting.[91, 113–124] The abnormality disappears soon after they stop training.[117] One case of

---

iIn one case, only after swallowing hot food or liquids.[110]

Table 15.1 **PRINCIPAL CAUSES OF ATRIOVENTRICULAR BLOCK**

Idiopathic progressive fibrosis of the conducting system
  Coronary heart disease
  Acute myocardial infarction
  Chronic coronary heart disease
Congenital heart disease
  Congenital complete atrioventricular block
  Atrial septal defect
  Corrected transposition of the great vessels
Aortic and mitral valve disease
Infections
  Lyme disease
  Infective endocarditis
  Chagas myocarditis
Rheumatological disease
  Acute rheumatic fever
  Rheumatoid arthritis
Cardiomyopathy
  Alcoholic
  Amyloidosis
  Congestive
  Hemochromatosis
  Hypertrophic
  Sarcoidosis
Cardiac surgery
Cardiac catheterization
Drugs
  Adenosine
  Antiarrhythmic drugs
  Digitalis
Endocrine and metabolic disorders
  Hyperkalemia
  Hyperthyroidism
Tumors

high-grade block causing syncope developed during exercise in a triathlon athlete.[125] A few healthy adults develop first-, second-, or rarely third-degree atrioventricular block during sleep.[126–128j]

Fibrosis of Conducting Tissue

Idiopathic progressive fibrosis of the atrioventricular conducting system is the most common cause of acquired chronic atrioventricular block.[12, 129–132] This condition should be suspected in patients with no evidence of clinical heart disease other than the arrhythmia.[133–135k]

Acute Myocardial Infarction[136–140]

First-degree atrioventricular block occurs in 8.5%, second-degree atrioventricular block in 4.8%, and complete atrioventricular block in 7.1% of patients with acute myocardial infarction who are admitted to coronary care units.[141–169l] Complete heart block develops in 10% of patients with inferior myocardial infarctions[142, 158, 166, 170–180m] and in 2% of those with anterior myocardial infarctions.[158, 160, 174n]

When compared with patients who do not develop atrioventricular block during myocardial infarction, those with block are older,[168, 175, 178, 180–182] and they are more likely to be women[181, 182] and to have the following:

---

jFour of 50 male medical students had PR intervals as long as 0.33 second, and 3 developed second-degree block.[127]
kWhen the presence of organic heart disease cannot be established, arrhythmias may be described as being due to electrical heart disease,[133] and conduction disturbances may be attributed to primary conduction disease[135] or idiopathic heart block.[134]
lFirst-degree atrioventricular block, in 238 of 2,812 patients in 10 series,[142, 145–147, 153–155, 157, 158, 163] second-degree atrioventricular block, in 149 of 3,112 patients in 11 series,[142, 145–147, 153–158, 163] and third-degree atrioventricular block, in 458 of 6,433 patients in 21 series.[142, 143, 145–149, 151, 153–158, 160–165, 167] In another very large, multihospital series from the Worcester, Massachusetts metropolitan area,[169] 5.8% of 4,762 patients with acute myocardial infarction developed complete heart block. The rate did not substantially change during six of the years from 1975 to 1988. Some investigators combined second- and third-degree block in their reports, and these results are not included.[144, 150, 152, 159]
All series reported results from continuous electrocardiographic monitoring. However, the amount of attention given to the electrocardiographic strips varied, and true incidences may be higher. The occurrence of third-degree atrioventricular block is probably the most accurate. Fleeting periods of PR prolongation[166] and second-degree block can easily be missed and, even when noted, may not have been reported in patients who also developed complete block.
The incidence of atrioventricular block discovered in patients with acute myocardial infarction before continuous monitoring became available was much lower. For example, in a report from 1938, second- and third-degree block could be observed in only 3.2% of 375 cases.[141] The same authors reported that the incidence of complete block during myocardial infarction was about 1.5% from 1923 to 1938.[141]
mIn inferior myocardial infarction, 602 of 5,142 patients in 10 series.[142, 158, 171–175, 178, 180] The range was 8% to 24%. In other series in which the highest degree of block is designated as advanced or high-grade and includes both second- and third-degree block, the incidence was 17%—91 of 529 patients.[166, 170, 176, 177] A review of 2,559 patients with inferior infarctions from 16 series revealed that 19% developed second- or third-degree atrioventricular block.[179]
nIn anterior myocardial infarction, 16 of 863 cases.[158, 160, 174]

- Atrial fibrillation.[183]
- Bundle branch block.[178, 180, 183, 184]
- Higher levels of serum glutamic-oxaloacetic transaminase[168, 175] and total creatine phosphokinase.[178, 180, 185]
- Left ventricular failure,[178, 180–182] pulmonary edema,[186] and cardiomegaly.[181]
- Killip class greater than 1.[183]
- Reduced left ventricular and right ventricular function.[175, 177, 178, 180o]
- Right ventricular infarction.[176, 187]
- Sustained hypotension.[186]
- Ventricular tachycardia and ventricular fibrillation.[186]

The syndrome of right ventricular infarction increases the incidence of atrioventricular block beyond that expected with other inferior infarctions.[176, 187p] Pre-infarction angina reduces threefold the likelihood of having complete block during right ventricular infarction.[188] Block rarely accompanies non–Q-wave (subendocardial) infarction.[189]

Thrombolytic therapy does not affect the incidence of heart block during acute inferior myocardial infarction.[190] Those who develop block are more likely to be women[182] and to be in Killip class 2 or greater.[182]

Onset of atrioventricular block. Fourteen percent of patients with inferior myocardial infarction and 2% of those with anterior myocardial infarction have atrioventricular block when examined in mobile coronary care units within 2 hours after the beginning of symptoms.[152] The arrhythmia appears in 41% of patients with acute infarction who will develop high-grade atrioventricular block by the time they are admitted to the hospital. By the end of 24 hours, 61% of those who develop block will have done so.[147, 158, 163, 166, 170, 173, 175, 178, 189, 191q] Most of the remaining cases appear by the end of the fifth day.[147, 158, 163, 166, 170, 173, 175, 178]

Complete atrioventricular block appears most often during the first hospital day.[163] High-grade atrioventricular block that develops within 6 to 24 hours after the onset of inferior myocardial infarction tends to end sooner—often lasting for only a few minutes to no longer than 1 hour—than when it appears later.[166, 173, 191r] When block develops early, high-grade block usually appears suddenly without noticeable first-degree block beforehand; in later block, PR prolongation often precedes higher degrees of block.[166]

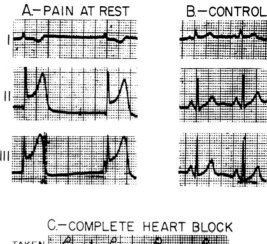
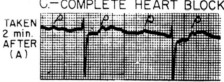

FIGURE 15.1 **Prinzmetal's variant angina (A)** producing complete atrioventricular block **(C)**. Lead I, II, and III tracings taken about an hour after onset of pain **(B)**. (Adapted from Prinzmetal M, Kennamer R, Merliss R, Wada T, Bor N. Angina pectoris: a variant form of angina pectoris. Am J Med 1959; 27:375–388, with permission.)[202]

Chronic Coronary Heart Disease

Although acute myocardial infarction is an important cause of transient atrioventricular block, chronic coronary heart disease infrequently produces persistent complete atrioventricular block.[52–54, 61, 62, 129, 192–200s]

Angina pectoris. Transient atrioventricular block rarely occurs in patients with standard angina pectoris,[201] but all degrees of block may develop during episodes of variant angina caused by coronary vasospasm (Fig. 15.1).[202–214]

Congenital Heart Disease

Congenital complete atrioventricular block.[2, 55, 57, 215–219] Most children and adults with congenital complete heart block have no structural heart disease. However, about 30% of children with the arrhythmia diagnosed at birth have structural heart disease,[55] most frequently[55]

- Endomyocardial fibrosis.
- Atrioventricular inversion.
- Atrioventricular septal defects.

---

oWomen may[178] or may not[175, 180] develop heart block more frequently than men with inferior myocardial infarction. A history of previous myocardial infarctions does not appear to increase the likelihood of developing heart block with inferior myocardial infarction.[178, 180]

pA high degree of atrioventricular nodal block developed in 14 (48%) of 29 patients with right ventricular infarction but in only 5 (13%) of 38 patients with inferior infarction and no right ventricular involvement.[176]

qOne hundred seventeen (41%) of 285 cases on admission,[147, 163, 175, 191] and 293 (61%) of 480 cases by 24 hours.[147, 158, 166, 170, 173, 175, 178, 189]

rEarly versus late atrioventricular block has been defined by time[166, 173] and by electrocardiographic signs.[191]

sFor example, in 25 patients with acquired nonsurgical complete heart block, coronary arteriography revealed significant obstruction in only 6 patients.[199] In 30 other patients with complete heart block, severe coronary disease was observed in 13.[200] Until the 1960s, when investigators discovered the importance of fibrosis of the conduction system, most observers thought that coronary heart disease was the principal cause of atrioventricular block.[52–54, 61, 62, 192–195, 197] Maurice Campbell, however, recognized, in 1944, that many of his patients who had what he called myocardial disease often had little coronary disease.[61]

Congenital heart block also occurs in association with long QT syndrome,[220-222] hydrops fetalis,[223, 224] and neonatal lupus syndrome.[225, 226]

The mothers of about half[227] the children with congenital complete heart block have, when their affected children are born, connective tissue disease, most frequently lupus erythematosus but also primary Sjögren's syndrome or undifferentiated autoimmune syndrome.[58, 88, 220, 227-240t] Nevertheless, clinical disturbances of atrioventricular conduction are uncommon among the children of women with systemic lupus erythematosus.[241]

Atrial septal defect. The PR interval is often slightly,[242-247] and rarely greatly,[243, 248] prolonged in patients with secundum atrial septal defects. It exceeded 0.22 second in 18% in one group of children and adults.[249] PR intervals in children with atrial septal defect are often less than 0.2 second but are longer than those in children of similar age without heart disease.[250-252]

Corrected transposition of the great vessels.[253-261] Atrioventricular block of all degrees appears in more than 75% of patients with congenitally corrected transposition of the great vessels,[2] and spontaneous complete atrioventricular block develops in 21%.[262u] Complete atrioventricular block is present at birth in 4% and develops at a rate of about 2% per year. Atrioventricular block appears in more than twice as many patients with intact ventricular septa than in those with ventricular septal defects,[262] although one report suggested that corrected transposition, ventricular septal defect, and atrioventricular block forms a "clinical triad."[263]

Miscellaneous conditions. Atrioventricular block appears in some patients with atrioventricular canal[264-266v] and Ebstein's anomaly of the tricuspid valve.[267-270] Partial atrioventricular block occurs rarely in association with the congenital long QT interval syndrome.[271]

Valve Disease

Atrioventricular block, usually only PR interval prolongation, occasionally occurs in mitral valve prolapse,[272, 273] although one group of investigators reported that up to 10% of patients have first-degree block.[274] In what is probably a unique setting, atrial pacing exposed atrioventricular conduction in 11 members of a family with a high prevalence of mitral valve prolapse.[275]

A few patients with aortic stenosis, and less frequently mitral stenosis or regurgitation, develop heart block from extension of valvular calcification into the

conducting system.[276-279w] The presence of mitral annular calcification increases the likelihood that patients older than 60 years of age with aortic stenosis will develop heart block.[280] Atrioventricular conduction disturbances occur more often in patients with mitral annular calcification than in patients of similar age without this lesion.[281]

Infections

Lyme disease.[282] The heart is affected in about 8% of patients with Lyme disease, and transient atrioventricular block is the most frequently observed abnormality.[283-290x] Of those with block, 98% have first-degree block, 40% have Wenckebach periods, and 50% have complete block,[291] which develops when the PR interval during first-degree block exceeds 0.30 second.[283] Complete block rarely persists longer than 1 week,[292] and most patients regain normal conduction after successful treatment.[292]

Infective endocarditis. First- or second-degree block or both occurs in 6% and complete atrioventricular block occurs in about 3% of patients with active endocarditis on native valves.[293-295y] Heart block occurs more often with infection of the aortic valve than with infection of the mitral valve.[294, 295]

Myocarditis. Viral and nonspecific myocarditis occasionally produces atrioventricular block.[296-300] Atrioventricular block frequently develops in patients with Chagas disease.[301, 302] Cases of high-grade atrioventricular block have been reported in patients with chronic paragonimiasis, in which the trematode parasite *Paragonimus westermani* produces calcified granulomas in the heart,[303] and in *Toxoplasma* myocarditis.[304]

Other infections. Diphtheria[54, 192] and syphilis[61, 192] were formerly reported to produce either acute or chronic atrioventricular block. Atrioventricular block rarely complicates acute streptococcal tonsillitis in the absence of acute rheumatic fever.[305-307]

Rheumatological Diseases

Acute rheumatic fever. Acute rheumatic fever characteristically prolongs the PR interval when carditis develops.[305, 307-309] Atrioventricular block may be the first sign of rheumatic fever.[310]

First-degree atrioventricular block is the most frequent significant electrocardiographic abnormality in rheumatic fever[311] and appears in about 30% of patients within the first 2 weeks after the illness begins.[312] The overall incidence is greater[313, 314] and can reach 95% when electrocardiograms are taken frequent-

---

*t*In a series of 23 asymptomatic mothers of children born with congenital complete heart block, 11 (48%) eventually developed rheumatic complaints or fulfilled diagnostic criteria for a rheumatic disease.[227]

*u*From a series of 107 patients from the Mayo Clinic.[262]

*v*Most of the long PR intervals are caused, however, by prolonged conduction from the sinus node to the atrioventricular node.[265, 266]

*w*Second- or third-degree atrioventricular block complicated the course of 8 (2.1%) of 397 patients with aortic stenosis; first-degree block was present in 42 (11%) of them.[278]

*x*Eighteen of 20 patients (90%) with Lyme disease and cardiac involvement had some degree of atrioventricular block.[283]

*y*From two series of 353 episodes of bacterial endocarditis.[293, 295]

ly.[311, 315–317z] Second-degree block is occasionally observed, but complete block is rare.[311, 314, 318, 319aa]

Other conditions. Atrioventricular block develops occasionally in ankylosing spondylitis,[320–323] polymyositis,[324–326] progressive systemic sclerosis,[327, 328] Reiter syndrome,[329–333] rheumatoid arthritis,[334] and lupus erythematosus.[335–338]

Cardiomyopathy

Infiltrative cardiomyopathies such as amyloidosis,[339–342bb] familial amyloidosis with polyneuropathy,[343–346] hemochromatosis,[347–352] and sarcoidosis[353–368cc] produce atrioventricular block by replacement of the conducting system with the foreign material and the associated edema, necrosis, and fibrosis. Atrioventricular block seldom develops in patients with alcoholic cardiomyopathy[369] or congestive dilated cardiomyopathy, but it has been reported in patients with hypertrophic cardiomyopathy.[81, 370–372]

Cardiac Surgery

Heart block, usually transient and of varying degrees, develops after cardiac surgery from traumatic and ischemic damage to the atrioventricular conducting system. Replacement of the aortic valve is the cardiac operation that most frequently produces atrioventricular block in adults.[373–376] The arrhythmia less often follows replacement of the mitral valve[377] and develops more often with repeated valve surgery than after the first operation.[378]

Coronary artery bypass graft operations seldom produce atrioventricular block unless an acute myocardial infarction occurs during or soon after the operation.[dd] When it does occur, the preoperatively demonstrated lesions most likely to be found are in the left anterior descending coronary artery, compromising flow in the first perforator.[379] Atrioventricular block occasionally develops after cardiac transplantation but much less often than does sick sinus syndrome.[380, 381]

In children, postoperative heart block may follow surgical correction of such lesions as ventricular septal defect and tetralogy of Fallot.[382, 383] Improvements in

technique have reduced the incidence of atrioventricular block after cardiac surgery.[384]

Congenital heart disease.[385ee] Atrioventricular block develops after repair of several congenital lesions, particularly those in the region of the conducting system, including

- Endocardial cushion malformations, such as primum atrial septal defects and complete common atrioventricular canal.
- Ventricular septal defects occurring alone or with tetralogy of Fallot, complete transposition of the great arteries, and congenitally corrected transposition of the great arteries.
- Tricuspid valve abnormalities as in Ebstein's anomaly.

Atrioventricular block is usually temporary, presumably from local inflammation related to the operation, but occasionally the block persists. Permanent atrioventricular block can appear long after the operation and occurs most frequently in patients who had transient block soon after the operation.

Cardiac Catheterization

Intracardiac catheters, even the soft Swan-Ganz catheter,[386] occasionally produce temporary, and rarely permanent, atrioventricular block when passed through the right ventricle especially in patients with preexisting left bundle branch block.[387–395] Balloon dilatation of pulmonary valve stenosis produced permanent complete block in a 5-year-old child.[396]

Catheter Ablation

Interrupting or modifying conduction in the atrioventricular junction to treat various atrial and supraventricular tachyarrhythmias produces atrioventricular block either intentionally or as a complication of the treatment. Specifically, temporary[397–403] and, rarely, permanent[400–410] atrioventricular block may follow ablation of atrial foci in patients with atrial tachycardia[411] and atrioventricular nodal and accessory pathways in those with supraventricular tachycardia.

Drugs

Many drugs prescribed for patients with heart disease can produce atrioventricular block[412] (Table 15.2).

Adenosine. In addition to those listed in Table 15.2, adenosine can produce transient atrioventricular block[413] during thallium imaging.[414] Patients with syncope from atrioventricular block are more likely to develop block when given adenosine than are those with syncope due to sick sinus syndrome.[415] This re-

---

[z]Atropine sulfate temporarily restores normal PR intervals in most cases,[316, 317] a finding suggesting that at least part of the block may be due to the acute illness.

[aa]Of 508 patients with acute rheumatic fever, 12 developed Wenckebach second-degree atrioventricular block, and 3 developed complete atrioventricular block.[314]

[bb]Of 40 patients with amyloidosis studied at autopsy, 40% had some degree of atrioventricular block, and 13% had complete block.[342] Complete atrioventricular block developed during life in 25 of 89 (28%) patients with cardiac sarcoidosis whose hearts were studied at autopsy.[360]

[cc]In Japan, the majority of sarcoid-related deaths are cardiac, which was the presumptive cause of high-degree atrioventricular block in 10 (11.2%) of 89 Japanese patients, most of whom were women aged 40 to 69 years.[368]

[dd]I conclude this from my own experience and because writers discussing coronary artery bypass grafting rarely refer to heart block produced by the operation.

[ee]Interested readers should read the recent (1998) and fully referenced chapter on heart block after surgery for congenital heart disease by Natterson, Perloff, Klitzner, and Stephenson.[385]

| Table 15.2 | CARDIAC DRUGS THAT MAY PRODUCE ATRIOVENTRICULAR BLOCK[412] |

Antiarrhythmic drugs, by classes
  IA: disopyramide, quinidine, procainamide
  IC: flecainide, propafenone
  II: beta-adrenergic–blocking drugs, adrenergic blockers
  III: amiodarone, bretylium, sotalol
  IV: calcium-channel blockers (diltiazem and verapamil)
Digitalis

(From Bigger JT Jr, Hoffman BF. Antiarrhythmic drugs. In Gilman AG, Rall TW, Nies AS, Taylor P (eds). The Pharmacological Basis of Therapeutics. 8th ed. New York: Pergamon Press, 1990, p. 847.)

| Table 15.3 | TUMORS REPORTED TO PRODUCE ATRIOVENTRICULAR BLOCK[429–431] |

Arterial angioma[432]
Atrioventricular nodal tumors, including
    mesothelioma[433, 443–445, 449–452, 454, 455, 457–459]
Hemangioendothelioblastoma[434]
Hodgkin's disease[440]
Leukemia[435]
Lymphoma[460]
Malignant granular cell myoblastoma[456]
Malignant melanoma[446]
Malignancies metastatic to the heart[436–439, 441, 442, 447]
Reticulum cell sarcoma[448]
Rhabdomyosarcoma[453]

(Data from references 429, 430, and 431.)

sponse may have diagnostic value when determining the cause of syncope of unknown origin.

Interleukin-2. Given to a woman with metastatic renal cell carcinoma, interleukin-2 induced complete atrioventricular block.[416]

Lidocaine. By suppressing escape foci during atrioventricular block complicating inferior infarction, lidocaine, thought to be particularly safe to use during myocardial infarction, can produce severe bradycardia or asystole.[417] Lidocaine can also induce high degrees of atrioventricular block by prolonging conduction in His-Purkinje tissues.[418]

Endocrine and Metabolic Disorders

Hyperthyroidism[419–422] and hyperparathyroidism[423, 424] may occasionally produce atrioventricular block. Hyperkalemia[425] and hypermagnesemia may induce atrioventricular block.[426] Addison's disease often lengthens the PR interval and may contribute to the production of heart block.[427, 428ff]

Tumors[429–431]

Benign and malignant tumors that invade the heart may rarely produce atrioventricular block[432–460] (Table 15.3).

Sleep

The degree of atrioventricular block present when awake may increase during sleep; first- and second-degree block usually worsen during the rapid eye movement phase.[461] Obstructive apnea during sleep may produce atrioventricular block including complete block.[462–464]

Exercise

Exercise may occasionally produce, or worsen the degree of, atrioventricular block.[194, 465–472]

---

ffThe cause has never been established. Changes in autonomic tone or the slight increase in potassium produced by adrenal insufficiency may prolong atrioventricular nodal conduction. Appropriate treatment for Addison's disease shortens PR intervals, as does Cushing's disease.[428]

Miscellaneous Conditions

Atrioventricular block of varying degrees has been occasionally reported in several other conditions[370, 473–501] (Table 15.4).

OTHER ARRHYTHMIAS IN PATIENTS WITH HEART BLOCK

Sick Sinus Syndrome

Many patients with atrioventricular block have abnormalities of sinus nodal function that can be recognized clinically or after invasive study.[422, 502–509gg] Although some also develop chronotropic incompetence in which the sinus node no longer responds normally to exercise,[510] clinical sick sinus syndrome develops infrequently.[511] Sinus bradycardia, presumably reflecting sick sinus syndrome, and complete heart block may also occur simultaneously on a congenital basis.[505]

---

ggIn 59 patients studied with electrophysiological techniques, 42% with atrioventricular disease had sinoatrial disease, and 55% with sick sinus syndrome had some degree of atrioventricular block.[508] See Chapter 16 for further information about this association.

| Table 15.4 | OCCASIONAL CAUSES OF ATRIOVENTRICULAR BLOCK |

A patient drinking alcohol[481]
Carcinoid heart disease[498]
Echinococcosis[501]
Fabry disease[496, 497]
Gout[477]
Guillain-Barré syndrome[492]
Interventricular septal hydatid cyst[500]
Kearns-Sayre syndrome (myocardial fibrosis, atypical retinitis pigmentosa, and external ophthalmoplegia)[483, 490, 495]
Marfan syndrome[370]
Muscular dystrophy[485, 489, 493, 494a]
Myotonic dystrophy[474, 475, 482, 484, 485]
Obesity and sleep apnea[488]
Primary oxalosis[479]
Primary pulmonary hypertension[487]
Rejection after cardiac transplantation[499]
Sialorrhea[473]
Trauma[476, 478, 480, 486]
Wegener's granulomatosis[491]

aAmong 892 patients with chronic complete heart block, only 0.7% had neuromuscular disease.[485]

Atrial Fibrillation[hh]

Patients with rheumatic carditis are more likely to develop atrial fibrillation when first-degree atrioventricular block is present than when the PR interval is normal.[512]

Torsades de Pointes and QT Prolongation

The bradycardia of acquired complete atrioventricular block predisposes patients,[513, 514] women more often than men,[514] to torsades de pointes. Atrioventricular block can develop in patients with long QT intervals who may also have ventricular, including polymorphic ventricular, tachycardia.[515–518]

PATIENT HISTORY

Syncope

The most dramatic symptom associated with atrioventricular block is syncope, the essential event of the Morgagni-Adams-Stokes syndrome.[54, 62, 519] Paul Wood described such episodes with his characteristic flair:[520]

> Loss of consciousness is abrupt, without warning. If standing, the patient collapses, and lies limp, still, pale and pulseless, with fixed, dilated pupils—as if dead; breathing, however, continues. If the attack lasts long enough, i.e. for more than 10 seconds or so, twitchings commence, and may progress to convulsions; and if ventricular asystole continues for more than two or three minutes, recovery is rare. As a rule, however, ventricular beating is resumed after a few seconds, consciousness returns abruptly, and a vivid flush ensues. When an attack occurs in bed, the lack of warning, short duration of unconsciousness, and abrupt return of full possession of the faculties, may prevent a dull patient from being aware of the fit, and he may only notice the flush. The sequence of events, both symptomatically and objectively, is so characteristic as to make the diagnosis probable on the history alone.

First-degree block never produces syncope, second-degree block seldom causes it, and not every patient with chronic third-degree heart block develops it.[194, 521–523] As Paul White observed in the final (fourth) edition of his cardiology text:[521]

> Much has been written in the past about the *Morgagni-Adams-Stokes* syndrome, perhaps too much in view of its rarity.[ii]

Or as Charles K. Friedberg wrote in the last (1966) edition of his text:[524]

[hh]See Chapter 4 for detailed discussion of this combination.

[ii]If we restrict the definition of Morgagni-Adams-Stokes syndrome to those patients who faint because of complete heart block, then White's admonition remains correct. In patients with intrinsic heart disease, ventricular tachyarrhythmias cause syncope much more frequently than does complete heart block. For example, the cardiovascular cause of syncope in 71 elderly patients was ventricular tachycardia in 33 and complete atrioventricular block only in 5.[523] Of 186 patients with syncope and bifascicular block, atrioventricular block was implicated in 5 cases.[522] Whether to include episodes of syncope from causes other than heart block under the rubric of Adams-Stokes disease remains a point of some controversy among physicians with literary and historical proclivities.

It is important to stress that the Adams-Stokes syndrome is not an invariable consequence of complete heart block. . . . Adams-Stokes attacks have been reported to occur in 35 to 70 per cent of cases of complete heart block studied in various hospital series. But it is apparent that many asymptomatic patients with complete heart block would not be included in such statistics.

Adams-Stokes attacks occur with particular frequency when partial atrioventricular block becomes complete.[519] In some patients, however, syncope that developed during the transition between partial and complete heart block may cease when permanent block becomes established.[194, 525]

Syncope occurs more often when the QRS complexes of the escape beats in complete block are wide rather than narrow.[193] Accordingly, fainting is uncommon in patients with congenital complete heart block, most of whom have narrow QRS complexes,[193, 526–528] except in those with excessively slow ventricular rates[65] and idioventricular or multiform escape beats.[57, 529] Patients with congenital complete heart block rarely faint during exercise when the ventricular rate is relatively rapid.[530]

One must always remember that syncope in patients with complete heart block, whether or not they are being paced, is often caused by ventricular tachycardia or ventricular fibrillation, rather than by severe bradycardia or asystole.[531] In addition, neurocardiogenic influences commonly cause syncope. Certain features of the clinical history help one to decide whether the cause is an arrhythmia or neurocardiogenic[532] (Table 15.5).

Other Symptoms

During transient atrioventricular block, patients may experience dizziness[533] and lightheadedness. However, these symptoms occur so frequently and from so many different causes that they are seldom helpful by themselves in identifying patients with heart block.

The slow heart rate of chronic complete atrioventricular block can decrease cardiac output sufficiently to cause patients to develop dyspnea on exertion, weakness, faintness, and reduced cerebral function.[61] Congestive heart failure was present in 26 of 100 patients

Table 15.5	**SYMPTOMS AND FINDINGS SUGGESTING CAUSE OF SYNCOPE**[532]		
	Neurocardiogenic Syncope	
Atrioventricular Block or Ventricular Tachycardia		*Before Fainting*	*After Fainting*
Male gender		Blurred vision	Fatigue
Age >54 years		Lightheadedness	Nausea
<3 episodes of syncope		Nausea	Sweating
Warning of <6 seconds		Palpitations	Warmth
		Sweating	
		Warmth	

(From Calkins H, Shyr Y, Frumin H, Schork A, Morady F. The value of the clinical history in the differentiation of syncope due to ventricular tachycardia, atrioventricular block, and neurocardiogenic syncope. Am J Med 1995; 98:365–373.)

with heart block and Adams-Stokes syndrome,[197] and, occasionally, it is the predominant clinical feature of heart block.[197]

Up to 25% of patients with complete heart block report palpitations.[62] However, patients seldom have angina pectoris during complete atrioventricular block.[194]

Absence of symptoms. Some patients deny having any symptoms directly related to the arrhythmia, and complete heart block may be first discovered at routine physical examination.[52, 53, 61] As Maurice Campbell observed in 1944:[534]

> It is surprising and significant that so many patients with complete heart block seem relatively well and are able to lead quiet lives, almost normal for their age, providing that they do not suffer from Stokes-Adams attacks. One common type is the elderly man with gray hair and thickened arteries who has led a strenuous and sometimes intellectual life, often with hardly a day's illness.[jj]

Most patients with isolated congenital complete heart block are asymptomatic[65, 527] and have normal or almost normal physical working capacity.[535-537] Some engage in vigorous activities without symptoms[535, 538-540] and can sustain pregnancy through delivery without complication.[541-545]

PHYSICAL EXAMINATION

Heart block produces abnormal physical findings during physical examination[2, 215, 546, 547] because of the slow heart rate and the dissociation between atrial and ventricular contraction.[kk]

Arterial Pulse

The arterial pulse is more forceful or fuller and the upstroke is quicker in patients with complete heart block and otherwise normal hearts than in those with sinus rhythm. The systolic pressure is often higher, the diastolic pressure lower, and the pulse pressure greater when complete heart block is present.[52, 61, 62, 548] Although slower heart rates may be expected to produce larger pulse pressures in patients with complete heart block, one study suggested no significant relationship between the two findings.[52]

The amplitude of the arterial pulse may vary from beat to beat. The strongest pulse occurs after normal

---

[jj]According to two series from the 1950s, 50%[53] to 65%[52] of cases of complete heart block are first discovered during routine examinations. Most of the clinical literature that reports the symptoms of patients with complete block was published before the development of contemporary electrocardiographic monitoring and cardiac pacemakers. The use of pacing in patients discovered to have atrioventricular block but no syncope has probably changed the clinical presentation of complete block, but I have found no reports in the pacemaker era comparable to those of earlier times to confirm this impression.

[kk]Physicians report the physical examination of children and young adults with congenital complete heart block more fully than of older patients with acquired block. I have discussed the findings in both groups in this section.

atrial filling and filling of the ventricles and corresponds to PR intervals of about 0.12 to 0.31 second.[549] Atrial impulses may be transmitted to the peripheral arterial pulse.[550]

Venous Pulse

Atrioventricular block affects the size of the A wave that is produced by right atrial contraction and the relation between the A wave and the V wave that occurs during ventricular contraction. To time the waveforms accurately, one should gently palpate the carotid artery or listen to the heart while watching the venous pulses.

As the PR interval lengthens in first-degree atrioventricular block, the time between the A wave and the V wave lengthens. If the PR interval is sufficiently long, occurring usually between the QRS and T waves, constant giant A waves can appear as the right atrium contracts when the tricuspid valve is closed.[551]

When a ventricular beat is dropped during second-degree atrioventricular block, no V wave is seen. Large cannon A waves appear intermittently.

In complete heart block, the A waves occur more rapidly than the arterial pulse, without apparent correlation between the two. It is in complete block that cannon A waves are detected most frequently[215, 527, 552] (Fig. 15.2). This finding was reported for the first time in English by William Stokes in 1846:[552]

> A new symptom has appeared, namely, a very remarkable pulsation in the right jugular vein. This is most evident when the patient is lying down. The number of the reflex pulsations . . . are more than double the number of the manifest ventricular contractions. About every third pulsation is very strong and sudden, and may be seen at a distance; the remaining waves are much less distinct.

Heart Sounds

First sound. The amplitude of the first heart sound varies with different PR intervals[553] (Fig. 15.3). This

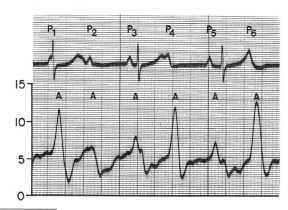

FIGURE 15.2 Large a waves in a patient with congenital complete heart block. When the right atrium contracts while the tricuspid valve is closed (P waves 1, 4, 6), large A waves appear in the right atrial tracing and in the jugular venous pulse. The pressure, recorded in the right atrium, is measured in millimeters of mercury. (Adapted from Ayers CR, Boineau JP, Spach MS. Congenital complete heart block in children. Am Heart J 1966; 72:381–390, with permission.)[215]

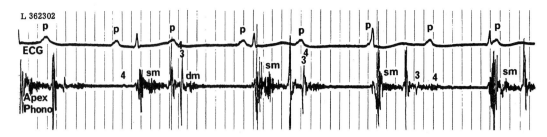

FIGURE 15.3 **Changing heart sounds and murmurs in complete heart block.** In this phonocardiographic record, the amplitude of the first and fourth heart sounds and the systolic murmurs (sm) depends on the relationship of the P waves and the QRS complexes. Notice the loud summation gallop associated with the fifth P wave when the third and fourth heart sounds occur at the same time. dm, diastolic murmur. (Adapted from Tavel ME. Variation of the systolic murmur of complete heart block. N Engl J Med 1966; 274:1298–1300, with permission.)[553]

may be difficult to discern in first-degree atrioventricular block. However, in Wenckebach second-degree block, the first heart sound clearly dims as the PR interval lengthens; then it suddenly returns to maximal intensity, as the *bruit de canon*,[194][u] when the first conducted beat occurs after the dropped beat. Rarely, the nonconducted beat is associated with a loud first sound from an atrial echo.[554]

In complete heart block, the varying intensity of the first sound is a characteristic feature of the physical examination.[527, 549, 555, 556][mm] The first sound is loudest when the PR interval is short and becomes softer as the PR interval lengthens.[549, 557, 558] In children, the first sound may intensify at PR intervals longer than 0.30 second.[558, 559] This finding is seldom observed in adults.[560] When the atria fibrillate, the loudness of the first heart sound does not change from beat to beat.[62, 561]

Second sound. The splitting of the second heart sound can indicate the location of the escape beats in complete heart block. Normal splitting suggests that the escape focus is in the atrioventricular junction, probably the bundle of His, and that the QRS complex has normal width.[561]

Idioventricular escape beats produce abnormal splitting.[561] Patients with escape beats in the form of left bundle branch block may have reversed splitting of the second heart sound, whereas physiological but widely split second sounds can be produced by escape beats that look like right bundle branch block.[562]

Third and fourth sounds. Fourth heart sounds, which coincide with atrial contraction, may be heard throughout diastole during complete heart block[550, 563] (see Fig. 15.3). Summation gallops can appear when atrial contraction occurs during rapid ventricular filling.

Murmurs

Functional systolic ejection murmurs are frequently heard in patients with complete heart block and otherwise normal hearts.[536] Careful auscultation reveals that the systolic murmur is louder during cycles when atrial contraction augments ventricular filling[553] (see Fig. 15.3). Apical diastolic murmurs, probably produced by the large stroke volume traversing the mitral valve,[527] are commonly heard in children with congenital complete heart block and occasionally in elderly adults with acquired complete block.[564, 565]

ELECTROCARDIOGRAPHY

Rates

Ventricular rate. The average ventricular rate of 610 patients with complete heart block was 40.1 beats per minute.[52, 54, 61, 62][nn] Rates of fewer than 20 to more than 89 beats per minute have been observed.

The ventricular rates of patients with acute myocardial infarction and complete atrioventricular block range from fewer than 30 beats per minute to greater than 70 beats per minute. Even with inferior infarcts, the escape rates may be lower than 40 beats per minute despite the general dogma that ventricular rates in such patients are not excessively slow.[566][oo]

The ventricular rates in children, whose complete heart block is usually congenital, are faster than in older patients with acquired block. The range is typically 45 to 60 beats per minute at rest.[57][pp] Asymptomatic adolescents and adults with complete congenital heart block have faster ventricular rates than those with syncope or other symptoms.[63] In one 19-year-old patient with complete heart block, presumably congenital, the ventricular rate was slower at night than during the day.[567] The ventricular rate of infants, children, and adults with congenital complete heart block characteristically decreases with increasing age[63, 530, 568] (Table 15.6).

---

[u]French for "cannon sound," so named because of its explosive quality.[194]

[mm]However, one is struck by the inconstant reporting of this and other physical signs of patients with heart block. For example, in a study of 61 infants and children with complete block, the intensity of the first heart sound changed in only 38 of 61 cases, and cannon A waves were seen in only 33.[555] Are these observations correct, or were the findings overlooked on physical examination?

[nn]From four series of patients without pacemakers.[52, 54, 61, 62]

[oo]Forty-two of 94 patients (44%) with complete block of dissociation and acute infarction, most inferior, had ventricular rates no greater than 40 beats per minute.[566]

[pp]Among 57 patients from a pediatric hospital, the average rate was 55 beats per minute.[555]

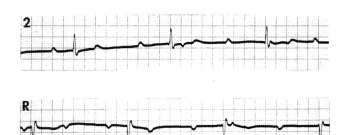

FIGURE 15.4 Ventriculoatrial conduction during complete atrioventricular block. Notice the inverted P wave that follows the second QRS complex in lead II and the upright P wave that follows the third QRS complex in R. These slightly premature beats are produced by abnormal atrial activation from the lower to the upper parts of the atria.

Table 15.6	VENTRICULAR RATES AT DIFFERENT AGES IN PATIENTS WITH CONGENITAL COMPLETE ATRIOVENTRICULAR BLOCK[530]	
Age (Years)		Ventricular Rate (Beats per Minute)
15		46
16–20		43
21–30		41
>40		39

(From Michaelsson M, Jonzon A, Riesenfeld T. Isolated congenital complete atrioventricular block in adult life: a prospective study. Circulation 1995; 92:442–449. By permission of the American Heart Association, Inc.)

Atrial rate. The rate of sinus rhythm is faster than, and bears no arithmetical relationship to, the ventricular rate in patients with complete heart block. Most data about atrial rates have been reported from patients with congenital complete heart block.[527, 545] Usually, the atrial rate is normal for the age of the patient.[256] In a group of seven patients, the atrial rate ranged from 64 to 136 beats per minute, and the average rate was 97 when the arrhythmia was discovered; the rate decreased to 82 beats per minute 22 years later.[568] The average atrial rate of 70 adults ranged from 73 beats per minute in those who were asymptomatic to 82 beats per minute in those with syncope.[63] The atrial rate often increases before and during Adams-Stokes attacks of short duration.[569, 570]

P Waves

The atria of most patients with heart block are in sinus rhythm, and the form of the P waves reflects atrial size or electrophysiological function. Thus, the P waves can indicate enlargement of either chamber, intra-atrial conduction disturbances, or ectopic origin.[2, 215] Electrocardiographic atrial enlargement is particularly frequent in symptomatic patients with congenital complete heart block.[65]

Atrial rhythm. The regularity of the PP intervals of patients with complete heart block can vary for several reasons: atrial premature beats, ventriculoatrial conduction, sinus arrhythmia (including ventriculophasic sinus arrhythmia), and synchronization.

- Retrograde conduction of ventricular impulses may disturb the atrial rhythm even in the presence of antegrade atrioventricular block.[571–593] This is an uncommon but well-documented finding and is recognized by the presence of premature, inverted P waves soon after the QRS complexes in the inferior electrocardiographic leads (Fig. 15.4).
- In ventriculophasic sinus arrhythmia, the PP intervals that contain QRS complexes are shorter than those that do not.[256, 594–598] It is the P waves after the QRS complexes that occur prematurely[599] (Fig. 15.5).
- In synchronization or *accrochage*[qq]—the term used when the finding is short-lived[600]—the sinus rhythm bears a specific, although different, relation to the independent ventricular rhythm. P waves develop a repetitive pattern of preceding, disappearing within, and following the QRS complexes.[600–602] Synchronization usually appears as isorhythmic dissociation in patients with accelerated junctional rhythms. The phenomenon, however, has been recorded with different degrees of atrioventricular block and slow ventricular rhythms.[602–607rr]

PR Interval

Abnormalities of PR intervals are the most characteristic electrocardiographic features of atrioventricular block.

First-degree atrioventricular block. In first-degree atrioventricular block, the PR interval is prolonged beyond the normal, age-related range when the patient

---

[qq]French for "hooking" or "hitching."
[rr]What appears to be synchronization on the surface electrocardiogram may be caused, in some cases, by retrograde conduction.[604]

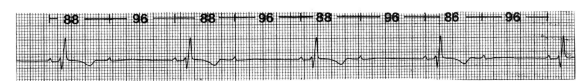

FIGURE 15.5 Ventriculophasic sinus arrhythmia. The intervals between the P waves, measured in hundredths of a second, are shorter when P waves enclose QRS complexes. The patient was an 88-year-old woman with congestive heart failure, 2:1 atrioventricular block, right bundle branch block, and left anterior fascicular block. Intracardiac electrocardiography located her block distal to the bundle of His.

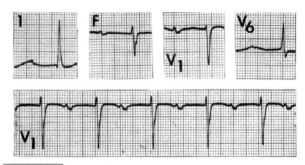

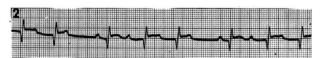

FIGURE 15.7 Type I second-degree atrioventricular block with Wenckebach periods in a patient with an acute inferior myocardial infarction. The third P wave starts a cycle. P waves 4 and 5 are longer than the previous interval. A QRS complex does not follow the sixth P wave. (From Kastor JA, Josephson ME. Treatment of atrioventricular block. In Fowler NO (ed). Cardiac Arrhythmias. Diagnosis and Treatment. 2nd ed. New York: Harper & Row, 1977, pp. 118–142, with permission.)[610]

FIGURE 15.6 First-degree atrioventricular block. The PR intervals are approximately 0.52 second.

is resting and has received no drugs that may affect atrioventricular conduction (Fig. 15.6). This usually means that the PR interval is longer than 0.21 second in adults and 0.18 second in children.[608] PR prolongation in first-degree atrioventricular block infrequently exceeds 0.30 second in asymptomatic subjects.[33] Each atrial beat activates the ventricles.

Electrocardiographers emphasize that the combination of sinus tachycardia and first-degree block may hide P waves within T waves. In such cases, the diagnosis of supraventricular tachycardia may be entertained incorrectly. Carotid sinus pressure should slow the sinus rate sufficiently to expose the P waves, or they may be recognized from unexpected notching of the T waves.[609]

Second-degree atrioventricular block. In atrioventricular block of the second degree, some of the P waves are not followed by QRS complexes. Two patterns of conduction may be discerned.[ss]

Type I second-degree atrioventricular block. This condition is usually recognized by the appearance of the

[ss]Called Mobitz type I and Mobitz type II second-degree atrioventricular block by those devoted to eponyms. Wenckebach periods occur during Mobitz type I block. (See Chap. 3.)

Wenckebach period or cycle, which consists of a group of sequentially and gradually prolonging PR intervals terminated by a P wave that does not conduct to the ventricles[610] (Fig. 15.7). Wenckebach periods have as few as three P waves and two QRS complexes or as many as 10 or more PR intervals before a QRS complex is missed. Typically, the following occur in Wenckebach cycles[611] (Fig. 15.8):

- The shortest PR interval follows and the longest PR interval precedes the ventricular pause; or, put another way, the first PR interval of a Wenckebach cycle is shorter than the last interval.
- Although the PR intervals progressively lengthen throughout a Wenckebach cycle, the increment, or the amount of additional prolonging of the PR intervals, decreases. This produces progressive shortening of the RR intervals.
- The pause is shorter than the PR intervals of any two consecutively conducted beats.

These features of Wenckebach cycles may be distorted by sinus arrhythmia,[612, 613] which can alter the RR spacing and the duration of the PR intervals,[614] and by autonomic tone, which can affect the function of the atrioventricular node as well as the sinoatrial node.

Wenckebach periods frequently evade the rules established for the typical cycle.[613, 615–617] Here are the

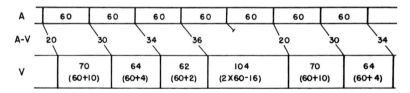

FIGURE 15.8 Diagram of Wenckebach period. Notice the progressive lengthening of the PR intervals in the first cycle from 0.20 to 0.36 second. In the V diagram, the QRS-QRS intervals shorten from 0.70 to 0.64 to 0.62 second because the increment of atrioventricular nodal block progressively decreases. The fifth P wave is blocked (indicated in the A-V box). The ventricular pause is 1.04 seconds, less than twice any of the shorter QRS-QRS intervals. The cycle then repeats. The shortest PR interval (0.20 sec) follows and the longest PR interval (0.36 sec) precede the ventricular pause. Letters (*left*) indicate atria (A), atrioventricular (A-V) node, and ventricles (V). Numbers are hundredths of a second. In this example, the atria beat at 100 beats per minute, with PP intervals of 0.60 second. (Adapted from Katz LN, Pick A. Clinical Electrocardiography. Part I. The Arrhythmias. Philadelphia: Lea & Febiger, 1956, with permission.)[611]

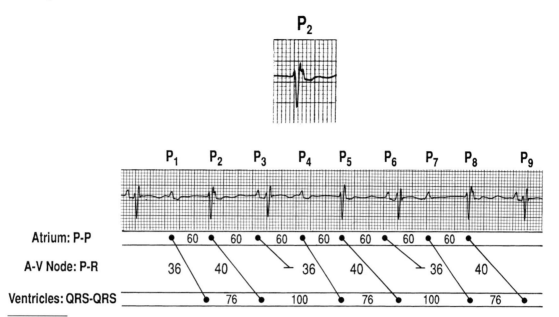

FIGURE 15.9 **Skipped P waves during type I second-degree atrioventricular block.** P_1 conducts with prolonged atrioventricular conduction. P_2, which appears at the end of the QRS complex, conducts with even more nodal delay. P_3 is blocked, and the cycle repeats. Atrial beats P_3 and P_6 may be misinterpreted as normally conducting beats. The enlargement of P_2 shows the P wave hugging the end of the QRS complex. (Numbers are hundredths of a second.)

most frequently observed atypical characteristics, listed in their order of frequency:[615tt]

- The length of the PR interval increases more in the last beat before the pause than in the preceding beat.[618]
- The length of the increase of the PR interval in the last beat before the pause is the largest increment of the cycle.
- The length of consecutive PR intervals repeats, rather than progressively lengthens, at least once during the cycle.
- The PR intervals sequentially decrease at least once during the cycle.
- The first increment of the PR intervals is not the largest increment of the cycle.

Very long PR intervals, which can exceed 0.80 second,[619, 620] appear in second-degree rather than first-degree atrioventricular block. Very slow conduction may produce a P wave preceding a QRS complex, to which it does not conduct despite an apparently normal PR interval. Accordingly, two P waves can appear between two QRS complexes in which the first P wave conducts with a very long PR interval and the second P wave is either blocked or conducts to the subsequent QRS complex, producing a skipped P wave[620–622] (Fig. 15.9).

Wenckebach periods may rarely appear during the

alternate beats of 2:1 atrioventricular block in which the PR intervals of the conducted beats progressively lengthen.[623] The presence of two levels of block may explain this phenomenon.[624, 625]

Type II second-degree atrioventricular block. This condition, which occurs much less often than type I block, is characterized by normal or slightly prolonged but unchanging PR intervals with unexpected nonconduction of one or more P waves[626, 627] (Fig. 15.10). The PR intervals before and after the blocked beats are not measurably different, and sinus arrhythmia does not significantly change the pattern.[628]

A few electrocardiographic events can confound the differentiation of type I from type II atrioventricular block:

- It may be difficult to decide from the electrocardiogram alone whether fixed 2:1

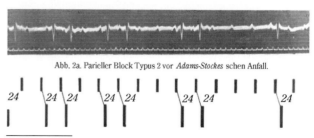

Abb. 2a. Parieller Block Typus 2 vor *Adams-Stockes* schen Anfall.

FIGURE 15.10 **Type II second-degree atrioventricular block.** This is the electrocardiographic tracing of one of the original cases described by Mobitz. In both the electrocardiogram and the diagram, the PR intervals are slightly prolonged at 0.24 second but do not change; the blocked P waves appear unpredictably. (Adapted from Mobitz W. Uber den partiellen Herzblok. Z Klin Med 1928; 107:450, with permission.)[626]

[tt]Atypical features appear so often[613, 616, 617] that one group has written that " 'typical Wenckebach periods' are the exception rather than rule."[615] They found that 86% of spontaneous Wenckebach periods demonstrated at least one atypical characteristic. Typical Wenckebach periodicity occurs most often with short cycles.[616] Atypical features are present in all cases when the P:QRS ratio is greater than 6:5.[615]

atrioventricular block should be classified as type I or type II[586, 628] (Fig. 15.11). At least two consecutively conducted P waves must be observed to make the diagnosis.

- When the last PR intervals of a Wenckebach cycle change little, type II block may be suspected.[617, 628, 629] Careful observation usually reveals that the first PR interval after the pause is shorter and that type I block is present.[630uu]
- Type II block may appear to be present when type I atrioventricular block develops transiently during an acute illness and as the sinus rhythm slows from vagotonia.[631]
- Nonpropagated or concealed His bundle or fascicular depolarizations can delay antegrade conduction and create the appearance of type I or type II block ("pseudo-atrioventricular block").[632–646] Patients may have both pseudo- and standard atrioventricular block.[641]

Patients with type II second-degree atrioventricular block frequently develop complete heart block, although in only a few patients with complete block have episodes of type II second-degree block been recorded.[627]

Third-degree atrioventricular block. When the atria and ventricles are totally dissociated, the P waves and QRS complexes appear without obvious correlation, and the PR intervals constantly change (Fig. 15.12).

QRS Complexes

Rhythm of ventricular complexes. In first-degree atrioventricular block, each QRS complex follows a P

[uu]This sequence has been called "pseudo-Mobitz II second-degree atrioventricular block."[617, 630]

2:1 A-V Nodal Block

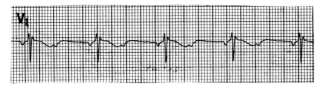

Infra-Nodal Block

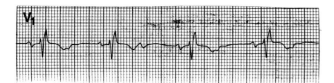

FIGURE 15.11 Two examples of 2:1 block. Top: Intracardiac electrocardiography showed the block to be within the atrioventricular node. The QRS width is normal at 0.84 second and the axis is −30 degrees. **Bottom:** This patient, who nearly fainted several times and was short of breath, had infranodal block. The QRS width was wider than normal at 0.13 second, and the axis was −30 degrees. The tracings demonstrate the similarity of electrocardiographic findings in 2:1 block, whatever its location. The right bundle branch block in the infranodal case provides a clue to the presence of trifascicular disease.

wave with prolonged intervals. Consequently, the atrial rhythm establishes the ventricular rhythm.

In type I second-degree atrioventricular block with Wenckebach periods, the RR intervals characteristically decrease as the PR intervals progressively prolong with successively shorter increments. No QRS complex appears after the nonconducted P wave.

In type II second-degree atrioventricular block, in which the PR interval of the conducted beats does not change, the atria establish the rhythm of the QRS complexes. No QRS complexes appear after the nonconducted P waves.

The ventricular rhythm in complete heart block is characteristically slow, regular,[647vv] and independent of atrial activity. Third-degree atrioventricular block may be chronic or paroxysmal. The onset of paroxysms is seldom recorded, but increasing[194, 545] and decreasing[481, 648, 649] atrial rates, even for brief periods, may worsen the amount of atrioventricular block and, in some cases, herald syncope.[650]

Premature ventricular beats that interrupt an idioventricular escape rhythm in patients with complete atrioventricular block can be followed by an interval, called the returning cycle, that may be longer than, or occasionally shorter than, the fundamental rate.[647] A fully compensatory pause is extremely rare. Returning cycles occur with approximately equal frequency as consistently prolonged, consistently unaltered, or consistently shortened intervals. Variable length of the returning cycles is the most common finding.

Form of conducted beats. The width of the QRS complexes is normal in most cases of first-degree and type I second-degree atrioventricular block, whereas intraventricular conduction disturbances characterize the QRS complexes of most cases of type II second-degree block. Atrioventricular block is more likely when bundle branch block complicates myocardial infarction.[651]

Form of escape beats. The QRS complexes may be narrow when originating in the atrioventricular junction or abnormally wide when arising from a junctional site with bundle branch block or from a ventricular site. The absence of normal septal waves may characterize the QRS complexes of some patients with block in the bundle of His.[652]

The duration of QRS complexes of adults with acquired complete heart block is 0.12 second or longer in 68% of cases,[193, 653, 654ww] whereas in congenital complete block they are usually narrow[57, 64, 536, 597, 655] (Fig. 15.13). The QRS complexes indicate left ventricular hypertrophy in over half of patients with congenital complete heart block.[57]

The duration of the QRS complexes of the escape

[vv]The ventricular rhythm was regular throughout prolonged observation in 50 of 120 cases of advanced atrioventricular block.[647] Irregularity was caused by ventricular premature beats in 39 cases; in the other patients, it was caused by uneven, slow discharge of a single ventricular pacemaker, temporary exit block of the idioventricular impulses, or capture of the ventricles by supraventricular impulses.

[ww]From 142 patients derived from three series.[193, 653, 654]

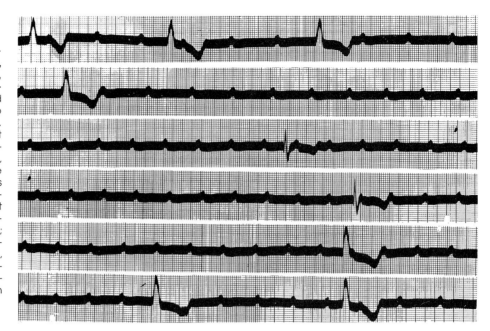

beats in the majority of patients with complete heart block complicating inferior myocardial infarction is narrow. However, these complexes are 0.12 second or longer in more than one-third of cases of block during inferior infarction[566, 656] and in almost all cases of anterior infarction.

The form of the idioventricular escape beats in complete heart block may indicate the site from which the beats originate. Those with the morphology of right bundle branch block are thought to arise from the left ventricle, and vice versa.[xx]

ST Segments and T Waves

Second- and third-degree atrioventricular block are more likely to complicate inferior myocardial in-

---

[xx]This presumption is based on "armchair reasoning" and, by inference, from mapping studies of patients with ventricular tachycardia but, to my knowledge, has not been established in the clinical electrophysiology laboratory or operating room.

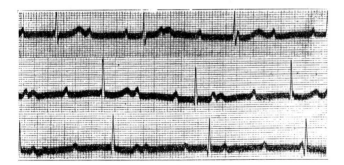

FIGURE 15.13 Congenital complete atrioventricular block. The ventricular rate is 43 beats per minute, and the atrial rate is 100 beats per minute. One sees complete atrioventricular dissociation. Intraventricular conduction is rapid, and the QRS complexes are narrow, as is typical in young children. This example of congenital complete heart block was the first published electrocardiographic record of the entity. (From White PD, Eustis RS, Kerr WJ. Congenital heart block. Am J Dis Child 1921; 22:299–306, with permission. Copyright 1921, American Medical Association.)[655]

farction when the ratio of the J point[yy] to the R wave is more than or equal to 0.5 millimeter in two or more leads.[182] ST segments and T waves in patients with heart block may be abnormal because of intrinsic cardiac disease, bundle branch block, or the origin of the ventricular beats. The T waves may be deeply inverted in some of the precordial leads of the electrocardiograms of children with congenital complete heart block and narrow QRS complexes.[536]

During first- and second-degree block, the ST segments are abnormal when the ventricles are ischemic, hypertrophied, or otherwise intrinsically diseased. When bundle branch block is present, conducted QRS complexes are characteristically followed by abnormal repolarization.

Because idioventricular escape beats in complete heart block activate and depolarize the ventricles abnormally, the ST and T waves are characteristically abnormal. The incidence of atrioventricular block is increased when the ST segments are elevated in lead V_{4R} indicating the presence of right ventricular infarction.[187]

QT Interval

Patients with atrioventricular block, ventricular premature beats, and QT intervals exceeding 0.60 second are at risk of developing polymorphic ventricular tachycardia.[517] The rate-corrected QT interval was prolonged in 59 (22%) of 273 children with congenital complete heart block. This finding occurred more often in children with symptoms, associated malformations, and slower ventricular rates.[657]

ELECTROCARDIOGRAM IN SINUS RHYTHM

Patients who develop atrioventricular block give evidence of predisposing factors in electrocardiographic

---

[yy]J point, the *junction* of the QRS complex and the ST segment.

signs of acute myocardial infarction, myocarditis, or enlargement of the cardiac chambers from congenital heart disease. However, the most important precursors of atrioventricular block are intraventricular conduction disturbances.

Fascicular and Bundle Branch Blocks[13, 14, 658]

Most patients with acquired complete atrioventricular block and idioventricular escape foci have reached this condition because of progressive block in the three fascicles of the intraventricular conduction system. Support for this conclusion is provided by the observation that conducted beats have bifascicular block in more than half of patients with transient or permanent complete heart block.[659–662zz]

When atrioventricular conduction is intact, we recognize these partial blocks by the electrocardiographic findings of

- Right bundle branch block.
- Left bundle branch block.
- Left anterior hemiblock, signifying block in the anterior division of the left bundle branch.
- Left posterior hemiblock, corresponding to block in the posterior division of the left bundle branch.

Bilateral bundle branch block produces the combination of right bundle branch block and left anterior hemiblock[659, 663, 664aaa] or right bundle branch and left posterior hemiblock. Most workers consider complete left bundle branch block to represent bifascicular block in which both divisions of the left bundle branch are at least partially diseased.

The patients with bifascicular block most likely to develop high degrees of atrioventricular block are older and have severe intrinsic heart disease.[135, 665] Bifascicular block can progress remorselessly in patients with Chagas disease, which produces continuing destruction of the conduction system.[13] Nevertheless, in other clinical settings, even though heart block may follow bifascicular block,[659, 666–670]

- Most patients with right bundle branch block, left anterior hemiblock, and no symptoms referable to bradycardia do not acquire advanced degrees of atrioventricular block,[671] even in such acute settings as noncardiac surgery.[672, 673]
- About 10% of patients with right bundle branch block and left posterior hemiblock develop a high degree of heart block.[665, 666, 674, 675bbb]
- Few patients with complete left bundle branch block and normal PR intervals develop complete atrioventricular block,[665] although the likelihood increases as the PR interval lengthens.[665]

Myocardial infarction.[676] Patients with bundle branch and fascicular blocks develop complete atrioventricular block during myocardial infarction more frequently than do patients with normal intraventricular conduction:[184, 677–679ccc]

- Right bundle branch block and left anterior hemiblock—38%.[680–688ddd]
- Right bundle branch block and left posterior hemiblock—37%.[681–683, 685, 688, 689eee]
- Left posterior hemiblock—18%.[683, 688, 689fff]
- Right bundle branch block—17%.[680, 682, 683, 685, 687, 688, 690ggg]
- Left bundle branch block—12%.[680, 682, 683, 688hhh]
- Left axis deviation—5%, a proportion that is not greater than that for all patients with myocardial infarction.[162, 683, 687, 688iii]

Bundle branch and fascicular blocks characteristically appear in many patients with anterior myocardial infarction who will eventually develop atrioventricular block[151, 682, 691] (Fig. 15.14). This progression is due to the widespread damage of the myocardium and underlying conducting tissue. Patients who acquire their bundle branch block with myocardial infarction are more likely to develop atrioventricular block than are patients whose intraventricular blocks were present before the acute infarction.[685]

Right Chest Leads

Atrioventricular block develops more often in patients with inferior infarction who have ST segment elevations or new QS waves in leads V_{3R} and V_{4R} than in those without these electrocardiographic changes[172] (Fig. 15.15). This finding probably reflects the higher incidence of block when the right ventricle is infarcted.[176]

DIFFERENTIAL DIAGNOSIS
Atrioventricular Dissociation

The PR intervals constantly change and no pattern can be established when atrioventricular dissociation due to complete heart block is present. Ventriculophasic sinus arrhythmia and synchronization may produce an apparent relationship between the P waves and the QRS complexes, but this is unaffected by antegrade conduction.

In atrioventricular dissociation, as the name implies, the atria and ventricles beat independently of each other either continuously or intermittently.[692] This independence may be produced by atrioventricular block or by accelerated junctional (His bundle) or

---

zzSixty-nine percent of 132 patients in three series.[659–661] Seventy-four percent of 67 patients with syncope caused by paroxysmal third-degree atrioventricular block had bifascicular block.[662]

aaaThe incidence of right bundle branch block and left axis deviation (left anterior hemiblock) was 0.5% in 47,500 hospital electrocardiograms.[659, 663] Of 5,204 working male Israeli civil servants, right bundle branch block and left anterior hemiblock appeared in 0.17%.[664]

bbbEight of 76 patients.[665, 666, 674, 675] The range was 0% to 20%.

cccAs reported before the development of thrombolysis and acute angioplasty for myocardial infarction.

dddOne hundred-three of 270 patients in nine series.[680–688]

eeeTwenty-one of 57 patients in six series.[681–683, 685, 688, 689]

fffTwo of 11 patients in three series.[683, 688, 689]

gggForty-nine of 287 patients in seven series.[680, 682, 683, 685, 687, 688, 690]

hhhTen of 84 patients in four series.[680, 682, 683, 688]

iiiSeven of 139 patients in four series.[162, 683, 687, 688]

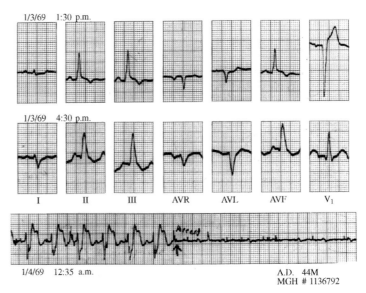

FIGURE 15.14 Complete atrioventricular block with ventricular asystole produced by extensive myocardial infarction. On admission to the hospital, the patient's electrocardiogram showed changes of an extensive anterior infarction (**top**) and an axis of +90 degrees. Three hours later, he developed right bundle branch block and left posterior hemiblock (**middle**). Cardiac arrest resulting from complete block occurred 8 hours later (**bottom**).

ventricular pacemakers that beat faster than the sinus pacemaker.

When an acclerated pacemaker in the junction or ventricles dominates the rhythm of the heart, antegrade atrioventricular conduction may still occur. This depends on the amount of antegrade block present and whether the P waves appear at the time in the cycle when their impulses may be conducted to the ventricles. When atrial capture occurs, the RR intervals are slightly shorter than the fundamental ventricular rhythm.

This phenomenon has been called "interference dissociation" or "atrioventricular dissociation with interference."[574, 693] A preferable phrase is "*atrioventricular dissociation with atrial capture.*"[692]

Sick Sinus Syndrome

Atrioventricular block and sinoatrial disease produce most abnormal bradyarrhythmias in humans. These conditions are seldom difficult to recognize electrocardiographically. In sinoatrial disease, the ventricular bradycardia is caused by the absence of organized atrial activity; in atrioventricular block, the slow heart rhythm develops while the atria are generating signals that could drive the ventricles if atrioventricular conduction were normal.

OTHER ELECTROCARDIOGRAPHIC STUDIES

Exercise Testing

The slightly prolonged PR intervals of otherwise healthy patients shorten into the normal range during exercise.[694] Exercise may, however, increase the degree of block in patients with abnormal conduction systems.[194, 465–468, 470–472, 695]

Congenital complete heart block. The ventricular rate in patients with complete congenital heart block

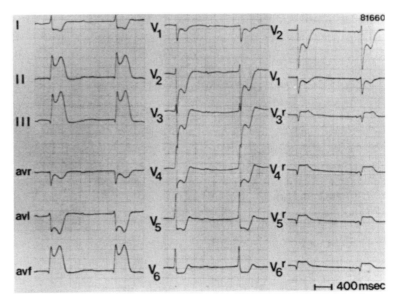

FIGURE 15.15 Acute inferoposterior myocardial infarction and a high degree of atrioventricular nodal block. Notice the evidence of right ventricular involvement in the ST segment elevations in leads V_{3R} through V_{6R}, the Q waves in leads V_{4R} through V_{6R}, and the depressions of the ST segments in leads V_1 and V_2. (From Braat SH, de Zwaan C, Brugada P, Coenegracht JM, Wellens HJJ. Right ventricular involvement with acute inferior wall myocardial infarction identifies high risk of developing atrioventricular nodal conduction disturbances. Am Heart J 1984; 107:1183–1187, with permission.)[176]

usually increases when patients exercise.[58, 535–537, 545, 696–698] For example, in 25 asymptomatic patients with isolated congenital heart block, the average ventricular rate rose from 49 beats per minute at rest to 97 beats per minute during exercise.[535, 698] The average atrial rate in 11 increased from 87 beats per minute to 168 beats per minute. Unlike the atrial rate, the ventricular rate does not increase smoothly and regularly. After exercise ceases, the ventricular rate returns to the resting rate more quickly than does the atrial rate.[535]

When compared with the normal response, the ventricular rate reached when exercising is subnormal, and the oxygen uptake is lower.[699] Thus, the hemodynamic adjustment to exercise of patients with congenital complete atrioventricular block is less than in patients with normal rhythm, and those with block have a higher than normal anaerobic/aerobic energy supply.[699]

Ventricular ectopic beats and accelerated idioventricular rhythm[465] develop during exercise in patients with complete congenital heart block more often than in healthy persons. The ectopy becomes more frequent and severe, whatever the heart rate, as age increases and when the width of the QRS complexes of the ventricular escape beats is prolonged.[535, 698]

Acquired complete heart block. The heart rate of patients with acquired block and idioventricular escape beats increases slightly, if at all, with exercise.[700–702]

Effects on degree of block. Exercise tends to reduce the amount of atrioventricular block when the QRS complexes in the conducted or escape beats have normal width, as in type I block, and to worsen the block when bundle branch block is present in the conducted beats,[466] as in type II block.[194, 467, 471, 644jjj]

Exercise-induced ischemia may rarely produce paroxysmal atrioventricular block.[468, 695, 703] A few patients without atrioventricular conduction disturbances at rest develop partial atrioventricular block not necessarily resulting from ischemia when they exercise.[126, 704]

Extended Monitoring[705]

Ambulatory monitoring reveals atrioventricular block to be the cause of syncope better than does exercise testing.[706] If 24 hours of monitoring does not supply the reason for suspected Adams-Stokes syndrome, longer recordings will seldom help.[707]

Extended electrocardiographic monitoring has shown when paroxysmal atrioventricular block is the cause of Adams-Stokes attacks[705, 708, 709] and

- All degrees of atrioventricular block appearing during sleep in symptomatic[126] and otherwise healthy subjects.[126–128]
- That patients with congenital complete heart block

---

jjjIn 44 patients with QRS complexes of less than 0.11 second, block improved in 62%, did not change in 24%, and worsened in 14%. In 16 patients with QRS complexes of 0.12 second or more, block improved in 13%, did not change in 44%, and worsened in 44%.[466]

and mean daytime heart rates lower than 50 beats per minute are more likely to develop excessive fatigue, presyncope, syncope, or sudden death than those with faster daytime heart rates. Some patients with slower rates also have nocturnal junctional exit block, little or no change in the ventricular rate with physical activity, and tachyarrhythmias.[710, 711]

- The patterns of atypical Wenckebach periods.[630]
- How transient or permanent complete atrioventricular block develops in symptomatic patients,[708] some of whom have bifascicular block.[661, 668]

How a 56-year-old woman with "presyncopal episodes," minimal mitral valve prolapse, first-degree atrioventricular block (PR interval, 160 milliseconds), right bundle branch block, and left anterior hemiblock, who died suddenly from complete atrioventricular block.[712]

Fetal Monitoring

Electrocardiographic monitoring reveals the presence of congenital complete atrioventricular block before birth.[713, 714]

ECHOCARDIOGRAPHY

Echocardiographic and Doppler studies have demonstrated

- That patients with inferior myocardial infarction are more likely to develop advanced atrioventricular block when left and right ventricular function is reduced.[177]
- Congenital complete heart block in the fetus.[715–723]
- The relationship between mitral and tricuspid valve closure and the intensity of the first heart sound during complete heart block.[556, 558, 724]
- That Doppler-determined arterial peak flow velocity in patients with complete heart block is greatest when the PR interval is 10 to 300 milliseconds long and least when atrial contraction occurs during ventricular systole.[725]

LABORATORY STUDIES

Chemistry

Maternal and infant antibodies.[220, 237, 239, 240, 726–732] All mothers of babies with congenital complete heart block have antibodies against the SSA/Ro antigen,[733] and some have antibodies against the SSB/La antigen ("autoantibody-associated congenital complete heart block").[227, 729] However, not all children of mothers with anti-SSA/Ro antibodies have congenital heart block. Anti-SSB/La antibodies correlate more closely with congenital complete heart block than do anti-SSA/Ro antibodies. All infants with congenital complete heart block and neonatal lupus erythematosus have anti-SSA/Ro and anti-SSB/La antibodies.[365]

Chest Radiography

Cardiomegaly is common in children with congenital complete heart block,[536] particularly in symptomatic patients.[65] The cardiothoracic ratio is greater than 55% in over half of patients with congenital block.[734] The chest radiography may reveal calcification of the valves or valve rings, which can contribute to the production of heart block.[132]

Nuclear Studies

Technetium pyrophosphate scintigraphy has revealed that atrioventricular block develops more frequently in patients with inferior myocardial infarction when the right ventricle is involved.[176] Radionuclide angiography has shown that right and left ventricular function is more likely to be decreased and infarct size is likely to be larger when block complicates inferior myocardial infarction.[177]

Left ventricular evaluation demonstrates that most patients with congenital complete heart block have normal resting cardiac index and ejection fraction but increased end-diastolic volume index.[735] The cardiac index usually increases with exercise.[735]

Cardiac Catheterization

Patients with inferior myocardial infarction and obstruction of their left anterior descending coronary arteries have a sixfold greater chance of developing atrioventricular block during the infarction than do patients without such obstruction.[736]

When contrast is used during catheterization, the presence of dye in the cardiac chambers in patients with complete heart block reveals that[737]

- As the atria contract during ventricular systole, the blood refluxes into all the afferent veins.
- The later in ventricular diastole that atrial systole occurs, the less completely the atria empty.
- When the atria contract a second time during the same ventricular diastole, little additional blood is forced into the ventricles.

HEMODYNAMICS

The hemodynamic consequences of complete heart block are due to the slow heart rate, the atrioventricular asynchrony,[738] and the extent of intrinsic valvular, myocardial, or other structural heart disease. In general, the circulation approaches the normal state more frequently in isolated congenital complete heart block than in acquired complete heart block, in which associated structural heart disease or the effects of aging on the heart may exert deleterious effects.

Congenital Complete Heart Block

In congenital complete heart block,[739] the cardiac output is usually normal.[527, 735, 740] This state is maintained, in spite of the slow ventricular rates, by increased stroke volume,[527, 735, 740] produced by the long period available for diastolic filling and the intermittent contribution of atrial contraction.

The characteristically increased end-diastolic volume[735] associated with slow heart rates produces the slight changes from normal observed in the intracardiac and extracardiac pressures. Pulmonary[527] and systemic arterial systolic pressures[536] are usually elevated from the ejection of the increased stroke volume. Pulmonary arterial and systemic arterial diastolic pressures are either normal or slightly decreased. The combination of increased systemic systolic and decreased diastolic pressures produces the characteristically increased pulse pressure.

Right ventricular, pulmonary arterial, and left ventricular systolic pressures are either normal or slightly increased.[527] Vena caval, right atrial, right ventricular end-diastolic, pulmonary artery wedge, left atrial mean, and left ventricular end-diastolic pressures are usually normal or slightly elevated.[527]

The amplitude of the A wave from atrial systole varies within the atrial chambers, as it does in the neck veins.[527, 741] The waves may reach 15 millimeters of mercury in the right atrium during ventricular systole.[597] A waves can be recorded in the right ventricular and in the pulmonary and brachial arterial pressure pulses.[597, 742] The cardiac output[537, 735, 740] and stroke volume[537] usually increase with exercise, but the end-diastolic volume does not change.[735]

Acquired Complete Heart Block

In most adults with chronic acquired complete atrioventricular block, the cardiac output is lower than normal because the slow heart rate is associated with a stroke volume that is either normal or decreased rather than increased, as it is in many patients with congenital complete heart block.[743–749] The systemic and pulmonary vascular resistances are characteristically higher than normal. Intracardiac right atrial, right ventricular end-diastolic and systolic, pulmonary arterial systolic, and left ventricular end-diastolic pressures may be elevated.[701, 743, 747, 750]

The cardiac output steadily rises in some but not all patients when pacing increases the ventricular rate to 70 to 90 beats per minute,[702, 744, 746–749, 751, 752] but the response is impaired.[747] At faster rates, the output rises no further and may decrease.[744, 748, 749, 752] As the heart rate rises, brachial artery pressure, left ventricular work, and central blood volume increase, and the stroke volume index, peripheral resistance, left ventricular ejection time, and intracardiac filling pressures decrease.[700, 702, 746, 748, 753] Raising the ventricular rate by pacing patients with heart block from acute myocardial infarction usually increases the cardiac output and systemic blood pressure and decreases the stroke volume and systemic vascular resistance.[754]

Pacing

Atrioventricular synchrony.[755] In patients with chronic heart block[748, 756–762] and heart block from acute myocardial infarction,[763] the reestablishment of atrioventricular synchrony by sequential or synchronous pacing[kkk] decreases elevated venous pressure and increases

- Arterial pressure (Fig. 15.16).
- Cardiac output.
- Ejection time.
- Exercise performance.
- Stroke volume.

The atrial contribution to ventricular filling in patients with heart block is greater when the ventricles are normal than when they are diseased.[764] Isolated atrial contractions lead to atriogenic reflux in some patients.[765]

Cardiac function depends on the duration of the PR interval[766] programmed into dual-chamber pacers.[761, 767–769] The cardiac output is even different if the atrium is sensed or paced at the same PR interval.[768]

Rate-responsive pacing. This type of pacing, in which the heart rate varies with physiological activity, improves exercise performance over fixed-rate ventricular pacing.[770] Furthermore, rate-responsive atrial synchronous pacing improves contractility[771] and cardiopulmonary performance[772] more than does rate-responsive ventricular pacing.

Atrial natriuretic peptide. Levels of this peptide, which is released from the atria and increased during tachycardia or on stretching from increased pressure or volume, are higher during ventricular pacing than during atrioventricular pacing and at faster pacing rates regardless of the pacing method.[773]

PATHOLOGY[774]

Atrioventricular block is caused by malfunction or destruction of the conducting tissues in the entrance to and within the body of the atrioventricular node, the penetrating and branching portions of the bundle of His, and the right and left bundle branches and their fascicles.[8, 775–778] Loss of some of the conducting cells at the branching points of the His bundle and the proximal portions of the bundle branches produces intra-His block.[779]

Acquired Atrioventricular Block

Fibrosis of the bundle branches and their fascicles and less often of the bundle of His[780] is the most common lesion producing chronic acquired heart block. This process, the cause of which is not known,[132lll] reveals itself on the surface electrocardiogram by the presence of bundle branch and fascicular blocks in conducted beats.[130] The usual pathological lesion is a sclerodegenerative replacement of both bundle branches.[130, 781mmm]

Coronary heart disease. Pathological studies reveal that acute or chronic coronary heart disease seldom produces chronic atrioventricular block.[782] For example, coronary heart disease could be incriminated as the probable cause in only 10 (15%) of 65 patients.[132] Some patients whose heart block was thought to be associated with chronic coronary disease had no history of myocardial infarction or angina.[132] Necropsy of a patient who developed type I second-degree block during Prinzmetal's angina revealed no significant parenchymal changes in the atrioventricular node of the penetrating or branching portions of the atrioventricular bundle.[211]

Coronary artery anatomy.[783–787] Branches of the left anterior descending coronary artery supply most of the right bundle branch and the anterior radiation of fascicle of the left bundle branch. The atrioventricular node and the bundle of His are perfused in 83% of patients from a branch of the right coronary artery just before it gives off the posterior descending branch.[788] In 17% of hearts, a branch of the left circumflex coronary artery supplies this area.[788] The posterior fascicle of the left bundle branch is supplied

---

[kkk]During sequential pacing, both the atria and ventricles are paced with an appropriate interval separating the two pacing signals, whereas in synchronous pacing, the atria are sensed and the ventricles are paced after a suitable PR interval.

[lll]Bilateral bundle branch fibrosis of unknown origin and without apparent myocardial disease was found in 26 (40%) of 65 patients in an autopsy series and was the most common cause of block in this group.[132]

[mmm]Jean Lenegre and Maurice Lev are uniquely associated with the pathology of bilateral bundle branch block and heart block. Lenegre's disease has been described as "an obscure sclero-degenerative process involving only the conduction system," and Lev's disease "is caused by an invasion of the conduction system from without—an involvement of the fascicles by fibrosis or calcification spreading from any of the fibrous structures adjacent to the conducting system."[781]

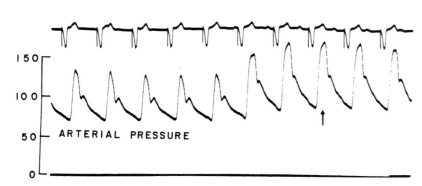

FIGURE 15.16 Hemodynamic effect of fixed-rate ventricular pacing. The systolic pressure is highest when the PR intervals indicate that the atria are contributing to ventricular filling. Shown are radial arterial pressure and electrocardiographic lead II. (From Leinbach RC, Chamberlain DA, Kastor JA, Harthorne JW, Sanders CA. A comparison of the hemodynamic effects of ventricular and sequential A-V pacing in patients with heart block. Am Heart J 1969; 78:502–508, with permission.)[757]

chiefly by the posterior descending coronary artery, which usually arises from the right coronary artery. Collateral anastomoses and individual variations distort this pattern in many patients.[786]

Acute myocardial infarction. The more frequent pathological cause of atrioventricular block in patients with inferior myocardial infarction appears to be necrosis of the atrial pre-nodal myocardial fibers rather than damage to the atrioventricular node or bundle of His itself.[785, 789, 790nnn] Many patients with block complicating inferior infarction have normal conduction systems or only small foci of necrosis in the atrioventricular node or the bundle branches[782, 791] and no acute necrosis, edema, or inflammation of the conducting system.[792] "Massive" necrosis is rare.[791] The transient character of the block and the lack of necrosis of the atrioventricular node may be explained in many patients by the arterial supply of the proximal conduction system by both the left anterior descending and right coronary arteries.[736] Patients may develop block because both their left anterior descending coronary arteries and the vessels supplying the inferior surface of the heart have at least some significant obstruction.[736]

Severe ischemic damage to both bundle branches and their ramifications is the typical pathological finding responsible for atrioventricular block that complicates the course of patients with anterior myocardial infarction.[793] The widespread extent of the associated myocardial damage explains the high mortality in these patients.[785, 791, 793] Severe bundle branch damage also characterizes the atrioventricular block that occurs in patients with combined anterior and inferior myocardial infarction.[791]

Acute infective endocarditis. The appearance of second-degree and complete atrioventricular block and right or left bundle branch block in patients with acute infective endocarditis strongly suggests the presence of an abscess of a valve ring, usually the aortic valve, which has extended into the atrioventricular node or bundle of His.[794–796]

Miscellaneous conditions. Pathological findings include the following:

- Thrombotic occlusion of the distal right coronary artery and the origin of the atrioventricular nodal artery and fibro-fatty changes in the atrioventricular conduction system were found in a patient with heart block and myotonic dystrophy.[482]

- In older patients, fatty replacement of the atrioventricular node and fibrotic changes of the ventricular septum can lead to atrioventricular block.[797]
- The atrioventricular node was almost completely replaced by granulation tissue in a 12-year-old girl who died from systemic lupus erythematosus and complete heart block.[336]
- Sarcoidosis produces focal fibromuscular dysplasia in the region of the atrioventricular node.[359]

Congenital Atrioventricular Block

In the few patients with congenital atrioventricular block[2, 798] who have come to necropsy, pathological findings included the following:

- Absence or deficiency of the connection between atrial muscle and the atrioventricular node[87, 238, 799–802] including necrosis of the central fibrous body.[803]
- Absence of the atrioventricular node.[229, 799, 801, 804]
- Separation of the atrioventricular node from the bundle of His.[775] Discontinuity between the atrioventricular node and the conduction axis is characteristic of children with congenital complete heart block and left isomerism.[805]
- Disruption of the bundle of His.[806]
- Abnormalities at the origins of the bundle branches or in the right or left bundle branch.[238, 801, 804, 806, 807]

Pathological processes at more than one level of the conducting system may also occur. Electron microscopy has revealed proliferation of mitochondria.[808]

Immunoglobulin G antibodies have been found[365] and, in a few cases, localized to the heart,[728, 809–811] specifically to the atrioventricular node[811] in infants with congenital complete heart block who have been born to mothers with lupus[811] or anti-Ro and anti-La antibodies.[237, 729, 812–814] These data strengthen the likelihood that some if not all cases of congenital complete heart block are due to the effects of antibodies passed transplacentally to the fetus from the mother, who often has systemic lupus erythematosus.

CLINICAL ELECTROPHYSIOLOGY[815–817]

The techniques of clinical electrophysiology, in particular the His bundle electrogram supplemented by programmed stimulation, can locate abnormalities of atrioventricular conduction.

His Bundle Electrocardiography

In a typical clinical electrophysiological study,[817] an electrode catheter is introduced, usually through the femoral vein, and advanced under fluoroscopic control into the right atrium. It is then positioned so that three discrete electrograms can be recorded from the electrodes on its tip. Each reflects activation of nearby structures: the A wave from the atrium, the H wave

---

nnnTwenty-nine of (97%) 30 hearts with atrioventricular block and inferior myocardial infarction had acute lesions in the atrial prenodal fibers, but only 11 (38%) of 29 showed changes in the atrioventricular node or the bundle of His. Lesions in the prenodal fibers were absent in 11 (79%) of 14 hearts from patients with inferior infarction and no atrioventricular block.[790] Other studies have also reported the importance of necrosis of the approaches to the atrioventricular node in acute atrioventricular block from ischemia.[785] Necrotic destruction of the atrioventricular node, however, does occur in patients who die with inferior myocardial infarctions and block.[789]

from the bundle of His, and the large V wave from the ventricles.

The intervals of time between the electrograms correspond to conduction from atrium to ventricles:[818–821] [ooo]

- The AH interval, normally 60 to 140 milliseconds, corresponds to conduction between the atrium and the bundle of His.
- The duration of the H deflection, normally 10 to 25 milliseconds, relates to conduction within the bundle of His.
- The HV interval, normally 35 to 55 milliseconds, reflects conduction from the bundle of His to the beginning of ventricular activation.
- The PA interval from the beginning of the P wave to the A wave on the His bundle electrode, normally 25 to 45 milliseconds, indicates conduction from the high to the low right atrium, where the bundle of His electrode rests.

Clinicopathological studies demonstrate a strong correlation between disease in the subdivisions of the atrioventricular conducting system and abnormalities in the corresponding intervals measured by His bundle electrocardiography.[789, 822–824]

Programmed Stimulation

Additional information about atrioventricular conduction may be derived by pacing the atrium, usually through another electrode catheter in the right atrium, or by introducing premature atrial beats with a programmed stimulator.[825–828]

Levels of Block

Excluding intra-atrial activation, we recognize, for clinical purposes, two regions of abnormal conduction:

- Within the atrioventricular node.
- Below the atrioventricular node, also called infranodal block, either within the bundle of His or in the bundle branch–fascicular system.

Abnormal conduction within the atrioventricular node gradually tends to worsen, whereas infranodal conduction, whether within the bundle of His or the bundle branches and fascicles, is prolonged only slightly before block develops.[ppp] Adults and children may have block at more than one level within the atrioventricular conduction system.[10, 508, 829–837]

Degrees of Atrioventricular Block

First-degree block. Prolonged PR intervals are usually due to block within the atrioventricular node and

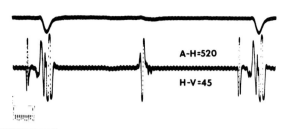

FIGURE 15.17   First-degree atrioventricular nodal block. The PR interval is exceedingly prolonged from delay in the atrioventricular node. This is confirmed by the long AH interval of 520 milliseconds in the His bundle electrogram. Infranodal conduction is normal, with an HV interval of 45 milliseconds. This patient also had Wenckebach periods.

are recognized in the His bundle electrogram by prolonged AH intervals[9, 591, 838–840] in the presence of but also particularly in the absence of bundle branch block[841] (Fig. 15.17).

Conduction within the infranodal system cannot be delayed greatly before beats are dropped, and, consequently, significantly prolonged HV intervals correspond to only slight lengthening of PR intervals on the electrocardiogram (Fig. 15.18). The PR interval may even be normal despite the presence of split His potentials—the sign of intra-His conduction delay[842, 843]—or prolongation of the HV interval.[209, 841, 844][qqq] Particularly when bifascicular block is present,

---

[qqq]For example, prolongation of the HV interval from 55 milliseconds, the upper limit of normal, to 80 milliseconds can indicate clinically important infranodal disease. Lengthening of the PR interval by 25 milliseconds (0.025 second) is barely noticeable on the surface electrocardiogram, and the PR interval may continue to appear normal.

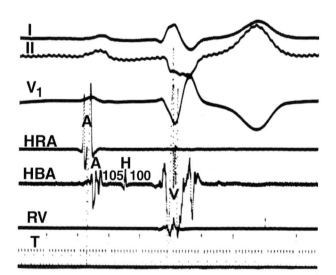

FIGURE 15.18   First-degree block from slow conduction below the atrioventricular node. The PR interval is 0.25 second. Conduction within the atrioventricular node is normal at 105 milliseconds, but infranodal conduction is greatly prolonged at 100 milliseconds. The right bundle branch block (V₁) and left anterior hemiblock (lead II) indicate the presence of trifascicular block. (From Kastor JA, Josephson ME. Treatment of atrioventricular block. In Fowler NO (ed). Cardiac Arrhythmias. Diagnosis and Treatment. 2nd ed. New York: Harper & Row, 1977, pp. 118–142, with permission.)[610]

[ooo]Many workers have developed ranges of normal values for the measurements made during clinical electrophysiological studies. The values I have listed are among those most frequently used. The normal intervals are shorter in children and lengthen with age.[818–821]

[ppp]The phrase "all or nothing" conduction is often applied to infranodal activation. The phrase is apt, although not precisely correct.

delayed infranodal conduction within the bundle of His[643, 843] or, more frequently within the bundle branches and fascicles, may contribute to first-degree block.[591, 840rrr]

Second-degree block. Type I second-degree atrioventricular block with Wenckebach cycles is usually due to block within the atrioventricular node and is recognized on the His bundle electrogram by progressively prolonging AH intervals.[6, 615, 616, 624, 838, 845–849sss] When a QRS complex is dropped, the A wave is not followed by an H or a V deflection.

The location of the disease in 2:1 second-degree block with narrow QRS complexes cannot be accurately estimated from the surface electrocardiogram. Intracardiac records have shown that the atrioventricular node[850] (Fig. 15.19) or the bundle of His (Fig. 15.20) may be at fault. Two-to-one block is particularly characteristic of block within the bundle of His, which is recognized electrophysiologically by prolongation or splitting of the H deflection.[851]

Type II second-degree atrioventricular block occurs almost always within the infranodal conduction system and is marked by prolonged HV intervals or prolonged or split His potentials.[838] When QRS complexes are dropped, the AH complex persists synchronously with the P waves of the electrocardiogram, but the V wave

---

[rrr]In 45 patients with first-degree atrioventricular block and narrow QRS complexes, the block was located in the atrioventricular nodal region in 87% and within the bundle of His in 13%.[591] In 73 patients with wide QRS complexes, the first-degree block was located in the atrioventricular nodal region in 22%, and below the node in 45% (12% within the bundle of His and 33% below the bundle of His) and in more than one location in one-third of the patients.[591]

[sss]His bundle electrocardiography with atrial pacing or programmed stimulation has helped provide electrophysiological explanations for alternating Wenckebach periodicity[624, 848, 849] and atypical Wenckebach cycles.[615, 616, 845, 847]

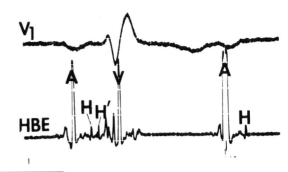

of ventricular activation is absent (Fig. 15.21). Two-to-one and 3:1 block, in which Wenckebach periods are not seen, are produced predominantly in the His-Purkinje system.[852ttt]

Block can occur in both the atrioventricular node and the infranodal tissues.[853] In one example, reduction of an abnormally prolonged HV interval produced a shortened PR interval of the second beat of a Wenckebach cycle.[854]

The width of the QRS complexes also helps to predict where atrioventricular block will be found on electrophysiological study. Narrow QRS complexes imply the absence of severe bundle branch disease, and block in these patients is usually located in the atrioventricular node when Wenckebach periods are present or in the bundle of His when 2:1 block or the type II pattern is seen. Block distal to His is likely when bundle branch block appears with 2:1 or type II block.[591, 852uuu]

Third-degree block. When complete heart block occurs in the atrioventricular node, atrial activation is identified by A waves, and the dissociated, independent ventricular activation is identified by HV units on the His bundle electrogram that correspond to each QRS complex on the surface electrocardiogram.[6, 838] The escape foci originate in the bundle of His, and

---

[ttt]In 141 cases of second-degree atrioventricular block,[591] type I block with Wenckebach periods occurred in 38%, type II block in 11%, and 2:1 or 3:1 block in 52%. The Wenckebach block was located in the atrioventricular node in 72%, within the bundle of His in 9%, and below the bundle of His in 19%. Type II block was found within the bundle of His in 20% and below the bundle of His in 80%. Two-to-one and 3:1 block without Wenckebach periods occurred within the atrioventricular node in 27%, within the bundle of His in 22%, and below the bundle of His in 51%.

[uuu]In those 141 patients with second-degree atrioventricular block[591] whose QRS complexes were narrow, second-degree block occurred within the atrioventricular node in 66%, within the bundle of His in 28%, and below the bundle of His in 6%. When the QRS complex was wide, block occurred within the atrioventricular node in 20%, within the bundle of His in 8%, and below the bundle of His in 72%.

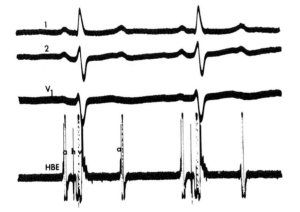

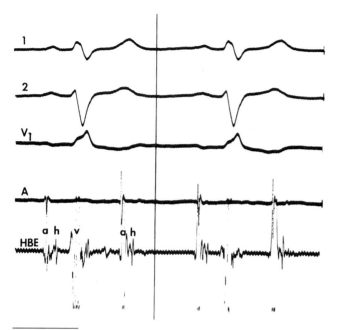

FIGURE 15.21   2:1 block below the bundle of His. The first beat is conducted with a prolonged HV interval. The second P wave, hidden within the T waves of lead V₁ and identified by the deflection in the atrial (A) and His bundle electrocardiograms (HBE), blocks after activating the bundle of His. The sequence is repeated in the next two atrial beats. Notice the presence of bifascicular block with right bundle branch block (V₁) and left anterior hemiblock (deep S wave in lead II). (From Kastor JA, Goldreyer BN, Moore EN, Spear JF. Re-entry: an important mechanism of cardiac arrhythmias. Cardiovasc Clin 1974; 6:111–135, with permission.)[850]

the QRS complexes are usually of normal width, unless concurrent bundle branch block is also present.

In patients in whom complete heart block develops within the infranodal system, the signal proceeds from the atrium to the atrioventricular node and the bundle of His.[6, 838, 855] Atrial activity is marked by P waves on the surface electrocardiogram and combined AH deflections in the His bundle electrogram. Only V waves appear with the QRS complexes (Fig. 15.22). The escape foci in most cases are idioventricular; consequently, the QRS complexes are abnormally wide because of their ectopic origin.

When complete infranodal atrioventricular block occurs within the bundle of His, H deflections may be split, with the first part following each A wave and the second part preceding each V wave.[652, 780, 856–858] The escape foci usually have narrow QRS complexes unless concurrent bundle branch block is present.[vvv]

Bundle Branch and Fascicular Blocks[859, 860]

Electrophysiological studies have helped to decipher the relationship between bundle branch and fascicular

---

[vvv]In 222 cases of complete block, the conduction abnormality was within the atrioventricular node in 21%, in the bundle of His in 18%, and in the bundle branches in 61%. When the QRS complex was narrow, 53% of blocks were within the atrioventricular node, and 47% were within the bundle of His.[591] When the QRS complex was wide, 11% of blocks were within the atrioventricular node, 5% were within the bundle of His, and 85% were below the bundle of His.

blocks and atrioventricular block.[861–863] The presence of organic heart disease strongly influences the course of patients with conduction system disease.

- In patients with bifascicular block,[www] the HV interval is more frequently prolonged, progression to heart block occurs more often, and death from heart disease is more likely when organic heart disease is present.[135] Similarly, when the HV interval is prolonged in patients with bifascicular block, organic heart disease occurs more often, total and sudden cardiac mortality rises, and progression to trifascicular block, although infrequent, is more likely.[864]
- The combination of first-degree atrioventricular block and bifascicular block is usually associated with prolonged HV intervals.[840]
- The mortality is higher in patients whose HV interval is longer than 80 milliseconds and who are symptomatic from heart disease and have bundle branch block.[865]
- The risk of progression in patients with bundle branch block to second- and third-degree atrioventricular block and to severe congestive heart failure rises when the HV interval is 70 milliseconds or more.[866, 867] The likelihood is particularly high when the interval exceeds 100 milliseconds.[867]
- Block distal to the bundle of His occurs more frequently when second-degree atrioventricular block is associated with left bundle branch block than with right bundle branch block.[852]
- Patients with left axis deviation in addition to left bundle branch block have longer AH, HV, and PR intervals, more myocardial disease, more advanced cardiac disease, and increased mortality than patients with left bundle branch block and normal axis.[868]

[www]Right bundle branch block and left anterior hemiblock, right bundle branch block and left posterior hemiblock, and left bundle branch block.

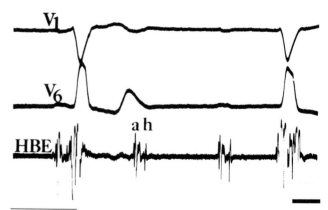

FIGURE 15.22   Third-degree block below the bundle of His. In the His bundle electrocardiogram (HBE), the second and third P waves are associated with A and H waves, but no evidence of conduction below the bundle of His can be seen. (From Kastor JA, Josephson ME. Treatment of atrioventricular block. In Fowler NO (ed). Cardiac Arrhythmias. Diagnosis and Treatment. 2nd ed. New York: Harper & Row, 1977, pp. 118–142, with permission.)[850]

- Fifty percent of patients with bundle branch block and syncope have HV intervals of 70 milliseconds or longer infranodal block during atrial pacing, or inducible monomorphic ventricular tachycardia.[869]
- The AH interval lengthens as people with bifascicular block and organic heart disease age.[870]
- When rapid atrial pacing produces block distal to the bundle of His in patients with bundle branch[871] or bifascicular block,[872] the risk of progression to atrioventricular block or sudden death is high.
- Patients with acute anteroseptal myocardial infarction and bifascicular block develop complete heart block more frequently when the HV interval is prolonged.[566, 844xxx]
- When anterior myocardial infarction produces right bundle branch block from block within the bundle of His,[yyy] the HV intervals are usually normal, but the clinical course is frequently complicated by progression to complete atrioventricular block, sustained ventricular tachycardia, or ventricular fibrillation.[873]

Levels of Block: Clinical Features

Coronary heart disease and myocardial infarction. Atrioventricular block due to inferior myocardial infarction usually occurs within the atrioventricular node, and this is identified by prolonged AH intervals during first- and second-degree block or dissociation between A waves and HV complexes during complete block.[209, 566, 691, 789] Intra-His block due to inferior myocardial infarction has been occasionally documented through the finding of split His potentials.[858] The block from anterior myocardial infarction develops within the infranodal conduction system. Each P wave is associated with A and H waves and the dissociated V wave with each QRS complex.[566, 691, 789zzz]

In a patient with Prinzmetal's angina, transient first-, second-, and third-degree atrioventricular block prolonged the AH interval, thus localizing the block to the atrioventricular node.[211] The atrioventricular nodes of patients with obstruction of their right coronary arteries, whether or not they have had previous myocardial infarctions, do not conduct as well as the nodes of patients without such pathological processes.[874] Thus, patients with significant disease of their right coronary arteries have latent defects in atrioventricular conduction.

The HV intervals of patients with ischemic cardiomyopathy and no bundle branch block are usually normal. The infranodal conduction system is seldom clinically affected by this condition.[875]

Idiopathic congestive cardiomyopathy. The HV interval is frequently prolonged in patients with idiopathic congestive cardiomyopathy, a finding suggesting that the pathological process is diffuse and affects both the myocardium and the conducting system.[875aaaa] There is an inverse relation between ventricular function and HV intervals in these patients. The HV interval tends to be prolonged as the ejection fraction decreases.[875]

Congenital atrioventricular block. Most cases of isolated congenital complete atrioventricular block are due to disease within or near the atrioventricular node; consequently, the A wave is dissociated from the HV pair.[6, 58, 801, 876–878bbbb] QRS complexes are characteristically narrow because bundle branch block is rarely present. Congenital block occurs within the atrioventricular node when it is due to congenitally corrected transposition of the great vessels. Less frequently, congenital block occurs within the bundle of His and is associated with split His potentials.[58, 877–879] When congenital block occurs within the infra-Hisian system, it produces AH coupling with a V wave associated with each escape beat; the QRS complexes are wide.

Intracardiac measurements can be abnormal in some patients with congenital heart disease and 1:1 atrioventricular conduction. The AH intervals are slightly,[252, 880–883] and occasionally greatly,[248] prolonged in patients with atrial septal and endocardial cushion defects.[265, 266, 884] Ebstein's anomaly of the tricuspid valve[269] and ostium primum atrial septal defect[880] can cause abnormally long HV intervals.

Ventricular escape rhythms. Ventricular escape rates tend to be slower in adults with block distal to the bundle of His than in those with atrioventricular nodal or intra-Hisian block[58, 134] (Table 15.7). An escape rhythm reliably activates the ventricles in a majority of patients whose bundles of His have been ablated.[885] However, artificial pacemakers suppress the discharge of intrinsic escape foci in many of these patients, so that syncope can occur from temporary ventricular standstill when a pacemaker suddenly fails.

Syncope. Electrophysiological studies can help to define a cardiac cause of syncope. It is seldom heart block; ventricular tachyarrhythmias are elicited much more commonly.[522, 523, 886, 887] Even in patients with chronic bifascicular block, electrophysiological studies show that high-grade atrioventricular block is seldom the cause of syncope.[522] However, when atrioventricular

---

[xxx]One of 18 patients developed complete block when the HV interval was normal, whereas 12 of 16 progressed to third-degree block when the HV interval was prolonged. The PR interval does not necessarily help in revealing the risk. It was normal in 18 of 19 patients with normal HV intervals, but the PR interval was long in only half of those with prolonged HV intervals.[566] AH intervals, shortened by increased sympathetic tone, help to make the PR interval appear "normal."

[yyy]Bundle branch block from lesions in the bundle of His is recognized electrophysiologically when pacing the bundle of His makes the bundle branch block disappear.

[zzz]The block was localized within the atrioventricular node in 24 (96%) of 25 patients with inferior myocardial infarction and was infranodal in each of 10 patients with anteroseptal infarction.[566]

[aaaa]The HV interval was prolonged in all but 1 of 18 patients with congestive cardiomyopathy and bundle branch block. Even in those with normal QRS complexes, 59% had prolonged HV intervals.[875]

[bbbb]Electrophysiological study of 16 children with congenital complete heart block localized the block to the atrioventricular node in 11 (69%), within the bundle of His in 3 (19%), and below the His bundle in 2 (13%).[58]

Table 15.7 **VENTRICULAR RATES DURING COMPLETE ATRIOVENTRICULAR BLOCK**[a]

Location of Block	Adults[134]			Children[58]	
	Number of Patients	Beats per Minute (Mean)	Beats per Minute (Range)	Number of Patients	Beats per Minute (Mean)
Atrioventricular node	17	44	32–61	11	60
Intra-His	8	45	32–54	3	45
Infra-His	22	35	15–45	2	44

[a]In two series of adults and children. In the adults, when the ventricular escape rates were faster than 50 beats per minute, block occurred only in the atrioventricular node or bundle of His. Ventricular rates slower than 30 beats per minute were observed only in patients with infra-Hisian block.

block does produce syncope, it is more often due to trifascicular disease than to block within the node or the bundle of His.[134, 630, 852, 871]cccc

When there is no clinical evidence of heart disease, electrophysiological studies are seldom helpful; healthy persons rarely faint or become dizzy from atrioventricular block.[888]dddd

Congestive heart failure. Congestive heart failure occurs more frequently in patients with second-degree atrioventricular nodal block than in those with type II second-degree block[630] and bundle branch block.[852] The incidence of heart failure, however, does not seem to correlate with the site of block in patients with advanced or complete heart block.[134]

Miscellaneous causes. The HV intervals are longer in patients with than in patients without *hypertension*. Infranodal conduction correlates closely with left ventricular mass.[889] The atrioventricular block produced by *Lyme disease* is usually located within the node[283, 286, 288] and only rarely in the infranodal region.[288]

Mechanical *trauma* of the conducting system by electrode catheters can produce intra-Hisian and type II second-degree block in patients with preexisting left bundle branch block.[394] A stab wound of the chest produced a ventricular septal defect plus complete heart block within the bundle of His.[480]

Atrioventricular nodal block with prolonged AH intervals developed in a patient with *hypothermia*. The AH intervals returned to normal after warming.[890]

Other Electrophysiological Observations

Ventriculoatrial conduction. Retrograde conduction from ventricles to atria, which can be produced rela-

tively easily in many patients with normal atrioventricular conduction, occurs occasionally in those with high-grade antegrade block.[571–574, 576, 577, 579–587, 589–593, 855, 891, 892] As one would expect, retrograde conduction occurs more often when antegrade conduction is intact.[583, 584, 588, 892]eeee During complete block, the phenomenon seems to depend on the presence of antegrade block in the bundle branches and fascicles and on preservation of retrograde conduction through the bundle of His and atrioventricular node.[581, 585, 588–590, 592, 593, 855]ffff The signal from the ventricular focus presumably reaches the intact bundle of His through intramyocardial conduction after bypassing the blocked bundle branches and fascicles.[581, 585, 589, 592]

Effects of atrial rate. As atrial pacing increases the heart rate in normal patients, the PR and AH intervals become progressively prolonged until Wenckebach periods appear. When conduction in the atrioventricular node is depressed, Wenckebach block appears at slower atrial paced rates than in patients with normal atrioventricular nodal function.[893]

The HV interval of the normal infranodal conduction system does not usually change with different atrial rates. However, rapid atrial rates produced by pacing or drugs such as atropine can elicit clinically significant infranodal block,[825, 871, 894] particularly in the presence of acute myocardial ischemia.[895] Block distal to His that can be induced by atrial pacing predicts progression of block and possible cardiac arrest in some patients.[872] By measuring the "RR index," one can estimate whether atrioventricular block occurs in the atrioventricular node or His-Purkinje system.[896]gggg

Fast atrial pacing may rarely *facilitate* infranodal conduction in those infrequent instances when the block is bradycardia-dependent and develops at slower rather than faster rates.[897] Decreasing the sinus rate either spontaneously or by maneuvers such as carotid sinus pressure may increase block in the atrioventricular node through hypervagotonia or in abnormal infranodal tissues through the mechanism of bradycardia-dependent block.[894, 898–902]

Provocative drug testing. The function of the infranodal conduction system in patients with bifascicular block and syncope can be tested by administering drugs such as disopyramide[903] that prolong conduction distal to the bundle of His. As with rapid atrial pacing,

cccc In 49 adults with high-grade block, syncope occurred in 29% when the block was in the atrioventricular node, in 25% when it was the bundle of His, and in 63% when it was below the bundle of His.[134]

dddd In 34 patients with syncope or "presyncope," all of whom had normal electrocardiograms, ambulatory electrocardiographic recording, or treadmill testing, electrophysiological study provided diagnoses that led to appropriate therapy that relieved symptoms in only 4 patients (11.8%).[888] None had atrioventricular block as the cause of their symptoms.

eeee In 200 patients studied electrophysiologically, retrograde conduction was present in 34 (68%) of 50 with normal antegrade conduction and in 66 (44%) of 150 with delayed antegrade conduction.[588]

ffff Retrograde conduction was present in 2 of 13 patients (15%) with complete trifascicular atrioventricular block but in none of 12 patients with third-degree block within the atrioventricular node or bundle of His.[588]

gggg The RR index is the ratio of the pacing-induced RR interval immediately before the block less the RR interval just after the block divided by the RR interval immediately before the block. An RR index of 0.85 or more has a sensitivity of 100% and a specificity of 99% for the identification of atrioventricular block localized to the His-Purkinje system. Smaller ratios favor atrioventricular nodal block.[896]

the HV interval may lengthen or ventricular beats may be dropped.[904] Such patients have a greater risk of developing second- or third-degree infranodal block, and a positive test suggests that their syncope may have been due to heart block.

Stability of escape foci. Pathological depression of escape foci that normally prevent syncope at exceedingly slow heart rates during complete atrioventricular block can develop at all levels of the conduction system, even in patients whose block is proximal to the bundle of His.[134, 905] Ventricular pacing sometimes suppresses escape foci and further depresses abnormal antegrade conduction.[906]

When pacemakers installed for high degrees of atrioventricular block are turned off, an intrinsic escape focus adequate to prevent fainting or lightheadedness will appear in three-fourths of patients within 10 seconds.[907] Those who do not develop adequate escape foci may have[907]

- A relatively long history of conduction disturbance.
- Slower intraventricular conduction.
- Been taking antiarrhythmic drugs.

Exercise. Patients who develop atrioventricular block during exercise can have conduction abnormalities in the atrioventricular node or within or below the bundle of His.[472]hhhh

Ventriculophasic modulation of atrioventricular nodal conduction. Electrophysiological techniques demonstrate, during atrioventricular block, an effect on the atrioventricular node similar to ventriculophasic sinus arrhythmia.[908]

Concealed and supernormal conduction. Concealed conduction in atrioventricular block refers to the depression of conduction produced by blocked impulses that enter the conducting system from the ventricles or the atria.[586, 895, 905, 909–911] In supernormal conduction, depressed tissues appear unexpectedly to acquire the ability to conduct better. This phenomenon has been used to explain occasional cases of enhanced conductivity.[854, 912–919]iiii

Conduction through an atriofascicular pathway. This type of conduction substituted for a diseased atrioventricular conduction system in one patient.[920]

TREATMENT[610]

Cardiac pacing is the primary treatment for patients who have or may develop paroxysmal or chronic severe atrioventricular block. Although drugs were used be-

fore pacing became available, they are seldom employed now except when the block is temporary or in emergencies before pacemaking can be applied.

Physical Maneuvers

Carotid sinus pressure. Carotid sinus pressure decreases conduction within the atrioventricular node[899–901, 921] and, occasionally, within the infranodal system.[894, 899] The maneuver, therefore, does not have therapeutic value, although it may help to reveal electrophysiological features of the block and individual patients. As expected, carotid sinus pressure usually decreases the sinus rate even in patients with complete heart block.[922]

Precordial percussion. This form of percussion ("thumpversion") can stimulate ventricular contraction during asystole resulting from complete heart block.[923, 924]

Drugs

Much of this discussion has historical rather than contemporary application.

Aminophylline. Aminophylline temporarily improves atrioventricular conduction in some patients with inferior myocardial infarction and heart block unrelieved by atropine.[925–928]jjjj

Amyl nitrite. Amyl nitrite, inhaled as required, produced 1:1 atrioventricular conduction in a patient with complete atrioventricular block and syncope.[929]

Antiarrhythmic drugs. Antiarrhythmic drugs should not be given to patients without pacemakers who have second- or third-degree atrioventricular block. Although some of these agents are vagolytic and may facilitate atrioventricular nodal conduction, they usually increase block in the infranodal regions and may worsen the conduction disturbance. Antiarrhythmic drugs also suppress ventricular escape foci and may produce Adams-Stokes attacks and cardiac arrest. If the ventricular rate is protected by a pacemaker, antiarrhythmic drugs may be administered to suppress tachyarrhythmias.

Atropine.[930] Atropine and related drugs such as belladonna reduce heart block within the atrioventricular node when the cause is hypervagotonia.[35, 473, 825, 900, 921, 931, 932] Consequently, atropine can relieve atrioventricular block during inferior myocardial infarction[152, 933–936] (Fig. 15.23), but not when the block is due to ischemia of the node.[166, 191, 925–927]kkkk The drug seldom directly affects infranodal conduction.[825, 937]

---

hhhhAmong 14 patients with exercise-induced block, conduction abnormalities were located in the atrioventricular node in 4, within the His bundle in 7, and distal to the His bundle in 3.[472]

iiiiElectrophysiologists have discovered that the interaction of various components of the conducting system can explain many of the electrocardiographic findings previously ascribed to supernormal atrioventricular conduction. The phrase is seldom employed now.[919]

---

jjjjAminophylline is a competitive antagonist of adenosine, a drug that decreases atrioventricular nodal conduction.

kkkkBoth vagotonia and ischemia may account for block in the early and late phases of inferior infarction. Authorities differ about which is more important.[166, 927]

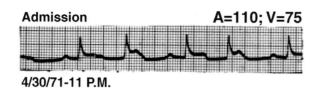

Admission   **A=110; V=75**

4/30/71-11 P.M.

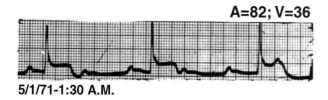

A=82; V=36

5/1/71-1:30 A.M.

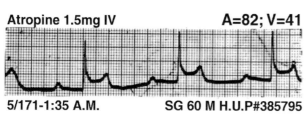

Atropine 1.5mg IV   **A=82; V=41**

5/171-1:35 A.M.   **SG 60 M H.U.P#385795**

Lead 2

FIGURE 15.23 Atropine reducing block in the atrioventricular node. The patient had an inferior myocardial infarction. Top: Wenckebach periods. **Middle:** Complete block. **Bottom:** After administration of 1.5 mg of atropine, the amount of block was reduced to 2:1. Ischemia of the sinus and atrioventricular nodes maintains a relatively slow sinus rate and some degree of block despite the effects of the large dose of atropine. (From Kastor JA, Josephson ME. Treatment of atrioventricular block. In Fowler NO (ed). Cardiac Arrhythmias. Diagnosis and Treatment. 2nd ed. New York: Harper & Row, 1977, pp. 118–142, with permission.)[850]

Vagolytic agents may *increase* the degree of atrioventricular block when the chronotropic effect on the sinus node exceeds its vagolytic effect on the atrioventricular node and thereby stresses the infranodal tissues.[833, 900, 929] By raising the sinus rate, atropine can also increase the amount of infranodal block in patients with type II second-degree block.[825] In patients with coronary disease, faster sinus rates may aggravate ischemia of the conduction system.[895] Blocking autonomic responses with atropine and propranolol causes little change in the rate of the ventricular rhythm in most patients with complete atrioventricular block.[938]

Beta-adrenergic agonists. Isoproterenol and other beta-adrenergic agonists increase the rate of escape foci in patients with atrioventricular block and may reduce the degree of block.[939–943] The drugs can also stabilize idioventricular pacemakers and may decrease the appearance of other ventricular beats. Inhaled isoproterenol[944] and a sustained-action preparation of isoproterenol that can be taken by mouth[945–949] produce similar effects. Isoproterenol shortens AH and HV intervals and may improve conduction both within and below[937] the atrioventricular node.[950] The beta-adrenergic agonists salbutamol[951] and isoproterenol,[952] administered intravenously to the mother, increase the heart

rate[951, 952] and improve ventricular function[951] in fetuses with congenital complete atrioventricular block.

Chlorothiazide. This diuretic improves atrioventricular conduction in patients with different degrees of heart block by producing hypokalemia.[953]

Corticosteroids. Corticosteroids shorten the PR interval about 20 milliseconds in patients without conduction system disease.[954] They also reduce the degree of atrioventricular block and the number of Adams-Stokes attacks in patients with acute block caused by myocardial infarction[955–957] and sarcoidosis[361] and in some patients whose block is chronic.[957–963]⁗ Prenatal administration of steroids does not prevent congenital complete heart block from developing in the children of women at risk of delivering babies with this arrhythmia.[89, 240, 964]

Digitalis. Digitalis prolongs atrioventricular nodal conduction[6] and is therefore contraindicated in patients with partial block who do not have ventricular pacemakers.[921, 965]

Digoxin-specific Fab fragments. Fab fragments relieve atrioventricular block produced by digoxin in adults[966] and children.[967]

Potassium, glucose, and insulin. These three agents may relieve heart block produced by myocardial infarction.[968]

Sodium lactate. Sodium lactate can temporarily restore ventricular beating in cardiac arrest caused by complete heart block.[969]

Theophylline. This drug appears to have prevented further atrioventricular block in a patient whose arrhythmia developed from organ rejection after cardiac transplantation.[499]

Verapamil. This drug increases the rate of junctional pacemakers during complete atrioventricular block.[970]

Pacing[20, 815, 816, 971]

The principal contemporary method for treating acute and chronic atrioventricular block is cardiac pacemaking. In properly selected patients, the technique relieves symptoms and prolongs life. Cardiologists usually install DDD pacers in patients with sinus rhythm in the atria. By reestablishing atrioventricular synchrony, these units improve cardiac function and quality of life[755, 972] and are more cost-effective for the treatment

---

⁗None of these studies was controlled. Because normal conduction usually returns in patients who recover from inferior myocardial infarction, the value of corticosteroids in facilitating this process has not been unequivocally established. The action of steroids on atrioventricular conduction is clear, however; the drugs decrease the PR intervals in patients in sinus rhythm.[954]

of atrioventricular block[973] than ventricular (VVI) pacers.[mmmm]

Deciding when to pace patients to relieve symptoms, however, is much easier than deciding when to pace them to prolong life. The following general rules help in deciding when to install pacemakers:

- Block within the atrioventricular node is less likely to be associated with slow ventricular rates and progression to complete block and possible cardiac arrest than is block within the bundle of His or the bundle branch–fascicular system.
- Temporary pacing is required when heart block complicates anterior infarctions but is less often necessary during inferior infarctions.
- Most asymptomatic patients with congenital complete heart block and no structural heart disease do not receive permanent pacemakers. However, their use in this group is increasing.

Symptoms. Pacing, which usually relieves symptoms produced by atrioventricular block, should be employed when the physician is certain that the complaints have been produced by the slow heart rate.[522, 669] However, reaching this conclusion may be difficult when the block is paroxysmal and is not present on the 12-lead electrocardiogram. Under such circumstances, the physician should try to document symptoms that occur at the time of block by extended electrocardiographic monitoring, exercise testing, or electrophysiological study.

Symptoms typical of atrioventricular block may develop from many, often benign, causes. As emphasized throughout this chapter, syncope is seldom caused by atrioventricular block and is rarely caused by paroxysmal block. Furthermore, shortness of breath, decreased exercise tolerance, and reduced mental function are usually manifestations of heart disease other than bradycardia. However, partial or complete block may worsen the effects of heart failure or ischemia, and pacing, in such cases, can help improve function.[974nnnn]

Acquired atrioventricular block in adults.[975oooo] Most patients who acquire chronic complete atrioventricular block receive pacemakers, because few escape symptoms produced by bradycardia, congestive failure, ventricular ectopy, or prolonged asystole[975] (Table 15.8).

[mmmm]See the earlier section on hemodynamics.

[nnnn]Most cardiologists know of patients with bradycardia caused by heart block whose relatively minor symptoms such as lightheadedness, decreased physical energy, and slightly reduced mental function were improved by cardiac pacemaking. One of my favorite examples was observed by Dr. Doris J. W. Escher, one of the pioneers in the clinical development of pacemakers. The patient was a physician who had lost interest in the intellectual aspects of his profession after complete atrioventricular block developed. On insertion of a pacemaker, his excitement for learning and his desire to read medical journals returned.[974]

[oooo]The American College of Cardiology/American Heart Association Task Force on Practice Guidelines (Committee on Pacemaker Implantation) published revised guidelines in 1998 for permanent cardiac pacemaking, which I have summarized in Tables 15.8, 15.9, and 15.10.[975]

| Table 15.8 | **PERMANENT PACING FOR ADULTS WITH ACQUIRED ATRIOVENTRICULAR BLOCK NOT DUE TO RECENT MYOCARDIAL INFARCTION**[975] |

Indicated (class I)
1. Third-degree atrioventricular block at any anatomical level, associated with one or more of the following:
   - Symptoms produced by the bradyarrhythmia.
   - Arrhythmias or other medical conditions requiring drugs that produce bradycardia.
   - Documented asystole ≥3.0 seconds or any escape rate <40 beats per minute in awake, asymptomatic patients.
   - After catheter ablation of the atrioventricular junction.
   - Postoperative atrioventricular block not expected to resolve.
   - Neuromuscular disease with atrioventricular block.
2. Second-degree atrioventricular block, regardless of site, with symptoms from bradycardia.

Probably indicated (class IIa)
1. Asymptomatic complete heart block, at any anatomical site, with average ventricular rate, when awake, of 40 beats per minute or faster.
2. Asymptomatic, type I second-degree atrioventricular block.
3. Asymptomatic, type II second-degree block at intra- or infra-His level found incidentally at electrophysiological study for other indications.
4. First-degree atrioventricular block with symptoms suggesting pacemaker syndrome and documented alleviation of symptoms with temporary pacing.

Possibly indicated (class IIb)
1. First-degree atrioventricular block with PR intervals >0.30 second in patients with left ventricular dysfunction and symptoms of congestive heart failure in whom a shorter PR interval improves hemodynamic function.

Not indicated and possibly harmful (class III)
1. Asymptomatic first-degree atrioventricular block.
2. Asymptomatic type I second-degree atrioventricular nodal block.
3. Atrioventricular block expected to resolve and unlikely to recur (such as due to drug toxicity or Lyme disease).

(Adapted from Gregoratos G, Cheitlin MD, Conill A, et al. ACC/AHA guidelines for implantation of cardiac pacemakers and antiarrhythmia devices [Committee on Pacemaker Implantation]. Circulation 1998; 97:1325–1335. By permission of the American Heart Association, Inc.)
(Adapted from Dreifus LS, Fisch C, Griffin JC, Gillette PC, Mason JW, Parsonnet V. Guidelines for implantation of cardiac pacemakers and antiarrhythmia devices. J Am Coll Cardiol 1991; 18:1–13. Reprinted with permission from the American College of Cardiology.)

Withholding a pacemaker from an asymptomatic patient with acquired complete heart block demands a certain amount of fortitude in the physician, because few asymptomatic patients survive for extended periods. The decision not to pace such patients is based, at least in part, on reports written in the pre-pacemaker era about patients with complete heart block who lived comfortably for decades after discovery of the arrhythmia.[976pppp]

[pppp]The complete heart block of many of the asymptomatic patients with prolonged survival reported in the past may have been congenital. Paul White and Helen Donovan described two such patients, both of whom were women.[976] In one case, a physician observed a slow pulse rate when the patient was 12 years old. An electrocardiogram taken in 1916 when she was 24 years old confirmed complete block with a ventricular rate of 40 beats per minute. She was "still in quite good health at the age of 73 years . . . with complete atrioventricular dissociation throughout the entire interval." Electrocardiograms taken on the second patient in 1917 when she was 29 years old revealed complete heart block. She led a vigorous life and died suddenly at the age of 73.

Ventricular pacing relieves the symptoms and can prevent a potentially fatal cardiac arrest in patients with type II infranodal block in whom progression to complete block is particularly likely to occur.[627, 852] Type II second-degree atrioventricular block is an uncommon electrocardiographic finding, however, and the number of completely asymptomatic patients with this type of block is small.[627] On the rare occasions when this abnormality is detected in asymptomatic patients, an electrophysiological study should be performed to discover whether the block is due to infranodal disease; if it is, I advise that a pacemaker be inserted, because one cannot predict when infranodal type II block will progress to complete block.[977]

First-degree atrioventricular block with moderate PR interval prolongation rarely progresses to advanced degrees of heart block and in otherwise asymptomatic patients does not require treatment.[978] A few patients with severe myocardial failure, prolonged PR intervals, and sinus bradycardia may benefit from atrioventricular pacing whereby a normal PR interval and a faster rate can be established.

Patients with asymptomatic type I second-degree nodal block, often presenting with Wenckebach periods, do not need pacing unless they have associated symptom-producing myocardial disease.[979, 980qqqq] Symptomatic patients with block within the bundle of His usually receive pacemakers, although the prognosis for asymptomatic patients with only prolonged His potentials is favorable without pacing.[981]

Chronic bifascicular and trifascicular block[975] (Table 15.9). Pacing patients with bifascicular block and symptoms caused by intermittent complete heart block

---

qqqqThis is the general consensus.[979] However, one group found that the prognosis for patients with type I second-degree block is no more favorable than for those with type II. Those patients who were paced survived longer regardless of the type of second-degree block.[980]

Table 15.9	**PERMANENT PACING FOR ADULTS WITH CHRONIC BIFASCICULAR OR TRIFASCICULAR BLOCK**[975]

Indicated (class I)
 1. Intermittent third-degree atrioventricular block.
 2. Type II second-degree atrioventricular block.
Probably indicated (class IIa)
 1. Syncope not proved to be due to atrioventricular block when other likely causes, specifically ventricular tachycardia, have been excluded.
 2. Incidental finding at electrophysiological study of HV interval ≥100 milliseconds in asymptomatic patients.
 3. Incidental finding at electrophysiological study of pacing-induced nonphysiological infra-His block.
Not indicated and possibly harmful (class III)
 1. Asymptomatic fascicular block without atrioventricular block.
 2. Asymptomatic fascicular block with first-degree atrioventricular block.

(Adapted from Gregoratos G, Cheitlin MD, Conill A, et al. ACC/AHA guidelines for implantation of cardiac pacemakers and antiarrhythmia devices [Committee on Pacemaker Implantation]. Circulation 1998; 97:1325–1335. By permission of the American Heart Association, Inc.)

relieves the symptoms. Whether such patients will survive longer depends on the extent of intrinsic myocardial disease.

The combination of intermittent type II second-degree and bifascicular block strongly suggests that the lesion is below the bundle of His.[852] Progression to complete block is likely, and pacing is indicated.[852]

Even though syncope is infrequently due to atrioventricular block even in patients with multifascicular block, one should nevertheless study the conduction system of such patients who have fainted with extended electrocardiographic monitoring or exercise to learn whether type II second-degree block or complete block will appear. If these tests fail to reveal block, an electrophysiological study can be performed in which HV prolongation and pacing-induced infranodal block are sought.[135, 522, 864, 866, 867, 871, 982] When either of these is present, the likelihood rises that the symptoms are due to intermittent atrioventricular block, and pacemaking should be considered.[135, 864, 866] HV prolongation beyond 70 milliseconds in such patients is an independent risk factor for complete block, and if the interval is prolonged beyond 100 milliseconds, the risk is even higher.[867] Pacing prevents syncope that is caused by block but does not necessarily prolong life because many of these patients also have severe myocardial disease.[867]

Asymptomatic patients with bifascicular block develop second- and third-degree atrioventricular block more frequently than those without fascicular blocks,[671] but the rate of progression is slow,[522, 667, 669, 675, 983–985] and prophylactic pacing in patients is not needed even when such patients must have major operations.[672, 673, 986]

In the first decade after the development of His bundle electrocardiography, some investigators suggested that pacemaking could prolong the lives of patients with isolated prolongation of the HV interval without bifascicular or documented heart block who presented with intermittent neurological symptoms such as syncope or dizziness.[987] This theory has not been subsequently supported. Such patients, however, should be followed for changes in their electrocardiograms and should report symptoms that could be caused by conduction system disease.

During myocardial infarction.[139, 140, 159, 160, 164, 168, 171, 173, 209, 566, 656, 676, 683, 684, 844, 988–1007rrrr] When heart block complicates acute infarction, temporary ventricular pacing is usually used if any of the following develop:

• Adams-Stokes attacks.
• Bifascicular block or alternating bundle branch block, because sudden progression to complete infranodal block may follow.[165, 209, 566, 656, 683, 684, 844, 1000, 1001, 1003, 1004, 1008–1010] Those patients who acutely develop bifascicular block during myocardial

---

rrrrThe indications for temporary pacing for atrioventricular block during myocardial infarction have not been rigorously investigated. At this time, controlled studies would be difficult and probably unethical.[159, 160, 164, 171, 173, 209, 566, 656, 676, 683, 684, 844, 988–992, 994–1007]

infarction and prolonged HV intervals have the highest risk of progressing to complete block.[566, 844]
- Congestive heart failure.
- Hypotension.
- Ventricular ectopy.
- Ventricular rate of less than about 50 beats per minute.

By reestablishing the atrial contribution to ventricular filling, temporary synchronous or sequential atrioventricular pacing increases cardiac output in patients with myocardial infarction and heart block but does not, by itself, improve survival.[763, 1011]

After myocardial infarction[975, 1012] (Table 15.10). Because atrioventricular block usually resolves spontaneously in patients with inferior infarction who survive the acute event, permanent pacing is seldom needed for such patients. For the few patients who survive anterior myocardial infarction complicated by atrioventricular block, permanent pacemaking is employed when second- or third-degree block persists. Permanent pacing is often considered for patients with myocardial infarctions, usually anterior, associated with transient atrioventricular block and new, persistent bilateral bundle branch block.[1004, 1009, 1013, 1014] The risk that these patients may progress to high degrees of atrioventricular block is greater when HV intervals are prolonged.[1015–1017ssss] Patients who have persistent

---

ssss However, several studies suggest that pacing may not improve the survival of patients with persistent bundle branch or bifascicular block that developed during their infarction.[1015–1017] These patients, who are more likely to die of ventricular tachyarrhythmias produced by their severe myocardial dysfunction than from cardiac arrest resulting from atrioventricular block, may require implantation of implantable cardioverter-defibrillators.

| Table 15.10 | **PERMANENT PACING AFTER THE ACUTE PHASE OF MYOCARDIAL INFARCTION**[975] |

Indicated (class I)
1. Persistent second-degree infranodal atrioventricular block with bilateral bundle branch block or third-degree infranodal atrioventricular block.
2. Transient second- or third-degree infranodal atrioventricular block with associated bundle branch block.
3. Persistent and symptomatic second- and third-degree atrioventricular block.

Possibly indicated (class IIb)
1. First-degree atrioventricular block with PR intervals >0.30 second in patients with left ventricular dysfunction and symptoms of congestive heart failure in whom a shorter PR interval improves hemodynamic function.

Not indicated and possibly harmful (class III)
1. Transient atrioventricular block in the absence of intraventricular conduction defects.
2. Transient atrioventricular block in the presence of isolated left anterior fascicular block.
3. Acquired left anterior fascicular block in the absence of atrioventricular block.
4. Persistent first-degree atrioventricular block in the presence of bundle branch block that is old or for which the age cannot be determined.

(Adapted from Gregoratos G, Cheitlin MD, Conill A, et al. ACC/AHA guidelines for implantation of cardiac pacemakers and antiarrhythmia devices [Committee on Pacemaker Implantation]. Circulation 1998; 97:1325–1335. By permission of the American Heart Association, Inc.)

unifascicular block or bifascicular block with normal infranodal conduction are not usually paced.

After cardiac surgery.[1018] Pacing is occasionally required to treat atrioventricular block that develops after cardiac surgery. Atrioventricular sequential or synchronous pacing can improve cardiac function in some children after correction of congenital heart lesions better than ventricular pacing alone.[1019]

Congenital complete heart block.[2, 975, 1020ttt] *Children.* Children with congenital complete heart block who faint or who develop congestive heart failure or dangerous ventricular ectopy should be paced.[2, 58, 63, 65, 134, 215, 256, 300, 545, 555, 1021–1025uuuu] As expected, children with structural congenital heart disease in addition to the block often need pacemakers.[58] Most children[vvvv] with autoantibody-associated congenital complete heart block need pacemakers.[227]

Children with congenital complete heart block and ventricular rates greater than 50 to 60 beats per minute rarely, if ever, faint or die from the arrhythmia;[251, 711, 1026] consequently, they do not need pacemakers if they are otherwise asymptomatic.[1, 2, 251, 711, 1027] Asymptomatic children, however, should be paced whose

- Average heart rate when awake is less than 50 beats per minute.[251, 711]
- Randomly detected rate is less than 45 beats per minute.[1]
- Junctional escape mechanism is unstable.[711wwww]

Pacemakers, however, have not yet been proved to prevent syncope and to prolong the life of children with congenital complete heart block who develop ventricular ectopy on Holter monitoring or during exercise testing.[65, 251, 710]

Rate-responsive ventricular pacing, rather than atrioventricular synchronous pacing, which requires two electrodes, provides adequate hemodynamic function for most children with congenital complete heart block.[1028] Fetuses with hydrops and congenital complete heart block may benefit from transplacental anticongestion treatment[1029] or from placement of a pacing electrode inserted through the mother's abdomen and uterus.[1030]

---

ttt The American College of Cardiology/American Heart Association Task Force on Practice Guidelines (Committee on Pacemaker Implantation) also prepared a detailed review in 1998 about pacing in children and adolescents.[975]

uuuu The comprehensive joint review of the Association of European Paediatric Cardiologists, published in 1981, reported that 65 of 425 patients (15%) with isolated congenital complete heart block received pacemakers.[63]

vvvv Pacemakers were required for 37 (67%) of 55 such children, 27 within 3 months after birth.[227]

wwww This advice, summarized in an authoritative text on pediatric arrhythmias,[1] has not, to my knowledge, been supported by specific studies. The use of pacemakers for children who develop atrioventricular block after cardiac surgery is reviewed elsewhere, and the interested reader should consult these sources.[385, 1013] The ventricular rate of a 23-week fetus with congestive heart failure from congenital complete heart block temporarily increased when an electrode catheter was inserted into the fetal right ventricle with ultrasound guidance.[1027]

Adults. The likelihood that adults with congenital complete heart block will need pacing rises as they grow older.[64] This observation and the relatively high prevalence of clinical events has led one group[530] to advise prophylactic pacing for all, even asymptomatic, adults with congenital complete heart block to prevent[530]

- Unpredictable syncope with considerable mortality from first attacks.
- Gradually decreasing ventricular rate.
- Significant morbidity.
- Mitral regurgitation thought to be due to the slow ventricular rate producing overdistension of the left ventricle and papillary muscles.

This advice,[530, 1020] however, is not universally accepted. Others suggest pacing only those young adults who develop such symptoms as dyspnea and dizziness.[1031]

During cardiac catheterization. Physicians frequently insert pacing catheters into the right ventricle during catheterization procedures in patients with bundle branch block because of concern that transient atrioventricular block may develop from bilateral bundle branch block produced by manipulation of the catheters.[387–395, 410] Pacing is seldom needed, according to the authors of one study, who suggest that ventricular fibrillation produced by the pacing electrode presents the greater risk.[1032]

Miscellaneous Conditions

Ventricular pacing, for as little as 1 minute,[1033] can so affect repolarization that when the pacing stops, the T waves of the spontaneous beats may be temporarily abnormal, a phenomenon called "cardiac memory."[1033, 1034] Plasmapheresis of a mother at risk of producing congenital complete atrioventricular block in her child did not prevent the arrhythmia from developing.[89]

PROGNOSIS[1035]

One observation made about complete atrioventricular block several decades ago[1036] is still relevant despite the therapeutic advance brought by pacemakers:[193, 866, 867, 1037]

Its prognosis depends upon the severity and duration but is *primarily determined by the accompanying heart disease.*[xxxx]

Obviously, pacemakers cannot repair the damage previously or subsequently inflicted on the myocardium by coronary disease, cardiomyopathy, or other pathological process.

Progression and Regression of Heart Block

Partial block may remain stable for years or decades or may progress quickly to higher degrees of block.[1038yyyy] Predicting the rate of change is hazardous.[1039]

Both acquired[61, 194, 1040] and congenital[2, 256, 548, 1040–1042] persistent complete block may spontaneously *decrease* in patients with[1041, 1043–1047zzzz] and without[194, 256, 548, 1040] pacemakers. Most patients, however, continue to depend on their pacemakers because the return of atrioventricular conduction is usually temporary.[1047]

Occasionally, permanent pacing can be discontinued, or a replacement need not be inserted when the battery expires.[1048] Dependence is less likely if implantation is preceded by

- Asymptomatic complete block of the atrioventricular node.[1048]
- Atrial fibrillation.[1046]
- Atrial flutter.[1046]
- Atrial tachycardia.[1046]
- Incomplete, especially type I, block.[1046]
- Symptomatic bradycardia.[1048]

Among the clinical reasons that a patient is likely to depend on the pacemaker are the following:

- Syncope occurred before the pacemaker was installed.
- The indication was complete block after cardiac surgery.[376]

Chronic Acquired Heart Block in Adults

Before pacemakers were available, fewer than half the patients survived for 1 year after their first Adams-Stokes attack caused by heart block, and the majority of all patients with electrocardiographic evidence of complete block died within 2 years.[1036, 1049, 1050aaaaa] Once effective pacemaking is established, survival depends on the extent of intrinsic noncardiac and cardiac diseases other than the conduction abnormality.[200, 1050] Hence, the prognosis is similar for paced patients with isolated block from idiopathic bundle branch fibrosis who are otherwise healthy and for similar patients without heart block.[200, 1051bbbbb] This finding includes patients from 65 to 79 years of age;[1052] however, survival is less for paced patients 80 years old or older than for controls.[1052]

---

xxxxAccording to Drs. Louis N. Katz and Alfred Pick in their renowned and, for its time (1956), highly sophisticated book on cardiac arrhythmias (italics by the authors).[1036]

yyyyCongenital complete heart block advanced from second- to third-degree in an infant with neonatal lupus syndrome.[1038]

zzzzSinus rhythm returned within 1 week in 14 of 58 patients (23%) with Adams-Stokes disease resulting from complete heart block, often within 1 day and usually after they received permanent ventricular pacemakers.[1043] In a woman with congenital complete atrioventricular block, normal conduction returned temporarily during two successive pregnancies.[1042]

aaaaaSome[1050] but not all[1049] investigators writing in the pre-pacemaker period reported that Adams-Stokes attacks specifically worsened the survival of patients with acquired complete heart block.

bbbbbSimilarly, patients with primary conduction system disease producing bifascicular block have a lower risk of death from cardiovascular disease and specifically cardiac arrest than those with similar electrocardiographic abnormalities and additional organic heart disease.[872]

Most patients who die of ischemic or cardiomyopathic heart disease in addition to complete heart block do so within the first year after pacemaker implantation. Thereafter, the survival of such patients is remarkably similar to the general population when matched for age and gender.[1053]

Myocardial Infarction

Second- and third-degree atrioventricular blocks increase the hospital mortality[168, 183] for both men and women.[1054] Between one-fifth and one-third of patients whose inferior myocardial infarctions are complicated by high degrees of atrioventricular block die during the acute period, three times more than those without block[168, 169, 178, 180, 186, 1055] (Fig. 15.24).[ccccc] Infarcted right ventricles increase hospital mortality when heart block complicates myocardial infarction.[180, 187ddddd] Death is

---

[ccccc]According to four of the largest series, 30% of 529 patients with high degrees of atrioventricular block died, compared with 10% of 3,447 patients without block.[178, 180, 1055] Each of these series was collected in coronary care units with pacemaking capability. In a multiyear (1980–1993), multihospital series conducted in Worcester, Massachusetts, the case-fatality rates were 49% among those with complete block and 16% of those without block.[169]

[ddddd]In 39 patients with complete block and inferior infarction, 41% who had right ventricular infarction died, but only 14% of those whose right ventricle was not affected. The development of complete atrioventricular block increased the mortality only slightly when right ventricular infarction was absent.[180] The diagnosis of right ventricular involvement in this report "was based on elevation of ST segment of 0.1 millivolt or more in right precordial leads V_{3R} and/or V_{4R} in patients with typical changes in inferior leads."[180]

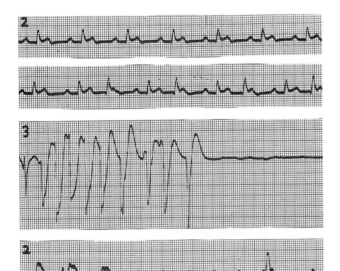

FIGURE 15.24 Death after acute inferior myocardial infarction and atrioventricular block. The top two tracings show the ST segment elevations in lead II that are characteristic of an acute inferior myocardial infarction. This patient had had previous anterior infarction. 2:1 block is present in the top tracing, and 3:2 Wenckebach periods are shown in the second. In the bottom two tracings, ventricular tachycardia appears, followed by asystole and complete block. The outcome from atrioventricular block after a second infarction, even if it is inferior, may be poor in patients who have had previous damage. (From Kitchen JB III, Kastor JA. Pacing in acute myocardial infarction: indications, methods, hazards, and results. Cardiovasc Clin 1975; 7:219–243, with permission.)[1005]

usually due to congestive heart failure and cardiogenic shock.[175, 178, 180] Despite successful thrombolysis, complications and hospital mortality are greater than in those who have not sustained heart block.[186]

As many as three-fourths of patients with anterior myocardial infarction and high degrees of atrioventricular block die.[148, 151, 158–160, 163, 992, 996, 1056eeeee] Widespread myocardial destruction producing cardiogenic shock and congestive heart failure characterize those who die.

Acutely developing bifascicular or trifascicular block, which often progresses to atrioventricular block of high degree, increases the mortality during acute myocardial infarction[666, 678, 680–683, 688, 1004, 1008, 1009, 1013, 1057–1060] by as much as twice.[683, 688, 1057–1059] Acute left anterior hemiblock alone does not adversely affect the prognosis,[162, 687, 1060] but patients who develop isolated left posterior hemiblock do not live as long as those without it.[689]

After Myocardial Infarction

When compared with survivors of inferior myocardial infarction without block, those with transient complete atrioventricular block have, when discharged from the hospital, similar

- Clinical characteristics.[1061]
- Left ventricular ejection fraction.[1061]
- Number of complex ventricular arrhythmias.[1061]
- Prognosis.[181, 183, 186, 1061–1063]

Accordingly, coronary arteriography need not be performed in the absence of other indications.[1061]

The prognosis of those few patients who survive acute, usually anterior myocardial infarction complicated by atrioventricular block of high degree is less favorable than the prognosis of those without block. Such patients have widespread myocardial destruction and die of ventricular tachyarrhythmias or congestive heart failure.

Cardiomyopathy

The presence of first- or second-degree atrioventricular block worsens the prognosis of patients with idiopathic dilated cardiomyopathy independently of other risk factors such as complex ventricular premature beats and reduced left ventricular ejection fraction.[1064]

Congenital Complete Heart Block[1065]

The prognosis for most patients with congenital complete heart block is excellent, except when the heart block was recognized in infancy or when other structural heart disease is present.[57, 58, 63–65, 217, 568, 597, 1026] At particularly high risk are children born with autoanti-

---

[eeeee]Of 94 patients with anterior infarction and high degrees of atrioventricular block, mostly complete, 71 (76%) died during the acute period. Most of these patients were treated in coronary care units with pacing utilized as determined by their physicians. I collected the data from eight series,[148, 151, 158, 160, 163, 992, 996, 1056] the largest of which had 35 patients.[996]

body-associated congenital complete heart block. One-third die in the early neonatal period.[227]

Poor prognostic signs in fetuses with congenital complete heart block include[723]

- Bradycardia with a heart rate of less than 55 beats per minute in early pregnancy or prenatal rapid decrease in heart rate.
- Hydrops.

Concern is rising about the risk of fatal cardiac arrest that may occur during the first episode of syncope in previously asymptomatic patients with congenital complete heart block. Six of 102 untreated patients in one large series died suddenly with no preceding symptoms.[55, 530]*fffff*

Type of Pacing

Patients with high-degree atrioventricular block and congestive heart failure live longer if they receive dual-chamber rather than ventricular demand pacers.[1066]

SUMMARY

Atrioventricular block of any degree seldom occurs in patients with normal hearts, although the PR interval lengthens as people age, and children and well-trained athletes may have asymptomatic PR prolongation. Complete heart block develops most commonly in older patients, more of whom are male than female. Patients with congenital block are more frequently female.

Idiopathic fibrosis of the conducting tissue accounts for most cases of acquired permanent atrioventricular block in adults. Acute myocardial infarction produces complete block in about 7% of patients, most of whom have inferior infarctions, often producing the syndrome of right ventricular infarction. Chronic coronary heart disease seldom produces heart block, with the notable exception of variant angina due to coronary vasospasm.

Atrioventricular block also develops in association with mitral and aortic valve disease, Lyme disease, infective endocarditis, some forms of myocarditis, acute rheumatic fever, and the infiltrative cardiomyopathies. Surgical correction of valve disease and of certain congenital anomalies may produce atrioventricular block, but the arrhythmia seldom develops after coronary artery bypass grafting. Many cardioactive drugs as well as hyperkalemia and hypermagnesemia may induce block.

Congenital complete atrioventricular block is an uncommon anomaly. Most children who survive have no other structural heart lesions. Mothers of babies with congenital complete heart block have antibodies directed against SSA/Ro or SSB/La antigens.

Syncope is the most characteristic symptom produced by complete atrioventricular block, but complaints arising from congestive failure and decreased cardiac output are frequent. Many patients with congenital heart block have no symptoms.

On physical examination, the dissociation between atrial and ventricular contraction in complete heart block produces large A waves in the venous pulse and variable intensity of the arterial pulse, the first heart sound, and systolic murmurs.

The electrocardiogram reveals first-degree atrioventricular block as prolonged PR intervals. Second-degree block is recognized by occasional nonconduction of P waves in the Wenckebach pattern or, in the Mobitz type II pattern, with fixed PR intervals in the conducted beats. In complete heart block, the P waves and QRS complexes are dissociated from each other. The ventricular rate is characteristically slow and regular. Narrow QRS complexes suggest that the block is located in the atrioventricular node or within the bundle of His. Wide complexes suggest that the block is below the atrioventricular junction. The rate of progression to higher degrees of block is unpredictable.

Bifascicular block usually precedes the appearance of high degrees of atrioventricular block in patients with chronic acquired conduction system disease. However, most patients with bifascicular block do not develop atrioventricular block. Patients with anterior myocardial infarctions characteristically demonstrate bundle branch or bifascicular block before they develop complete block.

When the heart is otherwise normal, as in most cases of congenital complete heart block, increased stroke volume can maintain a normal cardiac output. Intracardiac pressures are frequently slightly elevated. In adults with chronic acquired complete atrioventricular block, the cardiac output is usually lower than normal because the ventricles cannot generate an adequately increased stroke volume. The intracardiac pressures are frequently elevated to levels consistent with congestive failure. The cardiac output rises in some but not all patients when pacing increases the ventricular rate.

The clinical electrophysiological study can define the level of atrioventricular block, a finding that has important clinical implications. Block within the atrioventricular node may be transient and is unlikely to progress to high degrees of atrioventricular block and syncope. Patients with partial block within or below the bundle of His often develop complete block and potentially fatal symptoms.

Drugs are seldom used for chronic treatment of atrioventricular block, although atropine and adrenergic agonists may temporarily decrease the degree of block. Cardiac pacemakers, many of which change their rates in response to physiological requirements, are the preferred method for treating block that produces symptoms or threatens the patient's survival.

Once pacemaking has been established, the survival of patients with acquired atrioventricular block

---

*fffff*One authority writes: "In general terms, a less favorable prognosis is associated with one or more of the following: (1) lowered working capacity; (2) low ventricular rate response (increase <40 beats/min); (3) frequent ventricular ectopy during heavy work; (4) mean awake heart rate <50 beats/min; (5) junctional instability; and (6) long QT interval."[55]

depends primarily on the severity of the accompanying cardiac and noncardiac disease. The mortality that is seen when high degrees of atrioventricular block complicate inferior myocardial infarction is at least three times greater than in the absence of this arrhythmia. However, heart block adds no risk to survivors of inferior myocardial infarction. At least three-fourths of those with anterior infarction and acute atrioventricular block die. The prognosis is excellent for those children with congenital complete heart block who survive infancy and have no structural heart disease.

REFERENCES

1. Ross BA, Pinsky WW, Driscoll DJ. Complete atrioventricular block. In Gillette PC, Garson A (eds). Pediatric Arrhythmias. Electrophysiology and Pacing. Philadelphia: W B Saunders, 1990, pp. 306–316.
2. Perloff JK. The Clinical Recognition of Congenital Heart Disease. 4th ed. Philadelphia: W B Saunders, 1994.
3. Denes P. Conduction abnormalities: His-Purkinje disease. In Podrid PJ, Kowey PR (eds). Cardiac Arrhythmia. Mechanisms, Diagnosis and Management. Baltimore: Williams & Wilkins, 1995, pp. 1051–1071.
4. Kocovic DZ, Friedman PL. Atrioventricular nodal block. In Podrid PJ, Kowey PR (eds). Cardiac Arrhythmia. Mechanisms, Diagnosis and Management. Baltimore: Williams & Wilkins, 1995, pp. 1039–1050.
5. Rardon DP, Miles WM, Mitrani RD, Klein LS, Zipes DP. Atrioventricular block and dissociation. In Zipes DP, Jalife J (eds). Cardiac Electrophysiology. From Cell to Bedside. 2nd ed. Philadelphia: W B Saunders, 1995, pp. 935–942.
6. Damato AN, Lau SH, Helfant R, et al. A study of heart block in man using His bundle recordings. Circulation 1969; 39:297–305.
7. Scherlag BJ, Lau SH, Helfant RH, Berkowitz WD, Stein E, Damato AN. Catheter technique for recording His bundle activity in man. Circulation 1969; 39:13–18.
8. Sugiura M. Trifascicular block: electrophysiological and histological correlation study on atrioventricular block. Jpn Circ J 1976; 40:233–237.
9. Damato AN, Lau SH, Patton RD, Steiner C, Berkowitz WD. A study of atrioventricular conduction in man using premature atrial stimulation and His bundle recordings. Circulation 1969; 40:61–69.
10. Wit AL, Weiss MB, Berkowitz WD, Rosen KM, Steiner C, Damato AN. Patterns of atrioventricular conduction in the human heart. Circ Res 1970; 27:345–359.
11. Kennedy HL. Ambulatory Electrocardiography Including Holter Recording Technology. Philadelphia: Lea & Febiger, 1981.
12. Davies MJ. Pathology of Conducting Tissue of the Heart. New York: Appleton-Century-Crofts, 1971.
13. Rosenbaum MB, Elizari MV, Lazzari JO. The Hemiblocks. Orlando, FL: Tampa Tracings, 1970.
14. Rosenbaum MB, Elizari MV, Kretz A, Taratuto AL. Anatomical basis of AV conduction disturbances. Geriatrics 1970; 25:132–144.
15. Furman S, Escher DJW. Principles and Techniques of Cardiac Pacing. New York: Harper & Row, 1970.
16. Zoll PM. Historical development of cardiac pacemakers. Prog Cardiovasc Dis 1972; 14:421–429.
17. Siddons H, Sowton E. Cardiac Pacemakers. Springfield, IL: Charles C Thomas, 1974.
18. Chardack WM. Recollections: 1958–1961. Pacing Clin Electrophysiol 1981; 4:592–596.
19. Furman S. Recollections of the beginning of transvenous cardiac pacing. PACE 1994; 17:1697–1705.
20. Jeffrey K, Parsonnet V. Cardiac pacing, 1960–1985: a quarter century of medical and industrial innovation. Circulation 1998; 97:1978–1991.
21. Zoll PM. Resuscitation of the heart in ventricular standstill by external electric stimulation. N Engl J Med 1952; 247:768–771.
22. Weirich WL, Gott VL, Lillehei CW. The treatment of complete heart block by the combined use of a myocardial electrode and an artificial pacemaker. Surg Forum 1957; 8:360–363.
23. Furman S, Schwedel JB. An intracardiac pacemaker for Stokes-Adams seizures. N Engl J Med 1959; 261:943–948.
24. Glenn WWL, Mauro A, Longo E, Lavietes PH, Mackay FJ. Remote stimulation of the heart by radiofrequency transmission. N Engl J Med 1959; 261:948–951.
25. Chardack WM, Gage AA, Greatbatch W. Correction of complete heart block by a self-contained and subcutaneously implanted pacemaker. J Thorac Cardiovasc Surg 1961; 42:814–830.
26. Lagergren H, Johansson L. Intracardiac stimulation for complete heart block. Acta Chir Scand 1963; 125:562–566.
27. Escher DJW, Schwedel JB, Schwartz LS, Solomon N. Transvenous electrical stimulation of the heart II. Ann N Y Acad Sci 1964; 111:981–991.
28. Bluestone R, Davies G, Harris A, Leatham A, Siddons H. Long-term endocardial pacing for heart-block. Lancet 1965; 2:307–311.
29. Lemberg L, Castellanos A, Berkovits VB. Pacemaking on demand in AV block. JAMA 1965; 191:106–108.
30. Nathan DA, Center S, Wu CY, Keller W. An implantable, synchronous pacemaker for the long-term correction of complete heart block. Circulation 1963; 27:682–685.
31. Feruglio GA, Rickards AF, Steinbach K, Feldman S, Parsonnet V. Cardiac pacing in the world: a survey of the state of the art in 1986. PACE 1987; 10:768–777.
32. Manning GW. Electrocardiography in the selection of Royal Canadian Air Force aircrew. Circulation 1954; 10:401–412.
33. Johnson RL, Averill KH, Lamb LE. Electrocardiographic findings in 67,375 asymptomatic subjects. Am J Cardiol 1960; 6:153–177.
34. Perlman LV, Ostrander LD, Jr., Keller JB, Chiang BN. An epidemiologic study of first degree atrioventricular block in Tecumseh, Michigan. Chest 1971; 59:40–46.
35. Logue RB, Hanson JF. A study of 100 cases with prolonged P-R interval. Am J Med Sci 1944; 207:765–769.
36. Katz LN, Pick A. Clinical Electrocardiography. Part I. The Arrhythmias. Philadelphia: Lea & Febiger, 1956.
37. Erikssen J, Otterstad JE. Natural course of a prolonged PR interval and the relation between PR and incidence of coronary heart disease: a 7-year follow-up study of 1,832 apparently healthy men aged 40–59 years. Clin Cardiol 1984; 7:6–13.
38. Fox TT, Weaver JC, Francis RL. Further studies on electrocardiographic changes in old age. Geriatrics 1948; 3:35–41.
39. Rajala S, Kaltiala K, Haavisto M, Mattila K. Prevalence of ECG findings in very old people. Eur Heart J 1984; 5:168–174.
40. Dolgin M, Grossman M, Simon AJ, Sorter H, Katz LN. Cardiovascular survey of residents in a custodial institution for the aged. J Gerontol 1949; 4:39–47.
41. McNamara RJ. A study of the electrocardiogram in persons over seventy. Geriatrics 1949; 4:150–160.
42. Wosika PH, Feldman E, Chesrow EJ, Myers GB. Unipolar precordial and limb lead electrocardiograms in the aged. Geriatrics 1950; 5:131–141.
43. White PD. Heart Disease. 4th ed. New York, Macmillan, 1951.
44. Rodstein M, Brown M, Wolloch L. First-degree atrioventricular heart block in the aged. Geriatrics 1968; 23:159–165.
45. Mihalick MJ, Fisch C. Electrocardiographic findings in the aged. Am Heart J 1974; 87:117–128.
46. Scott O, Williams GJ, Fiddler GI. Results of 24-hour ambulatory monitoring of electrocardiogram in 131 healthy boys aged 10 to 13 years. Br Heart J 1980; 44:304–308.

47. Southall DP, Johnston F, Shinebourne EA, Johnston PG. 24-hour electrocardiographic study of heart rate and rhythm patterns in population of healthy children. Br Heart J 1981; 45:281–291.

48. Dickinson DF, Scott O. Ambulatory electrocardiographic monitoring in 100 healthy teenage boys. Br Heart J 1984; 51:179–183.

49. Clarke JM, Hamer J, Shelton JR, Taylor S, Venning GR. The rhythm of the normal human heart. Lancet 1976; 1:508–512.

50. Rajala S, Haavisto M, Kaltiala K, Mattila K. ECG findings and survival in very old people. Eur Heart J 1985; 6:247–252.

51. Shaw DB, Eraut D. Prevalence and morbidity of heart block in Devon. BMJ 1970; 1:144–147.

52. Ide LW. The clinical aspects of complete auriculoventricular heart block: a clinical analysis of 71 cases. Ann Intern Med 1952; 32:510–523.

53. Wright JC, Hejtmancik MR, Herrmann GR, Shields AH. A clinical study of complete heart block. Am Heart J 1956; 52:369–378.

54. Rowe JC, White PD. Complete heart block: a follow-up study. Ann Intern Med 1958; 49:260–270.

55. Michaelsson M. Congenital complete atrioventricular block. Prog Pediatr Cardiol 1995; 4:1–10.

56. Machado MV, Tynan MJ, Curry PV, Allan LD. Fetal complete heart block. Br Heart J 1988; 60:512–515.

57. Keith JD, Rowe RD, Vlad P. Heart Disease in Infancy and Childhood. New York: Macmillan, 1978.

58. Pinsky WW, Gillette PC, Garson A Jr, McNamara DG. Diagnosis, management, and long-term results of patients with congenital complete atrioventricular block. Pediatrics 1982; 69:728–733.

59. Iseri LT, Humphrey SB, Siner EJ. Prehospital brady-asystolic cardiac arrest. Ann Intern Med 1978; 88:741–745.

60. Ector H, Rolies L, De Geest H. Dynamic electrocardiography and ventricular pauses of 3 seconds and more: etiology and therapeutic implications. Pacing Clin Electrophysiol 1983; 6:548–551.

61. Campbell M. Complete heart block. Br Heart J 1944; 6:69–92.

62. Penton GB, Miller H, Levine SA. Some clinical features of complete heart block. Circulation 1956; 13:801–824.

63. Esscher E. Review article: congenital complete heart block. Acta Paediatr Scand 1981; 70:131–136.

64. Reid JM, Coleman EN, Doig W. Complete congenital heart block: report of 35 cases. Br Heart J 1982; 48:236–239.

65. Sholler GF, Walsh EP. Congenital complete heart block in patients without anatomic cardiac defects. Am Heart J 1989; 118:1193–1198.

66. Sarachek NS, Leonard JL. Familial heart block and sinus bradycardia: classification and natural history. Am J Cardiol 1972; 29:451–458.

67. Schaal SF, Seidensticker J, Goodman R, Wooley CF. Familial right bundle-branch block, left axis deviation, complete heart block, and early death: a heritable disorder of cardiac conduction. Ann Intern Med 1973; 79:63–66.

68. Morgans CM, Gray KE, Robb GH. A survey of familial heart block. Br Heart J 1974; 36:693–696.

69. Amat-y-Leon F, Racki AJ, Denes P, et al. Familial atrial dysrhythmia with A-V block. Circulation 1974; 50:1097–1104.

70. Lynch HT, Mohiuddin S, Moran J, et al. Hereditary progressive atrioventricular conduction defect. Am J Cardiol 1975; 36:297–301.

71. Waxman MB, Catching JD, Felderhof CH, Downar E, Silver MD, Abbott MM. Familial atrioventricular heart block: an autosomal dominant trait. Circulation 1975; 51:226–233.

72. Schneider MD, Roller DH, Morganroth J, Josephson ME. The syndromes of familial atrioventricular block with sinus bradycardia: prognostic indices, electrophysiologic and histopathologic correlates. Eur J Cardiol 1978; 7:337–351.

73. Ebisawa K, Nakayama T, Tanaka K, Shimada K. Familial atrioventricular heart block of adult onset: electrocardiogram and HLA typing analysis. Pacing Clin Electrophysiol 1995; 18:1276–1278.

74. Kahler RL, Braunwald E, Plauth WH, Morrow AG. Familial congenital heart disease. Am J Med 1966; 40:384–399.

75. Amarasingham R, Fleming HA. Congenital heart disease with arrhythmia in a family. Br Heart J 1967; 29:78–82.

76. Bizarro RO, Callahan JA, Feldt RH, Kurland LT, Gordon H, Brandenburg RO. Familial atrial septal defect with prolonged atrioventricular conduction; a syndrome showing the autosomal dominant pattern of inheritance. Circulation 1970; 41:677–683.

77. Bjornstad PG. Secundum type atrial septal defect with prolonged PR interval and autosomal dominant mode of inheritance. Br Heart J 1974; 36:1149–1154.

78. Emanuel R, O'Brien K, Somerville J, Jefferson K, Hedge M. Association of secundum atrial septal defect with abnormalities of atrioventricular conduction of left axis deviation: genetic study of 10 families. Br Heart J 1975; 37:1085–1092.

79. Pease WE, Nordenberg A, Ladda RL. Familial atrial septal defect with prolonged atrioventricular conduction. Circulation 1976; 53:759–762.

80. Maron BJ, Lipson LC, Roberts WC, Savage DD, Epstein SE. "Malignant" hypertrophic cardiomyopathy: identification of a subgroup of families with unusually frequent premature death. Am J Cardiol 1978; 41:1133–1140.

81. Louie EK, Maron BJ. Familial spontaneous complete heart block in hypertrophic cardiomyopathy. Br Heart J 1986; 55:469–474.

82. Wendkos MH, Study RS. Familial congenital complete A-V heart block. Am Heart J 1947; 34:138–142.

83. Wallgren G, Agorio E. Congenital complete A-V block in three siblings. Acta Paediatr 1960; 49:49–56.

84. Crittenden IH, Latta H, Ticinovich DA. Familial congenital heart block. Am J Dis Child 1964; 108:104–108.

85. Gazes PC, Culler RM, Taber E, Kelly TE. Congenital familial cardiac dysfunction defects. Circulation 1965; 32:32–34.

86. Gambetta M, Weese J, Ginsburg M, Shapiro D. Sick sinus syndrome in a patient with familial PR prolongation. Chest 1973; 64:520–523.

87. James TN, McKone RC, Hudspeth AS. De subitaneis mortibus. X. Familial congenital heart block. Circulation 1975; 51:379–388.

88. Winkler RB, Nora AH, Nora JJ. Familial congenital complete heart block and maternal systemic lupus erythematosis. Circulation 1977; 56:1103–1107.

89. Buyon J, Roubey R, Swersky S, et al. Complete congenital heart block: risk of occurrence and therapeutic approach to prevention. J Rheumatol 1988; 15:1104–1108.

90. Greenspahn BR, Denes P, Daniel W, Rosen KM. Chronic bifascicular block: evaluation of familial factors. Ann Intern Med 1976; 84:521–525.

91. Zehender M, Meinertz T, Keul J, Just H. ECG variants and cardiac arrhythmias in athletes: clinical relevance and prognostic importance. Am Heart J 1990; 119:1378–1391.

92. Kosinski D, Grubb BP. Syncope due to advanced atrioventricular block despite no demonstrable cardiac disease. Pacing Clin Electrophysiol 1997; 20:997–998.

93. Alexander HL, Bauerlein TC. The influence of posture on partial heart-block. Am Heart J 1936; 11:223–226.

94. Poel W. Cardiometric studies on children. Arch Intern Med 1942; 69:1040–1050.

95. Holmes CJH, Weill DR. Incomplete heart block produced by changes in posture. Am Heart J 1945; 30:291–298.

96. Scherf D, Dix JH. The effects of posture on A-V conduction. Am Heart J 1952; 43:494–506.

97. Manning GW, Sears GA. Postural heart block. Am J Cardiol 1962; 9:558–563.

98. Sumiyoshi M, Nakata Y, Mineda Y. Paroxysmal atrioventricular block induced during head-up tilt testing in an apparently healthy man. J Cardiovasc Electrophysiol 1997; 8:561–564.

99. Hart G, Oldershaw PJ, Cull RE, Humphrey P, Ward D. Syncope caused by cough-induced complete atrioventricular block. Pacing Clin Electrophysiol 1982; 5:564–566.

100. Saito D, Matsuno S, Matsushita K, et al. Cough syncope due to atrioventricular conduction block. Jpn Heart J 1982; 23:1015–1020.

101. Baron SB, Huang SK. Cough syncope presenting as Mobitz

type II atrioventricular block: an electrophysiologic correlation. Pacing Clin Electrophysiol 1987; 10:65–69.

102. Harrington JT Jr, DeSanctis RW. Hiccup-induced atrioventricular block. Ann Intern Med 1969; 70:105–106.

103. Weiss S, Ferris EB. Adams-Stokes syndrome with transient complete heart block of vagovagal reflex origin. Arch Intern Med 1934; 54:931–951.

104. Correll HL, Lindert MCF. Vagovagal syncope: report of a case apparently induced by digitalization. Am Heart J 1949; 37:446–454.

105. James AH, Oxon DM. Cardiac syncope after swallowing. Lancet 1958; 1:771–772.

106. Ragaza EP, Rectra EH, Pardi MT. Intermittent complete heart block associated with swallowing as a complication of acute myocardial infarction. Am Heart J 1970; 79:396–400.

107. Sapru RP, Griffiths PH, Guz A, Eisele J. Syncope on swallowing. Br Heart J 1971; 33:617–622.

108. Lichstein E, Chadda KD. Atrioventricular block produced by swallowing, with documentation by His bundle recordings. Am J Cardiol 1972; 29:561–563.

109. Drake CE, Rollings HE, Ham OE Jr, Heidary DH, Yeh TJ. Visually provoked complete atrioventricular block: an unusual form of deglutition syncope. Am J Cardiol 1984; 53:1408–1409.

110. Kunis RL, Garfein OB, Pepe AJ, Dwyer EM Jr. Deglutition syncope and atrioventricular block selectively induced by hot food and liquid. Am J Cardiol 1985; 55:613.

111. Gambetta M, Denes P, Childers RW. Vagally induced second degree A-V block Mobitz type I, and the hyporeactive SA node. Chest 1972; 62:152–155.

112. Sra J, Singh B, Blanck Z, Dhala A, Akhtar M. Sinus tachycardia with atrioventricular block: an unusual presentation during neurocardiogenic (vasovagal) syncope. J Cardiovasc Electrophysiol 1998; 9:203–207.

113. Cullen KJ, Collin R. Daily running causing Wenckebach heart-block. Lancet 1964; 2:729–730.

114. Smith WG, Cullen KJ, Thorburn IO. Electrocardiograms of marathon runners in 1962 Commonwealth Games. Br Heart J 1964; 26:469–476.

115. Sargin O, Alp C, Tansi C, Karaca L. Wenckebach phenomenon with nodal and ventricular escape in marathon runner. Chest 1970; 57:102–105.

116. Nakamoto K. Various types of second degree A-V node-ventricular block (block in block) observed in a case of complete A-V block with atrial fibrillation and bilateral bundle branch block. Jpn Circ J 1970; 34:1083–1092.

117. Meytes I, Kaplinsky E, Yahini JH, Hanne-Paparo N, Neufeld HN. Wenckebach A-V block: a frequent feature following heavy physical training. Am Heart J 1975; 90:426–430.

118. Gibbons LW, Cooper H, Martin RP, Pollock ML. Medical examination and electrocardiographic analysis of elite distance runners. Ann N Y Acad Sci 1977; 301:283–296.

119. Rasmussen V, Haunso S, Skagen K. Cerebral attacks due to excessive vagal tone in heavily trained persons: a clinical and electrophysiologic study. Acta Med Scand 1978; 204:401–405.

120. Zeppilli P, Fenici R, Sassara M, Pirrami MM, Caselli G. A-V block in top-ranking athletes: an old problem revisited. Am Heart J 1980; 100:281–292.

121. Viitasalo MT, Kala R, Eisalo A. Ambulatory electrocardiographic recording in endurance athletes. Br Heart J 1982; 47:213–220.

122. Viitasalo MT, Kala R, Eisalo A. Ambulatory electrocardiographic findings in young athletes between 14 and 16 years of age. Eur Heart J 1984; 5:2–6.

123. Huston TP, Puffer JC, Rodney WM. The athletic heart syndrome. N Engl J Med 1985; 313:24–32.

124. Kinoshita S, Konishi G. Atrioventricular Wenckebach periodicity in athletes: influence of increased vagal tone on the occurrence of atypical periods. J Electrocardiol 1987; 20:272–279.

125. Hurwitz JL, Conley MJ, Wharton JM, Prystowsky EN. Syncope secondary to paroxysmal high grade AV block in a heavily trained man. Pacing Clin Electrophysiol 1991; 14:994–999.

126. Lipski J, Cohen L, Espinoza J, Motro M, Dack S, Donoso E.

127. Brodsky M, Wu D, Denes P, Kanakis C, Rosen KM. Arrhythmias documented by 24-hour continuous electrocardiographic monitoring in 50 male medical students without apparent heart disease. Am J Cardiol 1977; 39:390–395.

Value of Holter monitoring in assessing cardiac arrhythmias in symptomatic patients. Am J Cardiol 1976; 37:102–107.

128. Gymoese E, Vilhemsen R, Damgaard Andersen J, Sandoe E. Circadian variation in heart block and Adams-Stokes disease: an autonomic nervous system effect. In Sandoe E, Julian DG, Bell JW (eds). Management of Ventricular Tachycardia—role of Mexiletine. Amsterdam: Excerpta Medica, 1978, pp. 170–177.

129. Zoob M, Smith KS. The aetiology of complete heart block. BMJ 1963; 2:1149–1153.

130. Lenegre J. Etiology and pathology of bilateral bundle branch block in relation to complete heart block. Prog Cardiovasc Dis 1964; 6:409–444.

131. Davies MJ, Redwood D, Harris A. Heart block and coronary artery disease. BMJ 1967; 3:342–343.

132. Harris A, Davies M, Redwood D, Leatham A, Siddons H. Aetiology of chronic heart block: a clinico-pathological correlation in 65 cases. Br Heart J 1969; 31:206–218.

133. Kastor JA. Electrical disorders of the heart. JAMA 1973; 224:1031–1033.

134. Rosen KM, Dhingra RC, Loeb HS, Rahimtoola SH. Chronic heart block in adults: clinical and electrophysiological observations. Arch Intern Med 1973; 131:663–672.

135. Dhingra RC, Wyndham C, Bauernfeind R, et al. Significance of chronic bifascicular block without apparent organic heart disease. Circulation 1979; 60:33–39.

136. James TN. Arrhythmias and conduction disturbances in acute myocardial infarction. Am Heart J 1962; 64:416–426.

137. Meltzer LE, Kitchell JB. The incidence of arrhythmias associated with acute myocardial infarction. Prog Cardiovasc Dis 1966; 9:50–63.

138. Kastor JA. Atrioventricular block during myocardial infarction. In Parrillo JE (ed). Current Therapy in Critical Care Medicine. Philadelphia: B.C. Decker, 1987, pp. 88–91.

139. Rosenfeld LE. Bradyarrhythmias, abnormalities of conduction, and indications for pacing in acute myocardial infarction. Cardiol Clin 1988; 6:49–61.

140. Wellens HJJ. Right ventricular infarction. N Engl J Med 1993; 328:1036–1038.

141. Master AM, Dack S, Jaffe HL. Partial and complete heart block in acute coronary artery occlusion. Am J Med Sci 1938; 196:513–529.

142. Julian DG, Valentine PA, Miller GG. Disturbances of rate, rhythm and conduction in acute myocardial infarction: a prospective study of 100 consecutive unselected patients with the aid of electrocardiographic monitoring. Am J Med 1964; 37:915–927.

143. Fluck DC, Olsen E, Pentecost BL, et al. Natural history and clinical significance of arrhythmias after acute cardiac infarction. Br Heart J 1967; 29:170–189.

144. Killip T III, Kimball JT. Treatment of myocardial infarction in a coronary care unit: a two year experience with 250 patients. Am J Cardiol 1967; 20:457–464.

145. Langhorne WH. The coronary care unit: a year's experience in a community hospital. JAMA 1967; 201:92–95.

146. Lawrie DM, Goddard M, Greenwood TW, et al. A coronary care unit in the routine management of acute myocardial infarction. Lancet 1967; 2:109–114.

147. Lown B, Vasaux C, Hood WB Jr, Fakhro AM, Kaplinsky E, Roberge G. Unresolved problems in coronary care. Am J Cardiol 1967; 20:494–508.

148. MacMillan RL, Brown KWG, Peckham GB, Kahn O, Hutchison DB, Paton M. Changing perspectives in coronary care. Am J Cardiol 1967; 20:451–456.

149. Restieaux N, Bray C, Bullard H, et al. 150 patients with cardiac infarction treated in a coronary unit. Lancet 1967; 1:1285–1289.

150. Stock E, Goble A, Sloman G. Assessment of arrhythmias in myocardial infarction. BMJ 1967; 2:719–723.

151. Stock RJ, Macken DL. Observations on heart block during

continuous electrocardiographic monitoring in myocardial infarction. Circulation 1968; 38:993–1005.

152. Adgey AA, Geddes JS, Mulholland HC, Keegan DA, Pantridge JF. Incidence, significance, and management of early bradyarrhythmia complicating acute myocardial infarction. Lancet 1968; 2:1097–1101.

153. Day HW. Acute coronary care: a five year report. Am J Cardiol 1968; 21:252–257.

154. Grier GS, McClellan JE. Effectiveness of a large community coronary care unit. South Med J 1968; 61:429–433.

155. Norris RM. Acute coronary care. N Z Med J 1968; 67:470–476.

156. Sloman G, Stannard M, Goble AJ. Coronary care unit: a review of 300 patients monitored since 1963. Am Heart J 1968; 75:140–143.

157. Wyman MG, Hammersmith L. Coronary care in the small community hospital. Dis Chest 1968; 53:584–591.

158. Brown RW, Hunt D, Sloman JG. The natural history of atrioventricular conduction defects in acute myocardial infarction. Am Heart J 1969; 78:460–466.

159. Norris RM. Heart block in posterior and anterior myocardial infarction. Br Heart J 1969; 31:352–356.

160. Kostuk WJ, Beanlands DS. Complete heart block associated with acute myocardial infarction. Am J Cardiol 1970; 26:380–384.

161. Chaturvedi NC, Shivalingappa G, Shanks B, et al. Myocardial infarction in the elderly. Lancet 1972; 1:280–282.

162. Kincaid DT, Botti RE. Significance of isolated left anterior hemiblock and left axis deviation during acute myocardial infarction. Am J Cardiol 1972; 30:797–800.

163. Simon AB, Steinke WE, Curry JJ. Atrioventricular block in acute myocardial infarction. Chest 1972; 62:156–161.

164. Rotman M, Wagner GS, Wallace AG. Bradyarrhythmias in acute myocardial infarction. Circulation 1972; 45:703–721.

165. Jones ME, Terry G, Kenmure AC. Frequency and significance of conduction defects in acute myocardial infarction. Am Heart J 1977; 94:163–167.

166. Feigl D, Ashkenazy J, Kishon Y. Early and late atrioventricular block in acute inferior myocardial infarction. J Am Coll Cardiol 1984; 4:35–38.

167. Lamas GA, Muller JE, Turi ZG, et al. A simplified method to predict occurrence of complete heart block during acute myocardial infarction. Am J Cardiol 1986; 57:1213–1219.

168. McDonald K, O'Sullivan JJ, Conroy RM, Robinson K, Mulcahy R. Heart block as a predictor of in-hospital death in both acute inferior and acute anterior myocardial infarction. Q J Med 1990; 74:277–282.

169. Goldberg RJ, Zevallos JC, Yarzebski J, et al. Prognosis of acute myocardial infarction complicated by complete heart block (the Worcester heart attack study). Am J Cardiol 1992; 69:1135–1141.

170. Courter SR, Moffat J, Fowler NO. Advanced atrioventricular block in acute myocardial infarction. Circulation 1963; 27:1034–1042.

171. Rotman M, Wagner GS, Waugh RA. Significance of high degree atrioventricular block in acute posterior myocardial infarction: the importance of clinical setting and mechanism of block. Circulation 1973; 47:257–262.

172. Barrillon A, Chaignon M, Guize L, Gerbaux A. Premonitory sign of heart block in acute posterior myocardial infarction. Br Heart J 1975; 37:2–8.

173. Gupta PK, Lichstein E, Chadda KD. Heart block complicating acute inferior wall myocardial infarction. Chest 1976; 69:599–604.

174. Biddle TL, Ehrich DA, Yu RN, Hodges M. Relation of heart block and left ventricular dysfunction in acute myocardial infarction. Am J Cardiol 1977; 39:961–966.

175. Tans AC, Lie KI, Durrer D. Clinical setting and prognostic significance of high degree atrioventricular block in acute inferior myocardial infarction: a study of 144 patients. Am Heart J 1980; 99:4–8.

176. Braat SH, de Zwaan C, Brugada P, Coenegracht JM, Wellens HJJ. Right ventricular involvement with acute inferior wall myocardial infarction identifies high risk of developing atrioventricular nodal conduction disturbances. Am Heart J 1984; 107:1183–1187.

177. Strasberg B, Pinchas A, Arditti A, et al. Left and right ventricular function in inferior acute myocardial infarction and significance of advanced atrioventricular block. Am J Cardiol 1984; 54:985–987.

178. Nicod P, Gilpin E, Dittrich H, Polikar R, Henning H, Ross J Jr. Long-term outcome in patients with inferior myocardial infarction and complete atrioventricular block. J Am Coll Cardiol 1988; 12:589–594.

179. Berger PB, Ryan TJ. Inferior myocardial infarction. Circulation 1990; 81:401–411.

180. Mavric Z, Zaputovic L, Matana A, et al. Prognostic significance of complete atrioventricular block in patients with acute inferior myocardial infarction with and without right ventricular involvement. Am Heart J 1990; 119:823–828.

181. Behar S, Zissman E, Zion M, et al. Complete atrioventricular block complicating inferior acute wall myocardial infarction: short- and long-term prognosis. Am Heart J 1993; 125:1622–1627.

182. Birnbaum Y, Sclarovsky S, Herz I, et al. Admission clinical and electrocardiographic characteristics predicting in-hospital development of high-degree atrioventricular block in inferior wall acute myocardial infarction. Am J Cardiol 1997; 80:1134–1138.

183. Dubois C, Pierard LA, Smeets JP, Carlier J, Kulbertus HE. Long-term prognostic significance of atrioventricular block in inferior acute myocardial infarction. Eur Heart J 1989; 10:816–820.

184. Melgarejo-Moreno A, Galcera-Tomas J, Garcia-Alberola A, et al. Incidence, clinical characteristics, and prognostic significance of right bundle-branch block in acute myocardial infarction: a study in the thrombolytic era. Circulation 1997; 96:1139–1144.

185. Opolski G, Kraska T, Ostrzycki A, Zielinski T, Korewicki J. The effect of infarct size on atrioventricular and intraventricular conduction disturbances in acute myocardial infarction. Int J Cardiol 1986; 10:141–147.

186. Clemmensen P, Bates ER, Califf RM, et al. Complete atrioventricular block complicating inferior wall acute myocardial infarction treated with reperfusion therapy. Am J Cardiol 1991; 67:225–230.

187. Zehender M, Kasper W, Kauder E, et al. Right ventricular infarction as an independent predictor of prognosis after acute inferior myocardial infarction. N Engl J Med 1993; 328:981–988.

188. Shiraki H, Yoshikawa T, Anzai T, et al. Association between preinfarction angina and a lower risk of right ventricular infarction. N Engl J Med 1998; 338:941–947.

189. Jackson AE, Bashour FA. Cardiac arrhythmias in acute myocardial infarction. I. Complete heart block and its natural history. Dis Chest 1967; 51:31–38.

190. Berger PB, Ruocco NA Jr, Ryan TJ, Frederick MM, Jacobs AK, Faxon DP. Incidence and prognostic implications of heart block complicating inferior myocardial infarction treated with thrombolytic therapy: results from TIMI II. J Am Coll Cardiol 1992; 20:533–540.

191. Sclarovsky S, Strasberg B, Hirshberg A, Arditi A, Lewin RF, Agmon J. Advanced early and late atrioventricular block in acute inferior wall myocardial infarction. Am Heart J 1984; 108:19–24.

192. Graybiel A, White PD. Complete auriculo-ventricular dissociation: a clinical study of seventy-two cases with a note on a curious form of auricular arrhythmia frequently observed. Am J Med Sci 1936; 192:334–344.

193. Kay HB. Ventricular complexes in heart block. Br Heart J 1948; 10:177–187.

194. Gilchrist AR. Clinical aspects of high-grade heart block. Scott Med J 1958; 3:53–75.

195. Johansson BW. Adams-Stokes syndrome. Am J Cardiol 1961; 8:76–93.

196. Ellis FH, Manning PC, Connolly DC. Treatment of Stokes-Adams disease. Mayo Clin Proc 1964; 39:945–953.

197. Friedberg CK, Donoso E, Stein WG. Nonsurgical acquired heart block. Ann N Y Acad Sci 1964; 111:835–847.

198. Harris A. Treatment of heart block. Curr Med Drugs 1965; 6:3–19.

199. Begg FR, Magovern GJ, Cushing WJ, Kent EM, Fisher DL. Selective cine coronary arteriography in patients with complete heart block. J Thorac Cardiovasc Surg 1969; 57:9–16.

200. Ginks W, Leatham A, Siddons H. Prognosis of patients paced for chronic atrioventricular block. Br Heart J 1979; 41:633–636.

201. Chiche P, Haiat R, Steff P. Angina pectoris with syncope due to paroxysmal atrioventricular block: role of ischaemia: report of two cases. Br Heart J 1974; 36:577–581.

202. Prinzmetal M, Kennamer R, Merliss R, Wada T, Bor N. Angina pectoris: a variant form of angina pectoris. Am J Med 1959; 27:375–388.

203. Botti RE. A variant form of angina pectoris with recurrent transient complete heart block. Am J Cardiol 1966; 17:443–446.

204. Gianelly R, Mugler F, Harrison DC. Prinzmetal's variant of angina pectoris with only slight coronary atherosclerosis. Calif Med 1968; 108:129–132.

205. Gillilan RE, Hawley RR, Warbasse JR. Second degree heart block occurring in a patient with Prinzmetal's variant angina. Am Heart J 1969; 77:380–382.

206. Whiting RB, Klein MD, Vander Veer J, Lown B. Variant angina pectoris. N Engl J Med 1970; 282:709–712.

207. Cosby RS, Giddings JA, See JR, Mayo M. Variant angina. Am J Med 1972; 53:739–742.

208. Macalpin RN, Kattus AA, Alvaro AB. Angina pectoris at rest with preservation of exercise capacity. Circulation 1973; 47:946–958.

209. Harper R, Hunt D, Vohra J, Peter T, Sloman G. His bundle electrogram in patients with acute myocardial infarction complicated by atrioventricular or intraventricular conduction disturbances. Br Heart J 1975; 37:705–710.

210. Wiener L, Kasparian H, Duca PR, et al. Spectrum of coronary arterial spasm: clinical, angiographic and myocardial metabolic experience in 29 cases. Am J Cardiol 1976; 38:945–955.

211. Bharati S, Dhingra RC, Lev M, Towne WD, Rahimtoola SH, Rosen KM. Conduction system in a patient with Prinzmetal's angina and transient atrioventricular block. Am J Cardiol 1977; 39:120–125.

212. Bodenheimer MM, Banka VS, Helfant RH. Relation between the site of origin of ventricular premature complexes and the presence and severity of coronary artery disease. Am J Cardiol 1977; 40:865–869.

213. Kerin NZ, Rubenfire M, Naini M, Wajszczuk WJ, Pamatmat A, Cascade PN. Arrhythmias in variant angina pectoris: relationship of arrhythmias to ST-segment elevation and R-wave changes. Circulation 1979; 60:1343–1350.

214. Araki H, Koiwaya Y, Nakagaki O, Nakamura M. Diurnal distribution of ST-segment elevation and related arrhythmias in patients with variant angina: a study by ambulatory ECG monitoring. Circulation 1983; 67:995–1000.

215. Ayers CR, Boineau JP, Spach MS. Congenital complete heart block in children. Am Heart J 1966; 72:381–390.

216. Esscher EB. Congenital complete heart block in adolescence and adult life: a follow-up study. Eur Heart J 1981; 2:281–288.

217. Camm AJ, Bexton RS. Congenital complete heart block. Eur Heart J 1984; 5:115–117.

218. Olah KS, Gee H. Antibody mediated complete congenital heart block in the fetus. Pacing Clin Electrophysiol 1993; 16:1872–1879.

219. Cobbe SM. Congenital complete heart block. BMJ 1983; 286:1769–1770.

220. Scott JS, Maddison PJ, Taylor PV, Esscher E, Scott O, Skinner RP. Connective-tissue disease, antibodies to ribonucleoprotein, and congenital heart block. N Engl J Med 1983; 309:209–212.

221. Case CL, Gillette PC. Conduction system disease in a child with long QT syndrome. Am Heart J 1990; 120:984–986.

222. Solti F, Szatmary L, Vecsey T, Renyi-Vamos F Jr, Bodor E. Congenital complete heart block associated with QT prolongation. Eur Heart J 1992; 13:1080–1083.

223. Altenburger KM, Jedziniak M, Roper WL, Hernandez J.

224. Holzgreve W, Curry CJ, Golbus MS, Callen PW, Filly RA, Smith JC. Investigation of nonimmune hydrops fetalis. Am J Obstet Gynecol 1984; 150:805–812.

Congenital complete heart block associated with hydrops fetalis. J Pediatr 1977; 91:618–620.

225. Lockshin MD, Gibofsky A, Peebles CL, Gigli I, Fotino M, Hurwitz S. Neonatal lupus erythematosus with heart block: family study of a patient with anti-SS-A and SS-B antibodies. Arthritis Rheum 1983; 26:210–213.

226. Lee LA, Weston WL. New findings in neonatal lupus syndrome. Am J Dis Child 1984; 138:233–236.

227. Waltuck J, Buyon JP. Autoantibody-associated congenital heart block: outcome in mothers and children. Ann Intern Med 1994; 120:544–551.

228. Hull D, Binns BA, Joyce D. Congenital heart block and widespread fibrosis due to maternal lupus erythematosus. Arch Dis Child 1966; 41:688–690.

229. Chameides L, Truex RC, Vetter V, Rashkind WJ, Galioto FM Jr, Noonan JA. Association of maternal systemic lupus erythematosus with congenital complete heart block. N Engl J Med 1977; 297:1204–1207.

230. McCue CM, Mantakas ME, Tingelstad JB, Ruddy S. Congenital heart block in newborns of mothers with connective tissue disease. Circulation 1977; 56:82–90.

231. Berube S, Lister G, Toews WH, Creasy RK, Heymann MA. Congenital heart block and maternal systemic lupus erythematosus. Am J Obstet Gynecol 1978; 130:595–596.

232. Esscher E, Scott JS. Congenital heart block and maternal systemic lupus erythematosus. BMJ 1979; 1:1235–1238.

233. Hardy JD, Solomon S, Banwell GS, Beach R, Wright V, Howard FM. Congenital complete heart block in the newborn associated with maternal systemic lupus erythematosus and other connective tissue disorders. Arch Dis Child 1979; 54:7–13.

234. Nolan RJ, Shulman ST, Victorica BE. Congenital complete heart block associated with maternal mixed connective tissue disease. J Pediatr 1979; 95:420–422.

235. Stephensen O, Cleland WP, Hallidie-Smith K. Congenital complete heart block and persistent ductus arteriosus associated with maternal systemic lupus erythematosus. Br Heart J 1981; 46:104–106.

236. Paredes RA, Morgan H, Lachelin GC. Congenital heart block associated with maternal primary Sjögren's syndrome: case report. Br J Obstet Gynaecol 1983; 90:870–871.

237. Taylor PV, Scott JS, Gerlis LM, Esscher E, Scott O. Maternal antibodies against fetal cardiac antigens in congenital complete heart block. N Engl J Med 1986; 315:667–672.

238. Ho SY, Esscher E, Anderson RH, Michaelsson M. Anatomy of congenital complete heart block and relation to maternal anti-Ro antibodies. Am J Cardiol 1986; 58:291–294.

239. Buyon JP, Ben-Chetrit E, Karp S, et al. Acquired congenital heart block: pattern of maternal antibody response to biochemically defined antigens of the SSA/Ro-SSB/La system in neonatal lupus. J Clin Invest 1989; 84:627–634.

240. Petri M, Watson R, Hochberg MC. Anti-Ro antibodies and neonatal lupus. Rheum Dis Clin North Am 1989; 15:335–360.

241. Goble MM, Dick M II, McCune WJ, Ellsworth J, Sullivan DB, Stern AM. Atrioventricular conduction in children of women with systemic lupus erythematosus. Am J Cardiol 1993; 71:94–98.

242. de Oliveira JM, Zimmerman HA. The electrocardiogram in interatrial septal defects and its correlation with hemodynamics. Am Heart J 1958; 55:369–382.

243. Waggoner DM, Wallace AG. Congenital partial heart block. Arch Intern Med 1968; 122:66–68.

244. Sobrino JA, deLombera F, Del Rio A, et al. Atrioventricular nodal dysfunction in patients with atrial septal defect. Chest 1982; 81:477–482.

245. Bagger JP, Thomsen PE, Bjerregaard P, Gotzsche H, Rasmussen K. Intracardiac electrography in patients before and after surgical repair of secundum atrial septal defect. J Electrocardiol 1984; 17:347–352.

246. Ho SY, Rossi MB, Mehta AV, Hegerty A, Lennox S, Anderson RH. Heart block and atrioventricular septal defect. Thorac Cardiovasc Surg 1985; 33:362–365.

247. Bink-Boelkens MT, Meuzelaar KJ, Eygelaar A. Arrhythmias after repair of secundum atrial septal defect: the influence of surgical modification. Am Heart J 1988; 115:629–633.

248. Reichek N, Jackson L, Ronan JA Jr, Perloff JK. Advanced congenital first-degree atrioventricular block: a His bundle electrocardiographic study. Arch Intern Med 1972; 130:765–767.

249. Barber JM, Magidson O, Wood P. Atrial septal defect; with special reference to the electrocardiogram, the pulmonary artery pressure and the second heart sound. Br Heart J 1950; 12:277–292.

250. Anderson PAW, Rogers MC, Canent RV, Spach MS. Atrioventricular conduction in secundum atrial septal defects. Circulation 1973; 48:27–31.

251. Karpawich PP, Gillette PC, Garson A Jr, Hesslein PS, Porter CB, McNamara DG. Congenital complete atrioventricular block: clinical and electrophysiologic predictors of need for pacemaker insertion. Am J Cardiol 1981; 48:1098–1102.

252. Shiku DJ, Stijns M, Lintermans JP, Vliers A. Influence of age on atrioventricular conduction intervals in children with and without atrial septal defect. J Electrocardiol 1982; 15:9–13.

253. Schiebler GL, Edwards JE, Burchell HB, DuShane JW, Ongley PA, Wood EH. Congenital corrected transposition of the great vessels: a study of 33 cases. Pediatrics 1962; 27:851–888.

254. Honey M. The diagnosis of corrected transposition of great vessels. Br Heart J 1963; 25:313–333.

255. Rotem CE, Hultgren HN. Corrected transposition of the great vessels without associated defects. Am Heart J 1965; 70:305–318.

256. Kangos JJ, Griffiths SP, Blumenthal S. Congenital complete heart block: a classification and experience with 18 patients. Am J Cardiol 1967; 20:632–638.

257. Friedberg DZ, Nadas AS. Clinical profile of patients with congenital corrected transposition of the great arteries. N Engl J Med 1970; 282:1053–1059.

258. Gillette PC, Reitman MJ, Mullins CE, Williams RL, Dawson JT, McNamara DG. Electrophysiology of ventricular inversion. Br Heart J 1974; 36:971–980.

259. Gillette PC, Busch U, Mullins CE, McNamara DG. Electrophysiologic studies in patients with ventricular inversion and "corrected transposition." Circulation 1979; 60:939–945.

260. Amikam S, Lemer J, Kishon Y, Riss E, Neufeld HN. Complete heart block in an adult with corrected transposition of the great arteries treated with permanent pacemaker. Thorax 1979; 34:547–549.

261. Daliento L, Corrado D, Buja G, John N, Nava A, Thiene G. Rhythm and conduction disturbances in isolated, congenitally corrected transposition of the great arteries. Am J Cardiol 1986; 58:314–318.

262. Huhta JC, Maloney JD, Ritter DG, Ilstrup DM, Feldt RH. Complete atrioventricular block in patients with atrioventricular discordance. Circulation 1983; 67:1374–1377.

263. Walker WJ, Denton MC, Cooley A, McNamara DG, Moser RH. Corrected transposition of the great vessels, atrioventricular heart block, and ventricular septal defect. Circulation 1958; 17:249–254.

264. Levy MJ, Cuello L, Tuna N, Lillehei CW. Atrioventricularis communis. Am J Cardiol 1964; 14:587–598.

265. Waldo AL, Kaiser GA, Bowman FO, Malm JR. Etiology of prolongation of the P-R interval in patients with an endocardial cushion defect: further observations on internodal conduction and the polarity of the retrograde P wave. Circulation 1973; 48:19–26.

266. Jacobsen JR, Gillette PC, Corbett BN, Rabinovitch M, McNamara DG. Intracardiac electrography in endocardial cushion defects. Circulation 1976; 54:599–603.

267. Genton E, Blount SG. Fundamentals of clinical cardiology; the spectrum of Ebstein's anomaly. Am Heart J 1967; 73:395–425.

268. Lowe KG, Emslie-Smith D, Robertson PGC, Watson H. Scalar, vector, and intracardiac electrocardiograms in Ebstein's anomaly. Br Heart J 1968; 30:617–629.

269. Kastor JA, Goldreyer BN, Josephson ME, et al. Electrophysiologic characteristics of Ebstein's anomaly of the tricuspid valve. Circulation 1975; 52:987–995.

270. Oh JK, Holmes DR Jr, Hayes DL, Porter CB, Danielson GK. Cardiac arrhythmias in patients with surgical repair of Ebstein's anomaly. J Am Coll Cardiol 1985; 6:1351–1357.

271. Scott WA, Dick M II. Two:one atrioventricular block in infants with congenital long QT syndrome. Am J Cardiol 1987; 60:1409–1410.

272. Rizzon P, Antonelli G, Biasco G, Brindicci G, DiBiase M. Chronic juvenile AV nodal dysfunction associated with mitral valve prolapse. Eur J Cardiol 1978; 8:589–598.

273. Ware JA, Magro SA, Luck JC, et al. Conduction system abnormalities in symptomatic mitral valve prolapse: an electrophysiologic analysis of 60 patients. Am J Cardiol 1984; 53:1075–1078.

274. Chandraratna PA, Ribas-Meneclier C, Littman BB, Samet P. Conduction disturbances in patients with mitral valve prolapse. J Electrocardiol 1977; 10:233–236.

275. Leichtman D, Nelson R, Gobel FL, Alexander CS, Cohn JN. Bradycardia with mitral valve prolapse: a potential mechanism of sudden death. Ann Intern Med 1976; 85:453–457.

276. Yater WM, Cornell VH. Heart block due to calcareous lesions of the bundle of His. Ann Intern Med 1935; 8:777–789.

277. Harris AM, Sleight P, Drew CE. The diagnosis and treatment of aortic stenosis complicated by heart block. Br Heart J 1965; 27:560–565.

278. Lombard JT, Selzer A. Valvular aortic stenosis: a clinical and hemodynamic profile of patients. Ann Intern Med 1987; 106:292–298.

279. Kremer R. Arrhythmias in the natural history of aortic stenosis. Acta Cardiol 1992; 47:135–140.

280. Nair CK, Aronow WS, Stokke K, Mohiuddin SM, Thomson W, Sketch MH. Cardiac conduction defects in patients older than 60 years with aortic stenosis with and without mitral anular calcium. Am J Cardiol 1984; 53:169–172.

281. Nair CK, Runco V, Everson GT, et al. Conduction defects and mitral annulus calcification. Br Heart J 1980; 44:162–167.

282. Olson LJ, Okafor EC, Clements IP. Cardiac involvement in lyme disease: manifestations and management. Mayo Clin Proc 1986; 61:745–749.

283. Steere AC, Batsford WP, Weinberg M, et al. Lyme carditis: cardiac abnormalities of Lyme disease. Ann Intern Med 1980; 93:8–16.

284. Bedell SE, Pastor BM, Cohen SI. Symptomatic high grade heart block in Lyme disease. Chest 1981; 79:236–237.

285. Jacobs JC, Rosen JM, Szer IS. Lyme myocarditis diagnosed by gallium scan. J Pediatr 1984; 105:950–952.

286. Reznick JW, Braunstein DB, Walsh RL, et al. Lyme carditis: electrophysiologic and histopathologic study. Am J Med 1986; 81:923–927.

287. Meyer LK, Swenson DB. Lyme carditis: high-grade heart block in Lyme disease. Minn Med 1987; 70:345–346.

288. van der Linde MR, Crijns HJ, Lie KI. Transient complete AV block in Lyme disease: electrophysiologic observations. Chest 1989; 96:219–221.

289. Gildein HP, Gunther S, Mocellin R. Complete heart block in a 9 year old girl caused by borreliosis. Br Heart J 1993; 70:88–90.

290. Greenberg YJ, Brennan JJ, Rosenfeld LE. Lyme myocarditis presenting as fascicular tachycardia with underlying complete heart block. J Cardiovasc Electrophysiol 1997; 8:323–324.

291. van der Linde MR, Crijns HJ, de Koning J, et al. Range of atrioventricular conduction disturbances in Lyme borreliosis: a report of four cases and review of other published reports. Br Heart J 1990; 63:162–168.

292. McAlister HF, Klementowicz PT, Andrews C, Fisher JD, Feld M, Furman S. Lyme carditis: an important cause of reversible heart block. Ann Intern Med 1989; 110:339–345.

293. Wang K, Gobel F, Gleason DF, Edwards JE. Complete heart block complicating bacterial endocarditis. Circulation 1972; 46:939–947.

294. Dinubile MJ. Heart block during bacterial endocarditis: a review of the literature and guidelines for surgical intervention. Am J Med Sci 1984; 287:30–32.

295. Dinubile MJ, Calderwood SB, Steinhaus DM, Karchmer AW. Cardiac conduction abnormalities complicating native valve active infective endocarditis. Am J Cardiol 1986; 58:1213–1217.

296. Whitehead R. Isolated myocarditis. Br Heart J 1965; 27:220–230.

297. Johnson JL, Lee LP. Complete atrioventricular heart block secondary to acute myocarditis requiring intracardiac pacing. J Pediatr 1971; 78:312–316.

298. Lim CH, Toh CC, Chia BL, Low LP. Stokes-Adams attacks due to acute nonspecific myocarditis. Am Heart J 1975; 90:172–178.

299. Kirmser R, Umbach R, Rowett D, Ross A. Complete heart block due to acute nonspecific carditis. Chest 1977; 71:682–684.

300. Mahoney LT, Marvin WJ Jr, Atkins DL, Clark EB, Lauer RM. Pacemaker management for acute onset of heart block in childhood. J Pediatr 1985; 107:207–211.

301. Rosenbaum MB, Alvarez AJ. The electrocardiogram in chronic chagasic myocarditis. Am Heart J 1955; 50:492–527.

302. Hagar JM, Rahimtoola SH. Chagas' heart disease in the United States. N Engl J Med 1991; 325:763–768.

303. Morrison WL, Petch MC. Heart block and paragonimiasis. Br Heart J 1988; 60:530–531.

304. Shee JC. Stokes-Adams attacks due to *Toxoplasma* myocarditis. Br Heart J 1964; 26:151–153.

305. Jones TD. The diagnosis of rheumatic fever. JAMA 1944; 126:481–484.

306. Rantz LA, Spink WW, Boisvert PJ. Abnormalities in the electrocardiogram following hemolytic *Streptococcus* sore throat. Arch Intern Med 1946; 77:66–79.

307. Caraco J, Arnon R, Raz I. Atrioventricular block complicating acute streptococcal tonsillitis. Br Heart J 1988; 59:389–390.

308. Bland EF, Jones TD. Rheumatic fever and rheumatic heart disease: a twenty year report on 1,000 patients followed since childhood. Circulation 1951; 4:836–843.

309. Mirowski M, Rosenstein BJ, Markowitz M. A comparison of atrioventricular conduction in normal children and in patients with rheumatic fever, glomerulonephritis, and acute febrile illnesses. Pediatrics 1964; 33:334–340.

310. White PD. Acute heart block occurring as the first sign of rheumatic fever. Am J Med Sci 1916; 152:589–591.

311. Friedberg CK. Diseases of the Heart. 3rd ed. Philadelphia: WB Saunders, 1966, p. 1344.

312. Anonymous. Paul Wood's Diseases of the Heart and Circulation. 3rd ed. Philadelphia: J B Lippincott, 1968, pp. 17–18.

313. Blackman NS, Hamilton CI. Serial electrocardiographic changes in young adults with acute rheumatic fever: report of 62 cases. Ann Intern Med 1948; 29:416–431.

314. Clarke M, Keith JD. Atrioventricular conduction in acute rheumatic fever. Br Heart J 1972; 34:472–479.

315. Rothschild MA, Sacks B, Libman E. The disturbances of the cardiac mechanism in subacute endocarditis and rheumatic fever. Am Heart J 1927; 2:356–374.

316. Bruenn HG. The mechanism of impaired auriculoventricular conduction in acute rheumatic fever. Am Heart J 1937; 13:413–425.

317. Robinson R. Effect of atropine upon the prolongation of the P-R interval found in acute rheumatic fever and certain vagotonic persons. Am Heart J 1945; 29:378–383.

318. White PD. Heart Disease. New York: Macmillan, 1951, p. 368.

319. Anonymous. Paul Wood's Diseases of the Heart and Circulation. 3rd ed. Philadelphia: J B Lippincott, 1968, p. 588.

320. Bottiger LE, Edhag O. Heart block in ankylosing spondylitis and uropolyarthritis. Br Heart J 1972; 34:487–492.

321. Bulkley BH, Roberts WC. Ankylosing spondylitis and aortic regurgitation: description of the characteristic cardiovascular lesion from study of eight necropsy patients. Circulation 1973; 48:1014–1027.

322. Nitter-Hauge S, Otterstad JE. Characteristics of atrioventricular conduction disturbances in ankylosing spondylitis (Mb. Bechterew). Acta Medica Scand 1981; 210:197–200.

323. Bergfeldt L. HLA b27-associated rheumatic diseases with severe cardiac bradyarrhythmias: clinical features and prevalence in 223 men with permanent pacemakers. Am J Med 1983; 75:210–215.

324. Henderson A, Cumming WJ, Williams DO, Hudgson P. Cardiac complications of polymyositis. J Neurol Sci 1980; 47:425–428.

325. Kehoe RF, Bauernfeind R, Tommaso C, Wyndham C, Rosen KM. Cardiac conduction defects in polymyositis: electrophysiologic studies in four patients. Ann Intern Med 1981; 94:41–43.

326. Stern R, Godbold JH, Chess Q, Kagen LJ. ECG abnormalities in polymyositis. Arch Intern Med 1984; 144:2185–2189.

327. Roberts NK, Cabeen WR Jr, Moss J, Clements PJ, Furst DE. The prevalence of conduction defects and cardiac arrhythmias in progressive systemic sclerosis. Ann Intern Med 1981; 94:38–40.

328. Follansbee WP, Curtiss EI, Rahko PS, et al. The electrocardiogram in systemic sclerosis (scleroderma): study of 102 consecutive cases with functional correlations and review of the literature. Am J Med 1985; 79:183–192.

329. Neu LT, Reider RA, Mack RE. Cardiac involvement in Reiter's disease: report of a case with review of the literature. Ann Intern Med 1960; 53:215–220.

330. Rossen RM, Goodman DJ, Harrison DC. A-V conduction disturbances in Reiter's syndrome. Am J Med 1975; 58:280–284.

331. Ruppert GB, Lindsay J, Barth WF. Cardiac conduction abnormalities in Reiter's syndrome. Am J Med 1982; 73:335–340.

332. Hassel D, Heinsimer J, Califf RM, Benson A, Rice J, German L. Complete heart block in Reiter's syndrome. Am J Cardiol 1984; 53:967–968.

333. Nielsen H. Complete heart block in Reiter's syndrome. Acta Cardiol 1986; 41:451–455.

334. Cathcart ES, Spodick DH. Rheumatoid heart disease. N Engl J Med 1962; 266:959–964.

335. Moffitt GR. Complete atrioventricular dissociation with Stokes-Adams attacks due to disseminated lupus erythematosus: report of a case. Ann Intern Med 1965; 63:299–304.

336. Bharati S, de la Fuente DJ, Kallen RJ, Freij Y, Lev M. Conduction system in systemic lupus erythematosus with atrioventricular block. Am J Cardiol 1975; 35:299–304.

337. Hover AR, Koppes GM. Atrial standstill and complete heart block in systemic lupus erythematosus. Chest 1979; 76:230–231.

338. Bilazarian SD, Taylor AJ, Brezinski D, Hochberg MC, Guarnieri T, Provost TT. High-grade atrioventricular heart block in an adult with systemic lupus erythematosus: the association of nuclear RNP (U1 RNP) antibodies, a case report, and review of the literature. Arthritis Rheum 1989; 32:1170–1174.

339. Brandt K, Cathcart ES, Cohen AS. A clinical analysis of the course and prognosis of 42 patients with amyloidosis. Am J Med 1968; 44:955–969.

340. Buja LM, Khoi NB, Roberts WC. Clinically significant cardiac amyloidosis. Am J Cardiol 1970; 26:394–405.

341. Ridolfi RL, Bulkley BH, Hutchins GM. The conduction system in cardiac amyloidosis: clinical and pathologic features of 23 patients. Am J Med 1977; 62:677–686.

342. Roberts WC, Waller BF. Cardiac amyloidosis causing cardiac dysfunction: analysis of 54 necropsy patients. Am J Cardiol 1983; 52:137–146.

343. Gozo EG Jr, Cosnow I, Cohen HC, Okun L. The heart in sarcoidosis. Chest 1971; 60:379–388.

344. Olofsson BO, Andersson R, Furberg B. Atrioventricular and intraventricular conduction in familial amyloidosis with polyneuropathy. Acta Med Scand 1980; 208:77–80.

345. Eriksson P, Karp K, Bjerle P, Olofsson BO. Disturbances of

cardiac rhythm and conduction in familial amyloidosis with polyneuropathy. Br Heart J 1984; 51:658–662.

346. Eriksson P, Boman K, Jacobsson B, Olofsson BO. Cardiac arrhythmias in familial amyloid polyneuropathy during anaesthesia. Acta Anaesthesiol Scand 1986; 30:317–320.

347. James TN. Pathology of the cardiac conduction system in hemochromatosis. N Engl J Med 1964; 271:92–94.

348. Aronow WS, Meister L, Kent JR. Atrioventricular block in familial hemochromatosis treated by permanent synchronous pacemaker. Arch Intern Med 1969; 123:433–435.

349. Schellhammer PF, Engle MA, Hagstrom JWC. Histochemical studies of the myocardium and conduction system in acquired iron-storage disease. Circulation 1967; 35:631–637.

350. Buja LM, Roberts WC. Iron in the heart. Am J Med 1971; 51:209–221.

351. Vigorita VJ, Hutchins GM. Cardiac conduction system in hemochromatosis: clinical and pathologic features of six patients. Am J Cardiol 1979; 44:418–423.

352. Short EM, Winkle RA, Billingham ME. Myocardial involvement in idiopathic hemochromatosis: morphologic and clinical improvement following venesection. Am J Med 1981; 70:1275–1279.

353. Simkins S. Boeck's sarcoid with complete heart block mimicking carotid sinus syncope. JAMA 1951; 146:270–276.

354. Phinney AO. Sarcoid of the myocardial septum with complete heart block: report of two cases. Am Heart J 1961; 62:270–276.

355. Duvernoy WF, Garcia R. Sarcoidosis of the heart presenting with ventricular tachycardia and atrioventricular block. Am J Cardiol 1971; 28:348–352.

356. McTaggart DR. Sarcoidosis with cardiac involvement. Med J Aust 1973; 2:689–690.

357. Fawcett FJ, Goldberg MJ. Heart block resulting from myocardial sarcoidosis. Br Heart J 1974; 36:220–223.

358. Fleming HA. Sarcoid heart disease. Br Heart J 1974; 36:54–68.

359. James TN. Clinicopathologic correlations: de subitaneis mortibus. XXV. Sarcoid heart disease. Circulation 1977; 56:320–326.

360. Roberts WC, McAllister HA Jr, Ferrans VJ. Sarcoidosis of the heart: a clinicopathologic study of 35 necropsy patients (group 1) and review of 78 previously described necropsy patients (group 11). Am J Med 1977; 63:86–108.

361. Lash R, Coker J, Wong BY. Treatment of heart block due to sarcoid heart disease. J Electrocardiol 1979; 12:325–329.

362. Bharati S, Lev M, Denes P, et al. Infiltrative cardiomyopathy with conduction disease and ventricular arrhythmia: electrophysiologic and pathologic correlations. Am J Cardiol 1980; 45:163–173.

363. Sekiguchi M, Numao Y, Imai M, Furuie T, Mikami R. Clinical and histopathological profile of sarcoidosis of the heart and acute idiopathic myocarditis: concepts through a study employing endomyocardial biopsy. I. Sarcoidosis. Jpn Circ J 1980; 44:249–263.

364. Thunell M, Bjerle P, Stjernberg N. ECG abnormalities in patients with sarcoidosis. Acta Med Scand 1983; 213:115–118.

365. Silverman E, Mamula M, Hardin JA, Laxer R. Importance of the immune response to the Ro/La particle in the development of congenital heart block and neonatal lupus erythematosus. J Rheumatol 1991; 18:120–124.

366. Sharma OP, Maheshwari A, Thaker K. Myocardial sarcoidosis. Chest 1993; 103:253–258.

367. Shammas RL, Movahed A. Sarcoidosis of the heart. Clin Cardiol 1993; 16:462–472.

368. Yoshida Y, Morimoto S, Hiramitsu S, Tsuboi N, Hirayama H, Itoh T. Incidence of cardiac sarcoidosis in Japanese patients with high-degree atrioventricular block. Am Heart J 1997; 134:382–386.

369. Bashour TT, Fahdul H, Cheng TO. Electrocardiographic abnormalities in alcoholic cardiomyopathy: a study of 65 patients. Chest 1975; 68:24–27.

370. Bear ES, Tung MY, Bordiuk J. Marfan's syndrome with complete heart block and junctional rhythm. JAMA 1971; 217:335–337.

371. Touboul P, Kirkorian G, Atallah G, Cahen P, de Zuloaga C, Moleur P. Atrioventricular block and preexcitation in hypertrophic cardiomyopathy. Am J Cardiol 1984; 53:961–963.

372. Rosen KL, Cameron RW, Bigham PJ, Neish SR. Hypertrophic cardiomyopathy presenting with third degree atrioventricular block. Tex Heart Inst J 1997; 24:372–375.

373. Williams JF, Morrow AG, Braunwald E. The incidence and management of "medical" complications following cardiac operations. Circulation 1965; 32:608–619.

374. Gannon PG, Sellers RD, Kanjuh VI, Edwards JE, Lillehei CW. Complete heart block following replacement of the aortic valve. Circulation 1966; 33(Suppl I):I-152–I-161.

375. Shean FC, Austen WG, Buckley MJ, Mundth ED, Scannell JG, Daggett WM. Survival after Starr-Edwards aortic valve replacement. Circulation 1971; 44:1–8.

376. Lin MH, Young ML, Wu JM, Wolff GS. Developmental changes of atrioventricular nodal recovery properties. Am J Cardiol 1997; 80:1178–1182.

377. Smith R, Grossman W, Johnson L, Segal H, Collins J, Dalen J. Arrhythmias following cardiac valve replacement. Circulation 1972; 45:1018–1023.

378. Jaeger FJ, Trohman RG, Brener S, Loop F. Permanent pacing following repeat cardiac valve surgery. Am J Cardiol 1994; 74:505–507.

379. Mosseri M, Meir G, Lotan C, et al. Coronary pathology predicts conduction disturbances after coronary artery bypass grafting. Ann Thorac Surg 1991; 51:248–252.

380. Cataldo R, Olsen S, Freedman RA. Atrioventricular block occurring late after heart transplantation: presentation of three cases and literature review. Pacing Clin Electrophysiol 1996; 19:325–330.

381. Woodard DA, Conti JB, Mills RM, Williams RM, Curtis AB. Permanent atrial pacing in cardiac transplant patients. PACE 1997; 20:2398–2404.

382. Hurwitz RA, Riemenschneider TA, Moss AJ. Chronic postoperative heart block in children. Am J Cardiol 1968; 21:185–189.

383. Marin-Garcia J, Moller JH. Sudden death after operative repair of tetralogy of Fallot. Br Heart J 1977; 39:1380–1385.

384. Rousou JA, Meeran MK, Engelman RM, Breyer RH, Lemeshow S. Does the type of venous drainage or cardioplegia affect postoperative conduction and atrial arrhythmias? Circulation 1985; 72:259–263.

385. Natterson PD, Perloff JK, Klitzner TS, Stevenson WG. Electrophysiologic abnormalities: unoperated occurrence and postoperative residua and sequelae. In Perloff JK, Child JS (eds). Congenital Heart Disease in Adults. 2nd ed. Philadelphia: WB Saunders, 1998, pp. 316–345.

386. Thomson IR, Dalton BC, Lappas DG, Lowenstein E. Right bundle-branch block and complete heart block caused by the Swan-Ganz catheter. Anesthesiology 1979; 51:359–362.

387. Goldman IR, Blount SG, Friedlich AL, Bing RJ. Electrocardiographic observations during cardiac catheterization. Bull Johns Hopkins Hosp 1950; 86:141–168.

388. Fraser RS, Macaulay WD, Rossall RE. Arrhythmias induced during intracardiac catheterization. Am Heart J 1962; 64:439–443.

389. Wennevold A, Christiansen I, Lindeneg O. Complications in 4,413 catheterizations of the right side of the heart. Am Heart J 1965; 69:173–180.

390. Gault JH, Ross J, Braunwald E. Persistent atrioventricular dissociation with block and nodal rhythm after cardiac catheterization. Am Heart J 1966; 71:690–694.

391. Stein PD, Mahur VS, Herman MV, Levine HD. Complete heart block induced during cardiac catheterization of patients with pre-existent bundle-branch block: the hazard of bilateral bundle-branch block. Circulation 1966; 34:783–791.

392. McIntosh HD. Arrhythmias. Circulation 1968; 37–38(Suppl III):III-27–III-35.

393. Patton RD, Bordia A, Ballantyne F, Ryan GF, Goldstein S, Heinle RA. Bundle-of-His recording of complete heart block during cardiac catheterization: electrophysiologic documentation of bilateral bundle branch block. Am Heart J 1971; 81:108–113.

394. Jacobson LB, Scheinman M. Catheter-induced intra-Hisian and intrafascicular block during recording of His bundle electrograms. Circulation 1974; 49:579–584.

395. Kimbiris D, Dreifus LS, Linhart JW. Complete heart block occurring during cardiac catheterization in patients with preexisting bundle branch block. Chest 1974; 65:95–97.

396. Lo RN, Lau KC, Leung MP. Complete heart block after balloon dilatation for congenital pulmonary stenosis. Br Heart J 1988; 59:384–386.

397. Wathen M, Natale A, Wolfe K, Yee R, Newman D, Klein G. An anatomically guided approach to atrioventricular node slow pathway ablation. Am J Cardiol 1992; 70:886–889.

398. Jentzer JH, Goyal R, Williamson BD, et al. Analysis of junctional ectopy during radiofrequency ablation of the slow pathway in patients with atrioventricular nodal reentrant tachycardia. Circulation 1994; 90:2820–2826.

399. Teixeira OH, Balaji S, Case CL, Gillette PC. Radiofrequency catheter ablation of atrioventricular nodal reentrant tachycardia in children. Pacing Clin Electrophysiol 1994; 17:1621–1626.

400. Fenelon G, d'Avila A, Malacky T, Brugada P. Prognostic significance of transient complete atrioventricular block during radiofrequency ablation of atrioventricular node reentrant tachycardia. Am J Cardiol 1995; 75:698–702.

401. Chen SA, Chiang CE, Tai CT, et al. Transient complete atrioventricular block during radiofrequency ablation of slow pathway for atrioventricular nodal reentrant tachycardia. Am J Cardiol 1996; 77:1367–1370.

402. Schaffer MS, Silka MJ, Ross BA, Kugler JD. Inadvertent atrioventricular block during radiofrequency catheter ablation: results of the Pediatric Radiofrequency Ablation Registry. Pediatric Electrophysiology Society. Circulation 1996; 94:3214–3220.

403. Basta MN, Krahn AD, Klein GJ, Rosenbaum M, Le Feuvre C, Yee R. Safety of slow pathway ablation in patients with atrioventricular node reentrant tachycardia and a long fast pathway effective refractory period. Am J Cardiol 1997; 80:155–159.

404. Jackman WM, Wang XZ, Friday KJ, et al. Catheter ablation of accessory atrioventricular pathways (Wolff-Parkinson-White syndrome) by radiofrequency current. N Engl J Med 1991; 324:1605–1611.

405. Fujimura O, Schoen WJ, Kuo CS, Leonelli FM. Delayed recurrence of atrioventricular block after radiofrequency ablation of atrioventricular node reentry: a word of caution. Am Heart J 1993; 125:901–904.

406. Swartz JF, Tracy CM, Fletcher RD. Radiofrequency endocardial catheter ablation of accessory atrioventricular pathway atrial insertion sites. Circulation 1993; 87:487–499.

407. Greene TO, Huang SK, Wagshal AB, et al. Cardiovascular complications after radiofrequency catheter ablation of supraventricular tachyarrhythmias. Am J Cardiol 1994; 74:615–617.

408. Scheinman MM. Patterns of catheter ablation practice in the United States: results of the 1992 NASPE survey. North American Society of Pacing and Electrophysiology. Pacing Clin Electrophysiol 1994; 17:873–875.

409. Epstein LM, Lesh MD, Griffin JC, Lee RJ, Scheinman MM. A direct midseptal approach to slow atrioventricular nodal pathway ablation. Pacing Clin Electrophysiol 1995; 18:57–64.

410. Stamato NJ, Eddy SL, Whiting DJ. Transient complete heart block during radiofrequency ablation of a left lateral bypass tract. Pacing Clin Electrophysiol 1996; 19:1351–1354.

411. Lin JL, Huang SKS, Lai LP, Ko WC, Tseng YZ, Lien WP. Clinical and electrophysiological characteristics and long-term efficacy of slow-pathway catheter ablation in patients with spontaneous supraventricular tachycardia and dual atrioventricular node pathways without inducible tachycardia. J Am Coll Cardiol 1998; 31:855–860.

412. Bigger JT Jr, Hoffman BF. Antiarrhythmic drugs. In Gilman AG, Rall TW, Nies AS, Taylor P (eds). The Pharmacological Basis of Therapeutics. 8th ed. New York: Pergamon Press, 1990, pp. 840–873.

413. Lai WT, Lee CS, Wu JC, Sheu SH, Wu SN. Effects of verapamil, propranolol, and procainamide on adenosine-induced negative dromotropism in human beings. Am Heart J 1996; 132:768–775.

414. Lee J, Heo J, Ogilby JD, Cave V, Iskandrian B, Iskandrian AS. Atrioventricular block during adenosine thallium imaging. Am Heart J 1992; 123:1569–1574.

415. Brignole M, Gaggioli G, Menozzi C, et al. Adenosine-induced atrioventricular block in patients with unexplained syncope: the diagnostic value of ATP testing. Circulation 1997; 96:3921–3927.

416. Vaitkus PT, Grossman D, Fox KR, McEvoy MD, Doherty JU. Complete heart block due to interleukin-2 therapy. Am Heart J 1990; 119:978–980.

417. Kuo CS, Reddy CP. Effect of lidocaine on escape rate in patients with complete atrioventricular block. B. Proximal His bundle block. Am J Cardiol 1981; 47:1315–1320.

418. Gupta PK, Lichstein E, Chadda KD. Lidocaine-induced heart block in patients with bundle branch block. Am J Cardiol 1974; 33:487–492.

419. Blizzard JJ, Rupp JJ. Prolongation of the P-R interval as a manifestation of thyrotoxicosis. JAMA 1960; 173:143.

420. Stern MP, Jacobs RL, Duncan GW. Complete heart block complicating hyperthyroidism. JAMA 1970; 212:2117–2119.

421. Campus S, Rappelli A, Malavasi A, Satta A. Heart block and hyperthyroidism: report of two cases. Arch Intern Med 1975; 135:1091–1095.

422. Kramer MR, Shilo S, Hershko C. Atrioventricular and sinoatrial block in thyrotoxic crisis. Br Heart J 1985; 54:600–602.

423. Crum WB, Till HJ. Hyperparathyroidism with Wenckebach's phenomenon. Am J Cardiol 1960; 6:838–840.

424. Muggia AL, Stjernholm M, Houle T. Complete heart block with thyrotoxic myocarditis: report of a case. N Engl J Med 1970; 283:1099–1100.

425. Tiberti G, Bana G, Bossi M. Complete atrioventricular block with unwidened QRS complex during hyperkalemia. PACE 1998; 21:1480–1482.

426. Mudge GH, Weiner IM. Agents affecting volume and composition of body fluids. In Gilman AG, Rall TW, Nies AS, Taylor P (eds). Goodman and Gilman's The Pharmacological Basis of Therapeutics. 8th ed. New York: Pergamon Press, 1990, pp. 682–707.

427. Somerville W, Levine HD, Thorn GW. The electrocardiogram in Addison's disease. Medicine 1951; 30:43–79.

428. Lown B, Arons WL, Ganong WF, Vazifdar JP, Levine SA. Adrenal steroids and auriculoventricular conduction. Am Heart J 1955; 50:760–769.

429. Harvey WP. Clinical aspects of cardiac tumors. Am J Cardiol 1968; 21:328–343.

430. Nadas AS, Ellison RC. Cardiac tumors in infancy. Am J Cardiol 1968; 21:363–366.

431. Davies MJ. Pathology of Conducting Tissue of the Heart. New York: Appleton-Century-Crofts, 1971, pp. 118–119.

432. Grant RT, Camp PD. A case of complete heart block due to an arterial angioma. Heart 1932; 16:137–142.

433. Perry CB, Rogers H. Lymphangio-endothelioma of the heart causing complete heart block. J Pathol 1934; 39:281–284.

434. Amsterdam HJ, Grayzel DM, Louria AL. Hemangio-endothelioblastoma of the heart. Am Heart J 1949; 37:291–300.

435. Dresdale DT, Spain D, Perez-Pina F. Heart block and leukemic cell infiltration of interventricular septum of heart. Am J Med 1949; 6:530–533.

436. Cohen GU, Perry TM, Evans JM. Neoplastic invasion of the heart and pericardium. Ann Intern Med 1955; 42:1238–1245.

437. Kellaway G, Gardner DL. Metastatic reticulum cell sarcoma of the heart causing complete heart block. Scott Med J 1959; 4:575–580.

438. Hanfling SM. Metastatic cancer to the heart: review of the literature and report of 127 cases. Circulation 1960; 22:474–483.

439. Buckberg GD, Fowler NO. Complete atrioventricular block due to cardiac metastasis of bronchogenic carcinoma. Circulation 1961; 24:657–661.

440. Goggio AF, Harkness JT, Palmer WS. Stokes-Adams syndrome in Hodgkin's granuloma. JAMA 1961; 176:687–689.

441. James TN. Metastasis of hypernephroma to atrioventricular node. N Engl J Med 1962; 266:705–708.
442. Tamura K, Oguro M, Aoki Y, Kawabe A, Mashima T, Oguro C. Bilateral bundle branch block due to cardiac metastasis of pulmonary carcinoma. Jpn Heart J 1963; 4:294–300.
443. Wolf PL, Bing R. The smallest tumor which causes sudden death. JAMA 1965; 194:674–675.
444. Kaminsky NI, Killip T III, Alonso DR, Hagstrom JW. Heart block and mesothelioma of the atrioventricular node. Am J Cardiol 1967; 20:248–254.
445. Barr JR, Pollock P. Inclusion cyst of the myocardium in a patient with complete heart block. Can Med Assoc J 1968; 98:52–53.
446. Glancy DL, Roberts WC. The heart in malignant melanoma; a study of 70 autopsy cases. Am J Cardiol 1968; 21:555–571.
447. Malaret GE, Aliaga P. Metastatic disease to the heart. Cancer 1968; 22:457–466.
448. Kaplan A, Cohen J. Restrictive cardiomyopathy as the presenting feature of reticulum cell sarcoma. Am Heart J 1969; 77:307–314.
449. Hopkinson JM, Newcombe CP. Heart block due to epithelial heterotopia. J Pathol 1971; 104:218–220.
450. Lafargue RT, Hand AM, Lev M. Mesothelioma (coelothelioma) of the atrioventricular node. Chest 1971; 59:571–574.
451. Manion WC, Nelson WP, Hall RJ, Brierty RE. Benign tumor of the heart causing complete heart block. Am Heart J 1972; 83:535–542.
452. Bharati S, Bicoff JP, Fridman JL, Lev M, Rosen KM. Sudden death caused by benign tumor of the atrioventricular node. Arch Intern Med 1976; 136:224–228.
453. Thiene G, Miraglia G, Menghetti L, Nava A, Rossi L. Multiple lesions of the conduction system in a case of cardiac rhabdomyosarcoma with complex arrhythmias. Chest 1976; 70:378–381.
454. James TN, Galakhov I. De subitaneis mortibus. XXVI. Fatal electrical instability of the heart associated with benign congenital polycystic tumor of the atrioventricular node. Circulation 1977; 56:667–678.
455. Ross MJ. Heart block, sudden death, and atrioventricular node mesothelioma. Am J Dis Child 1977; 131:1209–1211.
456. Kubac G, Doris I, Ondro M, Davey PW. Malignant granular cell myoblastoma with metastatic cardiac involvement: case report and echocardiogram. Am Heart J 1980; 100:227–229.
457. Hellemans IM, van Hemel NM, Kooyman CA. Atrioventricular block in childhood caused by mesothelioma. Pacing Clin Electrophysiol 1981; 4:216–220.
458. Nishida K, Kamijima G, Nagayama T. Mesothelioma of the atrioventricular node. Br Heart J 1985; 53:468–470.
459. Strauss WE, Asinger RW, Hodges M. Mesothelioma of the AV node: potential utility of pacing. Pacing Clin Electrophysiol 1988; 11:1296–1298.
460. Otsuji Y, Arima N, Fujiwara H, Saito K, Kisanuki A, Tanaka H. Reversible complete atrioventricular block due to malignant lymphoma. Eur Heart J 1994; 15:407–408.
461. Otsuka K, Ichimaru Y, Yanaga T, Sato Y. Studies of arrhythmias by 24-hour polygraphic recordings: relationship between atrioventricular block and sleep states. Am Heart J 1983; 105:934–940.
462. Guilleminault C, Connolly SJ, Winkle RA. Cardiac arrhythmia and conduction disturbances during sleep in 400 patients with sleep apnea syndrome. Am J Cardiol 1983; 52:490–494.
463. Rama PR, Sharma SC. Sleep apnea and complete heart block. Clin Cardiol 1994; 17:675–677.
464. Grimm W, Hoffmann J, Menz V, et al. Electrophysiologic evaluation of sinus node function and atrioventricular conduction in patients with prolonged ventricular asystole during obstructive sleep apnea. Am J Cardiol 1996; 77:1310–1314.
465. Gooch AS. Exercise testing for detecting changes in cardiac rhythm and conduction. Am J Cardiol 1972; 30:741–746.
466. Moulopoulos SD, Darsinos J, Sideris DA. Atrioventricular block response to exercise and intraventricular conduction at rest. Br Heart J 1972; 34:998–1004.
467. Bakst A, Goldberg B, Schamroth L. Significance of exercise-induced second degree atrioventricular block. Br Heart J 1975; 37:984–986.
468. Rozanski JJ, Castellanos A, Sheps D, Pozen R, Myerberg RJ. Paroxysmal second-degree atrioventricular block induced by exercise. Heart Lung 1980; 9:887–890.
469. Den Dulk K, Bouwels L, Lindemans F, Rankin I, Brugada P, Wellens HJJ. The Activitrax rate responsive pacemaker system. Am J Cardiol 1988; 61:107–112.
470. Peller OG, Moses JW, Kligfield P. Exercise-induced atrioventricular block: report of three cases. Am Heart J 1988; 115:1315–1317.
471. Chokshi SK, Sarmiento J, Nazari J, Mattioni T, Zheutlin T, Kehoe R. Exercise-provoked distal atrioventricular block. Am J Cardiol 1990; 66:114–116.
472. Sumiyoshi M, Nakata Y, Yasuda M, et al. Clinical and electrophysiologic features of exercise-induced atrioventricular block. Am Heart J 1996; 132:1277–1281.
473. Chesler E, Schamroth L. The Wenckebach phenomenon associated with sialorrhoea. Br Heart J 1957; 19:577–580.
474. Petkovich NJ, Dunn M, Reed W. Myotonia dystrophica with A-V dissociation and Stokes-Adams attacks: a case report and review of the literature. Am Heart J 1964; 68:391–396.
475. Bulloch RT, Davis JL, Hara M. Dystrophia myotonica with heart block: a light and electron microscopic study. Arch Pathol 1967; 84:130–140.
476. Sims BA, Geddes JS. Traumatic heart block. Br Heart J 1969; 31:140–142.
477. Virtanen KS, Halonen PI. Total heart block as a complication of gout. Cardiology 1969; 54:359–363.
478. Sustaita HS, Balsara RK, Niguidula FN, Davila JC. Penetrating wounds of the heart. Chest 1970; 57:340–343.
479. Coltart DJ, Hudson RE. Primary oxalosis of the heart: a cause of heart block. Br Heart J 1971; 33:315–319.
480. Rosen KM, Heller R, Ehsani A, Rahimtoola SH. Localization of site of traumatic heart block with His bundle recordings: electrophysiologic observations regarding the nature of "split" H potentials. Am J Cardiol 1972; 30:412–417.
481. Goodfriend MA, Barold SS. Tachycardia-dependent and bradycardia-dependent Mobitz type II atrioventricular block within the bundle of His. Am J Cardiol 1974; 33:908–913.
482. Kennel AJ, Titus JL, Merideth J. Pathological findings in the atrioventricular conduction system in myotonic dystrophy. Mayo Clin Proc 1974; 49:838–842.
483. Clark DS, Myerburg RJ, Morales AR, Befeler B, Hernandez FA, Gelband H. Heart block in Kearns-Sayre syndrome: electrophysiologic-pathologic correlation. Chest 1975; 68:727–730.
484. Griggs RC, Davis RJ, Anderson DC, Dove JT. Cardiac conduction in myotonic dystrophy. Am J Med 1975; 59:37–42.
485. Lambert CD, Fairfax AJ. Neurological associations of chronic heart block. J Neurol Neurosurg Psychiatry 1976; 39:571–575.
486. Brennan JA, Field JM, Liedtke AJ. Reversible heart block following nonpenetrating chest trauma. J Trauma 1979; 19:784–788.
487. Kanemoto N, Sasamoto H. Arrhythmias in primary pulmonary hypertension. Jpn Heart J 1979; 20:765–775.
488. Kerin NZ, Edelstein J, Goldberg LB, Louridas G. Cardiac dysrhythmias associated with obesity and sleep apnea. Cardiovasc Med 1979; 4:1167–1172.
489. Prystowsky EN, Pritchett EL, Roses AD, Gallagher J. The natural history of conduction system disease in myotonic muscular dystrophy as determined by serial electrophysiologic studies. Circulation 1979; 60:1360–1364.
490. Roberts NK, Perloff JK, Kark RA. Cardiac conduction in the Kearns-Sayre syndrome (a neuromuscular disorder associated with progressive external ophthalmoplegia and pigmentary retinopathy): report of 2 cases and review of 17 published cases. Am J Cardiol 1979; 44:1396–1400.
491. Forstot JZ, Overlie PA, Neufeld GK, Harmon CE, Forstot SL. Cardiac complications of Wegener granulomatosis: a case report of complete heart block and review of the literature. Semin Arthritis Rheum 1980; 10:148–154.
492. Greenland P, Griggs RC. Arrhythmic complications in the

Guillain-Barre syndrome. Arch Intern Med 1980; 140:1053–1055.

493. Perloff JK. Cardiac rhythm and conduction in Duchenne's muscular dystrophy: a prospective study of 20 patients. J Am Coll Cardiol 1984; 3:1263–1268.

494. Hassan AB, Abinader EG, Goldhammer EI, Malouf S. Complete heart block and trigeminal neuralgia. Neurology 1987; 37:1089–1090.

495. Kenny D, Wetherbee J. Kearns-Sayre syndrome in the elderly: mitochondrial myopathy with advanced heart block. Am Heart J 1990; 120:440–443.

496. Suzuki M, Goto T, Kato R, Yamauchi K, Hayashi H. Combined atrioventricular block and sinus node dysfunction in Fabry's disease. Am Heart J 1990; 120:438–440.

497. Ikari Y, Kuwako K, Yamaguchi T. Fabry's disease with complete atrioventricular block: histological evidence of involvement of the conduction system. Br Heart J 1992; 68:323–325.

498. Pellikka PA, Tajik J, Khandheria BK, et al. Carcinoid heart disease: clinical and echocardiographic spectrum in 74 patients. Circulation 1993; 87:1188–1196.

499. Haught WH, Bertolet BD, Conti JB, Curtis AB, Mills RM Jr. Theophylline reverses high-grade atrioventricular block resulting from cardiac transplant rejection. Am Heart J 1994; 128:1255–1257.

500. Agarwal DK, Agarwal R, Barthwal SP. Interventricular septal hydatid cyst presenting as complete heart block. Heart 1996; 75:266.

501. Ozdemir M, Diker E, Aydogdu S, Goksel S. Complete heart block caused by cardiac echinococcosis and successfully treated with albendazole. Heart 1997; 77:84–85.

502. Rokseth R, Hatle L. Prospective study on the occurrence and management of chronic sinoatrial disease, with follow-up. Br Heart J 1974; 36:582–587.

503. Onat A, Domanic N, Onat T. Sick sinus syndrome in an infant: severe disturbance of impulse formation and conduction involving the S-A node and the A-V junctional tissue. Eur J Cardiol 1974; 2:79–83.

504. Frey WG III, Grant JL. Chronic binodal block with Wenckebach phenomenon. J Electrocardiol 1975; 8:363–368.

505. Stopfkuchen H, Jungst BK. Congenital sinus bradycardia combined with congenital total atrioventricular block. Eur J Pediatr 1977; 125:219–224.

506. Tan AT, EE BK, Mah PK, Choo MH, Chia BL. Diffuse conduction abnormalities in an adolescent with familial sinus node disease. Pacing Clin Electrophysiol 1981; 4:645–649.

507. Vallin H, Edhag O. Associated conduction disturbances in patients with symptomatic sinus node disease. Acta Med Scan 1981; 210:263–270.

508. Rasmussen K, Myhre ES, Gunnes P, Wang H. Multilevel disease of the conduction system. Eur Heart J 1983; 4:73–78.

509. Barak M, Herschkowitz S, Shapiro I, Roguin N. Familial combined sinus node and atrioventricular conduction dysfunctions. Int J Cardiol 1987; 15:231–239.

510. Gwinn N, Leman R, Kratz J, White JK, Zile MR, Gillette P. Chronotropic incompetence: a common and progressive finding in pacemaker patients. Am Heart J 1992; 123:1216–1219.

511. Morsi A, Lau C, Nishimura S, Goldman BS. The development of sinoatrial dysfunction in pacemaker patients with isolated atrioventricular block. PACE 1998; 21:1430–1434.

512. Altschule MD. The relation between prolonged P-R interval and auricular fibrillation in patients with rheumatic heart disease. Am Heart J 1939; 18:1–7.

513. Kurita T, Ohe T, Marui N, Aihara N, Takaki H, Kamakura S, and others. Bradycardia-induced abnormal QT prolongation in patients with complete atrioventricular block with torsades de pointes. Am J Cardiol 1992; 69:628–633.

514. Kawasaki R, Machado C, Reinoehl J, et al. Increased propensity of women to develop torsades de pointes during complete heart block. J Cardiovasc Electrophysiol 1995; 6:1032–1038.

515. Steinbrecher UP, Fitchett DH. Torsade de pointes: a cause of syncope with atrioventricular block. Arch Intern Med 1980; 140:1223–1226.

516. Sharma S, Nair KG, Gadekar HA. Romano-Ward prolonged QT syndrome with intermittent T wave alternans and atrioventricular block. Am Heart J 1981; 101:500–501.

517. Strasberg B, Kusniec J, Erdman S, et al. Polymorphous ventricular tachycardia and atrioventricular block. Pacing Clin Electrophysiol 1986; 9:522–526.

518. Van Hare GF, Franz MR, Roge C, Scheinman MM. Persistent functional atrioventricular block in two patients with prolonged QT intervals: elucidation of the mechanism of block. Pacing Clin Electrophysiol 1990; 13:608–618.

519. Anonymous. Paul Wood's Disease of the Heart and Circulation. 3rd ed. Philadelphia: JB Lippincott, 1968, pp. 239–249.

520. Anonymous. Paul Wood's Diseases of the Heart and Circulation. 3rd ed. Philadelphia: JB Lippincott, 1968, p. 245.

521. White PD. Heart Disease. New York: Macmillan, 1951, p. 939.

522. Dhingra RC, Denes P, Wu D, et al. Syncope in patients with chronic bifascicular block: significance, causative mechanisms, and clinical implications. Ann Intern Med 1974; 81:302–306.

523. Kapoor W, Snustad D, Peterson J, Wieand HS, Cha R, Karpf M. Syncope in the elderly. Am J Med 1986; 80:419–428.

524. Friedberg CK. Diseases of the Heart. 3rd ed. Philadelphia: WB Saunders, 1966, p. 599.

525. Landergren J, Bioerck G. The clinical assessment and treatment of complete heart block and Adams-Stokes attacks. Medicine 1963; 42:171–196.

526. Nichamin SJ. Stokes-Adams syndrome associated with complete congenital heart block in infancy and childhood. Pediatrics 1948; 1:327–330.

527. Paul MH, Rudolph AM, Nadas A. Congenital complete atrioventricular block: problems of clinical assessment. Circulation 1958; 18:183–190.

528. Begg TB, Thompson WRM. Stokes-Adams attacks in pregnancy. Br Heart J 1961; 23:729–732.

529. Molthan ME, Miller RA, Hastreiter AR, Paul MH. Congenital heart block with fatal Adams-Stokes attacks in childhood. Pediatrics 1962; 30:32–41.

530. Michaelsson M, Jonzon A, Riesenfeld T. Isolated congenital complete atrioventricular block in adult life: a prospective study. Circulation 1995; 92:442–449.

531. Jensen G, Sigurd B, Sandoe E. Adams-Stokes seizures due to ventricular tachydysrhythmias in patients with heart block: prevalence and problems of management. Chest 1975; 67:43–48.

532. Calkins H, Shyr Y, Frumin H, Schork A, Morady F. The value of the clinical history in the differentiation of syncope due to ventricular tachycardia, atrioventricular block, and neurocardiogenic syncope. Am J Med 1995; 98:365–373.

533. Van Durme JP. Tachyarrhythmias and transient cerebral ischemic attacks. Am Heart J 1975; 89:538–540.

534. Campbell M. Complete heart block. Br Heart J 1944; 6:71.

535. Ikkos D, Hanson JS. Response to exercise in congenital complete atrioventricular block. Circulation 1960; 22:538–590.

536. Moss AJ. Congenital complete AV block. Lancet 1961; 81:542–547.

537. Taylor MR, Godfrey S. Exercise studies in congenital heart block. Br Heart J 1972; 34:930–935.

538. Campbell M. Congenital complete heart block. Br Heart J 1943; 5:15–18.

539. Turner LB. Asymptomatic congenital complete heart block in an Army Air Force pilot. Am Heart J 1947; 34:426–431.

540. Mathewson FAL, Harvie FH. Complete heart block in an experienced pilot. Br Heart J 1957; 19:253–258.

541. Barton RM, LaDue CN. Complete heart block in a case of pregnancy. Am J Med 1948; 4:447–451.

542. Mowbray R, Bowley CC. Congenital complete heart block complicating pregnancy. J Obstet Gynaecol Br Emp 1948; 55:438–441.

543. Ziegler AM. Pregnancy with complete congenital heart block. Am J Obstet Gynecol 1951; 62:445–446.

544. Kenmure AC, Cameron AJ. Congenital complete heart block in pregnancy. Br Heart J 1967; 29:910–912.

545. McHenry MM. Factors influencing longevity in adults with congenital complete heart block. Am J Cardiol 1972; 29:416–421.

546. Harvey WP, Ronan JA Jr. Bedside diagnosis of arrhythmias. Prog Cardiovasc Dis 1966; 8:419–445.

547. Perloff JK. Physical Examination of the Heart and Circulation. 2nd ed. Philadelphia: W B Saunders, 1982, pp. 103–140.

548. Campbell M, Thorne MG. Congenital heart block. Br Heart J 1956; 18:90–102.

549. Wolferth CC, Margolies A. The influence of auricular contraction on the first heart sound and the radial pulse. Arch Intern Med 1930; 46:1048–1071.

550. Merrill JM, France R. Double atrial sounds and peripheral atrial impulses in a patient with complete heart block. Ann Intern Med 1963; 58:867–871.

551. Berman ND, Waxman MB. Cannon waves with A-V association. Am Heart J 1976; 91:643–644.

552. Stokes W. Observations in some cases of permanently slow pulse. In Willius FA, Keys TE (eds). Classics of Cardiology. New York: Dover, 1941, pp. 462–469.

553. Tavel ME. Variation of the systolic murmur of complete heart block. N Engl J Med 1966; 274:1298–1300.

554. Ali N. Loud first heart sound with long P-R intervals. Am J Cardiol 1975; 35:435–438.

555. Nakamura FF, Nadas AS. Complete heart block in infants and children. N Engl J Med 1964; 270:1261–1268.

556. Shah PM, Kramer DH, Gramiak R. Influence of the timing of atrial systole on mitral valve closure and on the first heart sound in man. Am J Cardiol 1970; 26:231–237.

557. Beard OW, Decherd GM. Variations in the first heart sound in complete A-V block. Am Heart J 1947; 34:809–816.

558. Zaky A, Steinmetz E, Feigenbaum H. Role of atrium in closure of mitral valve in man. Am J Physiol 1969; 217:1652–1659.

559. Shearn MA, Tarr E, Rytand DA. The significance of changes in amplitude of the first heart sound in children with A-V block. Circulation 1953; 7:839–846.

560. Rytand DA. An analysis of the variable amplitude of the first heart sound in complete heart block. Stanford Med Bull 1948; 6:187–197.

561. Martinez-Lopez JI. The second heart sound in complete atrioventricular block. South Med J 1970; 63:254–257.

562. Haber E, Leatham A. Splitting of heart sounds from ventricular asynchrony in bundle-branch block, ventricular ectopic beats, and artificial pacing. Br Heart J 1965; 27:691–696.

563. Kincaid-Smith P, Barlow J. The atrial sound and the atrial component of the first heart sound. Br Heart J 1959; 21:470–478.

564. Rytand DA. An auricular diastolic murmur with heart block in elderly patients. Am Heart J 1946; 32:579–598.

565. Jelveh M, Berger M, Goldberg E. The genesis of the diastolic murmur of complete heart block: phono-echocardiographic observations. Circulation 1978; 53:747–750.

566. Lie KI, Durrer D. Conduction disturbances in acute myocardial infarction. In Narula OS (ed). Cardiac Arrhythmias. Electrophysiology, Diagnosis and Management. Baltimore: Williams & Wilkins, 1979, pp. 140–163.

567. Christ JE, Hoff HE. An analysis of the circadian rhythmicity of atrial and ventricular rates in complete heart block. J Electrocardiol 1975; 8:69–72.

568. Campbell M, Emanuel R. Six cases of congenital complete heart block followed for 34–40 years. Br Heart J 1967; 29:577–587.

569. Parkinson J, Papp C, Evans W. The electrocardiogram of the Stokes-Adams attack. Br Heart J 1941; 3:171–199.

570. Bredikis YI, Kostenko IG. The auricular rhythm in patients with the Morgagni-Adams-Stokes syndrome before and after electrical cardiac stimulation. Bull Experimental Biol Med 1964; 55:375–377.

571. Cohn AE, Fraser FR. The occurrence of auricular contractions in a case of incomplete and complete heart-block due to stimuli received from the contracting ventricles. Heart 1919; 5:141–145.

572. Wolferth CC, McMillan TM. Observations on the mechanism of relatively short intervals in ventriculoauricular and auriculoventricular sequential beats during high grade heart-block. Am Heart J 1929; 4:521–544.

573. Winternitz M, Langendorf R. Auriculoventricular block with ventriculoauricular response. Am Heart J 1944; 27:301–321.

574. Marriott HJL. Interactions between atria and ventricles during interference-dissociation and complete A-V block. Am Heart J 1957; 53:884–889.

575. Adams CW. Retrograde atrial conduction with complete heart block following implantation of an internal ventricular pacemaker. Chest 1963; 43:544–545.

576. Gubbay ER, Mora CA. Retrograde conduction and isorhythmic dissociation in heart block. Am Heart J 1964; 68:166–172.

577. Louvros N, Costeas F. Retrograde activation of atria in auriculoventricular block; an electrocardiographic demonstration. Arch Intern Med 1964; 116:778–779.

578. Scherf D, Cohen J, Orphanos RP. Retrograde activation of atria in atrioventricular block. Am J Cardiol 1964; 13:219–225.

579. Langendorf R, Pick A. Atrioventricular (A-V) block with ventriculoatrial (V-A) response: relation of unidirectional to type II (Mobitz) A-V block and to bilateral bundle-branch block. Circulation 1966; 33–34(Suppl III):III-152.

580. Castillo C, Samet P. Retrograde conduction in complete heart block. Br Heart J 1967; 29:553–558.

581. Kastor JA, Sanders CA, Harthorne JW, Sulit YQM, Leinbach RC, Schulman CL. Retrograde conduction during cardiac catheterization and in patients with heart block. Circulation 1967; 35–36(Suppl II):II-156–II-157.

582. Fletcher E, Morton P. Atrioventricular dissociation with intact retrograde conduction. Br Heart J 1968; 30:458–463.

583. Kastor JA, Sanders CA, Leinbach RC, Harthorne JW. Factors influencing retrograde conduction: study of 30 patients during cardiac catheterization. Br Heart J 1969; 31:580–587.

584. Goldreyer BN, Bigger JT Jr. Ventriculo-atrial conduction in man. Circulation 1970; 41:935–946.

585. Gupta PK, Haft JI. Retrograde ventriculoatrial conduction in complete heart block: studies with His bundle electrography. Am J Cardiol 1972; 30:408–411.

586. Langendorf R, Cohen H, Gozo EG Jr. Observations on second degree atrioventricular block, including new criteria for the differential diagnosis between type I and type II block. Am J Cardiol 1972; 29:111–119.

587. Cohen SI, Smith LK, Aroesty JM, Voukydis P, Morkin E. Concealed retrograde conduction in complete atrioventricular block. Circulation 1974; 50:496–498.

588. Schuilenburg RM. Patterns of V-A conduction in the human heart in the presence of normal and abnormal A-V conduction. In Wellens HJJ, Lie KI, Janse MJ (eds). The Conduction System of the Heart. Structure, Function and Clinical Implications. Philadelphia: Lea & Febiger, 1976, pp. 485–503.

589. Takeshita A, Tanaka S, Nakamura M. Study of retrograde conduction in complete heart block using His bundle recordings. Br Heart J 1974; 36:462–467.

590. Touboul P, Huerta F, Delahaye JP. Retrograde conduction in complete atrioventricular block study using His bundle recordings. Br Heart J 1976; 38:706–711.

591. Puech P, Grolleau R, Guimond C. Incidence of different types of A-V block and their localization by His bundle recordings. In Wellens HJJ, Lie KI, Janse MJ (eds). The Conduction System of the Heart: Structure, Function and Clinical Implications. Philadelphia: Lea & Febiger, 1976, pp. 467–484.

592. Khalilullah M, Singhal N, Gupta U, Padmavati S. Unidirectional complete heart block. Am Heart J 1979; 97:608–612.

593. Inoue T, Kobayashi K, Fukuzaki H. Ventriculo-atrial conduction in patients with normal and impaired atrioventricular conduction. Jpn Heart J 1985; 26:707–714.

594. Parsonnet AE, Miller R. Heart block. The influence of

ventricular systole upon the auricular rhythm in complete and incomplete heart block. Am Heart J 1944; 27:676–687.

595. Roth IR, Kisch B. The mechanism of irregular sinus rhythm in auriculoventricular heart block. Am Heart J 1948; 36:257–276.

596. Rosenbaum MB, Lepeschkin E. The effect of ventricular systole on auricular rhythm in auriculoventricular block. Circulation 1955; 11:240–261.

597. Donoso E, Braunwald E, Jick S, Grishman A. Congenital heart block. Am J Med 1956; 20:869–878.

598. Katz LN, Pick A. Clinical Electrocardiography. Part I. The Arrhythmias. Philadelphia: Lea & Febiger, 1956, p. 583.

599. Katz LN, Pick A. Clinical Electrocardiography. Part I. The Arrhythmias. Philadelphia: Lea & Febiger, 1956, p. 538.

600. Marriott HJL. Atrioventricular synchronization and accrochage. Circulation 1956; 14:38–43.

601. Schubart AF, Marriott HJL, Gorten RJ. Isorhythmic dissociation. Am J Med 1958; 24:209–214.

602. Jacobs DR, Donoso E, Friedberg CK. A-V dissociation: a relatively frequent arrhythmia: analysis of thirty cases with detailed discussion of the etiologic differential diagnosis. Medicine 1961; 40:101–117.

603. Segers M, Lequime J, Denolin H. Synchronization of auricular and ventricular beats during complete heart block. Am Heart J 1947; 33:685–691.

604. Waldo AL, Vitikainen KJ, Harris PD, Malm JR, Hoffman BF. The mechanism of synchronization in isorhythmic A-V dissociation: some observations on the morphology and polarity of the P wave during retrograde capture of the atria. Circulation 1968; 38:880–898.

605. Fletcher E, Morton P, Murtagh JG, Bekheit S. Atrioventricular dissociation with accrochage. Br Heart J 1971; 33:572–577.

606. Christ JE, Hoff HE. An analysis of atrioventricular synchronization in complete A-V block. J Electrocardiol 1973; 6:53–62.

607. Izumi K, Ota S, Yoshikawa K, Otomi S, Sato T. Complete AV block simulating 2:1 incomplete AV block: a possible case of 2:1 AV synchronization. J Electrocardiol 1973; 6:359–366.

608. Bellet S. Clinical Disorders of the Heart Beat. 3rd ed. Philadelphia: Lea & Febiger, 1971, p. 325.

609. Katz LN, Pick A. Clinical Electrocardiography. Part I. The Arrhythmias. Philadelphia: Lea & Febiger, 1956, pp. 560–561.

610. Kastor JA, Josephson ME. Treatment of atrioventricular block. In Fowler NO (ed). Cardiac Arrhythmias. Diagnosis and Treatment. 2nd ed. New York: Harper & Row, 1977, pp. 118–142.

611. Katz LN, Pick A. Clinical Electrocardiography. Part I. The Arrhythmias. Philadelphia: Lea & Febiger, 1956, p. 159.

612. Katz LN, Pick A. Clinical Electrocardiography. Part I. The Arrhythmias. Philadelphia: Lea & Febiger, 1956, p. 551.

613. Kupfer JM, Kligfield P. A generalized description of Wenckebach behavior with analysis of determinants of ventricular cycle-length variation during ambulatory electrocardiography. Am J Cardiol 1991; 67:981–986.

614. Katz LN, Pick A. Clinical Electrocardiography. Part I. The Arrhythmias. Philadelphia: Lea & Febiger, 1956, p. 575.

615. Denes P, Levy L, Pick A, Rosen KM. The incidence of typical and atypical A-V Wenckebach periodicity. Am Heart J 1975; 89:26–31.

616. Friedman HS, Gomes JAC, Haft JI. An analysis of Wenckebach periodicity. J Electrocardiol 1975; 8:307–315.

617. el-Sherif N, Aranda J, Befeler B, Lazzara R. Atypical Wenckebach periodicity simulating Mobitz II AV block. Br Heart J 1978; 40:1376–1383.

618. Dressler W, Swiller SL. Atypical Wenckebach periods with dropped atrial beats. Am J Cardiol 1958; 2:575–578.

619. Faulkner JM. An extraordinary degree of partial heart-block. Am Heart J 1935; 10:969–973.

620. Myerburg RJ, Goodman JS, Marriott HJL. Atypical forms of the Wenckebach phenomenon. Am J Cardiol 1963; 11:418–423.

621. Katz LN, Pick A. Clinical Electrocardiography. Part I. The Arrhythmias. Philadelphia: Lea & Febiger, 1956, p. 574.

622. Katz LN, Pick A. Clinical Electrocardiography. Part I. The Arrhythmias. Philadelphia: Lea & Febiger, 1956, p. 592.

623. Halpern MS, Nau GJ, Levi RJ, Elizari MV, Rosenbaum MB. Wenckebach periods of alternate beats: clinical and experimental observations. Circulation 1973; 48:41–49.

624. Amat-y-Leon F, Chuquimia R, Wu D, et al. Alternating Wenckebach periodicity: a common electrophysiologic response. Am J Cardiol 1975; 36:757–763.

625. Elencwajg B, Zaman L, Rozanski JJ, Myerburg RJ, Castellanos A. Transverse dissociation of the human His bundle. Pacing Clin Electrophysiol 1982; 5:323–328.

626. Mobitz W. Uber den partiellen Herzblock. Z Klin Med 1928; 107:450.

627. Donoso E, Adler LN, Friedberg CK. Unusual forms of second-degree atrioventricular block, including Mobitz type-II block, associated with the Morgagni-Adams-Stokes syndrome. Am Heart J 1964; 67:150–157.

628. Barold SS, Friedberg HD. Second degree atrioventricular block: a matter of definition. Am J Cardiol 1974; 33:311–315.

629. Rosen KM, Loeb HS, Gunnar RM, Rahimtoola SH. Mobitz type II block without bundle-branch block. Circulation 1971; 44:1111–1119.

630. Lange HW, Ameisen O, Mack R, Moses JW, Kligfield P. Prevalence and clinical correlates of non-Wenckebach, narrow-complex second-degree atrioventricular block detected by ambulatory ECG. Am Heart J 1988; 115:114–120.

631. Massie B, Scheinman MM, Peters R, Desai J, Hirschfeld D, O'Young J. Clinical and electrophysiologic findings in patients with paroxysmal slowing of the sinus rate and apparent Mobitz type II atrioventricular block. Circulation 1978; 58:305–314.

632. Langendorf R, Mehlman JS. Blocked (nonconducted) A-V nodal premature systoles imitating first and second degree A-V block. Am Heart J 1947; 34:500–506.

633. Rosen KM, Rahimtoola SH, Gunnar RM. Pseudo A-V block secondary to premature nonpropagated His bundle depolarizations: documentation by His bundle electrocardiography. Circulation 1970; 42:367–373.

634. Cannom DS, Gallagher JJ, Goldreyer BN, Damato AN. Concealed bundle of His extrasystoles simulating nonconducted atrial premature beats. Am Heart J 1972; 83:777–779.

635. Eugster GS, Godfrey CC, Brammell HL, Pryor R. Pseudo A-V block associated with A-H and H-V conduction defects. Am Heart J 1973; 85:789–796.

636. Castellanos A, Befeler B, Myerburg RJ. Pseudo AV block produced by concealed extrasystoles arising below the bifurcation of the His bundle. Br Heart J 1974; 36:457–461.

637. Bonner AJ, Zipes DP. Lidocaine and His bundle extrasystoles. His bundle discharge conducted with functional right or left bundle-branch block, or blocked entirely (concealed). Arch Intern Med 1976; 136:700–704.

638. Childers RW. The junctional premature beat: an instructional exercise in modes of concealment. J Electrocardiol 1976; 9:85–88.

639. Fisch C, Zipes DP, McHenry PL. Electrocardiographic manifestations of concealed junctional ectopic impulses. Circulation 1976; 53:217–223.

640. Abrams J, Dykstra JR. Pseudo A-V block secondary to concealed junctional extrasystoles: case report and review of the literature. Am J Med 1977; 63:434–440.

641. Rosen KM, Wu D, Bauernfeind RA, Ashley WW, Smith TM, Denes P. Occurrence of pseudoatrioventricular block and atrioventricular block in the same patient. Chest 1978; 73:211–214.

642. Belic N, Grais M, Singer DH, Cohen H. Pseudo atrioventricular block. Arch Intern Med 1979; 139:459–460.

643. Donzeau JP, Bernadet P, Bounhoure JP, Calazel P. His bundle block and concealed His bundle premature depolarization. Eur J Cardiol 1979; 9:13–20.

644. Freeman G, Hwang MH, Danoviz J, Moran JF, Gunnar RM. Exercise induced "Mobitz type II" second degree AV block

in a patient with chronic bifascicular block (right bundle
branch block and left anterior hemiblock). J Electrocardiol
1984; 17:409–412.

645. Wang K, Salerno DM. Pseudo AV block secondary to
concealed premature His bundle depolarizations. Am Heart
J 1991; 121:1236–1237.

646. Geelen P, Malacky T, Lorga A, Manios E, Brugada P. The
value of an electrophysiological study in a clear-cut case.
Pacing Clin Electrophysiol 1996; 19:1643–1645.

647. Fleischmann P, Pick A. Premature ventricular beats in
complete A-V dissociation: the returning cycle. Am Heart J
1962; 63:299–308.

648. Coumel P, Fabiato A, Waynberger M, Motte G, Slama R,
Bouvrain Y. Bradycardia-dependent atrioventricular block:
report of two cases of A-V block elicited by premature beats.
J Electrocardiol 1971; 4:168–177.

649. Castellanos A, Khuddus SA, Sommer LS, Sung RJ, Myerburg
RJ. His bundle recordings in bradycardia-dependent AV
block induced by premature beats. Br Heart J 1975;
37:570–575.

650. Ursell S, Habbab MA, el-Sherif N. Atrioventricular and
intraventricular conduction disorders: clinical aspects. In
el-Sherif N, Samet P (eds). Cardiac Pacing and Electrophysiology. Philadelphia: W B Saunders, 1991, pp. 140–157.

651. Sgarbossa EB, Pinski SL, Topol EJ, et al. Acute myocardial
infarction and complete bundle branch block at hospital
admission: clinical characteristics and outcome in the
thrombolytic era. J Am Coll Cardiol 1998; 31:105–110.

652. Berman ND. The surface electrocardiogram in complete
intra-His heart block. J Electrocardiol 1978; 11:151–158.

653. Narula OS, Samet P. Wenckebach and Mobitz type II A-V
block due to block within the His bundle and bundle
branches. Circulation 1970; 41:947–965.

654. Rosen KM, Loeb HS, Rahimtoola SH. Mobitz type II block
with narrow QRS complex and Stokes-Adams attacks. Arch
Intern Med 1973; 132:595–596.

655. White PD, Eustis RS, Kerr WJ. Congenital heart block. Am J
Dis Child 1921; 22:299–306.

656. Lie KI, Wellens HJJ, Schuilenburg RM, Durrer D.
Mechanism and significance of widened QRS complexes
during complete atrioventricular block in acute inferior
myocardial infarction. Am J Cardiol 1974; 33:833–839.

657. Esscher E, Michaelsson M. Q-T interval in congenital
complete heart block. Pediatr Cardiol 1983; 4:121–124.

658. Rosenbaum MB, Elizari MV, Lazzari JO, Nau GJ, Levi RJ,
Halpern MS. Intraventricular trifascicular blocks: review of
the literature and classification. Am Heart J 1969;
78:450–459.

659. Lasser RP, Haft JI, Friedberg CK. Relationship of right
bundle-branch block and marked left axis deviation (with
left parietal or peri-infarction block) to complete heart
block and syncope. Circulation 1968; 37:429–437.

660. Lopez JF. Electrocardiographic findings in patients with
complete atrioventricular block. Br Heart J 1968; 30:20–28.

661. Kulbertus H, Collignon P. Association of right bundle-
branch block with left superior or inferior intraventricular
block: its relation to complete heart block and Adams-Stokes
syndrome. Br Heart J 1969; 31:435–440.

662. Jensen G, Sigurd B, Meibom J, Sandoe E. Adams-Stokes
syndrome caused by paroxysmal third-degree atrioventricular
block. Br Heart J 1973; 35:516–520.

663. McAnulty JH, Kauffman S, Murphy E, Kassebaum DG,
Rahimtoola SH. Survival in patients with intraventricular
conduction defects. Arch Intern Med 1978; 138:30–35.

664. Siegman-Igra Y, Yahini JH, Goldbourt U, Neufeld HN.
Intraventricular conduction disturbances: a review of
prevalence, etiology, and progression for ten years within a
stable population of Israeli adult males. Am Heart J 1978;
96:669–679.

665. Wiberg TA, Richman HG, Gobel FL. The significance and
prognosis of chronic bifascicular block. Chest 1977;
71:329–334.

666. Scanlon PJ, Pryor R, Blount SG. Right bundle-branch block
associated with left superior or inferior intraventricular
block: associated with acute myocardial infarction.
Circulation 1970; 42:1135–1142.

667. DePasquale NP, Bruno MS. Natural history of combined
right bundle branch block and left anterior hemiblock
(bilateral bundle branch block). Am J Med 1973;
54:297–303.

668. Kulbertus HE. The magnitude of risk of developing
complete heart block in patients with LAD-RBBB. Am Heart
J 1973; 86:278–280.

669. McAnulty JH, Rahimtoola SH, Murphy E, et al. Natural
history of "high-risk" bundle-branch block: final report of a
prospective study. N Engl J Med 1982; 307:137–143.

670. Homcy CJ. Atrioventricular block. In Eagle KA, Haber E,
DeSanctis RW, Austen WG (eds). The Practice of Cardiology.
2nd ed. Boston: Little, Brown, 1989, pp. 274–277.

671. Pine MB, Oren M, Ciafone R, et al. Excess mortality and
morbidity associated with right bundle branch and left
anterior fascicular block. J Am Coll Cardiol 1983;
1:1207–1212.

672. Kunstadt D, Punja M, Cagin N, Fernandez P, Levitt B,
Yuceoglu YZ. Bifascicular block: a clinical and
electrophysiologic study. Am Heart J 1973; 86:173–181.

673. Pastore JO, Yurchak PM, Janis KM, Murphy JD, Zir LM. The
risk of advanced heart block in surgical patients with right
bundle branch block and left axis deviation. Circulation
1978; 57:677–680.

674. Varriale P, Kennedy RJ. Right bundle branch block and left
posterior fascicular block. Am J Cardiol 1972; 29:459–465.

675. Dhingra RC, Denes P, Wu D, et al. Chronic right bundle
branch block and left posterior hemiblock: clinical,
electrophysiologic and prognostic observations. Am J Cardiol
1975; 36:867–879.

676. Klein RC, Vera Z, Mason DT. Intraventricular conduction
defects in acute myocardial infarction: incidence, prognosis,
and therapy. Am Heart J 1984; 108:1007–1013.

677. Scheidt S, Killip T. Bundle-branch block complicating acute
myocardial infarction. JAMA 1972; 222:919–924.

678. Basualdo CAE, Haraphongse M, Rossall RE. Intraventricular
blocks in acute myocardial infarction. Chest 1975; 67:75–78.

679. Dubois C, Pierard LA, Smeets JP, Foidart G, Legrand V,
Kulbertus HE. Short- and long-term prognostic importance
of complete bundle-branch block complicating acute
myocardial infarction. Clin Cardiol 1988; 11:292–296.

680. Norris RM, Croxson MS. Bundle branch block in acute
myocardial infarction. Am Heart J 1970; 79:728–733.

681. Godman MJ, Alpert BA, Julian DG. Bilateral bundle-branch
block complicating acute myocardial infarction. Lancet 1971;
2:345–347.

682. Scheinman M, Brenman B. Clinical and anatomic
implications of intraventricular conduction blocks in acute
myocardial infarction. Circulation 1972; 46:753–760.

683. Atkins JM, Leshin SJ, Blomqvist G, Mullins CB. Ventricular
conduction blocks and sudden death in acute myocardial
infarction. N Engl J Med 1973; 288:281–284.

684. Stephens MR, Fadayomi MO, Davies GJ, Muir JR. The
clinical features and significance of bifascicular block
complicating acute myocardial infarction. Eur J Cardiol
1975; 3:289–296.

685. Lie KI, Wellens HJJ, Schuilenburg RM. Bundle branch block
and acute myocardial infarction. In Wellens HJJ, Lie KI,
Janse MJ (eds). The Conduction System of the Heart.
Philadelphia: Lea & Febiger, 1976, p. 37.

686. Ritter WS, Atkins JM, Blomqvist CG, Mullins CB. Permanent
pacing in patients with transient trifascicular block during
acute myocardial infarction. Am J Cardiol 1976; 38:205–208.

687. Otterstad JE, Gundersen S, Anderssen N. Left anterior
hemiblock in acute myocardial infarction: incidence and
clinical significance in relation to the presence of bundle
branch block and to the absence of intraventricular
conduction defects. Acta Med Scand 1978; 203:529–534.

688. Domenighetti G, Perret C. Intraventricular conduction
disturbances in acute myocardial infarction: short- and long-
term prognosis. Eur J Cardiol 1980; 11:51–59.

689. Rizzon P, Rossi L, Baissus C, Demoulin JC, DiBiase M. Left
posterior hemiblock in acute myocardial infarction. Br Heart
J 1975; 37:711–720.

690. Ricou F, Nicod P, Gilpin E, Henning H, Ross J. Influence of

right bundle branch block on short- and long-term survival after acute anterior myocardial infarction. J Am Coll Cardiol 1991; 17:858–863.

691. Rosen KM, Loeb HS, Chuquimia R, Sinno MZ, Rahimtoola SH, Gunnar RM. Site of heart block in acute myocardial infarction. Circulation 1970; 42:925–933.

692. Pick A. A-V dissociation. A proposal for a comprehensive classification and consistent terminology. Am Heart J 1963; 66:147–150.

693. Schott A. Atrioventricular dissociation with and without interference. Prog Cardiovasc Dis 1960; 2:444–464.

694. Graybiel A, McFarland RA, Gates DC, Webster FA. Analysis of the electrocardiograms obtained from 1,000 young healthy aviators. Am Heart J 1944; 27:524–549.

695. Den Dulk K, Brugada P, Braat S, Heddle B, Wellens HJJ. Myocardial bridging as a cause of paroxysmal atrioventricular block. J Am Coll Cardiol 1983; 1:965–969.

696. Holmgren A, Karlberg P, Pernow B. Circulatory adaptation at rest and during muscular work in patients with complete heart block. Acta Med Scand 1959; 164:119–130.

697. Corne RA, Mathewson FA. Congenital complete atrioventricular heart block: a 25 year follow-up study. Am J Cardiol 1972; 29:412–415.

698. Winkler RB, Freed MD, Nadas AS. Exercise-induced ventricular ectopy in children and young adults with complete heart block. Am Heart J 1980; 99:87–92.

699. Reybrouck T, Vanden Eynde B, Dumoulin M, Van der Hauwaert LG. Cardiorespiratory response to exercise in congenital complete atrioventricular block. Am J Cardiol 1989; 64:896–899.

700. Benchimol A, Li YB, Dimond G, Voth RB, Roland AS. Effect of heart rate, exercise, and nitroglycerin on the cardiac dynamics in complete heart block. Circulation 1963; 28:510–519.

701. Bevegard S, Jonsson B, Karlof I, Lagergren H, Sowton E. Effect of changes in ventricular rate on cardiac output and central pressures at rest and during exercise in patients with artificial pacemakers. Cardiovasc Res 1967; 1:21–33.

702. Gobel FL, Medina JR, Guenter CA, Wang Y. Immediate hemodynamic response of patients with atrioventricular block and cardiac failure to transvenous pacing. Circulation 1969; 39:64–71.

703. Gooch AS, McConnell D. Analysis of transient arrhythmias and conduction disturbances occurring during submaximal treadmill exercise testing. Prog Cardiovasc Dis 1970; 13:293–307.

704. Woelfel AK, Simpson RJ Jr, Gettes LS, Foster JR. Exercise-induced distal atrioventricular block. J Am Coll Cardiol 1983; 2:578–581.

705. Johansson BW. Long-term ECG in ambulatory clinical practice. Analysis and 2-year follow-up of 100 patients studied with a portable ECG tape recorder. Eur J Cardiol 1977; 5:39–48.

706. Boudoulas H, Schaal SF, Lewis RP, Robinson JL. Superiority of 24-hour outpatient monitoring over multi-stage exercise testing for the evaluation of syncope. J Electrocardiol 1979; 12:103–108.

707. Abdon NJ, Johansson BW, Lessem J. Predictive use of routine 24-hour electrocardiography in suspected Adams-Stokes syndrome: comparison with cardiac rhythm during symptoms. Br Heart J 1982; 47:553–558.

708. Tzivoni D, Stern S. Pacemaker implantation based on ambulatory ECG monitoring in patients with cerebral symptoms. Chest 1975; 67:274–278.

709. Abdon NJ. Frequency and distribution of long-term ECG-recorded cardiac arrhythmias in an elderly population: with special reference to neurological symptoms. Acta Med Scand 1981; 209:175–183.

710. Levy AM, Camm AJ, Keane JF. Multiple arrhythmias detected during nocturnal monitoring in patients with congenital complete heart block. Circulation 1977; 55:247–253.

711. Dewey RC, Capeless MA, Levy AM. Use of ambulatory electrocardiographic monitoring to identify high-risk patients with congenital complete heart block. N Engl J Med 1987; 316:835–839.

712. Medina-Ravell V, Rodriguez-Salas L, Castellanos A, Myerburg RJ. Death due to paroxysmal atrioventricular block during ambulatory electrocardiographic monitoring. Pacing Clin Electrophysiol 1989; 12:65–69.

713. Sokol RJ, Hutchison P, Krouskop RW, Brown EG, Reed G, Vasquez H. Congenital complete heart block diagnosed during intrauterine fetal monitoring. Am J Obstet Gynecol 1974; 120:1115–1117.

714. Shenker L. Fetal cardiac arrhythmias. Obstet Gynecol Surv 1979; 34:561–572.

715. Madison JP, Sukhum P, Williamson DP, Campion BC. Echocardiography and fetal heart sounds in the diagnosis of fetal heart block. Am Heart J 1979; 98:505–509.

716. Kleinman CS, Hobbins JC, Jaffe CC, Lynch DC, Talner NS. Echocardiographic studies of the human fetus: prenatal diagnosis of congenital heart disease and cardiac dysrhythmias. Pediatrics 1980; 65:1059–1067.

717. Allan LD, Anderson RH, Sullivan ID, Campbell S, Holt DW, Tynan M. Evaluation of fetal arrhythmias by echocardiography. Br Heart J 1983; 50:240–245.

718. Kleinman CS, Donnerstein RL, Jaffe CC, et al. Fetal echocardiography: a tool for evaluation of in utero cardiac arrhythmias and monitoring of in utero therapy: analysis of 71 patients. Am J Cardiol 1983; 51:237–243.

719. Allan LD, Crawford DC, Anderson RH, Tynan M. Evaluation and treatment of fetal arrhythmias. Clin Cardiol 1984; 7:467–473.

720. Arbeille PH, Paillet CH, Chantepie B, Berger CH, Pourcelot L. In utero ultrasonic diagnosis of atrioventricular block. J Cardiovasc Ultrasonogr 1984; 3:313–316.

721. Crawford D, Chapman M, Allan L. The assessment of persistent bradycardia in prenatal life. Br J Obstet Gynaecol 1985; 92:941–944.

722. Steinfeld L, Rappaport HL, Rossbach HC, Martinez E. Diagnosis of fetal arrhythmias using echocardiographic and Doppler techniques. J Am Coll Cardiol 1986; 8:1425–1433.

723. Groves AM, Allan LD, Rosenthal E. Outcome of isolated congenital complete heart block diagnosed in utero. Heart 1996; 75:190–194.

724. Burggraf GW, Craige E. The first heart sound in complete heart block: phono-echocardiographic correlations. Circulation 1974; 50:17–24.

725. Benchimol A, Maia IG, Gartlan JL, Franklin D. Telemetry of arterial flow in man with a Doppler ultrasonic flowmeter. Am J Cardiol 1968; 22:75–84.

726. Gawkrodger DJ, Beveridge GW. Neonatal lupus erythematosus in four successive siblings born to a mother with discoid lupus erythematosus. Br J Dermatol 1984; 111:683–687.

727. Singsen BH, Akhter JE, Weinstein MM, Sharp GC. Congenital complete heart block and SSA antibodies: obstetric implications. Am J Obstet Gynecol 1985; 152:655–658.

728. Deng JS, Bair LW Jr, Shen-Schwarz S, Ramsey-Goldman R, Medsger T Jr. Localization of Ro (SS-A) antigen in the cardiac conduction system. Arthritis Rheum 1987; 30:1232–1238.

729. Taylor PV, Taylor KF, Norman A, Griffiths S, Scott JS. Prevalence of maternal Ro (SS-A) and La (SS-B) autoantibodies in relation to congenital heart block. Br J Rheumatol 1988; 27:128–132.

730. Alexander E, Buyon JP, Provost TT, Guarnieri T. Anti-Ro/SS-A antibodies in the pathophysiology of congenital heart block in neonatal lupus syndrome, an experimental model: in vitro electrophysiologic and immunocytochemical studies. Arthritis Rheum 1992; 35:176–189.

731. Li JM, Horsfall AC, Maini RN. Anti-La (SS-B) but not anti-Ro52 (SS-A) antibodies cross-react with laminin: a role in the pathogenesis of congenital heart block? Clin Exp Immunol 1995; 99:316–324.

732. Smeenk RJ. Immunological aspects of congenital atrioventricular block. Pacing Clin Electrophysiol 1997; 20:2093–2097.

733. Meilof JF, Frohn-Mulder IM, Stewart PA, et al. Maternal autoantibodies and congenital heart block: no evidence for

the existence of a unique heart block-associated anti-Ro/SS-A autoantibody profile. Lupus 1993; 2:239–246.

734. Keith JD, Rowe RD, Vlad P. Heart Disease in Infancy and Childhood. 3rd ed. New York: Macmillan, 1978, p. 291.

735. Manno BV, Hakki AH, Eshaghpour E, Iskandrian AS. Left ventricular function at rest and during exercise in congenital complete heart block: a radionuclide angiographic evaluation. Am J Cardiol 1983; 52:92–94.

736. Bassan R, Maia IG, Bozza A, Amino JG, Santos M. Atrioventricular block in acute inferior wall myocardial infarction: harbinger of associated obstruction of the left anterior descending coronary artery. J Am Coll Cardiol 1986; 8:773–778.

737. Lind J, Wegelius C, Lichtenstein H. The dynamics of the heart in complete A-V block. Circulation 1954; 10:195–200.

738. Samet P, Bernstein WH, Nathan DA, Lopez A. Atrial contribution to cardiac output in complete heart block. Am J Cardiol 1965; 16:1–10.

739. Scarpelli EM, Rudolph AM. The hemodynamics of congenital heart block. Prog Cardiovasc Dis 1964; 6:327–342.

740. Thilenius OG, Chiemmongkoltip P, Cassels DE, Arcilla RA. Hemodynamics studies in children with congenital atrioventricular block. Am J Cardiol 1972; 30:13–18.

741. Samet P, Jacobs W, Bernstein WH, Shane R. Hemodynamic sequelae of idioventricular pacemaking in complete heart block. Am J Cardiol 1963; 11:594–599.

742. Howarth S. Atrial waves on arterial pressure records in normal rhythm, heart block, and auricular flutter. Br Heart J 1954; 16:171–176.

743. Stack MF, Rader B, Sobol BJ, Farber SJ, Eichna LW. Cardiovascular hemodynamic functions in complete heart block and the effect of isopropylnorepinephrine. Circulation 1958; 17:526–536.

744. Gaal PG, Goldberg SJ, Linde LM. Cardiac output as a function of ventricular rate in a patient with complete heart block. Circulation 1964; 30:592–596.

745. McGregor M, Klassen GA. Observations on the effect of heart rate on cardiac output in patients with complete heart block at rest and during exercise. Circ Res 1964; 15(Suppl II):II-215–II-224.

746. Samet P, Bernstein WH, Meadow A, Nathan DA. Effect of alterations in ventricular rate on cardiac output in complete heart block. Am J Cardiol 1964; 14:477–482.

747. Segel N, Hudson WA, Harris P, Bishop JM. The circulatory effects of electrically induced changes in ventricular rate at rest and during exercise in complete heart block. J Clin Invest 1964; 43:1541–1550.

748. Benchimol A, Duenas A, Liggett MS, Dimond EG. Contribution of atrial systole to the cardiac function at a fixed and at a variable ventricular rate. Am J Cardiol 1965; 16:11–21.

749. Rowe GG, Stenlund RR, Thomsen JH, Terry W, Querimit AS. Coronary and systemic hemodynamic effects of cardiac pacing in man with complete heart block. Circulation 1969; 40:839–845.

750. Benchimol A, Ellis JG, Dimond EG, Wu T-L. Hemodynamic consequences of atrial and ventricular arrhythmias in man. Am Heart J 1965; 70:775–788.

751. Johansson BW, Karnell J, Malm A, Sievers J, Swedberg J. Electrocardiographic studies in patients with an artificial pacemaker. Br Heart J 1963; 25:514–524.

752. Sowton E. Haemodynamic studies in patients with artificial pacemakers. Br Heart J 1964; 26:737–746.

753. Benchimol A, Li YB, Dimond EG. Cardiovascular dynamics in complete heart block at various heart rates. Circulation 1964; 30:542–553.

754. Lassers BW, Julian DG. Artificial pacing in management of complete heart block complicating acute myocardial infarction. BMJ 1968; 2:142–146.

755. Sutton R, Citron P. Electrophysiological and haemodynamic basis for application of new pacemaker technology in sick sinus syndrome and atrioventricular block. Br Heart J 1979; 41:600–612.

756. Palmero HA. Complete heart block and the role of atrial activity. Am Heart J 1965; 70:449–454.

757. Leinbach RC, Chamberlain DA, Kastor JA, Harthorne JW, Sanders CA. A comparison of the hemodynamic effects of ventricular and sequential A-V pacing in patients with heart block. Am Heart J 1969; 78:502–508.

758. Fananapazir L, Bennett DH, Monks P. Atrial synchronized ventricular pacing: contribution of the chronotropic response to improved exercise performance. Pacing Clin Electrophysiol 1983; 6:601–608.

759. Faerestrand S, Ohm OJ. A time-related study of the hemodynamic benefit of atrioventricular synchronous pacing evaluated by Doppler echocardiography. Pacing Clin Electrophysiol 1985; 8:838–848.

760. Rediker DE, Eagle KA, Homma S, Gillam LD, Harthorne JW. Clinical and hemodynamic comparison of VVI versus DDD pacing in patients with DDD pacemakers. Am J Cardiol 1988; 61:323–329.

761. Occhetta E, Piccinino C, Francalacci G, et al. Lack of influence of atrioventricular delay on stroke volume at rest in patients with complete atrioventricular block and dual chamber pacing. Pacing Clin Electrophysiol 1990; 13:916–926.

762. Leonelli FM, Wang K, Youssef M, Hall R, Brown D. Systolic and diastolic effects of variable atrioventricular delay in patients with complete heart block and normal ventricular function. Am J Cardiol 1997; 80:294–298.

763. Chamberlain DA, Leinbach RC, Vassaux CE, Kastor JA, DeSanctis RW, Sanders CA. Sequential atrioventricular pacing in heart block complicating acute myocardial infarction. N Engl J Med 1970; 282:577–582.

764. Gillespie WJ, Greene DG, Karatzas NB, Lee GD. Effect of atrial systole on right ventricular stroke output in complete heart block. BMJ 1967; 1:75–79.

765. Rutishauser W, Wirz P, Gander M, Luthy E. Atriogenic diastolic reflux in patients with atrioventricular block. Circulation 1966; 34:807–817.

766. Forfang K, Otterstad JE, Ihlen H. Optimal atrioventricular delay in physiological pacing determined by Doppler echocardiography. Pacing Clin Electrophysiol 1986; 9:17–20.

767. Haskell RJ, French WJ. Optimum AV interval in dual chamber pacemakers. Pacing Clin Electrophysiol 1986; 9:670–675.

768. Janosik DL, Pearson AC, Buckingham TA, Labovitz AJ, Redd RM. The hemodynamic benefit of differential atrioventricular delay intervals for sensed and paced atrial events during physiologic pacing. J Am Coll Cardiol 1989; 14:499–507.

769. Mehta D, Gilmour S, Ward DE, Camm AJ. Optimal atrioventricular delay at rest and during exercise in patients with dual chamber pacemakers: a non-invasive assessment by continuous wave Doppler. Br Heart J 1989; 61:161–166.

770. Rossi P, Rognoni G, Occhetta E, et al. Respiration-dependent ventricular pacing compared with fixed ventricular and atrial-ventricular synchronous pacing: aerobic and hemodynamic variables. J Am Coll Cardiol 1985; 6:646–652.

771. Ausubel K, Steingart RM, Shimshi M, Klementowicz P, Furman S. Maintenance of exercise stroke volume during ventricular versus atrial synchronous pacing: role of contractility. Circulation 1985; 72:1037–1043.

772. Vogt P, Goy JJ, Kuhn M, Leuenberger P, Kappenberger L. Single versus double chamber rate responsive cardiac pacing: comparison by cardiopulmonary noninvasive exercise testing. Pacing Clin Electrophysiol 1988; 11:1896–1901.

773. Noll B, Krappe J, Goke B, Maisch B. Influence of pacing mode and rate on peripheral levels of atrial natriuretic peptide (ANP). Pacing Clin Electrophysiol 1989; 12:1763–1768.

774. Anonymous. Aetiology of complete heart-block. Lancet 1968; 1:731–732.

775. Lev M. The anatomic basis for disturbances in conduction and cardiac arrhythmias. Prog Cardiovasc Dis 1959; 2:360–369.

776. Lev M. Anatomic basis for atrioventricular block. Am J Med 1964; 37:742–748.

777. Lev M, Bharati S. Atrioventricular and intraventricular conduction disease. Arch Intern Med 1975; 135:405–410.

778. Sugiura M, Iizuka H, Okawa S, Okada R. Histological studies on the conduction system in 8 cases of AV conduction disturbances. Jpn Heart J 1970; 11:460–469.

779. Nakazato Y, Nakata Y, Tokano T, et al. Intra-His bundle block corresponds with interruption of the branching portion of the His bundle. PACE 1994; 17:1124–1133.

780. Bharati S, Lev M, Wu D, Denes P, Dhingra R, Rosen KM. Pathophysiologic correlations in two cases of split His bundle potentials. Circulation 1974; 49:615–623.

781. Marriott HJL, Myerburg RJ. Recognition of cardiac arrhythmias and conduction disturbances. In Hurst JW, Schlant RC (eds). The Heart Arteries and Veins. 7th ed. New York: McGraw-Hill, 1990, p. 522.

782. Titus JL. Cardiac arrhythmias. I. Anatomy of the conduction system. Circulation 1973; 47:170–177.

783. James TN. Anatomy of the coronary arteries in health and disease. Circulation 1965; 32:1020–1033.

784. James TN. The coronary circulation and conduction system in acute myocardial infarction. Prog Cardiovasc Dis 1968; 10:410–449.

785. Lev M, Kinare SG, Pick A. The pathogenesis of atrioventricular block in coronary disease. Circulation 1970; 42:409–425.

786. Van der Hauwaert LG, Stroobandt R, Verhaeghe L. Arterial blood supply of the atrioventricular node and main bundle. Br Heart J 1972; 34:1045–1051.

787. Frink RJ, James TN. Normal blood supply to the human His bundle and proximal bundle branches. Circulation 1973; 47:8–18.

788. Kennel AJ, Titus JL. The vasculature of the human atrioventricular conduction system. Mayo Clinic Proc 1972; 47:562–566.

789. Hunt D, Lie JT, Vohra J, Sloman G. Histopathology of heart block complicating acute myocardial infarction: correlation with the His bundle electrogram. Circulation 1973; 48:1252–1261.

790. Bilbao FJ, Zabalza IE, Vilanova JR, Froufe J. Atrioventricular block in posterior acute myocardial infarction: a clinicopathologic correlation. Circulation 1987; 75:733–736.

791. Sutton R, Davies M. The conduction system in acute myocardial infarction complicated by heart block. Circulation 1968; 38:987–992.

792. Hackel DB, Wagner G, Ratliff NB, Cies A, Estes EH. Anatomic studies of the cardiac conducting system in acute myocardial infarction. Am Heart J 1972; 83:77–81.

793. Becker AE, Lie KI, Anderson RH. Bundle-branch block in the setting of acute anteroseptal myocardial infarction: clinicopathological correlation. Br Heart J 1978; 40:773–782.

794. Meshel JC, Wachtel HL, Graham J. Bacterial endocarditis presenting as heart block. Am J Med 1970; 48:254–255.

795. Kleid JJ, Kim ES, Brand B, Eckles S, Gordon GM. Heart block complicating acute bacterial endocarditis. Chest 1972; 61:301–303.

796. Arnett EN, Roberts WC. Valve ring abscess in active infective endocarditis: frequency, location, and clues to clinical diagnosis from the study of 95 necropsy patients. Circulation 1976; 54:140–145.

797. Bharati S, Lev M. The pathologic changes in the conduction system beyond the age of ninety. Am Heart J 1992; 124:486–496.

798. Lev M. Conduction system in congenital heart disease. Am J Cardiol 1968; 21:619–627.

799. Lev M, Benjamin JE, White PD. A histopathologic study of the conduction system in a case of complete heart block of 42 years' duration. Am Heart J 1958; 55:198–214.

800. Smithells RW, Outon EB. Congenital heart block. Arch Dis Child 1959; 34:223–227.

801. Lev M, Silverman J, Fitzmaurice FM, Paul MH, Cassels DE, Miller RA. Lack of connection between the atria and the more peripheral conduction system in congenital atrioventricular block. Am J Cardiol 1971; 27:481–490.

802. James TN, St. Martin E, Willis PW III, Lohr TO. Apoptosis as a possible cause of gradual development of complete heart block and fatal arrhythmias associated with absence of the AV node, sinus node, and internodal pathways. Circulation 1996; 93:1424–1438.

803. Sotelo-Avila C, Rosenberg HS, McNamara DG. Congenital heart block due to a lesion in the conduction system. Pediatrics 1970; 45:640–650.

804. Miller RA, Mehta AB, Rodriguez-Coronel A, Lev M. Congenital atrioventricular block with multiple ectopic pacemakers: electrocardiographic and conduction system correlation. Am J Cardiol 1972; 30:554–558.

805. Ho SY, Fagg N, Anderson RH, Cook A, Allan L. Disposition of the atrioventricular conduction tissues in the heart with isomerism of the atrial appendages: its relation to congenital complete heart block. J Am Coll Cardiol 1992; 20:904–910.

806. Lev M, Cuadros H, Paul MH. Interruption of the atrioventricular bundle with congenital atrioventricular block. Circulation 1971; 43:703–710.

807. Lev M, Paul MH, Cassels DE. Complete atrioventricular block associated with atrial septal defect of the fossa ovalis (secundum) type: a histopathologic study of the conduction systems. Am J Cardiol 1967; 19:266–274.

808. Ludatscher R, Amikam S, Roguin N, Gellei B, Riss E. Electron microscopical study of myocardial biopsy material in congenital heart block. Br Heart J 1975; 37:561–569.

809. Litsey SE, Noonan JA, O'Connor WN, Cottrill CM, Mitchell B. Maternal connective tissue disease and congenital heart block: demonstration of immunoglobulin in cardiac tissue. N Engl J Med 1985; 312:98–100.

810. Lee LA, Coulter S, Erner S, Chu H. Cardiac immunoglobulin deposition in congenital heart block associated with maternal anti-Ro autoantibodies. Am J Med 1987; 83:793–796.

811. Ishibashi-Ueda H, Yutani C, Imakita M, Kanzaki T, Utsu M, Chiba Y. An autopsy case of congenital complete heart block in a newly born of a mother with systemic lupus erythematosus. Pediatr Cardiol 1988; 9:157–161.

812. Reed BR, Lee LA, Harmon C, et al. Autoantibodies to SS-A/Ro in infants with congenital heart block. J Pediatr 1983; 103:889–891.

813. Harley JB, Kaine JL, Fox OF, Reichlin M, Gruber B. Ro (SS-A) antibody and antigen in a patient with congenital complete heart block. Arthritis Rheum 1985; 28:1321–1325.

814. Reichlin M, Friday K, Harley JB. Complete congenital heart block followed by anti-Ro/SSA in adult life: studies of an informative family. Am J Med 1988; 84:339–344.

815. Kastor JA. Atrioventricular block. N Engl J Med 1975; 292:462–465.

816. Kastor JA. Atrioventricular block. N Engl J Med 1975; 292:572–574.

817. Josephson ME. Clinical Cardiac Electrophysiology. Techniques and Interpretations. 2nd ed. Philadelphia: Lea & Febiger, 1993, pp. 96–116.

818. Abella JB, Teixeira OHP, Misra KP, Hastreiter AR. Changes of atrioventricular conduction with age in infants and children. Am J Cardiol 1972; 30:876–883.

819. Roberts N, Olley P. His bundle electrogram in children: statistical correlation of the atrioventricular conduction times in children with their age and heart rate. Br Heart J 1972; 34:1099–1101.

820. Wolff GS, Freed MD, Ellison RC. Bundle of His recordings in congenital heart disease. Br Heart J 1973; 35:805–810.

821. Shiku DJ, Stijns M, Lintermans JP, Vliers A. Atrioventricular conduction and right atrial volume in children with and without secundum atrial septal defects. Br Heart J 1981; 46:69–73.

822. Rosen KM, Rahimtoola SH, Bharati S, Lev M. Bundle branch block with intact atrioventricular conduction: electrophysiologic and pathologic correlations in three cases. Am J Cardiol 1973; 32:783–793.

823. Bharati S, Lev M, Dhingra RC, Chuquimia R, Towne WD, Rosen KM. Electrophysiologic and pathologic correlations in two cases of chronic second degree atrioventricular block with left bundle branch block. Circulation 1975; 52:221–229.

824. Ohkawa S, Sugiura M, Itoh Y, et al. Electrophysiologic and histologic correlations in chronic complete atrioventricular block. Circulation 1981; 64:215–231.

825. Haft JI, Weinstock M, DeGuia R. Electrophysiologic studies in Mobitz type II second degree heart block. Am J Cardiol 1971; 27:682–686.

826. Damato AN, Varghese PJ, Caracta AR, Akhtar M, Lau SH. Functional 2:1 A-V block within the His-Purkinje system: simulation of type II second-degree A-V block. Circulation 1973; 47:534–542.
827. Batsford WP, Akhtar M, Caracta AR, Josephson ME, Seides SF, Damato AN. Effect of atrial stimulation site on the electrophysiological properties of the atrioventricular node in man. Circulation 1974; 50:283–292.
828. Amat-y-Leon F, Denes P, Wu D, Pietras RJ, Rosen M. Effects of atrial pacing site on atrial and atrioventricular nodal function. Br Heart J 1975; 37:576–582.
829. Mandel WJ, Lozano J, Carrasco H, Hayakawa H. Coexisting intra- and subnodal block: an unusual abnormality of atrioventricular conduction. Am Heart J 1971; 82:586–592.
830. Dhingra RC, Rosen KM, Rahimtoola SH. Wenckebach periods with repetitive block: evaluation with His bundle recording. Am Heart J 1973; 86:444–448.
831. Kosowsky BD, Latif P, Radoff AM. Multilevel atrioventricular block. Circulation 1976; 54:914–921.
832. Brusca A, Rosettani E, Mangiardi L, Bonamini R, Orzan F. Atypical 2nd degree AV block due to bilateral bundle branch block with Wenckebach phenomenon and concealed conduction in the bundle branch system. Eur J Cardiol 1977; 5:183–199.
833. Castellanos A, Garcia HG, Rozanski JJ, Zaman L, Pefkaros K, Myerburg RJ. Atropine-induced multilevel block in acute inferior myocardial infarction: a possible indication for prophylactic pacing. Pacing Clin Electrophysiol 1981; 4:528–537.
834. Roy D, Waxman HL, Buxton AE, Josephson ME. Horizontal and longitudinal dissociation of the A-V node during atrial tachycardia. Pacing Clin Electrophysiol 1983; 6:569–576.
835. Sherron P, Torres-Arraut E, Tamer D, Garcia OL, Wolff GS. Site of conduction delay and electrophysiologic significance of first-degree atrioventricular block in children with heart disease. Am J Cardiol 1985; 55:1323–1327.
836. Young ML, Gelband H, Wolff GS. Atrial pacing-induced alternating Wenckebach periodicity and multilevel conduction block in children. Am J Cardiol 1986; 57:135–141.
837. Castellanos A, Cox MM, Fernandez PR, et al. Mechanisms and dynamics of episodes of progression of 2:1 atrioventricular block in patients with documented two-level conduction disturbances. Am J Cardiol 1992; 70:193–199.
838. Narula OS, Scherlag BJ, Javier RP, Hildner FJ, Samet P. Analysis of the A-V conduction defect in complete heart block utilizing His bundle electrograms. Circulation 1970; 41:437–448.
839. Narula OS, Cohen LS, Samet P, Lister JW, Scherlag B, Hildner FJ. Localization of A-V conduction defects in man by recording of the His bundle electrogram. Am J Cardiol 1970; 25:228–237.
840. Rosen KM, Rahimtoola SH, Chuquimia R, Loeb HS, Gunnar RM. Electrophysiological significance of first degree atrioventricular block with intraventricular conduction disturbance. Circulation 1971; 43:491–502.
841. Ranganathan N, Dhurandhar R, Phillips JH, Wigle ED. His bundle electrogram in bundle-branch block. Circulation 1972; 45:282–294.
842. Schuilenburg RM, Durrer D. Conduction disturbances located within the His bundle. Circulation 1972; 45:612–628.
843. McAnulty JH, Murphy E, Rahimtoola SH. Prospective evaluation of intra-Hisian conduction delay. Circulation 1979; 59:1035–1039.
844. Lie KI, Wellens HJJ, Schuilenburg RM, Becker AE, Durrer D. Factors influencing prognosis of bundle branch block complicating acute antero-septal infarction: the value of His bundle recordings. Circulation 1974; 50:935–941.
845. Castillo C, Maytin O, Castellanos A Jr. His bundle recordings in atypical A-V nodal Wenckebach block during cardiac pacing. Am J Cardiol 1971; 27:570–576.
846. Lightfoot PR, Sasse L, Mandel WJ, Hayakawa H. His bundle electrograms in healthy adolescents with persistent second degree A-V block. Chest 1973; 63:358–362.
847. el-Sherif N, Scherlag BJ, Lazzara R. Pathophysiology of second-degree atrioventricular block: a unified hypothesis. Am J Cardiol 1975; 35:421–434.
848. Littmann L, Svenson RH. Concealed reentry: a mechanism of atrioventricular nodal alternating Wenckebach periodicity. Circulation 1981; 65:1269–1275.
849. Littmann L, Svenson RH. Atrioventricular alternating Wenckebach periodicity: conduction patterns in multilevel block. Am J Cardiol 1982; 49:855–862.
850. Kastor JA, Goldreyer BN, Moore EN, Spear JF. Re-entry: an important mechanism of cardiac arrhythmias. Cardiovasc Clin 1974; 6:111–135.
851. Schuilenburg RM, Durrer D. Problems in the recognition of conduction disturbances in the His bundle. Circulation 1975; 51:68–74.
852. Dhingra RC, Denes P, Wu D, Chuquimia R, Rosen KM. The significance of second degree atrioventricular block and bundle branch block: observations regarding site and type of block. Circulation 1974; 49:638–646.
853. Castellanos A, Sung RJ, Mallon SM, Bloom MG, Myerburg RJ. Effects of proximal intra-atrial Wenckebach on distal atrioventricular nodal, and His-Purkinje, block with special reference to the theory of alternating Wenckebach periods. Am Heart J 1978; 95:228–234.
854. Pinski SL, Tchou PJ, Trohman RG. Paradoxical shortening of the second PR interval during 3:2 atrioventricular nodal block. J Cardiovasc Electrophysiol 1996; 7:1091–1094.
855. Schuilenburg RM, Durrer D. Observations on atrioventricular conduction in patients with bilateral bundle-branch. Circulation 1970; 41:967–979.
856. Gupta PK, Lichstein E, Chadda K. Electrophysiological features of complete AV block within the His bundle. Br Heart J 1973; 35:610–615.
857. Gupta PK, Lichstein E, Chadda KD. Chronic His bundle block: clinical, electrocardiographic, electrophysiological, and follow-up studies on 16 patients. Br Heart J 1976; 38:1343–1349.
858. Rizzon P, DiBiase M. Intra-His bundle block in acute myocardial infarction: report of two cases. J Electrocardiol 1977; 10:197–200.
859. Peters RW, Scheinman MM, Sauve MJ, Williams K, Desai J, Abbott J. Bundle branch block: anatomic, electrophysiologic and clinical correlates. In Rapoport E (ed). Cardiology Update. Review for Physicians. New York: Elsevier Biomedical, 1983, pp. 219–240.
860. Jordaens L. Are there any useful investigations that predict which patients with bifascicular block will develop third degree atrioventricular block? Heart 1996; 75:542–543.
861. Kastor JA. Cardiac electrophysiology: hemiblocks and stopped hearts. N Engl J Med 1978; 299:249–251.
862. Anonymous. Partial heart-block: can His-bundle electrography predict progression? Lancet 1978; 2:820–821.
863. Bauernfeind RA, Welch WJ, Brownstein SL. Distal atrioventricular conduction system function. Cardiol Clin 1986; 4:417–428.
864. Dhingra RC, Palileo E, Strasberg B, et al. Significance of the HV interval in 517 patients with chronic bifascicular block. Circulation 1981; 64:1265–1271.
865. Dhingra RC, Denes P, Wu D, et al. Prospective observations in patients with chronic bundle branch block and marked H-V prolongation. Circulation 1976; 53:600–604.
866. Scheinman MM, Peters RW, Modin G, Brennan M, Mies C, O'Young J. Prognostic value of infranodal conduction time in patients with chronic bundle branch block. Circulation 1977; 56:240–244.
867. Scheinman MM, Peters RW, Suave MJ, et al. Value of the H-Q interval in patients with bundle branch block and the role of prophylactic permanent pacing. Am J Cardiol 1982; 50:1316–1322.
868. Dhingra RC, Amat-y-Leon F, Wyndham C, Sridhar SS, Wu D, Rosen KM. Significance of left axis deviation in patients with chronic left bundle branch block. Am J Cardiol 1978; 42:551–556.
869. Morady F, Higgins J, Peters RW, et al. Electrophysiologic testing in bundle branch block and unexplained syncope. Am J Cardiol 1984; 54:587–591.

870. Dhingra RC, Wyndham C, Deedwania PC, et al. Effect of age on atrioventricular conduction in patients with chronic bifascicular block. Am J Cardiol 1980; 45:749–756.

871. Petrac D, Radic B, Birtic K, Gjurovic J. Prospective evaluation of infrahisal second-degree AV block induced by atrial pacing in the presence of chronic bundle branch block and syncope. Pacing Clin Electrophysiol 1996; 19:784–792.

872. Dhingra RC, Wyndham C, Bauernfeind R, et al. Significance of block distal to the His bundle induced by atrial pacing in patients with chronic bifascicular block. Circulation 1979; 60:1455–1464.

873. Cortadellas J, Cinca J, Moya A, Rius J. Clinical and electrophysiologic findings in acute ischemic intra-Hisian bundle-branch block. Am Heart J 1990; 119:23–29.

874. de Soyza NDB, Bissett JK, Kane JJ, Murphy ML. Latent defects of atrioventricular conduction in right coronary artery disease. Am Heart J 1974; 87:164–169.

875. Probst P, Pachinger O, Murad AA, Leisch F, Kaindl F. The HQ time in congestive cardiomyopathies. Am Heart J 1979; 97:436–441.

876. Kelly DT, Brodsky SJ, Mirowski M, Krovetz LJ, Rowe RD. Bundle of His recordings in congenital complete heart block. Circulation 1972; 45:277–281.

877. Rosen KM, Mehta A, Rahimtoola SH, Miller RA. Sites of congenital and surgical heart block as defined by His bundle electrocardiography. Circulation 1971; 44:833–841.

878. Karpawich PP, Antillon JR, Cappola PR, Agarwal KC. Pre- and postoperative electrophysiologic assessment of children with secundum atrial septal defect. Am J Cardiol 1985; 55:519–521.

879. Nasrallah AT, Gillette PC, Mullins CE. Congenital and surgical atrioventricular block within the His bundle. Am J Cardiol 1975; 36:914–920.

880. Levin AR, Haft JI, Engle MA, Ehlers KH, Klein AA. Intracardiac conduction intervals in children with congenital heart disease: comparison of His bundle studies in 41 normal children and 307 patients with congenital cardiac defects. Circulation 1977; 55:286–294.

881. Clark EB, Kugler JD. Preoperative secundum atrial septal defect with coexisting sinus node and atrioventricular node dysfunction. Circulation 1982; 65:976–980.

882. Bolens M, Friedli B. Sinus node function and conduction system before and after surgery for secundum atrial septal defect: an electrophysiologic study. Am J Cardiol 1984; 53:1415–1420.

883. Ruschhaupt DG, Khoury DG, Thilenius OG, Replogle RL, Arcilla RA. Electrophysiologic abnormalities of children with ostium secundum atrial septal defect. Am J Cardiol 1984; 53:1643–1647.

884. Goodman DJ, Harrison DC, Cannom DS. Atrioventricular conduction in patients with incomplete endocardial cushion defect. Circulation 1974; 49:631–637.

885. Schmidinger H, Probst P, Schneider B, Weber H, Kaliman J. Subsidiary pacemaker function in complete heart block after His-bundle ablation. Circulation 1988; 78:893–898.

886. Ezri M, Lerman BB, Marchlinski FE, Buxton AE, Josephson ME. Electrophysiologic evaluation of syncope in patients with bifascicular block. Am Heart J 1983; 106:693–697.

887. Bass EB, Elson JJ, Fogoros RN, Peterson J, Arena VC, Kapoor WN. Long-term prognosis of patients undergoing electrophysiologic studies for syncope of unknown origin. Am J Cardiol 1988; 62:1186–1191.

888. Gulamhusein S, Naccarelli GV, Ko PT, et al. Value and limitations of clinical electrophysiologic study in assessment of patients with unexplained syncope. Am J Med 1982; 73:700–705.

889. Coste P, Clementy J, Besse P, Bricaud H. Left ventricular hypertrophy and ventricular dysrhythmic risk in hypertensive patients: evaluation by programmed electrical stimulation. J Hypertens Suppl 1988; 6:S116–S118.

890. Jacob AI, Lichstein E, Ulano SD, Chadda KD, Gupta PK, Werner BM. A-V block in accidental hypothermia. J Electrocardiol 1978; 11:399–402.

891. Scherf D, Cohen J. The Atrioventricular Node and Selected Cardiac Arrhythmias. New York: Grune & Stratton, 1964, pp. 208–225.

892. Levy S, Corbelli JL, Labrunie P, et al. Retrograde (ventriculoatrial) conduction. Pacing Clin Electrophysiol 1983; 6:364–371.

893. Danzig R, Alpern H, Swan HJC. The significance of atrial rate in patients with atrioventricular conduction abnormalities complicating acute myocardial infarction. Am J Cardiol 1969; 24:707–712.

894. Jonas EA, Kosowsky BD, Ramaswamy K. Complete His-Purkinje block produced by carotid sinus massage: report of a case. Circulation 1974; 50:192–197.

895. el-Sherif N, Scherlag BJ, Lazzara R, Hope R, Williams DO, Samet P. The pathophysiology of tachycardia-dependent paroxysmal atrioventricular block after acute myocardial ischemia: experimental and clinical observations. Circulation 1974; 50:515–528.

896. Englund A. The RR index test for the differentiation of atrioventricular nodal block from His-Purkinje block during incremental atrial pacing in patients with bifascicular block. Eur Heart J 1997; 18:311–317.

897. Wu D, Deedwania P, Dhingra RC, Engleman RM, Rosen KM. Electrophysiologic observations in a patient with bradycardia-dependent atrioventricular block. Am J Cardiol 1978; 42:506–512.

898. Rosenbaum MB, Elizari MV, Levi RJ, Nau GJ. Paroxysmal atrioventricular block related to hypopolarization and spontaneous diastolic depolarization. Chest 1973; 63:678–688.

899. Castellanos A, Sung RJ, Cunha D, Myerburg RJ. His bundle recordings in paroxysmal atrioventricular block produced by carotid sinus massage. Br Heart J 1974; 36:487–491.

900. Mangiardi LM, Bonamini R, Conte M, et al. Bedside evaluation of atrioventricular block with narrow QRS complexes: usefulness of carotid sinus massage and atropine administration. Am J Cardiol 1982; 49:1136–1145.

901. Zaman L, Moleiro F, Rozanski JJ, Pozen R, Myerburg RJ, Castellanos A. Multiple electrophysiologic manifestations and clinical implications of vagally mediated AV block. Am Heart J 1983; 106:92–99.

902. Denes P, Murabit I, Ezri M, Eybel C. Tachycardia- and bradycardia-dependent atrioventricular block: observations regarding the mechanism of block. J Am Coll Cardiol 1987; 9:446–449.

903. Englund A, Bergfeldt L, Rosenqvist M. Disopyramide stress test: a sensitive and specific tool for predicting impending high degree atrioventricular block in patients with bifascicular block. Br Heart J 1995; 74:650–655.

904. Bergfeldt L, Rosenqvist M, Vallin H, Edhag O. Disopyramide induced second and third degree atrioventricular block in patients with bifascicular block: an acute stress test to predict atrioventricular block progression. Br Heart J 1985; 53:328–334.

905. Aravindakshan V, Surawicz B, Daoud FS. Depression of escape pacemakers associated with rapid supraventricular rate in patients with atrioventricular block. Circulation 1974; 50:255–259.

906. Wald RW, Waxman MB. Depression of distal AV conduction following ventricular pacing. Pacing Clin Electrophysiol 1981; 4:84–91.

907. Rosenheck S, Bondy C, Weiss AT, Gotsman MS. Comparison between patients with and without reliable ventricular escape rhythm in the presence of long standing complete atrioventricular block. PACE 1993; 16:272–276.

908. Skanes AC, Tang ASL. Ventriculophasic modulation of atrioventricular nodal conduction in humans. Circulation 1998; 97:2245–2251.

909. Langendorf R. Concealed A-V conduction: the effect of blocked impulses on the formation and conduction of subsequent impulses. Am Heart J 1948; 35:542–552.

910. Langendorf R, Pick A. Causes and mechanisms of ventricular asystole in advanced A-V block. In Surawicz B, Pellegrino ED (eds). Sudden Cardiac Death. New York: Grune & Stratton, 1964, pp. 97–108.

911. Langendorf R, Pick A, Edelist A, Katz LN. Experimental

demonstration of concealed AV conduction in the human heart. Circulation 1965; 32:386–393.

912. Pick A, Fishman AP. Observations in heart block: supernormality of A-V and intraventricular conduction and ventricular parasystole under the influence of epinephrine. Acta Cardiol 1950; 5:270–287.

913. Mack I, Langendorf R, Katz LN. The supernormal phase of recovery of conduction in the human heart. Am Heart J 1947; 34:374–389.

914. Pick A, Langendorf R, Katz LN. The supernormal phase of atrioventricular conduction. I. Fundamental mechanisms. Circulation 1962; 26:388–404.

915. Dolara A, Cammilli L. Supernormal excitation and conduction; electrocardiographic observations during subthreshold stimulation in two patients with implanted pacemaker. Am J Cardiol 1968; 21:746–752.

916. Hernandez-Pieretti O, Morales-Rocha J, Barcelo JE. Supernormal phase of conduction in human heart demonstrated by subthreshold pacemakers. Br Heart J 1969; 31:553–558.

917. Damato AN, Lau SH. Concealed and supernormal atrioventricular conduction. Circulation 1971; 43:967–970.

918. Gallagher JJ, Damato AN, Varghese PJ, Caracta AR, Josephson ME, Lau SH. Alternative mechanisms of apparent supernormal atrioventricular conduction. Am J Cardiol 1973; 31:362–371.

919. Ward DE, Camm AJ. Clinical Electrophysiology of the Heart. Baltimore: Edward Arnold, 1987, pp. 52–53.

920. Mecca A, Telfer A, Lanzarotti C, Olshansky B. Symptomatic atrioventricular block in an atriofascicular pathway inserting into the left bundle branch without apparent atrioventricular node function. J Cardiovasc Electrophysiol 1997; 8:922–926.

921. Jick H, Linenthal AJ. Reversible Wenckebach type atrioventricular block associated with severe coronary artery disease. Circulation 1959; 20:262–266.

922. Carlsten A, Heyman F. Effect of brief carotid-sinus pressure on atrial and ventricular rhythms in complete heart block. Acta Med Scand 1965; 177:281–286.

923. Scherf D, Bornemann C. Thumping of the precordium in ventricular standstill. Am J Cardiol 1960; 5:30–40.

924. Michael TAD, Stanford RL. Precordial percussion in cardiac asystole. Lancet 1963; 1:699.

925. Wesley RC Jr, Lerman BB, DiMarco JP, Berne RM, Belardinelli L. Mechanism of atropine-resistant atrioventricular block during inferior myocardial infarction: possible role of adenosine. J Am Coll Cardiol 1986; 8:1232–1234.

926. Shah PK, Nalos P, Peter T. Atropine resistant post infarction complete AV block: possible role of adenosine and improvement with aminophylline. Am Heart J 1987; 113:194–195.

927. Strasberg B, Bassevich R, Mager A, Kusniec J, Sagie A, Sclarovsky S. Effects of aminophylline on atrioventricular conduction in patients with late atrioventricular block during inferior wall acute myocardial infarction. Am J Cardiol 1991; 67:527–528.

928. Goodfellow J, Walker PR. Reversal of atropine-resistant atrioventricular block with intravenous aminophylline in the early phase of inferior wall acute myocardial infarction following treatment with streptokinase. Eur Heart J 1995; 16:862–865.

929. Lawrence JS, Forbes GW. Paroxysmal heart block and ventricular standstill. Br Heart J 1944; 6:53–60.

930. Schweitzer P, Mark H. The effect of atropine on cardiac arrhythmias and conduction. Am Heart J 1980; 100:255–261.

931. Damato AN, Lau SH, Helfant RH, Stein E, Berkowitz WD, Cohen SI. Study of atrioventricular conduction in man using electrode catheter recordings of His bundle activity. Circulation 1969; 39:287–296.

932. Strasberg B, Lam W, Swiryn S, et al. Symptomatic spontaneous paroxysmal AV nodal block due to localized hyperresponsiveness of the AV node to vagotonic reflexes. Am Heart J 1982; 103:795–801.

933. Webb SW, Adgey AA, Pantridge JF. Autonomic disturbance at onset of acute myocardial infarction. BMJ 1972; 3:89–92.

934. Christiansen I, Haghfelt T, Amtorp O. Complete heart block in acute myocardial infarction: drug therapy. Am Heart J 1973; 85:162–166.

935. Chadda KD, Lichstein E, Gupta PK, Choy R. Bradycardia-hypotension syndrome in acute myocardial infarction: reappraisal of the overdrive effects of atropine. Am J Med 1975; 59:158–164.

936. Scheinman MM, Thorburn D, Abbott JA. Use of atropine in patients with acute myocardial infarction and sinus bradycardia. Circulation 1975; 52:627–633.

937. Markel ML, Miles WM, Zipes DP, Prystowsky EN. Parasympathetic and sympathetic alterations of Mobitz type II heart block. J Am Coll Cardiol 1988; 11:271–275.

938. Finucane JF, Gialafos J. Role of autonomic nervous system in chronic complete heart block. Br Heart J 1974; 36:1028–1030.

939. Schumacher EE, Schmock CL. The control of certain cardiac arrhythmias with isopropylnorepinephrine. Am Heart J 1954; 48:933–940.

940. Robbin SR, Goldfein S, Schwartz MJ, Dack S. Adams-Stokes syndrome. Am J Med 1955; 18:577–590.

941. Chandler D, Clapper MI. Complete atrioventricular block treated with isoproterenol hydrochloride. Am J Cardiol 1959; 3:336–342.

942. Schwartz SP, Schwartz LS. The Adams-Stokes syndrome during normal sinus rhythm and transient heart block. I. The effects of Isuprel on patients with the Adams-Stokes syndrome during normal sinus rhythm and transient heart block. Am Heart J 1959; 57:849–861.

943. Kalusche D, Roskamm H. Tachycardia-dependent second degree AV-block in a patient with right bundle branch block. J Electrocardiol 1987; 20:169–175.

944. Stamler JS, Rodgers C, Hirano I, Brezinski D, Sharma GV. Treatment of complete heart block with inhaled beta-agonists. Am Heart J 1992; 124:1093–1095.

945. Dack S, Robbin SR. Treatment of heart block and Adams-Stokes syndrome with sustained-action isoproterenol. JAMA 1961; 176:505–512.

946. Fleming HA, Mirams JA. A clinical trial of a sustained-action preparation of isoprenaline in the treatment of heart-block. Lancet 1963; 2:214–217.

947. Bluestone R, Harris A. Treatment of heart-block with long-acting isoprenaline. Lancet 1965; 1:1299–1301.

948. Nissen NI, Thomsen AC. Oral treatment of A-V block and other bradycardias with sustained action isoprenaline. Br Heart J 1965; 27:926–931.

949. Redwood D. Conservative treatment of chronic heart block. BMJ 1969; 1:26–29.

950. Dhingra RC, Winslow E, Pouget JM, Rahimtoola SH, Rosen KM. The effect of isoproterenol on atrioventricular and intraventricular conduction. Am J Cardiol 1973; 32:629–636.

951. Groves AM, Allan LD, Rosenthal E. Therapeutic trial of sympathomimetics in three cases of complete heart block in the fetus. Circulation 1995; 92:3394–3396.

952. Schmidt KG, Ulmer HE, Silverman NH, Kleinman CS, Copel JA. Perinatal outcome of fetal complete atrioventricular block: a multicenter experience. J Am Coll Cardiol 1991; 17:1360–1366.

953. Tobian L. Prevention of Stokes-Adams seizures with chlorothiazide. N Engl J Med 1961; 265:623–628.

954. Singh RG, Kassir M, Roistacher N, Lerman BB, Kligfield P. Acceleration of atrioventricular conduction during corticosteroid therapy. Am Heart J 1993; 125:1432–1434.

955. Phelps MD, Lindsay JD. Cortisone in Stokes-Adams disease secondary to myocardial infarction. N Engl J Med 1957; 256:204–208.

956. Dall JLC. The effect of steroid therapy on normal and abnormal atrioventricular conduction. Br Heart J 1964; 26:537–543.

957. Aber CP, Jones EW. Corticotrophin and corticosteroids in the management of acute and chronic heart block. Br Heart J 1965; 27:916–925.

958. Litchfield JW, Manley KA, Polak A. Stokes-Adams attacks treated with corticotrophin. Lancet 1958; 1:935–938.

959. Caramelli Z, Tellini RR. Treatment of atrioventricular block with prednisone. Am J Cardiol 1960; 5:263–265.

960. Friedberg CK, Kahn M, Scheuer J, Bleifer S, Dack S. Adams-Stokes syndrome associated with chronic heart block. JAMA 1960; 172:1146–1152.

961. Perry EL, Jaeck JL. Use of corticosteroids in Stokes-Adams syndrome. Ann Intern Med 1960; 53:589–599.

962. Pay BW, Waverley. Adrenocortical steroids in intermittent heart-block. BMJ 1961; 2:139–142.

963. Verel D, Mazurkie SJ, Rahman F. Prednisone in the treatment of Adams-Stokes attacks. Br Heart J 1963; 25:709–712.

964. Buyon JP, Swersky SH, Fox HE, Bierman FZ, Winchester RJ. Intrauterine therapy for presumptive fetal myocarditis with acquired heart block due to systemic lupus erythematosus: experience in a mother with a predominance of SS-B (La) antibodies. Arthritis Rheum 1987; 30:44–49.

965. Schwartz SP, Schwartz LS. The Adams-Stokes syndrome during normal sinus rhythm and transient heart block. Arch Intern Med 1960; 106:138–149.

966. Antman EM, Wenger TL, Butler VP, Haber E, Smith TW. Treatment of 150 cases of life-threatening digitalis intoxication with digoxin-specific Fab antibody fragments. Circulation 1990; 81:1744–1752.

967. Woolf AD, Wenger T, Smith TW, Lovejoy FH Jr. The use of digoxin-specific Fab fragments for severe digitalis intoxication in children. N Engl J Med 1992; 326:1739–1744.

968. Mittra B. Potassium, glucose, and insulin in treatment of heart block after myocardial infarction. Lancet 1966; 2:1438–1441.

969. Bellet S, Wasserman F, Brody JI. Molar sodium lactate: its effect in complete atrioventricular heart block and cardiac arrest occurring during Stokes-Adams seizures and in the terminal state. N Engl J Med 1955; 253:891–900.

970. Schwartz JB, Nielsen AP, Griffin JC. Concentration-dependent enhancement of junctional pacemaker activity by verapamil in man. Circulation 1985; 71:450–457.

971. Kusumoto FM, Goldschlager N. Cardiac pacing. N Engl J Med 1996; 334:89–98.

972. Menozzi C, Brignole M, Moracchini PV, et al. Intrapatient comparison between chronic WIRr and DDD pacing in patients affected by high degree AV block without heart failure. Pacing Clin Electrophysiol 1990; 13:1816–1822.

973. Sutton R, Bourgeois I. Cost benefit analysis of single and dual chamber pacing for sick sinus syndrome and atrioventricular block: an economic sensitivity analysis of the literature. Eur Heart J 1996; 17:574–582.

974. Escher DJ. Personal communication.

975. Gregoratos G, Cheitlin MD, Conill A, et al. ACC/AHA guidelines for implantation of cardiac pacemakers and antiarrhythmia devices (Committee on Pacemaker Implantation). Circulation 1998; 97:1325–1335.

976. White PD, Donovan H. Hearts. Their Long Follow-up. Philadelphia: W B Saunders, 1967, pp. 274–278.

977. Vera Z, Mason DT, Fletcher RD, Awan NA, Massumi RA. Prolonged His-Q interval in chronic bifascicular block: relation to impending complete heart block. Circulation 1976; 53:47–55.

978. Mymin D, Mathewson FA, Tate RB, Manfreda J. The natural history of primary first-degree atrioventricular heart block. N Engl J Med 1986; 315:1183–1187.

979. Strasberg B, Amat-y-Leon F, Dhingra RC, et al. Natural history of chronic second-degree atrioventricular nodal block. Circulation 1981; 63:1043–1049.

980. Shaw DB, Kekwick CA, Veale D, Gowers J, Whistance T. Survival in second degree atrioventricular block. Br Heart J 1985; 53:587–593.

981. Lerman BB, Marchlinski FE, Kempf FC, Buxton AE, Waxman HL, Josephson ME. Prognosis in patients with intra-Hisian conduction disturbances. Int J Cardiol 1984; 5:449–460.

982. Touboul P, Tessier Y, Magrina J, Clement C, Delahaye JP. His bundle recording and electrical stimulation of atria in patients with Wolff-Parkinson-White syndrome type A. Br Heart J 1972; 34:623–630.

983. Denes P, Dhingra RC, Wu D, Wyndham CR, Amat-y-Leon F, Rosen KM. Sudden death in patients with chronic bifascicular block. Arch Intern Med 1977; 137:1005–1010.

984. McAnulty JH, Rahimtoola SH, Murphy ES, et al. A prospective study of sudden death in "high-risk" bundle-branch block. N Engl J Med 1978; 299:209–215.

985. Peters RW, Scheinman MM, Dhingra R, et al. Serial electrophysiologic studies in patients with chronic bundle branch block. Circulation 1982; 65:1480–1485.

986. Berg GR, Kotler MN. The significance of bilateral bundle branch block in the preoperative patient. Chest 1977; 59:62–67.

987. Altschuler H, Fisher JD, Furman S. Significance of isolated H-V interval prolongation in symptomatic patients without documented heart block. Am Heart J 1979; 97:19–26.

988. Bruce RA, Blackmon JR, Cobb LA, Dodge HT. Treatment of asystole or heart block during acute myocardial infarction with electrode catheter pacing. Am Heart J 1965; 69:460–469.

989. Paulk EA Jr, Hurst JW. Complete heart block in acute myocardial infarction: a clinical evaluation of the intracardiac bipolar catheter pacemaker. Am J Cardiol 1966; 17:695–706.

990. Epstein EJ, Coulshed N, McKendrick CS, Clarke J, Kearns WE. Artificial pacing by electrode catheter for heart block or asystole complicating acute myocardial infarction. Br Heart J 1966; 28:546–556.

991. Scott ME, Geddes JS, Patterson GC, Adgey AA, Pantridge JF. Management of complete heart block complicating acute myocardial infarction. Lancet 1967; 2:1382–1385.

992. Friedberg CK, Cohen H, Donoso E. Advanced heart block as a complication of acute myocardial infarction: role of pacemaker therapy. Prog Cardiovasc Dis 1968; 10:466–481.

993. Gregory JJ, Grance WJ. The management of sinus bradycardia, nodal rhythm and heart block for the prevention of cardiac arrest in acute myocardial infarction. Prog Cardiovasc Dis 1968; 10:505–517.

994. Lassers BW, Anderton JL, George M, Muir AL, Julian DG. Hemodynamic effects of artificial pacing in complete heart block complicating acute myocardial infarction. Circulation 1968; 38:308–323.

995. Beregovich J, Fenig S, Lasser J, Allen D. Management of acute myocardial infarction complicated by advanced atrioventricular block: role of artificial pacing. Am J Cardiol 1969; 23:54–65.

996. Julian DG, Lassers BW, Godman MJ. Pacing for heart block in acute myocardial infarction. Ann N Y Acad Sci 1969; 167:911–918.

997. Schluger J, Iraj I, Edson JN. Cardiac pacing in acute myocardial infarction complicated by complete heart block. Am Heart J 1970; 80:116–124.

998. Hatle L, Rokseth R. Conservative treatment of AV block in acute myocardial infarction: results in 105 consecutive patients. Br Heart J 1971; 33:595–600.

999. Watson CC, Goldberg MJ. Evaluation of pacing for heart block in myocardial infarction. Br Heart J 1971; 33:120–124.

1000. Gould L, Venkataraman K, Mohammad N, Gomprecht RF. Prognosis of right bundle-branch block in acute myocardial infarction. JAMA 1972; 219:502–503.

1001. Norris RM, Mercer CJ, Croxson MS. Conduction disturbances due to anteroseptal myocardial infarction and their treatment by endocardial pacing. Am Heart J 1972; 84:560–566.

1002. Resnekov L, Lipp H. Pacemaking and acute myocardial infarction. Prog Cardiovasc Dis 1972; 14:475–499.

1003. Lichstein E, Gupta PK, Chadda KD, Liu HM, Sayeek M. Findings of prognostic value in patients with incomplete bilateral bundle branch block complicating acute myocardial infarction. Am J Cardiol 1973; 32:913–917.

1004. Waugh RA, Wagner GS, Haney TL, Rosati RA, Morris JJ. Immediate and remote prognostic significance of fascicular block during acute myocardial infarction. Circulation 1973; 47:765–775.

1005. Kitchen JB III, Kastor JA. Pacing in acute myocardial infarction: indications, methods, hazards, and results. Cardiovasc Clin 1975; 7:219–243.

1006. Nimetz AA, Shubrooks SJ Jr, Hutter AM Jr, DeSanctis RW. The significance of bundle branch block during acute myocardial infarction. Am Heart J 1975; 90:439–444.

1007. Sugiura T, Iwasaka T, Takahashi N, et al. Factors associated with late onset of advanced atrioventricular block in acute Q wave inferior infarction. Am Heart J 1990; 119:1008–1013.

1008. Fenig S, Lichstein E. Incomplete bilateral bundle branch block and A-V block complicating acute anterior wall myocardial infarction. Am Heart J 1972; 85:38–44.

1009. Hindman MC, Wagner GS, JaRo M, et al. The clinical significance of bundle branch block complicating acute myocardial infarction. II. Indications for temporary and permanent pacemaker insertion. Circulation 1978; 58:689–699.

1010. Hollander G, Nadiminti V, Lichstein E, Greengart A, Sanders M. Bundle branch block in acute myocardial infarction. Am Heart J 1983; 105:738–743.

1011. Matangi MF. Temporary physiologic pacing in inferior wall acute myocardial infarction with right ventricular damage. Am J Cardiol 1987; 59:1207–1208.

1012. Barold SS. American College of Cardiology/American Heart Association Guidelines for pacemaker implantation after acute myocardial infarction: what is persistent advanced block at the atrioventricular node? Am J Cardiol 1997; 80:770–774.

1013. Ross DL. Approach to the patient with bundle branch block. In Wellens HJJ, Kulbertus HE (eds). What's New in Electrocardiography. Boston: Martinus Nijhoff, 1981, pp. 111–130.

1014. Edhag O, Bergfeldt L, Edvardsson N, Holmberg S, Rosenqvist M, Vallin H. Pacemaker dependence in patients with bifascicular block during acute anterior myocardial infarction. Br Heart J 1984; 52:408–412.

1015. Ginks WR, Sutton R, Oh W, Leatham A. Long-term prognosis after acute anterior infarction with atrioventricular block. Br Heart J 1977; 39:186–189.

1016. Watson RDS, Glover DR, Page AJF, et al. The Birmingham trial of permanent pacing in patients with intraventricular conduction disorders after acute myocardial infarction. Am Heart J 1984; 108:496–501.

1017. Pagnoni F, Finzi A, Valentini R, Ambrosini F, Lotto A. Long-term prognostic significance and electrophysiological evolution of intraventricular conduction disturbances complicating acute myocardial infarction. Pacing Clin Electrophysiol 1986; 9:91–100.

1018. Olshansky B, Kleinman B, Wilber DJ. Management of arrhythmias and conduction disturbances in the perioperative setting. In Naccarelli GV (ed). Cardiac Arrhythmias. A Practical Approach. Mount Kisco, NY: Futura Publishing Co., 1991, pp. 325–358.

1019. Scott WA. Temporary DDD pacing after surgically induced heart block. Am J Cardiol 1993; 71:1123–1124.

1020. Friedman RA. Congenital AV block: pace me now or pace me later? Circulation 1995; 92:283–285.

1021. Liu L, Griffiths SP, Gerst PH. Implanted cardiac pacemakers in children: a report of their application in five patients. Am J Cardiol 1967; 20:639–647.

1022. Trusler GA, Mustard WT, Keith JD. The role of pacemaker therapy in congenital complete heart block: report of three cases. J Thorac Cardiovasc Surg 1968; 55:105–111.

1023. Veracochea O, Zerpa F, Morales J, Hernandez O, Waich S. Pacemaker implantation in familial congenital A-V block complicated by Adams-Stokes attacks. Br Heart J 1967; 29:810–812.

1024. Martin TC, Arias F, Olander DS, Hoffman RJ, Marbarger JP, Maurer MM. Successful management of congenital atrioventricular block associated with hydrops fetalis. J Pediatr 1988; 112:984–986.

1025. Saxena A, Mathur A, Iyer KS, Talwar KK. Congenital complete heart block in a neonate. Am Heart J 1992; 123:1706–1707.

1026. Michaelsson M, Engle MA. Congenital complete heart block: an international study of the natural history. Cardiovasc Clin 1972; 4:85–101.

1027. Strasburger J, Carpenter R, Smith RT, Deter R, Garson A. Fetal transthoracic pacing for advanced hydrops fetalis secondary to complete atrioventricular block. PACE 1986; 9:295.

1028. Ragonese P, Guccione P, Drago F, Turchetta A, Calzolari A, Formigari R. Efficacy and safety of ventricular rate responsive pacing in children with complete atrioventricular block. Pacing Clin Electrophysiol 1994; 17:603–610.

1029. Harris JP, Alexson CG, Manning JA, Thompson HO. Medical therapy for the hydropic fetus with congenital complete atrioventricular block. Am J Perinatol 1993; 10:217–219.

1030. Carpenter RJ Jr, Strasburger JF, Garson A Jr, Smith RT, Deter RL, Engelhardt HT Jr. Fetal ventricular pacing for hydrops secondary to complete atrioventricular block. J Am Coll Cardiol 1986; 8:1434–1436.

1031. Besley DC, McWilliams GJ, Moodie DS, Castle LW. Long-term follow-up of young adults following permanent pacemaker placement for complete heart block. Am Heart J 1982; 103:332–337.

1032. Gilchrist IC, Cameron A. Chronic bundle branch block and use of temporary transvenous pacemakers during coronary arteriography. Cathet Cardiovasc Diagn 1988; 15:229–232.

1033. Goyal R, Syed ZA, Mukhopadhyay PS, et al. Changes in cardiac repolarization following short periods of ventricular pacing. J Cardiovasc Electrophysiol 1998; 9:269–280.

1034. Rosenbaum MB, Blanco HH, Elizari MV, Lazzari JO, Davidenko JM. Electrotonic modulation of the T wave and cardiac memory. Am J Cardiol 1982; 50:213–222.

1035. Johansson BW. Longevity in complete heart block. Ann N Y Acad Sci 1969; 167:1031–1037.

1036. Katz LN, Pick A. Clinical Electrocardiography. Part I. The Arrhythmias. Philadelphia: Lea & Febiger, 1956, p. 545.

1037. Peters RW, Scheinman MM, Modin C, O'Young J, Somelofski CA, Mies C. Prophylactic permanent pacemakers for patients with chronic bundle branch block. Am J Med 1979; 66:978–985.

1038. Geggel RL, Tucker L, Szer I. Postnatal progression from second- to third-degree heart block in neonatal lupus syndrome. J Pediatr 1988; 113:1049–1052.

1039. Young D, Eisenberg R, Fish B, Fisher JD. Wenckebach atrioventricular block (Mobitz type I) in children and adolescents. Am J Cardiol 1977; 40:393–399.

1040. Rytand DA, Stinson E, Kelly JJ Jr. Remission and recovery from chronic, established, complete heart block. Am Heart J 1976; 91:645–652.

1041. Tsuji A, Yanai J, Komai T, Sato M, Asaishi T, Fukuda T. Recovery from congenital complete atrioventricular block. Pediatr Cardiol 1988; 9:163–166.

1042. Holdright DR, Sutton GC. Restoration of sinus rhythm during two consecutive pregnancies in a woman with congenital complete heart block. Br Heart J 1990; 64:338–339.

1043. Sowton E. Artificial pacemaking and sinus rhythm. Br Heart J 1965; 27:311–318.

1044. Lichstein E, Ribas-Meneclier C, Naik D, Chadda KD, Gupta PK, Smith H Jr. The natural history of trifascicular disease following permanent pacemaker implantation: significance of continuing changes in atrioventricular conduction. Circulation 1976; 54:780–783.

1045. Edhag O, Rosenqvist M. Heart rhythm during permanent cardiac pacing. Br Heart J 1979; 42:182–185.

1046. Staessen J, Ector H, De Geest H. The underlying heart rhythm in patients with an artificial cardiac pacemaker. Pacing Clin Electrophysiol 1982; 5:801–807.

1047. Rosenqvist M, Edhag KO. Pacemaker dependence in transient high-grade atrioventricular block. Pacing Clin Electrophysiol 1984; 7:63–70.

1048. Iskos D, Lurie KG, Sakaguchi S, Benditt DG. Termination of implantable pacemaker therapy: experience in five patients. Ann Intern Med 1997; 126:787–790.

1049. Curd GW, Dennis EW, Jordan J, et al. Etiology of atrioventricular heart block: a study of its relevance to prognosis and pacemaker therapy. Cardiovasc Res Center Bull 1963; 1:63–70.

1050. Cosby RS, Lau F, Rhode R, Cafferky E, Mayo M. Complete heart block, prognostic value of electrocardiographic features and clinical complications. Am J Cardiol 1966; 17:190–193.

1051. Dhingra RC, Wyndham C, Amat-y-Leon F, et al. Incidence and site of atrioventricular block in patients with chronic bifascicular block. Circulation 1979; 59:238–246.

1052. Shen WK, Hammill SC, Hayes DL, et al. Long-term survival after pacemaker implantation for heart block in patients ≥65 years. Am J Cardiol 1994; 74:560–564.

1053. Siddons H. Deaths in long-term paced patients. Br Heart J 1974; 36:1201–1209.

1054. Greenland P, Reicher-Reiss H, Goldbourt U, Behar S, Israeli SPRINT investigators. In-hospital and 1-year mortality in 1,524 women after myocardial infarction: comparison with 4,315 men. Circulation 1991; 83:484–491.

1055. Tans AC, Lie KI. A-V nodal block in acute myocardial infarction. In Wellens HJJ, Lie KI, Janse MJ, (eds). The Conduction System of the Heart. Philadelphia: Lea & Febiger, 1976, pp. 655–661.

1056. Norris RM, Brandt PWT, Lee AJ. Mortality in a coronary-care unit analysed by a new coronary prognostic index. Lancet 1969; 1:278–281.

1057. Bauer GE, Julian DG, Valentine PA. Bundle-branch block in acute myocardial infarction. Br Heart J 1965; 27:724–730.

1058. Hindman MC, Wagner GS, JaRo M, et al. The clinical significance of bundle branch block complicating acute myocardial infarction. 1. Clinical characteristics, hospital mortality, and one-year follow-up. Circulation 1978; 58:679–688.

1059. Hunt D, Sloman G. Bundle-branch block in acute myocardial infarction. BMJ 1969; 1:85–88.

1060. Rizzon P, DiBiase M, Baissus C. Intraventricular conduction defects in acute myocardial infarction. Br Heart J 1974; 36:660–668.

1061. Nicod P, Gilpin E, Dittrich H, et al. Late clinical outcome in patients with early ventricular fibrillation after myocardial infarction. J Am Coll Cardiol 1988; 11:464–470.

1062. Lassers BW. First-year follow-up after recovery from acute myocardial infarction with complete heart-block. Lancet 1969; 1:1172–1174.

1063. Thygesen K, Haghfelt T, Steinmetz E, Nielsen BL. Long-term survival after myocardial infarction as related to early complications. Eur J Cardiol 1977; 6:41–51.

1064. Schoeller R, Andresen D, Buttner P, Oezcelik K, Vey G, Schroder R. First- or second-degree atrioventricular block as a risk factor in idiopathic dilated cardiomyopathy. Am J Cardiol 1993; 71:720–726.

1065. Michaelsson M, Riesenfeld T, Jonzon A. Natural history of congenital complete atrioventricular block. Pacing Clin Electrophysiol 1997; 20:2098–2101.

1066. Alpert MA, Curtis JJ, Sanfelippo JF, et al. Comparative survival after permanent ventricular and dual chamber pacing for patients with chronic high degree atrioventricular block with and without preexistent congestive heart failure. J Am Coll Cardiol 1986; 7:925–932.

Sick Sinus Syndrome[1-19a]

The sick sinus syndrome refers to a group of bradyarrhythmias caused by malfunction of the sinus node and surrounding tissues, often associated with supraventricular tachyarrhythmias and faulty escape mechanisms. Although the bradyarrhythmias that characterize patients with sick sinus syndrome have been known since the earliest days of electrocardiography, Bernard Lown first suggested that the condition qualifies as a clinical entity when he wrote, while describing the arrhythmias that follow cardioversion of atrial arrhythmias in 1967,[20b]

> The majority of abnormal rhythms immediately after cardioversion are atrial. . . . They generally represent one of three mechanisms: (1) delayed warm-up of the sinus node . . . ; (2) increased atrial automaticity . . . ; (3) the "sick sinus" syndrome, a defect in elaboration or conduction of sinus impulses characterized by chaotic atrial activity, changing P wave contour, bradycardia, interspersed with multiple and recurrent ectopic beats, with runs of atrial and nodal tachycardia.[20, 21c]

In a series of articles, the first of which appeared a year later, M. Irené Ferrer described and popularized the syndrome as our knowledge of its clinical, electrocardiographic, and electrophysiological features accumulated.[2, 4, 8, 14, 22] Other names for the same condition include

Lazy sinus syndrome.[23, 24]
Sinoatrial disease.
Sinoatrial dysfunction.
Sinus node dysfunction.
Sluggish sinus node syndrome.[25]

Many physicians refer to the condition simply as "sick sinus."

The frequent concurrence of atrial tachyarrhythmias with the characteristic bradyarrhythmias in the sick sinus syndrome led to adoption of the phrase "bradycardia-tachycardia syndrome" for such patients.[6, 26] In an article titled "The Syndrome of Alternating Bradycardia and Tachycardia," D. S. Short first described the combination in 1954[27] (Figs. 16.1 and 16.2):

> Among the large number of patients suffering from syncopal attacks who attended the National Heart Hospital during a four year period, there were four in whom examination revealed sinus bradycardia alternating with prolonged phases of auricular tachycardia. . . . The basic fault remains obscure but a concept of subnormal activity of the sino-auricular node would account for most features of the syndrome.[27]

Treatment in Short's day was pharmacological and inadequate, as he observed:

> Although an intravenous injection of atropine caused acceleration of the sinus rate to normal resting levels, no drug was found to have this effect when administered by mouth.[27]

The 1960s brought pacemakers, the most effective treatment for the bradyarrhythmias of the syndrome. Sick sinus syndrome subsequently became the leading indication for using pacemakers in the United States.[28–32]

PREVALENCE

Sick sinus syndrome was detected in 0.17% of 3,000 patients older than the age of 50 years attending a center for the detection of cardiovascular disease in

---

[a] Portions of this chapter are based on material in Chapter 9, "Sick Sinus Syndrome," by David G. Benditt and Stephen C. Remole[1] in the first edition of this book.

[b] In his definitive review of cardioversion.[20]

[c] Dr. Lown adds: "I observed three types of sinus activity following cardioversion: the active sinus, the somnolent sinus, and the sick sinus. The somnolent sinus was defined as depressed sinus node activity that was in effect a warming-up interlude generally of 20 to 30 seconds before a consistent sinus mechanism usurped pacemaking. The sick sinus syndrome was, of course, something quite different. The P-wave morphology was variable and quite erratic, the rhythm chaotic, with a host of mini diverse arrhythmias. An intraatrial lead divulged bizarre P-wave formations and no 2 P waves were alike. Furthermore, there were bursts of atrial tachycardia and flutter; and atrial fibrillation consistently recurred."[21]

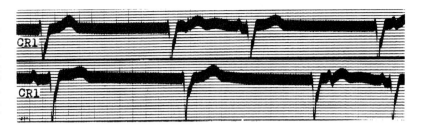

FIGURE 16.1 Sick sinus syndrome. This electrocardiogram from a 38-year-old woman with mitral valve disease shows what D. S. Short described in 1954 as ''sinus rhythm with wandering pacemaker and A-V nodal escape.'' The name ''sick sinus syndrome'' had not yet been adopted for this condition. (Adapted from Short DS. The syndrome of alternating bradycardia and tachycardia. Br Heart J 1954; 16:208–214, with permission.)[27]

Belgium.[33] Except for this figure, the prevalence of the syndrome is not known.

AGE

Adults develop sick sinus syndrome most often in the sixth and seventh decades of life[33–43d] (Fig. 16.3). However, the arrhythmia does appear in young adults,[28, 44–47] and it is the most frequent indication for pacing in patients 20 to 40 years of age.[28] Sick sinus syndrome rarely occurs spontaneously in children.[48, 49]

GENDER

Men and women are similarly affected by sick sinus syndrome.[35, 36, 38–43, 50, 51e]

---

[d] The average age, from seven series, of 1,034 patients with sick sinus syndrome when they came to medical attention was 67.2 years.[33, 34, 36, 40–43]

[e] Of 1,145 patients with sick sinus syndrome in eight series, 570 (50%) were men.[35, 36, 38–43, 50]

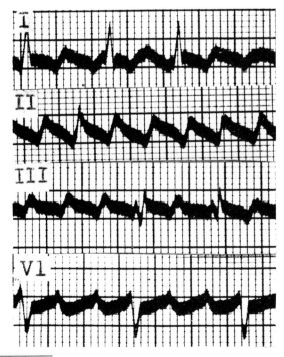

FIGURE 16.2 Atrial flutter in a 41-year-old woman without structural heart disease and periods of slow sinus rhythm, another of Short's cases (1954) of what we now call sick sinus syndrome. (Adapted from Short DS. The syndrome of alternating bradycardia and tachycardia. Br Heart J 1954; 16:208–214, with permission.)[27]

GENETICS

Most cases of sick sinus syndrome are acquired. However, occasionally, the condition or the arrhythmias that characterize it will appear in several family members, suggesting a genetic relationship.[52–68]

CLINICAL SETTING

Many, but far from all, patients with sick sinus syndrome have structural heart disease (Table 16.1). In many cases, one cannot be certain whether the cardiac disease that the patient may have causes the arrhythmia.

Coronary Heart Disease[69]

About 40% of adults with sick sinus syndrome have coronary heart disease, not unexpectedly, in view of the age of most of the patients.[35, 43f] Although sinoatrial block and sinus arrest[70–72] develop occasionally during acute myocardial infarction, and sinus bradycardia develops relatively often in patients with inferior infarctions, abnormally slow rhythms rarely persist after recovery.[71, 73, 74] Thus, acute myocardial infarction seldom produces sick sinus syndrome.

Cardiomyopathy

Idiopathic cardiomyopathy accounts for about 5% to 10% of cases of sick sinus syndrome;[35, 43] arrhythmo-

---

[f] Two-hundred seventeen (43%) of 507 patients in one large series[43] and 20 (35%) in an older but frequently quoted series of 56 patients[35] had coronary heart disease with their sick sinus syndrome.

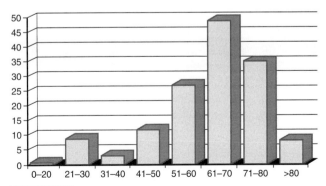

FIGURE 16.3 The age (horizontal axis) of 146 patients (vertical axis) with sick sinus syndrome. Sick sinus syndrome is most frequently diagnosed in older patients, most often those in their sixties (from two series of 146 patients).[35, 37] (From Benditt DG, Remole SC. Sick sinus syndrome. In Kastor JA (ed). Arrhythmias. Philadelphia: WB Saunders, 1994; pp. 225–249, with permission.)[1]

Table 16.1   ETIOLOGY OF HEART DISEASE IN PATIENTS WITH SICK SINUS SYNDROME FROM TWO SERIES[35, 43]

	Sgarbossa and Others[43]		Rubenstein and Others[35]	
Number of patients in series	507		56	
Diagnosis	No. of Patients	%	No. of Patients	%
Coronary heart disease	217	43	20	36
Valvular heart disease	61	12	—	—
Cardiomyopathy	35	7	3	5
Hypertension	—	—	4	7
Other	46	9	4	7
No structural heart disease	214	42	25	45

*a*Two hundred seventeen patients (43%) of those in the Sgarbossa series had hypertension, but this diagnosis was treated as a "concomitant disease."[43]

(Data from references 35 and 43.)

genic right ventricular dysplasia may produce the arrhythmia.[75] Sick sinus syndrome including atrial standstill appears as part of the cardiomyopathy that some patients with muscular and neuromuscular disease develop.[76–81]

Drugs[82]

Although many drugs used to treat patients with heart disease decrease the sinus rate, a few can produce sinoatrial block, sinus arrest, or severe sinus bradycardia[83–110] (Table 16.2).

Surgery

Congenital heart disease.[111, 112] Surgical repair of congenital heart disease is the most frequent cause of sick sinus syndrome in children[46, 113–137] (Table 16.3). Sick sinus syndrome also develops in adults after repair of congenital lesions, particularly atrial septal defect,[138] and the arrhythmia developed in a 48-year-old woman with mirror-image dextrocardia.[139]

Cardiac transplantation. The donor hearts in as many as 45%[140] of patients exhibit some abnormality of sinoatrial nodal function after cardiac transplantation.[140–152] The electrocardiogram usually shows sinus bradycardia or arrest with dependence on junctional

Table 16.2   DRUGS INCRIMINATED IN PRODUCING THE ARRHYTHMIAS OF SICK SINUS SYNDROME

Amiodarone[101, 103–105]
Clonidine[106]
Diltiazem[109]
Digitalis[83, 84, 93]
Lidocaine[86, 90–92] in a patient also taking amiodarone[100] and in another taking quinidine[89]
Lithium[94, 96, 102, 108]
Phenytoin[85, 87, 97]
Propranolol[95] and, presumably, other beta-adrenergic–blocking drugs
Quinidine[88, 98]
Sotalol[110]
Tocainide[107]
Verapamil[99]

escape rhythms or pacing to maintain systole. The frequency of these bradycardias decreases as surgical teams gain greater experience performing the operation.[152]

Factors that can increase the likelihood of developing the arrhythmias of sick sinus syndrome after cardiac transplantation include

- Prolonged ischemia of the donor heart.[147, 148]
- Surgical trauma.[148, 152]
- Antiarrhythmic drugs.[148]

Maze procedure. This operation to cure atrial fibrillation sometimes leaves patients with an inadequately functioning sinus node and the bradyarrhythmias of sick sinus syndrome.[153] The frequency of this complication, when produced by the operation itself, has decreased with improving surgical technique.[154]

After Cardioversion

When sinus rhythm does not return immediately after cardioversion,[155–158] sick sinus syndrome may develop. The arrhythmia most often appears in those patients whose atrial fibrillation has been long-lasting[20] or whose ventricular response is slow.[159]

No Structural Heart Disease

Many patients with sick sinus syndrome,[160] probably more than 40% of adults, have no discernible organic heart disease.[35, 161, 162] Most children who spontaneously develop sick sinus syndrome[163] have structurally normal hearts.[118, 164, 165]

Miscellaneous Conditions

Hypothyroidism[166] and thyrotoxicosis[33, 167–170] cause an occasional case of sick sinus syndrome. Sick sinus syndrome was the presenting diagnosis of a patient with reticulum cell sarcoma.[171]

Other Diagnoses

In view of the age of most patients with sick sinus syndrome, it is not surprising that many will have dis-

Table 16.3	SURGICAL OPERATIONS FOR REPAIR OF CONGENITAL HEART DISEASE THAT MAY PRODUCE SICK SINUS SYNDROME		
Congenital Lesion		**Surgical Procedure**	**Maximum Incidence Reported**
Transposition of the great arteries[46, 113, 114, 116–120, 122–124, 126, 127, 129, 131–133, 135]		Mustard	50%[124a]
Transposition of the great arteries[128, 132]		Senning	—
Atrial septal defect[114, 118, 138]		—	39%[114]
Tetralogy of Fallot[115, 121, 135, 136]		—	36%[136]
Various conditions[130, 134, 135, 137]		Fontan	—

[a]Improvements in surgical technique have decreased but not eliminated sick sinus syndrome after the Mustard procedure.[113, 116]

eases that directly or indirectly affect the heart. For example, the following were present among 308 patients with the arrhythmia:[43]

- Hypertension—43%.
- Cerebrovascular disease—20%.
- Diabetes—14%.
- Peripheral vascular disease—9%.

Extrinsic Versus Intrinsic Disease: Autonomic Influences

Some workers suggest that we consider sick sinus syndrome or sinus node dysfunction as intrinsic or extrinsic.[172] "Intrinsic disease" implies pathology of the structure and function of the sinus node, what most of us would call, under the proper circumstances, sick sinus syndrome. "Extrinsic disease" refers to the influence of autonomic tone on sinus nodal function that can mimic the features of intrinsic disease.

Temporary changes in autonomic tone, particularly hypervagotonia, can produce marked and symptomatic sinus bradycardia, sinoatrial block, and sinus arrest[173–195] (Table 16.4). Because these events are usually reversible, we are stretching the diagnosis by calling them manifestations of the sick sinus syndrome even though persistent vagal overactivity, others have suggested, may predispose to sick sinus syndrome.[196] It should be kept in mind, however, that sick sinus syndrome and hypervagotonia can coexist and can produce severe bradyarrhythmias and symptoms.

Stroke and Embolism[197]

Stroke, which complicates the course of some patients with sick sinus syndrome,[35, 78, 198–200] occurs more often in those with the bradycardia-tachycardia syndrome

Table 16.4	PROCEDURES AND EVENTS STIMULATING HYPERVAGOTONIA THAT CAN PRODUCE SEVERE BRADYARRHYTHMIAS

Carotid sinus pressure and carotid sinus hypersensitivity[183, 188]
Deep inspiration[192]
Excessive physical training[181]
Glossopharyngeal neuralgia[174, 176]
Sleep apnea[180, 182, 184–186, 189, 190, 193, 194]
Rapid eye movement sleep[194]
Swallowing[173, 177–179, 191, 195]
Diffuse esophageal spasm[175]

than in patients with sick sinus syndrome and no tachyarrhythmias,[201] whether or not they have atrioventricular block.[202] The risk of emboli persists even when pacing removes the risk from bradyarrhythmias,[201] or, as one would expect, when chronic atrial fibrillation replaces the bradycardia-tachycardia syndrome.[201]

In a series of 507 adults with sick sinus syndrome, stroke developed in 6.3% within 65 months.[162] The actuarial incidence was[162]

- Three percent at 1 year.
- Five percent at 5 years.
- Thirteen percent at 10 years.

Other factors that increase the likelihood of stroke in patients with sick sinus syndrome include

- Greater age.[201]
- Valvular heart disease.[162]
- History of cerebrovascular disease.[162]
- History of paroxysmal atrial fibrillation.[162]
- Ventricular pacing mode.[162]

SYMPTOMS

Lightheadedness, dizziness, and syncope most frequently bring patients with sick sinus syndrome to see their physicians.[33, 35, 37–40, 45, 161, 167, 203, 204] These symptoms, when due to arrhythmias, are usually caused by bradyarrhythmias[205, 206g] and appear more often in those without tachyarrhythmias.[35] Syncope, although the most dramatic symptom in the sick sinus syndrome,[33, 164, 207] occurs in a minority of adults[35, 36, 78] and children.[118h]

Palpitations in patients with sick sinus syndrome are usually produced by tachyarrhythmias and suggest the presence of the bradycardia-tachycardia syndrome.[35] The development of chronic atrial fibrillation relieves many patients of the symptoms produced by bradycardia and the bradycardia-tachycardia syndrome.[200, 208]

Patients with sick sinus syndrome may also complain of angina[36, 38, 40] or fatigue and other symptoms suggesting heart failure or decreased cardiac output.[35, 36, 38]

---

[g] One should keep in mind that the cause of most episodes of syncope associated with transient bradycardia is neurogenic and is seldom cardiogenic.[205]

[h] Although in one series of 100 patients with chronic sick sinus syndrome, three-fourths of whom had cerebral ischemic symptoms, the most common presenting feature was syncope in 34 of the cases.[78] See Chapter 15 for a fuller discussion of the clinical and electrophysiological evaluation of syncope.

Severe bradycardia may be discovered in some patients, however, who report no symptoms.[209]

PHYSICAL EXAMINATION

The physical examination of patients with the sick sinus syndrome usually reveals the findings of bradycardia.

Procedures

Carotid sinus pressure produces excessive bradycardia or prolonged atrial asystole in many patients with sick sinus syndrome[16, 210, 211] (Fig. 16.4). However, the response to postural changes and the Valsalva maneuver is usually normal in patients with this arrhythmia.[211]

ELECTROCARDIOGRAPHY[212]

Although bradyarrhythmias are the fundamental electrocardiographic characteristic of sick sinus syndrome, many patients also have the bradycardia-tachycardia syndrome.[6, 26, 213]

Bradyarrhythmias

The resting heart rate of patients with sick sinus syndrome is almost always less than that of control subjects.[214-216] Long pauses usually occur spontaneously and thus, contrary to common belief, are infrequently caused by suppression of a diseased sinus node by tachyarrhythmias.[217]

Sinus bradycardia, which originates in the sinus node at a rate of less than 50 beats per minute,[i] is the most common bradyarrhythmia of the sick sinus syndrome. However, most people with sinus bradycardia do not have the sick sinus syndrome. The resting heart rate of well-trained athletes and of some healthy children, adolescents, and adults may be as slow as 40 beats per minute.[218, 219]

Elderly patients may have sinus rates lower than 50 beats per minute without any evidence of depressed cardiac performance.[220j] Therefore, sinus bradycardia

---

[i] Formerly 60 beats per minute.
[j] In one series of seven asymptomatic subjects aged 67 to 79 years with heart rates between 41 and 51 beats per minute.[220]

should be taken as abnormal and consistent with sick sinus syndrome only when persistent bradycardia produces symptoms or interferes with normal activity.[24, 28, 44, 46, 48, 118, 221-226k] What appears to be sinus bradycardia can be a slow atrial escape rhythm in some patients with sick sinus syndrome.[204, 227]

Sinus pauses,[225, 228] *sinus arrest,*[39, 46, 48, 118, 163, 167, 192, 203, 209, 222, 224, 229, 230] (Fig. 16.5) and *atrial standstill,*[55, 56, 76, 77, 80, 81, 231-248l] characteristic arrhythmias of sick sinus syndrome, produce atrial and ventricular asystole of varying lengths. The sinus node stops discharging, no P waves from atrial activation appear, and the atria and ventricles stop beating until the sinus recovers or another pacemaker escapes and captures the heart. The duration of sinus pauses correlates poorly with symptoms and does not predict sudden death.[249]

Sinoatrial block[250] produces bradycardia by interfering with transmission of the sinus impulse to the atrial myocardium and ultimately to the ventricles.[36, 46, 48, 118, 167, 203, 204, 207, 222, 225, 229, 251-255] During the period of block, no P waves appear. Electrophysiologically, however, the sinus continues to discharge during sinoatrial block—a phenomenon producing a signal that can be recorded with intracardiac electrodes but, because of its low amplitude, does not appear in the electrocardiogram.

Electrocardiographers recognize three degrees of sinoatrial block that correspond to the three degrees of atrioventricular block (Fig. 16.6), as follows:

- *First-degree sinoatrial block* describes prolonged transmission of the signal generated by the sinus pacemaker to the atria. Because depolarization of the sinus node produces no deflection on the electrocardiogram, first-degree sinoatrial block remains, electrocardiographically, a theoretical or "armchair" rather than a manifest diagnosis.
- In *second-degree sinoatrial block,* some of the sinus impulses activate and some do not activate the atria. Applying the patterns of atrioventricular block, electrocardiographers separate second-degree

---

[k] Abnormal sinus bradycardia has also been defined by the inability of submaximal exercise or intravenous atropine (0.01 milligram/kilogram) to raise the heart rate by more than 20%.[118]
[l] Many of the cases of atrial standstill have been described in the literature as isolated arrhythmias and not as part of the sick sinus syndrome.

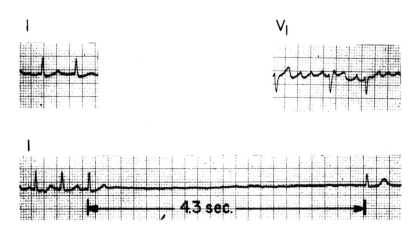

FIGURE 16.4 Asystole produced by carotid sinus pressure in a patient with the sick sinus syndrome and paroxysmal atrial fibrillation. This patient, who had repeatedly fainted for short periods of time, had paroxysmal atrial fibrillation and the bradycardia-tachycardia syndrome. **Top:** From leads I and V₁, coarse atrial fibrillation. **Bottom:** The patient became lightheaded as carotid sinus pressure produced a 4.3-sec pause of both atrial and ventricular activity. A junctional (His bundle) escape beat terminated the pause, which was then followed by sinus rhythm. The patient received a pacemaker that cured his syncope. The electrocardiograms illustrate the failure of escape foci, influenced in this case by carotid sinus pressure, to maintain an adequate heart rate in some patients with sick sinus syndrome.

FIGURE 16.5 Prolonged periods of sinus arrest or sinoatrial block in a 20-year-old patient with myocarditis producing asystole of sufficient duration to induce presyncope. **Top:** Lead II. **Bottom:** Lead III. (Adapted from Yabek SM, Swensson RE, Jarmakani JM. Electrocardiographic recognition of sinus node dysfunction in children and young adults. Circulation 1977; 56:235–239, by permission of the American Heart Association, Inc.)[118]

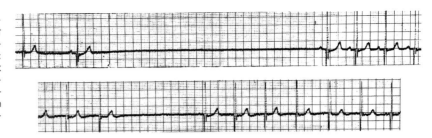

sinoatrial block into type I, with Wenckebach periods,[256] and type II. When Wenckebach periods develop, a common interval may be found that corresponds to the rhythm of the sinus pacemaker. Furthermore, the PP intervals shorten before the pause,[118] just as the RR intervals shorten in type I second-degree atrioventricular block. In type II second-degree sinoatrial block, the pauses are multiples of the sinus nodal discharge rate. Distinguishing between the two types of second-degree sinoatrial block seems to have little clinical significance.

- *Third-degree sinoatrial block* defines the condition in which none of the sinus impulses activate the atria. Consequently, the atria either become quiescent ("atrial standstill") or are driven by an atrial escape rhythm or a tachyarrhythmia such as atrial fibrillation.

Atrioventricular block[257] may coexist with sick sinus syndrome either when the patient is first examined[48, 49, 64, 65, 168, 203, 258] or later.[161, 259–264] Seventeen percent of patients show at least first-degree atrioventricular block when sick sinus syndrome is initially diagnosed.[261] During follow-up, 8% develop further amounts of atrioventricular block.[261] The number of patients who progress to high degrees of block, however, is relatively low—3% according to one study[264] and 4.5% in another.[265] The electrocardiograms of patients likely to develop atrioventricular block frequently show conduction system disease when sick sinus syndrome is first recognized.[260]

Tachyarrhythmias

Atrial fibrillation, the most common sustained tachyarrhythmia in patients with sick sinus syndrome,[36, 39] appears in 8% of patients when they first present with the syndrome[261] (see Fig. 16.4).[m] After patients with sick sinus syndrome receive pacemakers, chronic atrial fibrillation develops in[162n]

- Seven percent by 1 year.
- Sixteen percent by 5 years.
- Twenty-eight percent at 10 years.

Patients who eventually develop chronic atrial fibrillation are more likely, when sick sinus syndrome is first diagnosed, to be older,[162] to take antiarrhythmic drugs,[162] and to have

---

[m] From a comprehensive review published in 1986.[261]
[n] In a series of 507 patients who received pacemakers of various types for sick sinus syndrome.[162]

- Paroxysmal atrial fibrillation,[162, 260] particularly when the patient has had episodes for a long time[162] or if the paroxysms are prolonged.[162]
- Atrial enlargement on chest radiograph.[260]
- Ventricular, rather than atrial or atrioventricular, pacers.[162]

Atrial flutter with atrial tachycardia sometimes appears as the tachycardia component of the bradycardia-tachycardia syndrome in patients with sick sinus syndrome[36, 39, 204, 207, 266] (Figs. 16.7 and 16.8). Supraventricular tachycardia, sustained in dual pathways, may also coexist with sick sinus syndrome. *Supraventricular tachycardia*, sustained in dual atrioventricular nodal pathways, can coexist in patients with sick sinus syndrome.[267, 268] *Atrial dissociation* with atrial "flutter/fibrillation" and sinus rhythm were present simultaneously in a patient with sick sinus syndrome.[269]

P Waves

The P terminal force in lead V_1 is larger in patients with sick sinus syndrome and paroxysmal atrial fibrillation than in patients with sick sinus syndrome and no atrial fibrillation and in patients with other cardiac arrhythmias who do not have sick sinus syndrome or atrial fibrillation.[270]

OTHER ELECTROCARDIOGRAPHIC STUDIES

Ambulatory (Holter) Monitoring[16, 212]

Extended electrocardiographic monitoring reveals the arrhythmias of sick sinus syndrome in most, although not all,[271] patients suspected of having the disease. Ambulatory monitoring reveals sick sinus syndrome as the cause of syncope better than does exercise testing.[272]

Specifically, Holter monitoring can show

- The specific bradyarrhythmias that account for symptoms.[187, 206, 224, 226, 271, 273–275]
- That brief episodes of unsuspected atrial tachyarrhythmias frequently occur.[276]
- How slow heart rates can become during sleep.[277]
- That sinus arrest is a leading cause of ventricular pauses that last for 3 seconds or more.[228]
- That pauses are also caused, although less frequently, by atrial fibrillation with a slow ventricular response and, occasionally, by atrioventricular block.[228]

A. NORMAL

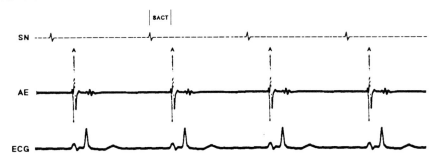

B. FIRST-DEGREE SA EXIT BLOCK

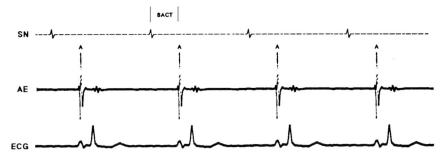

FIGURE 16.6 Normal and abnormal sinoatrial conduction. In each case, a (presumed) recording from the sinoatrial node (SN), an atrial electrogram (AE), and a surface electrocardiographic lead (ECG) are shown. **A,** Normal relationships. Note the prolonged interval from discharge of the sinus node to activation of the atria (SACT) in first-degree sinoatrial (SA) block **(B),** the prolonged intervals with the dropped atrial beat in second-degree block **(C),** and the sequence of two dropped atrial beats during the transient period of third-degree sinoatrial block **(D).** In the absence of electrophysiological recordings, we can only assume the presence of first-degree sinoatrial block when it occurs. (From Benditt DG, Remole SC. Sick sinus syndrome. In Kastor JA (ed). Arrhythmias. Philadelphia: WB Saunders, 1994; pp. 225–249, with permission.)[1]

C. SECOND-DEGREE SA EXIT BLOCK
    3:2 WENCKEBACH PERIODICITY

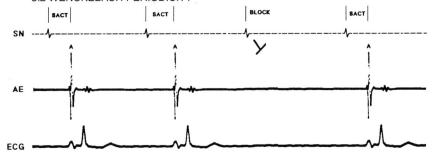

D. THIRD-DEGREE SA EXIT BLOCK

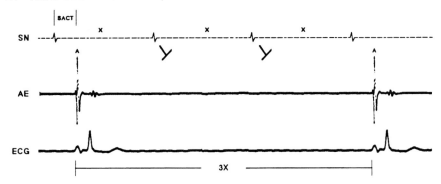

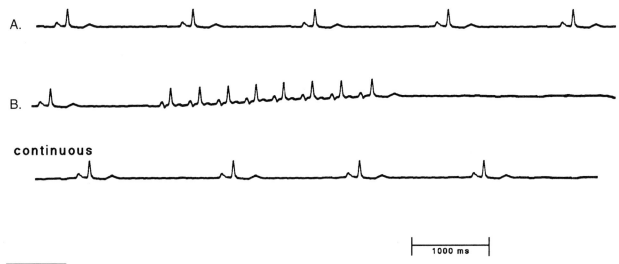

FIGURE 16.7 Bradycardia-tachycardia syndrome in a patient with slow sinus bradycardia. (A) The tachyarrhythmia is atrial tachycardia, bursts of which **(B)** suppress the abnormal sinus pacemaker and produce a sufficiently long period of asystole to account for lightheadedness. (From Benditt DG, Remole SC. Sick sinus syndrome. In Kastor JA (ed). Arrhythmias. Philadelphia: WB Saunders, 1994; pp. 225–249, with permission.)[1]

- That overdrive suppression by tachyarrhythmias does *not* produce most long sinus pauses.[217]
- That the disappearance of circadian periodicity is proportional to the severity of sinus nodal dysfunction and that intrinsic or extrinsic dysfunction can remove the normal circadian variation in these patients.[278]
- The character of arrhythmias, including sick sinus syndrome, after recovery from surgery for congenital heart disease.[137]

Exercise Testing[16, 279]

The maximum heart rate achieved by exercise is slower in patients with sick sinus syndrome than in healthy persons[215, 216, 280o] or matched controls.[214] Oxygen up-

---

[o] One hundred twenty-four beats per minute in seven patients with sick sinus syndrome versus 163 beats per minute in seven younger well-trained subjects without heart disease.[215]

take or consumption during exercise is probably lower than normal in those with sick sinus syndrome.[214, 215p] Atropine increases the heart rate of patients with sick sinus syndrome to normal resting levels but has little effect on the maximal heart rate during exercise.[214]

Signal-Averaged Electrocardiograms

The voltage (root mean square) of the initial 30 milliseconds of the filtered P wave is lower, and the duration of the initial low amplitude signals of the filtered P wave is longer, in patients with sick sinus syndrome than in age-matched control subjects[281] (Fig. 16.9).

HEMODYNAMICS

Carotid sinus massage and head-up tilt testing demonstrate that syncope in patients with sick sinus syndrome

---

[p] Although not all workers agree.[215]

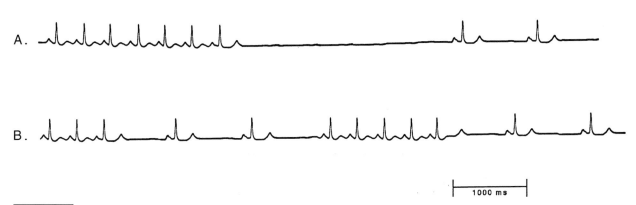

FIGURE 16.8 Bradycardia-tachycardia syndrome in another patient with atrial tachycardia and a prolonged pause resulting from sinus arrest or high-degree sinoatrial block occurring when the tachycardia terminates **(A)**. At other times, tachycardia was not followed by excessive bradycardia **(B)**. Bradyarrhythmias, tachyarrhythmias, or both may cause the symptoms of sick sinus syndrome. (From Benditt DG, Remole SC. Sick sinus syndrome. In Kastor JA (ed). Arrhythmias. Philadelphia: WB Saunders, 1994; pp. 225–249, with permission.)[1]

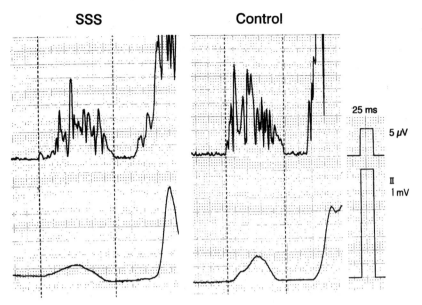

SSS　　　　　　**Control**

FIGURE 16.9 **Signal-averaged electrocardiogram** of P waves *(upper portion)* and electrocardiogram *(lower portion)* from patients with (SSS) and without (Control) sick sinus syndrome. The initial portion of the P wave has lower amplitude and longer duration in the patients with sick sinus syndrome. The *vertical dashed lines* indicate the beginning and end of the filtered P waves. (Adapted from Yamada T, Fukunami M, Kumagai K, et al. Detection of patients with sick sinus syndrome by use of low amplitude potentials early in filtered P wave. J Am Coll Cardiol 1996; 28:738–744, with permission.)[281]

is frequently caused by an abnormal neural reflex, most often cardioinhibitory, rather than solely by bradycardia.[282]

PATHOLOGY[283, 284] AND ANGIOGRAPHY

The microscopic appearance of the sinoatrial nodes of most patients with sick sinus syndrome is abnormal. The nodal tissue appears atrophic or fibrosed,[285] with total or subtotal destruction.[286] Extensive lesions, including fatty infiltration,[287–289] of the sinoatrial and atrioventricular nodes and of the approaches to both nodes[288, 290] are characteristic. Amyloid is sometimes present.[56, 67, 285]

The atria of patients with atrial standstill show arteriosclerosis, fibroelastosis, fatty infiltration, and vacuolar degeneration of the muscle cells.[291] The normal architecture of both the sinoatrial node and the atrial myocardium is affected by the bradycardia-tachycardia syndrome.[290] Other lesions in patients with the sick sinus syndrome or bradycardia-tachycardia syndrome include

- Chronic or acute lesions of the atrioventricular node, bundle of His, and its branches or their distal subdivisions.[286]
- Destruction, total or subtotal, of the areas of nodal-atrial continuity.[286]
- Inflammatory or degenerative changes of the nerves and ganglia surrounding the node.[286]
- Pathological changes in the atrial wall.[286]

Coronary Heart Disease

Necropsy and angiography show that coronary atherosclerosis is not responsible for most cases of sick sinus syndrome.[285, 292, 293] However, coronary arteriography reveals that, in patients with sick sinus syndrome who have had inferior myocardial infarctions, the sinoatrial artery or the vessels supplying it are more severely

obstructed[72] than in those with sick sinus syndrome and no history of inferior infarction.[294]

After Cardiac Surgery

When sinus dysfunction follows cardiac surgery, the following can be found at autopsy:[295]

- Bisection of the sinus node.
- Epicarditis adjacent to the sinus node.
- Hemorrhage in the node.
- Necrosis of sinus nodal tissue with fibrosis, foreign body reaction, vascular proliferation, and infiltration of neutrophils, lymphocytes, and plasma cells.
- Occlusion of the sinus nodal artery with organized thrombus.
- Suture material in or adjacent to the sinus node.
- Vasculitis.

Miscellaneous

Patients with polyarteritis nodosa and arrhythmias consistent with the sick sinus syndrome have pathological changes in the sinoatrial node.[296] The sinus node and conduction system were extensively involved with the tumor in a patient with reticulum cell sarcoma who presented with sick sinus syndrome.[171]

Although antibodies against human conducting tissue have been postulated to cause sick sinus syndrome,[297] at this writing, the etiologic cause of most cases of the syndrome is unknown. The sinus node does not show consistent pathological abnormalities in infants who die suddenly.[298]

ELECTROPHYSIOLOGY[5, 12, 16, 18, 19, 212, 279, 299–309]

Measurements of Sinoatrial Electrophysiological Function[310]

Several electrophysiological tests have been developed that measure sinoatrial nodal function in healthy persons and patients with sick sinus syndrome. These measurements become more abnormal as both healthy persons and patients with sick sinus syndrome age.[311] For the most part, the results are reproducible when the tests are repeated in the same patient.[312]

Sinoatrial conduction time. This value is the number of milliseconds from discharge of the sinus node until atrial activation begins. It can be measured directly by recording activation of the sinus node in the electrophysiology laboratory in adults[313–322] (Fig. 16.10) and children[323–325] and in the operating room.[326] The interval can be estimated indirectly by observing the responses to programmed atrial depolarization—the introduction of paced premature atrial beats at predetermined intervals from the previous spontaneous sinus beat[327–333]—or by atrial pacing.[331, 334] The data produced by the indirect method[314, 315, 320, 324, 335] correlate reasonably well, according to most investigators,[314, 315, 324q] with those obtained from the direct technique.

---

[q]But not so well according to others.[318, 320, 335] One group found "no significant correlation" among sinoatrial conduction times determined by the direct and indirect methods in their patients with sinus node dysfunction.[318]

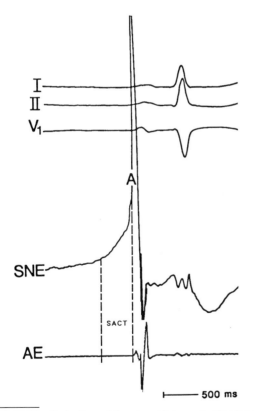

FIGURE 16.10 Derivation of the sinoatrial conduction time from an electrogram recorded directly from the sinus node. *Dashed vertical lines* indicate the onset of both the sinus node potential (SNE, *left*) and the local atrial electrogram *(right)*. The *interval between the dashed lines* is the sinoatrial conduction time. Tracings from *top* to *bottom* are electrocardiographic leads I, II, and V₁ and intracardiac electrograms from the sinus node (SNE) and the nearby right atrium (AE). (From Benditt DG, Remole SC. Sick sinus syndrome. In Kastor JA (ed). Arrhythmias. Philadelphia: WB Saunders, 1994; pp. 225–249, with permission.)[1]

Sinoatrial conduction time measured indirectly may be less than when measured directly,[316] especially in patients with a prolonged direct result.[332] Electrograms from the sinus node demonstrate that carotid sinus pressure in patients with hypersensitive carotid sinuses can produce temporary sinoatrial block and even sinus arrest in the absence of clinical disease of the sinus node.[188]

Sinus node recovery time. Pacing the atria faster than the sinus rate briefly suppresses the automaticity of the sinus pacemaker. The interval from the last paced beat to the first P wave is consequently longer—in other words, the rate is briefly slower—than the PP interval before the pacing was started.[336, 337r] The same phenomenon can be observed when a supraventricular tachyarrhythmia terminates[338] or after ventricular pacing in patients with intact ventriculoatrial conduction.[210] When studying sinus function in the electrophysiology laboratory, one usually measures atrial activation from an intra-atrial electrode.

This interval between the last nonsinus beat and the first sinus beat is called the "sinus node recovery time." Deducting the last sinus PP interval before pacing from the sinus node recovery time gives the "corrected" sinus node recovery time. The value of the sinus node recovery time differs if one measures the termination of the postpacing interval from the sinus node electrogram (direct method) or from the high right atrial electrogram (indirect method).[319]

Specific features of the sinus node recovery time include the following:

- The slower the sinus rate before pacing, the longer is the sinus node recovery time.[339]
- The faster the rate of pacing, the longer is the sinus node recovery time.[340] This relationship applies at paced rates less than a range of 120[339] to 150[340] impulses per minute. At faster rates, the postpacing interval progressively shortens.[339]
- The duration of pacing has little effect on the sinus node recovery time.[340]
- The corrected sinus node recovery time is longer in patients with organic heart disease and no clinical evidence of sick sinus syndrome than in healthy persons, and this difference is due to intrinsic abnormalities and not to extrinsic autonomic influences.[341]

Electrophysiological Findings in Patients with Sick Sinus Syndrome

Electrophysiological abnormalities of both automaticity in the sinus node and conduction from the node to the atria account for the bradyarrhythmias of sick sinus syndrome.[204] Such abnormal measurements of sinoatrial nodal function alone, however, do not make the diagnosis of sick sinus syndrome. One must seek

---

[r]This characteristic was first observed clinically by the effect of spontaneous premature beats on sinus rhythm.[336] The sinus node, however, is less susceptible to suppression than are subsidiary pacemakers.[337]

symptoms and demonstrate suitable clinical arrhythmias. Conversely, few patients who have normal electrophysiological measurements and a normal Holter monitor result have clinical sick sinus syndrome.[271]

Sinoatrial conduction. This conduction is characteristically prolonged in most patients with sick sinus syndrome[144, 225, 271, 316, 318, 325, 329, 342–345] (Table 16.5).[s] Recording electrograms from the sinus node show that many, if not most, prolonged pauses produced by atrial pacing in patients with sick sinus syndrome are caused by sinoatrial block rather than by suppression of sinus nodal automaticity.[204, 317, 319] Presumably, this is also the case clinically.

Prolonged sinoatrial conduction time, when measured in a general population, identifies those persons with a high likelihood of having electrocardiographic and electrophysiological abnormalities of sinus node and atrial function. Many of these people, however, may not yet have clinically significant sick sinus syndrome.[346] Sinoatrial conduction time increases as the sinus cycle length decreases (heart rate rises), and vice versa, both in patients with sick sinus syndrome and in normal healthy persons.[347]

Sinus node recovery time or corrected sinus node recovery time. This time is prolonged beyond the normal range in most,[115, 210, 225, 319, 348–361] although not all,[28, 354] patients with sick sinus syndrome.[t] Furthermore, the PP intervals *after* the first sinus beat are abnormally prolonged[339] ("secondary pauses") more often in patients with sick sinus syndrome than in healthy persons.[362] The intrinsic heart rate—the sinus rate after blockade of autonomic forces with atropine and propranolol—in patients with sick sinus syndrome and prolonged sinus node recovery time is abnormally slow.[363] Secondary pauses occur more frequently in those with abnormal intrinsic heart rates.[172]

Electrophysiological study shows that sinus node recovery time is prolonged in some children with secundum atrial septal defect *before* the lesion is surgically repaired.[364, 365] This observation suggests that the substrate for sick sinus syndrome can be present before operation, after which the arrhythmia may appear.[114, 118, 364] The operation can shorten sinus node recovery

time, presumably by decreasing the volume of the right atrium.[365]

Sinus node recovery time and sinoatrial conduction are prolonged in many children after the Mustard operation for transposition of the great arteries[122] and the Fontan procedure for repair of functional single ventricle.[134] There is a high incidence of recipient sinus node dysfunction in asymptomatic long-term survivors of cardiac transplantation.[366, 367]

Penetration of the sinus node by an ectopic slow atrial focus can suppress sinus node function in patients with sick sinus syndrome. This phenomenon, which may produce an electrocardiogram that looks like "sinus bradycardia,"[204, 227] probably constitutes an example of unidirectional block in which *entrance* to the sinoatrial node[368u] is preserved despite the presence of complete sinoatrial *exit* block.[204, 227] Consequently, sinoatrial entrance block does not correlate with the presence or absence of sick sinus syndrome.[369]

Many patients with persistent sinus bradycardia whose sinus node recovery time is abnormal later develop serious clinical disease of the sinus node.[370] Consequently, corrected sinus node recovery time can help to predict the fate of sinus function in patients with sick sinus syndrome who have received pacemakers. The function of the sinus pacemaker deteriorates more in those with severely prolonged corrected sinus node recovery time than in patients with syncope whose corrected sinus node recovery time is normal.[371]

Refractoriness. Refractoriness of the sinus node[323, 372] and the atria[373, 374] is prolonged in patients with sick sinus syndrome, particularly in those who also have atrial fibrillation or flutter.[373] During sinus rhythm, the duration and dispersion of refractoriness are greater in patients with sick sinus syndrome and atrial arrhythmias than in healthy persons or those with atrial arrhythmias and no sick sinus syndrome.[373] Refractoriness in the donor heart is not abnormal in patients who develop sick sinus syndrome after cardiac transplantation.[360]

Excitability. The atria are characteristically inexcitable during atrial standstill, and electrical stimulation cannot capture atria that have this arrhythmia.[55, 233, 237, 247, 291, 375]

Atrial electrograms. These electrograms are abnormally prolonged or fragmented in patients with sick

---

[s]Sinoatrial conduction is also prolonged in patients with severe stenosis proximal to the origin of the sinus nodal artery even in the absence of sick sinus syndrome.[345]

[t]Atropine may render abnormal the sinus node recovery time in some patients with sick sinus syndrome whose sinus node recovery time without the drug is normal.[349]

[u]Entrance block into the sinoatrial node can be demonstrated by electrophysiological testing.[368]

Table 16.5   MEAN SINOATRIAL CONDUCTION TIME (MILLISECONDS) IN ADULTS AND CHILDREN WITH AND WITHOUT SICK SINUS SYNDROME

	Normal		Sick Sinus Syndrome	
	No. of Patients	*Sinoatrial Conduction Time*	*No. of Patients*	*Sinoatrial Conduction Time*
28 adults[316]	16	87	12	135
27 children[325]	21	67	6	138

sinus syndrome.[376] Furthermore, the electrograms are more prolonged and fractionated in patients with both sick sinus syndrome and paroxysmal atrial fibrillation than in those without arrhythmia or with only paroxysmal atrial fibrillation.[377] One can record most abnormal electrograms from the high right atrium in patients with sick sinus syndrome and no tachyarrhythmias, but in those who also have paroxysmal atrial fibrillation, abnormal electrograms can be detected from other locations in that chamber.[378]

Sustained atrial fibrillation can be induced more easily in patients with sick sinus syndrome who have, than in those who do not have, abnormal atrial electrograms. These patients also have[379]

- Abnormally long duration of the P waves.
- Abnormally long duration of conduction within and between the atria.
- Greater sinus node dysfunction.

Patients with sick sinus syndrome who can be induced into atrial fibrillation respond to single atrial extrastimuli with repetitive atrial firing and fragmented atrial electrograms.[380]

Duration of sinus node depolarization. This parameter, which can be measured from sinus node electrograms, probably reflects both local action potentials and conduction within the node.[381] Severe sinus node dysfunction is likely if the duration of sinus node depolarization exceeds 200 milliseconds and is unlikely if the duration is less than 150 milliseconds.[381]

Effects of age. As patients with sick sinus syndrome age, intrinsic corrected sinus node recovery time and intrinsic sinoatrial conduction time increase.[382] However, basic heart rate, the rate with autonomic function intact, basic corrected sinus node recovery time, and basic sinoatrial conduction time in these patients do not change with age.[382]

Intrinsic Versus Extrinsic Abnormalities of Sinus Function

To learn whether sinus arrhythmias are caused by intrinsic disease of the sinus node or by the external effects of the autonomic nervous system, investigators block the autonomic system by administering atropine (0.04 milligram/kilogram) to eliminate parasympathetic influence and propranolol (0.2 milligram/kilogram) to block beta-adrenergic sympathetic effects. This produces the "intrinsic heart rate." All the electrophysiological measurements of intrinsic sinus nodal function in both normal patients and those with sick sinus syndrome lengthen progressively with age, whereas extrinsic function does not correlate with age.[383]

In patients with normal intrinsic function, autonomic blockade shortens corrected sinus node recovery time and sinoatrial conduction time,[384] and when bradyarrhythmias are due to external effects, the corrected sinus node recovery time and intrinsic heart rates are normal.[187, 363] Accordingly, these measure-

ments are normal in most patients with ventricular asystole due to obstructive sleep apnea[194] because the "sick sinus syndrome" in these patients is extrinsic and is due to autonomic tone.

Autonomic blockade reveals that intrinsic abnormalities of sinoatrial nodal function account for the bradyarrhythmias of most cases of sick sinus syndrome.[384v] Thus, such patients have prolonged corrected sinus node recovery time after autonomic blockade[187, 363, 384] and abnormal intrinsic heart rates.[363] However, the autonomic nervous system seems to play a major role in the genesis of sick sinus syndrome when the syndrome develops in children and young adults after surgical correction of congenital heart disease.[135] Autonomic activity, rather than intrinsic disease of the sinoatrial node, primarily influences sinoatrial conduction time.[384, 385]

Associated Electrophysiological Findings

Atrioventricular block. Although no electrocardiographic abnormality may be found, atrioventricular conduction, when evaluated electrophysiologically, is prolonged in as many as half the patients with sick sinus syndrome[165, 225, 359, 386, 387] or sinus bradycardia.[388] Conversely, many patients with bifascicular and trifascicular conduction disease have electrophysiological abnormalities of sinus nodal function.[389] These findings support the thesis that sick sinus syndrome, in many patients, is but one manifestation of a general pathological process involving many cardiac tissues with electrophysiological properties.[387, 390]

Patients presenting with sick sinus syndrome who have severe, infranodal conduction defects are the ones most likely to develop clinical atrioventricular block later.[260] However, high-grade atrioventricular block does not usually follow when conduction abnormalities are limited to the atrioventricular node.[260] Antiarrhythmic drugs account for much of the atrioventricular block that develops in those patients whose atrioventricular conduction is intact when sick sinus syndrome is first diagnosed.[391]

Retrograde ventriculoatrial conduction. This form of conduction, which can occur when patients with sick sinus syndrome have ventricular (VVI) pacemakers and normal antegrade atrioventricular conduction,[392] accounts, in part, for the increased incidence of atrial fibrillation in these patients when compared with those who have atrial (AAI) or atrioventricular (DDD) pacers.[264] In contrast, atrial fibrillation develops infrequently in patients with ventricular pacers inserted for atrioventricular block, in whom retrograde conduction is usually absent.[264]

Escape foci. Clinical observation and the results from rapid atrial pacing demonstrate that the escape foci in the bundle of His and ventricles that protect the heart from asystole frequently discharge abnormally late in patients with the sick sinus syndrome.[356, 387]

---

[v] Seventy-six percent according to one study.[384]

This accounts for the long periods of asystole that often characterize the disease and produce syncope and other troublesome symptoms (see Figs. 16.5 to 16.8).

Supernormal conduction. The greater the atrial conduction defects, the less frequently supernormal conduction occurs in the atria of patients with sick sinus syndrome.[393]

Wolff-Parkinson-White syndrome. Sinoatrial conduction is frequently prolonged in patients with Wolff-Parkinson-White syndrome and supraventricular tachycardia.[331] The reasons for this finding are unknown.

Effects of Drugs

Among their other effects, some drugs shorten and some prolong sinus node recovery time in patients with sick sinus syndrome[210, 394–404] (Table 16.6).

Atropine. This drug increases the heart rate in patients with sick sinus syndrome,[210, 225, 395, 405] as it does in healthy persons. Reports differ on whether atropine significantly affects sinoatrial conduction time in patients with sick sinus syndrome.[395, 405]

Digitalis. The potential side effects of digitalis do not necessarily prohibit its use in appropriate doses in patients with sick sinus syndrome.[398]

Isoproterenol. The expected increase in heart rate is less in patients with sick sinus syndrome and syncope given isoproterenol than in patients without syncope or in normal subjects.[406]

Lidocaine. This drug further increases corrected sinus node recovery time in some patients with sick sinus syndrome.[407]

Procainamide. This drug can prolong asystole, particularly after tachyarrhythmias, in patients with sick sinus syndrome.[400]

Propranolol. This drug increases the sinoatrial conduction time and decreases, sometime markedly and

dangerously, the heart rate of patients with sick sinus syndrome.[95, 408]

Sympatholytic agents. Agents such as methyldopa, clonidine, and guanethidine can precipitate severe bradycardia in patients with sick sinus syndrome.[408]

Theophylline.[409] This drug speeds the heart rate[403, 410, 411] and decreases the sinoatrial conduction time in young patients with symptomatic bradycardia and sinus arrest.[403]

Verapamil. This drug can prolong asystole in patients with sick sinus syndrome.[396] Thus, the drug should not be given to treat tachyarrhythmias in patients with the bradycardia-tachycardia syndrome who do not have pacemakers.

TREATMENT
Drugs

No drugs satisfactorily treat the chronic bradyarrhythmias of sick sinus syndrome.[203, 412w] A few drugs, however, can relieve the acute effects of severe bradyarrhythmia.

Atropine. Given intravenously, atropine increases the heart rate in most patients with sick sinus syndrome,[210, 395, 405] but it seldom raises the rate to as much as 90 beats per minute.[210, 405, 412]

Aminophylline. An antagonist of adenosine, aminophylline does not improve sinus nodal function.[413]

Theophylline. This drug suppresses sinus pauses, sinus bradycardia, and associated symptoms in some patients with sick sinus syndrome.[403, 410, 411] The drug has a similar effect on the symptoms produced by bradycardia during rejection of transplanted hearts.[414]

Anticoagulation. This treatment should be prescribed for all suitable patients with the bradycardia-tachycardia syndrome, whether or not they have pacemakers, because of the high incidence of thromboembolic disease in this group.[201, 202, 415]

Pacing[416–422x]

Pacing is the most effective means of treating the symptoms caused by the bradyarrhythmias of sick sinus syndrome.[28, 33–35, 37, 39, 50, 117, 130, 161, 213, 222, 253, 411, 423–434] Atrial (AAI) and atrioventricular (DDD) pacers are the preferred pacing modes for patients with sick sinus syn-

Table 16.6	**EFFECT OF DRUGS ON SINUS NODE RECOVERY TIME IN PATIENTS WITH SICK SINUS SYNDROME**

Drug	Sinus Node Recovery Time
Atropine	↓ [210, 395]
Digitalis	↓ [394, 398]
	↑ [404]
Disopyramide	↑ [399]
Flecainide	↑ [402]
Lidocaine	↓ [397]
Procainamide	↑ [400]
Quinidine	No effect[401]
Theophylline	↓ [403]
Verapamil	↑ [396]

<hr/>

[w]For treatment of the tachyarrhythmias, see the relevant chapters of this book.

[x]Dr. Bernard Lown, who coined the name "sick sinus syndrome," writes: "I regret the name, for the inference that others draw from it is that sick sinus syndrome automatically means implantation of a pacemaker, which I believe is unwarranted for many. One should let atrial fibrillation resume and thereby obviate that mechanical assist."[21]

drome in the absence of a chronic atrial arrhythmia.[145, 199, 259, 261, 262, 265, 280, 411, 424, 435–453] Dual-chamber pacing often improves the health-related quality of life more than does ventricular pacing[452] and is more cost-effective in patients with sick sinus syndrome.[448]

Atrial rate–responsive (AAIR) pacing responds to physiological requirements better than atrial inhibited (AAI) pacing,[454] although clinically, AAIR pacing adds little to the good effects of atrial inhibited pacing.[455] When atrial fibrillation prevents atrial sensing, dual-chamber rate adaptive (DDDR) pacers convert to physiologic ventricular (VVIR) pacing.[456]

Indications[457] (Table 16.7).[y] Pacing should be instituted in patients with sick sinus syndrome as soon as one has established that

- The symptoms are disabling or dangerous.
- The arrhythmias produce the symptoms; sinoatrial pauses of greater than 2 seconds, for example, may alarm the observer but produce no symptoms.[249]
- The arrhythmias are chronic and are not due to temporary hypervagotonia or drugs that may be discontinued.

Patients who develop escape rhythms throughout the period of postoperative hospitalization after cardiac transplantation and those with persistent postoperative heart rates of less than 70 beats per minute often need permanent pacing,[140] but those with mild abnormalities of sinus node function who are in sinus rhythms when discharged can usually be followed without pacemaker treatment.[458] No single factor reliably

---

[y]The American College of Cardiology/American Heart Association Task Force on Practice Guidelines (Committee on Pacemaker Implantation) has published (1998) guidelines for permanent cardiac pacemaking in patients with sick sinus syndrome, which I have summarized in Table 16.7.[457]

| Table 16.7 | PERMANENT PACING FOR PATIENTS WITH SINUS NODE DYSFUNCTION (SICK SINUS SYNDROME)[457] |

Indicated (Class I)[457]
    Sinus node dysfunction with documented symptomatic bradycardia, including frequent sinus pauses that produce symptoms
    Symptomatic chronotropic incompetence
Probably indicated (Class IIa)
    Sinus node dysfunction occurring spontaneously or because of necessary drug therapy with heart rate less than 40 beats per minute without documented correlation between symptoms and bradycardia
Possibly indicated (Class IIb)
    Heart rate consistently less than 30 beats per minute in awake, minimally symptomatic patients
Not indicated and possibly harmful (Class III)
    Asymptomatic sinus node dysfunction
    Sinus node dysfunction in patients with symptoms suggesting bradycardia unassociated with a slow heart rate
    Sinus node dysfunction with symptomatic bradycardia due to nonessential drug therapy

(Adapted from Gregoratos G, Cheitlin MD, Conill A, et al. ACC/AHA guidelines for implantation of cardiac pacemakers and antiarrhythmia devices [Committee on Pacemaker Implantation]. Circulation 1998; 97:1325–1335. By permission of the American Heart Association, Inc.)

predicts which patients with transplanted hearts will require permanent pacing.[140]

Atrial or atrioventricular pacing. When the atria are paced, the hemodynamic advantages of atrioventricular synchrony can be preserved, and the complications of retrograde ventriculoatrial conduction can be avoided.[z] The principal risk of atrial (AAI) pacing is asystole should atrioventricular block develop. Atrioventricular (DDD) pacing avoids this complication.

Atrial fibrillation.[459] This arrhythmia recurs less often or becomes chronic less frequently when patients with sick sinus syndrome receive atrial or atrioventricular pacing rather than ventricular pacing.[41, 162, 261, 264, 265, 439, 442, 446, 460–463] This advantage of atrial pacing affects only those patients who have paroxysmal atrial fibrillation *before* receiving the pacemaker,[162] but it applies whether or not they have atrioventricular block.[460] The pacing mode, however, is only one, and not necessarily the most important, factor determining which patients with sick sinus syndrome will develop atrial fibrillation.[162]

Stroke and thromboembolism. These conditions occur less often in patients with sick sinus syndrome when atrial or atrioventricular rather than ventricular pacing is used.[162, 261, 437, 442, 446, 462aa]

Congestive heart failure. Most,[41, 265, 453] but not all,[464] workers report that ventricular pacing, more than atrial pacing, favors the development of congestive heart failure and increases the cardiothoracic ratio on radiographs[442, 462] in patients with sick sinus syndrome.

Ventricular pacing. Ventricular (VVI), unlike atrial (AAI), pacing ensures an adequate ventricular rhythm in those relatively infrequent[263, 264, 438] occasions when clinical atrioventricular block develops in patients with sick sinus syndrome,[259] but at the cost of

- Atrial fibrillation.
- Emboli.
- Congestive failure.[41]
- Left ventricular performance.[465bb]

Atrioventricular (DDD) pacing reduces the likelihood of all these complications.

Chronic Atrial Fibrillation

The spontaneous development of persistent atrial fibrillation eliminates the symptoms of bradycardia in

---

[z]The hemodynamic consequences of the different types of pacing are discussed in Chapter 15.
[aa]1.6% with atrial pacing versus 13% with ventricular pacing during a period of 2½ years, according to a review of the literature published in 1986.[261]
[bb]Echocardiographic studies reveal that long-term ventricular pacing in patients with sick sinus syndrome increases left ventricular end-systolic dimension and permanently reduces left ventricular ejection fraction.[465] In the left atrium, VVI pacing decreases fractional shortening and increases diastolic dimension.[465]

patients with the sick sinus syndrome so long as high-grade atrioventricular block is not present.[200, 208, 391] However, because most of these patients have already received pacemakers, a therapeutic decision arises only when one must consider whether to replace a depleted or malfunctioning electrode or impulse generator.

PROGNOSIS[466]

Once pacemaking has been established, the prognosis for patients with isolated sick sinus syndrome is indistinguishable from that for the general population.[467, 468] Coexisting disease accounts for the excess mortality.[40, 160, 213, 469]

General mortality,[265, 463, 470] cardiac mortality,[442, 460] and death from stroke[460] are lower in patients with sick sinus syndrome who have atrial (AAI) or atrioventricular (DDD) than in those with ventricular (VVI) pacers. In all patients with sick sinus syndrome, survival at 5 years is better for those with atrial pacing who have no structural heart disease or coronary heart disease than for those with other forms of cardiac pathology.[461]

Factors present when pacemakers are implanted in patients with sick sinus syndrome that predict a poorer prognosis include

- Advanced age.[432, 471]
- Bradycardia-tachycardia syndrome rather than sinus bradycardia alone.[432]
- Congestive heart failure.[432, 471]
- Continuing symptoms.[40, 472]
- Coronary heart disease.[471]
- Hypertension.[471]

The life expectancy for paced patients with sick sinus syndrome exceeds that for paced patients with atrioventricular block,[473] even in those who are severely symptomatic.[466] The excess mortality for patients with atrioventricular block is related to age, pacing mode, and underlying heart disease.[473]

SUMMARY

Sick sinus syndrome encompasses those bradyarrhythmias due to malfunction of the sinus node that produce troubling or disabling symptoms. Many patients with sick sinus syndrome also have supraventricular tachyarrhythmias (bradycardia-tachycardia syndrome) and dysfunction of the normal escape mechanisms.

Although sick sinus syndrome affects a few children and young adults, it occurs with the greatest frequency in the sixth and seventh decades of life. Males and females are equally affected. Sick sinus syndrome is usually an acquired condition, but a few cases have a genetic basis.

Patients with sick sinus syndrome most often have coronary heart disease; a few have cardiomyopathy. Many, however, have no structural heart disease. Among children, cardiac surgery to repair congenital lesions, most frequently the Mustard procedure for transposition of the great arteries, produces most of the cases of sick sinus syndrome. Some adults develop

sick sinus syndrome from surgical closure of atrial septal defect. Sick sinus syndrome also appears in the donor heart of some patients after cardiac transplantation and occasionally after the Maze operation for atrial fibrillation. The function of the sinus node may be so affected by a long period of chronic atrial fibrillation that an adequate sinus rhythm may not appear following cardioversion. Vagotonia can transiently produce the bradyarrhythmias of sick sinus syndrome. Stroke and embolism are important complications of the bradycardia-tachycardia syndrome but not of sick sinus syndrome without tachyarrhythmias.

Bradyarrhythmias cause lightheadedness, dizziness, and fainting, the principal complaints of patients with sick sinus syndrome. Abnormal neural responses, rather than bradyarrhythmias alone, however, contribute to much of the syncope that affects many patients with sick sinus syndrome. Palpitations suggest that the patient has the bradycardia-tachycardia syndrome.

The standard or extended ambulatory electrocardiograms of patients with sick sinus syndrome characteristically show sinus bradycardia, sinoatrial block, sinus pauses, sinus arrest, or atrial standstill. Atrioventricular block may appear at the onset of sick sinus syndrome or may develop later in the course of the disease. The most common sustained tachyarrhythmia of patients with the bradycardia-tachycardia syndrome is atrial fibrillation. Sick sinus syndrome limits the heart rate that patients can achieve when exercising.

Sick sinus syndrome is associated with several pathological abnormalities in the atria and sinus nodes. However, the coronary arteries supplying these areas are infrequently occluded in patients with sick sinus syndrome.

On electrophysiological evaluation, sinoatrial conduction time, sinus node recovery time, and refractoriness of the sinus node and atria are characteristically prolonged. Atrial electrograms are prolonged and fractionated in many patients with sick sinus syndrome and particularly in those with atrial fibrillation. Electrophysiological studies show nonclinical atrioventricular conduction disease in many patients with sick sinus syndrome. However, only those with severe abnormalities are likely to develop atrioventricular block in the future.

Pacing is the most successful treatment for the symptoms produced by the bradyarrhythmias of sick sinus syndrome. However, one must be certain that the arrhythmias produce the symptoms before prescribing a pacemaker. When compared with ventricular pacing, atrial or atrioventricular pacing reduces the incidence of atrial fibrillation, stroke, and possibly congestive heart failure. Atrioventricular pacing also protects against the development of atrioventricular block and, consequently, has become the preferred pacing mode for most patients.

Use of appropriate pacemakers makes the prognosis of patients with sick sinus syndrome and no structural heart disease indistinguishable from the otherwise healthy general population. Coexisting disease accounts for any excess mortality. Patients who receive atrial or atrioventricular rather than ventricular pacers survive longer.

REFERENCES

1. Benditt DG, Remole SC. Sick sinus syndrome. In Kastor JA (ed). Arrhythmias. Philadelphia: WB Saunders, 1994; pp. 225–249.
2. Ferrer MI. The sick sinus syndrome in atrial disease. JAMA 1968; 206:645–646.
3. Lloyd-Mostyn RH, Kidner PH, Oram S. Sinu-atrial disorder including the brady-tachycardia syndrome: a review with addition of 11 cases. Q J Med 1973; 42:41–57.
4. Ferrer MI. The sick sinus syndrome. Circulation 1973; 47:635–641.
5. Goldreyer BN. Sinus node dysfunction: a physiologic consideration of arrhythmias involving the sinus node. Cardiovasc Clin 1974; 6:179–198.
6. Moss AJ, Davis RJ. Brady-tachy syndrome. Prog Cardiovasc Dis 1974; 16:439–454.
7. Scarpa WJ. The sick sinus syndrome. Am Heart J 1976; 92:648–660.
8. Ferrer MI. The sick sinus syndrome: its status after ten years. Chest 1977; 72:554–555.
9. Jordan JL, Yamaguchi I, Mandel WJ. The sick sinus syndrome. JAMA 1977; 237:682–684.
10. Bower PJ. Sick sinus syndrome. Arch Intern Med 1978; 138:133–137.
11. Kaplan BM. Sick sinus syndrome. Arch Intern Med 1978; 138:28.
12. Bigger JT Jr, Reiffel JA. Sick sinus syndrome. Annu Rev Med 1979; 30:91–118.
13. Ferrer MI. The primary pacemaker: functions, falterings, fate, and false alarms. Chest 1979; 75:376–379.
14. Ferrer MI. The etiology and natural history of sinus node disorders. Arch Intern Med 1982; 142:371–372.
15. Alpert MA, Flaker GC. Arrhythmias associated with sinus node dysfunction: pathogenesis, recognition, and management. JAMA 1983; 250:2160–2166.
16. Karagueuzian HS, Jordan JL, Sugi K, et al. Appropriate diagnostic studies for sinus node dysfunction. Pacing Clin Electrophysiol 1985; 8:242–254.
17. Kugler JD. Sinus node dysfunction. In Gillette PC, Garson A Jr (eds). Pediatric Arrhythmias. Electrophysiology and Pacing. Philadelphia: WB Saunders, 1990; pp. 250–300.
18. Josephson ME. Sinus node function. In Josephson ME (ed). Clinical Cardiac Electrophysiology. Techniques and Interpretations. 2nd ed. Philadelphia: Lea & Febiger, 1993; pp. 71–95.
19. Reiffel JA. Normal sinus rhythm and its variants (sinus arrhythmia, sinus tachycardia, sinus bradycardia), sinus node reentry, and sinus node dysfunction (sick sinus syndrome): mechanisms, recognition, and management. In Podrid PJ, Kowey PR (eds). Cardiac Arrhythmia. Mechanisms, Diagnosis and Management. Baltimore: Williams & Wilkins, 1995; pp. 752–767.
20. Lown B. Electrical reversion of cardiac arrhythmias. Br Heart J 1967; 29:469–489.
21. Lown B. Personal communication; 1997.
22. Ferrer MI. The natural history of the sick sinus syndrome. J Chron Dis 1972; 25:313–315.
23. Ginks WR. Lazy sinus syndrome. Proc R Soc Med 1970; 63:1307–1308.
24. Eraut D, Shaw DB. Sinus bradycardia. Br Heart J 1971; 33:742–749.
25. Tabatznik B, Mower MM, Samson EB, Prempree A. Syncope in the "sluggish sinus node syndrome." Circulation 1969; 39 and 40(Suppl III):III-200.
26. Kaplan BM, Langendorf R, Lev M, Pick A. Tachycardia-bradycardia syndrome (so-called "sick sinus syndrome"): pathology, mechanisms and treatment. Am J Cardiol 1973; 31:497–508.
27. Short DS. The syndrome of alternating bradycardia and tachycardia. Br Heart J 1954; 16:208–214.
28. Kay R, Estioko M, Wiener I. Primary sick sinus syndrome as an indication for chronic pacemaker therapy in young adults: incidence, clinical features, and long-term evaluation. Am Heart J 1982; 103:338–342.
29. Feruglio GA, Rickards AF, Steinbach K, Feldman S, Parsonnet V. Cardiac pacing in the world: a survey of the state of the art in 1986. PACE 1987; 10:768–777.
30. Parsonnet V, Bernstein AD, Galasso D. Cardiac pacing practices in the United States in 1985. Am J Cardiol 1988; 62:71–77.
31. Bernstein AD, Parsonnet V. Survey of cardiac pacing in the United States in 1989. Am J Cardiol 1992; 69:331–338.
32. Bernstein AD, Parsonnet V. Survey of cardiac pacing and defibrillation in the United States in 1993. Am J Cardiol 1996; 78:187–196.
33. Kulbertus HE, de Leval-Rutten F, Demoulin JC. Sino-atrial disease: a report on 13 cases. J Electrocardiol 1973; 6:303–312.
34. Easley RM Jr, Goldstein S. Sino-atrial syncope. Am J Med 1971; 50:166–177.
35. Rubenstein JJ, Schulman CL, Yurchak PM, DeSanctis RW. Clinical spectrum of the sick sinus syndrome. Circulation 1972; 46:5–13.
36. Sigurd B, Jensen G, Meibom J, Sandoe E. Adams-Stokes syndrome caused by sinoatrial block. Br Heart J 1973; 35:1002–1008.
37. Hartel G, Talvensaari T. Treatment of sinoatrial syndrome with permanent cardiac pacing in 90 patients. Acta Med Scand 1975; 198:341–347.
38. Gould L, Reddy CV, Becker WH. The sick sinus syndrome: a study of 50 cases. J Electrocardiol 1978; 11:11–14.
39. Kaul TK, Kumar EB, Thomson RM, Bain WH. Sinoatrial disorders, the "sick sinus" syndrome: experience with implanted cardiac pacemakers. J Cardiovasc Surg 1978; 19:261–266.
40. van Hemel NM, Schaepkens van Riempst AL, Bakema H, Swenne CA. Long-term follow-up after pacemaker implantation in sick sinus syndrome. Pacing Clin Electrophysiol 1981; 4:8–13.
41. Rosenqvist M, Brandt J, Schuller H. Atrial versus ventricular pacing in sinus node disease: a treatment comparison study. Am Heart J 1986; 111:292–297.
42. Brandt J, Anderson H, Fahraeus T, Schuller H. Natural history of sinus node disease treated with atrial pacing in 213 patients: implications for selection of stimulation mode. J Am Coll Cardiol 1992; 20:633–639.
43. Sgarbossa EB, Pinski SL, Maloney JD. The role of pacing modality in determining long-term survival in the sick sinus syndrome. Ann Intern Med 1993; 119:359–365.
44. Ikeme AC, D'Arbela PG, Somers K. The sick-sinus syndrome in Africans. Am Heart J 1975; 89:295–300.
45. Lister JW, Gosselin AJ, Swaye PS. Obscure syncope and the sick sinus syndrome. Pacing Clin Electrophysiol 1978; 1:68–79.
46. Yabek SM, Jarmakani JM. Sinus node dysfunction in children, adolescents, and young adults. Pediatrics 1978; 61:593–598.
47. Albin G, Hayes DL, Holmes DR Jr. Sinus node dysfunction in pediatric and young adult patients: treatment by implantation of a permanent pacemaker in 39 cases. Mayo Clin Proc 1985; 60:667–672.
48. Onat A, Domanic N, Onat T. Sick sinus syndrome in an infant: severe disturbance of impulse formation and conduction involving the S-A node and the A-V junctional tissue. Eur J Cardiol 1974; 2:79–83.
49. Stopfkuchen H, Jungst BK. Congenital sinus bradycardia combined with congenital total atrioventricular block. Eur J Pediatr 1977; 125:219–224.
50. Conde CA, Leppo J, Lipski J, et al. Effectiveness of pacemaker treatment in the bradycardia-tachycardia syndrome. Am J Cardiol 1973; 32:209–214.
51. Gulotta SJ, Gupta RD, Padmanabhan VT, Morrison J. Familial occurrence of sinus bradycardia, short PR interval,

intraventricular conduction defects, recurrent supraventricular tachycardia, and cardiomegaly. Am Heart J 1977; 93:19–29.

52. Bacos JM, Eagan JT, Orgain ES. Congenital familial nodal rhythm. Circulation 1960; 22:887–895.

53. Khorsandian RS, Moghadam AN, Muller OF. Familial congenital A-V dissociation. Am J Cardiol 1964; 14:118–124.

54. Wagner CW Jr, Hall RJ. Congenital familial atrioventricular dissociation: report of three siblings. Am J Cardiol 1967; 19:593–596.

55. Allensworth DC, Rice GJ, Lowe GW. Persistent atrial standstill in a family with myocardial disease. Am J Med 1969; 47:775–784.

56. Harrison WH Jr, Derrick JR. Atrial standstill: a review, and presentation of two new cases of familial and unusual nature with reference to epicardial pacing in one. Angiology 1969; 20:610–617.

57. Spellberg RD. Familial sinus node disease. Chest 1971; 60:246–251.

58. Livesley B, Catley PF, Oram S. Familial sinuatrial disorder. Br Heart J 1972; 34:668–670.

59. Gambetta M, Weese J, Ginsburg M, Shapiro D. Sick sinus syndrome in a patient with familial PR prolongation. Chest 1973; 64:520–523.

60. Caralis DG, Varghese PJ. Familial sinoatrial node dysfunction: increased vagal tone a possible aetiology. Br Heart J 1976; 38:951–956.

61. Nordenberg A, Varghese PJ, Nugent EW. Spectrum of sinus node dysfunction in two siblings. Am Heart J 1976; 91:507–512.

62. Lehmann H, Klein UE. Familial sinus node dysfunction with autosomal dominant inheritance. Br Heart J 1978; 40:1314–1316.

63. Mackintosh AF, Chamberlain DA. Sinus node disease affecting both parents and both children. Eur J Cardiol 1979; 10:117–122.

64. Tan AT, EE BK, Mah PK, Choo MH, Chia BL. Diffuse conduction abnormalities in an adolescent with familial sinus node disease. Pacing Clin Electrophysiol 1981; 4:645–649.

65. Barak M, Herschkowitz S, Shapiro I, Roguin N. Familial combined sinus node and atrioventricular conduction dysfunctions. Int J Cardiol 1987; 15:231–239.

66. Lorber A, Maisuls E, Palant A. Autosomal dominant inheritance of sinus node disease. Int J Cardiol 1987; 15:252–256.

67. Maeda S, Tanaka T, Hayashi T. Familial atrial standstill caused by amyloidosis. Br Heart J 1988; 59:498–500.

68. Surawicz B, Hariman RJ. Follow-up of the family with congenital absence of sinus rhythm. Am J Cardiol 1988; 61:467–469.

69. Rosenfeld LE. Bradyarrhythmias, abnormalities of conduction, and indications for pacing in acute myocardial infarction. Cardiol Clin 1988; 6:49–61.

70. Lippestad CT, Marton PF. Sinus arrest in proximal right coronary artery occlusion. Am Heart J 1967; 74:551–556.

71. Rokseth R, Hatle L. Sinus arrest in acute myocardial infarction. Br Heart J 1971; 33:639.

72. Kyriakidis M, Barbetseas J, Antonopoulos A, Skouros C, Tentolouris C, Toutouzas P. Early atrial arrhythmias in acute myocardial infarction: role of the sinus node artery. Chest 1992; 101:944–947.

73. Hatle L, Bathen J, Rokseth R. Sinoatrial disease in acute myocardial infarction: long-term prognosis. Br Heart J 1976; 38:410–414.

74. Parameswaran R, Ohe T, Goldberg H. Sinus node dysfunction in acute myocardial infarction. Br Heart J 1976; 38:93–96.

75. Nogami A, Adachi S, Nitta J, et al. Arrhythmogenic right ventricular dysplasia with sick sinus syndrome and atrioventricular conduction disturbance. Jpn Heart J 1990; 31:417–423.

76. Caponnetto S, Pastorini C, Tirelli G. Persistent atrial standstill in a patient affected with facioscapulohumeral dystrophy. Cardiology 1968; 53:341–350.

77. Baldwin BJ, Talley RC, Johnson C, Nutter DO. Permanent paralysis of the atrium in a patient with facioscapulohumeral muscular dystrophy. Am J Cardiol 1973; 31:649–653.

78. Fairfax AJ, Lambert CD. Neurological aspects of sinoatrial heart block. J Neurol Neurosurg Psychiatry 1976; 39:576–580.

79. Perloff JK. Neurological disorders and heart disease. In Braunwald E (ed). Heart Disease. A Textbook of Cardiovascular Medicine. 5th ed. Philadelphia: WB Saunders, 1997; pp. 1865–1886.

80. Antonio JH, Diniz MC, Miranda D. Persistent atrial standstill with limb girdle muscular dystrophy. Cardiology 1978; 63:39–46.

81. Woolliscroft J, Tuna N. Permanent atrial standstill: the clinical spectrum. Am J Cardiol 1982; 49:2037–2041.

82. Bigger JT Jr, Sahar DI. Clinical types of proarrhythmic response to antiarrhythmic drugs. Am J Cardiol 1987; 59:2E–9E.

83. Greenwood RJ, Finkelstein D, Monheit R. Sinoatrial heart block with Wenckebach phenomenon. Am J Cardiol 1961; 8:140–146.

84. Castellanos A, Lemberg L, Brown JP, Berkovits BV. An electrical digitalis tolerance test. Am J Med Sci 1967; 254:717–726.

85. Goldschlager AW, Karliner JS. Ventricular standstill after intravenous diphenylhydantoin. Am Heart J 1967; 74:410–412.

86. Lippestad CT, Forfang K. Production of sinus arrest by lignocaine. Br Med J 1971; 1:537.

87. Wood RA. Sinoatrial arrest: an interaction between phenytoin and lignocaine. Br Med J 1971; 1:645.

88. Grayzel J, Angeles J. Sino-atrial block in man provoked by quinidine. J Electrocardiol 1972; 5:289–294.

89. Jeresaty RM, Kahn AH, Landry AB Jr. Sinoatrial arrest due to lidocaine in a patient receiving quinidine. Chest 1972; 61:683–685.

90. Cheng TO, Wadhwa K. Sinus standstill following intravenous lidocaine administration. JAMA 1973; 223:790–792.

91. Parameswaran R, Kahn D, Monheit R, Goldberg H. Sinus bradycardia due to lidocaine: clinical-electrophysiologic correlations. J Electrocardiol 1974; 7:75–78.

92. Klein HO, Jutrin I, Kaplinsky E. Cerebral and cardiac toxicity of a small dose of lignocaine. Br Heart J 1975; 37:775–778.

93. Margolis JR, Strauss HC, Miller HC, Gilbert M, Wallace AG. Digitalis and the sick sinus syndrome: clinical and electrophysiologic documentation of severe toxic effect on sinus node function. Circulation 1975; 52:162–169.

94. Wellens HJJ, Cats VM, Duren DR. Symptomatic sinus node abnormalities following lithium carbonate therapy. Am J Med 1975; 59:285–287.

95. Strauss HC, Gilbert M, Svenson RH, Miller HC, Wallace AG. Electrophysiologic effects of propranolol on sinus node function in patients with sinus node dysfunction. Circulation 1976; 54:452–459.

96. Wilson JR, Kraus ES, Bailas MM, Rakita L. Reversible sinus-node abnormalities due to lithium carbonate therapy. N Engl J Med 1976; 294:1223–1224.

97. Zoneraich S, Zoneraich O, Siegel J. Sudden death following intravenous sodium diphenylhydantoin. Am Heart J 1976; 91:375–377.

98. Cohen IS, Jick H, Cohen SI. Adverse reactions to quinidine in hospitalized patients: findings based on data from the Boston Collaborative Drug Surveillance Program. Prog Cardiovasc Dis 1977; 20:151–163.

99. de Faire U, Lundman T. Attempted suicide with verapamil. Eur J Cardiol 1977; 6:195–198.

100. Keidar S, Grenadier E, Palant A. Sinoatrial arrest due to lidocaine injection in sick sinus syndrome during amiodarone administration. Am Heart J 1982; 104:1384–1385.

101. McGovern B, Garan H, Ruskin JN. Sinus arrest during treatment with amiodarone. Br Med J 1982; 284:160–161.

102. Montalescot G, Levy Y, Farge D, et al. Lithium causing a serious sinus-node dysfunction at therapeutic doses. Clin Cardiol 1984; 7:617–620.

103. Strasberg B, Davidson E, Berand M. Amiodarone-induced sinoatrial block. Int J Cardiol 1985; 8:214–216.

104. Veltri EP, Reid PR. Sinus arrest with intravenous amiodarone. Am J Cardiol 1986; 58:1110–1111.

105. Hoffmann A, Kappenberger L, Jost M, Burckhardt D. Effect of amiodarone on sinus node function in patients with sick sinus syndrome. Clin Cardiol 1987; 10:451–452.

106. Schwartz E, Friedman E, Mouallem M, Farfel Z. Sinus arrest associated with clonidine therapy. Clin Cardiol 1988; 11:53–54.
107. Gould LA, Betzu R, Vacek T, Muller R, Pradeep V, Downs L. Sinoatrial block due to tocainide. Am Heart J 1989; 118:851–853.
108. Rosenqvist M, Bergfeldt L, Aili H, Mathe AA. Sinus node dysfunction during long-term lithium treatment. Br Heart J 1993; 70:371–375.
109. Andrivet P, Beasly V, Kiger JP, vu Gnoc C. Complete sinus arrest during diltiazem therapy: clinical correlates and efficacy of intravenous calcium. Eur Heart J 1994; 15:350–354.
110. Pfammatter JP, Paul T, Lehmann C, Kallfelz HC. Efficacy and proarrhythmia of oral sotalol in pediatric patients. J Am Coll Cardiol 1995; 26:1002–1007.
111. Stevenson WG, Klitzner T, Perloff JK. Electrophysiologic abnormalities. Natural occurrence and postoperative residua and sequelae. In Perloff JK, Child JS (eds). Congenital Heart Disease in Adults. Philadelphia: WB Saunders, 1991; pp. 259–295.
112. Perry JC, Garson A. Arrhythmias following surgery for congenital heart disease. In Zipes DP, Jalife J (eds). Cardiac Electrophysiology. From Cell to Bedside. 2nd ed. Philadelphia: WB Saunders, 1995; pp. 838–848.
113. el-Said G, Rosenberg HS, Mullins CE, Hallman GL, Cooley DA, McNamara DG. Dysrhythmias after Mustard's operation for transposition of the great arteries. Am J Cardiol 1972; 30:526–532.
114. Greenwood RD, Rosenthal A, Sloss LJ, LaCorte M, Nadas AS. Sick sinus syndrome after surgery for congenital heart disease. Circulation 1975; 52:208–213.
115. Niederhauser H, Simonin P, Friedli B. Sinus node function and conduction system after complete repair of tetralogy of Fallot. Circulation 1975; 52:214–220.
116. Lewis AB, Lindesmith GG, Takahashi M, et al. Cardiac rhythm following the Mustard procedure for transposition of the great vessels. J Thorac Cardiovasc Surg 1977; 73:919–926.
117. Schiller MS, Levin AR, Haft JI, Engle MA, Ehlers KH, Klein AA. Electrophysiologic studies in sick sinus syndrome following surgery for D-transposition of the great arteries. J Pediatr 1977; 91:891–896.
118. Yabek SM, Swensson RE, Jarmakani JM. Electrocardiographic recognition of sinus node dysfunction in children and young adults. Circulation 1977; 56:235–239.
119. Egloff LP, Freed MD, Dick M, Norwood WI, Castaneda AR. Early and late results with the Mustard operation in infancy. Ann Thorac Surg 1978; 26:474–484.
120. Saalouke MG, Rios J, Perry LW, Shapiro SR, Scott LP. Electrophysiologic studies after Mustard's operation for D-transposition of the great vessels. Am J Cardiol 1978; 41:1104–1109.
121. Fox K, Evans T, Rowland E, Krikler D. "Bradycardia-tachycardia" syndrome 8 yr after correction of Fallot's tetralogy. Eur J Cardiol 1979; 10:109–115.
122. Gillette PC, Kugler JD, Garson A Jr, Gutgesell HP, Duff DF, McNamara DG. Mechanisms of cardiac arrhythmias after the Mustard operation for transposition of the great arteries. Am J Cardiol 1980; 45:1225–1230.
123. Southall DP, Keeton BR, Leanage R, et al. Cardiac rhythm and conduction before and after Mustard's operation for complete transposition of the great arteries. Br Heart J 1980; 43:21–30.
124. Bink-Boelkens MT, Velvis H, van der Heide JJ, Eygelaar A, Hardjowijono RA. Dysrhythmias after atrial surgery in children. Am Heart J 1983; 106:125–130.
125. Beerman LB, Neches WH, Fricker FJ, et al. Arrhythmias in transposition of the great arteries after the Mustard operation. Am J Cardiol 1983; 51:1530–1534.
126. Flinn CJ, Wolff GS, Dick M II, et al. Cardiac rhythm after the Mustard operation for complete transposition of the great arteries. N Engl J Med 1984; 310:1635–1638.
127. Ashraf MH, Cotroneo J, DiMarco D, Subramanian S. Fate of long-term survivors of Mustard procedure (inflow repair) for simple and complex transposition of the great arteries. Ann Thorac Surg 1986; 42:385–389.

128. Byrum CJ, Bove EL, Sondheimer HM, Kavey RE, Blackman MS. Hemodynamic and electrophysiologic results of the Senning procedure for transposition of the great arteries. Am J Cardiol 1986; 58:138–142.
129. Hayes CJ, Gersony WM. Arrhythmias after the Mustard operation for transposition of the great arteries: a long-term study. J Am Coll Cardiol 1986; 7:133–137.
130. Vince DJ, Tyers GF, Kerr CR. Transvenous atrial pacing in the management of sick sinus syndrome following surgical treatment of the univentricular heart: case report and review. Pacing Clin Electrophysiol 1986; 9:441–448.
131. Warnes CA, Somerville J. Transposition of the great arteries: late results in adolescents and adults after the Mustard procedure. Br Heart J 1987; 58:148–155.
132. Deanfield J, Camm J, Macartney F, et al. Arrhythmia and late mortality after Mustard and Senning operation for transposition of the great arteries. J Thorac Cardiovasc Surg 1988; 96:569–576.
133. Turina M, Siebenmann R, Nussbaumer P, Senning A. Long-term outlook after atrial correction of transposition of great arteries. J Thorac Cardiovasc Surg 1988; 95:828–835.
134. Kurer CC, Tanner CS, Vetter VL. Electrophysiologic findings after Fontan repair of functional single ventricle. J Am Coll Cardiol 1991; 17:174–181.
135. Marcus B, Gillette PC, Garson A Jr. Electrophysiologic evaluation of sinus node dysfunction in postoperative children and young adults utilizing combined autonomic blockade. Clin Cardiol 1991; 14:33–40.
136. Roos-Hesselink J, Perlroth MG, McGhie J, Spitaels S. Atrial arrhythmias in adults after repair of tetralogy of Fallot: correlations with clinical, exercise, and echocardiographic findings. Circulation 1995; 91:2214–2219.
137. Gardiner HM, Dhillon R, Bull C, de Leval MR, Deanfield JE. Prospective study of the incidence and determinants of arrhythmia after total cavopulmonary connection. Circulation 1996; 94(Suppl II):II-17–II-21.
138. Ohnishi S, Kasanuki H, Takamizawa K, Takao A, Hirosawa K. Long-term management of bradyarrhythmias following open heart surgery: surgical A-V block and sick sinus syndrome after surgery for secundum atrial septal defects treated with permanent cardiac pacing. Jpn Circ J 1986; 50:903–917.
139. Goyal SL, Lichestein E, Gupta PK, Chadda KD, Lajam F. Sick sinus syndrome requiring permanent pacemaker implantation in a patient with mirror-image dextrocardia. Chest 1976; 69:558–561.
140. Heinz G, Hirschl M, Buxbaum P, Laufer G, Gasic S, Laczkovics A. Sinus node dysfunction after orthotopic cardiac transplantation: postoperative incidence and long-term implications. Pacing Clin Electrophysiol 1992; 15:731–737.
141. Schroeder JS, Berke DK, Graham AF, Rider AK, Harrison DC. Arrhythmias after cardiac transplantation. Am J Cardiol 1974; 33:604–607.
142. Mackintosh AF, Carmichael DJ, Wren C, Cory-Pearce R, English TA. Sinus node function in first three weeks after cardiac transplantation. Br Heart J 1982; 48:584–588.
143. Romhilt DW, Doyle M, Sagar KB, et al. Prevalence and significance of arrhythmias in long-term survivors of cardiac transplantation. Circulation 1982; 66:1219–1222.
144. Bexton RS, Nathan AW, Camm AJ. Unusual sinus node response curves in two cardiac transplant recipients. Pacing Clin Electrophysiol 1986; 9:223–230.
145. Loria K, Salinger M, McDonough T, Frohlich T, Arentzen C. Activitrax AAIR pacing for sinus node dysfunction after orthotopic heart transplantation: an initial report. J Heart Transplant 1988; 7:380–384.
146. Zmyslinski RW, Warner MG, Diethrich EB. Symptomatic sinus node dysfunction after heart transplantation. Pacing Clin Electrophysiol 1988; 11:445–448.
147. Heinz G, Ohner T, Laufer G, Gasic S, Laczkovics A. Clinical and electrophysiologic correlates of sinus node dysfunction after orthotopic heart transplantation: observations in 42 patients. Chest 1990; 97:890–895.
148. Jacquet L, Ziady G, Stein K, et al. Cardiac rhythm disturbances early after orthotopic heart transplantation: prevalence and clinical importance of the observed abnormalities. J Am Coll Cardiol 1990; 16:832–837.

149. Miyamoto Y, Curtiss EI, Kormos RL, Armitage JM, Hardesty RL, Griffith BP. Bradyarrhythmia after heart transplantation: incidence, time course, and outcome. Circulation 1990; 82:313–317.
150. DiBiase A, Tse TM, Schnittger I, Wexler L, Stinson EB, Valantine HA. Frequency and mechanism of bradycardia in cardiac transplant recipients and need for pacemakers. Am J Cardiol 1991; 67:1385–1389.
151. Heinz G, Ohner T, Laufer G, Gossinger H, Gasic S, Laczkovics A. Demographic and perioperative factors associated with initial and prolonged sinus node dysfunction after orthotopic heart transplantation: the impact of ischemic time. Transplantation 1991; 51:1217–1224.
152. Heinz G, Kratochwill C, Schmid S, et al. Sinus node dysfunction after orthotopic heart transplantation: the Vienna experience 1987–1993. Pacing Clin Electrophysiol 1994; 17:2057–2063.
153. Cox JL, Boineau JP, Schuessler RB, Kater KM, Lappas DG. Five-year experience with the Maze procedure for atrial fibrillation. Ann Thorac Surg 1993; 56:814–823.
154. Cox JL, Jaquiss RD, Schuessler RB, Boineau JP. Modification of the Maze procedure for atrial flutter and atrial fibrillation. II. Surgical technique of the Maze III procedure. J Thorac Cardiovasc Surg 1995; 110:485–495.
155. Lemberg L, Castellanos A, Swenson J, Gosselin A. Arrhythmias related to cardioversion. Circulation 1964; 30:163–170.
156. Kleiger R, Lown B. Cardioversion and digitalis. II. Clinical studies. Circulation 1966; 33:878–887.
157. Kastor JA, DeSanctis RW. The electrical conversion of atrial fibrillation. Am J Med Sci 1967; 253:511–519.
158. Bjerkelund C, Orning OM. An evaluation of DC shock treatment of atrial arrhythmias. Acta Med Scand 1968; 184:481–491.
159. Paulk EA Jr, Hurst JW. Clinical problems of cardioversion. Am Heart J 1965; 70:248–274.
160. Boal BH, Kleinfeld MJ. A study of patients with the sick sinus syndrome with long-term survival. J Chronic Dis 1978; 31:501–505.
161. Breivik K, Ohm OJ, Segadal L. Sick sinus syndrome treated with permanent pacemaker in 109 patients: a follow-up study. Acta Med Scand 1979; 206:153–159.
162. Sgarbossa EB, Pinski SL, Maloney JD, et al. Chronic atrial fibrillation and stroke in paced patients with sick sinus syndrome: relevance of clinical characteristics and pacing modalities. Circulation 1993; 88:1045–1053.
163. Young D, Eisenberg RE. Symptomatic sinus arrest in a young girl. Arch Dis Child 1977; 52:331–334.
164. Scott O, Macartney FJ, Deverall PB. Sick sinus syndrome in children. Arch Dis Child 1976; 51:100–105.
165. Beder SD, Gillette PC, Garson A Jr, Porter CB, McNamara DG. Symptomatic sick sinus syndrome in children and adolescents as the only manifestation of cardiac abnormality or associated with unoperated congenital heart disease. Am J Cardiol 1983; 51:1133–1136.
166. Lee JK, Lewis JA. Myxoedema with complete A-V block and Adams-Stokes disease abolished with thyroid medication. Br Heart J 1962; 24:253–256.
167. Wan SH, Lee GS, Toh CC. The sick sinus syndrome: a study of 15 cases. Br Heart J 1972; 34:942–952.
168. Kramer MR, Shilo S, Hershko C. Atrioventricular and sinoatrial block in thyrotoxic crisis. Br Heart J 1985; 54:600–602.
169. Nakagawa S, Higa A, Kondoh H, Koiwaya Y, Tanaka K. Cyclic sinus node dysfunction in a patient with hyperthyroidism. Arch Intern Med 1985; 145:2126–2127.
170. Talley JD, Wathen MS, Hurst JW. Hyperthyroid-induced atrial flutter-fibrillation with profound sinoatrial nodal pauses due to small doses of digoxin, verapamil, and propranolol. Clin Cardiol 1989; 12:45–47.
171. Metzger AL, Goldbarg AN, Hunter RL. Sick sinus node syndrome as the presenting manifestation of reticulum cell sarcoma. Chest 1971; 60:602–604.
172. Desai JM, Scheinman MM, Strauss HC, Massie B, O'Young J. Electrophysiologic effects on combined autonomic blockade

173. James AH, Oxon DM. Cardiac syncope after swallowing. Lancet 1958; 1:771–772.
174. Kong Y, Heyman A, Entman ML, McIntosh HD. Glossopharyngeal neuralgia associated with bradycardia, syncope, and seizures. Circulation 1964; 30:109–113.
175. Kopald HH, Roth HP, Fleshler B, Pritchard WH. Vagovagal syncope: report of a case associated with diffuse esophageal spasm. N Engl J Med 1964; 271:1238–1241.
176. Khero BA, Mullins CB. Cardiac syncope due to glossopharyngeal neuralgia: treatment with a transvenous pacemaker. Arch Intern Med 1971; 128:806–808.
177. Tolman KG, Ashworth WD. Syncope induced by dysphagia: correction by esophageal dilatation. Am J Dig Dis 1971; 16:1026–1031.
178. Levin B, Posner JB. Swallow syncope: report of a case and review of the literature. Neurology 1972; 22:1086–1093.
179. Wik B, Hillestad L. Deglutition syncope. BMJ 1975; 3:747.
180. Tilkian AG, Guilleminault C, Schroeder JS, Lehrman KL, Simmons FB, Dement WC. Sleep-induced apnea syndrome: prevalence of cardiac arrhythmias and their reversal after tracheostomy. Am J Med 1977; 63:348–358.
181. Rasmussen V, Haunso S, Skagen K. Cerebral attacks due to excessive vagal tone in heavily trained persons: a clinical and electrophysiologic study. Acta Med Scand 1978; 204:401–405.
182. Shaw TR, Corrall RJ, Craib IA. Cardiac and respiratory standstill during sleep. Br Heart J 1978; 40:1055–1058.
183. Thormann J, Schwarz F, Ensslen R, Sesto M. Vagal tone, significance of electrophysiologic findings and clinical course in symptomatic sinus node dysfunction. Am Heart J 1978; 95:725–731.
184. Miller WP. Cardiac arrhythmias and conduction disturbances in the sleep apnea syndrome: prevalence and significance. Am J Med 1982; 73:317–321.
185. Zwillich C, Devlin T, White D, Douglas N, Weil J, Martin R. Bradycardia during sleep apnea: characteristics and mechanism. J Clin Invest 1982; 69:1286–1292.
186. Guilleminault C, Connolly SJ, Winkle RA. Cardiac arrhythmia and conduction disturbances during sleep in 400 patients with sleep apnea syndrome. Am J Cardiol 1983; 52:490–494.
187. Szatmary L, Czako E, Solti F, Szabo Z. Autonomic sinus node dysfunction and its treatment. Acta Cardiol 1984; 39:209–220.
188. Gang ES, Oseran DS, Mandel WJ, Peter T. Sinus node electrogram in patients with the hypersensitive carotid sinus syndrome. J Am Coll Cardiol 1985; 5:1484–1490.
189. Otsuka K, Sadakane N, Ozawa T. Arrhythmogenic properties of disordered breathing during sleep in patients with cardiovascular disorders. Clin Cardiol 1987; 10:771–782.
190. Peiser J, Ovnat A, Uwyyed K, Lavie P, Charuzi I. Cardiac arrhythmias during sleep in morbidly obese sleep-apneic patients before and after gastric bypass surgery. Clin Cardiol 1985; 8:519–521.
191. Golf S, Forfang K. Congenital swallowing-induced symptomatic heart block: a case report of a probably hereditary disorder. Pacing Clin Electrophysiol 1986; 9:602–605.
192. Strasberg B, Sclarovsky S, Arditti A, Lewin RF, Agmon J. Deep inspiration induced sinus arrest: an unusual manifestation in a patient with the sick sinus syndrome. J Electrocardiol 1986; 19:91–92.
193. Flemons WW, Remmers JE, Gillis AM. Sleep apnea and cardiac arrhythmias: is there a relationship? Am Rev Respir Dis 1993; 148:618–621.
194. Grimm W, Hoffmann J, Menz V, et al. Electrophysiologic evaluation of sinus node function and atrioventricular conduction in patients with prolonged ventricular asystole during obstructive sleep apnea. Am J Cardiol 1996; 77:1310–1314.
195. Antonelli D, Rosenfeld T. Deglutition syncope associated with carotid sinus hypersensitivity. Pacing Clin Electrophysiol 1997; 20:2282–2283.
196. Santinelli V, Chiariello M, Clarizia M, Condorelli M. Sick sinus syndrome: the role of hypervagotonia. Int J Cardiol 1984; 5:532–535.

in patients with sinus node disease. Circulation 1981; 63:953–960.

197. Alt E, Lehmann G. Stroke and atrial fibrillation in sick sinus syndrome. Heart 1997; 77:495–497.
198. Samarasinghe HH, Senanyake N. Permanent neurological deficits complicating sinoatrial block. Br Heart J 1973; 35:503–506.
199. Radford DJ, Julian DG. Sick sinus syndrome: experience of a cardiac pacemaker clinic. BMJ 1974; 3:504–507.
200. Krishnaswami V, Geraci AR. Permanent pacing in disorders of sinus node function. Am Heart J 1975; 89:579–585.
201. Fairfax AJ, Lambert CD, Leatham A. Systemic embolism in chronic sinoatrial disorder. N Engl J Med 1976; 295:190–192.
202. Bathen J, Sparr S, Rokseth R. Embolism in sinoatrial disease. Acta Med Scand 1978; 203:7–11.
203. Rokseth R, Hatle L. Prospective study on the occurrence and management of chronic sinoatrial disease, with follow-up. Br Heart J 1974; 36:582–587.
204. Wu DL, Yeh SJ, Lin FC, Wang CC, Cherng WJ. Sinus automaticity and sinoatrial conduction in severe symptomatic sick sinus syndrome. J Am Coll Cardiol 1992; 19:355–364.
205. Brignole M, Menozzi C, Bottoni N, et al. Mechanisms of syncope caused by transient bradycardia and the diagnostic value of electrophysiologic testing and cardiovascular reflexivity maneuvers. Am J Cardiol 1995; 76:273–278.
206. Hilgard J, Ezri MD, Denes P. Significance of ventricular pauses of three seconds or more detected on twenty-four-hour Holter recordings. Am J Cardiol 1985; 55:1005–1008.
207. Fujii J, Takahashi N, Kato K. The bradycardia-tachycardia syndrome. Treatment with cardiac drugs and adrenal corticosteroid. Jpn Heart J 1973; 14:414–431.
208. Vera Z, Mason DT, Awan NA, et al. Improvement of symptoms in patients with sick sinus syndrome by spontaneous development of stable atrial fibrillation. Br Heart J 1977; 39:160–167.
209. Marmor BM, Black MM. Unusual manifestations of severe sick sinus syndrome. Am Heart J 1980; 100:95–98.
210. Mandel WJ, Hayakawa H, Allen HN, Danzig R, Kermaier AI. Assessment of sinus node function in patients with the sick sinus syndrome. Circulation 1972; 46:761–769.
211. Bhandari S, Talwar KK, Kaul U, Bhatia ML. Value of physical and pharmacological tests in predicting intrinsic and extrinsic sick sinus syndrome. Int J Cardiol 1986; 12:203–212.
212. Schweitzer P, Mark H. The values and limitations of deductive analysis and electrophysiological testing in patients with sinoatrial arrhythmias. Pacing Clin Electrophysiol 1984; 7:403–420.
213. Aroesty JM, Cohen SI, Morkin E. Bradycardia-tachycardia syndrome: results in twenty-eight patients treated by combined pharmacologic therapy and pacemaker implantation. Chest 1974; 66:257–263.
214. Abbott JA, Hirschfeld DS, Kunkel FW, Scheinman MM, Modin G. Graded exercise testing in patients with sinus node dysfunction. Am J Med 1977; 62:330–338.
215. Holden W, McAnulty JH, Rahimtoola SH. Characterisation of heart rate response to exercise in the sick sinus syndrome. Br Heart J 1978; 40:923–930.
216. Johnston FA, Robinson JF, Fyfe T. Exercise testing in the diagnosis of sick sinus syndrome in the elderly: implications for treatment. Pacing Clin Electrophysiol 1987; 10:831–838.
217. Hattori M, Toyama J, Ito A, et al. Comparative evaluation of depressed automaticity in sick sinus syndrome by Holter monitoring and overdrive suppression test. Am Heart J 1983; 105:587–592.
218. Brodsky M, Wu D, Denes P, Kanakis C, Rosen KM. Arrhythmias documented by 24-hour continuous electro-cardiographic monitoring in 50 male medical students without apparent heart disease. Am J Cardiol 1977; 39:390–395.
219. Romano M, Clarizia M, Onofrio E, et al. Heart rate, PR, and QT intervals in normal children: a 24-hour Holter monitoring study. Clin Cardiol 1988; 11:839–842.
220. Agruss NS, Rosin EY, Adolph RJ, Fowler NO. Significance of chronic sinus bradycardia in elderly people. Circulation 1972; 46:924–930.
221. Burchfield RI, Menefee EE, Bryant GDN. Disease of the sinoatrial node associated with bradycardia, asystole, syncope, and paroxysmal atrial fibrillation. Circulation 1957; 16:20–26.
222. Chokshi DS, Mascarenhas E, Samet P, Center S. Treatment of sinoatrial rhythm disturbances with permanent cardiac pacing. Am J Cardiol 1973; 32:215–220.
223. Dighton DH. Sinus bradycardia: autonomic influences and clinical assessment. Br Heart J 1974; 36:791–797.
224. Lipski J, Cohen L, Espinoza J, Motro M, Dack S, Donoso E. Value of Holter monitoring in assessing cardiac arrhythmias in symptomatic patients. Am J Cardiol 1976; 37:102–107.
225. Strauss HC, Bigger JT Jr, Saroff AL, Giardina EG. Electrophysiologic evaluation of sinus node function in patients with sinus node dysfunction. Circulation 1976; 53:763–776.
226. Lichstein E, Aithal H, Jonas S, et al. Natural history of severe sinus bradycardia discovered by 24 hour Holter monitoring. Pacing Clin Electrophysiol 1982; 5:185–189.
227. Yeh SJ, Lin FC, Wu D. Complete sinoatrial block in two patients with bradycardia-tachycardia syndrome. J Am Coll Cardiol 1987; 9:1184–1188.
228. Ector H, Rolies L, De Geest H. Dynamic electrocardiography and ventricular pauses of 3 seconds and more: etiology and therapeutic implications. Pacing Clin Electrophysiol 1983; 6:548–551.
229. Lien WP, Lee YS, Chang FZ, Lee SY, Chen CM, Tsai HC. The sick sinus syndrome: natural history of dysfunction of the sinoatrial node. Chest 1977; 72:628–634.
230. Bashour TT, Chen F, Feeney J. Ischemic sinus node hibernation: resolution following angioplasty. Am Heart J 1991; 122:1156–1158.
231. Wada M, Takada C, Mise J. A case report of atrial standstill. Jpn Circ J 1966; 30:543–553.
232. Messinger WJ, Mirkinson AM. Permanent atrial standstill: eight-year observation of a patient. Arch Intern Med 1969; 124:211–214.
233. Patton RD, Damato AN, Berkowitz WD, Lau SH, Stein E. The electrically silent right atrium. J Electrocardiol 1970; 30:239–243.
234. Combs DT, Bellaci HF, Shively HH, Gregoratos G. Persistent atrial standstill. Am J Med 1974; 56:231–236.
235. Benchimol CB, Schlesinger P, Ginefra P, Barbosa S, Saad EA, Benchimol AB. Persistent atrial standstill. Acta Cardiol 1975; 30:313–322.
236. Kurokawa A, Kurita A, Kasai G, Kimura E. Persistent atrial standstill: report of three cases. J Electrocardiol 1975; 8:357–362.
237. Tanaka H, Atsuchi Y, Tanaka N, Nishi S, Kanehisa T. Persistent atrial standstill due to atrial inexcitability: an electrophysiological and histological study. Jpn Heart J 1975; 16:639–653.
238. Harris CL, Baldwin BJ. Permanent atrial paralysis. J Electrocardiol 1976; 9:81–84.
239. Amram SS, Vagueiro MC, Pimenta A, Machado HB. Persistent atrial standstill with atrial inexcitability. Pacing Clin Electrophysiol 1978; 1:80–89.
240. Csapo G, Weisswange A, Kalusche D, Schnellbacher K. Partial atrial standstill in sick sinus syndrome; intraatrial and AV nodal block with short PR interval. Eur J Cardiol 1978; 8:617–627.
241. Effendy FN, Bolognesi R, Bianchi G, Visioli O. Alternation of partial and total atrial standstill. J Electrocardiol 1979; 12:121–127.
242. Hover AR, Koppes GM. Atrial standstill and complete heart block in systemic lupus erythematosus. Chest 1979; 76:230–231.
243. Kanemoto N, Uchiyama F, Sasamoto H, et al. A case of persistent atrial standstill. Eur J Cardiol 1979; 9:175–180.
244. Levy S, Pouget B, Bemurat M, Lacaze JC, Clementy J, Bricaud H. Partial atrial electrical standstill: report of three cases and review of clinical and electrophysiological features. Eur Heart J 1980; 1:107–116.
245. Ward DE, Ho SY, Shinebourne EA. Familial atrial standstill and inexcitability in childhood. Am J Cardiol 1984; 53:965–967.
246. Wohlgelernter D, Otis CN, Batsford WP, Cabin HS. Myocarditis presenting with "silent" atrium and left atrial thrombus. Am Heart J 1984; 108:1557–1558.

247. Talwar KK, Dev V, Chopra P, Dave TH, Radhakrishnan S. Persistent atrial standstill: clinical, electrophysiological, and morphological study. Pacing Clin Electrophysiol 1991; 14:1274–1280.

248. Nakazato Y, Nakata Y, Hisaoka T, Sumiyoshi M, Ogura S, Yamaguchi H. Clinical and electrophysiological characteristics of atrial standstill. Pacing Clin Electrophysiol 1995; 18:1244–1254.

249. Mazuz M, Friedman HS. Significance of prolonged electrocardiographic pauses in sinoatrial disease: sick sinus syndrome. Am J Cardiol 1983; 52:485–489.

250. Scherf D. The mechanism of sinoatrial block. Am J Cardiol 1969; 23:769–770.

251. Muller OF, Finkelstein D. Adams-Stokes syndrome due to sinoatrial block. Am J Cardiol 1966; 17:433–436.

252. Rasmussen K. Chronic sinoatrial heart block. Am Heart J 1971; 81:39–47.

253. Obel IW, Cohen E, Millar RN. Chronic symptomatic sinoatrial block: a review of 34 patients and their treatment. Chest 1974; 65:397–402.

254. Dighton DH. Sinoatrial block. Autonomic influences and clinical assessment. Br Heart J 1975; 37:321–325.

255. Yeh SJ, Yamamoto T, Lin FC, Wang CC, Wu D. Repetitive sinoatrial exit block as the major mechanism of drug-provoked long sinus or atrial pause. J Am Coll Cardiol 1991; 18:587–595.

256. Schamroth L, Dove E. The Wenckebach phenomenon in sino-atrial block. Br Heart J 1966; 28:350–358.

257. Rowland E, Morgado F. Sino-atrial node dysfunction, atrioventricular block and intraventricular conduction disturbances. Eur Heart J 1992; 13:130–135.

258. Frey WG III, Grant JL. Chronic binodal block with Wenckebach phenomenon. J Electrocardiol 1975; 8:363–368.

259. Bertholet M, Demoulin JC, Fourny J, Kulbertus H. Natural evolution of atrioventricular conduction in patients with sick sinus syndrome treated by atrial demand pacing: a study of 26 cases. Acta Cardiol 1983; 38:227–232.

260. Rosenqvist M, Vallin H, Edhag O. Clinical and electro-physiologic course of sinus node disease: five-year follow-up study. Am Heart J 1985; 109:513–22.

261. Sutton R, Kenny RA. The natural history of sick sinus syndrome. Pacing Clin Electrophysiol 1986; 9:1110–1114.

262. Kallryd A, Kruse I, Ryden L. Atrial inhibited pacing in the sick sinus node syndrome: clinical value and the demand for rate responsiveness. Pacing Clin Electrophysiol 1989; 12:954–961.

263. Lemke B, Holtmann BJ, Selbach H, Barmeyer J. The atrial pacemaker: retrospective analysis of complications and life expectancy in patients with sinus node dysfunction. Int J Cardiology 1989; 22:185–193.

264. Grimm W, Langenfeld H, Maisch B, Kochsiek K. Symptoms, cardiovascular risk profile and spontaneous ECG in paced patients: a five-year follow-up study. Pacing Clin Electrophysiol 1990; 13:2086–2090.

265. Rosenqvist M, Brandt J, Schuller H. Long-term pacing in sinus node disease: effects of stimulation mode on cardiovascular morbidity and mortality. Am Heart J 1988; 116:16–22.

266. Bradlow BA. Supraventricular paroxysmal tachycardia interrupted by repeated episodes of total cardiac standstill with syncopal attacks. Chest 1970; 58:122–128.

267. Kreiner G, Frey B, Gossinger HD. Atrioventricular nodal reentry tachycardia in patients with sinus node dysfunction: electrophysiologic characteristics, clinical presentation, and results of slow pathway ablation. J Cardiovasc Electrophysiol 1998; 9:470–478.

268. Sung RJ. Can alteration of dual atrioventricular nodal pathway physiology be related to sinus node dysfunction? J Cardiovasc Electrophysiol 1998; 9:479–480.

269. Gomes JA, Kang PS, Matheson M, Gough WB Jr, el-Sherif N. Coexistence of sick sinus rhythm and atrial flutter-fibrillation. Circulation 1981; 63:80–86.

270. Liu Z, Hayano M, Hirata T, et al. Abnormalities of electrocardiographic P wave morphology and their relation to electrophysiological parameters of the atrium in patients with sick sinus syndrome. PACE 1998; 21:79–86.

271. Reiffel JA, Bigger JT Jr, Cramer M, Reid DS. Ability of Holter electrocardiographic recording and atrial stimulation to detect sinus nodal dysfunction in symptomatic and asymptomatic patients with sinus bradycardia. Am J Cardiol 1977; 40:189–194.

272. Boudoulas H, Schaal SF, Lewis RP, Robinson JL. Superiority of 24-hour outpatient monitoring over multi-stage exercise testing for the evaluation of syncope. J Electrocardiol 1979; 12:103–108.

273. Van Durme JP. Tachyarrhythmias and transient cerebral ischemic attacks. Am Heart J 1975; 89:538–540.

274. Grodman RS, Capone RJ, Most AS. Arrhythmia surveillance by transtelephonic monitoring: comparison with Holter monitoring in symptomatic ambulatory patients. Am Heart J 1979; 98:459–464.

275. Abdon NJ. Frequency and distribution of long-term ECG-recorded cardiac arrhythmias in an elderly population: with special reference to neurological symptoms. Acta Med Scand 1981; 209:175–183.

276. Crook BR, Cashman PM, Stott FD, Raftery EB. Tape monitoring of the electrocardiogram in ambulant patients with sinoatrial disease. Br Heart J 1973; 35:1009–1013.

277. Szatmary LJ. Autonomic blockade and sick sinus syndrome: new concept in the interpretation of electrophysiological and Holter data. Eur Heart J 1984; 5:637–648.

278. Alboni P, degli Uberti E, Codeca L, et al. Circadian variations of sinus rate in subjects with sinus node dysfunction. Chronobiologia 1982; 9:173–183.

279. Vera Z, Mason DT. Detection of sinus node dysfunction: consideration of clinical application of testing methods. Am Heart J 1981; 102:308–312.

280. Mitsuoka T, Kenny RA, Yeung TA, Chan SL, Perrins JE, Sutton R. Benefits of dual chamber pacing in sick sinus syndrome. Br Heart J 1988; 60:338–347.

281. Yamada T, Fukunami M, Kumagai K, et al. Detection of patients with sick sinus syndrome by use of low amplitude potentials early in filtered P wave. J Am Coll Cardiol 1996; 28:738–744.

282. Brignole M, Menozzi C, Gianfranchi L, Oddone D, Lolli G, Bertulla A. Neurally mediated syncope detected by carotid sinus massage and head-up tilt test in sick sinus syndrome. Am J Cardiol 1991; 68:1032–1036.

283. Shaw DB. The etiology of sino-atrial disorder (sick sinus syndrome). Am Heart J 1976; 92:539–540.

284. Rossi L. Histopathologic correlates of atrial arrhythmias. In Touboul P, Waldo AL (eds). Atrial Arrhythmias. Current Concepts and Management. St. Louis: Mosby–Year Book, 1990; pp. 27–40.

285. Evans R, Shaw DB. Pathological studies in sinoatrial disorder (sick sinus syndrome). Br Heart J 1977; 39:778–786.

286. Demoulin JC, Kulbertus HE. Histopathological correlates of sinoatrial disease. Br Heart J 1978; 40:1384–1389.

287. Balsaver AM, Morales AR, Whitehouse FW. Fat infiltration of myocardium as a cause of cardiac conduction defect. Am J Cardiol 1967; 19:261–265.

288. Bharati S, Nordenberg A, Bauernfiend R, et al. The anatomic substrate for the sick sinus syndrome in adolescence. Am J Cardiol 1980; 46:163–172.

289. Bharati S, Lev M. The pathologic changes in the conduction system beyond the age of ninety. Am Heart J 1992; 124:486–496.

290. Thery C, Gosselin B, Lekieffre J, Warembourg H. Pathology of sinoatrial node: correlations with electrocardiographic findings in 111 patients. Am Heart J 1977; 93:735–740.

291. Rosen KM, Rahimtoola SH, Gunnar RM, Lev M. Transient and persistent atrial standstill with His bundle lesions: electrophysiologic and pathologic correlations. Circulation 1971; 44:220–236.

292. Engel TR, Meister SG, Feitosa GS, Fischer HA, Frankl WS. Appraisal of sinus node artery disease. Circulation 1975; 52:286–291.

293. Shaw DB, Linker NJ, Heaver PA, Evans R. Chronic sinoatrial disorder (sick sinus syndrome): a possible result of cardiac ischaemia. Br Heart J 1987; 58:598–607.

294. Alboni P, Baggioni GF, Scarfo S, et al. Role of sinus node

artery disease in sick sinus syndrome in inferior wall acute myocardial infarction. Am J Cardiol 1991; 67:1180–1184.

295. Tung KS, James TN, Effler DB, McCormack LJ. Injury of the sinus node in open-heart operations. J Thorac Cardiovasc Surg 1967; 53:814–829.

296. James TN, Birk RE. Pathology of the cardiac conduction system in polyarteritis nodosa. Arch Intern Med 1966; 117:561–567.

297. Maisch B, Lotze U, Schneider J, Kochsiek K. Antibodies to human sinus node in sick sinus syndrome. Pacing Clin Electrophysiol 1986; 9:1101–1109.

298. Kozakewich HP, McManus BM, Vawter GF. The sinus node in sudden infant death syndrome. Circulation 1982; 65:1242–1246.

299. Mandel WJ, Laks MM, Obayashi K. Sinus node function; evaluation in patients with and without sinus node disease. Arch Intern Med 1975; 135:388–394.

300. Reiffel JA, Bigger JT Jr, Giardina EG. "Paradoxical" prolongation of sinus nodal recovery time after atropine in the sick sinus syndrome. Am J Cardiol 1975; 36:98–104.

301. Talano JV, Euler D, Randall WC, Eshaghy B, Loeb HS, Gunnar RM. Sinus node dysfunction: an overview with emphasis on autonomic and pharmacologic consideration. Am J Med 1978; 64:773–781.

302. Reiffel JA. Principles and applications of electrophysiologic testing of sinus node function. Cardiovasc Med 1979; January:97–111.

303. Scheinman MM, Strauss HC, Abbott JA. Electrophysiologic testing for patients with sinus node dysfunction. J Electrocardiol 1979; 12:211–216.

304. Wiener I. Current applications of clinical electrophysiologic study in the diagnosis and treatment of cardiac arrhythmias. Am J Cardiol 1982; 49:1287–1292.

305. Tonkin AM, Heddle WF. Electrophysiological testing of sinus node function. Pacing Clin Electrophysiol 1984; 7:735–748.

306. Reiffel JA. Electrophysiologic evaluation of sinus node function. Cardiol Clin 1986; 4:401–416.

307. Benditt DG, Gornick CC, Dunbar D, Almquist A, Pool-Schneider S. Indications for electrophysiologic testing in the diagnosis and assessment of sinus node dysfunction. Circulation 1987; 75(Suppl III):III-93–III-102.

308. Yee R, Strauss HC. Electrophysiologic mechanisms: sinus node dysfunction. Circulation 1987; 75:12–18.

309. Benditt DG, Sakaguchi S, Goldstein MA, Lurie KG, Gornick CC, Adler SW. Sinus node dysfunction: pathophysiology, clinical features, evaluation, and treatment. In Zipes DP, Jalife J (eds). Cardiac Electrophysiology. From Cell to Bedside. 2nd ed. Philadelphia: WB Saunders, 1995; pp. 1215–1247.

310. Reiffel JA, Bigger JT Jr. Current status of direct recordings of the sinus node electrogram in man. Pacing Clin Electrophysiol 1983; 6:1143–1150.

311. De Marneffe M, Gregoire JM, Waterschoot P, Kestemont MP. The sinus node function: normal and pathological. Eur Heart J 1993; 14:649–654.

312. Jewell GM, Magorien RD, Schaal SF, Leier CV. Autonomic tone of patients during an electrophysiological catheterization: the role of autonomic influences on the reproducibility of sinus node function studies. Am Heart J 1980; 99:51–57.

313. Hariman RJ, Krongrad E, Boxer RA, Weiss MB, Steeg CN, Hoffman BF. Method for recording electrical activity of the sinoatrial node and automatic atrial foci during cardiac catheterization in human subjects. Am J Cardiol 1980; 45:775–781.

314. Reiffel JA, Gang E, Gliklich J, et al. The human sinus node electrogram: a transvenous catheter technique and a comparison of directly measured and indirectly estimated sinoatrial conduction time in adults. Circulation 1980; 62:1324–1334.

315. Rakovec P, Jakopin J, Rode P, Kenda MF, Horvat M. Clinical comparison of indirectly and directly determined sinoatrial conduction time. Am Heart J 1981; 102:292–294.

316. Gomes JA, Kang PS, el-Sherif N. The sinus node electrogram in patients with and without sick sinus syndrome: techniques and correlation between directly measured and indirectly

estimated sinoatrial conduction time. Circulation 1982; 66:864–873.

317. Asseman P, Berzin B, Desry D, et al. Persistent sinus nodal electrograms during abnormally prolonged postpacing atrial pauses in sick sinus syndrome in humans: sinoatrial block vs overdrive suppression. Circulation 1983; 68:33–41.

318. Juillard A, Guillerm F, Chuong HV, Barrillon A, Gerbaux A. Sinus node electrogram recording in 59 patients: comparison with simultaneous estimation of sinoatrial conduction using premature atrial stimulation. Br Heart J 1983; 50:75–84.

319. Gomes JA, Hariman RI, Chowdry IA. New application of direct sinus node recordings in man: assessment of sinus node recovery time. Circulation 1984; 70:663–671.

320. Bethge C, Gebhardt-Seehausen U, Mullges W. The human sinus nodal electrogram: techniques and clinical results of intra-atrial recordings in patients with and without sick sinus syndrome. Am Heart J 1986; 112:1074–1082.

321. Zhang DL, Chen SL. A simple modified technique for recording sinus node electrogram. Cathet Cardiovasc Diagn 1988; 15:64–65.

322. Asseman P, Berzin B, Desry D, et al. Postextrasystolic sinoatrial exit block in human sick sinus syndrome: demonstration by direct recording of sinus node electrograms. Am Heart J 1991; 122:1633–1643.

323. Kerr CR. Effect of pacing cycle length and autonomic blockade on sinus node refractoriness. Am J Cardiol 1988; 62:1192–1196.

324. Young ML, Atkins DL. Correlation between directly measured and indirectly estimated sinoatrial conduction time in children. Am J Cardiol 1988; 62:1197–1201.

325. Zhang DL, Chen SL, Xi YA, Zhou XN. Recording of the electrocardiogram from the sinus node and direct measurement of the sinuatrial conduction time in children. Int J Cardiol 1989; 23:207–213.

326. Hariman RJ, Krongrad E, Boxer RA, Bowman FO Jr, Malm JR, Hoffman BF. Methods for recording electrograms of the sinoatrial node during cardiac surgery in man. Circulation 1980; 61:1024–1029.

327. Strauss HC, Saroff AL, Bigger JT Jr, Giardina EGV. Premature atrial stimulation as a key to the understanding of sinoatrial conduction in man: presentation of data and critical review of the literature. Circulation 1973; 47:86–93.

328. Bigger JT Jr. A simple, rapid method for the diagnosis of first degree sinoatrial block in man. Am Heart J 1974; 87:731–733.

329. Breithardt G, Seipel L, Loogen F. Sinus node recovery time and calculated sinoatrial conduction time in normal subjects and patients with sinus node dysfunction. Circulation 1977; 56:43–50.

330. Kugler JD, Gillette PC, Mullins CE, McNamara DG. Sinoatrial conduction in children: an index of sinoatrial node function. Circulation 1979; 59:1266–1276.

331. Rakovec P, Rode P, Jakopin J, Horvat M. Latent sinoatrial conduction disturbances in symptomatic patients with Wolff-Parkinson-White syndrome. Pacing Clin Electrophysiol 1983; 6:2–7.

332. Reiffel JA, Gang E, Livelli F, Gliklich J, Bigger JT Jr. Indirectly estimated sinoatrial conduction time by the atrial premature stimulus technique: patterns of error and the degree of associated inaccuracy as assessed by direct sinus node electrography. Am Heart J 1983; 106:459–463.

333. Satoh S, Kanatsuka H, Kyono H, et al. A new indirect method for measurement of sinoatrial conduction time and sinus node return cycle. Jpn Heart J 1985; 26:335–348.

334. Narula OS, Shantha N, Vasquez M, Towne WD, Linhart JW. A new method for measurement of sinoatrial conduction time. Circulation 1978; 58:706–714.

335. Zhang D, Chen S. Comparison of indirect and direct sinoatrial conduction time by synchronous sinus node electrogram. Int J Cardiol 1988; 1988:381–386.

336. Pick A, Langendorf R, Katz LN. Depression of cardiac pacemakers by premature impulses. Am Heart J 1951; 41:49–57.

337. Jordan J, Yamaguchi I, Mandel WJ, McCullen AE. Comparative effects of overdrive on sinus and subsidiary pacemaker function. Am Heart J 1977; 93:367–374.

338. Gang ES, Reiffel JA, Livelli FD Jr, Bigger JT Jr. Sinus node recovery times following the spontaneous termination of supraventricular tachycardia and following atrial overdrive pacing: a comparison. Am Heart J 1983; 105:210–215.

339. Kulbertus HE, Leval-Rutten F, Mary L, Casters P. Sinus node recovery time in the elderly. Br Heart J 1975; 37:420–425.

340. Mandel W, Hayakawa H, Danzig R, Marcus HS. Evaluation of sino-atrial node function in man by overdrive suppression. Circulation 1971; 44:59–66.

341. Alboni P, Pirani R, Filippi L, et al. Latent abnormalities of sinus node function in patients with organic heart disease and normal sinus node on clinical basis. J Electrocardiol 1984; 17:385–391.

342. Masini G, Dianda R, Graziina A. Analysis of sino-atrial conduction in man using premature atrial stimulation. Cardiovasc Res 1975; 9:498–508.

343. Steinbeck G, Luderitz B. Comparative study of sinoatrial conduction time and sinus node recovery time. Br Heart J 1975; 37:956–962.

344. Engel TR, Bond RC, Schaal SF. First-degree sinoatrial heart block: sinoatrial block in the sick-sinus syndrome. Am Heart J 1976; 91:303–310.

345. Jordan J, Yamaguchi I, Mandel WJ. Characteristics of sinoatrial conduction in patients with coronary artery disease. Circulation 1977; 55:569–574.

346. Dhingra RC, Amat-y-Leon F, Wyndham C, et al. Clinical significance of prolonged sinoatrial conduction time. Circulation 1977; 55:8–15.

347. Reiffel JA, Bigger JT Jr, Konstam MA. The relationship between sinoatrial conduction time and sinus cycle length during spontaneous sinus arrhythmia in adults. Circulation 1974; 50:924–934.

348. Narula OS, Samet P, Javier RP. Significance of the sinus-node recovery time. Circulation 1972; 45:140–158.

349. Gupta PK, Lichstein E, Chadda KD, Badui E. Appraisal of sinus nodal recovery time in patients with sick sinus syndrome. Am J Cardiol 1974; 34:265–270.

350. Toyama J, Ito A, Sawada K, Ito T, Tanahashi Y. Overdrive suppression in diagnosis of sick sinus syndrome. J Electrocardiol 1975; 8:209–216.

351. Okimoto T, Ueda K, Kamata C, Yoshida H, Ohkawa SI. Sinus node recovery time and abnormal postpacing phase in the aged patients with sick sinus syndrome. Jpn Heart J 1976; 17:290–301.

352. Scheinman MM, Kunkel FW, Peters RW, et al. Atrial pacing in patients with sinus node dysfunction. Am J Med 1976; 61:641–649.

353. Evans TR, Callowhill EA, Krikler DM. Clinical value of tests of sino-atrial function. Pacing Clin Electrophysiol 1978; 1:2–7.

354. Lien WP, Lee YS, Chang FZ, Chen JJ. Electrophysiologic manifestations in so-called "sick sinus syndrome." Jpn Circ J 1978; 42:195–206.

355. Scheinman MM, Strauss HC, Abbott JA, et al. Electrophysiologic testing in patients with sinus pauses and/or sinoatrial exit block. Eur J Cardiol 1978; 8:51–60.

356. Lien WP, Chen JJ, Wu TL, Chang FZ. Automaticity of subsidiary pacemakers of patients with dysfunction of the sinus node. Chest 1980; 78:747–752.

357. Reiffel JA, Gang E, Bigger JT Jr, Livelli F Jr, Rolnitzky L, Cramer M. Sinus node recovery time related to paced cycle length in normals and patients with sinoatrial dysfunction. Am Heart J 1982; 104:746–752.

358. Szatmary L, Medvedowsky JL, Barnay C, Coste A, Pisapia A. Electrophysiological effect of overdrive suppression and combined autonomic blockade with propranolol and atropine in patients with sinus node dysfunction. Eur Heart J 1982; 3:47–55.

359. Bellinder G, Nordlander R, Pehrsson SK, Astrom H. Atrial pacing in the management of sick sinus syndrome: long-term observation for conduction disturbances and supraventricular tachyarrhythmias. Eur Heart J 1986; 7:105–109.

360. Heinz G, Laufer G, Hirschl M, et al. Postoperative sinus node dysfunction in the transplanted heart: impaired automaticity but normal refractoriness. Chest 1992; 101:603–606.

361. Bergfeldt L, Vallin H, Rosenqvist M, Insulander P, Nordlander R, Astrom H. Sinus node recovery time assessment revisited: role of pharmacologic blockade of the autonomic nervous system. J Cardiovasc Electrophysiol 1996; 7:95–101.

362. Benditt DG, Strauss HC, Scheinman MM, Behar VS, Wallace AG. Analysis of secondary pauses following termination of rapid atrial pacing in man. Circulation 1976; 54:436–441.

363. Jordan JL, Yamaguchi I, Mandel WJ. Studies on the mechanism of sinus node dysfunction in the sick sinus syndrome. Circulation 1978; 57:217–223.

364. Clark EB, Kugler JD. Preoperative secundum atrial septal defect with coexisting sinus node and atrioventricular node dysfunction. Circulation 1982; 65:976–980.

365. Bolens M, Friedli B. Sinus node function and conduction system before and after surgery for secundum atrial septal defect: an electrophysiologic study. Am J Cardiol 1984; 53:1415–1420.

366. Bexton RS, Nathan AW, Hellestrand KJ, et al. Electrophysiological abnormalities in the transplanted human heart. Br Heart J 1983; 50:555–563.

367. Bexton RS, Nathan AW, Hellestrand KJ, et al. Sinoatrial function after cardiac transplantation. J Am Coll Cardiol 1984; 3:712–723.

368. Goldreyer BN, Damato AN. Sinoatrial-node entrance block. Circulation 1971; 44:789–802.

369. Reiffel JA, Gang E, Livelli F Jr, Gliklich J, Bigger JT Jr. Clinical and electrophysiologic characteristics of sinoatrial entrance block evaluated by direct sinus node electrography: prevalence, relation to antegrade sinoatrial conduction time, and relevance to sinus node disease. Am Heart J 1981; 102:1011–1014.

370. Gann D, Tolentino A, Samet P. Electrophysiologic evaluation of elderly patients with sinus bradycardia: a long-term follow-up study. Ann Intern Med 1979; 90:24–29.

371. Vardas PE, Fitzpatrick A, Ingram A, et al. Natural history of sinus node chronotropy in paced patients. Pacing Clin Electrophysiol 1991; 14:155–160.

372. Kerr CR, Strauss HC. The measurement of sinus node refractoriness in man. Circulation 1983; 68:1231–1237.

373. Luck JC, Engel TR. Dispersion of atrial refractoriness in patients with sinus node dysfunction. Circulation 1979; 60:404–412.

374. Michelucci A, Padeletti L, Fradella GA, Monizzi D, Giomi A, Fantini F. Effects of pharmacologic autonomic blockade on atrial electrophysiologic properties in normal subjects and in patients with sinus node disease. Int J Cardiol 1985; 8:437–449.

375. Talwar KK, Radhakrishnan S, Chopra P. Myocarditis manifesting as persistent atrial standstill. Int J Cardiol 1988; 20:283–286.

376. Centurion OA, Fukatani M, Konoe A, et al. Electrophysiological abnormalities of the atrial muscle in patients with sinus node dysfunction without tachyarrhythmias. Int J Cardiol 1992; 37:41–50.

377. Tanigawa M, Fukatani M, Konoe A, Isomoto S, Kadena M, Hashiba K. Prolonged and fractionated right atrial electrograms during sinus rhythm in patients with paroxysmal atrial fibrillation and sick sinus node syndrome. J Am Coll Cardiol 1991; 17:403–408.

378. Centurion OA, Fukatani M, Konoe A, et al. Different distribution of abnormal endocardial electrograms within the right atrium in patients with sick sinus syndrome. Br Heart J 1992; 68:596–600.

379. Centurion OA, Isomoto S, Fukatani M, et al. Relationship between atrial conduction defects and fractionated atrial endocardial electrograms in patients with sick sinus syndrome. Pacing Clin Electrophysiol 1993; 16:2022–2033.

380. Centurion OA, Shimizu A, Isomoto S, et al. Repetitive atrial firing and fragmented atrial activity elicited by extrastimuli in the sick sinus syndrome with and without abnormal atrial electrograms. Am J Med Sci 1994; 307:247–254.

381. Reiffel JA, Zimmerman G. The duration of the sinus node depolarization on transvenous sinus node electrograms can identify sinus node dysfunction and can suggest its severity. Pacing Clin Electrophysiol 1989; 12:1746–1756.

382. Kuga K, Yamaguchi I, Sugishita Y, Ito I. Assessment by

autonomic blockade of age-related changes of the sinus node function and autonomic regulation in sick sinus syndrome. Am J Cardiol 1988; 61:361–366.

383. De Marneffe M, Gregoire JM, Waterschoot P, Kestemont MP. The sinus node and the autonomic nervous system in normals and in sick sinus patients. Acta Cardiol 1995; 50:291–308.

384. Sethi KK, Jaishankar S, Balachander J, Bahl VK, Gupta MP. Sinus node function after autonomic blockade in normals and in sick sinus syndrome. Int J Cardiol 1984; 5:707–719.

385. Kang PS, Gomes JA, el-Sherif N. Differential effects of functional autonomic blockade on the variables of sinus nodal automaticity in sick sinus syndrome. Am J Cardiol 1982; 49:273–282.

386. Rosen KM, Loeb HS, Sinno MZ, Rahimtoola SH, Gunnar RM. Cardiac conduction in patients with symptomatic sinus node disease. Circulation 1971; 43:836–844.

387. Vallin H, Edhag O. Associated conduction disturbances in patients with symptomatic sinus node disease. Acta Med Scand 1981; 210:263–270.

388. Narula OS. Atrioventricular conduction defects in patients with sinus bradycardia: analysis by His bundle recordings. Circulation 1971; 44:1096–1110.

389. Wyse DG, McAnulty JH, Rahimtoola SH, Murphy ES. Electrophysiologic abnormalities of the sinus node and atrium in patients with bundle branch block. Circulation 1979; 60:413–420.

390. Rasmussen K, Myhre ES, Gunnes P, Wang H. Multilevel disease of the conduction system. Eur Heart J 1983; 4:73–78.

391. van Mechelen R, Segers A, Hagemeijer F. Serial electrophysiologic studies after single chamber atrial pacemaker implantation in patients with symptomatic sinus node dysfunction. Eur Heart J 1984; 5:628–636.

392. van Mechelen R, Hagemeijer F, de Boer H, Schelling A. Atrioventricular and ventriculoatrial conduction in patients with symptomatic sinus node dysfunction. Pacing Clin Electrophysiol 1983; 6:13–21.

393. Centurion OA, Isomoto S, Shimizu A, et al. Supernormal atrial conduction and its relation to atrial vulnerability and atrial fibrillation in patients with sick sinus syndrome and paroxysmal atrial fibrillation. Am Heart J 1994; 128:88–95.

394. Engel TR, Schaal SF. Digitalis in the sick sinus syndrome: the effects of digitalis on sinoatrial automaticity and atrioventricular conduction. Circulation 1973; 48:1201–1207.

395. Breithardt G, Seipel L, Both A, Loogen F. The effect of atropine on calculated sinoatrial conduction time in man. Eur J Cardiol 1976; 4:49–57.

396. Carrasco HA, Fuenmayor A, Barboza JS, Gonzalez G. Effect of verapamil on normal sinoatrial node function and on sick sinus syndrome. Am Heart J 1978; 96:760–771.

397. Dhingra RC, Deedwania PC, Cummings JM, et al. Electrophysiologic effects of lidocaine on sinus node and atrium in patients with and without sinoatrial dysfunction. Circulation 1978; 57:448–454.

398. Vera Z, Miller RR, McMillin D, Mason DT. Effects of digitalis on sinus nodal function in patients with sick sinus syndrome. Am J Cardiol 1978; 41:318–323.

399. LaBarre A, Strauss HC, Scheinman MM, et al. Electrophysiologic effects of disopyramide phosphate on sinus node function in patients with sinus node dysfunction. Circulation 1979; 59:226–235.

400. Goldberg D, Reiffel JA, Davis JC, Gang E, Livelli F, Bigger JT Jr. Electrophysiologic effects of procainamide on sinus function in patients with and without sinus node disease. Am Heart J 1982; 103:75–79.

401. Vera Z, Awan NA, Mason DT. Assessment of oral quinidine effects on sinus node function in sick sinus syndrome patients. Am Heart J 1982; 103:80–84.

402. Vik-Mo H, Ohm OJ, Lund-Johansen P. Electrophysiologic effects of flecainide acetate in patients with sinus nodal dysfunction. Am J Cardiol 1982; 50:1090–1094.

403. Benditt DG, Benson DW Jr, Kreitt J, et al. Electrophysiologic effects of theophylline in young patients with recurrent symptomatic bradyarrhythmias. Am J Cardiol 1983; 52:1223–1229.

404. Bolognesi R, Benedini G, Ferrari R, Visioli O. Inhibitory effect of acute and chronic administration of digitalis on the sick sinus node. Eur Heart J 1986; 7:334–340.

405. Dhingra RC, Amat-y-Leon F, Wyndham C, et al. Electrophysiologic effects of atropine on sinus node and atrium in patients with sinus nodal dysfunction. Am J Cardiol 1976; 38:848–855.

406. Ogawa H, Inoue T, Miwa S, Fujimoto T, Ohnishi Y, Fukuzaki H. Heart rate responses to autonomic drugs in sick sinus syndrome: correlation with syncope and electrophysiologic data. Jpn Circ J 1991; 55:15–23.

407. Ishii Y, Mitsuda H, Eno S, et al. Electrophysiological effects of lidocaine in sick sinus syndrome. Jpn Heart J 1980; 21:27–34.

408. Scheinman MM, Strauss HC, Evans GT, Ryan C, Massie B, Wallace A. Adverse effects of sympatholytic agents in patients with hypertension and sinus node dysfunction. Am J Med 1978; 64:1013–1020.

409. Watt AH. Sick sinus syndrome: an adenosine-mediated disease. Lancet 1985; 1:786–788.

410. Saito D, Matsubara K, Yamanari H, et al. Effects of oral theophylline on sick sinus syndrome. J Am Coll Cardiol 1993; 21:1199–1204.

411. Alboni P, Menozzi C, Brignole M, et al. Effects of permanent pacemaker and oral theophylline in sick sinus syndrome. The THEOPACE study: a randomized controlled trial. Circulation 1997; 96:260–266.

412. Sauerwein HP, Roos JC, Becker AE, Dunning AJ. The sick sinus syndrome. Acta Med Scand 1976; 199:467–473.

413. Lai WT, Lai HM, Lin CT, Sheu SH, Hwang YS. Is sick sinus syndrome an adenosine-mediated disease? Effects of intravenous aminophylline on sick sinus node function after pharmacologic autonomic blockade. Chest 1991; 99:887–891.

414. Ellenbogen KA, Szentpetery S, Katz MR. Reversibility of prolonged chronotropic dysfunction with theophylline following orthotopic cardiac transplantation. Am Heart J 1988; 116:202–206.

415. Simonsen E, Nielsen JS, Nielsen BL. Sinus node dysfunction in 128 patients: a retrospective study with follow-up. Acta Med Scand 1980; 208:343–348.

416. Moss AJ. Therapeutic uses of permanent pervenous atrial pacemakers: a review. J Electrocardiol 1975; 8:373–380.

417. Camm AJ, Katritsis D. Ventricular pacing for sick sinus syndrome: a risky business? Pacing Clin Electrophysiol 1990; 13:695–699.

418. Sutton R. Pacing in atrial arrhythmias. Pacing Clin Electrophysiol 1990; 13:1823–1827.

419. Sgarbossa EB, Pinski SL. Pacemaker therapies for atrial fibrillation. Prim Cardiol 1994; 20:16–20.

420. Mason JW, Hlatky MA. Do patients prefer physiologic pacing? N Engl J Med 1998; 338:1147–1148.

421. Andersen HR, Nielsen JC. Pacing in sick sinus syndrome: need for a prospective, randomized trial comparing atrial with dual chamber pacing. PACE 1998; 21:1175–1179.

422. Ovsyshcher IE, Hayes DL, Furman S. Dual-chamber pacing is superior to ventricular pacing: fact or controversy? Circulation 1998; 97:2368–2370.

423. Adelman AG, Wigle ED. The bradycardia, tachycardia, asystole syndrome: treatment by a pacemaker. Can Med Assoc J 1969; 100:75–77.

424. Kastor JA, DeSanctis RW, Leinbach RC, Harthorne JW, Wolfson IN. Long-term pervenous atrial pacing. Circulation 1969; 40:535–544.

425. Sandoe E, Flensted-Jensen E. Adams-Stokes seizures in patients with attacks of both tachy- and bradycardia, a therapeutical challenge. Acta Med Scand 1969; 186:111–116.

426. Fowler NO, Fenton JC, Conway GF. Syncope and cerebral dysfunction caused by bradycardia without atrioventricular block. Am Heart J 1970; 80:303–312.

427. Rokseth R, Hatle L, Gedde-Dahl D, Foss PO. Pacemaker therapy in sino-atrial block complicated by paroxysmal tachycardia. Br Heart J 1970; 32:93–98.

428. Bayley TJ. Long-term ventricular pacing in treatment of sinoatrial block. BMJ 1971; 3:456–458.

429. Morgan CV, Orcutt TW, Collins HA, Killen DA. Permanent cardiac pacing for sinoatrial bradycardia. J Thorac Cardiovasc Surg 1972; 63:453–457.

430. Matsuura Y, Yamashina H, Mishima H, Futakawa S, Sekiguchi Y, Takizawa I. Treatment of sick sinus syndrome with permanent cardiac pacemaker (sick sinus syndrome and artificial pacemaker). J Cardiovasc Surg 1977; 18:447–452.

431. Amikam S, Riss E. Natural history of sick sinus syndrome following permanent pacemaker implantation. Isr J Med Sci 1979; 15:889–893.

432. Simon AB, Zloto AE. Symptomatic sinus node disease: natural history after permanent ventricular pacing. Pacing Clin Electrophysiol 1979; 2:305–314.

433. Leclercq JF, Rosengarten MD, Delcourt P, Attuel P, Coumel P, Slama R. Prevention of intra-atrial reentry by chronic atrial pacing. Pacing Clin Electrophysiol 1980; 3:162–170.

434. Frank R, Petitot JC, Touil F, Lascault G, Fontaine G. Pacemaker indications and selection in sick sinus syndrome. In Touboul P, Waldo AL (eds). Atrial Arrhythmias. Current Concepts and Management. St. Louis: Mosby–Year Book, 1990; pp. 392–399.

435. Joseph SP, White J. Long-term atrial pacing for sinus node disease with output-terminal programmable pacemakers. J Thorac Cardiovasc Surg 1979; 78:292–297.

436. Sutton R, Citron P. Electrophysiological and haemodynamic basis for application of new pacemaker technology in sick sinus syndrome and atrioventricular block. Br Heart J 1979; 41:600–612.

437. Stone JM, Bhakta RD, Lutgen J. Dual chamber sequential pacing management of sinus node dysfunction: advantages over single-chamber pacing. Am Heart J 1982; 104:1319–1327.

438. Hayes DL, Furman S. Stability of AV conduction in sick sinus node syndrome patients with implanted atrial pacemakers. Am Heart J 1984; 107:644–647.

439. Markewitz A, Schad N, Hemmer W, Bernheim C, Ciavolella M, Weinhold C. What is the most appropriate stimulation mode in patients with sinus node dysfunction? Pacing Clin Electrophysiol 1986; 9:1115–1120.

440. Mast EG, van Hemel NM, Bakema L, Derksen B, Defauw JA. Is chronic atrial stimulation a reliable method for single chamber pacing in sick sinus syndrome? Pacing Clin Electrophysiol 1986; 9:1127–1130.

441. Attuel P, Pellerin D, Mugica J, Coumel P. DDD pacing: an effective treatment modality for recurrent atrial arrhythmias. Pacing Clin Electrophysiol 1988; 11:1647–1654.

442. Sasaki Y, Shimotori M, Akahane K, et al. Long-term follow-up of patients with sick sinus syndrome: a comparison of clinical aspects among unpaced, ventricular inhibited paced, and physiologically paced groups. Pacing Clin Electrophysiol 1988; 11:1575–1583.

443. Swiatecka G, Lubinski A, Raczak G, Stanke A, Juzwa A, Kubica J. Transesophageal programmed atrial pacing as a method of selecting patients with sick sinus syndrome for permanent atrial pacing. Pacing Clin Electrophysiol 1988; 11:1655–1661.

444. Zanini R, Facchinetti AI, Gallo G, Cazzamalli L, Bonandi L, Dei Cas L. Morbidity and mortality of patients with sinus node disease: comparative effects of atrial and ventricular pacing. Pacing Clin Electrophysiol 1990; 13:2076–2079.

445. Benditt DG, Wilbert L, Hansen R, et al. Late follow-up of dual-chamber rate-adaptive pacing. Am J Cardiol 1993; 71:714–719.

446. Andersen HR, Thuesen L, Bagger JP, Vesterlund T, Thomsen PE. Prospective randomised trial of atrial versus ventricular pacing in sick-sinus syndrome. Lancet 1994; 344:1523–1528.

447. Lau CP, Tai YT, Leung WH, Wong CK, Lee P, Chung FL. Rate adaptive pacing in sick sinus syndrome: effects of pacing modes and intrinsic conduction on physiological responses, arrhythmias, symptomatology and quality of life. Eur Heart J 1994; 15:1445–1455.

448. Sutton R, Bourgeois I. Cost benefit analysis of single and dual chamber pacing for sick sinus syndrome and atrioventricular block: an economic sensitivity analysis of the literature. Eur Heart J 1996; 17:574–582.

449. Andersen HR, Nielsen JC, Thomsen PEB, et al. Long-term follow-up of patients from a randomised trial of atrial versus ventricular pacing for sick-sinus syndrome. Lancet 1997; 350:1210–1216.

450. Vardas PE, Simantirakis EN, Parthenakis FI, Chrysostomakis SI, Skalidis EI, Zuridakis EG. AAIR versus DDDR pacing in patients with impaired sinus node chronotropy: an echocardiographic and cardiopulmonary study. Pacing Clin Electrophysiol 1997; 20:1762–1768.

451. Woodard DA, Conti JB, Mills RM, Williams RM, Curtis AB. Permanent atrial pacing in cardiac transplant patients. PACE 1997; 20:2398–2404.

452. Lamas GA, Orav EJ, Stambler BS, et al. Quality of life and clinical outcomes in elderly patients treated with ventricular pacing as compared with dual-chamber pacing. N Engl J Med 1998; 338:1097–1104.

453. Nielsen JC, Andersen HR, Thomsen PEB, et al. Heart failure and echocardiographic changes during long-term follow-up of patients with sick sinus syndrome randomized to single-chamber atrial or ventricular pacing. Circulation 1998; 97:987–995.

454. Rosenqvist M, Aren C, Kristensson BE, Nordlander R, Schuller H. Atrial rate-responsive pacing in sinus node disease. Eur Heart J 1990; 11:537–542.

455. Haywood GA, Katritsis D, Ward J, Leigh-Jones M, Ward DE, Camm AJ. Atrial adaptive rate pacing in sick sinus syndrome: effects on exercise capacity and arrhythmias. Br Heart J 1993; 69:174–178.

456. Sgarbossa EB, Pinski SL, Castle LW, Trohman RG, Maloney JD. Incidence and predictors of loss of pacing in the atrium in patients with sick sinus syndrome. Pacing Clin Electrophysiol 1992; 15:2050–2054.

457. Gregoratos G, Cheitlin MD, Conill A, et al. ACC/AHA guidelines for implantation of cardiac pacemakers and antiarrhythmia devices (Committee on Pacemaker Implantation). Circulation 1998; 97:1325–1335.

458. Heinz G, Kratochwill C, Killer-Strametz J, et al. Benign prognosis of early sinus node dysfunction after orthotopic cardiac transplantation. PACE 1998; 21:422–429.

459. Lamas GA, Estes NM III, Schneller S, Flaker GC. Does dual chamber or atrial pacing prevent atrial fibrillation? The need for a randomized controlled trial. Pacing Clin Electrophysiol 1992; 15:1109–1113.

460. Santini M, Alexidou G, Ansalone G, Cacciatore G, Cini R, Turitto G. Relation of prognosis in sick sinus syndrome to age, conduction defects and modes of permanent cardiac pacing. Am J Cardiol 1990; 65:729–735.

461. Stangl K, Seitz K, Wirtzfeld A, Alt E, Blomer H. Differences between atrial single chamber pacing (AAI) and ventricular single chamber pacing (VVI) with respect to prognosis and antiarrhythmic effect in patients with sick sinus syndrome. Pacing Clin Electrophysiol 1990; 13:2080–2085.

462. Sasaki Y, Furihata A, Suyama K, et al. Comparison between ventricular inhibited pacing and physiologic pacing in sick sinus syndrome. Am J Cardiol 1991; 67:771–774.

463. Hesselson AB, Parsonnet V, Bernstein AD, Bonavita GJ. Deleterious effects of long-term single-chamber ventricular pacing in patients with sick sinus syndrome: the hidden benefits of dual-chamber pacing. J Am Coll Cardiol 1992; 19:1542–1549.

464. Sgarbossa EB, Pinski SL, Trohman RG, Castle LW, Maloney JD. Single-chamber ventricular pacing is not associated with worsening heart failure in sick sinus syndrome. Am J Cardiol 1994; 73:693–697.

465. Costeas C, Kassotis J, Blitzer M, Reiffel JA. Rhythm management in atrial fibrillation: with a primary emphasis on pharmacological therapy. II. PACE 1998; 21:742–752.

466. Rasmussen K. Chronic sinus node disease: natural course and indications for pacing. Eur Heart J 1981; 2:455–459.

467. Shaw DB, Holman RR, Gowers JI. Survival in sinoatrial disorder (sick-sinus syndrome). BMJ 1980; 280:139–141.

468. Alt E, Volker R, Wirtzfeld A, Ulm K. Survival and follow-up after pacemaker implantation: a comparison of patients with sick sinus syndrome, complete heart block, and atrial fibrillation. Pacing Clin Electrophysiol 1985; 8:849–855.

469. Skagen K, Hansen JF. The long-term prognosis for patients with sinoatrial block treated with permanent pacemaker. Acta Med Scand 1975; 199:13–15.

470. Alpert MA, Curtis JJ, Sanfelippo JF, et al. Comparative survival following permanent ventricular and dual-chamber pacing for

patients with chronic symptomatic sinus node dysfunction with and without congestive heart failure. Am Heart J 1987; 113:958–965.

471. Simon AB, Janz N. Symptomatic bradyarrhythmias in the adult: natural history following ventricular pacemaker implantation. Pacing Clin Electrophysiol 1982; 5:372–383.

472. Wohl AJ, Laborde NJ, Atkins JM, Blomqvist CG, Mullins CB. Prognosis of patients permanently paced for sick sinus syndrome. Arch Intern Med 1976; 136:406–408.

473. Zanini R, Facchinetti A, Gallo G, et al. Survival rates after pacemaker implantation: a study of patients paced for sick sinus syndrome and atrioventricular block. Pacing Clin Electrophysiol 1989; 12:1065–1069.

Index

Note: Page numbers in *italics* indicate figures; those with an n indicate footnotes; those with a t indicate tables.